Reza Shaker · Peter C. Belafsky
Gregory N. Postma · Caryn Easterling
Editors

Principles of Deglutition

A Multidisciplinary Text for
Swallowing and its Disorders

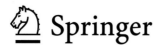 Springer

Editors
Reza Shaker
Division of Gastroenterology
  and Hepatology
Medical College of Wisconsin
Milwaukee, Wisconsin, USA

Gregory N. Postma
Center for Voice, Airway
  and Swallowing Disorders
Department of Otolaryngology
Georgia Health Sciences University
Augusta, Georgia, USA

Peter C. Belafsky
Department of Otolaryngology/
  Head and Neck Surgery
University of California
Davis Medical Center
Sacramento, California, USA

Caryn Easterling
Department of Communication Sciences
  and Disorders
University of Wisconsin-Milwaukee
Milwaukee, Wisconsin, USA

ISBN 978-1-4614-3793-2   ISBN 978-1-4614-3794-9 (eBook)
DOI 10.1007/978-1-4614-3794-9
Springer New York Heidelberg Dordrecht London

Library of Congress Control Number: 2012943384

Printed on acid-free paper

Springer is part of Springer Science+Business Media (www.springer.com)

Preface

Deglutology, like no other medical field, is in need of convergence of many contributory disciplines to develop a transdisciplinary model to further improve patient care, advance research, and facilitate education.

Despite steady progress in recent years, various aspects of *Deglutology* have evolved within various medical disciplines resulting in fragmentation of expertise, knowledge, and skills which not only have hampered the progress of the field but also have resulted in the fragmented and inconsistent patterns of care for patients with dysphagia.

The need to remedy this problem was recognized over 2 decades ago, and the initial step toward a resolution resulted in the publication of the Dysphagia Journal and the formation of the Dysphagia Research Society (DRS). Over the past 25 years, the Dysphagia Journal and the DRS have been committed to removing the specialty barriers while providing a platform for interdisciplinary interaction and collaboration.

The vision for the "Principles of Deglutition," with over 100 contributing experts from 12 disciplines, is the convergence of knowledge from various fields involved in the care of dysphagic patients and deglutition research to help the development of the transdisciplinary model so badly needed for the evolution of deglutology.

We envision the future *Deglutologist* as a professional with a diverse background, whose initial and foundational knowledge and skills are derived from varied disciplines. In addition they will be equipped with the converged multidisciplinary knowledge and skills necessary to address the deglutition disorders in its entirety providing all the critical pieces of the puzzle that compromises the health and quality of life for so many with dysphagia.

Milwaukee, WI, USA   Reza Shaker
Sacramento, CA, USA   Peter C. Belafsky
Augusta, GA, USA   Gregory N. Postma
Milwaukee, WI, USA   Caryn Easterling

Contents

Part IV   Pharyngeal Phase of Deglutition

Part V   UES and Its Deglutitive Function

Part VI   Esophageal Phase of Deglutition

Part VII   Esophageal Motility and Its Deglutitive Function

Part VIII   Oral/Pharyngeal Phase Dysphagia

Contributors

Stewart I. Adam, MD Department of Otolaryngology, Yale New Haven Hospital, New Haven, CT, USA

Jacqueline Allen, MBChB, FRACS Department of Otolaryngology, North Shore Hospital, Takapuna, Auckland, New Zealand

Andreea Antonescu-Turcu, MD Medical College of Wisconsin, Milwaukee, WI, USA

Peter C. Belafsky, MD, MPH, PhD Department of Otolaryngology/ Head and Neck Surgery, University of California, Davis Medical Center, Sacramento, CA, USA

William L. Berger, MD Division of Gastroenterology and Hepatology, Medical College of Wisconsin, Clement J. Zablocki VA Medical Center, Milwaukee, WI, USA

Detlef Bieger, Dr.Med Faculty of Medicine, Memorial University, Health Science Centre, St. John's, NL, Canada

Margareta Bülow, PhD Diagnostic Centre of Imaging and Functional Medicine, Skåne University Hospital, Malmö, Sweden

Miguel Burch, MD Department of Surgery, Cedars-Sinai Medical Center, Los Angeles, CA, USA

Lindsay D. Clendaniel, PhD Department of Psychology, Children's Hospital, New Orleans, New Orleans, LA, USA

Jeffrey L. Conklin, MD Department of Gastroenterology and Hepatology, Cedars-Sinai Medical Center, Los Angeles, CA, USA

Ian J. Cook, MBBS, MD(Syd), FRACP Department of Gastroenterology and Hepatology, St George Hospital, Kogarah, Australia

Seth Dailey, MD Division of Otolaryngology Head and Neck Surgery, University of Wisconsin Hospital and Clinics, Madison, WI, USA

Michel Dallaporta, PhD Physiologie Neurovegatative (PNV), Faculte Des Sciences St. Jerome, University Aix-Marseille Paul Cezanne, Avenue Escadrille Normandie-Niemen, Marseille, France

Stephanie K. Daniels, PhD Communication Sciences and Disorders, University of Houston, Houston, TX, USA

Roberto Oliveira Dantas, MD Department of Medicine, University Hospital of Ribeirão Preto, Capitão Osório Junqueira, São Paulo, Brazil

Amy L. Delaney, PhD, CCC-SLP SLP Program Specialist-Feeding and Swallowing Research, Children's Hospital of Wisconsin, Medical College of Wisconsin, Milwaukee, WI, USA

Sameer Dhalla, MD Division of Gastroenterology and Hepatology, Johns Hopkins Hospital, Baltimore, MD, USA

Nicholas Evans Diamant, MDCM, FRCP(C) Department of Medicine/Gastroenterology, Kingston General Hospital, Kingston, Ontario, Canada

Kulwinder S. Dua, MD, FACP, FRCP (Edinburgh), FRCP (London), FASGE Department of Medicine, Division of Gastroenterology and Hepatology, Medical College of Wisconsin, Milwaukee, WI, USA

André Duranceau, MD Division of Thoracic Surgery, Department of Surgery, Université de Montréal, Centre Hospitalier de l'Université de Montréal, Montréal, QC, Canada

Caryn Easterling, PhD, CCC, BRS-S, ASHAF Fellow Department of Communication Sciences and Disorders, University of Wisconsin-Milwaukee, Milwaukee, WI, USA

Olle Ekberg, MD, PhD Diagnostic Centre of Imaging and Functional Medicine, Skåne University Hospital, Malmö, Malmö, Sweden

Gary W. Falk, MD, MS Department of Medicine/Division of Gastroenterology, Perelman School of Medicine at the University of Pennsylvania, Hospital of the University of Pennsylvania, Philadelphia, PA, USA

D. Gregory Farwell, MD, FACS Department of Otolaryngology Head and Neck Surgery, University of California, Davis, Sacramento, CA, USA

Allison R. Gallaugher, MA Communication Sciences and Disorders, University of Houston, Houston, TX, USA

Eric Gaumnitz, MD Division of Gastroenterology and Hepatology, University of Wisconsin School of Medicine and Public Health, Madison, WI, USA

Samer Gawrieh, MD Division of Gastroenterology and Hepatololgy, Froedtret Hospital, Medical College of Wisconsin, Milwaukee, WI, USA

Ian C. Grimes, MD Division of Gastroenterology and Hepatology, University of Wisconsin School of Medicine and Public Health, Madison, WI, USA

C. Prakash Gyawali, MD Division of Gastroenterology, St. Louis, MO, USA

Shaheen Hamdy, PhD, FRCP Salfaord Royal NHS Foundation Trust, School of Translational Medicine—Inflammation Sciences, University of Manchester, Salford, Greater Manchester, UK

Ingo F. Herrmann, MD, PhD ENT Department, Reflux Center Düsseldorf, Düsseldorf, Nordrhein-Westfalen, Germany

Ikuo Hirano, MD Division of Gastroenterology, Northwestern University Feinberg School of Medicine, Chicago, IL, USA

Walter J. Hogan, MD Division of Gastroenterology and Hepatology, Froedtert Hospital, Milwaukee, WI, USA

Toshitaka Hoppo, MD, PhD Department of Cardiothoracic Surgery, University of Pittsburgh Medical Center, Pittsburgh, PA, USA

Maggie-Lee Huckabee, PhD Swallowing Rehabilitation Research Lab at the Van der Veer Institute, The University of Canterbury, Christchurch, New Zealand

Louise Hughes, BSLT (hons) Department of Speech and Language Therapy, The Princess Margaret Hospital, Canterbury District Health Board, Christchurch, New Zealand

John Hodges, MBBS, MD, FRCP Neuroscience Research, Randwick, Sydney, NSW, Australia

Matthew R. Hoffman, BS Division of Otolaryngology—Head and Neck Surgery, University of Wisconsin Hospital and Clinics, Madison, WI, USA

Thomas Hummel, MD Department of Otorhinolaryngology, Technical University of Dresden Medical School, Smell and Taste Clinic, Dresden, Germany

Paul E. Hyman, MD Lousiana State University, Children's Hospital, New Orleans, LA, USA

Manabu Ikeda, MD, PhD Department of Neuropsychiatry, Kumamoto University, Kumamoto, Japan

Elizabeth R. Jacobs, MD, MBA Pulmonary and Critical Care Medicine, Medical College of Wisconsin, Milwaukee, WI, USA

Sudarshan R. Jadcherla, MD, FRCP, (Irel), DCH, AGAF Sections of Neonatology, Pediatric Gastroenterology and Nutrition, The Neonatal and Infant Feeding Disorders Program, Neonatal Nutrition Program, Neonatal Occupational and Physical Therapy Program, Nationwide Children's Hospital, Columbus, OH, USA

Safwan Jaradeh, MD Professor of Neurology and Neurological Sciences, Stanford University Medical Center, Stanford, CA, USA

André Jean, MD, DSc Physiologie Neurovegatative (PNV), Faculte Des Sciences St. Jerome, University Aix-Marseille Paul Cezanne, Avenue Escadrille Normandie-Niemen, Marseille, France

Blair A. Jobe, MD, FACS Cardiothoracic Surgery, University of Pittsburgh Medical Center, Pittsburgh, PA, USA

Eric Johnson, MD Division of Gastroenterology and Hepatology, University of Wisconsin School of Medicine and Public Health, Madison, WI, USA

Peter J. Kahrilas, MD Department of Gastroenterology, Northwestern University Hospital, Chicago, IL, USA

Robert T. Kavitt, MD Division of Gastroenterology, Hepatology and Nutrition, Vanderbilt University Medical Center, Nashville, TN, USA

Martijn P. Kos, MD, PhD Department of Otorhinolaryngology, Waterland Hospital, Purmerend, The Netherlands

Braden Kuo, MD, BSc, MSc Department of Gastroenterology, Harvard Medical School, Massachusetts General Hospital, MGH Digestive Healthcare Center, Boston, MA, USA

Vladimir M. Kushnir, MD Division of Gastroenterology, Barnes Jewish Hospital/ Washington University School of Medicine, St. Louis, MO, USA

Monika A. Kwiatek, PhD Department of Medicine, Northwestern Memorial Hospital, Chicago, IL, USA

Ivan M. Lang, DVM, PhD Medicine: Division of Gastroenterology and Hepatology, Milwaukee, WI, USA

Cathy Lazarus, PhD, CCC-SLP, BRS-S, ASHA Fellow Department of Otorhinolaryngology Head and Neck Surgery, Beth Israel Medical Center, New York, NY, USA

Department of Otorhinolaryngology Head & Neck Surgery, Albert Einstein College of Medicine, New York, NY, USA

Steven B. Leder, PhD Department of Surgery, Surgery, Section of Otolaryngology, Yale University School of Medicine, New Haven, CT, USA

Rebecca J. Leonard, AB, MS, PhD Department of Otolaryngology/HNS, University of California, Davis, Medical Center/Health System, Sacramento, CA, USA

Catherine Rees Lintzenich, MD Department of Otolaryngology, Wake Forest School of Medicine, Medical Center Boulevard, Winston Salem, NC, USA

Christy L. Ludlow, PhD Communication Sciences and Disorders, James Madison University, Harrisonburg, VA, USA

Hans F. Mahieu, MD, PhD Department of Otorhinolaryngology, Meander Medical Center, Amersfoort, The Netherlands

Georgia A. Malandraki, PhD, CCC-SLP Department of Biobehavioral Sciences, Program of Speech and Language Pathology, Teachers College, Columbia University, New York, NY, USA

Thomas Mandl, MD, PhD Department of Rheumatology, Skåne University Hospital Malmö, Malmö, Sweden

Bonnie Martin-Harris, PhD, CCC-SLP, BRS-S, ASHA, Fellow MUSC Evelyn Trammell Institute for Voice and Swallowing, Doctoral Program in Health and Rehabilitation Science, Otolaryngology-Head and Neck Surgery, College of Health Professions, Medical University of South Carolina, Charleston, SC, USA

Benson T. Massey, MD, FACP Division of Gastroenterology and Hepatology, Medical College of Wisconsin, Milwaukee, WI, USA

Denis M. McCarthy, MD, PhD Department of Medicine, Division of Gastroenterology and Hepatology, University of New Mexico Health Sciences Center, Albuquerque, NM, USA

Tim McCulloch, MD Otolaryngology Division of the Department of Surgery, University of Wisconsin, Madison, WI, USA

David H. McFarland, PhD École d'orthophonie et d'audiologie, Faculté de médicine, Université de Montréal, Montréal, QC, Canada

Paul Menard-Katcher, MD Division of Gastroenterology, Raymond and Ruth Perelman School of Medicine of the University of Pennsylvania, Philadelphia, PA, USA

Ravinder Mittal, MD Department of Medicine, University of California San Diego and San Diego VA Health Care Center, San Diego, CA, USA

Arthur J. Miller, PhD Division of Orthodontics, Department of Orofacial Sciences, School of Dentistry, University of California at San Francisco, San Francisco, CA, USA

Michele P. Morrison Department of Otolaryngology, Naval Medical Center Portsmouth, Portsmouth, VA, USA

Joseph A. Murray, MD Division of Gastroenterology and Hepatology, Mayo Clinic, Rochester, MN, USA

Vikneswaran Namasivayam, MBBS, MRCP Department of Gastroenterology and Hepatology, Singapore General Hospital, Singapore, Singapore

Winfried Neuhuber, MD Institute of Anatomy, University of Erlangen-Nuremberg, Erlangen, Germany

Linda Nguyen, MD Division of Gastroenterology and Hepatology, Stanford University School of Medicine, Stanford, CA, USA

Jeffrey B. Palmer, MD Physical Medicine and Rehabilitation, Johns Hopkins Hospital, Baltimore, MD, USA

John Pandolfino, MD, MSCI Department of Medicine, Northwestern Memorial Hospital, Chicago, IL, USA

Pankaj J. Pasricha, MD Division of Gastroenterology and Hepatology, Stanford University, Stanford, CA, USA

William G. Paterson, BSc, MD, FRCPC Division of Gastroenterology, Hotel Dieu Hospital, Department of Medicine, Hotel Dieu Hospital and Kingston General Hospital, Kingston, Ontario, Canada

Jeffrey H. Peters, MD Department of Surgery, University of Rochester, Rochester, NY, USA

Patrick R. Pfau, MD Division of Gastroenterology and Hepatology, University of Wisconsin School of Medicine and Public Health, Madison, WI, USA

Gregory N. Postma, MD Center for Voice, Airway and Swallowing Disorders, Department of Otolaryngology, Georgia Health Sciences University, Augusta, GA, USA

Mark Reichelderfer, MD Division of Gastroenterology and Hepatology, University of Wisconsin School of Medicine and Public Health, Madison, WI, USA

Joel E. Richter, MD Department of Medicine, Temple University School of Medicine, Philadelphia, PA, USA

JoAnne Robbins, PhD, CCC-SLP, BRS-S Department of Medicine and Wm. S. Middleton Memorial Veterans Hospital, University of Wisconsin, Madison, WI, USA

Sabine Roman, MD, PhD Digestive Physiology, Hospices Civils de Lyon and Claude Bernard University, Hopital E Herriot, Lyon, France

John C. Rosenbek, PhD Speech, Language Hearing Sciences, University of Florida, Gainesville, FL, USA

Colin Rudolph, MD, PhD Global Medical Affairs, Mead Johnson Nutrition, Evansville, IN, USA

Carmel Ryan, BA, Dip Ed School of Communication Disorders and Deafness, Kean University, Union, NJ, USA

Erica A. Samuel, MD Division of Gastroenterology and Hepatology, Medical College of Wisconsin, Milwaukee, WI, USA

Clarence T. Sasaki, MD Department of Surgery-Otolaryngology, Yale Comprehensive Cancer Center, Yale New Haven Hospital, New Haven, CT, USA

Anisa Shaker, MD Division of Gastroenterology, Washington University School of Medicine/Barnes Jewish Hospital/Internal Medicine, St. Louis, MO, USA

Reza Shaker, MD Division of Gastroenterology and Hepatology, Digestive Disease Center, Clinical and Translational Science Institute, Medical College of Wisconsin, Milwaukee, WI, USA

C. Blake Simpson, MD Department of Otorhinolaryngology—Head and Neck Surgery, Medical Arts and Research Center, San Antonio, TX, USA

Robert M. Siwiec, MD Division of Gastroenterology and Hepatology, Medical College of Wisconsin, Milwaukee, WI, USA

Stuart Jon Spechler, MD Division of Gastroenterology, Dallas VA Medical Center, UT Southwestern Medical Center at Dallas, Dallas, TX, USA

Kyle Staller, MD Department of Internal Medicine, Massachusetts General Hospital, Boston, MA, USA

Debra M. Suiter, PhD Department of Speech Pathology, Speech-Language Pathologist, VA Medical Center-Memphis, Surgical Service, Memphis, TN, USA

Rade Tomic, MD Department of Medicine, Division of Pulmonary and Critical Care, Froedtert Hospital, Medical College of Wisconsin, Milwaukee, WI, USA

Michelle S. Troche, PhD Department of Speech, Language, and Hearing Sciences, University of Florida, Gainesville, FL, USA

Michael F. Vaezi, MD, PhD, MSc (Epi) Division of Gastroenterology, Hepatology and Nutrition, Vanderbilt University Medical Center, Nashville, TN, USA

Dipesh H. Vasant, MB, ChB, MRCP School of Translational Medicine—Inflammation Sciences, University of Manchester, Eccles Old Road, Salford, Greater Manchester, England, UK

Mikhail Wadie, MD Department of Otolaryngology, Yale New Haven Hospital, New Haven, CT, USA

Kenneth K. Wang, MD Department of Gastroenterology and Hepatology, Mayo Clinic, Rochester, MN, USA

Candice L. Wilshire, MD Division of Thoracic and Foregut Surgery, University of Rochester School of Medicine and Dentistry, Rochester, NY, USA

Carol-Leigh Wilson, MA Communication Sciences and Disorders, University of Houston, Houston, TX, USA

Kaicheng Lawrence Yen, MD, PhD Department of Otolaryngology Head and Neck Surgery, University of California, Davis, Sacramento, CA, USA

Part I

General Aspects of Deglutition

Overview of Deglutition and Digestion

Arthur J. Miller

Abstract

The gastrointestinal tract, also defined as the digestive tract, or alimentary tract, is a system in the body designed to take in food and liquids, decrease and modify the food through mechanical and chemical digestion to absorb the end products through the mucosal epithelial cells that line the intestine, primarily in the small intestine. Swallowing refers to the functions of the oral, pharyngeal, and esophageal regions that begin the process of ingestion and digestion, and transport the food to the stomach where the bolus is transformed into chyme that is further broken down in the stomach and the small intestine. Accessory organs work with the digestive tract and include the tongue, salivary glands, pancreas, liver, and gallbladder. The final products eliminated contain mostly fiber and bacteria.

Keywords

Gastrointestinal tract • Digestion • Swallowing • Dysphagia rehabilitation • Deglutition

Introduction

The gastrointestinal system or digestive system refers to one of the several systems in the body like the cardiovascular, respiratory, and renal systems [1]. The gastrointestinal tract refers to a system in the higher order animals in which food and water intake is processed to extract the needed nutrients and retain the water while removing the fiber and some bacteria. The gastrointestinal tract develops early in the animal kingdom with multicellular animals, and the development of this internalized digestive system provides a mechanism for animals to support a larger body size [2]. The gastrointestinal system, also defined as the alimentary tract, is a long muscular tube in the humans extending 15–18 ft with multiple accessory organs that include the tongue, teeth, and salivary glands of the oral cavity as well as the pancreas, liver, and gallbladder (Fig. 1.1). Most of these accessory organs secrete into the gastrointestinal tract except for the tongue

A.J. Miller, PhD (✉)
Division of Orthodontics, Department of Orofacial Sciences, School of Dentistry, University of California at San Francisco, San Francisco, CA, USA
e-mail: art.miller@ucsf.edu

R. Shaker et al. (eds.), *Principles of Deglutition: A Multidisciplinary Text for Swallowing and its Disorders*, DOI 10.1007/978-1-4614-3794-9_1, © Springer Science+Business Media New York 2013

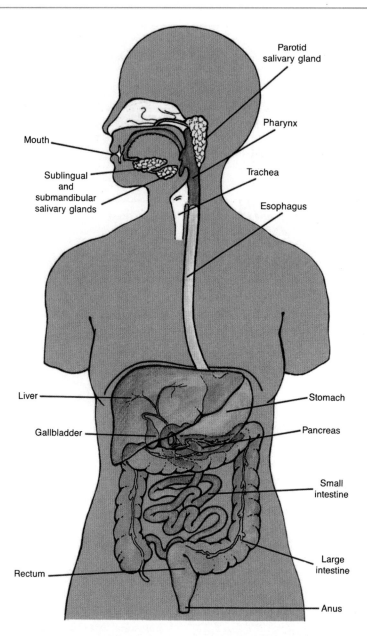

Fig. 1.1 A schematic of the entire gastrointestinal system which includes the oral, pharyngeal, and esophageal regions that connect to the stomach, small and large intestine, and colon. Accessory organs include the salivary glands, teeth, and tongue of the oral region as well as the pancreas, liver, and gall bladder that secrete into the small intestine. From A. Vander et al. Human physiology: the mechanisms of body function, 8th ed. New York: McGraw Hill; 2001 with permission

and teeth, which are vital to digestion and the transport of food. The gastrointestinal system is critical to maintaining water balance in the body as the combination of daily water intake with secretions by the salivary glands, stomach, intestines, pancreas, and liver into the gastrointestinal lumen means much water must be reabsorbed to prevent serious water loss to the body. Dysfunction of the gastrointestinal tract in maintaining this secreted water results in severe dehydration and death and is one of the leading reasons for high mortality worldwide.

While the gastrointestinal system has been called the digestive tract, digestion is but one of its four major functions which include ingestion, digestion, absorption, and defense. Food is ingested through the oral cavity and digested mechanically in the oral cavity and stomach as well as digested by enzymes secreted in the oral cavity, stomach, intestine, and from the pancreas's exocrine portion. Once the mechanical and chemical digestion breaks down the food to its fundamental building chemicals, these sugars, amino acids, and fatty acids are absorbed across the epithelial cells lining the mucosa lumen, mostly in the small intestine.

The neural control of the gastrointestinal system is not entirely dependent on the autonomic nervous system as are other internal systems like the cardiovascular or renal systems. The gastrointestinal system has the somatic type of innervation for the oral cavity, pharynx, and part of the rostral esophagus in the humans in which motoneurons in cranial motor nuclei directly innervate the striated muscles. Proceeding more caudally in the esophagus, the neural control switches to the autonomic nervous system, which innervates smooth muscles complemented by local neural reflexes and hormonal modulation [4, 5]. The autonomic nervous system controls the remainder of the gastrointestinal system beginning with the more caudal esophagus through the stomach, small intestine, large intestine, and colon [6].

The autonomic nervous system works through a series of ganglia in the gastrointestinal wall and these ganglia compose the enteric nervous system. The enteric nervous system is composed of a series of ganglionic nerve plexi that extend from the esophagus to the rectum and contain over a million neurons. These ganglionic plexuses are either located in the submucosal region below the epithelial cells that compose the mucosa or between the circular and longitudinal muscle layers and defined as the myenteric plexus [7]. The neurons in these ganglia provide a highly independent local control for the gastrointestinal system independent of the autonomic neurons proceeding from the brain stem. Cells in the gastrointestinal tract beginning with the stomach secrete a variety of hormones which can affect secretion of enzymes and motility (i.e., gastrin, cholecystokinin, secretin), and include many peptides that are also transmitters in the central nervous system. Secretin was the first hormone discovered by physiologists.

Four Major Functions

Ingestion

Ingestion refers to several functions which begin with bringing the food into the mouth by incising, biting, or sipping the food and/or liquid [8, 9]. The tongue, cheek, and lip muscles maneuver the food, and the complex process begins in which the food is manipulated to soften it, transport it to the posterior teeth for mastication, and further manipulate it for additional chewing until smaller sizes are achieved, sufficient for the tongue to transport the boluses toward the pharynx [10, 11]. The different functions of digestion include an initial oral preparatory phase. During this period, the masticated food becomes smaller material. During the oral manipulation, the salivary glands secrete fluids with enzymes that can begin the digestion phase that involves the breaking down of the food to smaller particles and their primary elements. Digestion begins in the oral cavity with both alpha amylase, which with initiates the chemical breakdown of starches, and lipase, which begins some digestion of fats. Once the food reaches the pharyngeal mucosa, it induces pharyngeal swallowing. More recent evidence suggests that the oral phase of swallowing may be more tightly bound to the pharyngeal phase of swallowing so that the two may be considered one continuous motor act [12].

Digestion

Digestion involves breaking food into smaller particles, and this occurs both mechanically and chemically. Mastication occurs in both the oral cavity with the teeth, and in the stomach with powerful muscles continually massaging the food into a sticky-like substance called chyme that must proceed through a narrow passage to enter the small intestine. Chewing with the teeth and contraction of the gastrointestinal muscles in the stomach mechanically convert food to products that can be absorbed. Complementing the mechanical breakdown of the food is the chemical digestion of food products to their ultimate elements and involves enzymes that are secreted by the salivary glands (i.e., amylase, lipase), stomach (pepsinogen), and pancreas as well as by cells lining the gastrointestinal lumen. Starches are converted to monosaccharides, proteins become dipeptides and amino acids, and fats become monoglycerides and free fatty acids so they can pass from the lumen of the gastrointestinal tract through the mucosal epithelial cells of the small intestine to the capillaries of the cardiovascular system and to the lymph glands. Some fats involve an additional action through emulsion to assist in their digestion. It is interesting to note that 50 % of the average Western diet is composed of starches. The average diet in the industrialized countries contains almost double the protein required by the body daily. Fiber comes from the carbohydrates, cellulose and pectin, and is not digested, but does absorb water creating a bulk form that stimulates intestinal motility.

Absorption

Absorption refers to the process by which the products of digestion are taken from the gastrointestinal lumen into the blood and lymph glands. Nutrients, water, and electrolytes move across the epithelial cells primarily in the small intestine, and water also moves across the epithelium of the small and large intestine and colon. The epithelial cells transport the fundamental elements of each of the three broad categories of food, carbohydrates, proteins, and lipids, using a variety of membrane protein carriers that move the sugars, amino acids, and fatty acids into the epithelial cells. The absorption of sugars and amino acids occurs more in the middle level of the small intestine (i.e., jejunum), while most fatty acids, vitamins, and ions like calcium are absorbed in the upper small intestine (i.e., duodenum). Bile salts are reabsorbed in the lower small intestine (i.e., ileum).

Defense

The gastrointestinal tract mucosa is the largest surface area of the body exposed to the environment, far more than the skin due to its numerous invaginations and deep pits of mucosa beginning with the stomach and proceeding caudally through the intestines. The gastrointestinal tract needs to protect the body against ingested viruses, bacteria, and toxins. The salivary glands secrete some lysozymes while the stomach has special epithelial cells that secrete hydrogen ions in the form of hydrochloric acid (HCl) which lowers the pH of the stomach lumen to highly acidic levels, thus killing many bacteria and viruses.

Four major functions of the gastrointestinal tract
- Ingestion
- Digestion
- Absorption
- Defense

Deglutition

The gastrointestinal tract is complex with varied functions from the oral cavity to the colon so that experts in the field often specialize in particular subfunctions and regions of the gastrointestinal tract. This two volume series is dedicated to experts and specialists that work in the field of swallowing and its disorders. This includes specialists in radiology, esophageal and stomach disorders, and otolaryngologists, as well as speech pathologists who have focused on swallowing versus the vocalization functions of the oral, pharyngeal, and laryngeal regions. As is true in so many fields, the clinicians who treat the patients often are ahead of the science that provides the basic understanding of the underlying mechanisms. Trial-and-error approaches through caregivers to patients with dysphagia often provide the next level of new diagnostic and treatment modalities. It can be the caregiver who provides the next level of innovation. Such dedicated people working in

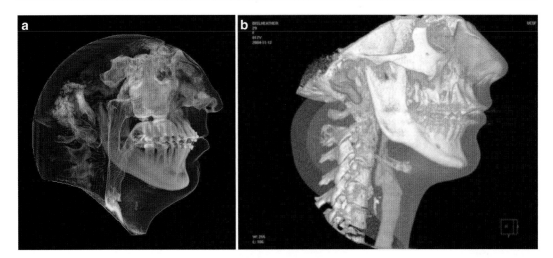

Fig. 1.2 A lateral view of an adult from a cone beam computed tomography (CBCT) scan which allows illustrating bone, such as the mandible, as well as the facial profile and airway. The CBCT scan was completed with a Hitachi MercuRay unit (Hitachi, Tokyo, Japan) with a 9.6 s scan. The software that develops the images is Anatomage In Vivo (Anatomage, San Jose, CA, USA)

swallowing and dysphagia continually search the fundamental research to provide a basis for their work, and the interaction among basic scientists, clinician scientists, and clinicians provides an effective method to improve health care.

Oral Phase of Swallowing

The oral phase of swallowing refers to transporting the food broken by chewing toward the pharynx and may be an integral part of the pharyngeal swallow [13]. In the oral phase, the tongue develops a squeezing-like action, analogous to squeezing a tube of toothpaste, as the bolus is held between the tongue and palate [9]. The bolus is pushed posteriorly to the opening of the pharynx. The oral phase integrates with ingestion and chewing so that the oral cavity is performing multiple and different motor functions with a purpose of decreasing the initial food to a size that can be swallowed through the pharynx and esophagus. The complex interaction of these different motor responses requires extended sensory feedback and coordination of the central nervous system [14]. The contribution of the different cortical regions to controlling regions of the brain stem which have groups of interneurons (i.e., central

pattern generators) that induce sequences of recruitment of motoneurons in different cranial motor nuclei for chewing and pharyngeal swallowing remains to be fully elucidated.

The oral phase of swallowing relates to a complex set of motor movements which coordinate the tongue, mandible, and hyoid bone (Fig. 1.2). The oral phase is one aspect of a series of oral movements that include incising, transporting food to the posterior teeth, mastication or chewing food to break it down to smaller sizes, and then moving the small boluses posteriorly toward the oropharynx with squeezing-like actions of the tongue with the palate [15]. These separate movement patterns are coordinated to process the original food to boluses of smaller size through chewing, and then manipulating the small boluses so they can be transported posteriorly toward the pharynx. The oral phase is tied to the pharyngeal phase in that it moves food posteriorly and caudally into the pharynx setting up a sensory input that triggers the pharyngeal swallow. Most of the actions of the oral cavity in transporting food to the posterior teeth, chewing, and then propelling the bolus posteriorly are unconsciously conducted based on continued sensory feedback from the oral region, but can be consciously controlled for each individual motor response. The tongue and palate have some of the

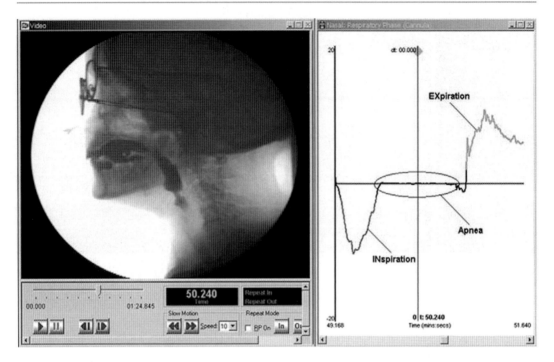

Fig. 1.3 A videofluoroscopic lateral view of an adult swallowing a barium bolus while sensors pick up changes in airflow depicting inspiration and expiration. From B. Martin-Harris et al. Otolaryngol Head Neck Surg 2005;133(2):234–40 with permission

highest density of touch and pressure sensory fibers which provide complex input that is processed and further characterized in terms of texture, shape, and size [16]. Sensory fibers responding to changes in temperature also innervate the oral cavity and provide information as to the relative level of bolus temperatures.

> Ingestion includes:
> - Bringing the food or liquid into the oral cavity
> - Manipulation of the food with saliva as part of the oral preparatory stage
> - Transporting the food to the posterior teeth for oral mastication
> - Transporting the food to the pharynx; the oral phase of swallowing

Pharyngeal Phase of Swallowing

The pharynx is unique in the gastrointestinal tract as it provides a conduit for two distinct functions which have to be separated: the passage of air and the transport of boluses of food and liquids [17]. The pharynx functions for the majority of a 24-h period as a respiratory conduit to provide passage of air during both inspiration and expiration (Fig. 1.3). Normally, in quiet resting conditions, most human subjects breathe in (i.e., inspire) through their nasal passages into the pharynx and through the vocal cords into the trachea to move a bolus of air into the alveoli of the lungs for gas exchange with the surrounding capillaries. Expiration involves expelling a portion of this air. In contrast, during eating and drinking, the central nervous system shifts the function of the pharynx to become a conduit for passing food and liquid to the esophagus [18]. The pharyngeal phase of swallowing refers to the transport of the bolus through the pharynx into the esophagus during which the normal respiratory function of the pharynx ceases. Aspiration of food and liquids into the trachea toward the lungs as well as rostrally into the nasopharynx and nasal passages is prevented by coordinated activity of muscles around the pharynx as the pharynx elevates and then peristaltically contracts to move the food

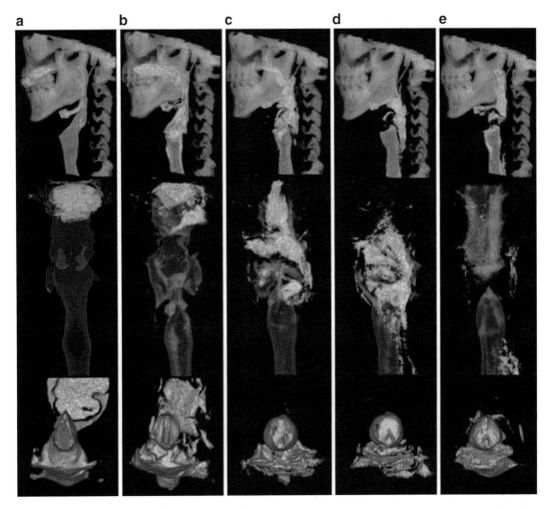

Fig. 1.4 Example of a swallow by one individual in which the entire volume of the bolus is depicted in real time at 0.1, 2.0, 2.2, 2.3, and 2.4 s (**a**–**e**) after the start of swallowing using a 320-detector-row multislice CT scanner from Aquilion One, Toshiba Medical Systems. The upper row demonstrates the *lateral view* while the middle row shows the *anterior view*, and the lower row depicts the *inferior view*. The contrast medium is depicted in *yellow* and the airway is *blue*. From N. Fujii et al. Dysphagia 2011;26(2):99–107 with permission

caudally. Peristaltic contractions occur with the pharynx and esophagus, and can occur in the stomach, which begins to demonstrate additional types of contraction patterns. The smooth muscles of the intestines do not demonstrate peristaltic contractions as seen with the pharynx or esophagus but rather have complex motor responses such as segmentation and migrating motor responses.

The pharyngeal phase of swallowing has been defined clinically with videofluoroscopy as well as with manometric measurements. New approaches are now providing three-dimensional imaging in real time for each swallow (Fig. 1.4) as well as cross-sectional views (Fig. 1.5) [19]. Pressure measurements are now possible in three dimensions with high-resolution manometry (Fig. 1.6). The pharyngeal phase of swallowing can be defined by its biomechanical properties and modeled [21]. Computer models have been developed to demonstrate how the tongue, jaw, and hyoid bone can move with contraction of specific muscles and are beginning to include the pharyngeal muscles (Fig. 1.7) [22].

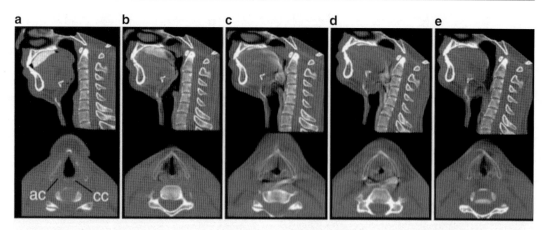

Fig. 1.5 Example of a swallow by one individual in which the entire volume of the bolus is depicted in real time in midsagittal (*upper*) and axial (*lower*) images at 0.1, 2.0, 2.2, 2.3, and 2.4 s (**a–e**) after the start of swallowing. The changes in the soft tissue and the movement of the hyoid bone and larynx, and the position of the contrast medium are shown. Abbreviations are: *ac* arytenoid cartilage; *cc* cricoid cartilage. From N. Fujii et al. Dysphagia 2011;26(2):99–107 with permission

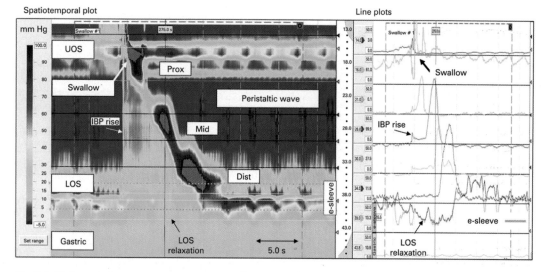

Fig. 1.6 High-resolution manometric measurement shows the esophageal pressure activity from the pharynx to the stomach. The spatiotemporal plot shows what the line pressure measures show. Time is shown on the horizontal axis while the distance from the nares is depicted on the vertical axis. The images are acquired by a 36 channel SSI Manoscan 360 unit. Abbreviations: *UOS* upper esophageal sphincter, *LOS* lower esophageal sphincter, *prox* proximal, *mid* midsection, *dist* distal. From M.R. Fox and A.J. Bredenoord. Gut 2008;57(3):405–23 with permission

Esophageal Phase of Swallowing

The esophagus is isolated from the pharynx by the upper esophageal sphincter and from the stomach by the lower esophageal sphincter [23]. The opening of these sphincters is tightly timed to open as boluses of food and water reach them.

The upper esophageal sphincter, or pharyngo-esophageal sphincter, is normally closed and then relaxes during pharyngeal swallowing, and then closes again as the food moves caudally in the esophagus toward the stomach [24]. The upper one-third of the human esophagus is composed of striated muscle which is under direct control of

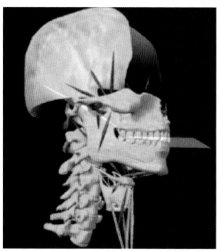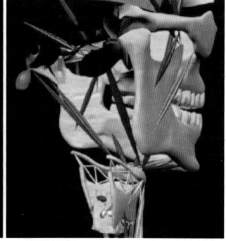

Fig. 1.7 A computer model of the craniofacial region with muscles simulated to determine the movement of the mandible and hyoid bone. From I. Stavness et al. An integrated dynamic jaw and laryngeal model constructed from CT data. Berlin: Springer; 2006:169–77 with permission

motoneurons located in the nucleus ambiguus, one of the cranial motor nuclei involved with swallowing [25–28]. The lower two-thirds of the human esophagus is composed of smooth muscle innervated by motoneurons located in ganglia, not in the brain stem [29]. The preganglionic neurons are located in the dorsal motor nucleus of the vagus nerve in the brain stem and send their axons through the vagus nerve to the ganglia in the gastrointestinal tract [28]. Despite the transition from striated muscles to smooth muscles in the esophagus and the shift in the location of the type of motoneuron, the esophagus demonstrates a peristaltic contraction sequence progressing caudally during the esophageal swallowing [7, 30–33]. Peristalsis is a coordinated pattern of muscle contractions and relaxation that is a wave-like activity [17]. It begins in the pharynx and proceeds caudally through the esophagus. The strength of the peristaltic contraction depends upon sensory feedback evident when food is present. The volume of a bolus can enhance the contraction of the muscles in the pharyngeal phase of swallowing and increase the intensity of esophageal contraction. The presence of a bolus in the esophagus can induce secondary peristalsis without primary initiation from central nervous system.

Saliva

Saliva refers to the secretions from three major glands (i.e., parotid, submandibular, and sublingual) and several additional glands that express their alkaline fluid into the oral cavity and partially into the pharynx. The three major glands secrete 95 % of the saliva which is composed of water, proteins, and electrolytes [34]. The submandibular and sublingual glands secrete a fluid higher in proteins than the parotid glands so that it is a thicker consistency. Saliva is higher in bicarbonate (HCO_3^-) than plasma, which accounts for the higher pH of saliva than blood. Saliva has multiple functions including neutralizing acids secreted by oral bacteria as well as acid that regurgitates from the stomach. Saliva includes some antibodies to bacteria and lyso-zymes that digest bacterial walls. Saliva also cools hot foods ingested. Enzymes secreted by the salivary glands begin the digestion phase. Alpha-amylase degrades starches into disaccharides and begins the process of carbohydrate digestion that continues in the stomach and is then complemented by amylase secreted by the pancreas into the small intestine.

The salivary glands are like most of the tissues in the gastrointestinal tract below the upper esophagus in which the autonomic nervous system innervates these target tissues. In contrast, the striated muscles of the tongue, pharynx, larynx, and upper esophageal regions have motoneurons innervating the muscles, and the cell bodies of the motoneurons reside in the brain stem in cranial motor nuclei (i.e., hypoglossal, nucleus ambiguus) [35]. Autonomic innervation means that both the sympathetic and parasympathetic nervous systems, which differ anatomically and use different transmitters in their postganglionic neurons, can innervate the same target organs. The salivary glands are unique in that both the sympathetic and parasympathetic nervous systems enhance their secretions, in contrast to their antagonistic roles with the rest of the gastrointestinal system. The sympathetic induces smaller volumes of saliva that are richer in proteins, while parasympathetic innervation enhances the volume of salivary secretion primarily by vasodilatation of the vessels near the fundamental units of the salivary gland, the acinar and duct cells.

Control of the Gastrointestinal Tract

Secretions and motor movements of much of the gastrointestinal tract, beginning with the stomach and proceeding caudally, are controlled by the autonomic nervous system and the enteric nervous system. The autonomic neural control has been defined by three phases: cephalic, gastric, and intestinal. The cephalic phase refers to the inducement of secretions like saliva into the oral cavity, acid into the stomach, and pancreatic enzymes and liver bile into the small intestine before the food reaches the organ. The sight, smell, or thought of food will induce this active autonomic drive. The gastric and intestinal phases refer to how various food products will further alter secretions in the stomach and intestine when the food is at those sites. Saliva secretion is affected by both a preoral stimulation as well as when the food is in the oral cavity.

Oral Cavity

The oral cavity is unique in the gastrointestinal tract as it has the tongue as an organ that transports food and liquid anteriorly and posteriorly as well as manipulates the food with the cheek muscles in order for the posterior teeth to masticate [10, 11]. The tongue is composed of extrinsic and intrinsic striated muscles that can alter their shape and position to manipulate food boluses. The tongue has the ability to alter shape and modify its force of contraction in speech, mastication, respiration, and in both the oral and pharyngeal phases of swallowing [36]. Control of the muscles that retract the tongue as compared to the one muscle that protrudes (i.e., genioglossus) the tongue is often reflexively determined.

The oral and pharyngeal cavities also have a unique set of sensory fibers that respond to different types of chemicals which range from sweet to sour, bitter, and salty [14, 37–39]. These taste sensory fibers have terminal endings with receptors that respond to specific chemicals, and while covering much of the tongue surface, also innervate the palate and pharyngeal mucosa. These taste sensory fibers synapse in the brain stem within the nucleus tractus solitarius more rostrally than the sensory fibers that directly trigger pharyngeal swallowing. Sour boluses enhance salivation and affect the pharyngeal phase of swallowing suggesting that some sensory fibers responding to certain chemicals facilitate or directly trigger the pharyngeal swallow [40].

Integrating the Cortex and Brain Stem in Control of Pharygneal Swallowing

The neural control of swallowing changes through the three phases of swallowing [41]. The oral phase depends upon multiple cortical sites that interact with regions of the brain stem which have interneuron groups dedicated to sequential contraction of mandibular, tongue, and hyoid muscles. A region of the brain stem near the trigeminal motor nucleus controls the sequence of jaw muscles that provide a cyclic contraction that moves the jaw in chewing-like or fictive movements [42, 43]. The timing and intensity of these jaw muscle contractions can be modified by stimulating specific regions of the cortex. Excellent work in the awake monkey using microstimulation and microelectrode recording depicts how the cortex

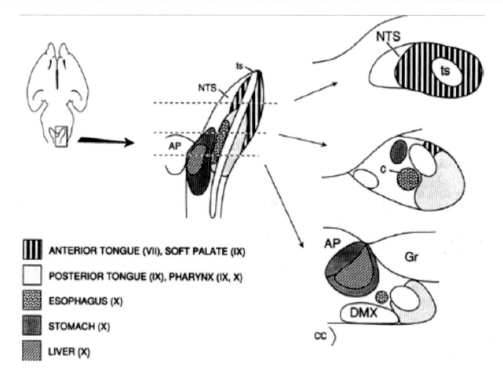

ANTERIOR TONGUE (VII), SOFT PALATE (IX)

POSTERIOR TONGUE (IX), PHARYNX (IX, X)

ESOPHAGUS (X)

STOMACH (X)

LIVER (X)

Fig. 1.8 Schematic of the nucleus tractus solitarius located in the brain stem and the location of sensory inputs from different regions of the gastrointestinal tract. The schematic shows the distribution of primary afferents from the alimentary canal to the dorsomedial medulla of the rat. Most of the esophageal afferents project to the central subnucleus. Abbreviations include: *DMX* dorsal motor nucleus of the vagus nerve, *AP* area postrema, *Gr* gracile nucleus, *cc* central canal. From E.T. Cunningham and P.E. Sawchenko. Dysphagia 1990;5(1):35–51 with permission

is organized to control the tongue muscles and swallowing [44]. The concepts of cortical and brain stem interaction, and the contribution of each, have changed most with the pharyngeal swallow [45]. Several studies have shown that the brain stem has a region of the nucleus tractus solitarius with neurons that discharge in various sequences like the muscles recruited from multiple motoneuron pools in several cranial motor nuclei, and that, in some species, there is a more ventral region which transmits the timing discharges to different motoneuron pools (Fig. 1.8) [46]. The concept that the cortex is vitally involved with the brain stem in controlling swallowing is well documented [47]. The studies in the brain stem suggest that groups of interneurons can be triggered to discharge in sequence to control a multimotor output that has a sequence [46]. Such groups of interneurons have been well studied in invertebrate nervous systems and are well documented in the mammalian CNS including sites controlling jaw movements as well as pharyngeal swallowing [48–50]. Such groups of interneurons are represented in the nucleus tractus solitarius and are triggered into sequential all or none action by specific sensory inputs [51, 52].

Sensory feedback from the oral and pharyngeal region can modify the intensity of the pharyngeal swallowing phase indicating that sensory input probably synapses centrally in both the brain stem and cortex, particularly as related to the volume of the bolus being swallowed [53]. Cortical studies of subjects swallowing both spontaneously and on command [54, 55], as well as studies of patients with dysphagia induced by a cortical stroke [56, 57], have implicated several cortical and subcortical sites [58].

Once the bolus begins to enter the pharynx, it triggers a region of the nucleus tractus solitarius

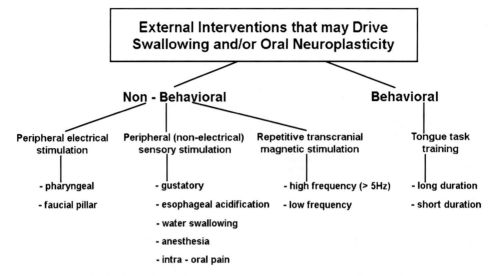

Fig. 1.9 Schematic indicating how rehabilitation might be approached using external interventions. From R.E. Martin. Dysphagia 2009;24(2):218–29 with permission

which sets up a sequence that proceeds to recruit motoneurons in multiple cranial motor nuclei [46]. The esophageal phase depends upon a sequential triggering of interneurons within a specific subnucleus of the nucleus tractus solitarius. The esophageal phase depends on coordination of output from the dorsal motor nucleus of the vagus, which provides the preganglionic neurons that innervate the ganglia in the esophagus to excite the postganglionic neurons innervating the smooth muscle portion.

Rehabilitation in Dysphagia

Dysphagia refers to multiple swallowing disorders which have different etiologies [59]. Some of these disorders relate to peripheral mechanisms that can be assisted by surgical approaches. However, damage to the central nervous system, as in a cortical infarct, raises the issue of how to replace a permanently damaged region of the cortex [60]. Rehabilitation requires retraining the remaining central neural pathways through exercise and practicing motor movements with the concept that the central nervous system will strengthen remaining alternative pathways to facilitate a motor action or accomplish the motor

response originally controlled by the damaged region with the lost neurons (Fig. 1.9) [61–65]. Stimulation of the cortex directly, as with electrical or magnetic fields, can alter the representation of the muscles or motor movement in that sensorimotor cortex [66]. Increasing sensory input to the cortex in a damaged central nervous system can also reorganize a cortical site [67–69]. Taste may also affect cortical activity of the swallowing pathway in the normal subject [70]. Rehabilitation can also work through strengthening the end organ, the target tissue or muscles, which become stronger and develop more force with repeated exercise against high loads [71, 72], or become more fatigue resistant with increased frequency of use which enhances blood supply to the muscle and muscle fibers and alters their mitochondrial number to be more oxidative fibers.

Exercising muscles of the tongue and oropharyngeal region through vocal exercises can improve the use of these muscles in swallowing. Practicing specific tongue movements can improve the tongue movements in swallowing. Electrical stimulation to submental muscles with inserted intramuscular fine wires allows a patient to improve her/his elevation of the larynx through recruitment of a suprahyoid muscle [73, 74]. Transcranial magnetic stimulation applied to the cortex can affect the learning of motor movements [75]. Much of the future studies in swallowing and dysphagia will concentrate on mechanisms and approaches to rehabilitate swallowing in a damaged nervous system [76].

Rehabilitation of patients with dysphagia may involve:

- Triggering the cephalic phase of control of salivation
- Stimulating oral sensory sites with stimuli that could include taste, water, sour solutions, temperature, touch/pressure, and air pulses
- Repeatedly stimulating oropharyngeal and hypopharyngeal sensory sites with sour stimuli, air puffs, or moving touch stimuli
- Selectively stimulating the cortex with transcranial magnetic stimulation
- Training tongue and pharyngeal muscles through exercise

References

1. Code CF, Schlegel JF. Handbook of physiology. In: Code CF, editor. Handbook of physiology, vol. IV. Washington DC: American Physiological Society; 1968.
2. Roberts DJ. Molecular mechanisms of development of the gastrointestinal tract. Dev Dyn. 2000;219(2): 109–20.
3. Vander A, Sherman J, Luciano D. Human physiology: the mechanisms of body function. 8th ed. New York: McGraw Hill; 2001.
4. Conklin JL. Control of esophageal motor function. Dysphag Fall. 1993;8(4):311–7.
5. Massey BT. Physiology of oral cavity, pharynx, and upper esophageal sphincter. GI Motility Online. 2006;doi:10.1038/gimo2(May 16, 2006).
6. Cunningham Jr ET, Sawchenko PE. Central neural control of esophageal motility: a review. Dysphagia. 1990;5(1):35–51.
7. Janssens J, De Wever I, Vantrappen G, Hellemans J. Peristalsis in smooth muscle esophagus after transfection and bolus deviation. Gastroenterology. 1976; 71(6):1004–9.
8. Hiiemae KM, Palmer JB. Food transport and bolus formation during complete feeding sequences on foods of different initial consistency. Dysphag Winter. 1999;14(1):31–42.
9. Hiiemae KM, Palmer JB. Tongue movements in feeding and speech. Crit Rev Oral Biol Med. 2003;14(6): 413–29.
10. Palmer JB, Hiiemae KM, Liu J. Tongue-jaw linkages in human feeding: a preliminary videofluorographic study. Arch Oral Biol. 1997;42(6):429–41.
11. Palmer JB, Hiiemae KM, Matsuo K, Haishima H. Volitional control of food transport and bolus formation during feeding. Physiol Behav. 2007;91(1): 66–70.
12. Martin-Harris B, Michel Y, Castell DO. Physiologic model of oropharyngeal swallowing revisited. Otolaryngol Head Neck Surg. 2005;133(2):234–40.
13. Hiiemae KM, Crompton AW, Hiiemae KM, Crompton AW. Mastication, food transport, and swallowing. In: Hildebrand MBD, Liem KF, et al., editors. Functional vertebrate morphology. Cambridge, MA: Harvard University Press; 1985. p. 262–90.
14. Sweazey R, Bradley R. Response characteristics of lamb trigeminal neurons to stimulation of the oral cavity and epiglottis with different sensory modalities. Brain Res Bull. 1989;22:883–91.
15. Hiiemae KTA, Crompton A. Intra oral food transport: the fundamental mechanism of feeding. In: Carlson DS, McNamara J, editors. Muscle adaptation in the Craniofacial Region. Ann Arbor, Michigan: Center for Human Growth and Development; 1978. p. 181–208.
16. Sweazey RD, Bradley RM. Response characteristics of lamb pontine neurons to stimulation of the oral cavity and epiglottis with different sensory modalities. J Neurophysiol. 1993;70:1168–80.
17. Kahrilas PJ. Pharyngeal structure and function. Dysphag Fall. 1993;8(4):303–7.
18. Jafari S, Prince RA, Kim DY, Paydarfar D. Sensory regulation of swallowing and airway protection: a role for the internal superior laryngeal nerve in humans. J Physiol. 2003;550(Pt 1):287–304.
19. Fujii N, Inamoto Y, Saitoh E, et al. Evaluation of swallowing using 320-detector-row multislice CT. Part I: Single- and multiphase volume scanning for three-dimensional morphological and kinematic analysis. Dysphagia. 2011;26(2):99–107.
20. Fox MR, Bredenoord AJ. Oesophageal high-resolution manometry: moving from research into clinical practice. Gut. 2008;57(3):405–23.
21. Kahrilas PJ, Lin S, Chen J, Logemann JA. Three-dimensional modeling of the oropharynx during swallowing. Radiology. 1995;194(2):575–9.
22. Stavness I, Hannam AG, Lloyd JE, Fall CH. An integrated dynamic jaw and laryngeal model constructd from CT data. In: Harders M, Szekely G, eds. Berlin: Springer; 2006:169–77.
23. Kahrilas PJ, Dodds WJ, Dent J, Logemann JA, Shaker R. Upper esophageal sphincter function during deglutition. Gastroenterology. 1988;95(1):52–62.
24. Lang IM, Dantas RO, Cook IJ, Dodds WJ. Videoradiographic, manometric, and electromyographic analysis of canine upper esophageal sphincter. Am J Physiol. 1991;260(6 Pt 1):G911–9.
25. Altschuler SM, Bao XM, Bieger D, Hopkins DA, Miselis RR. Viscerotopic representation of the upper

alimentary tract in the rat: sensory ganglia and nuclei of the solitary and spinal trigeminal tracts. J Comp Neurol. 1989;283(2):248–68.

26. Altschuler SM, Bao XM, Miselis RR. Dendritic architecture of nucleus ambiguus motoneurons projecting to the upper alimentary tract in the rat. J Comp Neurol. 1991;309(3):402–14.

27. Broussard DL, Altschuler SM. Central integration of swallow and airway-protective reflexes. Am J Med. 2000;108(Suppl 4a):62S–7.

28. Broussard DL, Altschuler SM. Brainstem viscerotopic organization of afferents and efferents involved in the control of swallowing. Am J Med. 2000;108(Suppl 4a):79S–86.

29. Lang IM, Dean C, Medda BK, Aslam M, Shaker R. Differential activation of medullary vagal nuclei during different phases of swallowing in the cat. Brain Res. 2004;1014(1–2):145–63.

30. Roman C, Orengo M, Tieffenbach L. [Electromyographic study of esophageal smooth muscle in cats]. J Physiol (Paris). 1969;61 Suppl 2:390.

31. Roman C, Tieffenbach L. [Esophageal smooth muscle motility after bivagotomy. Electromyographic study (E.M.G)]. J Physiol (Paris). 1971;63(8):733–62.

32. Roman C, Tieffenbach L. Recording the unit activity of vagal motor fibers innervating the baboon esophagus. J Physiol (Paris). 1972;64(5):479–506.

33. Janssens J, Vantrappen G, Hellemans J. Neural control of primary esophageal peristalsis. Gastroenterology. 1978;74(4):801–3.

34. Pedersen AM, Bardow A, Jensen SB, Nauntofte B. Saliva and gastrointestinal functions of taste, mastication, swallowing, and digestion. Oral Dis. 2002;8:117–29.

35. Sawczuk A, Mosier KM. Neural control of tongue movement with respect to respiration and swallowing. Crit Rev Oral Biol Med. 2001;12(1):18–37.

36. Miller AJ. Oral and pharyngeal reflexes in the mammalian nervous system: their diverse range in complexity and the pivotal role of the tongue. Crit Rev Oral Biol Med. 2002;13(5):409–25.

37. Sweazey R, Bradley R. Responses of neurons in the lamb nucleus tractus solitarius to stimulation of the caudal oral cavity and epiglottis with different stimulus modalities. Brain Res. 1989;480:133–50.

38. Sweazey R, Bradley R. Central connections of the lingual-tonsillar branch of the glossopharyngeal nerve and the superior laryngeal nerve in lamb. J Comp Neurol. 1986;245:471–82.

39. Sweazey R, Bradley R. Response of lamb nucleus of the solitary tract neurons to chemical stimulation of the epiglottis. Brain Res. 1988;439:195–210.

40. Kajii Y, Shingai T, Kitagawa J, et al. Sour taste stimulation facilitates reflex swallowing from the pharynx and larynx in the rat. Physiol Behav. 2002;77(2–3):321–5.

41. Lang IM. Brain stem control of the phases of swallowing. Dysphagia. 2009;24(3):333–48.

42. Lund JP. Mastication and its control by the brain stem. Crit Rev Oral Biol Med. 1991;2(1):33–64.

43. Lund JP, Kolta A. Generation of the central masticatory pattern and its modification by sensory feedback. Dysphagia. 2006;21(3):167–74.

44. Huang CS, Hiraba H, Murray GM, Sessle BJ. Topographical distribution and functional properties of cortically induced rhythmical jaw movements in the monkey (Macaca fascicularis). J Neurophysiol. 1989;61(3):635–50.

45. Hamdy S, Mikulis DJ, Crawley A, et al. Cortical activation during human volitional swallowing: an event-related fMRI study. Am J Physiol. 1999;277(1 Pt 1):G219–25.

46. Jean A. Brainstem control of swallowing: localization and organization of the central pattern generator for swallowing. In: Taylor A, editor. Neurophysiology of the Jaws and Teeth. London: MacMillan Press; 1990.

47. Daniels SK, Corey DM, Fraychinaud A, DePolo A, Foundas AL. Swallowing lateralization: the effects of modified dual-task interference. Dysphagia. 2006;21(1):21–7.

48. Tell F, Fagni L, Jean A. Neurons of the nucleus tractus solitarius, in vitro, generate bursting activities by solitary tract stimulation. Exp Brain Res. 1990;79:436–40.

49. Tell F, Jean A. Bursting discharges evoked in vitro, by solitary tract stimulation or application of N-methyl-D-aspartate, in neurons of the rat nucleus tractus solitarii. Neurosci Lett. 1991;124:221–4.

50. Marder E, Bucher D. Central pattern generators and the control of rhythmic movements. Curr Biol. 2001;11(23):R986–96.

51. Theurer JA, Czachorowski KA, Martin LP, Martin RE. Effects of oropharyngeal air-pulse stimulation on swallowing in healthy older adults. Dysphagia. 2009;24(3):302–13.

52. Doty R. Influence of stimulus pattern on reflex deglutition. Am J Physiol. 1951;166:142–55.

53. Kahrilas PJ, Logemann JA. Volume accommodation during swallowing. Dysphagia. 1993;8(3):259–65.

54. Martin RE, Goodyear BG, Gati JS, Menon RS. Cerebral cortical representation of automatic and volitional swallowing in humans. J Neurophysiol. 2001;85(2):938–50.

55. Soros P, Inamoto Y, Martin RE. Functional brain imaging of swallowing: an activation likelihood estimation meta-analysis. Hum Brain Mapp. 2009;30(8):2426–39.

56. Robbins J, Levin RL. Swallowing after unilateral stroke of the cerebral cortex: preliminary experience. Dysphagia. 1988;3(1):11–7.

57. Robbins J, Levine RL, Maser A, Rosenbek JC, Kempster GB. Swallowing after unilateral stroke of the cerebral hemisphere. Arch Phys Med Rehabil. 1993;74:1295–300.

58. Martin RE, Kemppainen P, Masuda Y, Yao D, Murray GM, Sessle BJ. Features of cortically evoked swallowing in the awake primate (Macaca fascicularis). J Neurophysiol. 1999;82(3):1529–41.

59. Cook IJ. Diagnostic evaluation of dysphagia. Nat Clin Pract Gastroenterol Hepatol. 2008;5(7):393–403.
60. Martin RE. Neuroplasticity and swallowing. Dysphagia. 2009;24(2):218–29.
61. Butefisch CM, Davis BC, Wise SP, et al. Mechanisms of use-dependent plasticity in the human motor cortex. Proc Natl Acad Sci U S A. 2000;97(7):3661–5.
62. Fridman EA, Hanakawa T, Chung M, Hummel F, Leiguarda RC, Cohen LG. Reorganization of the human ipsilesional premotor cortex after stroke. Brain. 2004;127(Pt 4):747–58.
63. Hamdy S. The organisation and re-organisation of human swallowing motor cortex. Suppl Clin Neurophysiol. 2003;56:204–10.
64. Hamdy S, Aziz Q, Rothwell JC, et al. Recovery of swallowing after dysphagic stroke relates to functional reorganization in the intact motor cortex. Gastroenterology. 1998;115(5):1104–12.
65. Taub E, Uswatte G, Morris DM. Improved motor recovery after stroke and massive cortical reorganization following Constraint-Induced Movement therapy. Phys Med Rehabil Clin N Am. 2003;14(1 Suppl): S77–91. ix.
66. Hummel F, Cohen LG. Improvement of motor function with noninvasive cortical stimulation in a patient with chronic stroke. Neurorehabil Neural Repair. 2005;19(1):14–9.
67. Teismann IK, Steinstrater O, Warnecke T, et al. Tactile thermal oral stimulation increases the cortical representation of swallowing. BMC Neurosci. 2009;10:71.
68. Hamdy S, Aziz Q, Rothwell JC, Hobson A, Barlow J, Thompson DG. Cranial nerve modulation of human cortical swallowing motor pathways. Am J Physiol. 1997;272(4 Pt 1):G802–8.
69. Hamdy S, Aziz Q, Rothwell JC, Hobson A, Thompson DG. Sensorimotor modulation of human cortical swallowing pathways. J Physiol. 1998;506(Pt 3):857–66.
70. Babaei A, Kern M, Antonik S, et al. Enhancing effects of flavored nutritive stimuli on cortical swallowing network activity. Am J Physiol Gastrointest Liver Physiol. 2010;299(2):G422–9.
71. Robbins J, Kays SA, Gangnon RE, et al. The effects of lingual exercise in stroke patients with dysphagia. Arch Phys Med Rehabil. 2007;88(2):150–8.
72. Robbins J, Gangnon RE, Theis SM, Kays SA, Hewitt AL, Hind JA. The effects of lingual exercise on swallowing in older adults. J Am Geriatr Soc. 2005;53(9): 1483–9.
73. Burnett TA, Mann EA, Cornell SA, Ludlow CL. Laryngeal elevation achieved by neuromuscular stimulation at rest. J Appl Physiol. 2003;94(1): 128–34.
74. Burnett TA, Mann EA, Stoklosa JB, Ludlow CL. Self-triggered functional electrical stimulation during swallowing. J Neurophysiol. 2005;94(6):4011–8.
75. Hamdy S, Xue S, Valdez D, Diamant NE. Induction of cortical swallowing activity by transcranial magnetic stimulation in the anaesthetized cat. Neurogastroenterol Motil. 2001;13(1):65–72.
76. Robbins J, Butler SG, Daniels SK, et al. Swallowing and dysphagia rehabilitation: translating principles of neural plasticity into clinically oriented evidence. J Speech Lang Hear Res. 2008;51(1):S276–300.

Gustation, Olfaction, and Deglutition

2

Carmel Ryan and Thomas Hummel

Abstract

Interactions occur between the chemical senses and swallowing, in particular retronasal and orthonasal olfaction, as well as gustatory and trigeminal factors. The swallow is impacted differentially by mixed sensory stimuli, including the addition of visual stimuli, and manipulation of bolus taste and temperature. Studies have investigated the impact of these sensory manipulations on the disordered swallow, particularly for disorders of the pharyngeal stage. A variety of populations with swallowing disorders have responded to treatments using chemosensory stimulation. However, it remains unclear whether the key facilitator for improvement of the disordered swallow is olfactory, gustatory, or trigeminal. A combination of stimuli seems to be indicated.

Keywords

Eating • Nutrition • Olfaction • Smell • Swallow

Swallowing and Deglutition

Swallowing encompasses the act of placing food/liquid into the mouth, and deglutition, which is the actual movement of the bolus (ball of food/liquid) from the oral cavity to the stomach. In addition to the oral cavity, the pharynx, larynx, and esophagus are involved in the swallowing process [1]. Swallowing is a complex process involving careful coordination of several muscles, in a finely balanced action involving both sensory and motor systems. It is a basic reflex that is modified consciously by the swallower [2]. Swallowing involves activation in several areas of the cortex called the "cortical swallowing network" [3], and requires activation of several cranial nerves, including the trigeminal, glossopharyngeal, and vagal nerves [2].

There are four stages to the normal swallow: the oral preparatory phase, the oral transit phase, the pharyngeal phase, and the esophageal phase [1]. The *oral preparatory phase* begins with recognizing the food/liquid on its utensil

C. Ryan
Kean University, School of Communication
Disorders and Deafness, Union, NJ, USA

T. Hummel, MD (✉)
Technical University of Dresden Medical School,
Smell and Taste Clinic, Department of
Otorhinolaryngology, Dresden, Germany
e-mail: thummel@mail.zih.tu-dresden.de

approaching the mouth, placement in the mouth, and then processing of the food/liquid by the oral structures (tongue, teeth, and jaw, with the involvement of the lips, cheeks, hard and soft palate). The *oral phase* initiates when the tongue moves the food/liquid (known as the bolus) posteriorly, ready for the pharyngeal swallow; this involves complex coordination so that the bolus is well formed and positioned for the next stage without premature leakage into the pharynx. This stage ends and the *pharyngeal phase* occurs when the bolus is moved through the pharynx to the esophagus. Then in the *esophageal stage* the bolus is passed through the esophagus to the stomach [1].

Each phase can vary slightly in duration and nature, depending on the type and quantity of input (food or liquid); for the swallow to occur, typically something (food, liquid, or saliva) must be in the mouth. The first two stages are under voluntary control by the swallower, whereas the latter two stages are under involuntary control, although there must be voluntary initiation of swallowing for it to begin [1].

Swallowing is modulated by factors such as age and gender. *With age* it changes in a number of ways, with many senile changes seen as a normal consequence [1, 4]. People in their 60s are thought to experience a longer oral phase and slower/less efficient clearance of the bolus, more often with residue in the pharynx; older people also take longer to trigger the swallow [5]. By the 1970s and 1980s, the larynx is lower in the neck, and arthritic changes affect the bone/cartilage structures, reducing flexibility, and strength of movements, resulting in multiple swallows to clear residue from the pathways [1]. As well as changes to the anatomical and physiological components, there are changes to the peripheral and central (cortical) functions during the swallow [5]. *Gender* has also been considered a factor, perhaps influenced by bolus size, or anatomical size differences, although no clear patterns have been established [1, 4]. It should be noted that there are also neurophysiological changes with increased age; not only do older adults have later onset of the pharyngeal swallow and increased residue in the pharynx, but they show an increase in the number of cortical regions involved during swallowing [5].

The respiratory system is also intimately involved in the act of deglutition. As the pharyngeal phase of swallowing occurs, respiration is paused [1]. Typically it is the exhalation phase of respiration that is interrupted by swallowing; this is thought to be an additional safeguard, so that if there should be any residue in the airway, exhalation will help to clear it [1].

As the bolus is moved posteriorly during the oral stage of the swallow, sensory information is sent from receptors in the tongue and oropharynx to the brain to trigger the pharyngeal swallow [1]. The point in the swallowing mechanism at which the pharyngeal swallow is triggered is thought to be when the head of the bolus reaches where the tongue base crosses the lower edge of the mandible (or jaw) [1].

Interactions Between the Chemical Senses and Swallowing

Most people are familiar with "orthonasal" olfaction, where odorants reach the olfactory epithelium during sniffing [6]. Less familiar is "retronasal" olfaction which allows us to perceive odor during eating and drinking when odors reach the olfactory epithelium by passing from the mouth through the pharynx to the olfactory cleft [7, 33]. Thus the major difference between orthonasal smelling and retronasal smelling is the direction of airflow. Interestingly, the olfactory receptors react differently depending on the direction of airflow which may be a basis for the differentiation between ortho- and retronasal smells [8, 36]. Specifically, odors bind differentially to the epithelium in a chromatographic way related to the direction of the airflow, from front to back or vice versa [9]. Both smell systems, along with the gustatory and trigeminal systems interact with the motor system and our cognitive status to form our perception of flavor [8] with the major purpose to control the intake of foods/drinks into the body.

Similar to the swallowing process, chemosensory function is subject to both *age* and *gender*.

Specifically, the olfactory, trigeminal, and gustatory systems have been shown to deteriorate with aging [10, 34]. Also, the chemosensory systems interact tightly with each other. Interestingly, these interactions occur very early in the processing of this information, likely at a subcortical level [11–13, 30], often in the form of a mutual amplification of the perceived intensity. However, the opposite may also be possible [14]. When people lose olfactory sensitivity they seem to lose trigeminal [15] and gustatory sensitivity as well, [2] which has been explained largely by the loss of mutual amplification.

The chemical senses also influence swallowing (for review, see [16]). Welge-Lüßen et al. [17] examined the effects of paired olfactory and gustatory stimuli on swallowing. They were interested in the differential effects of orthonasal versus retronasal presentation of an odor. Both the frequency and the speed of swallowing were significantly enhanced using retronasal presentation. Another study [18] investigated the question whether ortho- or retronasal stimulation has a specific effect on taste-related perceptions with regard to the various phases of the swallowing process. The authors presented ortho- and retronasal olfactory stimuli while subjects received oral stimuli of two different consistencies at the same time (milk, milk plus thickener). Among other dimensions subjects rated the "creaminess" of the oral stimulus. Interestingly, significant effects for creaminess were only found for retronasal stimuli, and here the effect was most pronounced during the phase when swallowing occurred compared to other phases (no oral stimulus, mouth filling, movement of oral stimulus). Thus, creaminess of the oral stimulus was rated highest during a phase where the retronasal stimulus actually could reach the nasal cavity—which was not possible during other phases.

A central-nervous connection between retronasal olfactory stimulation and swallowing may be established through brain areas [19] related to mastication and oral activity which are activated by retronasal olfactory stimulation to a much higher degree compared to orthonasal stimulation (see also [20]).

There is also some evidence that taste, and here especially sour [4, 5, 21–23], plays a certain role in the initiation of swallowing. For clarification, taste as opposed to retronasal olfaction relates to sensations like sweet, sour, salty, bitter, and umami, while retronasal olfaction relates to flavor, e.g., cherry or chocolate.

Effects of Mixed Sensory Stimuli on Swallowing

The use not only of olfactory but also of visual stimuli was found to enhance salivation which helps evoke the swallow in normal adults [2]. Babaei et al. [3] investigated the effects on cortical activity of presentation of concurrent gustatory, olfactory, and visual stimuli. They found the activity of the cortical swallowing network enhanced; however, the study design did not allow the separation of the specific effects of each of the sensory stimuli within this network.

In addition, temperature stimuli (different temperatures of the bolus) have been studied in terms of their effect on swallowing [16]. It was found that it affected sensory perception with 50° being optimum. In addition, the authors of this study found that participants preferred sweet tasting foods rather than bitter or sour foods.

Theurer and coauthors investigated delivering pulses of air to the oropharyngeal region, to see what effect this would have on swallowing. In the first study with younger adults they found a significant effect on frequency of the swallow, and all subjects reported an irrepressible urge to swallow in response to the stimulation [24]. They went on to check responses in a group of healthy older adults, and again found a significant effect on swallowing, although this group did not report the urge to swallow what the younger subjects did [1].

Chemosensory Stimulation in Swallowing Disorders

Sensory stimulation to trigger the swallow in patients with dysphagia has been explored with some success [23, 25]. However, the potential effectiveness of olfactory stimulation alone remains a largely unexplored area. In addition, much of the contemporary research does not clearly delineate the effects of different sensory stimuli, such as smell and taste.

A number of alterations to the bolus have been tried to facilitate triggering of the pharyngeal swallow—a cold bolus, a larger size of bolus, a textured bolus, a strong flavored bolus, or a bolus that required chewing [1]. Thickened liquids and thick foods are also thought to facilitate triggering of the pharyngeal swallow [1]. One study [24] found that a sour bolus of lemon–barium sulfate mixture significantly improved a number of swallowing parameters, including decreasing pharyngeal delay. In this study the stimulant combined elements of taste and smell, so the exact cause remains unclear.

Thin liquids associated with aspiration have been replaced with thickened liquids, but patients may dislike the taste/texture and limit their fluid intake, consequently increasing the chance of dehydration. Pelletier and Lawless [5] experimented with a bolus of citrus (sour) plus sucrose (sweet) to see if it would improve swallow function in patients suffering from neurogenic oropharyngeal dysphagia without the negative effects of a sour only bolus. Only the sour bolus improved the swallow, as measured by less aspiration and penetration. Which mechanism was triggered is unclear—it may have been taste, trigeminal stimulation, or a combination of the two at work here; similarly, what was responsible for inhibiting an effect in the sweet–sour mixture is also unknown [5].

In terms of taste stimulants, sour seems to be consistently effective in improving a number of parameters of the swallow, including latency of triggering the swallow in typical adults [10]. While lemon flavor is used to stimulate swallowing by some clinicians, there seems to be no clear evidence to support its use [10].

According to Theurer et al. [24] four studies looked at oropharyngeal stimulation using sensory stimulants; thermal–tactile stimulation (TTS) had short-term effects, as did a sour bolus, but with no reduction in aspiration in dysphagic patients. Sciortino et al. [23] explored the three elements in TTS separately in all possible combinations (tactile/thermal/gustatory) to isolate

what is the most effective, and found that all three were needed to improve swallow latency. These researchers point to the need for studies looking for any long-term effects of these techniques [24, 26, 27] as well as effects of varying the intensity, frequency, and treatment duration of TTS [27].

A recently published study by South et al. [28] looked for the effect of gum chewing on the frequency and latency of the swallow in patients with Parkinson's disease (PD), who are known to have reduced saliva management. They found that chewing gum helped PD patients normalize rate and latency of saliva swallows, although more research is needed to evaluate long-term effects.

Olfactory stimuli were one part of a sensory stimulation plan evaluated by Lippert et al. [27] with patients in a coma. They used acoustic, tactile, olfactory, gustatory, and kinesthetic stimulants in combination and found effects on the heart rate, respiration, and head and eye movements of the comatose patients. They recommend use of tactile and acoustic input, which had the biggest effects in early stages, followed by use of the other stimuli as coma depth decreases.

Ebihara and colleagues [31, 32] significantly improved the timing of the swallow in the post-stroke patients in their study. They used black pepper oil presented nasally to successfully stimulate the swallow. The swallowing reflex was triggered via delivery of a bolus of distilled water through the nasal catheter (see also [21]).

A randomized, controlled study using elderly at-risk patients investigated the potential of having the patient dissolve a capsaicin troche (tablet with a center hole to prevent choking) in their mouth each day. This study resulted in significant improvement in swallowing reflex, both between subjects and within subjects [29] (see also [35]). However, it required considerable effort from caregivers to have the patient do this every day, and would not be suitable for patients with cognitive impairments, or patients that could not suck and dissolve the troche [32]. In their study published in 2010, Yamasaki and colleagues [2] investigated the potential of capsiate, considered a nonpungent alternative to capsaicin, to trigger the pharyngeal swallow in elderly patients with aspiration pneumonia. No patients reported experiencing unpleasant feelings, supporting the nonpungency of capsiate. They timed the "latent time of swallowing reflex" (LTSR) from the time of injection of stimulus material into a nasal catheter to the onset of swallowing and found a significant improvement in time of the swallow for higher strengths (10 and 100 nM). They proposed that potential benefits could be achieved for this population with injection of capsiate into liquids or food; the research has not been done with this method of delivery, however. Further studies in this area should also determine if any positive results endure beyond termination of the study condition.

Conclusions

Chemosensory stimulation appears to facilitate deglutition. However, currently it is unclear whether the olfactory, gustatory, or trigeminal stimuli play a special role in this process. From a therapeutic angle it seems that the chemical senses play a role in deglutition, but they play this role best in combination with other sensory stimuli.

References

1. Theurer J, Czachorowski K, Martin L, Martin R. Effects of oropharyngeal air-pulse stimulation on swallowing in healthy older adults. Dysphagia. 2009;24:302–13.
2. Steele CM, Miller AJ. Sensory input pathways and mechanisms in swallowing: a review. Dysphagia. 2010;25:323–33.
3. Babaei A, Kern M, Antonik S, Mepani R, Ward B, Douglas Li S-J, Hyde J, Shaker R. Enhancing effects of flavored nutritive stimuli on cortical swallowing network activity. Am J Physiol Gastrointest Liver Physiol. 2010;299:G422–9.
4. Cola PC, Gatto AR, Silva RG, Spadotto AA, Schelp AO, Henry MA. The influence of sour taste and cold temperature in pharyngeal transit duration in patients with stroke. Arq Gastroenterol. 2010;47:18–21.
5. Pelletier C, Lawless H. Effect of citric acid and citric acid-sucrose mixtures on swallowing in neurogenic oropharyngeal dysphagia. Dysphagia. 2003;18: 231–41.
6. Shepherd GM. Smell images and the flavor system in the human brain. Nature. 2006;444(16):316–21.
7. Logemann JA. Evaluation and treatment of swallowing disorders. 2nd ed. Austin: Pro Ed; 1998.
8. Scott JW, Acevedo HP, Sherrill L, Phan M. Responses of the rat olfactory epithelium to retronasal air flow. J Neurophysiol. 2007;97:1941–50.
9. Yamasaki M, Ebihara S, Ebihara T, Yamanda S, Arai H, Kohzuki M. Effects of capsiate on the triggering of the swallowing reflex in elderly patients with aspiration pneumonia. Geriatr Gerontol Int. 2010;10: 107–9.
10. Pelletier C. Chemosenses, aging, and oropharyngeal dysphagia. Top Geriatr Rehabil. 2007;23(3):249–68.
11. Frasnelli J, Hummel T. Interactions between the chemical senses: trigeminal function in patients with olfactory loss. Int J Psychophysiol. 2007;65:177–81.
12. Kobal G, Hummel C. Cerebral chemosensory evoked potentials elicited by chemical stimulation of the human olfactory and respiratory nasal mucosa. Electroencephalogr Clin Neurophysiol. 1988;71: 241–50.
13. Welge-Lüssen A, Drago J, Wölfensberger M, Hummel T. Gustatory stimulation influences the processing of intranasal stimuli. Brain Res. 2005;1038:69–75.
14. Cichero J, Murdoch B. Acoustic signature of the normal swallow: characterization by age, gender, and bolus volume. Ann Otol Rhinol Laryngol. 2002; 111:623–32.
15. Landis BN, Scheibe M, Weber C, Berger R, Brämerson A, Bende M, Nordin S, Hummel T. Chemosensory interaction: acquired olfactory impairment is associated with decreased taste function. J Neurol. 2010;257:1303–8.
16. Yamamura K, Kitagawa J, Kurose M, Sugino S, Takatsujih H, Mostafeezur R, Hossain Z, Yamada Y, et al. Neural mechanisms of swallowing and effects of taste and other stimuli on swallow initiation. Biol Pharm Bull. 2010;33:1786–90.
17. Welge-Lüssen A, Ebnother M, Wölfensberger M, Hummel T. Swallowing is differentially influenced by retronasal compared with orthonasal stimulation in combination with gustatory stimuli. Chem Senses. 2009;6:499–502.
18. Cain WS. Bilateral interaction in olfaction. Nature. 1977;268:50–3.
19. Small DM, Gerber JC, Mak YE, Hummel T. Differential neural responses evoked by orthonasal versus retronasal odorant perception in humans. Neuron. 2005;47:593–605.
20. Abdul Wahab N, Jones R, Huckabee M. Effects of olfactory and gustatory stimuli on neural excitability for swallowing. Physiol Behav. 2010;101:568–75.
21. Hamdy S, Jilani S, Price V, Parker C, Hall N, Power M. Modulation of human swallowing behaviour by thermal and chemical stimulation in health and after brain injury. Neurogastroenterol Motil. 2003;15: 69–77.
22. Logemann JA, Pauloski BR, Colangelo L, Lazarus C, Fujiu M, Kahrilas PJ. Effects of a sour bolus on

oropharyngeal swallowing measures in patients with neurogenic dysphagia. J Speech Hear Res. 1995;38: 556–63.

23. Sciortino K, Liss JM, Case JL, Gerritsen KG, Katz RC. Effects of mechanical, cold, gustatory, and combined stimulation to the human anterior faucial pillars. Dysphagia. 2003;18:16–26.

24. Theurer J, Bihari F, Barr A, Martin R. Oropharyngeal stimulation with air-pulse trains increases swallowing frequency in healthy adults. Dysphagia. 2005;20: 254–60.

25. Miyaoka Y, Haishima K, Takagi M, Haishima H, Asari J, Yamada Y. Influences of thermal and gustatory characteristics on sensory and motor aspects of swallowing. Dysphagia. 2006;21:38–48.

26. Regan J, Walshe M, Tobin WO. Immediate effects of thermal-tactile stimulation on timing of swallow in idiopathic Parkinson's disease. Dysphagia. 2010;25(3): 207–15.

27. Teismann I, Steinsträter O, Warnecke T, Suntrup S, Ringelstein E, Pantev C, Dziewas R. Tactile thermal oral stimulation increases the cortical representation of swallowing. BMC Neurosci. 2009;10:71. http://www.biomedcentral.com/1471-2202/10/71.

28. South A, Somers S, Jog M. Gum chewing improves swallow frequency and latency in Parkinson patients. Neurology. 2010;74:1198–202.

29. Humbert I, Fitzgerald J, McLaren D, Johnson S, Porcaro E, Kosmatka K, Hind J, Robbins J. Neurophysiology of swallowing: effects of age and bolus type. Neuroimage. 2009;44:982–91.

30. Bult JHF, de Wijk RA, Hummel T. Investigations on multimodal sensory integration: texture, taste, and ortho- and retronasal olfactory stimuli in concert. Neurosci Lett. 2007;411:6–10.

31. Ebihara T, Ebihara S, Maruyama M, Kobayashi M, Itou A, Aria H, Sasaki H. A randomized trial of olfactory stimulation using plack pepper oil in older people with swallowing dysfunction. J Am Geriatr Soc. 2006;54(9):1401–6.

32. Ebihara T, Takahashi H, Ebihara S, Okazake T, Sasaki T, Watando A, Nemoto M, Sasaki H. Capsaicin troche for swallowing dysfunction in older people. J Am Geriatr Soc. 2005;53:824–8.

33. Halpern BP. Retronasal olfaction. In: Squire LR, editor. Encyclopedia of neuroscience. 8th ed. Oxford: Academic; 2009. p. 297–304.

34. Hummel T, Heilmann S, Murphy C. Age-related changes of chemosensory functions. In: Rouby C, Schaal B, Dubois D, Gervais R, Holley A, editors. Olfaction, taste and cognition. New York: Cambridge University Press; 2002. p. 441–56.

35. Lippert A, Grüner M, Terhaag D. Multimodal early onset stimulation (MEOS) in rehabilitation after brain injury. Brain Inj. 2000;14(6):585–94.

36. Mozell MM. Evidence for sorption as a mechanism of the olfactory analysis of vapours. Nature. 1964;203: 1181–2.

Coordination of Deglutition and Respiration

3

Bonnie Martin-Harris and David H. McFarland

Abstract

Respiratory–swallowing coordination is vital for airway protection and other aspects of swallowing function. Perturbations in coordinative mechanisms have been linked to disordered swallowing in susceptible patients. We provide a general overview of respiratory–swallowing interactions in adults discussing neural control systems, reconfigurations of shared muscle systems, timing of the initiation of swallowing processes within the respiratory cycle, disorders of coordination and potential mechanisms, and directions of future clinical and basic research. Importance is given to the normal timing of the initiation of swallowing during the expiratory phase of the breathing cycle at mid to low lung volumes. The airway protection and potential mechanical advantages of this coordinative relationship are highlighted. Potential differences in coordinative synchrony related to task and subject factors are reviewed and set the stage for additional experimental inquiry. Future directions related to re-training of appropriate respiratory–swallowing mechanisms to improve swallowing function disrupted by various clinical pathologies are introduced.

Keywords

Swallowing • Dysphagia • Respiration • Respiratory–swallow pattern • Airway protection • Aspiration

Introduction

The sensorimotor mechanisms driving the synergy of swallowing activate contraction of muscle groups that generate pressures. These pressures facilitate bolus containment, airway protection, and passage of ingested material through the upper aerodigestive tract. Swallowing, like many complex motor behaviors, relies on multiple cross-system interactions. One salient example is

B. Martin-Harris, PhD, CCC-SLP, BRS-S, ASHA Fellow (✉)
Medical University of South Carolina, 135 Rutledge Avenue, MSC 550, Charleston, SC 29424, USA
e-mail: harrisbm@musc.edu

D.H. McFarland, PhD
École d'orthophonie et d'audiologie, Faculté de médicine, Université de Montréal, C.P. 6128, Succ. Centre-Ville, Montréal, QC, Canada, H3C 2J7

R. Shaker et al. (eds.), *Principles of Deglutition: A Multidisciplinary Text for Swallowing and its Disorders*,
DOI 10.1007/978-1-4614-3794-9_3, © Springer Science+Business Media New York 2013

the coordinated neural and functional interactions between respiration and swallowing. Respiration and swallowing must be tightly coordinated because they share a common pathway, the pharynx, and airway protection must be assured. Much work has been directed to identifying the neural mechanisms underlying the coordination of breathing and swallowing (and chewing) using both human and nonhuman animal models. Both behaviors are regulated by brain stem central pattern generators (CPG), and multifunctional CPG interneurons may underlie the requisite cross-system interactions [1].

In the periphery, breathing and swallowing share many common structures. Muscles of the lips, face, tongue, palate, pharynx, larynx, and esophagus all show respiratory and swallowing-related activity, and there must be precise "switching" of activity states for appropriate function. Coordinated coupling of respiration and swallowing may be disrupted by various diseases or other medical conditions and may be intentionally manipulated during behavioral therapeutic approaches to improve swallowing function in dysphagic patients [2–10].

Respiratory-related activity has been recorded from the cricopharyngeus, genioglossus, styloglossus, and stylopharyngeus muscles during resting quiet inspiration [11–14], with the latter serving to stiffen the airway to protect against upper airway collapse during the generation of negative inspiratory pressures [15]. Clearly, these muscle groups also play essential roles in oral bolus propulsion and oropharyngeal clearance. The tongue serves a crucial role in swallowing by maintaining, manipulating, and transporting the food and/or liquid bolus [2, 16]. In addition to its critical role in bolus propulsion, the base of the tongue has also been described as the ventral wall of the respiratory pharynx and critical to airway patency during quiet breathing [2]. Respiratory-related activity has been recorded from the genioglossus that is time locked to diaphragm contraction [17]. The larynx obviously serves crucial functional roles during both breathing and swallowing. It assures a patent airway during respiration and airway protection during swallowing through vocal fold closure and progressive

superior–anterior hyolaryngeal movement [18, 19]. The sternothyroid and omohyoid muscles also demonstrate dual respiratory and swallowing roles. They assist in returning the larynx to rest following hyolaryngeal excursion during swallowing and serve to stabilize the larynx during quiet inspiration [20, 21].

The cricopharyngeal (CP) muscle—the primary anatomic and functional component of the pharyngoesophageal segment (PES)—is tonically active during the inspiratory phase of the breathing cycle to prevent inspired air from entering the esophagus and stomach [22]. The CP muscle then relaxes and becomes compliant to accommodate bolus flow during PES opening. The velopharyngeal (VP) port is open during respiration but elevates and fully retracts at maximal contraction during the swallow to prevent entry of ingested material into the nasal cavity [23].

Normal Breathing and Swallowing Coordination

Given that breathing and swallowing (and other airway protective behaviors, such as coughing) share these common muscles and structures, it is obvious that upper airway structures must be rapidly and precisely reconfigured for appropriate function. Respiration and swallowing share neural elements that are "switched" for task-specific functionality. Brainstem pattern generators and multifunctional interneuron networks presumably underlie these cross-system interactions and network reconfigurations [1]. Respiration is a rhythmic continuous behavior while swallowing is induced either through food and/or liquid ingestion or occurs spontaneously in response to saliva or other secretions during wakefulness or sleep. Respiration is inhibited to accommodate swallowing and the respiratory rhythm is reset [24–27]. The perturbing effects of swallowing on the respiratory rhythm are generally limited to the co-occurring respiratory cycle in normal subjects, but sequential or successive swallows are common, further increasing respiratory perturbation [24]. Mastication and swallowing can put significant burdens on respiratory control and stability in respiratory compromised patients, such as those with chronic obstructive pulmonary disease (COPD) [28, 29].

Given the necessity of airway protection, it is not surprising that the relatively brief respiratory inhibition to accommodate swallowing (sometimes referred to as "deglutition" apnea) occurs at rather specific moments in the respiratory cycle. In nonhuman animal species, swallowing occurs primarily during the inspiratory phase of the breathing cycle (e.g., McFarland and Lund [25]). In contrast, swallowing tends to occur during the expiratory phase of the breathing cycle in infant and adult humans observed during wakefulness and sleep [9, 30–33]. Whole body posture while feeding and upper airway anatomical differences between adult humans and other animal species may contribute to these coordinative differences [30]. When adult humans adopt a feeding position more similar to nonhuman animal species, swallowing shifts occur more in the early expiratory and inspiratory phases of the breathing cycle. This is more similar to other animal species [30].

Respiratory–swallowing coordination has been explored from a variety of different perspectives using both adult and infant human and nonhuman animal models. Nonhuman animal models have elaborated fundamental neural control elements and the reconfiguration of respiratory networks to accommodate swallowing [1, 34]. Some adult work has been directed to further exploring control properties at a fundamental level, but most has been directed towards understanding respiratory–swallowing coordination from a clinical perspective, either by providing normative data or in exploring "disordered" respiratory swallowing coordination. Human studies can be further divided into those that have studied liquids (single or sequential) [6, 31, 33, 35–38], solids [24, 26, 39–41], and/or spontaneously occurring swallowing of saliva or other secretions during wakefulness and sleep [42, 43]. This is an important distinction as swallowing dynamics and potentially respiratory swallowing coordination are influenced by bolus properties including volume and viscosity [37, 44, 45]. Further, swallowing (and mastication) and its coordination with respiration is influenced by experimental

task and subject factors. Asking subjects to hold boluses in their mouths and other experimental tasks, such as sequential swallowing, may result in changes in respiratory rhythm and stability (for example, inspiration prior to swallowing and partial vocal fold adduction and other protective elements) that may influence respiratory control and respiratory–swallowing coordination [6]. This should be kept in mind when comparing results across studies and particular attention should be given to instructions and tasks demanded of experimental subjects.

Although this provides a very "high-level" introduction to the literature surrounding respiratory–swallowing coordination, we will now turn our attention to providing more detail of experimental findings from adult humans and use our own work with liquid (Martin-Harris) and solid (McFarland) food swallowing under "natural" swallowing conditions as examples. Despite some experimental differences and discrepancies, as mentioned previously, a clear picture of respiratory swallowing coordination is emerging that suggests that most—but not all—swallows are initiated in the expiratory phase of the breathing cycle, with the respiratory inhibition to accommodate swallowing immediately proceeded and followed by expiratory airflow [11, 26, 29, 34, 35, 46]. When studying liquid swallows during synchronized observations of respiratory flow and videofluoroscopic images of swallowing and bolus movements, investigators have often used a pattern characterization scheme originally developed by Martin-Harris and modified slightly for different experimental contexts (Fig. 3.1). Using this pattern analysis, Martin-Harris and colleagues [32, 33] have found that self-paced liquid swallows from a cup are typically the "E–E" pattern, that is, they occur in the expiratory phase of the breathing cycle and are followed by a brief exhalation. As illustrated in Fig. 3.2, this expiratory–expiratory, or E–E pattern, was present in over 75% of the swallows of 76 healthy adults across the age spectrum in the large-scale study by Martin-Harris et al. [32]. This pattern was followed in frequency of occurrence by I–E, or when swallowing was immediately preceded by inspiratory and followed by expiratory flow

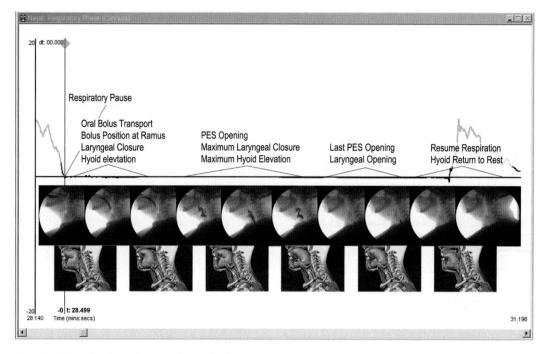

Fig. 3.1 The timeline derived from simultaneous videofluorographic and nasal airflow recordings illustrating the phases of respiration surrounding swallowing and the temporal relationships between the respiratory pause and functional groupings of swallowing events. From B. Martin-Harris et al. Arch Otolaryngol Head Neck Surg 2005;131:762–70 with permission

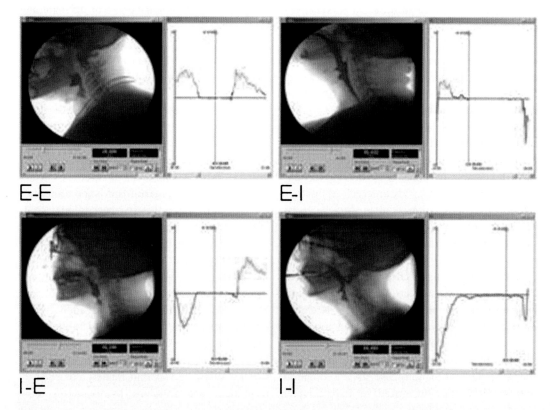

Fig. 3.2 Examples of four respiratory–swallow phase patterns recorded during liquid swallows

(20%). The two least frequently occurring patterns were E–I (4%), when swallowing was preceded by expiratory activity but immediately followed by inspiratory flow, and I–I (1%), when swallowing occurred during and was followed by inspiratory flow [32].

McFarland and colleagues have studied respiratory–swallowing coordination of solid food boluses and factors that influence this coordination from within a general motor control perspective [24]. Coordination was assessed by determining the timing of a physiological marker of the pharyngeal swallow or by looking at the timing of the occurrence of the respiratory inhibition to accommodate swallowing. As mentioned previously, swallowing perturbs the ongoing respiratory rhythm, and these analyses were directed towards determining the respiratory phase and volume of these deviations to accommodate swallowing. Similar techniques have been used for decades to characterize phase-related perturbations in a variety of rhythmic behaviors including mastication, respiration, and locomotion. These "phase" analyses reveal highly similar findings to those described above for liquid swallowing. Swallowing was consistently observed to occur in the expiratory phase of the breathing cycle, and more than 50% occur in the second half of the expiratory phase of the quiet breathing cycle [24]. It is also interesting to note that there was a tendency for swallows to occur later in the respiratory cycle (at lower quiet breathing lung volumes) for terminal swallows (those that occur at the end of a masticatory sequence) versus interposed swallows (those that occur within a masticatory sequence) [24].

As mentioned previously, our data for both liquid and solid food boluses from our laboratories are in general agreement with most published work in this area. An important question is why does the respiratory inhibition to accommodate swallowing appear to occur consistently during the expiratory phase of the breathing cycle in adult humans? This is intuitively obvious since, although respiration is always inhibited to accommodate swallowing, swallowing surrounded by expiratory flow is "safer" in contrast to inspiratory flow before or after swallowing, which could lead to food and liquid entering the lungs. This may

be particularly important when there is disordered timing of swallowing with respiration or the respiratory pause may be shortened, both of which places disordered patients at greater risk of inspiratory aspiration of food and liquids. Further, expiration prior to other swallowing events may encourage medialization (i.e., partially adducted) of the true vocal fold–arytenoid complex. This laryngeal posture may promote an advantageous starting point for further airway protection (Fig. 3.3) [31, 35]. This medial glottic position has also been observed during laryngeal descent in the late stage of the swallow and associated with a brief expiration depicted in the flow and kinematic data. It would appear that liquid swallows initiated at mid to low lung volumes would serve to facilitate this potentially protective, slightly adducted vocal fold position.

It has also been suggested that swallowing at particular phase and volumes of the respiratory cycle may impart additional mechanical and/or airway protective benefits as contrasted to other moments in the coordinative range. One such mechanical advantage may be the facilitation of laryngeal elevation and CP sphincter opening, both crucial aspects of normal swallowing function. Previous work has shown that diaphragm contraction, which continues well into the expiratory phase of the breathing cycle to assure adequate gas exchange [47], exerts a downward pull or "traction" on tracheal and laryngeal structures [11, 48]. The position of the human larynx remains relatively stable during quiet breathing, despite these "traction" forces placed on the diaphragm through co-contraction of suprahyoid muscles [11, 48]. At mid to low expiratory lung volumes, laryngeal elevators would not be working against active diaphragmatic contraction, which may explain why swallows typically occur in this volume range in many experimental contexts [3, 24, 30, 49].

Additional experimental attention has been given to the potential importance of subglottal pressure as a control variable related to swallowing–respiratory phase/volume relationships. Subglottal pressure, or the force against the adducted vocal folds, is related to expiratory drive as the result of active respiratory forces and passive recoil properties of the lungs/thorax (determined by lung

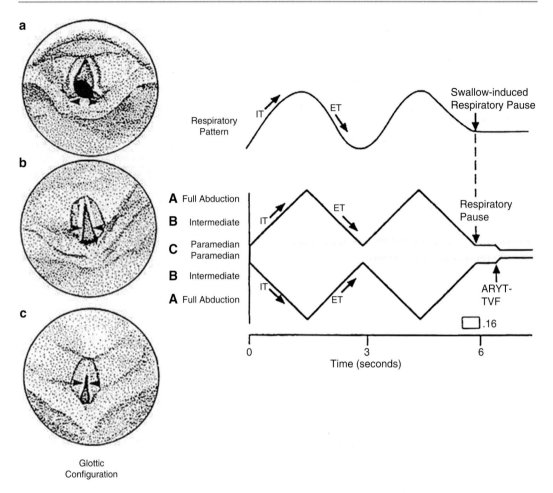

Fig. 3.3 Glottic configuration associated respiratory phases and swallowing: a. Inspiration-Full Abduction, b. Exhalation-Intermediate, c. Exhalation-Paramedian. Changes in respiratory glottic configuration that occurred in subjects. The arytenoid-true vocal fold (ARYT-TVF) complex assumed a fully abducted configuration during inspiration (IT) and an intermediate or paramedian posi-

tion during expiration (ET). The ARYT-TVF complex remained fixed in the end exhalatory glottic position at the onset of the swallow-induced respiratory cessation. Further medial displacement of the ARYT-TVF complex usually began .16 seconds after swallow-induced cessation onset and was not associated with a change in the flat respiratory trace

volume). Some authors have proposed that we swallow at lung volumes higher than end tidal breathing expiratory levels to take advantage of passive recoil forces and increased subglottal pressure. Increased subglottal pressure may be potentially beneficial for airway protective mechanisms, such as cough, in the advent of disturbances to normal coordination and laryngeal penetration or aspiration [50, 51]. There is some intriguing evidence that thin liquids are swallowed at higher lung volumes (still within the quiet breathing range) when contrasted to thin and thick paste consistencies—presumably as a

preparatory precautionary mechanism in case additional expiratory pressures are needed for airway clearance. Thin liquids obviously place greater demands on respiratory—swallowing coordination as they may be more easily aspirated. Liquids, particularly larger volumes, flow at fast velocities and require rapid accommodation by pharyngeal contraction and laryngeal valving to close and prevent airway entry and open the PES [19].

Sequential liquid swallows in particular may place additional demands on coordination [31, 35, 36, 50, 52]. A study by Dozier et al. [6]

showed a significant increase in the occurrence of inspiration surrounding spontaneous, sequential swallows of larger volumes when compared to small volume liquid swallows. This finding along with observations of laryngeal vestibular opening between swallows in a sequence, points to the potential for increased risk of aspiration when compared to a small volume, single swallowing task. It is interesting to note that previous investigators have observed sequential and/or successive swallows of solid food boluses, which had cumulative effects in perturbing respiratory control and stability and prolonging the durations of co-occurring respiratory cycles [24, 25]. These data suggest that respiratory–swallowing coordination is somewhat flexible within a relatively restricted range of respiratory volumes and phases, and perhaps coordinative demands vary depending upon the nature of the swallowed bolus. This issue deserves further experimental attention as it has both fundamental and clinical implications.

Few studies have examined the integration of respiration, mastication, and swallowing behavior. McFarland and Lund [24] found that mastication could have profound perturbing effects on the respiratory rhythm in some subjects—even to the extent of producing a long period of apnea. Like the McFarland study, Palmer et al. [40, 41] also reported abrupt changes in breathing pattern during eating. The chewed bolus aggregated in the valleculae as breathing was maintained, which may place additional coordinative demands of breathing and swallowing. These data suggest respiratory–swallowing coordination is flexible and "sensitive" to changing peripheral conditions in feeding and swallowing. The normally precise coordination between breathing and swallowing also indicates swallowing control mechanisms are receiving respiratory volume and phase information from pulmonary or other respiratory-related sensory mechanisms. Such feedback is obviously used by and/or influencing the multifunctional brainstem interneuronal networks that coordinate breathing and swallowing [49]. Additional studies of "natural" eating and drinking behavior are essential to further understand the influence

of these "peripheral" influences of food type and feeding task on respiratory–swallowing coordination.

Aging Effects on Respiratory–Swallowing Coordination

Fragile patients on the extreme ends of the age continuum fall victim to swallowing disorders, aspiration, and aspiration pneumonia. Respiratory–swallowing coordination, like other aspects of swallowing physiology, appears to be influenced by the aging process [32, 44, 50, 51]. For example, there is some evidence of pattern shifts from the more typical pattern (E–E) to the (I–E, E–I, or I–I) pattern with advancing age [32, 44, 51]. Although they have not been associated with any overt swallowing disturbances, they may predispose older patients to the negative effects of disease or damage, such as stroke [53], Parkinson disease [54], COPD [30, 31, 55–59], and head and neck cancer [60], on swallowing function. The respiratory pause to accommodate swallowing has also been shown to nearly double in duration during liquid swallowing in older individuals [34] that may "tax" coordinative mechanisms and significantly influence respiratory control and stability, which ultimately may increase the risk of airway compromise—particularly in patients with COPD.

Swallowing Impairment and "Disordered" Respiratory-Swallow Coordination

There is obviously a strong neural imperative of appropriate respiratory–swallowing coordination. "Normal" respiratory–swallowing phase relationships have been observed in laryngectomized patients despite major mechanical alterations to the upper airway and the fact that airway protection is not necessary [52]. Therefore, the occurrence of particular and/or stable respiratory–swallow patterns may be a clinical marker of the integrity of neural control mechanisms, and of airflow and mechanical events that are crucial for safe and efficient swallowing. Emerging data are pointing to disruptions in this stable coupling between respiration and swallowing under certain physiologic conditions, such as normal aging, presence of neurologic disease, cancers of the head and neck, various swallowing tasks, and compensatory postures.

Our collaborative work suggests partial surgical ablation of the oropharynx and/or various combinations of radiation and chemotherapy change normal respiratory–swallowing phase relationships [60]. This may be due to three related factors: (1) impairments within the swallowing system (e.g., oropharyngeal swallow delay, incomplete tongue base retraction, impaired anterior motion of the hyoid and larynx all leading to incomplete opening of the PES) that may impact coordination with breathing, (2) impairments within the respiratory system (e.g., obstruction, restriction) that may impact coordination with swallowing, and/or (3) problems in breathing–swallowing coordination that extends beyond these systems (e.g., neural control). These multiple potential origins of difficulty stress the necessity of examining both "within" and "across" systems and mechanisms of swallowing function. It also creates a research imperative for further exploring the nature of respiratory–swallowing interaction in health and disease.

Conclusions

Clinical and experimental evidence support the existence of neurophysiologic, structural, and functional interdependence between respiration and swallowing. Health care professionals who treat patients with swallowing disorders are able to modify abnormal swallowing physiology using compensatory techniques that involve peripheral alterations in both breathing and swallowing. New recording technologies, methods, and analyses emerging from cross-sectional, cohort studies will be applied to similar patient groups over the natural history of diseases and conditions. These future studies will lead to improved understanding of respiratory–swallowing relationships and the potential functional relevance of these relationships on swallowing impairment, pulmonary status, and quality of life. Although the phenomena of breathing and swallowing coordination or the respective disruption in this coordination would appear to have substantial influence on the safety and efficiency of swallowing, this hypothesis has not yet been adequately tested. Studies are warranted to determine the relationship of breathing and swallowing coordination on overall swallowing impairment and health of various patient populations with dysphagia. Clinical studies of the impact of neurologic, pulmonary, and oncologic diseases on the coordination of breathing and swallowing are emerging. Some clinical scientists are also developing and testing novel interventions with potential for cross-system respiratory–swallowing advantages to reduce swallowing impairment and improve overall swallowing function [61]. Our research, conducted independently in our respective laboratories, has established an ideal backdrop for exploring the presence and effect of cross-system respiratory–swallowing impairments on swallowing system impairment (Fig. 3.4).

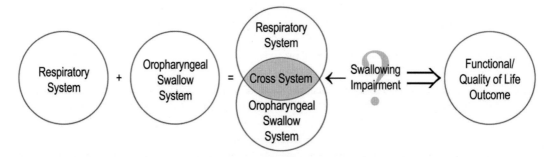

Fig. 3.4 Theoretical model of cross-system, respiratory–swallowing impairment

Studies are warranted and currently underway to test whether or not retraining stable coupling is feasible, as well as to test the effect of respiratory–swallowing phase training alone or in combination with traditional swallowing treatments on the recovery of swallowing dysfunction.

References

1. Jean A. Brain stem control of swallowing: neuronal network and cellular mechanisms. Physiol Rev. 2001; 81:929–69.
2. Logemann JA. Rehabilitation of oropharyngeal swallowing disorders. Acta Otorhinolaryngol Belg. 1994; 48:207–15.
3. Martin-Harris B. Clinical implications of respiratory-swallowing interactions. Curr Opin Otolaryngol Head Neck Surg. 2008;16:194–9.
4. Ayuse T, Ishitobi S, Kurata S, et al. Effect of reclining and chin-tuck position on the coordination between respiration and swallowing. J Oral Rehabil. 2006; 33:402–8.
5. Butler SG, Stuart A, Pressman H, et al. Preliminary investigation of swallowing apnea duration and swallow/respiratory phase relationships in individuals with cerebral vascular accident. Dysphagia. 2007;22: 215–24.
6. Dozier TS, Brodsky MB, Michel Y, et al. Coordination of swallowing and respiration in normal sequential cup swallows. Laryngoscope. 2006;116:1489–93.
7. Martin-Harris B BM, Michel Y, Gillespie MB, Day TA. Aberrant breathing and swallowing patterns in patients treated for oropharyngeal cancer. 6th International Conference on Head and Neck Cancer; 2004; Washington, DC.
8. Kelly BN, Huckabee ML, Jones RD, et al. The first year of human life: coordinating respiration and nutritive swallowing. Dysphagia. 2007;22:37–43.
9. Nixon GM, Charbonneau I, Kermack AS, et al. Respiratory-swallowing interactions during sleep in premature infants at term. Respir Physiol Neurobiol. 2008;160:76–82.
10. Terzi N, Orlikowski D, Aegerter P, et al. Breathing-swallowing interaction in neuromuscular patients: a physiological evaluation. Am J Respir Crit Care Med. 2007;175:269–76.
11. Andrew BL. The nervous control of the cervical oesophagus of the rat during swallowing. J Physiol. 1956;134:729–40.
12. Sauerland EK, Mitchell SP. Electromyographic activity of the human Genioglossus muscle in response to respiration and to positional changes of the head. Bull Los Angeles Neurol Soc. 1970;35:69–73.
13. Lowe AA, Sessle BJ. Tongue activity during respiration, jaw opening, and swallowing in cat. Can J Physiol Pharmacol. 1973;51:1009–11.
14. Adachi S, Lowe AA, Tsuchiya M, et al. Genioglossus muscle activity and inspiratory timing in obstructive sleep apnea. Am J Orthod Dentofacial Orthop. 1993;104:138–45.
15. Berne RM, Levy M, Koeppen BM, Stanton BA. Physiology. St Louis: Mosby; 1998.
16. Shedd D, Scatliff J, Kirchner JA. The buccopharyngeal propulsive mechanism in human deglutition. Surgery. 1960;48:846–53.
17. van Lunteren E, Dick TE. Intrinsic properties of pharyngeal and diaphragmatic respiratory motoneurons and muscles. J Appl Physiol. 1992;73:787–800.
18. Ekberg O, Sigurjonsson SV. Movement of the epiglottis during deglutition. A cineradiographic study. Gastrointest Radiol. 1982;7:101–7.
19. Logemann JA, Kahrilas PJ, Cheng J, et al. Closure mechanisms of laryngeal vestibule during swallow. Am J Physiol. 1992;262:G338–44.
20. Zemlin W. Speech and hearing science: anatomy and physiology. Boston: Allyn & Bacon; 1997.
21. Kennedy J, Kent R. Anatomy and physiology of deglutition and related functions. Semin Speech Lang. 1985;6:257–72.
22. Atkinson M, Kramer P, Wyman SM. The dynamics of swallowing. I. Normal pharyngeal mechanisms. J Clin Invest. 1957;36:581–8.
23. Matsuo K, Metani H, Mays KA, et al. Effects of respiration on soft palate movement in feeding. J Dent Res. 2010;89:1401–6.
24. McFarland DH, Lund JP. Modification of mastication and respiration during swallowing in the adult human. J Neurophysiol. 1995;74:1509–17.
25. McFarland DH, Lund JP. An investigation of the coupling between respiration, mastication, and swallowing in the awake rabbit. J Neurophysiol. 1993;69: 95–108.
26. Paydarfar D, Eldridge FL, Kiley JP. Resetting of mammalian respiratory rhythm: existence of a phase singularity. Am J Physiol. 1986;250:R721–7.
27. Paydarfar D, Gilbert RJ, Poppel CS, et al. Respiratory phase resetting and airflow changes induced by swallowing in humans. J Physiol. 1995;483(Pt 1):273–88.
28. Cvejic L, Harding R, Churchward T, et al. Laryngeal penetration and aspiration in individuals with stable COPD. Respirology. 2010;16:269–75.
29. Martin-Harris B. Optimal patterns of care in patients with chronic obstructive pulmonary disease. Semin Speech Lang. 2000;21:311–21.
30. McFarland DH, Lund JP, Gagner M. Effects of posture on the coordination of respiration and swallowing. J Neurophysiol. 1994;72:2431–7.
31. Martin BJ. The Influence of Deglutition on Respiration. Evanston: Northwestern University; 1991. [unpublished dissertation]
32. Martin-Harris B, Brodsky MB, Michel Y, et al. Breathing and swallowing dynamics across the adult lifespan. Arch Otolaryngol Head Neck Surg. 2005;131:762–70.
33. Martin-Harris B, Brodsky MB, Price CC, et al. Temporal coordination of pharyngeal and laryngeal

dynamics with breathing during swallowing: single liquid swallows. J Appl Physiol. 2003;94:1735–43.

34. Doty R. Neural organization of deglutition. In: Code C, editor. Handbook of physiology. Washington, DC: Am Phys Soc; 1968. p. 1861–902.

35. Martin BJ, Logemann JA, Shaker R, et al. Coordination between respiration and swallowing: respiratory phase relationships and temporal integration. J Appl Physiol. 1994;76:714–23.

36. Preiksaitis HG, Mills CA. Coordination of breathing and swallowing: effects of bolus consistency and presentation in normal adults. J Appl Physiol. 1996;81: 1707–14.

37. Butler SG, Postma GN, Fischer E. Effects of viscosity, taste, and bolus volume on swallowing apnea duration of normal adults. Otolaryngol Head Neck Surg. 2004;131:860–3.

38. Perlman AL, Ettema SL, Barkmeier J. Respiratory and acoustic signals associated with bolus passage during swallowing. Dysphagia. 2000;15:89–94.

39. Matsuo K, Hiiemae KM, Gonzalez-Fernandez M, et al. Respiration during feeding on solid food: alterations in breathing during mastication, pharyngeal bolus aggregation, and swallowing. J Appl Physiol. 2008;104:674–81.

40. Palmer JB, Rudin NJ, Lara G, et al. Coordination of mastication and swallowing. Dysphagia. 1992;7: 187–200.

41. Palmer JB, Hiiemae KM. Eating and breathing: interactions between respiration and feeding on solid food. Dysphagia. 2003;18:169–78.

42. Sonies BC, Ship JA, Baum BJ. Relationship between saliva production and oropharyngeal swallow in healthy, different-aged adults. Dysphagia. 1989;4:85–9.

43. Dua KS, Bajaj JS, Rittmann T, et al. Safety and feasibility of evaluating airway-protective reflexes during sleep: new technique and preliminary results. Gastrointest Endosc. 2007;65:483–6.

44. Hiss SG, Treole K, Stuart A. Effects of age, gender, bolus volume, and trial on swallowing apnea duration and swallow/respiratory phase relationships of normal adults. Dysphagia. 2001;16:128–35.

45. Leow LP, Huckabee ML, Sharma S, et al. The influence of taste on swallowing apnea, oral preparation time, and duration and amplitude of submental muscle contraction. Chem Senses. 2007;32:119–28.

46. Perlman AL, He X, Barkmeier J, et al. Bolus location associated with videofluoroscopic and respirodeglutometric events. J Speech Lang Hear Res. 2005;48:21–33.

47. Agostoni E, Mead J. Statics of the respiratory system. In: Fenn WO, Rahn H, editors. Handbook of physiology.

Washington, DC: American Physiological Society; 1964. p. 387–409.

48. Mitchinson AG, Yoffey JM. Respiratory displacement of larynx, hyoid bone and tongue. J Anat. 1947;81 :118–20. 111.

49. Charbonneau I, Lund JP, McFarland DH. Persistence of respiratory-swallowing coordination after laryngectomy. J Speech Lang Hear Res. 2005;48:34–44.

50. Wheeler Hegland KM, Huber JE, Pitts T, et al. Lung volume during swallowing: single bolus swallows in healthy young adults. J Speech Lang Hear Res. 2009;52:178–87.

51. Diez Gross R, Atwood CW, Grayhack JP, Shaiman S. Lung volume effects on pharyngeal swallowing physiology. J Appl Physiol. 2003;95:2211–7.

52. Hirst LJ, Ford GA, Gibson GJ, et al. Swallow-induced alterations in breathing in normal older people. Dysphagia. 2002;17:152–61.

53. Selley WG, Flack FC, Ellis RE, Brooks WA. Respiratory patterns associated with swallowing: Part 1. The normal adult pattern and changes with age. Age Ageing. 1989;18:173–6.

54. Leslie P, Drinnan MJ, Ford GA, et al. Swallow respiration patterns in dysphagic patients following acute stroke. Dysphagia. 2002;17:202–7.

55. Pinnington LL, Mudhiddin KA, Ellis RE, Playford ED. Non-invasive assessment of swallowing and respiration in Parkinson's disease. J Neurol. 2000;247: 773–7.

56. Shaker R, Li Q, Ren J, et al. Coordination of deglutition and phases of respiration: effect of aging, tachypnea, bolus volume, and chronic obstructive pulmonary disease. Am J Physiol. 1992;263:G750–5.

57. Good-Fratturelli MD, Curlee RF, Holle JL. Prevalence and nature of dysphagia in VA patients with COPD referred for videofluoroscopic swallow examination. J Commun Disord. 2000;33:93–110.

58. Mokhlesi B, Logemann JA, Rademaker AW, et al. Oropharyngeal deglutition in stable COPD. Chest. 2002;121:361–9.

59. Stein M, Williams AJ, Grossman F, et al. Cricopharyngeal dysfunction in chronic obstructive pulmonary disease. Chest. 1990;97:347–52.

60. Brodsky MB, McFarland DH, Dozier TS, et al. Respiratory-swallow phase patterns and their relationship to swallowing impairment in patients treated for oropharyngeal cancer. Head Neck. 2010; 32:481–9.

61. Sapienza CM, Wheeler K. Respiratory muscle strength training: functional outcomes versus plasticity. Semin Speech Lang. 2006;27:236–44.

Airway Protective Mechanisms, Reciprocal Physiology of the Deglutitive Axis

4

Anisa Shaker and Reza Shaker

Abstract

In the setting of shared embryonic origin and anatomical continuity, the upper airway, aerodigestive tract and the esophagus participate in an elaborate stimulatory mechanism that in response to either mechanical or acid stimulation enhances the barriers against entry of gastric content into the pharynx and trachea, clear the pharyngeal content and closes the glottis, and increases the tracheal mucus secretion whereby enhancing the airway protection. Parallel to this stimulatory mechanism there exist a number of inhibitory reflexes. This results in relaxation of the lower esophageal sphincter and inhibition of primary and secondary esophageal peristalsis potentially weakening the airway protection against aspiration of gastric contents. Overall balance of these mechanisms and conditions associated with the recruitment of involved reflexes comprise the reciprocal physiology of the upper airway and upper GI tract which are the topic of ongoing investigations.

This chapter provides a concise description of these mechanisms which are involved in protection of the airway against aspiration during transit of material through deglutitive axis.

Keywords

Airway protective mechanisms • Reciprocal physiology • Deglutitive axis • Esophago-UES contractile reflex • Esophago-glottal closure reflex • Pharyngeal reflexive swallow

A. Shaker, MD
Internal Medicine/Division of Gastroenterology,
Washington University School of Medicine/Barnes
Jewish Hospital, 660 S. Euclid Avenue Campus,
Box 8124, St. Louis, MO 63105, USA

R. Shaker, MD (✉)
Division of Gastroenterology and Hepatology,
Digestive Disease Center, Clinical and Translational
Science Institute, Medical College of Wisconsin,
9200 W. Wisconsin Avenue, Milwaukee, WI 53226, USA
e-mail: rshaker@mcw.edu

Airway compromise resulting in aspiration may occur in relation to swallowing or gastro-esophago-pharyngeal reflux. The mechanisms that protect against aspiration involve the pharynx, upper esophageal sphincter [1], esophageal body, glottis and vocal cords, and the airway. These structures not only physically help prevent aspiration, but they are also the site of initiation of an

R. Shaker et al. (eds.), *Principles of Deglutition: A Multidisciplinary Text for Swallowing and its Disorders*, 35
DOI 10.1007/978-1-4614-3794-9_4, © Springer Science+Business Media New York 2013

elaborate system of reflexes that enhances the pressure barriers and sphincteric mechanisms against aspiration. All together these mechanisms can be divided into two major groups: basal and response. The basal mechanisms are constantly present without the need for stimulation, such as the lower and upper esophageal sphincter which provide a pressure barrier between stomach and esophagus and between esophagus and pharynx, respectively, helping to prevent entry of gastric content into the esophagus and from esophagus into the pharynx. Other examples of basal mechanism include the capacity of the esophagus to hold material without allowing it to escape into the pharynx and the capacity of the pharynx to contain certain volumes before their spillage into the airway. Response mechanisms, on the other hand, become activated in response to certain stimuli, such as distention or surface contact. There are at least nine response mechanisms identified that result in volume clearance of the pharynx and esophagus (such as reflexive pharyngeal swallow (RPS) and secondary esophageal peristalsis) or accentuate the upper esophageal sphincter pressure barrier such as esophago-UES, pharyngo-UES and laryngo-UES contractile reflexes or induce closure of the vocal cords and introitus to the trachea such as esophago-glottal, pharyngo-glottal, laryngo-laryngeal reflexes. The sum effects of various combinations of the basal and response mechanisms help prevent pharyngeal reflux and laryngeal aspiration of swallowed and reflux materials. In other words, the airway protective mechanism against aspiration is multi-factorial and involves a delicate and reciprocal interaction between upper gastrointestinal and upper airway tracts. It is noteworthy that in addition to airway protective reflexes which are universally stimulatory, there are a number of inhibitory reflexes that emanate from the esophagus, pharynx and the larynx which either relax the lower and upper esophageal sphincters or inhibit progression of the primary and secondary esophageal peristalsis. These inhibitory reflexes will not be described in detail here and will only be alluded to in descriptive figures. Since the UES and LES are covered in detail in subsequent chapters, these two mechanisms will not be covered either and the readers are referred to those chapters for a comprehensive description.

Esophago-UES Contractile Reflex

The UES is one of the components of the airway protective mechanism against the entry of gastroesophageal refluxate into the aerodigestive tract. It contributes by maintaining a high-pressure zone between the esophagus and the pharynx. However, the magnitude of pressure within UES is quite variable. It decreases significantly during sleep and periods of calmness and increases with wakefulness and excitation. In addition, the resting basal pressure of the UES is significantly lower in the elderly when compared to the young. Therefore, it is conceivable that the pressure of the gastroesophageal refluxate may overcome the UES pressure if it occurs during periods of low UES pressure. Hence, UES function as an anti-aspiration mechanism has been of great interest. Indeed the first description of UES response to esophageal distension appeared in 1957 by Creamer and Schlegel [2].

Since then, a large body of literature at the basic and clinical science level has emerged that suggests the existence of a complex reflex circuitry determining the UES pressure response to esophageal distention depending on the type and number of activated mucosal, submucosal and muscular receptors and their relative concentration and location in relationship to the UES. These studies show that not only the physical properties of the distending agent such as gastroesophageal refluxate play a role in the activation of these reflex circuitries, but also the spatial orientation of the esophagus through influencing the distention and affecting the proximal extension of the refluxate significantly affects the UES pressure response.

Esophageal and UES pressure response to esophageal distention, namely generation of secondary peristalsis and contraction of UES, has been described as early as 33 weeks of gestational age [3]. This response is preserved through the life span but aging selectively affects these responses. In that, while UES contractile response to balloon distention remains intact, generation of secondary peristalsis in response to generalized distension of esophagus such as those induced by air injection decreases significantly in subjects over 70 years. This decrease is associated with a significant increase in UES relaxation response to air distention [4].

Differential UES response to proximal and distal esophageal stimulations by air injection has been reported in humans [5, 6]. In a human model of UES contraction induced by mid-esophageal balloon distention, which also served to separate the esophagus into proximal and distal compartments, experiments have shown that UES relaxation response is more common after proximal esophageal air insufflations and its contraction is more prevalent due to distal air insufflation [5]. On the other hand, earlier studies have shown that in humans UES contractile response to slow intra-esophageal fluid infusion is augmented by acidity and proximity of the liquid to the UES [6].

In a study of 321 postprandial reflux events (identified by the development of abrupt intra-esophageal pressure increases with a pH drop) an overwhelming majority of events, 99 and 100 %, of all reflux events irrespective of pH drop were associated with an abrupt increase in UES pressure among GERD patients and controls, respectively. The average percentage of maximum UES pressure increase over pre-reflux values ranged between 66 and 96 % in control subjects and 34 and 122 % in patients [7].

Studies of the UES pressure change during 109 Transient Lower Esophageal Sphincter Relaxations (TLESR), the main mechanism of gastroesophageal reflux (GER) events, have shown that UES relaxation is the predominant response during upright position which is characteristically associated with the presence of air in the refluxate and UES contraction is the predominant response during recumbent position mainly associated with liquid refluxate. These studies support the notion that the UES relaxation or contraction response during TLESR is related to the posture and constituents of the refluxate [8].

In a series of sleep studies, the response of the UES to simulated proximal reflux event by slow intra-esophageal infusion of distilled water was evaluated [9]. Findings indicate that esophageal UES contractile reflex can be elicited in stage II and REM but is preempted by arousal in slow-wave sleep (Fig. 4.1). It was also found that the threshold volume for eliciting this reflex was significantly lower in REM sleep compared to stage II sleep and awake state suggesting a heightened sensitivity during REM sleep. These studies confirm that although UES pressure progressively declines with deeper stages of sleep it can still reflexively contract during REM despite generalize hypotonia. Interestingly in these studies, provocation of secondary esophageal peristalsis paralleled that of the esophago-UES contractile reflex.

Studies of the mechanisms of reflexes induced by esophageal distension in cats [10] indicate that the differential relaxation and contractile responses of the upper esophageal sphincter to the regional and generalized distention of the esophagus induced either by physiologic or simulated reflux events are mediated by vagal afferent fibers and interplay of mucosal and deep mechanoreceptor activation.

Based on these findings, it is surmised that UES pressure response to esophageal distention induced by reflux of gastric content is multifactorial. These factors include spatial orientation of the esophagus, rate and magnitude of proximal intra-esophageal pressure increase, physical property and volume of the refluxate. Variations in the combination of these factors result in variation in the UES pressure response to reflux events. As such generalization of UES response under a given set of circumstances representing only a limited number of factors is best avoided.

Esophago-Glottal Closure Reflex

Abrupt esophageal distention occurs commonly during GER, thereby generating a circumstance favorable to esophagopharyngeal regurgitation

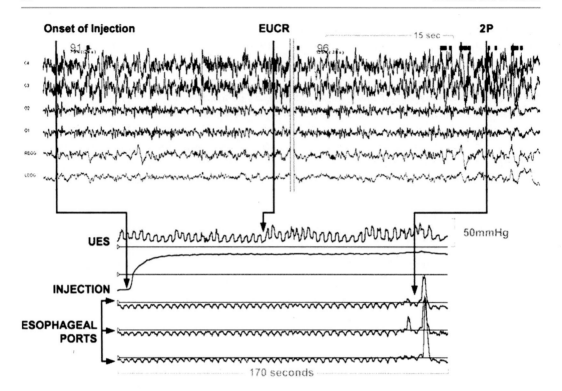

Fig. 4.1 An example of elicitation of EUCR and 2P in stage II sleep. Manometry: As seen following infusion of 3.8 mL water at the rate of 2.7 mL/min into the proximal esophagus, the UES pressure rose from 8 to 20 mmHg (esophago-UES contractile reflex; EUCR). This pressure increase continues until the development of secondary peristalsis (2P) 74 s later. EEF: Central (C3 or C4) and occipital (O1 or O2) deviations. EOG activity from *right* and *left* eye (recorded from the outer canthi). Stage II is characterized by K complexes (an initial negative sharp wave followed by a positive component) and sleep spindles (episodic, rhythmical complexes occurring with frequency of 7–14 cycles per second grouped in sequences lasting 1–2 s). There are no eye movements, and EMG activity is decreased compared with the "awake" state. From J. Bajaj et al. Gastroenterology 2006;130:17–25 with permission

and laryngeal aspiration of gastric refluxate. Large-volume GER episodes may cause an instantaneous increase in intraesophageal pressure that might overcome the UES. This circumstance potentially leaves the upper airway vulnerable to aspiration.

Studies in humans and animal models have documented the existence of an esophagoglottal closure reflex [11, 12]. The function of this reflex is to adduct the vocal cords and, thereby, close the introitus to the trachea in response to abrupt esophageal distention. To evoke the reflex, esophageal distention may involve the entire body of the esophagus, such as the distention caused by air insufflation, or it may be regional, such as distention caused by a short balloon. In either case, the distention must be abrupt to evoke the reflex. The prime candidate for the sensory signal for this reflex is the stretch receptors present in the body of the esophagus. The afferent nerves run in the vagus nerve, carrying the sensory impulse to the brainstem. The efferent fibers are likely vagal motor fibers to the larynx that traverse the recurrent laryngeal nerve and stimulate the adductor muscles of the glottis. The target muscles include all or some of the glottal adductors. Bilateral cervical vagotomy in a feline model abolishes this reflex [12].

Vocal cord adduction results from contractions of glottal adductor muscles. These muscles include thyroarytenoid that is also an isometric tensor of the cords, cricothyroid (also an isometric tensor), lateral cricoarytenoid, and, finally, the unpaired interarytenoid muscle that closes the posterior gap in the glottis. Except for the cricothyroid muscle, which is innervated by the external division of the superior laryngeal nerve, all adductor muscles are innervated by the recurrent laryngeal nerve. Because the posterior glottal gap becomes closed on direct viewing, we suggest that, in addition to the lateral cricoarytenoid muscles, the interarytenoid muscle is also involved. Since the glottis, in response to esophageal distention, shortens and narrows, we also suggest that the thyroarytenoid muscles have a strong participation in the reflex.

Reflex connections between the digestive tract and the respiratory system have been reported previously [13]. Such studies generally focus on a reflex connection between acid-sensitive receptors in the esophagus and pulmonary bronchi, such that refluxed acid may induce bronchiolar spasm. Coordination of the digestive and respiratory systems during swallowing is well established [1, 14, 15]. The esphagoglottic reflex is an example of close coordination between digestive and respiratory systems during reflux. This reflex seems to be a simple reflex whereby a mechanical stretch of the esophagus provokes a brief closure response of the vocal cords. The physiologic role of the esophagoglottal closure reflex could be postulated to be one of the airway protective mechanisms operative during retrograde esophageal transit, such as during belching, GER, regurgitation, and possibly vomiting.

Studies have also documented that this reflex is evoked during spontaneous GER episodes [16]. Other studies have shown that this reflex is absent in about half of the patients over the age of 70 years. The function of this reflex in patients with esophagitis or supraesophageal complication of GERD has not been evaluated as yet. Study in cats, however, has demonstrated that acute experimental esophagitis either completely abolishes this reflex or results in significant reduction in its frequency of activation [17]. In addition, treatment of esophageal mucosa with Lidocaine or capsaicin as well as removal of esophageal mucosa or intravenous injection of baclofen in cats blocks or inhibits, whereas thoracic vagotomy completely blocks this reflex [10].

Pharyngeal Reflexive Swallow

The primary swallow acts as one of the major airway protective mechanisms by keeping the aerodigestive tract free of debris and residue. It is usually a voluntary act but may also occur subconsciously. Previous studies have shown that mechanical stimulation of the pharyngeal wall in animals [18] and injection of water into the pharynx in humans [19, 20] also trigger swallowing (pharyngeal swallow). This additional stimulus to the initiation of swallowing may play a role in airway protection from pharyngeal reflux of gastric contents, as well as inadvertent spillage of oral contents into the pharynx, during the preparatory phase of swallowing. Recent studies [21] have characterized the pharyngeal swallow and determined the threshold volume of liquid required to trigger this type of swallowing in young and elderly volunteers. These studies [19–22] have shown that the swallowing mechanism in humans can be readily activated by water stimulation of the pharynx. They also showed that swallows triggered by direct stimulation of the pharynx are different from volitional or primary swallows by not inducing sequential contact of the proximal tongue with the hard palate known to occur during primary swallows (Table 4.1). In this regard, the pharyngeal swallow could be com-

Table 4.1 Comparison of the biomechanical events during primary and pharyngeal swallow

Events	Primary swallow	Pharyngeal swallow
Lingual peristalsis	+	−
Tongue base movement	+	+
Oral volume clearance	+	−
Pharyngeal volume clearance	+	+
Hyoid bone movement	+	+
Velo pharyngeal contact	+	+
Vocal cord closure	+	+
Aryepiglottal descent	+	+
Laryngeal elevation	+	+
Vestibular closure	+	+

From Shaker R, et al. The American Journal of Medicine. 2000;108:8S–14S

Table 4.2 Function of various elements involved in belching and swallowing

Events	Vestibular closure			Epiglottal descent	Laryngeal elevation	Hyoid movement		
	VC-AD	Supraglottic	Subepiglottic			Anterior	Superior	Inferior
Swallowing	+	+	+	+	+	+	+	−
Esopahgeal belch without increase in intragastric pressure	+	−	−	−	−	+	±	±
Esophageal belch with increase in intragastric pressure	+	+	−	−	−	+	±	±
Gastric belch without increase in intragastric pressure	+	−	−	−	−	+	±	±
Gastric belch with increase in intragastric pressure	+	+	−	−	−	+	±	±

VC-AD vocal cord adduction, +=present, −=absent
From R. Shaker Dysphagia. 1993;8:326–330 with permission

pared to secondary esophageal peristalsis, which usually spares the activation of the peristaltic wave from areas proximal to the point of stimulation [23–25]. For this reason, the term "secondary swallow" is used interchangeably with pharyngeal swallow. Except for lingual peristalsis and transit of oral bolus, the rest of the deglutitive biomechanical events during both types of swallows were found to be similar (Table 4.2).

A significantly larger volume of liquid is required to trigger a pharyngeal swallow in the elderly [21]. From a functional point of view, we speculate that pharyngeal swallows may help prevent aspiration by two mechanisms: (1) Activating the swallow-induced glottal closure (this, in turn, seals off the airway and prevents possible aspiration of material that may either fall into the pharynx inadvertently during the preparatory phase of swallowing, or enter the pharynx during large volume GER episodes) and (2) clearing the pharynx of materials that enter it during reflux from the esophagus.

The demonstrated need for larger volumes to trigger pharyngeal swallow in elderly patients could potentially have clinical implications. In the interval between the entry of sub-threshold volumes of gastric content into the pharynx and occurrence of a primary swallow, the material may be inhaled into the airway. This possibility is further enhanced by the fact that the rate of

spontaneous swallowing in the elderly is lower than in the young [26, 27].

Several areas within the oropharyngeal cavity have been shown to be sensitive for elicitation of the swallowing reflex. Stimulation of the anterior faucial pillars, the tongue, and the epiglottis, as well as the larynx and the posterior pharyngeal wall [28, 29], has been shown to trigger swallowing.

It has been shown previously that the spontaneous (primary) swallow occurs infrequently during stable sleep [26, 27, 30]. The stimulation of pharyngeal swallow during sleep has not been studied systematically. However, its nocturnal activation can potentially play an important role in preventing the contact of refluxed gastric content with laryngeal structures and its subsequent aspiration. A preliminary study [30] evaluating the effect of pharyngeal water stimulation on airway protective reflexes in sleep suggests three types of response: arousal followed by swallow was the predominant response followed by cough and arousal followed by swallow and the least frequent was swallow followed by arousal.

Pharyngo-UES Contractile Reflex

Pharyngeal mechanical stimulation in cats [31] and water stimulation in humans [32] result in an increase in the resting tone of the UES, the phar-

yngo-UES contractile reflex (PUCR). It is speculated that it functions as an airway-protective
mechanism whereby retrograde entry of small
volumes of liquid into the pharynx from the
stomach results in augmentation of UES tone,
reducing the chance of further regurgitation into
the pharynx. During slow, continuous water
injection into the pharynx, the UES pressure
increases precipitously before the occurrence of
the pharyngeal swallow. In the young group in
the supine position during the slow continuous
injection, the UES pressure increased from a
basal pressure of 50 ± 7 to a pressure of
94 ± 9 mmHg, which is a 76 ± 16 % increase
($P < 0.05$). In the elderly, although similar trend
existed, the pressure difference was not statistically significant. These findings are similar for
the upright position.

The afferent limb of the PUCR is thought to
be mediated by the glossopharyngeal nerves. In
animal studies, cutting the glossopharyngeal
nerve blocked the PUCR but did not block the
esophago-UES contractile reflex or the responses
of the thyropharyngeus or cricopharyngeus muscles during swallowing [31]. The efferent limb of
the PUCR is mediated by the pharyngoesophageal nerves (somato-motor nerves) that branch
from the vagal trunk just rostral to the nodose
ganglion [33]; transection of this nerve eliminated basal tone of the cricopharyngeus muscle
and blocked the cricopharyngeus muscle response
to all reflex stimuli: PUCR, esophago-UES contractile reflex, and swallowing, but did not block
the response of thyropharyngeus muscle during
swallowing. Transection of the vagus nerves at
the cervical level (i.e., below the nodose ganglion) had no effect on the PUCR but blocked the
esophago-UES contractile reflex, which indicated that the recurrent laryngeal nerve (which
branches from the vagal trunk in the thoracic
cavity) serves no role in this reflex [31]. It is possible, however, that activation of these pharyngeal receptors may affect laryngeal muscle
activity that may be medicated through the recurrent laryngeal nerves [34].

A recent study was conducted on the effect of
volume, temperature and anesthesia on the PUCR
in humans [17]. Pharyngeal water injection at a
threshold volume of 0.1 ± 0 mL invariably
resulted in a significant increase in the UES pressure in all subjects. This pressure increase was
significantly lower than that for triggering a pharyngeal swallow. The results were similar for
slow continuous injection. Topical 4 % anesthetic
applied to the pharyngeal mucosa completely
abolished this reflex.

Pharyngo-UES Contractile Reflex in Patients with Posterior Laryngitis

In a recent study [35], 14 consecutive patients
with posterior laryngitis (48 ± 6 years) and 13
normal healthy volunteers (53 ± 6 years) were
studied using concurrent pharyngeal water stimulation and UES manometry. The threshold volume required to evoke the PUCR in the laryngitis
group (0.4 ± 0.05 mL) was significantly higher
than that of the control (0.2 ± 0.04 mL) ($P < 0.05$).
Following stimulation of the PUCR, the maxi-
mum post-injection pressure in patients
(75 ± 6 mmHg) was similar to that of the controls
(78 ± 6 mmHg). Because of a significantly lower
pre-injection UES pressure value in laryngitis
patients when compared to normal controls, the
percentage increase in UES pressure following
stimulation of the reflex in the laryngitis group
(99 ± 15 %) was significantly higher than that of
controls (55 ± 11 %) ($P < 0.05$). It was concluded
that, when compared to normal controls, a
significantly larger volume of liquid is required
to trigger this reflex in posterior laryngitis
patients. When triggered, the maximum UES
pressure induced by the PUCR is similar between
the two groups. These findings suggest an alteration of the afferent limb of the reflex in posterior
laryngitis patients, most probably at the level of
the pharyngeal receptors. However, whether this
alteration is a primary defect or secondary to the
effect of pharyngeal acid reflux is not determined. Study findings also indicate that when
triggered, the response of the target organ—
namely, the UES in the patient group—is similar
to that of the controls, indicating the intact function of the efferent limb and central control of
the reflex.

Although the finding of a significantly larger threshold volume required to trigger the pharyngo-UES reflex has physiologic significance, its clinical implications are currently undetermined because the difference of the threshold volume between controls and patients is small. However, it documents a significant difference in one of the proposed airway protective mechanisms against reflux of gastric content into the pharynx in a patient group with presumed reflux-induced laryngeal abnormalities.

Pharyngo-Glottal Adduction Reflex

Recent studies have shown that injection of minute amounts of water into the pharynx results in brief closure of the vocal cords [36, 37]. Gradual entry of liquid into the pharynx induced partial adduction of the cords. It is postulated that this adduction response is a part of the complex protective mechanisms that protect the airway from retrograde aspiration. On the other hand, studies have clearly shown the activation of this reflex during the preparatory phase of swallowing as the bolus overflows into the pharynx while mastication is in progress [38]. Entry of the oral content into the pharynx before swallowing is initiated induces a partial adduction of the cords believed to reduce the chance of aspiration by decreasing the glottis opening to the trachea. The threshold volume that stimulates this glottal adduction was found to be significantly smaller than that required to trigger an irrepressible pharyngeal swallow but similar to that required to induce a PUCR. Recent evidence suggests that a significantly larger volume of liquid is needed to trigger a pharyngoglottal reflex in the elderly when compared to the young. Although preserved, a significantly larger volume of water is required to stimulate this reflex by rapid pulse injection in the elderly, suggesting some deterioration in this age group. The pharyngoglottal closure reflex induced by rapid pulse injection is absent in dysphagic patients with predeglutitive aspiration, suggesting its contribution to airway protection against aspiration [39].

Effect of Alcohol and Cigarette Smoking on Pharyngeal Airway Protective Reflexes

Integrity of the aerodigestive reflexes is important in protecting the airways against aspiration injury. Alcoholics are at risk of developing aspiration pneumonia during an episode of severe alcohol intoxication. It is plausible that the depressant effect of alcohol on the central nervous system blunts the airway protective reflexes that may then predispose those with alcohol intoxication to aspiration of gastric contents. It is also not uncommon for cigarette smokers to have recurrent laryngeal and pulmonary disorders. Recent studies have shown that acute and chronic cigarette smoking can adversely affect the elicitation of Pharyngo-glottal, PUCR and RPS [40, 41], thereby predisposing cigarette smokers to risks of aspiration. Indeed recent studies have confirmed aspiration in smokers lacking intact aerodigestive reflexes [42]. As smokers are given nicotine patches to help them quit smoking, it is important to know whether this adverse effect of smoking on the aerodigestive reflexes is secondary to the local effect of cigarette smoke on the pharynx, due to gastroesophagopharyngeal reflux, or to the effect of systemic nicotine.

Acute alcohol exposure can adversely affect the triggering of PUCR and RPS [43] effects of alcohol can weaken the airway protective mechanisms against aspiration and may have implications in the pathogenesis of pneumonia after acute alcohol intoxication. This deleterious effect of alcohol appears to be secondary to a systemic effect of alcohol rather than its local effect on the pharynx [43]. Similarly, like previous studies [40, 41], acute cigarette smoking further increased the threshold volume required to trigger these reflexes, whereas no such adverse effect was seen after a nicotine patch was applied. This finding suggests that the negative effect of smoking on these reflexes may be due to a local effect of smoking on the pharynx rather than a systemic action of nicotine. Hence, preparations that deliver systemic nicotine to help quit smoking like nicotine patches may be used without compromising the aerodigestive reflexes.

It is conceivable that concurrent use of tobacco and alcohol may have an additive deleterious effect on the aerodigestive reflexes.

Pharyngeal Safe Volume and Its Relation to Airway Protective Reflexes

Comparison between the maximum capacity of fluid that can safely dwell in the hypopharynx (i.e., hypopharyngeal safe volume) before spilling into the larynx and the threshold volumes required to trigger pharyngo-glottal closure reflex (PGCR) PUCR and RPS has been reported recently [44]. These studies have shown that in healthy young individuals the threshold volume for eliciting aerodigestive reflexes by pharyngo water stimulation is significantly smaller than the maximum capacity of the hypopharynx to safely hold contents without spilling into the airway (Fig. 4.2). These studies also showed that by abolishing these reflexes with pharyngeal anesthesia the safe volume can be exceeded without being able to trigger these reflexes resulting in

laryngeal spillage. These observations directly demonstrate the protective role of the aerodigestive reflexes. This notion has been supported in a study of chronic cigarette smokers in whom the pharyngeal airway protective reflexes are shown to be defective. In these studies, pharyngeal water infusion resulted in laryngeal spillage in 12 of the 15 smokers with absent RPS. In addition, pharyngeal anesthesia abolishing the RPS in non-smokers resulted in laryngeal spillage. Of note, none of the non-smokers were found to develop laryngeal spillage before pharyngeal anesthesia [42]. Interestingly, pharyngeal safe volume in healthy young individuals as well as smokers has been reported to be less than 1 mL [42]. This finding has clinical ramification in post-deglutitive residue and its potential aspiration.

Mechanisms of Airway Protection During Belching

Belching is defined as voiding of gas from the stomach and esophagus through the mouth. However, it is known that distention of the esophagus by water may also initiate an esophageal

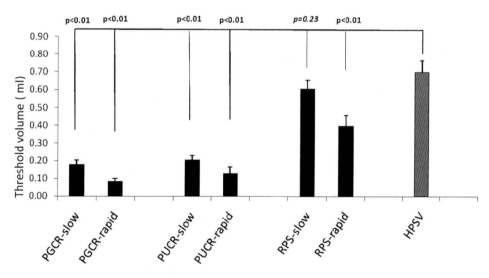

Fig. 4.2 The threshold volume for triggering PGCR, pharyngo-UES contractile reflex (PUCR), and reflexive pharyngeal swallow (RPS) by slow and rapid injections before pharyngeal anesthesia was 0.18±0.02 and 0.09±0.02 mL, 0.20±0.020 and 0.13±0.04 mL, and 0.61±0.04 and 0.4±0.06 mL, respectively. All of the above volumes were significantly smaller than the maximum volume that can safely dwell in the hypopharynx hypopharyngeal safe volume (HPSV) of 0.70±0.06 mL ($P<0.01$) except for the threshold volume to elicit RPS during slow perfusion, which was not significantly different from HPSV ($P=0.23$). From K. Dua et al. Am J Physiol Gastrointest Liver Physiol 2011;301:G197–G202 with permission

belching that does not involve gas reflux from the stomach. Ventilation of gastric or esophageal gas across the UES into the pharynx may be accompanied by entry of food particles, acid mist, etc., into the hypopharynx, and lead to aspiration.

Recent studies indicate that the glottis is actively involved in the belch reflex by activation of its closure mechanism [45]. They also indicate the existence of a close coordination between the UES and glottal function during belching. These studies also show that the glottal closure mechanism is activated and the vocal cords become closed before UES relaxation and its subsequent opening during belching (Table 4.2). One may hypothesize that the same coordination may exist during regurgitation and vomiting.

Glottal function during belching consists of the following sequences: (1) vocal cord adduction concurrent with the adduction of arytenoids, resulting in full closure of the introitus to trachea—onset of vocal cord adduction occurs 0.1 ± 0.08 s after onset of intra-esophageal pressure increase, due to air injection; (2) anterior/caudad movements of the glottis; and (3) opening of the UES that is either slit-like or triangular [45].

During some belches, the adducted arytenoids approximate the base of epiglottis, whereby closing the supraglottic portion of laryngeal vestibule. Supraglottic closure of the laryngeal vestibule, when present, is associated with an increase in intragastric pressure. Glottal function during gastric belches is similar to its function during esophageal belching.

Glottal closure and its precedence to the UES relaxation and opening during belching is an important protective function against aspiration of food particles, acid mist, and gastric content that maybe regurgitated into the pharynx during belching and could be aspirated into the trachea. Glottal closure during belching in humans is in sharp contrast to the glottal function in ruminants in which the glottis remains open during belching, resulting in tracheal reflux of gastric gas [46].

The time interval between the onset of vocal cord adduction and their complete closure, as well as the time interval between the onset of their abduction to their return to resting open position during belching, is fixed and indicates that the closure and opening of the cords during belching is preprogrammed by a stereotypical neural program. On the other hand, the duration of complete cord closure during belching is modified according to the volume of belched air.

We suggest that the neural pathway of glottal closure during belching begins with the vagus innervating the stretch receptors in the esophageal wall that carries the signal to the brainstem. The efferent vagal fibers, through recurrent laryngeal nerve, carry the signal to the glottal adductor muscles—interarytenoid, lateral cricoarytenoid and thyroarytenoid. We also suggest that the signals carried by the vagus to the brainstem from the esophageal wall stretch receptors stimulate supra- and infrahyoid muscles through ansa cervicalis and result in UES opening. A comparison of the functions of the various elements involved in belching and swallowing is shown in Table 4.2.

Glottal closure is an integral component of both esophageal and gastric belch reflexes and prevents aspirations of regurgitated material into the airway. The glottal closure mechanism during belching has two tiers of closure: vocal cord closure and aryepiglottic approximation. Glottal and UES functions are closely coordinated during belching.

Laryngo-Upper Esophageal Sphincter Contractile Reflex

The UES pressure response to laryngeal air stimulations documented the existence of a laryngo UES contractile reflex (Fig. 4.3). Significant reduction in the frequency stimulation of this reflex in elderly subjects compared with young subjects has been reported [47].

The laryngo UES contractile reflex can be elicited by stimulus intensity as low as an air pulse of 6 mmHg pressure with 50-ms duration. However, this ultrashort stimulation in awake humans is not reliable because the frequency of elicitation of the reflex with this stimulus is very low. This is most probably caused by the difficulty in maintaining a constant distance between the air delivery system and the targeted site.

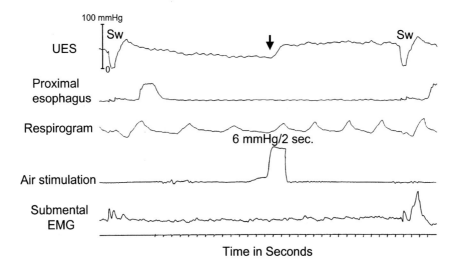

Fig. 4.3 An example of the UES pressure response to laryngeal air stimulation of 6 mmHg with 2-s duration in a young volunteer. As seen, UES pressure abruptly increased from about 30 mmHg and reached 60 mmHg after an air simulation delivered to the interarytenoid area. The poststimulation pressure continued until the subject swallowed by demand. From O. Kawamura et al. Gastroenterology 2004;127:57–64 with permission

Using longer duration pulses of at least 2-s duration improves reliability. When laryngeal mucosa is stimulated by 2-s continuous air stimulation, elicitation of this reflex increased to about 80 % of the trials and is significantly higher than those by air stimulations of shorter duration.

The afferent arm of this reflex in humans is the laryngeal mechanoreceptor and internal division of the superior laryngeal nerve [48], a branch of the vagus nerve. The efferent arm is the vagus nerve [49], including the superior laryngeal nerve and recurrent laryngeal nerve, although the glossopharyngeal nerve cannot be excluded because it serves branches into the pharyngeal plexus. The central pathway for this reflex is probably different from those of deglutition because the contractile response to the stimulation of this reflex is the opposite of the relaxation response of the UES to volitional, subconscious and reflexive or pharyngeal swallow. This reflex is different from the PUCR that is triggered by stimulation of mechanoreceptors in the posterior pharyngeal wall [31, 32] although the effector organ and efferent arc are the same for both the reflexes, the sensory field and afferent arc are different in that the PUCR is mediated via the glossopharyngeal [31] nerve with possible contribution from the superior laryngeal nerve.

Earlier studies have shown that air stimulation of the larynx also has an inhibitory effect on the lower esophageal sphincter [50, 51], it is conceivable that activation of the laryngo-UES contractile reflex may counteract the possible consequences of the inhibitory effect of laryngeal stimulation on the lower esophageal sphincter, namely, pharyngeal reflux of gastric content by increasing the UES pressure. In addition, although highly speculative at this stage, this reflex may be activated during pharyngeal reflux events by contact of regurgitated material with the laryngeal mucosa and by inducing an augmentation of UES resting pressure, possibly preventing further entry of refluxate into the pharynx and larynx. It is conceivable that deterioration of this reflex in elderly subjects may negatively affect airway protection against aspiration in this age group, especially during nighttime reflux events with the subject in the supine position when the airway is most vulnerable.

Paradoxical and absent UES response to laryngeal stimulation in a small group of patients with UES dysphagia has been reported [47] and suggests the possibility of alteration of the laryngo-UES contractile reflex in disease conditions. The potential groups exhibiting this alteration other than dysphagic patients may include those with reflux-induced laryngeal and pulmonary compli- cations. The paradoxical response of the UES to laryngeal air stimulation, observed in patients with UES dysphagia, suggests changes in the brain stem control of this reflex inducing inhibition of the efferent nerves instead of their stimulation.

It is surmised that, afferent signals originating from the larynx induce contraction of the UES (the laryngo-UES contractile reflex). Frequency elici- tation of this reflex is significantly lower in elderly subjects compared with young subjects, while the magnitude of change in UES pressure remains unchanged, indicating a deleterious effect of aging on the afferent arm of this reflex. The laryngo-UES contractile reflex is more reproducibly elicited by 2-s air stimulations than stimuli of shorter dura- tions. The laryngo-UES contractile reflex is altered in some patients with UES dysphagia.

Phonation-Induced UES Contractile Reflex

Activation of airway-protective mechanisms in response to respiratory function with potential for causing reflux events such as phonation and cough has been recently studied [52].

Phonation requires rapid opening and closing of the vocal folds to interrupt the air stream [15], accompanied by an increase in subglottal tracheal pressure believed to be generated by contraction of the diaphragm, simultaneously causing an increase in intra-abdominal pressure. This minimal sub- glottal pressure is necessary to drive the vocal cords into vibration. The fundamental frequency of a voice depends on the rapidity of vocal fold vibration, pharyngeal dimensions and vocal fold length among others [53]. Whenever the subglottal pressure is increased, the vocal fold vibrates faster and fundamental voice frequency is increased [15]. This phenomenon, especially during high-fre- quency vocalization such as that seen in profes- sional singers, can potentially predispose to GER, a recognized clinical problem in this group [54].

The effect of phonation on the intraluminal pressures of the esophagus and its sphincters was characterized by using concurrent manometry, voice recording, and videofluoroscopy in young,

healthy volunteers (Fig. 4.4a). The study findings indicate that during phonation there develops a significantly higher pressure increase within the UES compared with the esophagus, LES, and stomach. In contrast, study findings indicate that phonation induces similar pressure increases within the stomach, LES, and esophagus (Fig. 4.4b).

Although the phonation-induced intrathoracic and intra-abdominal pressure increases have been described previously, the observed disproportion- ately higher UESP increase during phonation has not been previously reported. Two mechanisms could be envisaged for this disproportionately higher pressure increase seen in the UES com- pared with the rest of the gastrointestinal tract dur- ing phonation: (1) mechanical squeeze of the sphincter by surrounding structures such as poste- rior movement of the larynx pressing the sphincter against the spine and (2) neuromuscular reflex mechanisms resulting in UES muscle contraction. Using concurrent videofluoroscopy during phona- tion, the excursion of the laryngeal apparatus was evaluated in these studies and the absence of its posterior movement documented, ruling out the first possibility. This finding supports the notion of a contractile UES response to phonation.

In that, phonation induces a significant increase in UESP. This UESP increase is significantly higher than that of the stomach, esophagus and LES indicating the existence of a phonation-induced UES contractile reflex.

Upper Esophageal Sphincter and Gastroesophageal Junction Pressures in Obstructive Apnea Patients

Recent studies have shown that during apnea epi- sodes in patients with obstructive sleep apnea (OSA) upper esophageal sphincter and gastroe- sophageal junction pressure changes act to pre- vent gastroesophageal and esophagopharyngeal reflux [55]. It has been thought that patients with OSA have more reflux events than healthy sub- jects [56]. In patients with OSA, end-inspiratory intraesophageal pressure progressively decreases during periods of apnea [57]. Moreover, nasal continuous positive airway pressure (CPAP)

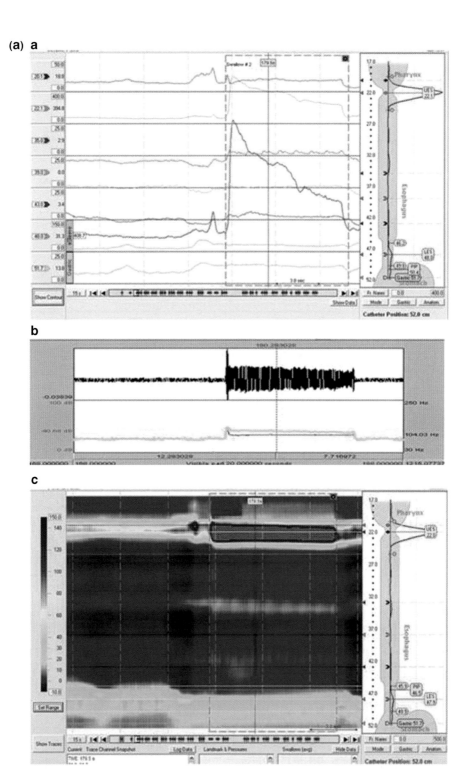

Fig. 4.4 (a) Example of concurrent manometry *line tracing* (a), voice recording (b), and contour plot (c) during high-pitch "ä" sound using ManoView and Praat software programs, respectively. *Dashed frame* in the manometry *line* tracing (a) demarcates a single trail of high-pitch "ä". *Brown* tracing represents eSleeve showing *upper* esophageal sphincter (UES) maximum pressure. Corresponding voice recording is showing in (b); *green* and *blue lines* represent pitch and amplitude, respectively, of high-pitch ä during this particular trial. On *right* of plot are three pitch values: *bottom*, floor of viewable pitch range (75 Hz); *top*, ceiling of pitch range (500 Hg); and *middle*, pitch value at cursor. On *left* of plot: *bottom*, floor (0 dB); *top*, ceiling (100–150 dB) of viewable intensity range; and middle,

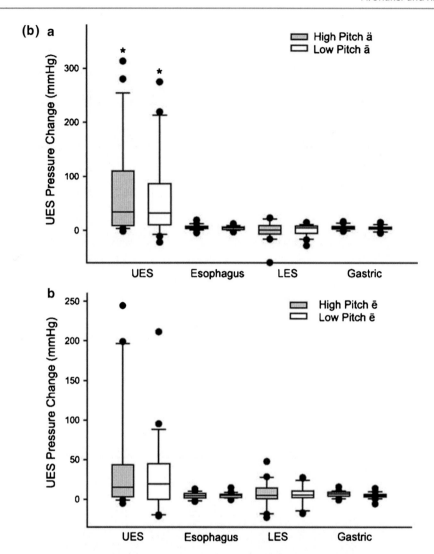

Fig. 4.4 (continued) intensity value at cursor (c): example of a manometric contour plot. (**b**) Effect of phonation on luminal pressure of esophagus and its sphincters. Median pressure changes over prephonation pressure during phonation of high- and low-pitch ä and c in stomach, esophagus, UES, and *lower* esophageal sphincter (LES) are shown. Median UES pressure (UESAP) increasing during ä (a) and c (b) for both *high* and *low* pitches was significantly higher than that of esophagus, LES, and stomach (*P<0.005). From L. Perera et al. Am J Physiol Gastrointest Liver Physiol 2008;294:G885–G891 with permission

reduces nocturnal GER events in patients with OSA [58]. Taken together, these findings suggest that the decrease in intraesophageal pressure during OSA could potentially facilitate GER events.

This notion was investigated in a study of 542 OSA events in patients with OSA without GERD, and 448 OSA events in patients with OSA and GERD. The findings indicate that over the course of the apneic events, progressive changes occur in the intraesophageal, UES, and GEJ pressures, resulting

in the intraesophageal pressure at the end-inspiratory phase at the end of OSA to be significantly lower than that at the beginning of OSA. In contrast, both the UES and GEJ pressures at the end-inspiratory phase at the end of OSA were found to be significantly higher than those at the beginning of OSA.

It was observed that despite a decrease in intraesophageal pressure during OSA events, compensatory changes in UES and GEJ pressures acted to prevent patients with OSA with

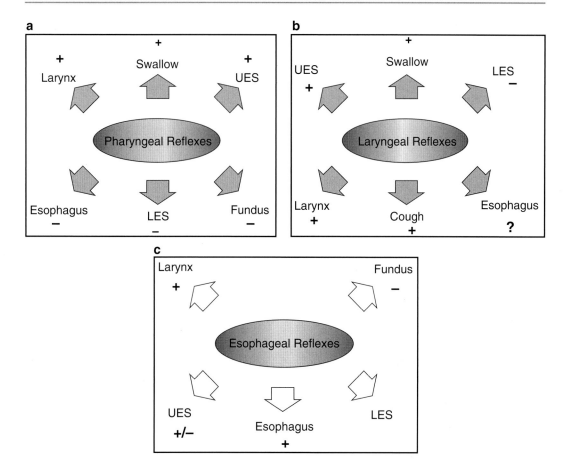

Fig. 4.5 (**a–c**) Summary figures showing excitatory and inhibitory reflexes emanating from pharynx (**a**), larynx (**b**), and esophagus (**c**). *Positive sign* indicates stiluation while *negative sign* indicates inhibition and unknown response is indicated by a *question mark*

and without GERD from having either acid or nonacid reflux events during periods of apnea.

Summary

In summary, there are a number of mechanisms including at least nine reflexes identified that either augment the UES pressure barrier, close the airway or clear the esophagus and pharynx from liquid or solid volumes. The reflex mechanisms may be activated as a result of pressure events associated with antegrade as well as retrograde transit of material through the pharyngoesophageal axis. Available evidence indicates that one or several of these reflexes may be stimulated in response to a single stimulus, such as stimulation of secondary peristalsis, esophago-UES contractile and esophageal closure reflex in response to esophageal distension or stimulation of the pharyngo-UES and pharyngoglottal closure reflexes as a consequence of stimulation of the pharyngeal mucosa. Aging, alcohol use, and smoking seem to adversely affect these reflexes. Emerging studies suggest the impairment of these reflexes in some conditions involving the aero-digestive tract, such as posterior laryngitis or predeglutitive aspiration. As mentioned earlier, in addition to protective reflexes, there are inhibitory reflexes that are triggered by the stimulation of the esophagus, pharynx, and the larynx. Summary representation of all the known inhibitory and excitatory esophageal, pharyngeal, and laryngeal reflexes is presented in Fig. 4.5a–c.

References

1. Curtis DJ, et al. Timing in the normal pharyngeal swallow. Prospective selection and evaluation of 16 normal asymptomatic patients. Invest Radiol. 1984;19(6):523–9.
2. Creamer B, Schlegel J. Motor responses of the esophagus to distention. J Appl Physiol. 1957;10(3):498–504.
3. Jadcherla SR, et al. Esophageal body and upper esophageal sphincter motor responses to esophageal provocation during maturation in preterm newborns. J Pediatr. 2003;143(1):31–8.
4. Ren J, et al. Effect of aging on the secondary esophageal peristalsis: presbyesophagus revisited. Am J Physiol. 1995;268(5 Pt 1):G772–9.
5. Aslam M, Kern M, Shaker R. Modulation of oesophago-UOS contractile reflex: effect of proximal and distal esophageal distention and swallowing. Neurogastroenterol Motil. 2003;15(3):323–9.
6. Gerhardt DC, et al. Human upper esophageal sphincter. Response to volume, osmotic, and acid stimuli. Gastroenterology. 1978;75(2):268–74.
7. Torrico S, et al. Upper esophageal sphincter function during gastroesophageal reflux events revisited. Am J Physiol Gastrointest Liver Physiol. 2000;279(2):G262–7.
8. Babaei A, Bhargava V, Mittal RK. Upper esophageal sphincter during transient lower esophageal sphincter relaxation: effects of reflux content and posture. Am J Physiol Gastrointest Liver Physiol. 2010;298(5):G601–7.
9. Bajaj JS, et al. Influence of sleep stages on esophago-upper esophageal sphincter contractile reflex and secondary esophageal peristalsis. Gastroenterology. 2006;130(1):17–25.
10. Lang IM, Medda BK, Shaker R. Mechanisms of reflexes induced by esophageal distension. Am J Physiol Gastrointest Liver Physiol. 2001;281(5):G1246–63.
11. Shaker R, et al. Esophagoglottal closure reflex: a mechanism of airway protection. Gastroenterology. 1992;102(3):857–61.
12. Shaker R, et al. Identification and characterization of the esophagoglottal closure reflex in a feline model. Am J Physiol. 1994;266(1 Pt 1):G147–53.
13. Wright RA, Miller SA, Corsello BF. Acid-induced esophagobronchial-cardiac reflexes in humans. Gastroenterology. 1990;99(1):71–3.
14. Shaker R, et al. Coordination of deglutitive glottic closure with oropharyngeal swallowing. Gastroenterology. 1990;98(6):1478–84.
15. Sasaki CT, Isaacson G. Functional anatomy of the larynx. Otolaryngol Clin North Am. 1988;21(4):595–612.
16. Shaker R, et al. Glottal function during postprandial gastroesophageal reflux. Gastroenterology. 1993;104(4):A581.
17. Ren J, et al. Effect of acute eosphagitis on the esophagoglottal closure reflex in a feline model. Gastroenterology. 1995;108(4):A677.
18. Paterson WG, Rattan S, Goyal RK. Experimental induction of isolated lower esophageal sphincter relaxation in anesthetized opossums. J Clin Invest. 1986;77(4):1187–93.
19. Nishino T, et al. Depression of the swallowing reflex during sedation and/or relative analgesia produced by inhalation of 50% nitrous oxide in oxygen. Anesthesiology. 1987;67(6):995–8.
20. Nishino T. Swallowing as a protective reflex for the upper respiratory tract. Anesthesiology. 1993;79(3):588–601.
21. Shaker R, et al. Effect of aging, position, and temperature on the threshold volume triggering pharyngeal swallows. Gastroenterology. 1994;107(2):396–402.
22. Ebihara T, et al. Capsaicin and swallowing reflex. Lancet. 1993;341(8842):432.
23. Paterson WG, Hynna-Liepert TT, Selucky M. Comparison of primary and secondary esophageal peristalsis in humans: effect of atropine. Am J Physiol. 1991;260(1 Pt 1):G52–7.
24. Christensen J, Lund GF. Esophageal responses to distension and electrical stimulation. J Clin Invest. 1969;48(2):408–19.
25. Paterson WG. Neuromuscular mechanisms of esophageal responses at and proximal to a distending balloon. Am J Physiol. 1991;260(1 Pt 1):G148–55.
26. Lichter I, Muir RC. The pattern of swallowing during sleep. Electroencephalogr Clin Neurophysiol. 1975;38(4):427–32.
27. Lear CS, Flanagan Jr JB, Moorrees CF. The frequency of deglutition in man. Arch Oral Biol. 1965;10:83–100.
28. Hollshwandner CH, Brenman HS, Friedman MH. Role of afferent sensors in the initiation of swallowing in man. J Dent Res. 1975;54(1):83–8.
29. Storey AT. Interactions of alimentary and upper respiratory tract reflexes, in mastication and swallowing. Toronto: University of Toronto Press; 1976. p. 22–36.
30. Dent J, et al. Mechanism of gastroesophageal reflux in recumbent asymptomatic human subjects. J Clin Invest. 1980;65(2):256–67.
31. Medda BK, et al. Characterization and quantification of a pharyngo-UES contractile reflex in cats. Am J Physiol. 1994;267(6 Pt 1):G972–83.
32. Shaker R, et al. Characterization of the pharyngo-UES contractile reflex in humans. Am J Physiol. 1997;273(4 Pt 1):G854–8.
33. McClure RC, Dallman MJ, Garrett PG. Cat anatomy. Philadelphia, PA: Lea & Febiger; 1973.
34. Bartlett D. Upper airway motor systems. Handbook of physiology, the respiratory system, control of breathing. Bethesda, MD: American Physiological Society; 1986.
35. Ulualp SO, et al. Pharyngo-UES contractile reflex in patients with posterior laryngitis. Laryngoscope. 1998;108(9):1354–7.
36. Ren J, et al. Glottal addcution response to pharyngeal water simulation: evidence for a pharyngoglottal closure reflex. Gastroenterology. 1994;106(4–2):A558.

37. Shaker R, et al. Pharyngoglottal closure reflex: identification and characterization in a feline model. Am J Physiol. 1998;275(3 Pt 1):G521–5.
38. Dua KS, et al. Coordination of deglutitive glottal function and pharyngeal bolus transit during normal eating. Gastroenterology. 1997;112(1):73–83.
39. Shaker R, et al. Pharyngoglottal closure reflex: characterization in healthy young, elderly and dysphagic patients with predeglutitive aspiration. Gerontology. 2003;49(1):12–20.
40. Dua K, et al. Effect of chronic and acute cigarette smoking on the pharyngo-upper oesophageal sphincter contractile reflex and reflexive pharyngeal swallow. Gut. 1998;43(4):537–41.
41. Dua K, et al. Effect of chronic and acute cigarette smoking on the pharyngoglottal closure reflex. Gut. 2002;51(6):771–5.
42. Dua K, et al. Protective role of aerodigestive reflexes against aspiration: study on subjects with impaired and preserved reflexes. Gastroenterology. 2011;140(7):1927–33.
43. Dua KS, et al. Effect of systemic alcohol and nicotine on airway protective reflexes. Am J Gastroenterol. 2009;104(10):2431–8.
44. Dua K, et al. Pharyngeal airway protective reflexes are triggered before the maximum volume of fluid that the hypopharynx can safely hold is exceeded. Am J Physiol Gastrointest Liver Physiol. 2011;301(2):G197–202.
45. Shaker R, et al. Mechanisms of airway protection and upper esophageal sphincter opening during belching. Am J Physiol. 1992;262(4 Pt 1):G621–8.
46. Dougherty RW, et al. Studies of pharyngeal and laryngeal activity during eructation in ruminants. Am J Vet Res. 1962;23:213–9.
47. Kawamura O, et al. Laryngo-upper esophageal sphincter contractile reflex in humans deteriorates with age. Gastroenterology. 2004;127(1):57–64.
48. Sasaki CT, Weaver EM. Physiology of the larynx. Am J Med. 1997;103(5A):9S–18.
49. Sasaki CT. Understanding the motor innervation of the human cricopharyngeus muscle. Am J Med. 2000;108(Suppl 4a):38S–9.
50. Ulualp SO, et al. Topography of the aerodigestive tract sensory field mediating lower esopahgeal sphincter relaxation. Gastroenterology. 1999;116:A1095.
51. Noordzij JP, et al. The effect of mechanoreceptor stimulation of the laryngopharynx on the oesophago-gastric junction. Neurogastroenterol Motil. 2000;12(4):353–9.
52. Perera L, et al. Manometric evidence for a phonation-induced UES contractile reflex. Am J Physiol Gastrointest Liver Physiol. 2008;294(4):G885–91.
53. Jiang J, Lin E, Hanson DG. Vocal fold physiology. Otolaryngol Clin North Am. 2000;33(4):699–718.
54. Cammarota G, et al. Reflux symptoms in professional opera choristers. Gastroenterology. 2007;132(3):890–8.
55. Kuribayashi S, et al. Upper esophageal sphincter and gastroesophageal junction pressure changes act to prevent gastroesophageal and esophagopharyngeal reflux during apneic episodes in patients with obstructive sleep apnea. Chest. 2010;137(4):769–76.
56. Berg S, Hoffstein V, Gislason T. Acidification of distal esophagus and sleep-related breathing disturbances. Chest. 2004;125(6):2101–6.
57. Zamagni M, et al. Respiratory effort. A factor contributing to sleep propensity in patients with obstructive sleep apnea. Chest. 1996;109(3):651–8.
58. Kerr P, et al. Nasal CPAP reduces gastroesophageal reflux in obstructive sleep apnea syndrome. Chest. 1992;101(6):1539–44.

Part II

Central Control of Deglutition

Cerebral Cortical Control of Deglutition

Dipesh H. Vasant and Shaheen Hamdy

Abstract

The human swallowing musculature is coordinated centrally through a multidimensional hierarchy of deglutative centres both in the cerebral cortex and brain stem. The cortex has an important role in initiation of the volitional swallow and has a role in all three phases of deglutition. Developments in technology, particularly functional brain imaging, have seen a fuller delineation of the human swallowing network and studies have shown that this system is adaptable to stimuli and subject to plastic change both to internal and external inputs. There is evidence to suggest cortical functional asymmetry, with a dominant swallowing hemisphere in healthy individuals, and when this is affected by stroke, with the non-dominant hemisphere clinically thought to be relevant in re-organisation and recovery of swallowing function. Finally, there is now considerable interest in neuromodulatory-based techniques in driving this brain re-organisation after cerebral injury.

Keywords

Cerebral cortex • Swallowing • Deglutition • Cortical control • Plasticity

Introduction

Normal deglutition is a dynamic, sensorimotor process involving 26 pairs of muscles, four cranial nerve motor nuclei and peripheral afferent inputs.

D.H. Vasant, MB ChB, MRCP • S. Hamdy, PhD, FRCP(✉)
Salford Royal Foundation Trust, School of Translational Medicine—Inflammation Sciences, University of Manchester, Eccles Old Road, Salford, Greater Manchester, England, UK
e-mail: Shaheen.Hamdy@manchester.ac.uk

This coordination in healthy individuals is vital for ensuring safe transport of ingested material from the mouth to the stomach for digestion without compromising the airway. The clinical relevance of the central control mechanism involved in swallowing is highlighted when considering brain injuries such as acute cerebral cortical or brain stem strokes that commonly disrupt central coordination resulting in oropharyngeal dysphagia which can lead to serious complications such as aspiration pneumonia [1].

Historically it was believed that the central neural control of swallowing was almost entirely

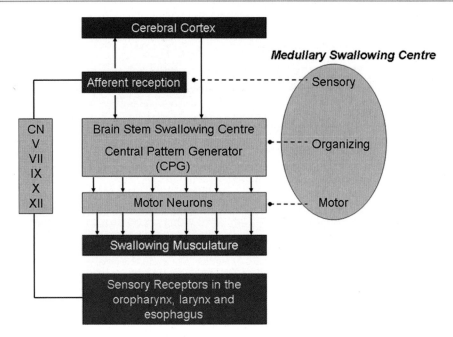

Fig. 5.1 The multidimensional model of central neural control in human swallowing. From N.E. Diamant Nat Med 1996;2:1190 with permission

dependent on brain stem reflexive mechanisms [2]. We now understand that deglutition is a dynamic process which can be initiated volitionally via the cerebral cortex and controlled by the central nervous system in a "multidimensional fashion" [2–4]. Normal swallowing has both volitional and reflexive components as illustrated in Fig. 5.1, which highlights the multidimensional levels of neural control of swallowing. In particular there is emphasis on descending cortical inputs to the brain stem, in association with sensory feedback which can influence cortical activity and hence motor output to swallowing musculature via the central pattern generator. This chapter will begin by discussing the evidence for the role of higher cortical centres and subcortical regions in the control of swallowing, in particular evidence from non-invasive cortical stimulation techniques and functional brain imaging which have revolutionised our understanding of human deglutition (Fig. 5.1).

Early evidence implicating regions of the cerebral cortex and the brain stem in the neural control of swallowing was based on neurophysiological observations in animals such as the seminal studies by Miller and Sherrington [5, 6]. Thereafter, Penfield et al. using direct electrical brain stimulation in anaesthetised humans during neurosurgery demonstrated that stimulation to certain parts of the cerebral cortex can induce swallowing [7]. In more recent times, studies using non-invasive cortical stimulation techniques have mapped areas of the cortex representing human swallowing musculature [8, 9]. Other evidence indicating cortical involvement came from reports of dysphagic stroke patients without brainstem disease with only unilateral cortical involvement [10–12]. In the past decade, significant advances in neuroscientific research using functional brain imaging techniques have improved our understanding of swallowing neurophysiology and the functional neuroanatomy of the brain structures involved in swallowing. We now have a better understanding of the recovery of swallowing after stroke and these developments have generated much interest in translational research looking at adjunctive neuromodulatory treatments for dysphagia after brain injury.

The Cerebral Cortex and Unravelling the Neurophysiology of Swallowing

Swallowing muscle activity in response to non-invasive cortical stimulation can be studied in detail in intact man, using non-invasive transcranial magnetic stimulation (TMS) and assessing pharyngeal and oesophageal motor evoked potentials by way of an intraluminal catheter and electromyography (EMG) recordings. Hamdy et al. used these methods to probe cortical projections to the pharynx and reported that muscle groups involved in swallowing are represented bilaterally, but asymmetrically in the human motor and premotor cortex areas in somatotopic fashion with the mylohyoid lateral and the pharynx more medial [9]. This important finding of asymmetric bilaterality which was *independent* of handedness was thought to indicate that humans have a dominant swallowing hemisphere and this may explain oropharyngeal dysphagia in patients with hemispheric stroke if the dominant side is involved [13]. Numerous studies using functional brain imaging have also observed functional asymmetry in the swallowing cortex, with the left hemisphere being most frequently cited. Additive to these assumptions, Mistry et al. reported evidence for functional asymmetry using inhibitory frequencies ("virtual lesions") of TMS applied to human pharyngeal motor cortices [14]. In the diseased state, Hamdy and colleagues have shown evidence for increased cortical excitability in the unaffected cerebral hemisphere following unilateral dysphagic stroke with this type of re-organisation in the pharyngeal motor cortex being associated with swallowing recovery [15]. Consequently, there is now considerable interest in cortical stimulation-based techniques being used to drive brain re-organisation in human swallowing motor cortex [16].

The above-mentioned TMS studies for the first time provided a clear description of cortical maps of cerebral areas involved in the corticobulbar pathway; demonstrating that multiple regions of the cerebral cortex could be stimulated to induce motor responses in swallowing musculature.

However, this did not give any information about the functional relevance of these corticofugal projections to swallowing function [9]. Functional magnetic resonance imaging (fMRI) is now widely available to researchers and has been extensively used to assess cortical regions involved in swallowing [17–22]. Techniques have now improved to reduce motion artefact. Both fMRI and positron emission tomography (PET) demonstrate changes in cortical function by way of altered regional cerebral blood flow but fMRI is often preferred given the absence of exposure to ionising radiation and it has excellent spatial resolution (Figs. 5.2 and 5.3). The main limitation of fMRI is that due to poor temporal resolution it is not possible to accurately follow the sequence of activations during execution of a sequential task such as swallowing. This is where magnetic encephalography (MEG) has proved useful (Fig. 5.4). Table 5.1 illustrates the advantages and limitations for each of these brain imaging techniques in investigating human swallowing pathways. Table 5.2 shows the main cortical and subcortical regions that have been identified as active during swallowing by each of these scanning modalities.

A recent meta-analysis has combined functional brain imaging data during swallowing from ten studies, including a total of 98 subjects. Based on these combined data, the authors have reported activity likelihood estimations (ALE) in cortical regions [23]. It was determined that during volitional water swallows, 12 cortical areas had significant ALE (Fig. 5.5). The left and right sensorimotor cortex, right inferior parietal lobe and right insula were found to have the highest ALE. A systematic review including 14 studies using fMRI in healthy subjects during swallowing showed similar data [24]. The primary motor cortex was again found to be the most prevalent region of activation, followed by the primary sensory cortex (S1, Brodmann's area (BA) 3, 2, 1). The insula and anterior cingulate cortex (BA32, 33) were also commonly activated during swallowing. Other cerebral sites are activated during swallowing but not consistently with some variability in studies and in individuals [25].

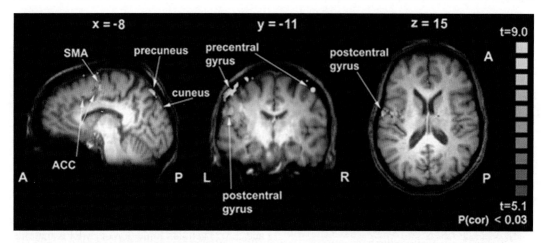

Fig. 5.2 Functional MRI during volitional swallowing. This functional MRI shows blood oxygenation level-dependent (BOLD) responses to voluntary saliva swallow (**a**), voluntary tongue elevation (**b**) and voluntary finger–thumb opposition (**c**) tasks. Talairach–Tournoux plane coordinate is displayed above each brain image. *ACC* anterior cingulate cortex, *SMA* supplementary motor area. From R.E. Martin et al. J Neurophysiol 2004;92:2428–493 with permission

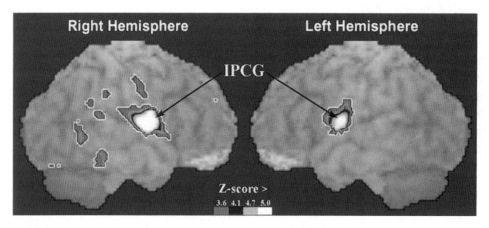

Fig. 5.3 Positron emission tomography (PET). Here, regional cerebral blood flow (rCBF) is superimposed on surface renderings of the lateral surface of the brain during swallowing. Cortical activation is seen at the precentral gyrus and other lateral cortical regions. The strongest activations localise to the inferior precentral gyrus (IPCG). In the right hemisphere, this focus extends into the adjacent inferior postcentral gyrus. Additional foci are seen in the right hemisphere within the inferior, superior and middle temporal gyri. From D. Zald et al. Ann Neurol 1999;46(3):281–86 with permission

Cortical Involvement in the Oral Phase of Deglutition

Initiation of swallowing is a voluntary process after a conscious decision and involves the cerebral cortex [13, 26, 27]. The first anatomical phase of swallowing is the oral phase. Hamdy et al., in an event-related functional magnetic resonance imaging (fMRI) study, confirmed involvement of the caudolateral sensorimotor cortex in the initiation of swallowing [17]. Around one second before a volitional swallow a very short activation in the cingulate cortex has been demonstrated to occur which is thought to represent initiation and cognitive processing of

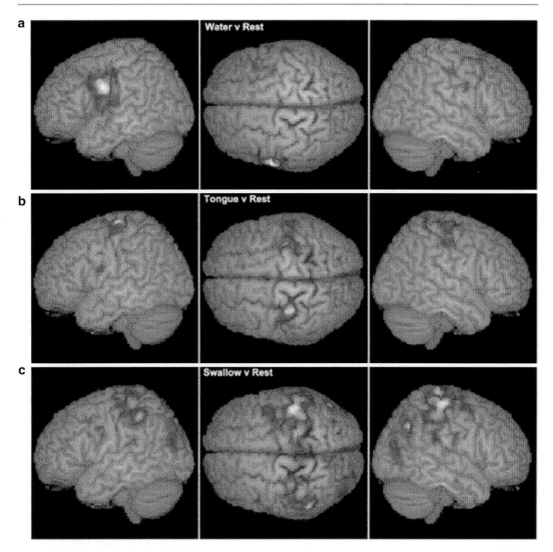

Fig. 5.4 Magnetoencephalography (MEG). These MEG images compare cortical activity associated with (**a**) infusion of water, (**b**) tongue thrusting and (**c**) swallowing. During swallowing significant activation is seen in the right superior postcentral gyri (BA3, 1, 2), the left paracentral lobule (BA6); inferior parietal lobule (BA40) in the right hemisphere was also significantly activated, as were the angular gyrus and supramarginal gyrus. From P.L. Furlong et al. Neuroimage 2004;22: 1147–155 with permission

the swallow. Moreover, just prior to a swallow, additional activations are seen in the anterior cingulate gyrus (BA24, 25, 32, 33) and supplementary motor areas of both hemispheres [28]. Further activity in the insula and inferior frontal gyrus appears to be associated with the pre-swallowing phase and continues up to the motor phases [29, 30]. The primary sensorimotor cortices together with the sensorimotor integration areas (BA5, 7) and primary motor cortex (BA4) appear to have a role planning and processing volitional swallowing. These activations do not occur during reflexive swallowing [25].

During the oral preparatory phase, the process of mastication sends sensory afferent information from the dorsum of the tongue and periodontal region that are important in regulating bolus consistency as well as lingual propulsive forces to aid transport to the pharynx [31]. This sensory input is thought to stimulate activity in the insula,

Table 5.1 Advantages and disadvantages of the different modalities used to study cortical involvement in swallowing

Imaging modality	Mode of detecting cortical activity during swallow	Advantages	Limitations
Transcranial magnetic stimulation (TMS)	• Electromagnetic fields used to induce activity in neural tissue below stimulator site • Pharyngeal response measured using electromyography (EMG)	• Non-invasive • Can be performed at bedside • Easier in dysphagic patients (no swallow required)	• Unable to assess functional neuroanatomy • Unable to study cortical activity during a swallowing task
Functional magnetic resonance imaging (fMRI)	• Alterations in cortical blood flow reflect changes in cortical activity • Blood oxygen level-dependent (BOLD)	• Detailed neuroanatomy (spatial resolution 2 mm) • Single-event-related approach gives specific cortical activity during a task and reduced motion-related artefact. • No exposure to ionising radiation	• Limited temporal resolution • Swallowing during scans can be difficult for dysphagic subjects
Positron emission tomography (PET)	• Alterations in cortical blood flow reflect changes in cortical activity • H2 15O injection to estimate blood flow	• Better spatial resolution in subcortical areas than fMRI	• Unable to use single-event-related approach • Temporal resolution inferior to fMRI • Ionising radiation exposure
Magnetoencephalo-graphy (MEG)	• Cortical neuronal activity shown by detection of postsynaptic magnetic fields	• Similar spatial resolution to fMRI and PET • Superior temporal resolution (milliseconds) • Can be used during motor task. • No exposure to ionising radiation	• Availability

Table 5.2 Summary of the main cortical and subcortical activations associated with swallowing, as identified by functional brain imaging studies

Brain region	PET	fMRI	MEG
Sensorimotor cortex	✓	✓	✓
Insula	✓	✓	
Anterior cingulate	✓	✓	✓
Posterior cingulate		✓	✓
Supplementary motor cortex	✓	✓	✓
Basal ganglia	✓	✓	
Cuneus	✓	✓	
Precuneus	✓	✓	✓
Temporal pole	✓	✓	
Orbitofrontal cortex	✓	✓	
Cerebellum	✓	✓	
Brainstem	✓	✓	

PET positron emission tomography
fMRI functional magnetic resonance imaging
MEG magnetoencephalography
[a]Reproduced with permission from *GI Motility Online* (2006) doi:10.1038/gimo8

amygdala and orbitofrontal cortex [32]. Cortical areas involved in tongue movements include the lateral pericentral cortex, frontoparietal operculum and Anterior Cingulate Cortex areas which are also known to be involved with swallowing. [18] This corticobulbar drive to the tongue muscles, submental, suprahyoid muscles is effected via cranial nerves V and XII [33]. Lamkadem et al., in a study involving direct brain stimulation in anaesthetised sheep, reported that stimulation of the chewing cortex inhibited initiation of reflex deglutition but did not halt progression once the process had started [34]. This suggests that whilst mastication is active, this inhibitory mechanism exists to ensure adequate preparation of the bolus before swallowing is initiated. fMRI studies have shown that mastication activates orofacial sensorimotor cortex and premotor cortex and both the posterior parietal and prefrontal cortical regions [32]. The physiological processes of olfaction and gustation also take place during the oral

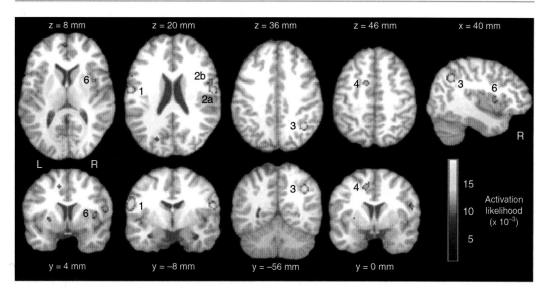

Fig. 5.5 Activation likelihood estimation (ALE) meta-analysis of brain activity associated with water swallowing. Significant activation clusters included the left precentral gyrus (1), right postcentral (2a) and inferior frontal gyrus (2b), right inferior parietal lobule (3), left cingulate gyrus (4) and right insula (6). From P. Soros et al. Human Brain Mapping 2009;30:2426–439 with permission

phase (further described in Chap. 2 of this book). Neurophysiological observations in animal studies and brain imaging during human swallowing indicate the cortical areas involved in gustation are the anterior/dorsal insula and the frontal operculum [35]. Recently, an interesting study by Babaei et al. using functional magnetic resonance imaging (fMRI) scanned the left cerebral cortex to compare the effects of different flavours (popcorn, lemon and milk chocolate) compared to water and saliva on the cortical swallowing network activity assessed by blood oxygenation level-dependent (BOLD) responses after each swallowing intervention. The results of this innovative study indicated that flavoured liquids compared to "inert" liquids led to significant increase in BOLD response both in anterior and posterior parts of the cingulate gyrus, prefrontal cortex, sensory/motor cortex but not in the insula [36]. These results may imply that in response to sensations such as taste, smell and visual sensations, the cortical swallowing network may be modulated and enhanced; however there were potential limitations of this study in particular the incomplete imaging of the whole brain. Mistry et al. have previously reported that there was no difference in excitability of the swallowing motor cortex when responses to bitter and sweet tastes were compared [37].

The Cerebral Cortex and the Pharyngeal Phase of Normal Deglutition

By the end of the oral phase of deglutition, the bolus is mobilised to the posterior aspect of the tongue towards the oropharynx. The pharyngeal phase of deglutition is then initiated and is believed to be semi-reflexive with its duration and muscular intensity regulated by pharyngeal sensory information [4]. This is emphasised when considering a study by Teismann et al. in which topical oropharyngeal anaesthesia led to pronounced decrease in activation in the primary motor and sensory cortex seen on MEG. The resulting impaired cortical activity manifested as reduced swallow speed and volume [38].

Arrival of the bolus in pharynx triggers a sequence of coordinated muscular events involving stabilisation of the closed mandible, hyoid bone movement and posterior tongue movements.

After the pharyngeal wall meets the tongue, the bolus is then propelled by waves of contraction. Laryngeal and hyoid movements serve to protect the airway and laryngeal movement facilitates opening of the upper esophageal sphincter (UES) [2]. There has been some debate about the role of the primary motor cortex (M1, precentral gyrus, BA4) in the seemingly more reflexive pharyngeal phase of swallowing. However, brain imaging studies have shown activation of M1 during the pharyngeal phase. Furlong et al. in an MEG study reported that during the motor phase of swallowing, the caudal region of the pericentral gyrus and regions of the sensorimotor cortex were also activated. These regions coincide with the topographic areas that Hamdy et al. described as corresponding to pharyngeal and oesophageal musculature using TMS [8, 39]. The superior premotor cortex also seems to be involved in the motor phase [17]. Doeltgen et al. investigated this recently using TMS over the motor cortex and measured surface EMG responses in submental musculature during swallowing conditions: volitional submental muscle contraction, volitional swallowing initiation and during the reflexive pharyngeal component of swallowing. The study showed corticobulbar excitability in the submental musculature was enhanced by volitional submental contraction but not by volitional swallowing and reflexive pharyngeal swallowing conditions. These results suggest that the primary motor cortex has a role in the control of swallowing [40]. Further evidence for the role of the cortex in pharyngeal swallowing comes from studies using pharyngeal electrical stimulation which has been shown to enhance corticobulbar excitability with enhancement of BOLD signal to fMRI during swallowing and reversal of focal inhibition in the pharyngeal motor cortex induced by low-frequency TMS [41, 42].

The anterior and posterior insula have been consistently activated during imaging studies. In a recent case report of an epileptic individual with a ganglionoma in the right posterior insular cortex, preoperative electrical stimulation in this specific area incidentally caused irregular and delayed swallowing, which the patient reported as a "stutter" in his swallow. These effects were frequency-dependent. The findings are similar to previous stimulation studies in the posterior insula [7]. The authors concluded that the posterior insula may be an important region in the cerebral cortical control possibly by affecting oropharyngeal–laryngeal sensory alterations leading to discomfort or constriction or interference with motor execution [43]. These case report observations, whilst of interest, require further investigation.

The Cerebral Cortex and the Esophageal Phase of Swallowing

The esophageal phase of deglutition is also reflexive and is triggered by bolus stimulation at the proximal esophagus. Sensory receptors here are thought to transmit this information via the superior laryngeal nerve (SLN) and recurrent laryngeal nerve (RLN) [44]. Once the cricopharyngeal muscles relax the bolus passes into the esophagus and primary peristaltic waves then transmit the bolus to the stomach.

The brain stem central pattern generator (CPG) has a crucial role in coordinating the time interval between the pharyngeal and esophageal phases of swallowing, to ensure efficient bolus transfer. This is achieved by separate neurally mediated excitatory and inhibitory mechanisms [44]. The inhibitory mechanism affects both the longitudinal and circular muscle layers of the esophageal wall [45]. This inhibition is important particularly after rapid sequential swallowing where it prevents the potentially obstructive situation of two unsynchronised esophageal peristaltic waves occurring at the same time [44]. Several animal studies have investigated this phenomenon and suggest that deglutitive inhibition is triggered by either SLN stimulation or pharyngeal mechanical stimulation, leading to inhibition of esophageal pre-motor neurones in the CPG, nucleus tractus solitarius (NTS) or the nucleus ambiguus (NA) [46–48].

Cerebral cortical areas which project to the esophageal musculature are more anterior and medial to the pharyngeal muscle representation [8]. In an fMRI study, Paine et al. compared cortical activations during swallowing after esophageal acid infusion to saline infusion. After saline infusion, predictable areas became active during swallowing (sensory and motor cortex, insula and putamen). After the acid infusion, it was noticed that subjects had reduction in activity in primary motor and sensorimotor association areas. The authors suggest that these inhibited cortical responses to painful visceral sensation could be due to a protective mechanism against swallowing a noxious substance such as acid [49]. These findings are in contradiction to another study of subliminal acid infusion into the esophagus where there was an enhancement of cortical activity associated with swallowing compared to a control buffer solution [50]. However, in both cases, these data support the view that chemosensory input from the esophagus has strong effects on cortical swallowing function, which may or may not be esophageal field-specific.

Ageing and Cortical Control of Swallowing

Pertinent to this review is the effect of aging on cortical swallowing function. There is literature to suggest that extreme age can alter the biomechanical behaviour of swallowing. A recent study by Humbert et al. compared cortical activation in healthy older subjects directly with younger subjects. The analysis showed that older subjects had more cortical activity in more regions compared to younger subjects using the same swallowing tasks, with higher activity in brain regions active during attention demanding tasks such as superior and middle frontal lobe activity. These results may imply that older people require more effort and hence more cortical input to maintain normal swallowing [51].

Conclusion

There have been considerable recent advances in our understanding of the cortical control of swallowing, driven in part by a massive expansion in knowledge through the advent of functional brain imaging in intact man. These observations, in association with more historic data from neurosurgical studies and explorations of the cerebral cortex in animal, have more fully delineated the cortical swallowing network and have shown that this system is adaptable to stimuli and subject to plastic change both to internal and external inputs.

Key Points

- Central control of swallowing is vital in preventing aspiration of ingested materials.
- The cerebral cortex has an important role in initiation and strong involvement in coordinating the normal swallow.
- Swallowing musculature is represented bilaterally but asymmetrically in the cerebral cortex.
- Lesions involving the "dominant" hemisphere may explain dysphagia after stroke and re-organisation of the contralateral (undamaged) hemisphere is thought be responsible for recovery of swallowing function.
- Functional brain imaging studies have shown activation of multiple cortical loci during normal human swallowing.
- Sensory input from the oropharynx, larynx and esophagus have an important modulatory role on cortical swallowing function.
- There is early evidence that advanced age can affect cortical activity levels during swallowing on functional brain imaging studies.

References

1. Martino R, et al. Dysphagia after stroke: incidence, diagnosis, and pulmonary complications. Stroke. 2005;36(12):2756–63.
2. Millers AJ. The neurobiology of swallowing and dysphagia. Dev Disabil Res Rev. 2008;14(2):77–86.
3. Martin RE, Sessle BJ. The role of the cerebral cortex in swallowing. Dysphagia. 1993;8(3):195–202.
4. Mistry S, Hamdy S. Neural control of feeding and swallowing. Phys Med Rehabil Clin N Am. 2008;19(4):709–28. Vii–viii.
5. Miller FR. The cortical paths for mastication and deglutition. J Physiol. 1920;53(6):473–8.

6. Miller FR, Sherrington CS. Some observations on the buccopharyngeal stage of reflex deglutition in the cat. Quart J Exp Physiol. 1916;9:147–86.

7. Penfield W, Boldrey E. Somatic motor and sensory representation in the cerebral cortex of man as studied by electrical stimulation. Brain. 1937;60:389–443.

8. Aziz Q, et al. The topographic representation of esophageal motor function on the human cerebral cortex. Gastroenterology. 1996;111(4):855–62.

9. Hamdy S, et al. The cortical topography of human swallowing musculature in health and disease. Nat Med. 1996;2(11):1217–24.

10. Barer DH. The natural history and functional consequences of dysphagia after hemispheric stroke. J Neurol Neurosurg Psychiatry. 1989;52(2):236–41.

11. Gordon C, Hewer RL, Wade DT. Dysphagia in acute stroke. Br Med J (Clin Res Ed). 1987;295(6595):411–4.

12. Meadows JC. Dysphagia in unilateral cerebral lesions. J Neurol Neurosurg Psychiatry. 1973;36(5):853–60.

13. Hamdy S, et al. Physiology and pathophysiology of the swallowing area of human motor cortex. Neural Plast. 2001;8(1–2):91–7.

14. Mistry S, et al. Unilateral suppression of pharyngeal motor cortex to repetitive transcranial magnetic stimulation reveals functional asymmetry in the hemispheric projections to human swallowing. J Physiol. 2007;585(Pt 2):525–38.

15. Hamdy S, et al. Recovery of swallowing after dysphagic stroke relates to functional reorganization in the intact motor cortex. Gastroenterology. 1998;115(5):1104–12.

16. Hamdy S. The organisation and re-organisation of human swallowing motor cortex. Suppl Clin Neurophysiol. 2003;56:204–10.

17. Hamdy S, et al. Cortical activation during human volitional swallowing: an event-related fMRI study. Am J Physiol. 1999;277(1 Pt 1):G219–25.

18. Martin RE, et al. Cerebral areas processing swallowing and tongue movement are overlapping but distinct: a functional magnetic resonance imaging study. J Neurophysiol. 2004;92(4):2428–43.

19. Martin R, et al. Cerebral cortical processing of swallowing in older adults. Exp Brain Res. 2007;176(1):12–22.

20. Toogood JA, et al. Discrete functional contributions of cerebral cortical foci in voluntary swallowing: a functional magnetic resonance imaging (fMRI) "Go, No-Go" study. Exp Brain Res. 2005;161(1):81–90.

21. Kern MK, et al. Cerebral cortical representation of reflexive and volitional swallowing in humans. Am J Physiol Gastrointest Liver Physiol. 2001;280(3):G354–60.

22. Mosier KM, et al. Lateralization of cortical function in swallowing: a functional MR imaging study. AJNR Am J Neuroradiol. 1999;20(8):1520–6.

23. Soros P, Inamoto Y, Martin RE. Functional brain imaging of swallowing: an activation likelihood estimation meta-analysis. Hum Brain Mapp. 2009;30(8):2426–39.

24. Humbert IA, Robbins J. Normal swallowing and functional magnetic resonance imaging: a systematic review. Dysphagia. 2007;22(3):266–75.

25. Hamdy S. Role of cerebral cortex in the control of swallowing. GI Motility Online (http://www.nature.com), 2006.

26. Miller AJ. Deglutition. Physiol Rev. 1982;62(1):129–84.

27. Palmer JB, et al. Volitional control of food transport and bolus formation during feeding. Physiol Behav. 2007;91(1):66–70.

28. Abe S, Wantanabe Y, Shintani M, Tazaki M, Takahashi M, Yamane GY, Ide Y, Yamada Y, Shimono M, Ishikawa T. Magnetoencephalographic study of the starting point of voluntary swallowing. Cranio. 2003;21(1):46–9.

29. Dziewas R, et al. Neuroimaging evidence for cortical involvement in the preparation and in the act of swallowing. Neuroimage. 2003;20(1):135–44.

30. Watanabe Y, et al. Cortical regulation during the early stage of initiation of voluntary swallowing in humans. Dysphagia. 2004;19(2):100–8.

31. Steele CM, Miller AJ. Sensory input pathways and mechanisms in swallowing: a review. Dysphagia. 2010;25(4):323–33.

32. Leopold NA, Daniels SK. Supranuclear control of swallowing. Dysphagia. 2010;25(3):250–7.

33. Ertekin C, Aydogdu I. Neurophysiology of swallowing. Clin Neurophysiol. 2003;114(12):2226–44.

34. Lamkadem M, et al. Stimulation of the chewing area of the cerebral cortex induces inhibitory effects upon swallowing in sheep. Brain Res. 1999;832(1–2):97–111.

35. Zald DH, Pardo JV. Cortical activation induced by intraoral stimulation with water in humans. Chem Senses. 2000;25(3):267–75.

36. Babaei A, et al. Enhancing effects of flavored nutritive stimuli on cortical swallowing network activity. Am J Physiol Gastrointest Liver Physiol. 2010;299(2):G422–9.

37. Mistry S, et al. Modulation of human cortical swallowing motor pathways after pleasant and aversive taste stimuli. Am J Physiol Gastrointest Liver Physiol. 2006;291(4):G666–71.

38. Teismann IK, et al. Functional oropharyngeal sensory disruption interferes with the cortical control of swallowing. BMC Neurosci. 2007;8:62.

39. Furlong PL, et al. Dissociating the spatio-temporal characteristics of cortical neuronal activity associated with human volitional swallowing in the healthy adult brain. Neuroimage. 2004;22(4):1447–55.

40. Doeltgen SH, et al. Task-dependent differences in corticobulbar excitability of the submental motor projections: Implications for neural control of swallowing. Brain Res Bull. 2011;84(1):88–93.

41. Fraser C, et al. Driving plasticity in human adult motor cortex is associated with improved motor function after brain injury. Neuron. 2002;34(5):831–40.

42. Jayasekeran V, et al. Adjunctive functional pharyngeal electrical stimulation reverses swallowing disability after brain lesions. Gastroenterology. 2010;138(5):1737–46.

43. Soros P, et al. Stuttered swallowing: electric stimulation of the right insula interferes with water swallowing. A case report. BMC Neurol. 2011;11(1):20.

44. Lang IM. Brain stem control of the phases of swallowing. Dysphagia. 2009;24(3):333–48.
45. Shi G, et al. Deglutitive inhibition affects both esophageal peristaltic amplitude and shortening. Am J Physiol Gastrointest Liver Physiol. 2003;284: G575–82.
46. Dong H, Loomis CW, Bieger D. Distal and deglutitive inhibition in the rat esophagus: role of inhibitory neurotransmission in the nucleus tractus solitarii. Gastroenterology. 2000;118(2):328–36.
47. Kruszewska B, Lipski J, Kanjhan R. An electrophysiological and morphological study of esophageal motoneurons in rats. Am J Physiol. 1994;266(2 Pt 2): R622–32.
48. Car A, Roman C, Zoungrana OR. Effects of atropine on the central mechanism of deglutition in anesthetized sheep. Exp Brain Res. 2002;142(4):496–503.
49. Paine PA, et al. Modulation of activity in swallowing motor cortex following esophageal acidification: a functional magnetic resonance imaging study. Dysphagia. 2008;23(2):146–54.
50. Kern M, et al. Effect of esophageal acid exposure on the cortical swallowing network in healthy human subjects. Am J Physiol Gastrointest Liver Physiol. 2009;297(1):G152–8.
51. Humbert IA, et al. Neurophysiology of swallowing: effects of age and bolus type. Neuroimage. 2009;44(3):982–91.

André Jean and Michel Dallaporta

Abstract

Deglutition, one of the most elaborate motor functions in mammals, depends on a CPG located in the medulla oblongata, which involves several brainstem motor nuclei and two main groups of interneurons. The DSG, located in a primary sensory nucleus, namely the NTS, contains the generator neurons involved in triggering, shaping and timing the sequential or rhythmic swallowing pattern. The VSG, located in the ventrolateral medulla, contains switching neurons that distribute the swallowing drive to the various pools of motoneurons. Both peripheral sensory inputs and supramedullary influences, such as the cortical ones, may shape the CPG activity in order to adapt the output of the network to the motor pattern required. Interestingly, signalling pathways involved in the control of food intake do also exert modulatory influences on the CPG. As regard the mechanisms at work in the CPG, they depend, very probably, on the pattern of intrinsic connections, with a crucial role of the inhibitory ones in shaping the sequential firing, as well as on the intrinsic cellular properties of swallowing neurons. Recent data indicate that the CPG may show some degree of flexibility, with neurons participating to the activity of other brainstem CPGs, providing interesting neuroplasticity capabilities.

Keywords

Brainstem control • Deglutition • Firing of brainstem swallowing neurons • Interneurons • Neural mechanisms • Swallowing pattern generator

Introduction

Swallowing in mammals, an alimentary function involving protection of the upper respiratory tract, is a complex but stereotyped motor sequence, with the implication that it involves a fixed behavioral pattern. It constitutes, however, one of the most elaborate motor functions, since it requires

A. Jean • M. Dallaporta (✉)
Faculte Des Sciences St. Jerome, Physiologie
Neurovegatative (PNV), University Aix-Marseille Paul
Cezanne, Avenue Escadrille Normandie-Niemen,
Marseille, France
e-mail: michel.dallaporta@univ-cezanne.fr

coordinating an extraordinary bilateral sequence of activation and inhibition among more than 25 pairs of muscles in the mouth, pharynx and larynx, plus the esophagus [1–5]. Interestingly, the whole motor sequence can be readily initiated by stimulating a single nerve, namely the internal branch of the superior laryngeal nerve (SLN), providing, therefore, a suitable model for studying the neurophysiological mechanisms underlying motor pattern generation [6–8].

As regards the motor pattern, neurophysiological studies have generally considered the swallowing sequence as having two phases: an oropharyngeal phase that constitutes an irreversible motor event, followed by an esophageal phase, corresponding to the primary peristalsis of the esophagus. Part of the swallowing sequence, namely esophageal peristalsis, can also be induced in the absence of the oropharyngeal phase of swallowing, and is called secondary peristalsis [2, 3, 9]. It is noteworthy that under the appropriate stimulus, such as long-lasting repetitive stimulation of the SLN, a pattern of rhythmic motor activities of swallowing can occur [3, 7]. In addition, SLN stimulation can elicit, in swallowing muscles, brief electromyographic responses with short latency, the so-called elementary reflexes [1, 6]. Finally, it should be stressed that muscles involved in swallowing may also be involved in several other motor behaviors, such as lapping, licking, sucking, chewing, respiration, emesis, and rumination [1–3, 9, 10]. In mammals, all muscles involved in the oropharyngeal phase are striated and are therefore driven by several pools of motoneurons located mainly in various cranial motor nuclei in the brainstem [1, 3, 5]. In some species, such as the dog, the esophageal muscle is entirely composed of striated fibers and is therefore also controlled by cranial motoneurons. In species such as cats, opossums, and primates, a variable portion of the lower esophagus is composed of smooth muscle fibers and is controlled by central preganglionic neurons and peripheral neurons of the enteric nervous system [2, 9, 11].

It is now clearly established, as originally postulated in the pioneer work by Meltzer [12], that the sequential and rhythmic patterns of swallowing are formed and organized by a central pattern generator (CPG). The CPG was previously described as a swallowing center, which can be subdivided into three systems: an afferent system corresponding to the central and peripheral inputs to the center, an efferent system corresponding to the outputs from the center, consisting of the various motoneuron pools involved in swallowing, and an organizing system, located in the medulla oblongata, corresponding to the interneuronal network that programs the motor pattern [1, 3, 13]. In fact, the concept of a swallowing center implies the idea of an anatomical localization, whereas that of a CPG is based on a more functional principle focusing on the activity of the various pools of neurons, i.e., motoneurons and interneurons, involved in the motor activity.

What Is Currently Known

Localization and Firing of Brainstem Swallowing Neurons: The Swallowing Pattern Generator

It was on the basis of microelectrode recordings that the swallowing-related neurons were identified, providing a general picture of the organization and functional principles of the swallowing CPG [7, 14–18]. In addition, lesion experiments, electrical brain stimulations, in situ microinjections of putative transmitters, anatomical tract tracing techniques, and more recently identification of c-fos expression in neurons have generally yielded fairly concordant results as regards the swallowing CPG [18–25].

Swallowing-related neurons are either (1) normally silent phasic neurons which present a burst of spikes, called "swallowing activity," occurring in a constant temporal relationship with the swallowing motor activity, or (2) spontaneously active neurons which exhibit a transient increase in their discharge frequency, or a phasic inhibition of their spontaneous discharge during swallowing [3, 7, 18]. Neurons have been classified into two main categories (Fig. 6.1b): oropharyngeal neurons, which fire before or during the oropharyngeal phase of swallowing, and esophageal neurons, which discharge during the esophageal

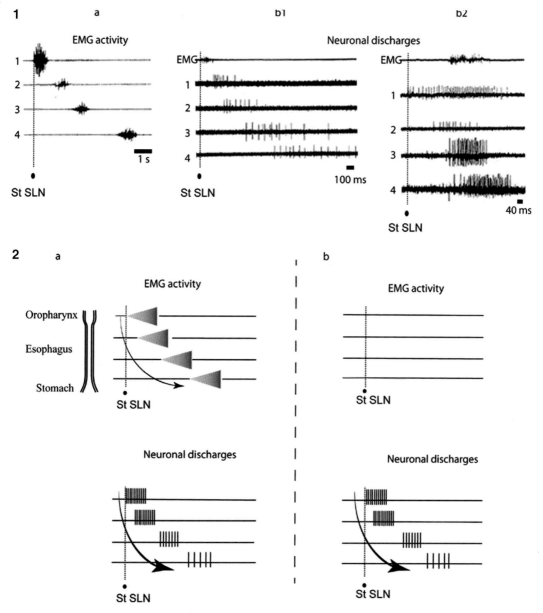

Fig. 6.1 Motor and neuronal swallowing patterns. (1a) typical swallowing sequence induced by electrical stimulation of the superior laryngeal nerve (SLN) with electromyographic (EMG) recordings, in sheep, from mylohyoid (1), upper (2) and lower (3) cervical esophagus and thoracic esophagus (4). (1b) sequential firing of several swallowing neurons recorded in the dorsal medulla (DSG) during swallowing induced by SLN stimulation. EMG: activity of the mylohyoid muscle, indicative of the onset of swallowing. In b1 and b2, are shown the firing patterns (1, 2, 3, 4) of different esophageal (b1) or oropharyngeal (b2) neurons. Note, in both cases, the firing in sequence with a more or less overlap between the neuronal activities, the differences in discharge duration between esophageal and oropharyngeal neurons, the lower discharge frequency for the esophageal neurons and the preswallowing activity in some oropharyngeal neurons (1 and 2 in b2). From Jean et al.; A. Jean. J Physiol Paris 1972a;64:227–68; A. Jean. Physiol Rev 2001;81:929–69 with permission. (2) schematic representation of both electromyographic (*red triangles*) and different neuronal discharges when swallowing is initiated by SLN stimulation, in physiological conditions (anesthetized animal in a) and after motor paralysis induced by curare injection (b). Note that during fictive swallowing the sequential activity of medullary swallowing neurons is still recorded, demonstrating the central nature of the burst firing. From A. Jean. J Physiol Paris 1972a;64:227–68; J.P. Kessler and A. Jean. Exp Brain Res 1985;57:256–63 with permission

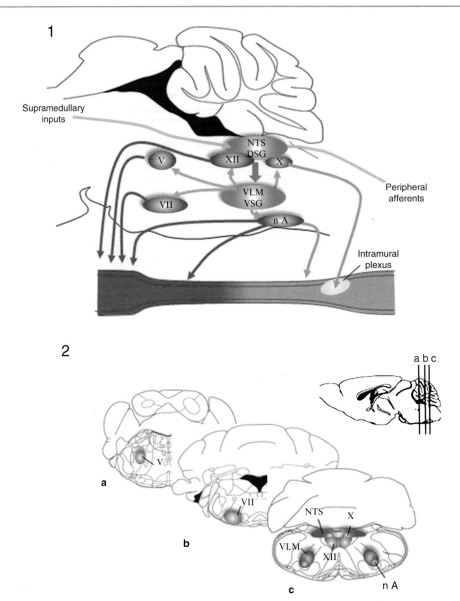

Fig. 6.2 The swallowing central pattern generator (CPG). The CPG is formed by two main groups of neurons (in *blue*) localized in the medulla: a DSG located within the nucleus tractus solitarii (NTS) and the adjacent reticular formation and a VSG located in the ventrolateral medulla adjacent to the nucleus ambiguus (nA). The DSG contains the swallowing generator neurons involved in triggering, shaping, and timing the swallowing motor pattern. The VSG contains switching neurons, driven by DSG neurons, which distribute the swallowing drive to the various pools of motoneurons and preganglionic neurons (in *red*) involved in swallowing. The CPG may be activated either by peripheral afferent inputs, such as those conducted within the superior laryngeal nerve, or supramedullary inputs, such as those coming from the cerebral cortex in the case of a voluntary swallow. In the case of smooth muscle esophagus, the central drive projects on intramural neurons (*yellow*). (1) a sagittal schematic representation with the main connections to date identified between the central neurons. (2) represents, on brainstem coronal sections, the rostro-caudal localization of the central pools of neurons (motoneurons and interneurons) involved in swallowing. (V: trigeminal motor nucleus, VII: facial nucleus, X: dorsal motor nucleus of the vagus nerve, XII: hypoglossal nucleus, nA: nucleus ambiguus). From Jean et al.; A. Jean. Physiol Rev 2001;81:929–69; A. Jean and M. Dallaporta. Electrophysiological characterization of the swallowing pattern generator: role of brainstem. GI Motility Online; 2006 with permission

peristalsis [3, 7]. In addition, brainstem swallowing neurons can be subdivided into motoneurons or preganglionic neurons, which provide innervation to the striated muscles or the esophageal smooth muscle, respectively, and interneurons forming the organizing system of the network that generates the sequential or rhythmic pattern of swallowing.

Motoneurons and Preganglionic Neurons

Swallowing motoneurons and preganglionic neurons are localized within the trigeminal (V), facial (VII), and hypoglossal (XII) motor nuclei, the nucleus ambiguus (IX, X), and the dorsal motor nucleus (DMX) of the vagus (X) and at the cervical spinal level between C1 and C3 (Fig. 6.2) [1, 3, 5, 13, 26]. It is noteworthy, however, that the main motor nuclei involved in the motor activity are the XII motor nucleus and the nucleus ambiguus. Indeed, most, if not all, of the motoneurons within these nuclei participate in swallowing [1, 3, 5]. As regards the innervation of the smooth muscle esophagus, the majority of the preganglionic neurons are located within the X DMX. They consist of two separate groups, one located in the rostral part of the DMX and the other in its caudal portion, providing, respectively, excitatory and inhibitory inputs to the esophageal smooth muscle and lower esophageal sphincter [27, 28].

Electrophysiological studies have shown that the later the neuron becomes active during swallowing, the longer it will fire and the lower its discharge frequency will be [7, 16]. Interestingly, intracellular recordings have shown that esophageal motoneurons, in the nucleus ambiguus, also receive, in addition to an excitatory drive, inhibitory inputs during swallowing [29]. Results also show that a central drive does exist for the smooth muscle esophagus and that in these species both the excitatory and inhibitory vagal pathways are involved in swallowing [4, 30–32].

Interneurons

Extensive microelectrode recordings, first performed on sheep [7, 14, 16, 17, 33] and subsequently on other species such as rat and cat [18, 34, 35], have shown that the swallowing neurons are located in two main brainstem areas (Fig. 6.2):

(1) in the dorsal medulla within the nucleus tractus solitarii (NTS) and in the adjacent reticular formation, where they form the dorsal swallowing group (DSG) and (2) in the ventrolateral medulla, just above the nucleus ambiguus, where they form the ventral swallowing group (VSG).

Within the NTS, oropharyngeal and esophageal neurons exhibit a typical sequential firing pattern which parallels the sequential motor pattern of deglutition [7, 13, 16]. Since these neurons are still active during fictive swallowing elicited in paralyzed animals, their bursting discharge cannot be due to peripheral afferent inputs generated by the muscular contraction, and actually corresponds to a central swallowing activity (Fig. 6.1-2) [7, 18, 36]. Therefore, NTS swallowing neurons are premotor neurons of the network that generates swallowing. It should be noted, however, that, to date, no central recordings have been performed on esophageal interneurons in species with a smooth muscle esophagus.

Interestingly, some oropharyngeal neurons exhibit a particular pattern of firing, starting long before the onset of the motor sequence (Fig. 6.1-1b). This continuous discharge, called "preswallowing activity," decreases and stops quite rapidly when no swallowing occurs, but continues and increases, turning into a bursting swallowing activity, when swallowing is initiated. This pattern of discharge suggests that these neurons are involved in the initiation of swallowing, and it has been postulated that they may constitute the trigger neurons in deglutition [3, 7, 37].

As regards the location of DSG neurons, it has emerged that the oropharyngeal neurons are situated rostro-caudally at the level of the intermediate-subpostremal portion of the NTS, within the medial part of the lateral NTS which overlaps the interstitial, intermediate, ventral, and to some extent, the ventrolateral subdivisions of the nucleus [3, 18, 19, 24, 25]. Interestingly, anatomical results have shown that both laryngeal and pharyngeal afferent fibers project mainly to the interstitial and intermediate subdivisions of the NTS in all the species studied [38, 39]. Moreover, recent experiments, using immunohistochemistry of the immediate early gene c-fos which reveals neurons activated during the motor sequence, also showed that these two subnuclei are mainly concerned with the oropharyngeal phase of swallowing [24, 25]. The DSG esophageal neurons are also situated at the level of the intermediate-subpostremal part of the NTS, between the tractus solitarius and the DMX, a region which probably corresponds to the centralis subdivision of the NTS in the rat [7, 20]. It is noteworthy that anatomical studies have shown that the esophageal afferent fibers end within this specific NTS subdivision, and that the subnucleus centralis is the main NTS subnucleus concerned with the esophageal phase of swallowing [24, 25].

In the ventrolateral medulla above the nucleus ambiguus, there is also a large population of oropharyngeal swallowing interneurons, forming the VSG [7, 13, 18, 40–42]. The burst firing behavior of the VSG neurons is very similar to that of the DSG neurons both in terms of sequential firing pattern and of discharge duration and frequency [7, 18]. VSG neurons are still active during fictive swallowing and, like DSG neurons, they belong to the neuronal network that generates swallowing. The existence of a large population of esophageal interneurons in the ventrolateral medulla is less clear. Bursting discharges in phase with esophageal peristalsis have been recorded in the medullary region above the nucleus ambiguous [16]. However, without any intracellular evidence, it is therefore not possible to clearly distinguish between motoneurons and actual interneurons [3, 16].

Connections Between Brainstem Groups of Swallowing Neurons

Although the detailed connections between functionally identified neurons within the CPG still remain to be mapped, results of electrophysiological and anatomical experiments have provided some information about the connections between the various groups of swallowing neurons [14, 15, 43, 44].

In addition to the swallowing burst, the swallowing-related neurons can exhibit, by stimulating the afferent fibers in the ipsilateral SLN or the vagus nerve, a short-latency synaptic response, in the form of a single spike. The latency of the synaptic response is variable, and clearly longer for swallowing neurons in the VSG (7–12 ms) than for those of the DSG (1–4 ms) [7, 18, 34, 36, 37]. Interestingly, the synaptic response initiated in swallowing neurons by stimulating a specific cortical area which induces swallowing is also shorter in the DSG (5–8 ms) than in the VSG neurons (10–16 ms) [17]. These results suggest that the neurons of the VSG are probably activated via neurons of the DSG. Indeed, regardless of the stimulated afferent pathway, the synaptic response of the VSG neurons is abolished after lesion of the DSG [13, 17]. Although no direct evidence is available, at the single cell level, that a connection of this kind exists between the DSG and VSG, several anatomical experiments have shown connections between the NTS region and the ventrolateral reticular formation surrounding the nucleus ambiguus, where swallowing neurons are located [3, 19, 20].

Electrophysiological experiments have shown that only oropharyngeal neurons within the brainstem VSG are connected to swallowing motoneurons in the V or XII motor nuclei [14, 15]. In addition, it has been established that, within the VSG, the same identified oropharyngeal neuron can project to several motor nuclei involved in swallowing [43, 45]. These electrophysiological data fit in well with those coming from anatomical studies, showing that the ventrolateral medullary region, which contains oropharyngeal neurons, is connected to the homologous contralateral medullary region and to V, VII, X, and XII motor nuclei, all of which are also involved in swallowing [44, 46]. Taken together, these data support the existence, within the swallowing network, of a trisynaptic circuit linking together the afferent fibers, the oropharyngeal neurons in the DSG, the VSG, and the motor nuclei (Fig. 6.2-1) [3]. Interestingly, it has been shown that the excitatory amino acids and their receptors are strongly involved at each synapse of this circuit [21, 23, 47, 48]. Nitrinergic transmission also has been shown to facilitate this circuitry [49].

As regards the esophageal neurons, neuroanatomical studies have shown that NTS neurons, located in the subnucleus centralis, send axon terminals in the rostral compact formation of the nucleus ambiguous where esophageal motoneurons are situated [20, 50]. A connection between the NTS subnucleus centralis and the DMX has also been shown to exist [51]. Glutamatergic and somatostatinergic transmission may be involved in this connection [21, 47, 48, 52, 53]. The NTS subnucleus centralis contains also nitrinergic and catecholaminergic neurons, which may be involved in the control of preganglionic vagal neurons [54–57].

During swallowing, the oropharyngeal and esophageal circuits are functionally linked in order to shape the entire motor sequence. There is no direct evidence available so far about connections between identified swallowing neurons belonging to the oropharyngeal and esophageal circuits. However, anatomical data, obtained with tract tracing techniques, show that such connections may exist between neurons located in the interstitial and centralis subnuclei of the NTS, where oropharyngeal and esophageal DSG neurons are located, respectively [50]. Interestingly, pharmacological experiments suggest that GABAergic and cholinergic transmission may be involved in the coupling of oropharyngeal and esophageal phases of swallowing [58–60]. NTS GABA-ergic neurons are also involved in the inhibition of swallowing following orofacial noxious stimulation [61].

Function of the Various Interneuronal Groups in the CPG

It has been established in several networks involved in fundamental motor behavior that, within a given CPG, all the neurons are not equal since some of them play a preeminent role [3, 62]. As regards swallowing, data already obtained suggest that neurons in the DSG are likely candidates to act as generator neurons in the initiation and organization of the sequential or rhythmic motor pattern [3, 4, 13, 63]. The swallowing network in mammals therefore provides a unique example of neurons located within a primary sensory relay, i.e., the NTS, which nevertheless play the role of generator neurons. Several lines of evidence support the "major" role of NTS neurons in swallowing [7, 18]: (1) NTS neurons exhibit a sequential or rhythmic firing pattern which parallels the motor pattern

[7, 18], (2) their firing remains unaltered after complete motor paralysis showing that it is an actual premotor activity centrally generated [7, 18, 36], (3) most, if not all, of the neurons, having a pre-swallowing activity, are located within the NTS, (4) both electrical and chemical stimulations of the brainstem show that the active points that trigger deglutition are situated only in the region of the solitary complex [8, 18, 21, 23, 48], (5) electrolytic lesion of the NTS results in the abolition, not only of the swallowing elicited by SLN stimulation, but also of that elicited by stimulating the swallowing cortical area [17], (6) fine lesions performed on sheep in the NTS region, which contains esophageal motility-controlling neurons, abolished the esophageal phase of swallowing without affecting the oropharyngeal phase, which indicates that some of the neurons actually involved in the generation of esophageal motility had been destroyed within the NTS [22]. Moreover, recent data, obtained with c-fos immunohistochemistry, confirm the prime role of NTS neurons in both the oropharyngeal and esophageal phases of swallowing [24, 25].

As regards the swallowing neurons in the ventrolateral medulla, the results available are consistent with the view that during swallowing, these neurons are driven by NTS neurons. As neurons of the VSG are connected to motoneurons, one of their functions probably consists in activating the motoneuronal pools during swallowing. The existence of neurons with collaterals to several pools of motoneurons also suggests that they may also participate in the coordination of the motoneuronal pools during swallowing [43–45]. Within the swallowing CPG, the ventral swallowing neurons act therefore very likely as switching neurons that distribute and coordinate the sequential or rhythmic drive generated in the dorsal group to the various pools of motoneurons involved in swallowing [13].

Adaptation of the Neuronal Swallowing Firing by Sensory Inputs

Although the swallowing motor sequence is centrally organized, it may change as a result of peripheral afferent information [64]. Direct evidence that

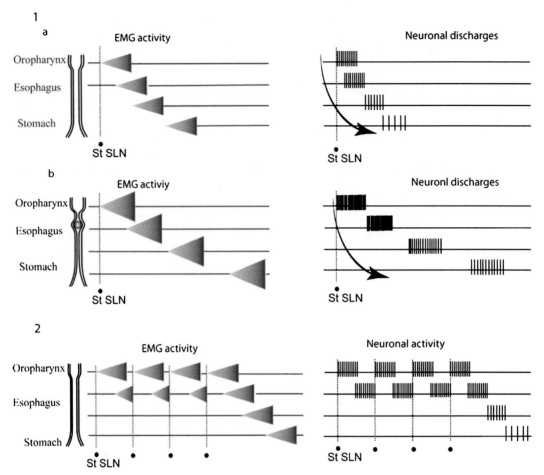

Fig. 6.3 Modulation of the motor and neuronal swallowing patterns. Although centrally generated, the swallowing motor sequence and the sequential firing of neurons may be adapted depending on peripheral afferent inputs and the activation of central inhibitory connections. (1) schematic representation of electromyographic (*red triangles*) and neuronal discharges during swallowing initiated by SLN stimulation, with (b) or without (a) the presence of a bolus within the swallowing tract. The presence of a swallowed bolus induced sensory feedback excitation, resulting in an increase of the EMG activity and the neuronal firing, both in frequency and duration, and a decrease in the velocity of the peristalsis. From A. Jean. J Physiol Paris 1972a;64:227–68; A. Jean. J Autonom Nerv Syst 1984;10:225–33 with permission. (2) schematic representation of rhythmic swallowing patterns, induced by repetitive stimulation of the superior laryngeal nerve (SLN). In these conditions, note that the sequential EMG or neuronal firing is interrupted when a new swallow is initiated and that only the last swallow of the series is complete, revealing the typical rostro-caudal inhibition during swallowing (deglutitive inhibition) which involves central inhibitory connections within the CPG. From A. Jean. J Physiol Paris 1972a;64:227–68; A. Jean. J Autonom Nerv Syst 1984;10:225–33; A. Jean. Physiol Rev 2001;81:929–69 with permission

sensory feedback intervenes during swallowing has also been provided by afferent nerve recordings, suggesting that continuous sensory feedback may influence the neurons of the CPG and thus modulate the central program [65–67]. Data obtained on swallowing neurons have shown that applying continuous stimulation to peripheral receptors by means of an inflated balloon can either induce a permanent activity in the neurons that are active during swallowing, or modify the bursting activity occurring during swallowing [7]. To be efficient, the distention must be performed more and more distally as the neuronal discharge occurs later and later during swallowing. Results showed that the burst firing activity of the neuron increases both in duration and frequency (Fig. 6.3-1); [3, 64]. The activation of peripheral receptors during swallowing therefore results in a decrease in the velocity of the peristalsis, which makes the duration of the whole sequence longer, and the muscular contraction more powerful. Sensory feedback can therefore be assumed to modify the central program, by adjusting the motor outputs depending on the contents of the tract [64].

In addition to the excitatory phenomena, the sensory inputs can also trigger inhibitory effects via central connections. The occurrence of these inhibitory phenomena has been fully confirmed by micro-electrode recordings showing that all esophageal neurons are strongly inhibited during the oropharyngeal stage of swallowing, so-called deglutitive inhibition, or during a pharyngeal distention which stimulated the peripheral receptors [7, 64, 68]. In addition, the activity of the esophageal neurons which fire during the contraction of the lower esophagus is also inhibited during an esophageal distention which stimulates receptors of the upper esophagus. The strength of the inhibition is variable depending on the size of the inflated balloon (degree of esophageal distension) [64]. These data indicate that the swallowing neurons controlling the distal regions of the swallowing tract are inhibited when neurons controlling the more proximal regions are excited. They support the idea that there may exist a rostro-caudal inhibition within the swallowing network, as suggested by the blockade of the esophageal peristalsis which occurs during rhythmic swallowing (Fig. 6.3-2); [3].

In addition to swallowing, recent data also show that sensory inputs from various oropharyngeal and esophageal receptors can mediate different types of reflexes, particularly in the esophagus, as well as motor activities such as belching, emesis, nausea, etc., demonstrating the role of sensory inputs not only on the central programming but also as potential therapeutic targets [69, 70].

Areas of Possible Future Research

What Are the Neural Mechanisms of Pattern Generation? (Network and Cellular Properties)

The central mechanisms that generate the bursting activity of swallowing neurons and their sequential or rhythmic firing behavior are still unknown.

All the results already obtained indicate, however, that, among the various groups of swallowing neurons, local mechanisms within the DSG, involving the connectivity and the synaptic interactions between NTS neurons, and their intrinsic properties, play a key role in pattern generation [3, 62, 71].

As regards the network organization, the swallowing CPG can be viewed as a linear-like chain of neurons based on the rostro-caudal anatomy of the swallowing tract. Since neurons of the NTS fire sequentially during swallowing, each neuron or group of neurons in this chain may control, through excitatory and inhibitory connections, more and more distal regions of the esophagus, and be responsible for the successive firing behavior via increasingly numerous polysynaptic connections (Fig. 6.4-1) [3, 64]. Several data suggest the inhibitory mechanisms may not only be responsible for delaying the onset of neuronal firing, but they may also contribute directly to the sequential excitation of the neurons via mechanisms such as disinhibition or post-inhibitory rebounds [3, 7]. Interestingly, disinhibition has been shown to exist within the swallowing network since blockade of GABA inhibitory transmission resulted in rhythmic oropharyngeal or esophageal motor events [60, 72–74].

Most of the data on the intrinsic properties of neurons liable to be involved in swallowing have been obtained in studies on brainstem slices and the link between the endogenous properties of neurons studied under these in vitro conditions and their possible role in swallowing pattern generation is far from being elucidated. Interestingly, within the peri-interstitial region of the NTS where swallowing-related neurons are situated, NTS neurons were found to have several endogenous properties, some of which seem to be relevant to swallowing pattern generation, such as delayed excitation, post-inhibitory rebound, and conditional pacemaker-like properties [75–77].

To further elucidate the intrinsic mechanisms underlying swallowing pattern generation, it will be useful to perform studies on other experimental models such as the isolated brainstem and the working heart–brainstem preparations or to initiate computational approaches and modeling natural

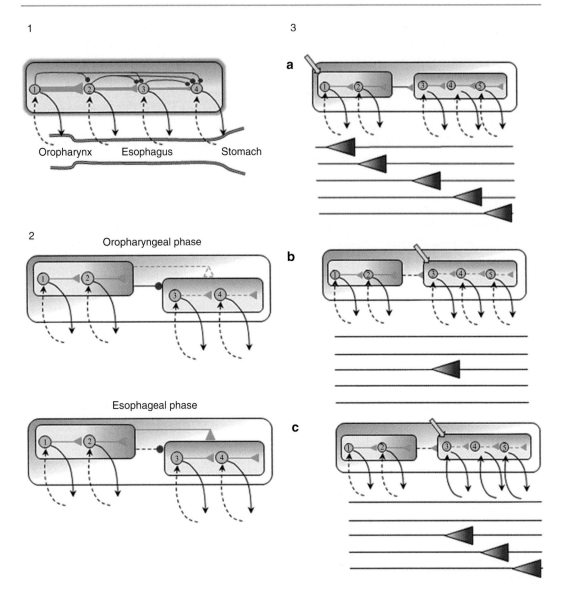

Fig. 6.4 Possible mechanisms of central pattern generation (1) the swallowing network can be viewed as a chain of neurons with excitatory (*green lines and triangles*) and inhibitory (*red lines and dots*) connections, and sensory feedback (*broken lines*). The excitatory inputs are less powerful along the chain, in contrast to the inhibitory influences, resulting in long periods of inhibition of neurons controlling more distal parts of the tract. (2) the CPG may be subdivided into an oropharyngeal and an esophageal networks. The esophageal net is first inhibited by the oropharyngeal net (*red dot*). This primary inhibition is followed by an excitatory action (*green triangle*), rendering possible the successive activation of esophageal neurons. From A. Jean and M. Dallaporta. Electrophysiological characterization of the swallowing pattern generator: role of brainstem. GI Motility Online; 2006 with permission. (3) when initiated (*yellow arrow*) at the beginning (oropharyngeal phase followed by an esophageal phase, i.e., primary peristalsis) the sequence can be generated without sensory feedback (a, *broken lines*). However, when initiated along the neuronal chain (i.e., secondary peristalsis), in general the sequence aborts without sensory feedback (b, *broken lines*) whereas it can progress with sensory feedback (c, *black lines*)

processes with artificial networks [78]. It will also be necessary to identify at the cellular level the action of neurotransmitters and neuromodulators and the types of receptors involved. This would provide valuable information about the possible sites of action for therapeutic agents.

Is There One Central Pattern Generator or Two Subnetworks for the Oropharyngeal and the Esophageal Phases of Swallowing?

Although swallowing is considered as a single patterned motor sequence, results indicate that unlike the all or none oropharyngeal sequence, the esophageal phase may show some lability suggesting that the central program controlling this phase may be less robust than that responsible for the oropharyngeal phase [2, 3, 9, 24, 79]. This difference is most striking in the case of secondary peristalsis of the esophagus, since peripheral afferent feedback has been shown to be essential for the propagation of the peristaltic wave [3, 9, 24, 79, 80]. These data suggest that the swallowing CPG can be subdivided into two subnetworks, an oropharyngeal and an esophageal net of neurons, each mediating the patterning of the respective phase of deglutition (Fig. 6.4-2). But they also suggest that the esophageal net is likely to have less robust central mechanisms and be more dependent on afferent inputs. This is puzzling from the patterning point of view. Indeed, the sole difference between primary and secondary peristalsis is that the latter lacks an oropharyngeal phase, and consequently is not accompanied by any oropharyngeal network activity. Therefore, the oropharyngeal net may serve as an intrinsic modulatory system, a mechanism which seems to play an important role in several CPGs [4, 81]. When the oropharyngeal net is activated, the esophageal net can program the peristaltic wave, whereas when it is inactive, as in the case of secondary peristalsis, the program requires peripheral influences (Fig. 6.4-2, 6.4-3). It may be supposed that the strong inhibition generated during the oropharyngeal stage of swallowing may be followed by a delayed excitation of the esophageal network, resulting in the sequential discharge of the neurons. Field potential recordings support such a hypothesis, since they show that the strong inhibition of esophageal neurons during the oropharyngeal phase is followed by a wave of excitation [3]. Interestingly, pharmacological data suggest that, within the DSG, GABA and acetylcholine might be involved in the fast inhibitory and the delayed excitatory actions,

respectively [3, 58–60]. Whatever the case, the linking between the oropharyngeal and esophageal phases of swallowing needs further studies. In addition, an important question which remains to be answered is whether the central nervous system of the species with a smooth muscle esophagus may include a network of neurons which is similar to that of the species with a striated esophagus, and if so, how this network functions. This issue is of particular relevance to our better understanding of the human esophagus the distal two-thirds of which is composed of smooth muscle.

What Is the Nature of the Swallowing CPG: Fixed or Flexible?

Swallowing, in particular its oropharyngeal stage, is a stereotyped motor behavior and the swallowing CPG has been classically viewed as a dedicated circuit, i.e., as a specific network of neurons which is hardwired so as to produce a sequence of excitation and inhibition which is always the same (Fig. 6.5-1) [1, 3, 5]. However, this view is now challenged in the light of numerous data obtained mainly on the central nervous system of invertebrates [82, 83]. In addition to being a classical dedicated network, most of the CPGs seem in fact to be either reorganizing or distributed circuits, and a single neural circuit can combine features typical of each of these different architectures, resulting in considerable functional plasticity. This is a particularly relevant point in the case of the swallowing CPG. The swallowing CPG is not an automatic, continuously functioning CPG, and the question arises as to whether the swallowing neurons are completely inactive when no swallowing occurs, or whether these neurons may have other functions. In invertebrates, it has been observed that swallowing depends on a pattern generator which is temporarily formed, preparatory to the production of the motor activity [84]. That is to say that when a given stimulus is delivered, a pool of appropriate neurons is activated and forms the swallowing CPG, whereas when no swallowing activity is required, these neurons are involved in other tasks (Fig. 6.5-2, 6.5-3).

Although there is no direct evidence in mammals that the swallowing CPG is flexible, recent

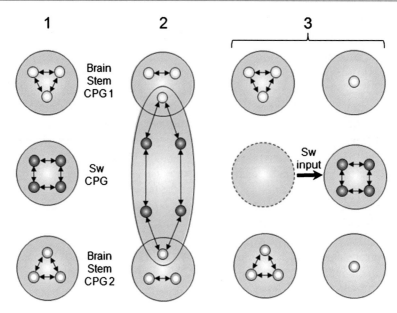

Fig. 6.5 Nature of the swallowing CPG (1) the swallowing CPG (Sw CPG) may be a dedicated circuit with neurons subserving only this function. The Sw CPG has connections with other CPGs (brainstem CPG 1, 2,…), such as those involved in respiration, mastication, etc.…, to ensure functional interactions under physiological conditions. (2) the swallowing CPG may be a reorganizing circuit consisting of pools of flexible neurons, i.e., neurons which can function in several CPGs involved in the organization of various kinds of motor behaviors. (3) alternatively, it is possible that the Sw CPG may be formed temporarily by neurons belonging previously to other CPGs. Following swallowing input, these neurons contribute to the newly formed swallowing CPG. From A. Jean and M. Dallaporta. Electrophysiological characterization of the swallowing pattern generator: role of brainstem. GI Motility Online; 2006 with permission

results have shown that, within the network, some neurons may participate in activities other than swallowing-related ones. It has been established that not only motoneurons but also interneurons can be involved in at least two different tasks, such as swallowing and respiration, swallowing and mastication, or swallowing and vocalization [36, 40–42, 45, 85, 86]. It can therefore be postulated that at least some of the components of the swallowing network are not dedicated to swallowing alone, but can also serve some purpose in other central networks or that, like in invertebrates, the swallowing CPG is formed temporarily [4]. In addition to neuroplasticity of supramedullary regions involved in swallowing, such as the cerebral cortex [87], the existence of some degree of plasticity within the CPG provides interesting capabilities in the whole swallowing circuitry for ability after injury and rehabilitation capabilities.

It seems likely, for future prospects, that by focusing research on populations of neurons with multiple recordings, with electrophysiological and/or optical methods, rather than single neuron recordings and by using brain imaging techniques, it will be possible to gain new insights into how the neurons of the mammalian CPGs can subserve multiple functions [88]. In addition, although swallowing is a vital function, some data have suggested that its underlying mechanisms may be not fixed at birth. Therefore, studies on the post-natal development of brainstem control of swallowing would be of particular interest to identify how the central nervous system operates to establish mature networks devoted to fundamental activities in the adult brain [89–91].

What Are the Mechanisms of Synchronization Between the Two Swallowing Hemi-CPGs?

It is noteworthy that the swallowing CPG consists of two hemi-CPGs, each located on one side of the medulla, which have to be tightly synchronized to organize the coordinated contraction of the bilateral muscles of the oropharyngeal region and of the esophagus [1, 3, 22, 92]. Microelectrode

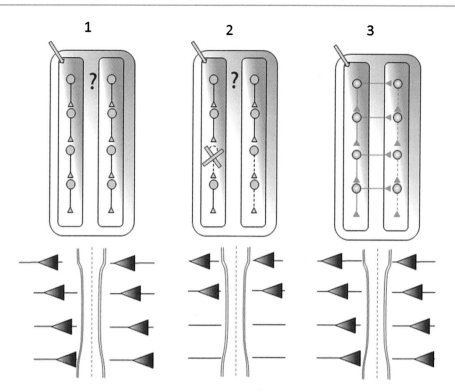

Fig. 6.6 Possible mechanisms of synchronization between the two hemi-CPGs. Although hypothetical, the mechanisms of synchronization are suggested by stimulating and lesions experiments. By contrast to physiological conditions, in experimental conditions, swallowing is generally initiated by stimulating only one SLN (*yellow arrow*) inducing a typical motor sequence bilaterally (1). Under the same experimental paradigm, when central lesions have been performed within the esophageal network in the ipsilateral CPG (*yellow cross*), it was surprising to observe that the motor sequence is blocked bilaterally (2), whereas the contralateral CPG is not lesioned and can initiate a complete swallowing sequence when activated by contralateral inputs (not represented). Therefore, it is suggested that, when swallowing is ipsilaterally initiated, it is within the ipsilateral CPG that the sequence is organized and generated, and that the synchronization between the two hemi-CPGs depends on ipsilateral inputs transferred "step by step" to the contralateral CPG which cannot organize and secure the sequence without these inputs (3). From A. Jean. J Physiol Paris 1972b;64:507–16 with permission

recordings have shown that in each case, a particular swallowing neuron produces a swallowing bursting discharge in response to stimulation of the ipsilateral as well as to that of the contralateral afferent fibers, regardless of the type of swallowing neuron tested. This indicates that at each step of the network operation, the entire population of neurons within the DSG, the VSG, or the motoneuronal pools is active.

However, the mechanisms underlying the synchronization of the two hemi-CPGs are not known, and this matter has not been well documented yet. It is likely that the peripheral afferent fibers do not play a crucial role, since lesion experiments have shown that splitting the medulla caudal to the obex, which interrupts the vagal afferent fibers crossing the midline through the solitary tract, does not affect swallowing [1, 92]. In addition, electrophysiological data show that the swallowing neurons receive a direct input (synaptic response) only via the ipsilateral afferent fibers.

Connections between central neurons, situated on each side of the brainstem, probably play a key role in the coordination of the two hemi-CPGs. Anatomical connections mediated by fibers crossing the midline have been found to exist between the two medullary regions where swallowing neurons are located, i.e., the DSG and VSG [44]. Interestingly, the results of unilateral lesion experiments performed on the NTS esophageal neuronal population have shown that upon stimulating the ipsilateral SLN, only an oropharyngeal stage of swallowing is elicited, whereas upon stimulating the contralateral nerve, a complete process of deglutition including the esophageal stage is initiated, indicating that swallowing NTS neurons play a crucial role in these synchronization processes [22]. These results suggest, in addition, that under ipsilateral stimulation conditions, the swallowing motor sequence is mainly generated in the ipsilateral hemi-CPG and that this CPG transfers the swallowing premotor signal to the contralateral CPG (Fig. 6.6) [7, 22, 37]. This may account in part for clinical observations in the context of dysphagia resulting from brain stem stroke in humans. For example, despite the existence of bilateral CPGs, patients suffering unilateral lateral medullary infarction (e.g., Wallenberg's syndrome) experience a markedly deranged or absent pharyngeal swallow [93–96]. Whatever the case, further experiments including selective lesion studies and tracing studies in animals are required to identify the pathways connecting left and right medullary CPG, respectively, and to elucidate the mechanisms underlying the synchronization of the two hemi-CPGs which is essential for the coordination of the muscular contraction, in order to better understand the functional consequences of stroke.

What About the Supramedullary Influences on Brainstem Swallowing Neurons?

The fact that an individual can swallow voluntarily shows that the medullary swallowing network can be activated by inputs from the cerebral cortex [1, 5, 17, 94, 97, 98]. In addition, several clinical reports have indicated that various cortical dysfunctions may result in dysphagia, swallowing impairments, or affect esophageal peristalsis [93–95]. These observations point out the involvement of supramedullary influences, since the peripheral afferent pathway and the CPG, which is localized in the caudal brainstem, seem to remain unaltered in these patients. Moreover, the numerous results obtained with classical stimulation experiments and new approaches such as cortical evoked potentials, transcranial magnetic stimulations, magnetoencephalographic recordings, and functional brain

imaging techniques, performed in animals and humans, show that several supramedullary structures may be responsible for various effects on swallowing, such as initiating the motor activity, or modulating the swallowing reflex [98–105]. However, most of the data available are difficult to interpret, since it is generally not a "pure" swallowing motor activity which is observed under these conditions, but more complex feeding behaviors, i.e., mastication and swallowing, or lapping, mastication and swallowing, or licking and swallowing, etc. In addition, it is difficult to identify among these effects those which are due to the afferent feedback and to distinguish between centrally organized movements and motor activities involving feedback phenomena.

In fact, very few studies have dealt with these central influences on the neurons of the CPG. As far as the supramedullary influences on swallowing and their action on brainstem neurons are concerned, all the results available so far have been obtained in studies on the cortical influences on swallowing [106]. Results indicate that most of the oropharyngeal neurons in the DSG were cortically activated with a shorter latency than those in the VSG which responded in smaller numbers [17]. Only the esophageal neurons in the DSG that fired during the contraction of the upper esophagus also responded to cortical stimulation [3, 17]. None of the esophageal neurons in the DSG, firing later during the contraction of the lower esophagus, or the esophageal neurons in the VSG were activated by cortical stimulation. Although a direct pathway from the cortex to motoneuronal pools involved in swallowing has been mapped, using tracing techniques, these results indicate that the cortical input to identified swallowing neurons mainly focuses on swallowing neurons in the DSG. The DSG neurons therefore receive convergent information from both cortical and peripheral inputs that trigger swallowing [3, 17]. Since only oropharyngeal and a few esophageal neurons respond to cortical stimulation, the cortical swallowing area may serve mainly to trigger deglutition and control the beginning of the motor sequence, after which the sequence might be carried out without any further cortical control.

In sheep, a population of sensory relay neurons firing in phase with the oropharyngeal stage of swallowing has been found to exist more rostrally in the pons [107, 108]. These neurons are thought to be involved in providing information from the oropharyngeal receptors to the higher nervous centers, in particular the cortical area [108]. Therefore, cortical neurons may belong to a ponto-cortico-medullary loop, so that upon receiving sensory information, they might control the activity of the CPG swallowing neurons as they fire successively, just as peripheral afferent fibers do [3]. It has been shown that cortical neurons in the swallowing cortical area of sheep are activated or inhibited during swallowing [109]. More recent findings on monkeys indicate that cortical areas associated with feeding behavior are involved in swallowing [94, 110]. However, changes in the firing activity of cortical neurons during swallowing have been shown to depend on sensory feedback, since they are abolished in paralyzed animals.

In any case, the supramedullary influences on swallowing, which have been only sparsely documented so far, require more thorough investigation. In particular, in the light of the numerous forebrain structures identified, with the functional brain imaging techniques, to be involved in swallowing. This would make it possible to specify the neuronal pathways involved and the role of these central influences in several pathological situations. Moreover, clinical observations, such as those following recovery after unilateral cortical stroke, suggest that cortical inputs to the medullary CPG exert very probably more complex modulatory influences than a simple triggering action and further experiments are needed to explore these possible modulatory effects [87, 102].

From Pattern Generation to Food Intake Behavior

Swallowing is an important motor component of feeding behavior since it is the last motor event before the entry of food into the digestive tract, therefore constituting the all or none motor sequence further allowing digestion, absorption, and nutrition.

The swallowing premotor neurons of the NTS are located in the caudal brainstem within the so-called dorsal vagal complex (DVC), which comprises, in addition to the NTS, two other interconnected nuclei: the area postrema, a neurohemal organ lining the fourth ventricle and the dorsal vagal motor nucleus of the vagus nerve containing cell bodies of efferent preganglionic vagal neurons [111, 112]. A growing body of evidence now supports the view that food intake control is not orchestrated by the hypothalamus, but is more widely distributed within the central nervous system, including the DVC which is a crucial integrator of satiety and adiposity signals [113–115]. The role of the DVC in the control of food intake put forward therefore the question to know whether or not the food intake signaling pathways can influence swallowing.

Recent results obtained in rats have shown that the adiposity signal, leptin, microinjected at physiological doses, within the DVC, inhibits the rhythmic swallowing elicited by SLN stimulation (Fig. 6.7) [116]. Interestingly, the inhibitory effect of leptin was not observed in leptin receptor-deficient Zucker rats. Whether this action on swallowing is part of the mechanisms through which leptin exerts its anorexigenic effect remains unclear, but these results clearly show that leptin inhibits ingestion by acting not only on the afferent and integrative components of the feeding networks but also on the premotor and motor networks of ingestive behavior.

Several lines of evidence have also shown that brain-derived neurotrophic factor (BDNF) and its high affinity receptor, tropomyosin-related kinase receptor type B (TrkB), constitutes an anorexigenic signaling pathway. Interestingly, recent results have provided evidence for an action of BDNF within the DVC where it may constitute a common downstream effector of the adiposity and satiety signals, leptin and CCK, and where it has been shown to act downstream the melanocortinergic signaling pathway [117–119]. In this connection, it has been shown that BDNF may also modulate swallowing in the DVC (Fig. 6.7) [72]. In anesthetized adult rats BDNF microinjections in the swallowing network within the DVC induce a rapid, transient, and dose-dependent inhibition

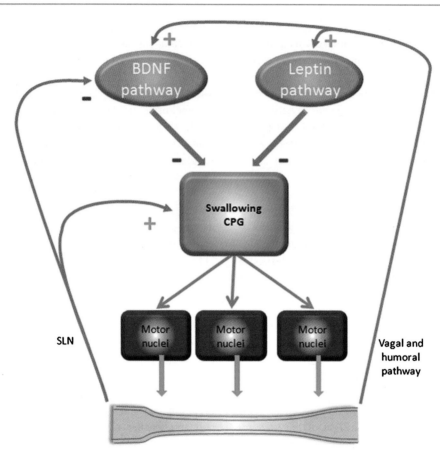

Fig. 6.7 Swallowing pattern generator and food intake. Recent results have shown inhibitory effects of anorexigenic signals, such as leptin and BDNF, on the swallowing CPG, revealing a direct action of these signals on the motor component of the ingestive behavior. Interestingly, it has been shown, in the case of BDNF signaling, that this anorexigenic pathway which can be activated either by hormonal pathway (adiposity signaling) or neural pathway (satiety reflex induced by sensory inputs coming from lower digestive tract) is inhibited by sensory inputs coming from the upper digestive tract, such as those running in the superior laryngeal nerve. Therefore, food intake signaling, such as BDNF, can modulate in the appropriate way the activity of the swallowing CPG. From B. Bariohay et al. Endocrinology 2005;146:5612–20; B. Bariohay et al. Am J Physiol Regul Integr Comp 2008;295:R1050–9 with permission

of the rhythmic swallowing initiated by repetitive SLN stimulation. The BDNF inhibitory effect is mediated via TrkB activation since it no longer occurs when TrkB receptors are antagonized by K-252a. In addition, the BDNF effects on swallowing are potentiated by GABA, since subthreshold doses of BDNF also inhibit swallowing when coinjected with subthreshold doses of GABA, suggesting a synergistic interaction between these two signaling substances. Interestingly, BDNF does not inhibit swallowing when coinjected with bicuculline, a GABA A receptor antagonist, thereby showing that GABAergic neurotransmission is an important downstream effector through

which BDNF inhibits swallowing. Therefore, the anorexigenic action of BDNF within the DVC may result from BDNF acting on the afferent and/ or integrative components of the feeding behavior networks, and it may also result from an action on the motor component of these networks.

In addition, it has been shown that the same SLN stimulation paradigm which induces rhythmic swallowing also induces a reduction in endogenous BDNF protein content within the DVC. These results suggest that prolonged stimulation of SLN could indeed favor food intake by reducing a BDNF-dependent anorexigenic tone. Within the caudal brainstem, BDNF protein content is both upregulated by adiposity and satiety signals and downregulated by the stimulation of SLN afferent fibers innervating the upper gastrointestinal tract. Therefore, within the DVC, BDNF can be considered as a common integrator for both positive and negative feedbacks triggered by the presence of food in the alimentary canal, as well as for adiposity signals, which places this anorexigenic factor in a key position for meal size control (Fig. 6.7) [72, 120].

Conclusion

Swallowing depends on a CPG located in the medulla oblongata, which involves several brainstem motor nuclei (V, VII, IX, X, XII) and two main groups of interneurons: a DSG in the NTS and a VSG located in the ventrolateral medulla above the nucleus ambiguus. Within the CPG, neurons in the DSG play the leading role in generating the swallowing pattern, while neurons in the VSG act as switching neurons, distributing the swallowing drive to the various motoneuronal pools. It is quite remarkable that a CPG for a fundamental motor activity should be located within a primary sensory nucleus, namely the NTS. As in the case of other CPGs, the functioning of the central network can be influenced by both peripheral and central inputs.

Little is known so far about the mechanisms at work in the CPG. The sequential burst firing of the swallowing neurons probably depends on the pattern of intrinsic connections within the swallowing network. Central inhibitory connections, in particular, are supposed to play a major role in the neuronal sequential firing. Intrinsic cellular properties, in particular those of NTS neurons, probably also contribute to determine the shaping and timing of the swallowing motor pattern. Interestingly, recent data indicate (1) that the swallowing CPG may show some degree of flexibility, suggesting that at least some of the swallowing neurons may belong to pools of neurons that are common to several brain stem CPGs, (2) that anorexigenic signaling pathways do exert modulatory influences on the brainstem CPG.

Several questions remain to be answered regarding the brain stem control of swallowing.

Although they are technically difficult, electrophysiological studies dealing with clearly identified swallowing neurons will be necessary to obtain significant insights into (1) the mechanisms underlying swallowing pattern generation, (2) the synchronization between the two hemi-CPGs, which has received little attention but is essential for the coordination of the muscular contraction, (3) the linking between the oropharyngeal and esophageal phases of swallowing, (4) the interplay between central and intrinsic networks in the case of the esophageal smooth muscle. The supramedullary influences on swallowing, which have been only sparsely documented so far, also require more thorough investigation, in particular in the light of the numerous forebrain structures identified, with the functional brain imaging techniques, to be involved in swallowing in order to specify the neuronal pathways involved and their different modulatory effects on the brainstem network.

Key Points

- Swallowing is a complex motor activity that is organized by a network of swallowing-related neurons which form the central swallowing pattern generator located in the medulla oblongata.
- Microelectrode recordings have shown that the swallowing network includes two main groups of interneurons: (1) a DSG in the NTS of the dorsomedial medulla and (2) a VSG, located in the ventrolateral medulla.
- The DSG contains the generator neurons involved in triggering, shaping, and timing the sequential or rhythmic swallowing pattern, and the VSG contains switching neurons that distribute the swallowing drive to the various pools of motoneurons involved in the motor activity.
- The location of the DSG within the NTS which is the primary sensory relay is convenient for peripheral input to shape the output of the network so that the swallowing movements correspond to the swallowed bolus.
- The sequential firing of the swallowing neurons depends on the neuronal circuitry, as well

as on the cellular properties of neurons. Within the network, inhibitory connections are thought to play a crucial role in the sequential firing of the neurons.

- VSG forms premotor neurons for oral and pharyngeal motor neurons, but esophageal premotor neurons may be located within the DSG. Both DSG and VSG receive cortical input that regulates their output.
- Recent studies suggest that there is considerable plasticity in the activity of the swallowing network and that the swallowing CPG activity is modulated by signaling pathways involved in the central control of food intake behavior.

References

1. Doty RW. Neural organization of deglutition. In: Code CF, editor. Handbook of physiology alimentary canal, vol. IV. Washington, DC: American Physiological Society; 1968. p. 1861–902.
2. Goyal RJ, Cobb BW. Motility of the pharynx, esophagus and esophageal sphincters. In: Johnson LR, editor. Physiology of the gastrointestinal tract. New York: Raven; 1981. p. 359–91.
3. Jean A. Brain stem control of swallowing: neuronal network and cellular mechanisms. Physiol Rev. 2001;81:929–69.
4. Jean A, Dallaporta M. Electrophysiological characterization of the swallowing pattern generator: Role of brainstem. In: Goyal R, Shaker R, editors. GI Motility Online. 2006, doi:10.1038/gimo74.
5. Miller AJ. Deglutition. Physiol Rev. 1982;62:129–84.
6. Doty RW. Influence of stimulus pattern on reflex deglutition. Am J Physiol. 1951;166:142–58.
7. Jean A. Localisation et activité des neurones déglutiteurs bulbaires. J Physiol Paris. 1972;64:227–68.
8. Miller AJ. Characteristics of the swallowing reflex induced by peripheral nerve and brain stem stimulation. Exp Neurol. 1972;34:210–22.
9. Roman C, Gonella J. Extrinsic control of digestive tract motility. In: Johnson LR, editor. Physiology of the gastrointestinal tract. 2nd ed. New York: Raven; 1987. p. 507–53.
10. Lang IM. Upper esophageal sphincter. In: Goyal R and Shaker R, editors. GI motility Online. 2006, 10.1038/gimo12.
11. Diamant NE. Physiology of esophageal motor function. In: Ongang A, editor. Gastroenterology clinics of North America, Motility disorders, vol. 18. Philadelphia: WB Saunders; 1989. p. 179–94.
12. Meltzer SJ. On the causes of the orderly progress of the peristaltic movements in the oesophagus. Am J Physiol. 1899;2:266–72.

13. Jean A. Brainstem control of swallowing: localization and organization of the central pattern generator for swallowing. In: Taylor A, editor. Neurophysiology of the jaws and teeth. London: Macmillan; 1990. p. 294–321.
14. Amri M, Car A, Jean A. Medullary control of the pontine swallowing neurones in sheep. Exp Brain Res. 1984;55:105–10.
15. Amri M, Car A. Projections from the medullary swallowing center to the hypoglossal motor nucleus: a neuroanatomical and electrophysiological study in sheep. Brain Res. 1988;441:119–26.
16. Jean A. Localisation et activité des motoneurones oesophagiens chez le mouton Etude par microélectrodes. J Physiol Paris. 1978;74:737–42.
17. Jean A, Car A. Inputs to the swallowing medullary neurons from the peripheral afferent fibers and the swallowing cortical area. Brain Res. 1979;178:567–72.
18. Kessler JP, Jean A. Identification of the medullary swallowing regions in the rat. Exp Brain Res. 1985;57:256–63.
19. Bao X, Wiedner EB, Altschuler SM. Transsynaptic localization of pharyngeal premotor neurons in rat. Brain Res. 1995;696:246–9.
20. Barrett RT, Bao X, Miselis RR, Altschuler SM. Brainstem localization of rodent esophageal premotor neurons revealed by transneuronal passage of pseudo-rabies virus. Gastroenterology. 1994;107:728–37.
21. Hashim MA, Bieger D. Excitatory amino acid receptor-mediated activation of solitarial deglutitive loci. Neuropharmacology. 1989;28:913–21.
22. Jean A. Effet de lésions localisées du bulbe rachidien sur le stade oesophagien de la déglutition. J Physiol Paris. 1972;64:507–16.
23. Kessler JP, Cherkaoui N, Catalin D, Jean A. Swallowing responses induced by microinjections of glutamate and glutamate agonists into the nucleus tractus solitarius of ketamine-anaesthetized rats. Exp Brain Res. 1990;83:151–8.
24. Lang IM, Dean C, Medda BK, Aslam M, Shaker R. Differential activation of medullary vagal nuclei during different phases of swallowing in the cat. Brain Res. 2004;1014:145–63.
25. Sang Q, Goyal RK. Swallowing reflex and brain stem neurons activated by superior laryngeal nerve stimulation in the mouse. Am J Physiol Gastrointest Liver Physiol. 2001;280:G191–200.
26. Lang IM. Brainstem control of the phases of swallowing. Dysphagia. 2009;24:333–48.
27. Collman PI, Tremblay L, Diamant NE. The central vagal efferent supply to the esophagus and lower esophageal sphincter of the cat. Gastroenterology. 1993;104:1430–8.
28. Rossiter CD, Norman WP, Jain M, Hornby PJ, Benjamin S, Gillis RA. Control of lower esophageal sphincter pressure by two sites in dorsal motor nucleus of the vagus. Am J Physiol Gastrointest Liver Physiol. 1990;259:G899–906.
29. Zoungrana OR, Amri M, Car A, Roman C. Intracellular activity of motoneurons of the rostral

nucleus ambiguous during swallowing in sheep. J Neurophysiol. 1997;77:909–22.

30. Gidda JS, Goyal RK. Swallow-evoked action potentials in vagal preganglionic efferents. J Neurophysiol. 1984;52:1169–80.

31. Miolan JP, Roman C. Activité des fibres vagales efférentes destinées à la musculature lisse du cardia du chien. J Physiol Paris. 1978;74:709–23.

32. Roman C, Tieffenbach L. Enregistrement de l'activité unitaire des fibres motrices vagales destinées à l'oesophage du Babouin. J Physiol Paris. 1972;64: 479–506.

33. Car A, Amri M. Activity of neurons located in the region of the hypoglossal motor nucleus during swallowing in sheep. Exp Brain Res. 1987;69:175–82.

34. Ootani S, Umezaki T, Shin T, Murata Y. Convergence of afferents from the SLN and GPN in cat medullary swallowing neurons. Brain Res Bull. 1995;37:397–404.

35. Sumi T. Neuronal mechanisms in swallowing. Pflugers Arch. 1964;278:467–77.

36. Saito Y, Ezure K, Tanaka I. Swallowing-related activities of respiratory and non-respiratory neurons in the nucleus of solitary tract in the rat. J Physiol London. 2002;540:1047–60.

37. Ciampini G, Jean A. Rôle des afférences glossopharyngiennes et trigéminales dans le déclenchement et le déroulement de la déglutition I Afférences glossopharyngiennes. J Physiol Paris. 1980;76:49–60.

38. Altschuler SM, Bao X, Bieger D, Hopkins DA, Miselis RR. Viscerotopic representation of the upper alimentary tract in the rat: sensory ganglia and nuclei of the solitary and spinal trigeminal tracts. J Comp Neurol. 1989;283:248–68.

39. Mrini A, Jean A. Synaptic organization of the interstitial subdivision of the nucleus tractus solitarii and of its laryngeal afferents in the rat. J Comp Neurol. 1995;355:221–36.

40. Chiao GZ, Larson CR, Yajima Y, Ko P, Kahrilas PJ. Neuronal activity in nucleus ambiguus during deglutition and vocalization in conscious monkeys. Exp Brain Res. 1994;100:29–38.

41. Oku Y, Tanaka I, Ezure K. Activity of bulbar respiratory neurons during fictive coughing and swallowing in the decerebrate cat. J Physiol London. 1994;480: 309–24.

42. Saito Y, Ezure K, Tanaka I. Activity of neurons in ventrolateral respiratory groups during swallowing in decerebrate rats. Brain Dev. 2003;25:338–45.

43. Amri M, Car A, Roman C. Axonal branching of medullary swallowing neurons projecting on the trigeminal and hypoglossal motor nuclei: demonstration by electrophysiological and fluorescent double labeling techniques. Exp Brain Res. 1990;81:384–90.

44. Jean A, Amri M, Calas A. Connections between the ventral medullary swallowing area and the trigeminal motor nucleus of the sheep studied by tracing techniques. J Autonom Nerv Syst. 1983;7:87–96.

45. Ezure K, Oku Y, Tanaka I. Location and axonal projection of one type of swallowing interneurons in cat medulla. Brain Res. 1993;632:216–24.

46. Cunningham Jr ET, Sawchenko PE. Dorsal medullary pathways subserving oromotor reflexes in the rat: implications for the central neural control of swallowing. J Comp Neurol. 2000;417: 448–66.

47. Kessler JP. Involvement of excitatory amino acids in the activity of swallowing-related neurons of the ventro-lateral medulla. Brain Res. 1993;603:353–7.

48. Kessler JP, Jean A. Evidence that activation of N-methyl-D-aspartate (NMDA) and non-NMDA receptors within the nucleus tractus solitarii triggers swallowing. Eur J Pharmacol. 1991;201:59–67.

49. Beyak MJ, Xue S, Collman PI, Valdez DT, Diamant NE. Central nervous system nitric oxide induces oropharyngeal swallowing and esophageal peristalsis in the cat. Gastroenterology. 2000;119:377–85.

50. Broussard DL, Lynn RB, Wiedner EB, Altschuler SM. Solitarial premotor neuron projections to the rat esophagus and pharynx: implications for control of swallowing. Gastroenterology. 1998;114:1268–75.

51. Rogers RC, Hermann GE, Travagli RA. Brainstem pathways responsible for oesophageal control of gastric motility and tone in the rat. J Physiol London. 1999;514:369–83.

52. Broussard DL, Bao X, Altschuler SM. Somatostatin immunoreactivity in esophageal premotor neurons of the rat. Neurosci Lett. 1998;250:201–4.

53. Cunningham Jr ET, Sawchenko PE. A circumscribed projection from the nucleus of the solitary tract to the nucleus ambiguus in the rat: anatomical evidence for somatostatin-28-immunoreactive interneurons subserving reflex control of oesophageal motility. J Neurosci. 1989;9:1668–82.

54. Beyak MJ, Collman PI, Xue S, Valdez DT, Diamant NE. Release of nitric oxide in the central nervous system mediates tonic and phasic contraction of the cat lower oesophageal sphincter. Neurogastroenterol Motil. 2003;15:401–7.

55. Gai W-P, Messenger JP, Yu YH, Gieroba ZJ, Blessing WW. Nitric oxide-synthesising neurons in the central subnucleus of the nucleus tractus solitarius provide a major innervation of the rostral nucleus ambiguus in the rabbit. J Comp Neurol. 1995;357:348–61.

56. Rogers RC, Travagli RA, Hermann GE. Noradrenergic neurons in the rat solitary nucleus participate in the esophageal-gastric relaxation reflex. Am J Physiol Regul Integr Comp Physiol. 2003;285:R479–89.

57. Wiedner EB, Bao X, Altschuler SM. Localization of nitric oxide synthase in the brain stem neural circuit controlling esophageal peristalsis in rats. Gastroenterology. 1995;108:367–75.

58. Bieger D. Muscarinic activation of rhombencephalic neurones controlling oesophageal peristalsis in the rat. Neuropharmacology. 1984;23:1451–64.

59. Car A, Roman C, Zoungrana OR. Effects of atropine on the central mechanism of deglutition in anesthetized sheep. Exp Brain Res. 2002;142:496–503.

60. Wang YT, Bieger D. Role of solitarial GABAergic mechanism in control of swallowing. Am J Physiol Regul Integr Comp Physiol. 1991;30:R639–46.

61. Tsujimura T, Kondo M, Kitagawa J, Tsuboi Y, Saito K, Tohara H, Ueda K, Sessle BJ, Iwata K. Involvement of ERK phosphorylation in brainstem neurons in modulation of swallowing reflex in rats. J Physiol. 2009;587:805–17.

62. Grillner S, Wallen P, Dale N, Brodin L, Buchanan J, Hill R. Transmitters, membrane properties and network circuitry in the control of locomotion in lamprey. Trends Neurosci. 1987;10:34–42.

63. Jean A, Kessler JP, Tell F. Nucleus tractus solitarii and deglutition: monoamines, excitatory amino acids and cellular properties. In: Baracco RA, Baracco RA, editors. Nucleus of the solitary tract. Boca Raton: CRC Press; 1994. p. 361–75.

64. Jean A. Control of the central swallowing program by inputs from the peripheral receptors. A review. J Autonom Nerv Syst. 1984;10:225–33.

65. Andrew BL. The nervous control of the cervical oesophagus of the rat during swallowing. J Physiol London. 1956;134:729–40.

66. Dong H, Loomis CW, Bieger D. Vagal afferent input determines the volume dependence of rat esophageal motility patterns. Am J Physiol Gastrointest Liver Physiol. 2001;281:G44–53.

67. Falempin M, Rousseau JP. Activity of lingual, laryngeal and oesophageal receptors in conscious sheep. J Physiol London. 1984;347:47–58.

68. Dong H, Loomis CW, Bieger D. Distal and deglutitive inhibition in the rat esophagus: role of inhibitory neurotransmission in the nucleus tractus solitarii. Gastroenterology. 2000;118:328–36.

69. Lang IM, Medda BK, Shaker R. Differential activation of pontomedullary nuclei by acid perfusion of different regions of the esophagus. Brain Res. 2010; 1352:94–107.

70. Lang IM, Medda BK, Shaker R. Differential activation of medullary vagal nuclei caused by stimulation of different esophageal mechanoreceptors. Brain Res. 1368:119–33.

71. Getting PA. Emerging principles governing the operation of neural networks. Annu Rev Neurosci. 1989;12:185–204.

72. Bariohay B, Tardivel C, Pio J, Jean A, Félix B. BDNF-TrkB signaling interacts with the GABAergic system to inhibit rhythmic swallowing in the rat. Am J Physiol Regul Integr Comp. 2008;295:R1050–9.

73. Harada H, Takakusaki K, Kita S, Matsuda M, Nonaka S, Sakamoto T. Effects of injecting GABAergic agents into the medullary reticular formation upon swallowing induced by the superior laryngeal nerve stimulation in decerebrate cats. Neurosci Res. 2005;51:395–404.

74. Sifrim D, Janssens J, Vantrappen G. A wave of inhibition precedes primary peristaltic contractions in the human esophagus. Gastroenterology. 1992;103: 876–82.

75. Tell F, Jean A. Activation of N-methyl-D-aspartate receptors induces endogenous rhythmic bursting activities in nucleus tractus solitarii neurons: an intracellular study on adult rat brainstem slices. Eur J Neurosci. 1991;3:1353–65.

76. Tell F, Jean A. Ionic basis for endogenous rhythmic patterns induced by activation of N-methyl-D-aspartate receptors in neurons of the rat nucleus tractus solitarii. J Neurophysiol. 1993;70:2379–90.

77. Tell F, Fagni F, Jean A. Neurons of the nucleus tractus solitarius, in vitro, generate busting activities by solitary tract stimulation. Exp Brain Res. 1990;79: 436–40.

78. Paton JF, Li YW, Kasparov S. Reflex response and convergence of pharyngoesophageal and peripheral chemoreceptors in the nucleus of the solitary tract. Neuroscience. 1999;93:143–54.

79. Roman C. Contrôle nerveux du péristaltisme oesophagien. J Physiol Paris. 1966;58:79–108.

80. Janssens J, Valembois P, Hellemans J, Vantrappen G, Pelemans W. Studies on the necessity of a bolus for the progression of secondary peristalsis in the canine oesophagus. Gastroenterology. 1974;67:245–51.

81. Katz PS, Frost WN. Intrinsic neuromodulation: altering neuronal circuits from within. Trends Neurosci. 1996;19:54–61.

82. Dickinson PS, Moulins M. Interactions and combinations between different networks in the stomatogastric nervous system. In: HarrisWarrick RM, Marder E, Selverston AI, Moulins M, editors. Dynamic biological networks, The stomatogastric nervous system. Cambridge: MIT Press; 1992. p. 139–60.

83. Morton DW, Chiel HJ. Neural architectures for adaptive behavior. Trends Neurosci. 1994;17:413–20.

84. Meyrand P, Simmers J, Moulins M. Construction of a pattern-generating circuit with neurons belonging to different networks. Nature. 1991;351:60–3.

85. Gestreau C, Milano S, Bianchi AL, Grélot L. Activity of dorsal respiratory group inspiratory neurons during laryngeal-induced fictive coughing and swallowing in decerebrate cats. Exp Brain Res. 1996;108:247–56.

86. Larson CR, Yajima Y, Ko P. Modification in activity of medullary respiratory-related neurons for vocalization and swallowing. J Neurophysiol. 1994;71:2294–304.

87. Martin RE. Neuroplasticity and Swallowing. Dysphagia. 2009;24:218–29.

88. Momose-Sato Y, Sato K. Optical recording of vagal pathway formation in the embryonic brainstem. Auton Neurosci Basic Clin. 2006;126–127:39–49.

89. Miller AJ, Dunmire CR. Characterization of the postnatal development of superior laryngeal nerve fibers in the postnatal kitten. J Neurobiol. 1976;7:483–94.

90. Sumi T. The nature and postnatal development of reflex deglutition in the kitten. Jap J Physiol. 1967;17:200–10.

91. Wallois F, Khater-Boidin J, Dusaussoy F, Duron B. Oral stimulations induce apnoea in newborn kittens. Neuroreport. 1993;4:903–6.

92. Doty RW, Richmond WH, Storey AT. Effect of medullary lesions on coordination of deglutition. Exp Neurol. 1967;17:91–106.

93. Ertekin C, Aydogdu I, Tarlaci S, Turman AB, Kiylioglu N. Mechanisms of dysphagia in suprabulbar palsy with lacunar infarct. Stroke. 2000;31:1370–6.

94. Martin RE, Sessle BJ. The role of the cerebral cortex in swallowing. Dysphagia. 1993;8:195–202.

95. Martino R, Terrault N, Ezerzer F, Mikulis D, Diamant NE. Dysphagia in a patient with lateral medullary syndrome: insight into the central control of swallowing. Gastroenterology. 2001;121:420–6.

96. Prosiegel M, Holing R, Heintze M, Wagner-Sonntag E, Wiseman K. The localization of central pattern generators for swallowing in humans—a clinical-anatomical study on patients with unilateral paresis of the vagal nerve, Avelli's syndrome, Wallenberg's syndrome, posterior fossa tumours and cerebellar hemorrhage. Acta Neurochir. 2005;93:85–8.

97. Bieger D, Hockman CH. Suprabulbar modulation of reflex swallowing. Expl Neurol. 1976;52:311–24.

98. Hamdy S, Aziz Q, Rothwell JC, Singh KD, Barlow J, Hughes DG, Tallis RC, Thompson DG. The cortical topography of human swallowing musculature in health and disease. Nat Med. 1996;2:1217–24.

99. Aziz Q, Rothwell JC, Barlow J, Thompson DG. Modulation of esophageal responses to magnetic stimulation of the human brain by swallowing and by vagal stimulation. Gastroenterology. 1995;109:1437–45.

100. Castell DO, Wood JD, Frieling T, Wright FS, Vieth RF. Cerebral electrical potentials evoked by balloon distention of the human esophagus. Gastroenterology. 1990;98:662–6.

101. Hamdy S, Mikulis DJ, Crawley A, Xue S, Lau H, Henry S, Diamant NE. Cortical activation during human volitional swallowing: an event-related fMRI study. Am J Physiol Gastrointest Liver Physiol. 1999;277:G219–25.

102. Leopold NA, Daniels SK. Supranuclear control of swallowing. Dysphagia. 2009;25:250–7.

103. Martin RE, Goodyear BG, Gati JS, Menon RS. Cerebral cortical representation of automatic and volitional swallowing in humans. J Neurophysiol. 2001;85:938–50.

104. Tougas G, Hudoba P, Fitzpatrick D, Hunt RH, Upton ARM. Cerebral-evoked potential responses following direct vagal and esophageal electrical stimulation in humans. Am J Physiol Gastrointest Liver Physiol. 1993;264:G486–91.

105. Valdez DT, Salapatek A, Niznik G, Linden RD, Diamant NE. Swallowing and upper esophageal sphincter contraction with transcranial magnetic-induced electrical stimulation. Am J Physiol Gastrointest Liver Physiol. 1993;264:G213–9.

106. Car A. La commande corticale du centre déglutiteur bulbaire. J Physiol Paris. 1970;62:361–86.

107. Car A, Jean A, Roman C. A pontine primary relay for the superior laryngeal nerve ascending projections. Exp Brain Res. 1975;22:197–210.

108. Jean A, Car A, Roman C. Comparison of activity in pontine versus medullary neurones during swallowing. Exp Brain Res. 1975;22:211–20.

109. Car A. Etude macrophysiologique et microphysiologique de la zone déglutitrice du cortex frontal. J Physiol Paris. 1977;73:945–61.

110. Martin RE, Murray GM, Kemppainen P, Masuda Y, Sessle BJ. Functional properties of neurons in the primate tongue primary motor cortex during swallowing. J Neurophysiol. 1997;78:1516–30.

111. Blessing WB. The lower brainstem and bodily homeostasis. New York: Oxford University Press; 1997.

112. Jean A. The nucleus tractus solitarius: neuroanatomic, neurochemical and functional aspects. Arch Int Physiol Biochim Biophys. 1991;99:A3–52.

113. Berthoud HR. Neural systems controlling food intake and energy balance in the modern world. Curr Opin Clin Nutr Metab Care. 2003;6:615–20.

114. Grill HJ. Distributed neural control of energy balance: contributions from hindbrain and hypothalamus. Obesity. 2006;14(5):216S–21.

115. Grill HJ, Kaplan JM. The neuroanatomical axis for control of energy balance. Front Neuroendocrinol. 2002;23:2–40.

116. Félix B, Jean A, Roman C. Leptin inhibits swallowing in rats. Am J Physiol Regul Integr Comp Physiol. 2006;291:R657–63.

117. Bariohay B, Lebrun B, Moyse E, Jean A. Brain-derived neurotrophic factor plays a role as an anorexigenic factor in the dorsal vagal complex. Endocrinology. 2005;146:5612–20.

118. Bariohay B, Roux J, Tardivel C, Trouslard J, Jean A, Lebrun B. Brain-derived neurotrophic factor/tropomyosin-related kinase receptor type B signaling is a downstream effector of the brainstem melanocortin system in food intake control. Endocrinology. 2009;150:2646–53.

119. Lebrun B, Bariohay B, Moyse E, Jean A. Brain-derived neurotrophic factor (BDNF) and food intake regulation: a minireview. Auton Neurosci. 2006;126–127:30–8.

120. Bailey EF. A tasty morsel: the role of the dorsal vagal complex in the regulation of food intake and swallowing. Am J Physiol Regul Integr Comp. 2008;295:R1048–9.

Brainstem Control of Deglutition: Brainstem Neural Circuits and Mediators Regulating Swallowing

7

Winfried Neuhuber and Detlef Bieger

Abstract

Swallowing requires coordination of several paired muscle groups in the head and neck including the diaphragm. Thus, motoneurons of the Vth, VIIth, IX through XIIth cranial, cervical spinal, and phrenic nerves are sequentially activated by a swallowing pattern generator (SPG) located in the lower brainstem for executing the oral, pharyngeal, and esophageal stages of swallowing. Independence of these stages from each other indicates distinct subcircuits, their coupling pointing to flexible links between them. Although intrinsically autonomous, the SPG depends on peripheral and suprabulbar afferents for proper functioning. Pivotal to both, integrating afferents and coordinating stage-specific subcircuits, are the nucleus tractus solitarii (NTS) with some of its subnuclei and their reciprocal interconnections with the brainstem reticular formation. This chapter provides a survey of the anatomical and functional organization of the SPG.

Keywords

c-fos • Crural diaphragm • Dorsal motor nucleus • Esophagus • Neuromodulation • Nucleus ambiguus • Nucleus of the solitary tract • Pharynx • Swallowing pattern generator • Transmitter

Introduction

To achieve the complex task of coordinating the activity of several dozen paired muscle groups, swallowing (deglutition) requires neural control mechanisms involving levels of the neuraxis extending from the spinal cord to the cortex. The brainstem has long been thought to harbor the central network generating the basic spatiotemporal pattern of deglutitive neuromuscular activity. As illustrated by the work of Bidder [1], Mosso [2], and Miller and Sherrington [3], much

W. Neuhuber, MD (✉)
Institute of Anatomy, University of Erlangen-Nuremberg,
Krankenhausstraße 9, Erlangen 91054, Germany
e-mail: winfried.neuhuber@anatomie1.med.uni-erlangen.de

D. Bieger, Dr. Med
Health Science Centre, Memorial University,
St. John's, NL, Canada A1B 3V6

R. Shaker et al. (eds.), *Principles of Deglutition: A Multidisciplinary Text for Swallowing and its Disorders*,
DOI 10.1007/978-1-4614-3794-9_7, © Springer Science+Business Media New York 2013

of the pioneering research on swallowing dealt with its properties as a brainstem reflex effecting bolus transport through the upper alimentary tract (UAT), along with protection of the airway and the middle ear. This view lingers on in clinical thinking to this day, but has undergone substantial evolution in contemporary experimental work.

More than 30 years ago, Doty [4] outlined a now classical but still relevant concept of the swallowing center that envisaged four salient features: (1) an intrinsic organization; (2) "peremptory" control over deglutitive motoneurons; (3) a mechanism for decoding afferent inputs; and (4) responsiveness to "central excitatory states." Thanks to recent advances in neuroanatomic, neurochemical, and pharmacologic methodology, a model of circuitry representing a structurally defined brainstem SPG has evolved, opening up new avenues toward elucidation of the underlying cellular mechanisms. The term "SPG" reflects the major conceptual reorientation toward the intrinsic operations of this system as an autonomous network. Although Doty's postulates have been validated in part, the need for further refinements has become evident, particularly with regard to the organization of sensory inputs and the neurochemical correlates of central network functions.

Although autonomous in its intrinsic operations, the SPG depends on sensory input from the periphery via primary afferent neurons for both the initiation of swallowing and accommodation of the motor pattern to size, consistency, and texture of the bolus. Afferents coursing in branches of cranial nerves V, VII, IX, and X transmit low threshold mechanical (tactile, proprioceptive, tension), thermal, and chemical (gustatory) information to their brainstem relay nuclei of the trigeminal sensory and solitary complexes [5]. Moreover, IX/Xth nerve afferents from sinoaortic chemoreceptors may convey excitatory drive to the SPG [6]. As these second-order neurons also mediate a variety of reflexes and motor patterns other than swallowing, specific properties of the afferent signal (e.g., impulse frequency and origin in a particular peripheral structure) or their central processing must determine an appropriate

and specific motor outcome (i.e., swallowing instead of retching or gagging). Remarkably, afferent signals from both the periphery and suprabulbar structures are capable of activating the SPG. Thus, a problem common to transfer of sensory information to motor networks, namely the decoding of coded neuronal information [7], as well as the integration of central commands, appears to be solved by the SPG in the same way as in other motor networks. Precisely how this task is accomplished is still unknown; however, second-order sensory neurons, in particular in the nucleus tractus solitarii (NTS), as well as higher-order solitarial and reticular neurons providing neuromodulatory inputs are thought to play a key role.

Pharmacologic approaches have provided first insights into the nature and potential diversity of chemical signals utilized by deglutitive neural circuits [5, 8]. Thus, Doty's hypothesized "central excitatory states" can now be related to neuromodulatory inputs into the SPG. Certain of these involve neuronal substrates and neurotransmitter systems extrinsic to the SPG and may operate as links in deglutitive pathways descending from the forebrain and diencephalon. On the other hand, neurons intrinsic to the SPG largely depend on excitatory amino acidergic transmission for fast information transfer but are also endowed with other messenger substances acting as cotransmitters.

This chapter surveys the current progress made in studies of deglutitive motor control in laboratory animals, particularly rodents, as these have yielded the most detailed neuroanatomical information to date. It represents an update of our previous review [9]. A book chapter by Miller et al. [5], a review by Jean [10] and his chapter in this book, and a recent review by Lang [11] may be consulted for broader coverage of the relevant literature and background information on suprabulbar and peripheral deglutitive pathways not dealt with here. The brainstem structures forming the SPG and its associated circuits will be considered under the broad headings of (1) neuroanatomic organization, (2) in vivo mapping studies, and (3) transmitter mechanisms.

Neuroanatomic Organization

General Features

The principal components of the SPG are defined in terms of both afferent and efferent connectivity. The former comprises primary sensory inputs that are capable of evoking either the deglutitive motor sequence (oral, pharyngeal, and esophageal stage) or secondary (bolus-induced) esophageal peristalsis; the latter represents the motoneuron pools innervating the muscle layers of the UAT. Each of the three successive stages—(1) bolus formation and presentation to pharynx, (2) pharyngeal propulsion and transit with airway closure, and (3) peristaltic transport through the esophagus—can be enacted quasi-independently, implying discrete neuroanatomic substrates of control or a capability of the SPG to function selectively in different subcircuits. The bilateral symmetry of afferent and efferent neural circuits imposes a functional "half-center" organization, represented on both sides of the brainstem [12].

The circuit diagrams presented below should be consulted extensively so as to enable the reader to navigate with greater ease through the maze of anatomic detail. For each deglutitive stage, the underlying organization will be discussed in terms of three integral components: viscerosensory afferents (input), premotoneuronal network (interneuronal throughput), and visceromotor efferents (output). In essence, the concept of stage-specific circuits derives from evidence demonstrating that the NTS subdivisions receiving viscerosensory afferent input from the UAT maintain viscerotopically organized connections with motoneurons that innervate muscle tunics in the corresponding pharyngeal and esophageal portions of the UAT. Interneuronal throughput in these subcircuits, especially that controlling the esophagus, is simpler than initially supposed, as NTS second-order sensory neurons engage the associated motoneuron pools with monosynaptic connections, in addition to relaying in the medullary reticular formation. This direct linkage implies a mandatory (i.e., peremptory) mode of motor control by at least some components of the SPG. Remarkably, the "tightness" of these premotor connections progresses from one deglutitive stage to the next.

Motoneurons

The principal pools of deglutitive motoneurons innervating striated musculature of the UAT reside in cranial nerve motor nuclei V, VII, IX/X (nucleus ambiguus, AMB), and XII, including the accessory portions of V and VII [5]. Those providing preganglionic innervation for smooth muscle layers of the esophageal body and lower esophageal sphincter are contained in the dorsal motor nucleus of the vagus (DMV) as part of the general visceral efferent column (GVEC), where they make up a rostral contingent projecting to excitatory, and a caudal group projecting to inhibitory, myenteric neurons [13–15]. Neck muscle motoneurons are located in the ventral horn of cervical spinal cord segments 1–3, in case of the spinal accessory nucleus down to segment C7 [16–19]. Motor axons supplying these facultative swallowing muscles reach their targets via the ansa cervicalis, accessory nerve, and short branches of cervical spinal nerves.

Motoneurons activated during deglutition participate in a wide range of other motor programs; that is, they are inherently multifunctional. At first glance, the topography of UAT efferents in the cranial motor nuclei V, VII, IX to XI, and XII does not reveal a deglutitive pattern; however, the myotopic organization and dendroarchitecture of the ambiguous complex ([20–22]; Fig. 7.1) exhibit features that may facilitate integration and coordination of deglutitive motor output. The existence of presumptive gap junctions between about 30 % of esophagomotor neurons in the rat nucleus ambiguus compact formation (AMBc) suggests an additional mechanism for synchronizing motor output [24]. In addition to cholinergic markers, esophageal motoneurons of the ambigual compact formation express other putative mediators with as yet unknown functions, including calcitonin gene-related peptide (CGRP), galanin, N-acetylaspartylglutamate, and

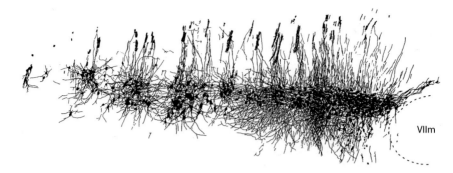

VIIm

Fig. 7.1 Cytodendroarchitecture of the rat ambiguus complex. Camera lucida reconstruction of serial oblique sagittal brainstem sections showing ambiguus neurons retrogradely labeled upon horseradish peroxidase application to the supranodose vagus nerve. Three main divisions are recognizable: a rostral compact formation of esophagomotor neurons (AMBc), a caudal loose formation (AMBl) of laryngomotor neurons, and an interposed semicompact formation (AMBsc) of chiefly pharyngomotor neurons. The AMBsc column continues into the rostral tip of the ambiguus complex overlying the facial motor nucleus (VIIm). Note dendritic radiations and bundling. Additional ventral most cell groups represent the AMB external formation of vagal preganglionic neurons. From W.W. Blessing et al. Brain Res 1984;322:346–50 with permission of Wiley and Sons

brain natriuretic peptide [25], as well as nitric oxide synthase (NOS; [26]).

Additional intricacies of esophageal motor control merit attention. All mammalian species, including rodents with a striated muscle esophagus, possess a full-length inner smooth muscle tube or tunica muscularis mucosae whose functional role remains to be clarified. The complex innervation of this structure by the myenteric plexus [25], the sympathetic nervous system [5], and spinal afferents [25, 27], along with the inferred inputs from the DMV, are consistent with a supportive role in bolus transport.

Another peculiarity is enteric coinnervation of striated esophageal muscle [28, 29]. Nitrergic and peptidergic myenteric neurons intermingle with cholinergic motor axons from AMBc neurons at esophageal motor endplates. Results from experiments with ex vivo vagus nerve-esophagus preparations suggest inhibitory modulation of vagally induced striated muscle contractions by nitrergic/peptidergic myenteric neurons [30–33]. Enteric coinnervation may also provide a pathway for DMV influence onto striated muscle of the esophagus [34]. However, the functional relevance of enteric coinnervation in vivo is still elusive.

A muscle that was largely neglected in considerations about neural control of swallowing until recently is the crural diaphragm. Clinical evidence and biomechanical reasoning indicated the crural diaphragm as an "external" lower esophageal sphincter which relaxes and contracts in concert with the "inner" lower esophageal sphincter [35, 36]. However, investigations on the neuronal basis of this coordination were only performed in the past few years. Besides a possible projection from deglutition-related brainstem nuclei to phrenic motoneurons in the cervical spinal cord which never has been rigorously tested, a more unorthodox vagal pathway from the DMV to the crural diaphragm was proposed based on both functional and retrograde transneuronal tracing studies in the ferret [37–39]. However, the retrograde tracing findings were not confirmed by anterograde tracing and have been interpreted by others as diffusion artifacts [40]. On the other hand, a peripheral reflex mechanism for esophago-diaphragmatic coordination was suggested [41].

Primary Afferents and Their Relay Nuclei

Transganglionic tracing studies have revealed the detailed somatotopy of primary afferent terminal fields in brainstem and spinal cord. Besides the well-known areas in the principal and spinal trigeminal nuclei, sensory neurons of the trigeminal ganglion also project to the NTS, particularly its lateral subnuclei [42, 43]. Proprioceptive neurons of the mesencephalic trigeminal nucleus send their axons to the trigeminal motor nucleus (Vm) and, via Probst's bundle, densely to the rhombencephalic parvicellular reticular formation (RFpc; [44, 45]), to the nucleus ambiguus [46], and to the hypoglossal nucleus [47]. Somatosensory, general, and special visceral (gustatory) afferents of the IXth and Xth cranial nerves terminate in specific subnuclei of the NTS with only little overlap, and in the paratrigeminal nucleus (PTN) [48–51]. Specifically, afferents from the soft palate, pharynx, and larynx terminate in the interstitial and intermediate subnuclei of the NTS (NTSis and NTSim, respectively) and in the PTN. Afferent terminals traced transganglionically from the superior laryngeal nerve (SLN), the major route of swallowing reflex afferents, are shown in Fig. 7.2.

Esophageal afferents are clustered in the central subnucleus of the NTS (NTSce; [48]). In general, afferents from cervical segments are represented rostral to those from thoracic and abdominal levels. Mucosal afferents from the upper cervical esophagus travel via the SLN to terminate in NTSis and NTSim, whereas muscular afferents coursing in the recurrent laryngeal nerve (RLN) reach the NTSce, similar to their counterparts from thoracic and abdominal esophagus ([53]; Fig. 7.3). The RLN also contains some afferents terminating in NTSis and NTSim, which may originate in the trachea [55].

Similar to the vagal efferent pathway to the crural diaphragm, there is also some indication for a vagal afferent innervation of the phrenicoesophageal ligament, i.e., the connective tissue tethering the esophagus to the crural diaphragm. In this case, electrophysiologic and retrograde tracing data were backened by anterograde tracing from the nodose ganglion showing terminal structures suggestive of mechanosensors [39].

Although there are monosynaptic connections between vagal primary afferents and general visceral efferent neurons of the DMV nerve [56–58], it is unknown if these include also esophageal or other swallowing-relevant afferents.

Functional studies in arterially perfused rat brainstem preparations suggest that stimulation of sinoaortic IX/Xth nerve chemoreceptor afferents can also elicit swallowing. This response may be mediated by neurons in the NTSim that receive convergent inputs from both pharyngoesophageal and chemoreceptor afferents [6, 59]. At first glance, this finding may be surprising, unless one takes into account that such a mechanism may constitute a defensive reflex for safeguarding airway patency.

Orofacial nociception, e.g., by injecting capsaicin into facial skin or tongue, inhibited reflex-induced swallowing in rat. This may be mediated via direct projections of trigeminal nociceptors to the NTS or via a relay in PTN and involves a GABAreceptor mechanism [54].

Ultrastructural studies demonstrate that terminals of afferents from the esophagus and the larynx form asymmetric synapses on dendrites of second-order neurons in the NTSce and NTSis [60, 61]. They may contact several dendrites, thus forming synaptic glomeruli. Primary afferents utilize glutamate as their main transmitter but apparently do not release nitric oxide (NO) from their central terminals. However, they often synapse on dendrites of nitrergic second-order neurons [62]. The NTSce neurons comprising the core region express neuronal nitric oxide synthase (nNOS), leu-enkephalin, and somatostatin [25, 63, 64] and, based on these markers, fall into different subpopulations. Noradrenergic neurons are found in its shell region [65].

The paucity of inhibitory synapses within the NTSce region would seem counterintuitive in light of functional evidence pointing to the existence of inhibitory processes operating at this level [66]. Moreover, the identification in NTSce neurons of alpha 1 subunit of gamma-aminobutyric acid (GABA). A receptor messenger RNA (mRNA) appears relevant in this context [67].

As noted above, connections between vagal second-order sensory neurons in the NTS and motoneurons are particularly tight in the case of ambigual neurons innervating muscles of the pharynx, larynx, and esophagus, the former two groups receiving monosynaptic inputs from interstitial and intermediate subnuclei and the latter from the central subnucleus. Ultrastructural analysis of synaptic contacts in the compact (AMBc),

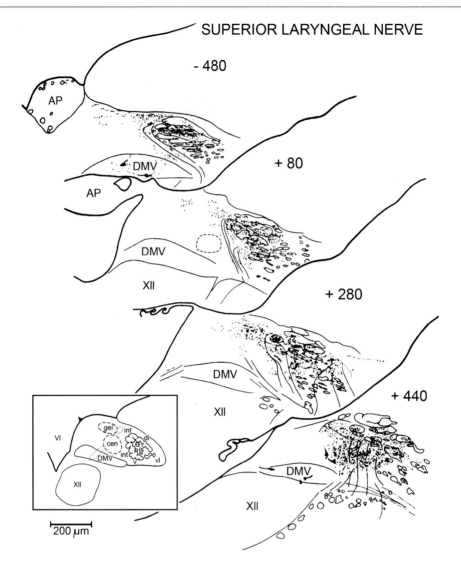

Fig. 7.2 Subnuclear divisions of rat nucleus tractus solitarii (insert at *lower left*) and distribution of central terminals of afferents coursing in the superior laryngeal nerve. Besides various afferents unrelated to deglutitive function, the SLN contains the majority of swallowing reflex afferents. The intrasolitarial distribution of transganglionically labeled terminals illustrated in this set of transverse sections overlaps with that revealed after tracer injections into the pharynx, larynx, or upper esophagus. Location of NTS subnucleus centralis (cen, core portion) is marked by dotted outline. Numbers indicate anterior–posterior distance (micrometers) from rostral edge of area postrema. *AP* area postrema, *DMV* dorsal motor nucleus of the vagus nerve, *NTS* nucleus tractus solitarii, *cen* central, *dl* dorsolateral, *gel* gelatinous, *int* intermediate, *is* interstitial, *v* ventral, *vl* ventrolateral subnucleus, IV—fourth ventricle, XII—hypoglossal motor nucleus. From W-Y Lu. Oesophageal premotor mechanisms in the rat. Ph.D. thesis, Memorial University of Newfoundland; 1996 with permission of Wiley and Sons

semicompact (AMBsc), and loose (AMBl) formations of the nucleus ambiguus, partly combined with tracer injections into the NTS, has revealed significant differences in the location of synapses on perikarya and dendrites, respectively, and types of synaptic vesicle [26, 68–71]. In the compact formation, almost all synapses are found on dendrites and contain small round clear vesicles (Gray's type I, presumptive excitatory). Pharyngeal and laryngeal motoneurons in the semicompact and loose formations, respectively, receive Gray's type I and type II (symmetric,

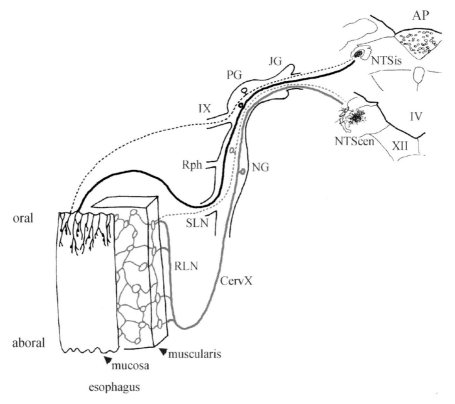

Fig. 7.3 Differential projection of vagal muscular and mucosal afferents from the rat upper esophagus. This summary diagram resulted from a combination of transganglionic tracing and selective neurectomy experiments. The majority of muscular afferents from intraganglionic laminar endings (IGLEs) course through the recurrent laryngeal nerve (RLN) and terminate in the central subnucleus of the solitary complex (NTScen) while a minority (stippled) takes the superior laryngeal nerve (SLN) route. In contrast, mucosal afferents travel through the SLN to the interstitial subnucleus (NTSis), some of them (stippled) reaching it via a branch of the glossopharyngeal nerve (IX). *AP* area postrema, *CervX* cervical vagus nerve, *IV*—fourth ventricle, *JG* jugular ganglion, *NG* nodose ganglion, *PG* petrosal ganglion, *Rph* pharyngeal branch of the vagus nerve. From Y.T. Wang and D. Bieger. Am J Physiol 1991;161:R639–46 with permission of Wiley and Sons

pleomorphic vesicles, presumptive inhibitory) at about equal numbers on both dendrites and somata. Synapses identified by anterograde tracing from the NTSce, NTSim, and NTSis concur with this general pattern. Solitario-ambigual neurons project also to small and medium-size nonmotoneurons of the nucleus ambiguus [69, 70]. Some of these neurons may project back to the NTS [45, 72]. Thus, premotor neuronal structures have mainly excitatory influences on the esophagus, whereas those for the pharynx and larynx are compatible with balanced excitatory/inhibitory inputs.

Moreover, there are significant projections from trigeminal (spinal and mesencephalic nuclei) and solitary complexes to the rhombencephalic RFpc [45, 73, 74], including Probst's nucleus and the intermediate reticular formation. It is reasonable to assume that premotor neurons in these reticular nuclei participate in afferent decoding and information processing.

Except for a few aberrant trigeminal and vagal fibers, primary afferents do not appear to project to the (rostral) reticular formation. However, second-order sensory projections from the NTS, spinal V, and PTN [75] reach the parabrachial area. In particular, the NTSim, but not the NTSce, sends a substantial projection to the parabrachial complex [76]. This pathway may account for the swallowing-associated activity described in the sheep dorsal pons ([34]; see Pontine Interneurons, below).

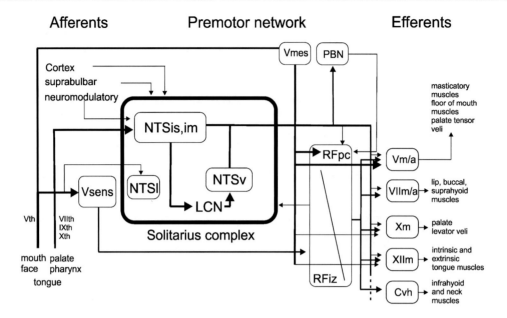

Afferents   Premotor network   Efferents

Oral stage subcircuit

Fig. 7.4 Proposed network circuit controlling the oral stage of swallowing. *Cvh* ventral horn of the first three cervical spinal segments, *LCN* local circuit neuron, *NTS* nucleus tractus solitarii, *NTSis* interstitial subnucleus, *NTSim* intermediate subnucleus, *NTSl* lateral subnucleus, *NTSv* ventral subnucleus, *PBN* parabrachial nuclei, *RFiz* reticular formation intermediate zone, *RFpc* reticular formation, *pars* parvicellularis, Vth—trigeminal nerve, Vm/a—motor/accessory nucleus of trigeminal nerve, Vmes—mesencephalic nucleus of trigeminal nerve, Vsens sensory nuclei of trigeminal nerve, VIIth—facial nerve, VIIm/a—motor/accessory nucleus of facial nerve, IXth—glossopharyngeal nerve, Xth—vagus nerve, Xm—nucleus ambiguus, XIIm—hypoglossal nucleus

Oral-Stage Subcircuit

Consisting of volitional and reflexive components (preparation, formation, and lingual propulsion of bolus), the oral stage [5] presents a less well-identified motor pattern as compared with the subsequent stages of swallowing. The network responsible for coordinating the oral stage provides integration with circuitry controlling mastication or drinking. Neuroanatomic evidence detailed below suggests a highly complex connectivity that overlaps only in some aspects with subcircuits thought to control the subsequent parts of the deglutitive sequence.

A proposed circuit model of the oral-stage network is presented in Fig. 7.4. As revealed by combined retrograde and anterograde tract tracing in the rat [73], the presumptive components of this subcircuit comprise portions of the rostral solitary complex, the rhombencephalic

parvicellular reticular formation (RFpc), and its projections to trigeminal (Vm), facial (VIIm), and hypoglossal (XIIm) motor nuclei. The RFpc subjacent to the dorsal vagal complex and lateral to the hypoglossal motor nucleus is implicated in deglutitive control because this region contains neurons that are active during the pharyngeal stage of deglutition (see below) and are likely to receive afferents from parts of the NTS receiving sensory inputs from the oral cavity [73]. The RFpc at the level of the rhombencephalon forms a sheet-like continuum extending in a ventro-rostro-lateral orientation toward the ventral vagal complex. Ventromedially it is flanked by the intermediate parvicellular reticular zone (RFiz), which includes a group of cholinergic neurons located just dorsomedial to the compact formation of the nucleus ambiguus [77, 78].

The projections from the RFpc [73] are bilateral and distributed preferentially to (1) jaw opener motoneurons in ventral Vm, (2) facial motoneurons in the dorsal intermediate subdivision innervating deep oral musculature (stylohyoid, posterior digastric), and (3) both protruder and retractor motoneurons in XIIm (ventral and dorsal subdivision, respectively). A mainly crossed projection to jaw closer motoneurons (dorsal division of Vm) originates from a group of large multipolar cells embedded in the RFpc, corresponding to the nucleus of Probst's tract. A defining feature of the RFpc neurons may be the formation of axon collaterals [79–82].

The inferred role in the control of oral-stage swallowing activity of connections between the RFpc and the rostral NTS [83] remains to be established. The same holds true for the presumed linkage with NTS subnuclei believed to form part of the SPG proper.

In the rat, Vm, VIIm, and XIIm also receive input from the NTS. However, these solitarial efferents, unlike those to the ambiguus complex, are relatively sparse [73, 82], although a preferential distribution to Vm jaw opener and accessory VIIm neurons is evident. In contrast, in the sheep, such connections are believed to be absent [10]. Instead, groups of interneurons in the ventral medullary reticular formation (putative "switching neurons" of Jean) are thought to operate as links between deglutitive NTS interneurons and motor neuron pools of the rostral rhombencephalon other than those projecting via the glossopharyngeal and vagus nerves. Anterograde [73, 84, 85] and retrograde [72, 73, 86] tracing studies in the rat implicate the periambigual parvicellular reticular formation as the presumptive location of ventral "switching" interneurons. A putative function of these premotor elements is coordination of deglutitive motor output within and between each half of the medulla.

Pharyngeal Stage Subcircuit

A proposed circuit model of the pharyngeal stage network is presented in Fig. 7.5. Based on anterograde [73, 84, 85] and retrograde transsynaptic [87, 88] tracing experiments, the solitarial interneurons projecting to buccopharyngeal stage

motoneurons, that is, pharyngeal and laryngeal motoneurons in the nucleus ambiguus, have been located in the intermediate, interstitial, and ventral NTS subnuclei (NTSim, NTSis, NTSv). Neurons in the NTSim are thought to provide premotor input to pharyngeal constrictor motoneurons in the semicompact formation [21] of the nucleus ambiguus. In addition, solitarial projections to trigeminal, facial, and hypoglossal motoneurons have been described in the rat [73, 82]. Retrograde transneuronal tracer studies using pseudorabies virus injections into rat pharyngeal muscles do not make specific mention of ventral reticular formation neurons [87]. It remains to be determined if all three NTS subnuclei play overlapping or distinct roles in deglutitive motor programming. For instance, chemostimulation maps (see Mapping Studies, below) do not unequivocally include the interstitial subnucleus as a site where swallowing responses can be triggered. Remarkably also, the NTSv is poorly supplied with UAT primary afferents [48]. In the cat, a newly defined ventromedial subnucleus of NTS (NTSvm; see c-fos/Fos mapping below) is involved in the pharyngeal stage [89]. It was suggested that NTSvm is equivalent to ventromedial parts of NTSce as defined in rodents [11].

Interconnections between these NTS subnuclei and the rhombencephalic RF probably enable the SPG to produce sequential inhibition and excitation of motoneurons and to ensure the bilateral coordination of the swallowing "half-centers." Connections, via NTSce or directly, with the GVEC of parasympathetic preganglionic neurons would represent the central link for swallowing-induced relaxation of the lower esophageal sphincter [90], sometimes regarded as the final stage of the swallowing sequence [12].

Esophageal Stage Subcircuit

A proposed circuit model of the esophageal stage network is presented in Fig. 7.6. Because esophageal peristalsis is held in abeyance during rapidly repeated oropharyngeal stage activity, or occurs independently, as in secondary (bolus-induced) peristalsis, it must be governed by a separate neural control circuit. Evidence from retrograde and anterograde neuroanatomic pathway tracing studies

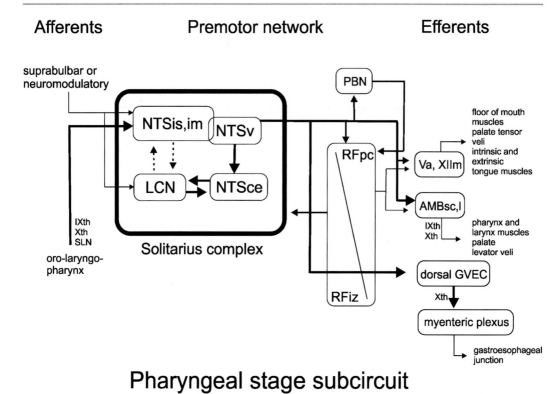

Afferents   **Premotor network**   **Efferents**

Pharyngeal stage subcircuit

Fig. 7.5 Proposed network circuit controlling the pharyngeal stage of swallowing. *AMBsc,l* semicompact and loose formation of nucleus ambiguus, *GVEC* general visceral efferent column, *LCN* local circuit neurons, *NTS* nucleus tractus solitarii, *NTSce* central subnucleus, *NTSis,im* interstitial and intermediate subnuclei, *NTSv* ventral subnucleus, *PBN* parabrachial nuclei, *RFiz* reticular formation intermediate zone, *RFpc* reticular formation pars parvicellularis, *SLN* superior laryngeal nerve, *Va*—accessory motor nucleus of trigeminal nerve, IXth—glossopharyngeal nerve, Xth—vagus nerve, XIIm—hypoglossal nucleus

supports this basic concept. Thus, the NTS subnucleus centralis receives a dense terminal projection from primary sensory vagal neurons innervating low-threshold mechanoreceptors in the esophagus [48] and, in turn, sends a massive projection to motoneurons of the compact formation of the nucleus ambiguus [64, 72, 88, 91], the source of special visceral efferents to the striated muscle tunic of the esophagus [21]. By comparison, projections from esophageal response loci in the NTS central subnucleus to the medullary reticular formation seem relatively sparse [84, 85], in agreement with anatomic anterograde tracing studies [73]. However, collateral projections to the RFiz were noted in another study using neurobiotin for extra- or juxtacellular labeling of functionally identified NTSce neurons [13].

The crucial question of whether the esophageal and the buccopharyngeal subcircuits are synaptically linked appears to have been resolved by viral tracing studies that demonstrate a projection from intermediate and interstitial subnuclei to the central subnucleus [20, 88]. However, the extent or strength of this linkage remains unclear. Thus, functional coupling between the buccopharyngeal and esophageal stages of swallowing may involve additional groups of NTS interneurons. Among these, cholinergic and GABA-ergic neurons are prime candidates (see Transmitter Mechanisms, below). In the cat, the newly defined NTSvm is now proposed as another possibility [89]. It is again worth noting that, in viral transneuronal retrograde tracing studies [88], NTSce neurons are visualized before neurons in the medullary RFpc and other brainstem structures

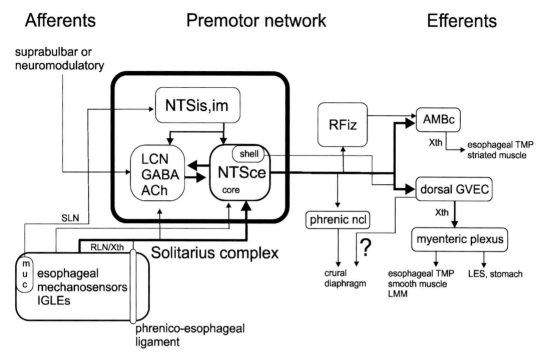

Esophageal stage subcircuit

Fig. 7.6 Proposed network circuit controlling the esophageal stage of swallowing. *ACh* acetylcholine, *AMBc* compact formation of nucleus ambiguus, *GABA* gamma-aminobutyric acid, *GVEC* general visceral efferent column, *IGLEs* intraganglionic laminar endings, *LCN* local circuit neurons, *LES* lower esophageal sphincter, *LMM* lamina muscularis mucosae, *muc* mucosa, *NTS* nucleus tractus solitarii, *NTSce* central subnucleus, *NTSis,im* interstitial and intermediate subnucleus, *phrenic ncl* phrenic nucleus, *RFiz* reticular formation intermediate zone, *RLN* recurrent laryngeal nerve, *SLN* superior laryngeal nerve, *TMP* tunica muscularis propria, Xth—vagus nerve

(nuclei of the spinal trigeminal tract, area postrema, locus ceruleus, subceruleus area, raphe nuclei, and midbrain central gray).

At present, information is incomplete regarding the connections between the solitarial subnuclei and vagal preganglionic neurons that control the motility of UAT smooth musculature. A group of noradrenergic neurons forming the shell region of the NTSce has been implicated in esophago-gastric reflex paths that trigger gastric relaxation during esophageal distension. These neurons reportedly send extensive projections to preganglionic neurons in the DMV nerve [13, 65], the source of general visceral efferents to UAT smooth musculature. Gastric relaxation may result from both alpha-1 adrenergic activation of DMV neurons projecting to gastric myenteric nitrergic neurons and alpha-2 mediated inhibition

of DMV neurons innervating gastric myenteric cholinergic neurons [92]. A similar mechanism may control the lower esophageal sphincter [37].

However, another anterograde tracing study of NTS efferents in the rat [73] suggests a paucity of connections with the DMV, but in view of contrary evidence from functional mapping studies [13, 65, 85], it seems reasonable to infer that the sites selected for tracer deposits missed some of the critical NTS subnuclei harboring deglutitive premotor neurons, including esophageal premotor neurons of the NTSce. This conclusion is further strengthened by data from "microchemostimulation" mapping studies (see Mapping Studies, below).

The current view of solitarial neurons as internuncial elements linking sensory input from and motoneuronal output to the UAT is no doubt somewhat simplistic. For example, intracellular staining of neurons in the NTS subnuclei intermedius and centralis ([52]; D. Bieger, unpublished observations) shows that, apart from their main axons projecting to the ambiguus complex, cells in these regions emit multiple axon collaterals that form extensive intrasolitary projections. Similarly, Rogers and coworkers [13, 65] have demonstrated the extensive dendritic arborizations of NTSce cells, which reach the ependyma overlying the NTS. In addition, other connections include crossed intersolitary projections [84], involving NTS subnuclei other than those receiving vagal input from the UAT, thereby forming additional local circuits. It is tempting to speculate that these intrasolitary networks play a role in coupling of the deglutitive stages, as well as in swallow-induced (deglutitive) and bolus-induced (distal) esophageal inhibition. Projections to the rostral parts of the GVEC of VIIth, IXth, and Xth nerve parasympathetic preganglionic neurons would provide a possible mechanism for coordinated activation of salivary and UAT mucous glands.

Functional Maps of Brainstem Deglutitive Pathways

Mapping of swallow-activated neuronal activity has been achieved by various means, including in vivo microelectrode extracellular recording, as well as by Fos immunocytochemistry. Deglutitive neural substrates have also been delineated by means of chemical microstimulation; for pertinent evidence see Transmitter Mechanisms, below. Apart from differences in sensitivity and specificity, these techniques have in common at least three limitations or caveats that need to be taken into account: (1) Neurons displaying activity during any particular stage of the swallowing sequence may not necessarily be involved in generating the deglutitive motor program but instead act as relays to other neural circuits serving different functions (e.g., breathing, coughing, vomiting, retching, as well as a variety of associated esophageal reflexes). (2) Deglutitive activation may be due to reafferent signals from the aerodi-

gestive tube. (3) Metabolic neuronal markers such as the c-fos signal cannot be detected in neurons undergoing synaptic inhibition, a process likely to play a significant role in deglutitive motor programming.

Microelectrode Studies

For detailed information on the functional typology and firing characteristics of dorsal and ventral swallowing group (DSG and VSG) neurons the reader should consult the chapter in this volume by Jean and Dallaporta. Here, only the most salient points will be covered. The majority of data on swallowing-related neurons in the mammalian brainstem come from extracellular recordings obtained in anesthetized or decerebrated animals [5, 10], including mainly the sheep, as well as the cat, rat, dog, and monkey. Intracellular recordings have been reported only recently and deal mainly with motoneurons (see below), except for two studies describing activity of interneurons in the cat [93] and rat NTS [6]. The most commonly used method for eliciting deglutition in these investigations is electrical stimulation of the SLN, resulting in reflexive activity involving chiefly the pharyngeal stage, with variable participation (or sometimes inhibition) of the esophageal stage. Based on these data, the preeminent role of the NTS and the periambigual reticular formation in deglutitive motor pattern generation was first established [10], thus providing a frame of reference for subsequent neuroanatomical investigations.

General features of swallowing neurons include (1) usual absence of a tonic (or resting) discharge and (2) a spike burst temporally correlated with deglutitive motor output. Other deglutitive neurons may show an accelerated resting discharge or phasic inhibition coinciding with swallow. Deglutitive neurons are furthermore excited by distention of that part of the UAT that contracts in phase with the swallowing neuronal discharge. Their general localization in the medulla oblongata to some extent overlaps with neurons involved in cardiorespiratory regulation [59].

Medullary Interneurons

These elements are characterized by two criteria: lack of antidromic activation with electrical stimulation of appropriate motor nerves, and a high spike rate [10]. Their two principal locations are (1) the NTS and subjacent RFpc; and (2) the ventrolateral reticular formation adjoining the nucleus ambiguus, representing the DSG and VSG. Additional loci are found in the immediate vicinity of motor nuclei of cranial nerves V, VII, and XII and of the principal sensory nucleus of the trigeminal nerve.

Specific NTS subnuclear localizations of DSG neurons were not determined in the original studies [10, 94]. However, their location in general overlaps with that of NTSis, NTSim, NTSv, and adjacent NTSvl. Burst discharges persist in the presence of neuromuscular paralysis (curarization), implying their central origin. Presumptive DSG interneurons of the rat NTS exhibit a predominantly excitatory convergence of inputs from pharyngoesophageal mechanoreceptors and IX/Xth nerve sinoaortic chemoreceptors [6].

The DSG neurons related to the esophageal stage of swallowing in the rat make up the main portion of the NTSce. More is known about their behavior during secondary peristalsis evoked by esophageal distention [13, 66, 95, 96] than during swallowing. Reflecting the potential diversity or complexity of the esophageal premotor control, responses to localized esophageal balloon distention reveal that at least three different types of neurons can be distinguished in the NTSce region [66]. One of these types would qualify as a local circuit neuron generating distal inhibition in the esophageal body or the stomach; the other types show either rhythmic or nonrhythmic discharges temporally correlated with distention-induced esophagomotor activity.

The VSG neurons have thus far only been identified for the oropharyngeal stage of swallowing. Compared with DSG neurons, they display longer synaptic latencies and lower instantaneous spike rates but have similar firing characteristics [10, 97]. Deglutitive interneurons are also located in or near trigeminal and hypoglossal motor nuclei.

Pontine Interneurons

Pontine interneurons are located in a region extending "rostrally to the VIIth nerve exit, above Vm at the level of the trigeminal principal sensory nucleus" [10]. Upon SLN stimulation, these spontaneously active cells produce a short-latency [1.5–4 millisecond (ms)] synaptic response. However, unlike that of DSG or VSG neurons, the deglutitive discharge of these cells is abolished by neuromuscular paralysis and, hence, likely to represent a response to sensory feedback from oropharyngeal receptors. Because these neurons can be antidromically driven from the ventral posteromedial nucleus of the thalamus, they would appear to form part of an ascending sensory pathway relaying in the parabrachial complex [75, 76]. In this context, a case report describing a patient with lateral medullary syndrome who presented, inter alia, with dysphagia could be of relevance [98]. MRI images (Fig. 7.1) show a small lesion in the caudal dorsolateral pons (erroneously identified as the dorsolateral medulla), which may have interrupted a pathway between the DSG and pontine interneurons.

Motoneurons

Information on the deglutitive activity of motoneurons comes mostly from extracellular recording experiments in sheep and rat [10, 94]. Motoneurons active during the pharyngeal stage produce low-frequency spike bursts at durations in the range of 50–200 ms and lack spontaneous activity. Short-latency (7–12 ms) activation is seen in pharyngeal stage motoneurons on stimulation of the ipsilateral afferent fibers in the SLN or IXth nerve, implying mediation via oligosynaptic pathways. In sheep, XIIm neurons produce deglutitive burst discharges at spike frequencies of 10–70 Hz, but only a minority of cells appears to receive oligosynaptic input via the SLN or lingual nerve [99].

Firing characteristics of esophageal stage motoneurons have been studied by (1) recording from the nucleus ambiguus [10], from which efferents to esophageal striated muscle arise; and (2) by means of single-fiber unit recordings from preganglionic vagal axons [100, 101] supplying the smooth muscle portions of the esophagus.

Burst discharges of nucleus ambiguus neurons exhibit a long duration (150–800 ms) with a low spike rate (10–40 Hz). Both parameters seem to correlate with the timing of the discharge; with increasing delay, burst duration lengthens and spike frequency decreases. In contrast, preganglionic fibers from the DMV to esophageal smooth muscle have discharge rates of 3–8 Hz with burst durations in the range of 1 s. Rat DMV neurons are either excited or inhibited by esophageal distention, depending on their localization (medial-rostral: inhibition; laterocaudal: excitation; [13]).

Intracellular recordings in the sheep rostral nucleus ambiguus have revealed a marked hyperpolarization of the membrane potential preceding the deglutitive spike burst; the apparent synaptic inhibition coincides with the oropharyngeal stage [102]. Intracellular recordings in cat XIIm styloglossal (tongue retractor) and genioglossal (tongue protruder) motoneurons [103] demonstrated simple excitatory postsynaptic potential (EPSPs) and complex EPSP-inhibitory postsynaptic potential (IPSP) sequences, respectively, during deglutition. Corresponding evidence for a centrally coordinated synaptic inhibition was first obtained in electromyography (EMG) studies showing a cessation of activity in certain "leading complex" motoneuronal pools preceding and following the deglutitive discharge ("bracketing inhibition") [12]. However, this inhibition does not involve all pharyngeal stage motoneurons.

c-fos/Fos Mapping

At present, the number of studies designed to visualize the deglutitive neural network by means of this metabolic marker technique is limited, and the data reported in the rat [104], mouse [105], and cat [89] do not present a coherent picture. Similar problems, inconsistencies, or apparent lack of specificity are found in studies of other functions (e.g., cardiovascular systems). The first study using this method [104] was carried out in ketamine/xylazine-anesthetized rats ($n=3$) subjected to prolonged stimulation of the RLN. Based on this report, putative swallow-associated cell activation in the rhombencephalic reticular

formation and solitary complex exhibits a rather poorly defined diffuse pattern. Moreover, the c-fos signal was absent in neurons supplying efferents to UAT striated or smooth musculature. These data conflict with neurophysiologic evidence and pharmacologic investigations considered below. It is thus doubtful that they can be interpreted as confirming earlier localizations of a "swallowing center" in the rostroventral medullary reticular formation [12, 106], which thus far has eluded detection by microelectrode recording.

Solitarius Complex

Pharyngeal stage-associated increases in Fos-positive neurons were reported in the feline [89] NTSim, NTSis, and NTSvm, but appeared to be absent in NTSv and NTSvl. As already noted, the latter two display deglutitive neural activity in sheep and rat. In the mouse, pharyngeal stage-associated elevations in c-fos expression were essentially confined to the NTSis and NTSim [105]. Conversely, in the cat [89], esophageal stage-associated c-fos elevations occurred in more widespread subnuclear divisions of the NTS (NTSce, NTSv, NTSdl, and NTSvl) than would be expected on the basis of either extracellular recording studies in rats and sheep or tract tracing studies in the rat (cf. Neuroanatomic Organization, above). This widespread activation, in particular of NTSvl, may relate to respiratory responses during the esophageal stage of swallowing [11]. In contrast, c-fos studies in the mouse [105] suggest a more restricted distribution of swallow- or esophageal stage-activated neurons in the interstitial, intermediate, and central subnuclei, even though the experimental protocol entailed electrical stimulation of the SLN, a procedure expected to activate also various vagal afferents involved in functions other than deglutition. Activation of the NTSce core region was not evident at intensities of SLN stimulation below the threshold for elicitation of primary peristalsis. In the rat [104], putative swallow-activated neurons showed a widespread relatively sparse distribution without a clear subnuclear pattern. In addition, both control and experimental animals exhibited activity in NTS areas overlapping rostrally with the subnucleus centralis, but erroneously identified as such at more caudal NTS levels. In rats subjected to repetitive esophageal distention, a c-fos signal was reported in group CA-2 noradrenergic neurons surrounding the NTSce and, to a lesser extent, in NTSce core neurons negative for nNOS [65]. A more diffuse activation was present in adjacent NTS subnuclei [65].

Dorsal Motor Nucleus of the Vagus

Pharyngeal stage-associated c-fos elevations were noted in the cat throughout the rostrocaudal extent of the nucleus, with preponderance in the dorsal aspect of the DMV and preferential involvement of small-sized presumptive interneurons [89]. Similarly, in the mouse [105], neurons activated by SLN electrical stimulation were located in both rostral and caudal parts of the nucleus; however, rostrally activation occurred only at a stimulus frequency sufficient to elicit swallowing. No data were reported in the rat studies [104].

Ambiguus Complex

Evidence of deglutitive c-fos activation was found in the dorsal subdivision of the cat nucleus ambiguus in association with pharyngeal stage activity, and in the ventral subdivision (at both caudal and rostral levels) following prolonged esophageal stage activity [89]. Direct interspecies comparison of these viscerotopic patterns is hampered by the divergent nomenclature applied to the nucleus ambiguus subdivisions in the cat and rat or mouse. However, it seems reasonable to infer that the feline ventral subdivision (so-called retrofacial nucleus) corresponds to the esophagomotor compact division of rodents, whereas the pharyngomotor semicompact subdivision of rodents is the homologue of the dorsal subdivision in the cat (cf. [107]). The pattern of Fos-activated neurons reported in the mouse ambiguus complex [105] agrees with the viscerotopic representation of the UAT motoneurons revealed by neuroanatomic tracer studies. In the rat [104], presumptive swallow-activated cells had a localization overlapping with that of the external formation of the nucleus ambiguus and the ventral respiratory group.

Rhombencephalic Reticular Formation

As evidenced by c-fos activation following repetitive swallowing activity in the mouse [105], the RFpc of the medulla oblongata would appear to receive deglutitive input through the appropriate NTS subnuclei. In the rat [104], a more widespread distribution of activated cells appeared to be evident in the RFpc, RFiz, periambigual RF, and centromedial gigantocellular RF. It should be noted, however, that "chemomicrostimulation" maps based on the use of excitatory amino acids (EAAs) in the rat do not support a role of neurons in these regions in generating deglutitive motor output (see next section).

Transmitter Mechanisms

Recent neuropharmacologic advances have provided a plethora of tools for probing the SPG, including agonists and antagonists acting at receptors for neurotransmitters or neuromediators. As evidenced by the elicitation of rhythmic (repetitive) swallowing in the anesthetized rat [8], the SPG responds with sustained excitation to a diversity of centrally acting pharmacologic stimuli. The stimulant efficacy of certain receptor agonists applied systemically or intraarterially approaches that of electrical stimulation of the SLN, the chief afferent route for elicitation of the swallowing reflex. In particular, "fictive" swallowing ensues upon localized chemostimulation of NTS areas receiving deglutitive reflex afferent input. Because primary afferent vagal input in both deglutitive subcircuits most probably utilizes glutamatergic transmission [91, 96, 108, 109], the effects of EAAs such as glutamate and certain of its analogues [kainate, quisqualate, and N-methyl-D-aspartate (NMDA)] should mimic those of glutamate (or aspartate) released endogenously either from peripheral vagal reflex afferent terminals in the solitarius complex or central afferents originating from rostral levels of the neuraxis (e.g., basal forebrain, hypothalamus, cortex). On the other hand, the excitatory actions of the monoamines and certain peptides would point to the involvement of suprabulbar neuromodulatory inputs converging on the SPG.

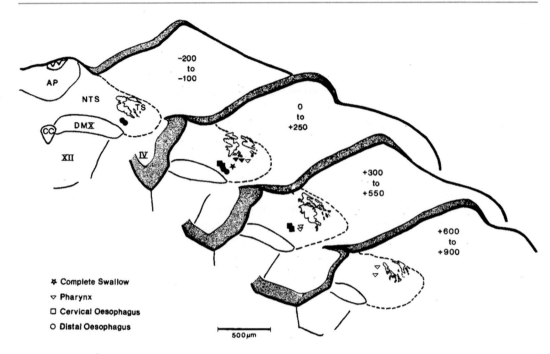

Fig. 7.7 Map of deglutitive response loci in the rat NTS as determined by pressure pulse microejection of L-glutamate or excitatory amino acid agonists. Sites included in this analysis typically yield stable highly reproducible responses with repeated stimulation and are distinctly localized. Open symbols denote single loci and filled symbols represent 2–4 overlapping loci from separate experiments. In the rostrocaudal series of transverse sections through the NTS, the distance from the obex is indicated in micrometers. *AP* area postrema, *CC* central canal, *NTS* nucleus tractus solitarii, *DMX* dorsal motor nucleus of the vagus, XII—hypoglossal nucleus, IV—fourth ventricle. From M. Amri et al. Brain Res 1991;548:144–55 with permission of Pergamon Press

Neuromodulatory inputs such as those mediated by serotonin and noradrenaline may operate at the NTS level to regulate the gain of synaptic responses to primary afferent input [8, 13].

Excitatory Amino Acids

Deglutitive excitant effects are obtained with EAA agonists acting at kainate, alpha-amino-3-hydroxy-5-methyl-4-isoxazole propionic acid (AMPA), NMDA, and the metabotropic receptor subtypes [54, 109–113]. Thus, all types of glutamate (EAA) receptor agonists appear capable of exciting the SPG at the NTS level. Because of their discrete neuroanatomic localization, organized nature, and potential rhythmicity, these responses have yielded important insights into the mode of operation of the SPG.

Mapping Studies

Due to their high efficacy, EAA agonists, including glutamate itself, can be used for constructing chemomicrostimulation maps of deglutitive functional organization within the solitarius complex (Fig. 7.7). Depending on the NTS locus being stimulated, a diversity of responses can be elicited, including the complete sequence, its pharyngeal or esophageal components, or fractions of the latter [85, 110, 111, 113]. In keeping with electrophysiologic evidence [94], deglutitive response loci controlling the complete swallowing sequence or its buccopharyngeal stage are clustered in an area coextensive with the intermediate and ventral subnuclei of the NTS [110, 111]. Other work [114], employing L-glutamate pulses in 100–500 times larger ejectate volumes, reported swallow response loci extending laterally into the interstitial and ventrolateral subnuclei.

Esophageal response loci are clustered in the NTSce [96, 110, 111], with sites mediating relaxation of the gastroesophageal junction lying in close proximity [113]. These observations strengthen the idea that the SPG network consists of spatially discrete, hierarchically organized modules.

Focal application of EAA agonists to the rat rostral nucleus ambiguus complex and adjacent ventral reticular formation typically elicits a single contraction of the esophagus, most probably reflecting direct excitation of motoneurons. Depending on the intraambigual site, the response may be stationary, more or less restricted to a particular segment, or propulsive and accompanied by a transient pharyngeal relaxation [33, 110]. The latter features suggest involvement of ventral swallowing group interneurons closely adjacent to motoneurons.

Interestingly, esophagomotor responses produced by application of ionotropic EAA agonists to the NTSce region are nonrhythmic in nature [111], even though afferent stimulation at the level of the distal esophagus may result in rhythmic peristalsis [66, 95]. The NTSce neurons have been shown to express mRNA for the NMDA-1 receptor [115]. The EAA agonist potency rank orders [111] are consistent with a prominent role for this receptor type in generating NTSce neuronal responses to synaptic input from peripheral afferents [96].

However, some evidence suggests that activation of metabotropic glutamate receptors (mGluRs) produces rhythmic responses [112]. This difference would be explained if afferent input via ionotropic EAA receptors were to initiate activation of higher order sensory interneurons, in particular cholinergic afferents to the NTS originating in the RFiz or the NTS itself, which would permit or facilitate repetitive activity of NTSce neurons. Alternatively, nonspecific EAA receptor stimulation may cause collateral activation of other transmitter systems with inhibitory (e.g., GABA, [54]) or as yet undefined (e.g., neurokinins, [116]) actions. Presynaptic mGluRs differentially modulate release of GABA at NTS second-order sensory neurons [117].

Gamma-Aminobutyric Acid

Studies using immunohistochemistry for glutamic acid decarboxylase (GAD), GABA, glycine, and, more recently, in situ hybridization for GAD67 and glycine transporter-2 have revealed widespread distribution of GABA-ergic neuronal cell bodies and terminals, which often colocalize glycine in the NTS of rat, cat, rabbit, and sheep [23, 118–123]. Most of the immunoreactive neurons were found in subnuclei surrounding the solitary tract and in NTSis. It is noteworthy that mixed GABA-glycine terminals coreleasing both transmitters were confined to lateral portions of the NTS [119]. Ultrastructural examination demonstrated mostly symmetric axodendritic synapses and the rare axoaxonic contact.

Enhancement of GABA-ergic transmission by systemic pharmacologic means results in inhibition of reflex deglutition in the anesthetized cat, an action persisting after decerebration and reversed by GABA antagonists [124]. In the rat, localized blockade of NTS GABAA receptors leads to overt excitation of the SPG. This mechanism of disinhibition accounts for the deglutitive stimulant action of the GABAA receptor blocker bicuculline and GABA chloride channel blocker picrotoxin [54, 66]. The underlying process of autoexcitation appears to involve NMDA receptors and cholinergic input to the NTSce. Thus, in subthreshold amounts delivered to this region, bicuculline converts S-glutamate-induced monophasic pharyngeal or esophageal responses into rhythmic ones, and promotes primary peristalsis [54]. With suprathreshold amounts, peristalsis-like activity ensues that is abolished by blockade of NTS muscarinic acetylcholine receptors [54].

Evidently, therefore, local GABA-ergic control provides a tonic background inhibition of the SPG that maintains both pharyngeal and esophageal stage premotor neurons in a quiescent state. Removal of this inhibition leads to sustained autoexcitation, with resultant rhythmic patterned motor output under control by these premotor neurons. It seems reasonable to infer that the underlying processes entail pacemaker-like oscillations of membrane potential in the constituent neuronal population [65, 125]. In pharyngeal-stage interneurons these are probably driven by NMDA receptors, and in esophageal-stage interneurons by coactivation of NMDA and muscarinic acetylcholine receptors [52, 113].

Furthermore, a GABAA receptor-mediated mechanism has been shown to operate at the NTS level in distal inhibition of the rat esophagus [66], that is, the cessation of peristalsis in aboral segments triggered by distention of the proximal esophagus.

Acetylcholine

Cholinergic transmission is required not only for translating motoneuronal impulses into deglutitive muscle activity but also for generating or shaping the central motor pattern of esophageal peristalsis. In the rat, both muscarinic (mAChR) and nicotinic (nAChR) receptors have been implicated, the former in NTS premotor control and the latter at the motoneuronal level. Stimulation of central nicotine receptors in the cat reportedly evokes full-length esophageal peristalsis [126]; however, the precise nature of this response and its neural substrates remain to be defined. In the rat, nicotine evokes rhythmic swallowing activity upon application to the NTS extraventricular surface (W.Y. Lu, personal communication), an action likely to result from release of other mediators, because indirect cholinergic stimulation by means of antiesterases produces inhibitory effects on rhythmic (fictive) swallowing activity [8]. In this species, NTS nicotinic receptor blockade fails to affect secondary peristalsis or NTSce neuronal responses to esophageal distention [96]. Although atropine is said to block esophageal peristalsis also in the sheep [10], available evidence from other species, including humans, does not clearly bear out a role of central mAChR [127, 128].

The rat NTSce contains a dense terminal field of cholinergic axons [77]; to date, the precise connectivity of these afferents has not been identified, particularly as regards the RFiz intermediate reticular nucleus [78]. One probable source is nearby choline acetyltransferase-immunoreactive neurons straddling the intermediate,

interstitial, and central subnuclei [77]. Cholinergic input mediated by mAChR plays important integrative functions of NTSce neurons, including (1) the coupling between the buccopharyngeal and esophageal stages of swallowing [54, 110] and (2) the generation of premotoneuronal firing patterns appropriate for the production of both propulsive and rhythmic esophagomotor output [95, 96, 113]. Coactivation of NMDA receptors appears to be essential.

More specifically, focal stimulation via mAChR of rat NTSce neurons [54, 110, 111, 113, 129] gives rise to patterned rhythmic esophagomotor activity, resembling bolus-induced peristalsis, whereas mAChR blockade impairs or eliminates different types of esophageal motor responses, irrespective of their mode of elicitation (reflex afferent stimulation or central pharmacologic interventions). Because mAChR blockade does not disrupt activation of NTSce neurons via vagal afferents [96], cholinergic transmission at this level may serve to gate throughput from reflex afferents to motoneurons. Esophageal premotor paralysis is accompanied by a loss of rhythmicity in NTSce neuron burst firing and absent spike activity in AMBc motoneurons.

Intracellular and whole cell patch recordings in medullary slice preparations have shown that AMBc neurons respond to focal muscarinic stimulation of the NTSce region with rhythmic depolarizing waves or bursts of EPSPs. This in vitro rhythm closely resembles that observed in vivo, suggesting that esophagomotor rhythm generation is a potentially intrinsic operation of the NTSce–AMBc circuitry [113]. Nonetheless, in the intact system, neuromuscular paralysis (curarization) severely impairs esophagomotor rhythmogenesis [95]. Reafferent feedback from vagal mechanoreceptors (esophageal intraganglionic laminar endings [IGLEs], [27, 130]) must therefore make a critical contribution to that process.

The nicotinic cholinoceptors present in AMBc neurons mediate a fast inward current and a spike burst discharge [33]. The same receptor generates an EPSP elicited by focal stimulation of the adjacent RFiz [86]. As yet the role of this input remains unclear, because blockade does not impair fictive peristalsis in vivo, nor does it alter EPSPs produced by electrical [86] or mAChR agonist [113] stimulation of the NTSce–AMBc pathway in slice preparations. Furthermore, nAChR-mediated excitation of ambiguus neurons is inhibited by somatostatin [131].

Other Neuromodulatory Inputs

The SPG of the rat is susceptible to excitation by several other neural messengers, such as serotonin (acting via 5-hydroxytryptamine-2A or -1 C receptors), norepinephrine (acting via alpha 1-adrenoceptors), thyroliberin, oxytocin, and vasopressin [8]. Monoaminergic inputs are likely to originate from diverse sources (intra-NTS, area postrema, raphe nuclei, locus ceruleus, and subceruleus group) [5, 8]. Some of the peptidergic afferents come from the paraventricular nucleus of the hypothalamus; other afferents may corelease peptides and monoamines. The diversity of these inputs reflects the range of functions (hunger, thirst, nausea, reward, sleep, etc.) that influence internal drive levels (central excitatory or inhibitory states) of the SPG. Moreover, these modulatory systems could serve as network links with other neural function generators, in particular those controlling feeding and respiration. A projection presumably subserving such integrative purposes originates from hypothalamic orexin neurons and provides virtually all NTS subnuclei relevant for deglutition with terminals [132]. Intriguingly, fourth ventricle orexin infusion resulted in particularly enhanced Fos expression in NTSce. However, swallowing induced by electrical stimulation of the SLN is significantly inhibited by orexin [133]. This suggests stimulation of inhibitory interneurons overriding excitatory mechanisms. Likewise, microinjection of the anorectic peptide leptin into the rat NTS appears to inhibit reflex-induced swallowing via a GABAergic mechanism [134]. On the other hand, NTS injections of the orexigenic peptide ghrelin may inhibit reflex swallowing [133] through reduced glutamate release from primary afferent terminals [135].

Neurotrophins represent another class of substances modulating swallowing. Injections of brain-derived neurotrophic factor (BDNF) into the NTS inhibited swallowing elicited by SLN stimulation through TrkB-mediated action on GABAergic neurons [136].

Important inferences as to the cellular basis of these neuromodulatory responses can be drawn from work on rat NTS gastric second-order sensory neurons [137]. As shown by in vitro imaging studies, these cells respond to alpha 1-receptor stimulation with slow Ca^{2+} oscillations (5/min) resulting from the interplay of inositol trisphosphate-mediated Ca^{2+} release and Ca^{2+}-adenosine triphosphatase (ATPase) storage pumps of the endoplasmic reticulum. Cyclical elevations of cytoplasmic Ca^{2+} may lead to augmented responsiveness to both viscerosensory input and background excitatory drives.

Subnucleus centralis neurons contain NOS [22, 138, 139] and receive nitrergic afferents from both peripheral (but see [62]) and central [140] sources. Preliminary evidence suggests that inhibition of NOS increases the responsiveness of centralis neurons to muscarinic activation [112] and blocks a crossed inhibition in which rhythmic esophagomotor activity induced by NTS mACh receptor stimulation on one side is suppressed by the identical stimulus applied contralaterally [141]. In cat, intracerebroventricular administration of the NOS inhibitor L-NMMA significantly reduced the number of reflex oropharyngeal swallows and the amplitude of peristalsis, particularly in the smooth muscle distal, and much less in the striated muscle proximal esophagus [142]. Thus, NO appears to be an important mediator in the SPG. The significantly different effects of NOS inhibition on striated and smooth muscle portions of the esophagus point to anatomically and chemically distinct control mechanisms for peristalsis in the proximal and distal esophagus.

Information transfer from NTS esophageal premotoneurons to ambigual compact formation (AMBc) motoneurons involves a complex interplay of glutamatergic fast transmission with somatostatin [143] and probably also nitric oxide.

Somatostatin-mediated modulation of NMDA receptors plays a critical role in motoneuronal ESPS generation and spike production [129]. The NTSce–AMBc pathway appears to carry predominantly excitatory fibers, suggesting that inhibitory inputs to esophageal motoneurons, such as that evidenced by deglutitive inhibition of esophageal peristalsis [66], arise either from other NTS subnuclei or from neurons in the bulbar reticular formation. Few, if any, of the fibers in this pathway project to the contralateral AMBc. The exact source of crossed projections from the NTS to the AMBc [84] remains to be identified. Besides a cholinergic nicotinic ACh receptor-mediated input, the RFiz is a likely source of glutamatergic EPSPs detected in AMBc neurons [86].

Outlook

An important general principle to emerge from the evidence described in the preceding section is the autonomy of the deglutitive coordination from peripheral sensory input under certain experimental conditions. Evidently, a discrete neurochemical stimulus impinging on what constitutes neuroanatomically Doty's "afferent portal" of the swallowing center [4, 12] can substitute for encoded sensory input to activate the complete, coordinated swallowing sequence. Because this form of afferent input does not provide specific timing cues, the central deglutitive network must have the capability of operating autonomously, that is, without or with only minimal afferent input. Clearly, however, the buccopharyngeal stage motor output is significantly modified by sensory feedback. Studies in the awake human have shown that motor timing of the initial stages of swallowing is regulated by bolus variables [144] and subglottic pressure or lung volume [145] as well as body posture [146]. Sensory input is of paramount importance in the esophageal stage of swallowing [11], the rat being no exception [95]. Yet certain aspects of motor programming such as rhythm generation

may be controlled centrally and remain functional in brainstem slice preparations [113, 125].

Some immediate challenges for future research arise from the neurochemical heterogeneity of NTSce neurons. For instance, do different neuronal phenotypes engage in specific functions in relation to (1) the regional variation in esophageal reflex motility; (2) the organization of premotor inhibitory processes; and (3) the diversity of projections within the dorsal vagal complex? A related intriguing issue is whether central commands to striated and smooth UAT musculature are channeled through the same premotor neuron pools. Similarly, it would be important to determine if some of the NTSim pharyngeal premotor neurons believed to project to esophageal premotor neurons of the NTSce are cholinergic in nature.

The nature of transmitters mediating deglutitive inhibition presents another enigma: if GABA- or glycinergic inhibition were not to contribute to intrinsic SPG operations at the NTS level, would these processes be confined to the RFpc/RFiz?

Finally, the issue of multifunctionality in swallowing interneurons [10], particularly those associated with the NTS, poses an unresolved problem. Given the potential diversity of interactions between the SPG and other medullary function generators, a high degree of sensory convergence and divergence of efferent output would be expected to occur at the level of second-order neurons, including those forming part of the SPG. Conceivably, neuromodulatory inputs impinging on the SPG network are required for channeling network function-specific patterns of excitation and inhibition through the SPG neuropil and associated local circuit neurons. In this manner, decoding of sensory input and stabilization of functionally dedicated circuits may be achieved. Besides "classical" neuromodulators, e.g., monoamines, elucidating the role of orexigenic and anorexigenic peptides and of neurotrophins in modulating swallowing represents an emerging field of research.

References

1. Bidder F. Beiträge zur Kenntniss der Wirkungen des Nervus laryngeus superior. Arch Anat Physiol Wissensch Med. 1856;322:492–507.
2. Mosso A. Über die Bewegungen der Speiserohre. Moleschotts Untersuch Naturlehre Menschen Thiere. 1876;11:327–49.
3. Miller FR, Sherrington CS. Some observations on the buccopharyngeal stage of reflex deglutition in the cat. Q J Exp Physiol. 1916;9:147–86.
4. Doty RW. The concept of neural centers. In: Fentress JC, editor. Simpler networks and behavior. Sunderland: Sinauer Associates; 1976. p. 251–65.
5. Miller AJ, Bieger D, Conklin J. Functional controls of deglutition. In: Perlman AL, Schulze-Delrieu K, editors. Deglutition and its disorders. San Diego: Singular; 1997. p. 43–97.
6. Paton JFR, Li Y-W, Kasparov S. Reflex response and convergence of pharyngoesophageal and peripheral chemoreceptors in the nucleus of the solitary tract. Neuroscience. 1999;93:143–54.
7. Salinas E, Abbott LF. Transfer of coded information from sensory to motor networks. J Neurosci. 1995;15:6461–74.
8. Bieger D. Neuropharmacologic correlates of deglutition: lessons from fictive swallowing. Dysphagia. 1991;6:147–64.
9. Bieger D, Neuhuber WL. Neural circuits and mediators regulating swallowing in the brainstem. GI Motility online. 2006;doi:10.1038/gimo74.
10. Jean A. Brain stem control of swallowing: neuronal networks and cellular mechanisms. Physiol Rev. 2001;81:929–69.
11. Lang IM. Brain stem control of the phases of swallowing. Dysphagia. 2009;24:333–48.
12. Doty RW. Neural organization of deglutition. In: Code CF, editor. Handbook of physiology, The alimentary canal, Section 6, vol IV. Washington, DC: American Physiological Society; 1968. p. 1861–902.
13. Rogers RC, Hermann GE, Travagli RA. Brainstem pathways responsible for oesophageal control of gastric motility and tone in the rat. J Physiol London. 1999;514:369–83.
14. Rossiter CD, Norman WP, Jain M, Hornby PJ, Benjamin S, Gillis RA. Control of lower esophageal sphincter pressure by two sites in dorsal motor nucleus of the vagus. Am J Physiol. 1990;259: G899–909.
15. Sang Q, Goyal RK. Lower esophageal sphincter relaxation and activation of medullary neurons by subdiaphragmatic vagal stimulation in the mouse. Gastroenterology. 2000;119:1600–9.
16. Gordon DC, Richmond FJ. Distribution of motoneurons supplying dorsal suboccipital and intervertebral muscles in the cat neck. J Comp Neurol. 1991;304:343–56.
17. Gottschall J, Neuhuber W, Müntener M, Mysicka A. The ansa cervicalis and the infrahyoid muscles of the rat. II. Motor and sensory neurons. Anat Embryol. 1980;159:59–69.
18. Krammer EB, Lischka MF, Egger TP, Riedl M, Gruber H. The motoneuronal organization of the spinal accessory nuclear complex. Adv Anat Embryol Cell Biol. 1987;103:1–62.
19. Richmond FJ, Scott DA, Abrahams VC. Distribution of motoneurons to the neck muscles, biventer cervicis, splenius and complexus in the cat. J Comp Neurol. 1978;181:451–63.
20. Altschuler SM. Laryngeal and respiratory protective reflexes. Am J Med. 2001;111(8A):90S–4.
21. Bieger D, Hopkins DA. Viscerotopic representation of the upper alimentary tract in the medulla oblongata of the rat: the nucleus ambiguus. J Comp Neurol. 1987;262:546–62.
22. Hopkins DA, Bieger D, DeVente J, Steinbusch HWM. Vagal efferent projections: viscerotopy, neurochemistry and effects of vagotomy. In: Holstege G, Bandler R, Saper CB, editors. The emotional motor system, Prog Brain Res. 107. p. 79–96.
23. Blessing WW, Oertel WH, Willoughby JO. Glutamic acid decarboxylase immunoreactivity is present in perikarya of neurons in nucleus tractus solitarius of rat. Brain Res. 1984;322:346–50.
24. Lewis DI. Dye-coupling between vagal motoneurones within the compact region of the adult rat nucleus ambiguus, in vitro. J Auton Nerv Syst. 1994;47:53–8.
25. Cunningham Jr ET, Sawchenko PE. Central neural control of esophageal motility: a review. Dysphagia. 1990;5:35–51.
26. Hopkins DA. Ultrastructure and synaptology of the nucleus ambiguus in the rat: the compact formation. J Comp Neurol. 1995;360:705–25.
27. Dütsch M, Eichhorn U, Wörl J, Wank M, Berthoud HR, Neuhuber WL. Vagal and spinal afferent innervation of the rat esophagus: a combined retrograde tracing and immunocytochemical study with special emphasis on calcium-binding proteins. J Comp Neurol. 1998;398:289–307.
28. Neuhuber WL, Wörl J, Berthoud HR, Conte B. NADPH-diaphorase-positive nerve fibers associated with motor end plates in the rat esophagus: evidence for co-innervation of striated muscle by enteric ganglia. Cell Tissue Res. 1994;276:23–30.
29. Wörl J, Neuhuber WL. Enteric co-innervation of motor endplates in the esophagus: state of the art ten years after. Histochem Cell Biol. 2005;123:117–30.
30. Boudaka A, Worl J, Shiina T, Neuhuber WL, Kobayashi H, Shimizu Y, Takewaki T. Involvement of TRPV1-dependent and -independent components in the regulation of vagally induced contractions in the mouse esophagus. Eur J Pharmacol. 2007;556:157–65.
31. Boudaka A, Wörl J, Shiina T, Shimizu Y, Takewaki T, Neuhuber WL. Galanin modulates vagally induced contractions in the mouse oesophagus. Neurogastroenterol Motil. 2009;21:180–8.
32. Izumi N, Matsuyama H, Ko M, Shimizu Y, Takewaki T. Role of intrinsic nitrergic neurons on vagally

mediated striated muscle contractions in the hamster oesophagus. J Physiol. 2003;551:287–94.

33. Wang YT, Neuman RS, Bieger D. Nicotinic cholinoceptor-mediated excitation in ambiguual motoneurons of the rat. Neuroscience. 1991;40: 759–67.

34. Neuhuber WL, Raab M, Berthoud HR, Worl J. Innervation of the mammalian esophagus. Adv Anat Embryol Cell Biol. 2006;185:1–73.

35. Mittal RK. The crural diaphragm, an external lower esophageal sphincter: a definitive study. Gastroenterology. 1993;105:1565–7.

36. Pickering M, Jones JFX. The diaphragm: two physiological muscles in one. J Anat. 2002;201:305–12.

37. Niedringhaus M, Jackson PG, Evans SRT, Verbalis JG, Gillis RA, Sahibzada N. Dorsal motor nucleus of the vagus: a site for evoking simultaneous changes in crural diaphragm activity, lower esophageal sphincter pressure, and fundus tone. Am J Physiol Regul Integr Comp Physiol. 2008;294:R121–31.

38. Niedringhaus M, Jackson PG, Pearson R, Shi M, Dretchen K, Gillis RA, Sahibzada N. Brainstem sites controlling the lower esophageal sphincter and crural diaphragm in the ferret: a neuroanatomical study. Auton Neurosci. 2008;144:50–60.

39. Young RL, Page AJ, Cooper NJ, Frisby CL, Blackshaw LA. Sensory and motor innervation of the crural diaphragm by the vagus nerves. Gastroenterology. 2010;138:1091–101.

40. Yates BJ, Smail JA, Stocker ST, Card JP. Transneuronal tracing of neural pathways controlling activity of diaphragm motoneurons in the ferret. Neuroscience. 1999;90:1501–13.

41. Liu J, Yamamoto Y, Schirmer BD, Ross RA, Mittal RK. Evidence for a peripheral mechanism of esophagocrural diaphragm inhibitory reflex in cats. Am J Physiol. 2000;278:G281–8.

42. Marfurt CF, Rajchert DM. Trigeminal primary afferent projections to "non-trigeminal" areas of the rat central nervous system. J Comp Neurol. 1991;355: 489–511.

43. Pfaller K, Arvidsson J. Central distribution of trigeminal and upper cervical primary afferents in the rat studied by anterograde transport of horseradish peroxidase conjugated to wheat germ agglutinin. J Comp Neurol. 1988;268:91–108.

44. Dessem D, Luo P. Jaw-muscle spindle afferent feedback to the cervical spinal cord in the rat. Exp Brain Res. 1999;128:451–9.

45. Mehler WR. Observations on the connectivity of the parvicellular reticular formation with respect to a vomiting center. Brain Behav Evol. 1983;23:63–80.

46. Zhang J, Yang R, Pendlebery W, Luo P. Monosynaptic circuitry of trigeminal proprioceptive afferents coordinating jaw movement with visceral and laryngeal activities in rats. Neuroscience. 2005;135:497–505.

47. Zhang J, Luo P, Pendlebury WW. Light and electron microscopic observations of a direct projection from mesencephalic trigeminal nucleus neurons to

hypoglossal motoneurons in the rat. Brain Res. 2001;917:67–80.

48. Altschuler SM, Bao X, Bieger D, Hopkins DA, Miselis RR. Viscerotopic representation of the upper alimentary tract in the rat: sensory ganglia and nuclei of the solitary and spinal trigeminal tracts. J Comp Neurol. 1989;283:248–68.

49. Hamilton RB, Norgren R. Central projections of gustatory nerves in the rat. J Comp Neurol. 1984;222:560–77.

50. Hayakawa T, Takanaga A, Maeda S, Seki M, Yajima Y. Subnuclear distribution of afferents from the oral, pharyngeal and laryngeal regions in the nucleus tractus solitarii of the rat: a study using transganglionic transport of cholera toxin. Neurosci Res. 2001;39:221–32.

51. Nomura S, Mizuno N. Central distribution of efferent and afferent components of the cervical branches of the vagus nerve: a HRP study in the cat. Anat Embryol (Berl). 1983;166:1–18.

52. Lu W-Y. Oesophageal premotor mechanisms in the rat. Ph.D. thesis, Memorial University of Newfoundland (1996).

53. Wank M, Neuhuber WL. Local differences in vagal afferent innervation of the rat esophagus are reflected by neurochemical differences at the level of sensory ganglia and by different brainstem projections. J Comp Neurol. 2001;435:41–59.

54. Wang YT, Bieger D. Role of solitarial GABA-ergic mechanisms in control of swallowing. Am J Physiol. 1991;161:R639–46.

55. Patrickson JW, Smith TE, Zhou S-S. Afferent projections of the superior and recurrent laryngeal nerves. Brain Res. 1991;539:169–74.

56. Neuhuber W, Sandoz PA. Vagal primary afferent terminals in the dorsal motor nucleus of the rat: are they making monosynaptic contact with preganglionic efferent neurons? Neurosci Lett. 1982;69:126–30.

57. Rinaman L, Card JP, Schwaber JS, Miselis RR. Ultrastructural demonstration of a gastric monosynaptic vagal circuit in the nucleus of the solitary tract. J Neurosci. 1989;9:1985–96.

58. Saha S, Batten TF, McWilliam PN. Glutamate-immunoreactivity in identified vagal afferent terminals of the cat: a study combining horseradish peroxidase tracing and postembedding electron microscopic immunogold staining. Exp Physiol. 1995;80:193–202.

59. Paton JFR, Kasparov S. Sensory channel specific modulation in the nucleus of the solitary tract. J Autonom Nerv Syst. 2000;80:117–29.

60. Hayakawa T, Takanaga A, Tanaka K, Maeda S, Seki M. Ultrastructure of the central subnucleus of the nucleus tractus solitarii and the esophageal afferent terminals in the rat. Anat Embryol. 2003;206:273–81.

61. Mrini A, Jean A. Synaptic organization of the interstitial subdivision of the nucleus tractus solitarii and of its laryngeal afferents in the rat. J Comp Neurol. 1995;355:221–36.

62. Atkinson L, Batten TF, Corbett EK, Sinfield JK, Deuchars J. Subcellular localization of neuronal nitric oxide synthase in the rat nucleus of the solitary tract in relation to vagal afferent inputs. Neuroscience. 2003;118:115–22.

63. Broussard DL, Bao X, Altschuler SM. Somatostatin immunoreactivity in esophageal premotor neurons of the rat. Neurosci Lett. 1998;250:201–4.

64. Cunningham Jr ET, Sawchenko PE. A circumscribed projection from the nucleus of the solitary tract to the nucleus ambiguus in the rat: anatomical evidence for somatostatin-28-immunoreactive interneurons subserving reflex control of esophageal motility. J Neurosci. 1989;9:1668–82.

65. Rogers RC, Travagli RA, Hermann GE. Noradrenergic neurons in the rat solitary nucleus participate in the esophageal-gastric relaxation reflex. Am J Physiol Integr Comp Physiol. 2003;285:R479–89.

66. Dong HH, Loomis CW, Bieger D. Distal and deglutitive inhibition in the rat esophagus: role of inhibitory neurotransmission in the nucleus tractus solitarii. Gastroenterology. 2000;118:328–36.

67. Broussard DL, Li X, Altschuler SM. Localization of GABAA alpha 1 mRNA subunit in the brainstem nuclei controlling esophageal peristalsis. Mol Brain Res. 1996;40:143–7.

68. Hayakawa T, Yajima Y, Zyo K. Ultrastructural characterization of pharyngeal and esophageal motoneurons in the nucleus ambiguus of the rat. J Comp Neurol. 1996;370:135–46.

69. Hayakawa T, Zheng JQ, Yajima Y. Direct synaptic projections to esophageal motoneurons in the nucleus ambiguus from the nucleus of the solitary tract of the rat. J Comp Neurol. 1997;381:18–30.

70. Hayakawa T, Zheng JQ, Seki M, Yajima Y. Synaptology of the direct projections from the nucleus of the solitary tract to pharyngeal motoneurons in the nucleus ambiguus of the rat. J Comp Neurol. 1998;393:391–401.

71. Saxon DW, Robertson GN, Hopkins DA. Ultrastructure and synaptology of the nucleus ambiguus in the rat: the semicompact and loose formations. J Comp Neurol. 1996;375:109–27.

72. Ross CA, Ruggiero DA, Reis DJ. Projections from the nucleus tractus solitarii to the rostral ventrolateral medulla. J Comp Neurol. 1985;242:511–34.

73. Cunningham Jr ET, Sawchenko PE. Dorsal medullary pathways subserving oromotor reflexes in the rat: implications for the central neural control of swallowing. J Comp Neurol. 2000;417:448–66.

74. Zerari-Mailly F, Pinganaud G, Dauvergne C, Buisseret P, Buisseret-Delmas C. Trigemino-reticulo-facial and trigemino-reticulo-hypoglossal pathways in the rat. J Comp Neurol. 2001;429:80–93.

75. Saxon DW, Hopkins DA. Efferent and collateral organization of paratrigeminal nucleus projections: an anterograde and retrograde fluorescent tracer study. J Comp Neurol. 1998;402:93–110.

76. Herbert H, Moga MM, Saper CB. Connections of the parabrachial nucleus with the nucleus of the solitary tract and the medullary reticular formation in the rat. J Comp Neurol. 1990;293:540–80.

77. Ruggiero DA, Giuliano R, Anwar M, Stornetta R, Reis DJ. Anatomical substrates of cholinergic-autonomic regulation in the rat. J Comp Neurol. 1990;292:1–53.

78. Tago H, McGeer PL, McGeer EG, Akiyama H, Hersh LB. Distribution of choline acetyltranferase immunopositive structures in the rat brainstem. Brain Res. 1989;495:271–97.

79. Amri M, Car A, Roman C. Axonal branching of medullary swallowing neurons projecting on the trigeminal and hypoglossal motor nuclei: demonstration by electrophysiological and fluorescent double labeling techniques. Exp Brain Res. 1990;81:384–90.

80. Li Y-Q, Takada M, Mizuno N. Premotor neurons projecting simultaneously to two orofacial motor nuclei by sending their branched axons. A study with a fluorescent retrograde double-labeling technique in the rat. Neurosci Lett. 1993;152:29–32.

81. Li Y-Q, Takada M, Mizuno N. Identification of premotor interneurons which project bilaterally to the trigeminal motor, facial and hypoglossal nuclei: a fluorescent retrograde double-labeling study in the rat. Brain Res. 1993;611:160–4.

82. Travers JB, Rinaman L. Identification of lingual motor control circuits using two strains of pseudorabies virus. Neuroscience. 2002;115:1139–51.

83. Beckman ME, Whitehead MC. Intramedullary connections of the rostral nucleus of the solitary tract in the hamster. Brain Res. 1991;557:265–79.

84. Hashim MA. Premotoneuronal organization of swallowing in the rat. Ph.D. thesis, Memorial University of Newfoundland (1989).

85. Hashim MA, Vyas D, Bieger D. Solitarial deglutitive efferents in the rat. Soc Neurosci Abstr. 1988;14:319.3.

86. Zhang M, Wang YT, Vyas DM, Neuman RS, Bieger D. Nicotinic cholinoceptor-mediated excitatory postsynaptic potentials in rat nucleus ambiguus. Exp Brain Res. 1993;96:83–8.

87. Bao X, Wiedner EB, Altschuler SM. Transsynaptic localization of pharyngeal premotor neurons in the rat. Brain Res. 1995;696:246–9.

88. Broussard DL, Lynn RB, Wiedner EB, Altschuler SM. Solitarial premotor projections to the rat esophagus and pharynx: implications for control of swallowing. Gastroenterology. 1998;144:1268–75.

89. Lang IM, Dean C, Medda BK, Aslam M, Shaker R. Differential activation of medullary vagal nuclei during different phases swallowing in the cat. Brain Res. 2004;1014:145–63.

90. Goyal RK, Padmanabhan R, San Q. Neural circuits in swallowing and abdominal vagal afferent-mediated lower esophageal sphincter relaxation. Am J Med. 2001;111(8A):95S–105.

91. Shihara M, Hori N, Hirooka Y, Eshima K, Akaike N, Takeshita A. Cholinergic systems in the nucleus of the solitary tract of rats. Am J Physiol. 1999;276: R1141–8.

92. Hermann GE, Travagli RA, Rogers RC. Esophageal-gastric relaxation reflex in rat: dual control of peripheral nitrergic and cholinergic transmission. Am J Physiol Regul Integr Comp Physiol. 2006;290:R1570–6.

93. Gestreau C, Milano S, Bianchi AL, Grélot L. Activity of dorsal respiratory group inspiratory neurons during laryngeal-induced fictive coughing and swallowing in decerebrate cats. Exp Brain Res. 1996;108:247–56.

94. Kessler JP, Jean A. Identification of the medullary swallowing regions in the rat. Exp Brain Res. 1985; 57:256–63.

95. Lu WY, Bieger D. Vagovagal reflex motility patterns of the rat esophagus. Am J Physiol Regul Integr Comp Physiol. 1998;274:R1425–35.

96. Lu WY, Bieger D. Vagal afferent transmission in the NTS mediating reflex responses of the rat esophagus. Am J Physiol Regul Integr Comp Physiol. 1998;274:R1436–45.

97. Jean A, Car A, Roman C. Comparison of activity in pontine vs. medullary neurones during swallowing. Exp Brain Res. 1975;22:211–20.

98. Martino R, Terrault N, Ezerzer F, Mikulis D, Diamant NE. Dysphagia in a patient with lateral medullary syndrome: insight into the central control of swallowing. Gastroenterology. 2001;121:420–6.

99. Amri M, Lamkadem M, Car A. Effects of lingual nerve and chewing cortex stimulation upon activity of the swallowing neurons located in the region of the hypoglossal motor nucleus. Brain Res. 1991; 548:144–55.

100. Gidda JS, Goyal RK. Swallow-evoked action potentials in vagal preganglionic efferents. J Neurophysiol. 1984;52:1169–80.

101. Roman C, Tieffenbach L. Enrégistrement de l'activité unitaire des fibres motrices vagales destinées à l'oesophage du Babouin. J Physiol Paris. 1972;64:479–506.

102. Zoungrana OR, Amri M, Car A, Roman C. Intracellular activity of motoneurons of the rostral nucleus ambiguus during swallowing in sheep. J Neurophysiol. 1997;77:909–22.

103. Tomume N, Takata M. Excitatory and inhibitory postsynaptic potentials in cat hypoglossal motoneurons during swallowing. Exp Brain Res. 1988; 71:262–72.

104. Amirali A, Tsai G, Schrader N, Weisz D, Sanders I. Mapping of brain stem neuronal circuitry active during swallowing. Ann Otol Rhinol Laryngol. 2001;110:502–13.

105. Sang Q, Goyal RK. Swallowing reflex and brain stem neurons activated by superior laryngeal nerve stimulation in the mouse. Am J Physiol Gastrointest Liver Physiol. 2001;280:G191–200.

106. Holstege G, Graveland G, Bijker-Biemond C, Schuddeboom I. Location of motoneurons innervat-ing soft palate, pharynx and upper esophagus. Anatomical evidence for a possible swallowing center in the pontine reticular formation. An HRP and autoradiographical tracing study. Brain Behav Evol. 1983;32:47–62.

107. Grélot L, Barillot JC, Bianchi AL. Central distribution of the efferent and afferent components of the pharyngeal branches of the vagus and glossopharyngeal nerves: an HRP study in the cat. Exp Brain Res. 1989;78:327–35.

108. Aylwin ML, Horowitz JM, Bonham AC. NMDA receptors contribute to primary visceral afferent transmission in the nucleus of the solitary tract. J Neurophysiol. 1997;77:2239–48.

109. Jean A, Kessler JP, Tell F. Nucleus tractus solitarii and deglutition: monoamines, excitatory acids and cellular properties. In: Baracco RA, editor. Nucleus of the solitary tract. Boca Raton: CRC Press; 1994. p. 355–69.

110. Bieger D. Muscarinic activation of rhombencephalic neurons controlling esophageal peristalsis in the rat. Neuropharmacology. 1984;23:1451–64.

111. Hashim MA, Bieger D. Excitatory amino acid receptor-mediated activation of solitarial deglutitive loci. Neuropharmacology. 1989;28:913–21.

112. Lu WY, Bieger D, Neuman RS. Does nitric oxide contribute to control of esophagomotor activity? Dysphagia. 1994;9:263.

113. Lu WY, Zhang M, Neuman RS, Bieger D. Fictive oesophageal peristalsis evoked by activation of muscarinic acetylcholine receptors in rat nucleus tractus solitarii. Neurogastroenterol Motil. 1997;9:247–56.

114. Kessler JP, Jean A. Evidence that activation of N-methyl-D-aspartate (NMDA) and non-NMDA receptors in the nucleus tractus solitarii trigger swallowing. Eur J Pharmacol. 1991;201:59–67.

115. Broussard DL, Wiedner EB, Li X, Altschuler SM. NMDAR1 mRNA expression in the brainstem circuit controlling esophageal peristalsis. Mol Brain Res. 1994;27:329–32.

116. Colin I, Blondeau C, Baude A. Neurokinin release in the rat nucleus of the solitary tract via NMDA and AMPA receptors. Neuroscience. 2002;115: 1023–33.

117. Young-Ho J, Bailey TW, Andresen MC. Cranial afferent glutamate heterosynaptically modulates GABA release onto second-order neurons via distinctly segregated metabotropic glutamate receptors. J Neurosci. 2004;24:9332–40.

118. Blessing WW. Distribution of glutamate decarboxylase-containing neurons in rabbit medulla oblongata with attention to intramedullary and spinal projections. Neuroscience. 1990;37:171–85.

119. Dufour A, Tell F, Kessler JP, Baude A. Mixed GABA-glycine synapses delineate a specific topography in the nucleus tractus solitarii of adult rat. J Physiol. 2010;588:1097–115.

120. Meeley MP, Ruggiero DA, Ishitsuka T, Reis DJ. Intrinsic gamma-aminobutyric acid neurons in the nucleus of the solitary tract and the rostral ventrolateral

medulla of the rat: an immunocytochemical and biochemical study. Neurosci Lett. 1985;58:83–9.

121. Saha S, Batten TF, McWilliam PN. Glycine-immunoreactive synaptic terminals in the nucleus tractus solitarii of the cat: ultrastructure and relationship to GABA-immunoreactive terminals. Synapse. 1999;33:192–206.

122. Sweazey RD. Distribution of GABA and glycine in the lamb nucleus of the solitary tract. Brain Res. 1996;737:275–86.

123. Tanaka I, Ezure K, Kondo M. Distribution of glycine transporter 2 mRNA-containing neurons in relation to glutamic acid decarboxylase mRNA-containing neurons in rat medulla. Neurosci Res. 2003;47:139–51.

124. Hockman CH, Weerasuriya A, Bieger D. GABA receptor-mediated inhibition of reflex deglutition in the cat. Dysphagia. 1996;11:209–15.

125. Tell F, Jean A. Ionic basis for endogenous rhythmic patterns induced by activation of N-methyl-D-aspartate receptors in neurons of the rat nucleus tractus solitarii. J Neurophysiol. 1993;70:2379–90.

126. Greenwood B, Blank E, Dodds WJ. Nicotine stimulates esophageal peristaltic contractions in cats by a central mechanism. Am J Physiol. 1992;262:G567–71.

127. Dodds WJ, Dent J, Hogan WJ, Arndorfer RC. Effect of atropine on esophageal motor function in humans. Am J Physiol. 1981;240:G290–6.

128. Paterson WG, Hynna-Liepert TT, Selucky M. Comparison of primary and secondary peristalsis in humans: effect of atropine. Am J Physiol Gastrointest Liver Physiol. 1991;260:G52–7.

129. Wang YT, Bieger D, Neuman RS. Activation of NMDA receptors is necessary for fast information transfer at brainstem vagal motoneurons. Brain Res. 1991;597:260–6.

130. Zagorodnyuk VP, Brookes SJ. Transduction sites of vagal mechanoreceptors in the Guinea pig esophagus. J Neuroscience. 2000;20:6249–55.

131. Wang YT, Neuman RS, Bieger D. Somatostatin inhibits nicotinic cholinoceptor mediated excitation in rat ambiguual motoneurons in vitro. Neurosci Lett. 1991;123:236–9.

132. Zheng H, Patterson LM, Berthoud HR. Orexin- A projections to the caudal medulla and orexin-induced c-Fos expression, food intake, and autonomic function. J Comp Neurol. 2005;485:127–42.

133. Kobashi M, Xuan SY, Fujita M, Mitoh Y, Matsuo R. Central ghrelin inhibits reflex swallowing elicited by activation of the superior laryngeal nerve in the rat. Regul Pept. 2010;160:19–25.

134. Félix B, Jean A, Roman C. Leptin inhibits swallowing in rats. Am J Physiol Regul Integr Comp Physiol. 2006;291:R657–63.

135. Cui RJ, Li X, Appleyard SM. Ghrelin inhibits visceral afferent activation of catecholamine neurons in the solitary tract nucleus. J Neurosci. 2011;31:3484–92.

136. Bariohay B, Tardivel C, Pio J, Jean A, Félix B. BDNF-TrkB signalling interacts with the GABAergic system to inhibit rhythmic swallowing in the rat. Am J Physiol Regul Integr Comp Physiol. 2008; 295:R1050–9.

137. Hermann GE, Nasse JS, Rogers RC. Alpha-1 adrenergic input to solitary nucleus neurones: calcium oscillations, excitation and gastric reflex control. J Physiol. 2005;562(2):553–68.

138. Broussard DL, Bao X, Li X, Altschuler SM. Co-localization of NOS and NMDAR receptor in esophageal premotor neurons of the rat. Neuroreport. 1995;6:2073–6.

139. Ohta A, Takagi H, Matsui T, Hamai Y, Iida S, Esumi H. Localization of nitric oxide synthase-immunoreactive neurons in the solitary nucleus and ventrolateral medulla oblongata of the rat: their relation to catecholaminergic neurons. Neurosci Lett. 1993;158:33–5.

140. Ruggiero DA, Mtui EP, Otake K, Anwar M. Central and primary visceral afferents to nucleus tractus solitarii may generate nitric oxide as a membrane-permeant neuronal messenger. J Comp Neurol. 1996; 364:51–67.

141. Lu WY, Bieger D, Neuman RS. Nitric oxide mediates crossed inhibition of rat esophageal premotoneurons. Dysphagia. 1995;10:137. abst.

142. Beyak MJ, Shuwen X, Collman PI, Valdez DT, Diamant NE. Central nervous system nitric oxide induces swallowing and esophageal peristalsis in the cat. Gastroenterology. 2000;119:377–85.

143. Wang YT, Zhang M, Neuman RS, Bieger D. Somatostatin regulates excitatory amino acid receptor-mediated fast excitatory postsynaptic potential components in vagal motoneurons. Neuroscience. 1993;53:7–9.

144. Shaker R, Ren J, Podvrsan B, Dodds WJ, Hogan WJ, Kern M, Hoffmann R, Hinz J. Effect of aging and bolus variables on pharyngeal and upper esophageal sphincter motor function. Am J Physiol. 1993;264:G427–32.

145. Gross DR, Atwood Jr CW, Grayhack JP, Shaiman S. Lung volume effects on pharyngeal swallowing physiology. J Appl Physiol. 2003;95:2211–7.

146. McFarland DH, Lund JP, Gagner M. Effects of posture on the coordination of respiration and swallowing. J Neurophysiol. 1994;72:2431–7.

147. Shiina T, Shimizu Y, Boudaka A, Wörl J, Takewaki T. Tachykinins are involved in local reflex modulation of vagally mediated striated muscle contractions in the rat esophagus via tachykinin NK1 receptors. Neuroscience. 2006;139:495–503.

148. Tsujimura T, Kondo M, Kitagawa J, Tsuboi Y, Saito K, Tohara H, Ueda K, Sessle BJ, Iwata K. Involvement of ERK phosphorylation in brainstem neurons in modulation of swallowing reflex in rats. J Physiol. 2009;587:805–17.

Part III

Preparatory/Oral Phase of Deglutition

Oral Phase Preparation and Propulsion: Anatomy, Physiology, Rheology, Mastication, and Transport

8

Koichiro Matsuo and Jeffrey B. Palmer

Abstract

The oral cavity is a chamber surrounded by and containing hard and soft tissues, notably the lips, cheeks, tongue, palate, and teeth. The oral cavity is the entrance to the digestive, vocal, and (at times) the respiratory tract. Thus, the structures of the oral cavity serve multiple functions in speaking, breathing, mastication and swallowing. Mastication, the initial phase of digestion, is the primary process of the oral preparatory phase of swallowing. Mastication is primarily controlled by motor pattern generators in the central nervous system and modified by internal factors such as dentition and saliva production and external factors such as food consistency. Coordinated motions of the jaws, tongue, soft palate, and hyoid bone reduce and moisten ingested food to render it suitable for swallowing, and transport food to the pharynx for bolus aggregation prior to swallowing. Saliva supports mastication by lubricating food during chewing, helping to forma bolus optimized for swallowing. Saliva also has protective functions for oral health. Food properties such as hardness, water content, flavor, and temperature modify masticatory performance and influence the initiation of swallowing.

Keywords

Oral phase preparation • Oral phase propulsion • Anatomy • Physiology • Rheology • Mastication • Transport

K. Matsuo
Department of Special Care Dentistry, Matsumoto Dental
University, 1780 Hirooka Gobara, Shiojiri,
Nagano, Japan
e-mail: kmatsuo@po.mdu.ac.jp

J.B. Palmer, MD (✉)
Physical Medicine and Rehabilitation, Johns Hopkins
Hospital, 600 North Wolfe Street, Phipps 160,
Baltimore, MD 21287, USA
e-mail: jpalmer@jhmi.edu

R. Shaker et al. (eds.), *Principles of Deglutition: A Multidisciplinary Text for Swallowing and its Disorders*,   117
DOI 10.1007/978-1-4614-3794-9_8, © Springer Science+Business Media New York 2013

Development, Anatomy and Physiology of the Oral Cavity

Anatomy of Structures

The oral cavity is a chamber surrounded by hard and soft tissues; the lips and cheeks form the anterior and lateral walls of the mouth. The upper and lower dental arches are inside the lips and cheeks. The mandible and suprahyoid muscles form the floor of the mouth and the tongue resides there. The oral cavity acts as the entrance of the digestive pathway as well as the vocal tract and, at times, the upper airway. Table 8.1 lists the innervation of the muscles of the oral cavity. Figure 8.1 shows the anatomy of the oral cavity.

The dental arches of the maxilla and mandible form the inside walls of the oral cavity. The teeth are important for mastication. The incisors cut (incise) ingested food, and the molars grind food. Masticatory muscles close the jaw and move it mediolaterally; the submental muscles open the jaw for chewing.

The roof of the oral cavity is formed by the hard and soft palate. The hard palate is anterior; it is the lower part of the maxilla. The posterior portion, the soft palate, consists of palatal muscles rather than bone. The posterior wall of the oral cavity is the fauces. The palatoglossal and palatopharyngeal arches form the fauces; these are folds of tissue surrounding the palatoglosssus and palatopharyngeus muscles. During nasal breathing at rest, the soft palate rests on the tongue surface. When the tongue and soft palate come into contact, they seal the oral cavity posteriorly, closing the fauces and separating the oral cavity from the pharynx [1]. During food processing and oropharyngeal food transport, the soft palate rises, opening the fauces and providing communication between the oral cavity and pharynx [2, 3]. The aroma of the masticated food is delivered from the oral cavity to the nasal cavity through the pharynx via shifts in air flow associated with masticatory jaw movement [4–6].

The hyoid bone plays a vital role in oral function. Muscles connecting the hyoid bone to the hard and soft tissues of the oral cavity, cranial bone, thyroid cartilage, and sternum enable jaw and tongue movements for mastication, swallowing, articulation, and breathing. The submental muscles

Table 8.1 Innervations of major muscles related to the oral cavity

Muscles	Cranial nerves	Muscles	Cranial nerves
Masticatory muscles		*Palatal muscles*	
Masseter	Trigeminal nerve (V)	Levator veli palatine	Pharyngeal plexus (IX, X)
Temporalis		Palatopharyngeous	
Lateral pterygoid		Palatoglossus	
Medial pterygoid		Uvulae	
		Tensor veli palatini	Trigeminal nerve (V)
Tongue muscles		*Pharyngeal muscles*	
Intrinsic tongue muscles	Hypoglossal nerve (XII)	Upper pharyngeal constrictor	Vagus nerve (X)
Genioglossus		Middle pharyngeal constrictor	
Hyoglossus		Cricophayrngeaus	
Styloglossus		Thyropharyngeus	
		Stylopharyngeus	Glossopharyngeal nerve (IX)
Supra-hyoid muscles		*Infra-hyoid muscles*	
Mylohyoid	Trigeminal nerve (V)	Thyrohyoid	Hypoglossal nerve (XII)
Anterior belly of digastric			
Posterior belly of digastric	Facial nerve (VII)	Sternohyoid	Cervical nerves (C1–C3)
Stylohyoid		Omohyoid	
Geniohyoid	Hypoglossal nerve (XII)	Sternothyroid	

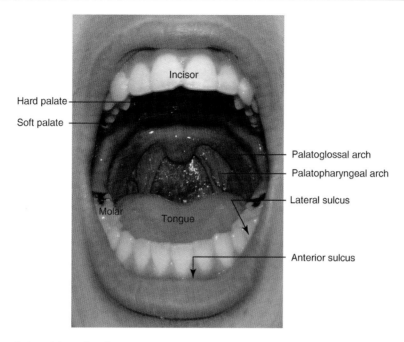

Fig. 8.1 *Frontal view* of the oral cavity

such as the mylohyoid, geniohyoid, and anterior belly of the digastric, running from the mandible to the hyoid bone, form the floor of the mouth. The tongue, resting on the floor on the mouth, is an isovolumic mass of muscle with no included bone or cartilage. The musculature of the tongue consists of extrinsic and intrinsic components; the former has mechanical connections to the mandible, hyoid, and cranial base, while the latter contains sets of intralingual muscle fiber bundles that have no connections to bony tissue. For mastication, swallowing, speech articulation, and breathing, the intrinsic and extrinsic tongue muscles produce a variety of movements and deformations of the isovolumic tongue associated with the motion of the other structures [7].

The lips and cheeks, which are composed of facial muscles, surround the outside of the dental arch. There are sulci between the jaws and lips and cheeks, called the anterior and lateral sulci. During chewing of food, the tongue and cheek push the food on the occlusal table during the time the jaw opens between closing strokes [8]. Partially masticated food can be accumulated in the lateral sulcus of the buccinator muscle is paralyzed.

Development of Anatomy

The anatomy of the oral cavity of infants is different from that of the adults and is more suitable for suckling rather than chewing (Fig. 8.2a). The infant has a flatter hard palate and fatty tissue in the buccinators to permit efficient generation of suction (subatmospheric pressure) for suckling. Teeth are not yet erupted in the infant so that the tongue is positioned between the upper and lower alveolar ridges. The volume of the oral cavity is small due to the lack of a dental arch, and the tongue fills the mouth. The location of the oral cavity relative to neighboring structures also differs between the infant and adult. The larynx and hyoid bone are higher in the neck in the infant, located posterior to the oral cavity. Because of high position of the larynx, the epiglottis is in contact with the soft palate (the so-called intranarial larynx that is typical of both adult and infantile anatomy in nonhuman mammals). The oral cavity does not directly communicate with the pharynx, and the larynx is open to the nasopharynx at rest. Thus, in between swallows, a soft tissue barrier separates the oral cavity and adjacent

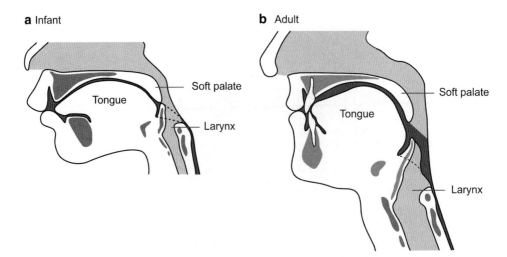

Fig. 8.2 Sagittal section of the oral cavity, pharynx, larynx in (**a**) infant and (**b**) adult human. (**a**) In infant human, the tongue and palate are flatter, and teeth are not erupted. The volume of the oral cavity is small and the tongue occupies the space. The larynx is high in position relative to the oral cavity. The epiglottis is in direct contact with the soft palate. (**b**) In adult human, the dentition of the maxilla and mandibular, and deeper hard palate increase the volume of the oral cavity and tongue. The larynx is lower in the neck, so the epiglottis loses contact with the soft palate

oropharynx from the nasopharynx and hypopharynx in the infant (but not the adult). During a swallow, the soft palate rises and opens the posterior oral cavity and oropharynx so the bolus can enter the hypopharynx.

The anatomy of the oral cavity in humans changes with development (Fig. 8.2b). With the growth of jaw bones, eruption of the teeth, and increase in the depth of the hard palate, the oral cavity increases its volume. Primary teeth erupt about 6 months after the birth, and the eruption is completed around 2 years of age. Permanent teeth are exchanged for the primary teeth from around 6 to 12 years of age. The relationship of the location of the oral cavity to the other structures changes with development. With increasing depth of the oral cavity and elongation of the neck, the larynx descends to a position lower in the neck. The contact of the soft palate and epiglottis is lost, and the soft tissue separation of the oral cavity and oropharynx from the hypophaynx is gone, so the oral cavity and oropharynx are open to the nasopharynx and hypopharynx.

Physiology

The oral cavity has multiple functions for mastication, swallowing, articulation, and breathing. Those physiological functions are controlled by the central nervous system and modulated by the input not only from receptors chiefly in the mouth but also in the nose, pharynx, and larynx.

Swallowing

During drinking of liquid and eating of solid food, the pharyngeal and esophageal stages have only minor differences (Fig. 8.3). The triturated bolus of solid food is more viscous than the typical bolus of liquid and contains particles of reduced solid food in suspension. Thus the work of swallowing can be greater and the pharyngeal and esophageal transit times longer. There is also a higher risk for retention of bits of triturated solid food in the oral and pharyngeal recesses after swallowing. The oral stage and the associated movements of food in the oral cavity and oropharynx are quite different in drinking and

(A) liquid swallow

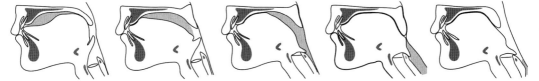

Fig. 8.3 Schematic drawings of normal swallowing of a liquid bolus. The bolus is held between the anterior surface of the tongue and hard palate, in a "swallow-ready" position. The oral cavity and pharynx are separated by posterior tongue–palate contact. When the swallow is initiated, the posterior tongue drops down and the soft palate rises, opening the fauces and permitting bolus flow from the oral cavity to the pharynx

eating. The physiology of drinking can be described with the four-stage model for swallowing a liquid bolus [9, 10]; intake of solid food will be described below.

When drinking liquid from a cup or by a straw, the liquid bolus is taken into the mouth and placed in the anterior part of the floor of the mouth or on the tongue surface until swallow initiation. Before the swallow is initiated, the lips and jaws are closed and the tongue holds the liquid bolus against the hard palate surrounded by the upper dental arch. Posteriorly, the fauces is sealed by the soft palate and tongue contact to prevent the liquid bolus leaking into the oropharynx before the swallow. Passage of a portion of the liquid bolus prior to swallow onset is relatively common, however, depending on bolus consistency (see Rheology below), especially in very young and elderly individuals and in a wide variety of diseases and disorders. In both infants and adults, the fauces open when the liquid bolus on the oral tongue surface is propelled to the oropharynx. When eating solid food, in contrast, the fauces are not sealed because the tongue and soft palate move continuously during mastication [3, 11], and the food bolus is moved to the pharynx prior to swallowing [12]. The details of mastication and oral food transport are described later in this chapter.

Articulation

Coordination of the movements of the jaw, tongue, lips and hyoid bone change the shape of the vocal tract to produce various speech sounds. The tongue plays the main role in articulation. The coordinated actions of intrinsic and extrinsic tongue muscles produce a variety of movements and deformations of the isovolumic tongue. There is kinematic linkage between the movements of the tongue and jaw during speech and feeding [7, 11]. Most of the extrinsic tongue muscles are attached directly to the jaw. Thus jaw motion has a substantial effect on the changes in shape and position of the tongue [13]. The tongue has dynamic motion during speech and swallowing, but the coordination of the movement among different regions within the tongue or to jaw movement is different between during speech and swallowing. The tongue surface elevates sequentially from anterior to posterior in a wavelike manner, propelling the food bolus during swallowing. Motions of the jaw, hyoid, and tongue are tightly linked during eating and swallowing, both temporally and spatially. This linkage is much looser during speech [14]. The hyoid bone plays a key role in mastication and swallowing; it has a role in jaw opening during mastication and in pulling the larynx forward during swallowing. During speech, however, the movement of the hyoid bone has relatively little influence on tongue movement. Tongue movement during feeding has tight temporospatial relationships with hyoid movement, but is more independent from hyoid movement during speech [7]. The range of motion of the hyoid during speech is smaller than during feeding [15]. Motions of the hyoid bone during swallowing in human infants have not been reported. In infant miniature pigs, there are minimal motions of the jaw and hyoid bone during both suckling and drinking [16].

Respiration

In breathing, air may flow through either the nose or the mouth, but flow is usually through the nose. The soft palate has a critical role in determining the route of airflow [1]. During oral breathing, the soft palate elevates to open the fauces, separating the nasal cavity from the pharyngeal airway [17]. During nasal breathing, the soft palate is lowered and rests on the tongue, dilating the velopharyngeal isthmus (retro-palatal airway) [18]. Complex activities of several palatal muscles determine the position of the palate in respiration. The two main muscles for determining palatal position are the levator veli palatini and the palatoglossus. Both muscles are active during oral and nasal breathing. However, the levator raises the soft palate during oral breathing and the palatoglossus lowers it during nasal breathing [19].

The tongue is also critical in controlling upper airway patency. The genioglossus is tonically active to maintain the tongue position in the oral cavity, and is phasically active in breathing, contracting during inspiration. Subatmospheric pressure in the upper airways during inspiration tends to collapse the airway by pulling the tongue posteriorly; this action is opposed by phasic contraction of the genioglossus muscle [20].

Rheology (Factors to Initiate the Pharyngeal Swallow)

Traditionally, it was thought that the food is held in the mouth during the oral preparatory phases, and that the pharyngeal phase of swallowing is triggered when the bolus head passes the fauces [10]. However, food properties, such as the texture, temperature, taste, and volume, alter the timing of the swallow initiation and bolus location at the time of the swallow initiation (Table 8.2). The determinants of swallow initiation have been studied extensively, but remain poorly understood.

In liquid swallows, viscosity is known to alter swallow initiation; modifying the viscosity of liquids is a mainstay of dysphagia rehabilitation. As bolus viscosity increases, the oral transit time is extended and the time of initiation of the pharyngeal swallow is correspondingly delayed

Table 8.2 Factors influencing swallow initiation

Factor	Effect on swallow initiation
Viscosity	High viscosity delays swallow initiation [21, 22]
Taste	Sour taste facilitates swallow initiation [23–25]
Chemesthesis	Menthol and capsaicin facilitate swallow initiation [26, 27]
Sequential drinking	Bolus leading edge is usually in the valleculae or hypopharynx before swallow initiation [28–34]. Swallow initiation can be delayed
Eating solid food	Bolus leading edge is usually in the oropharynx or valleculae before swallow initiation [2]
Eating two-phase food	The bolus leading edge is usually in the hypopharynx before swallow initiation [35]

[21, 36]. Adding a thickening agent to a liquid is a useful compensatory maneuver for some people with dysphagia. The higher viscosity slows bolus flow, thus reducing premature leakage of liquid from the oral cavity and enabling a bolus position higher in the pharynx at swallow initiation. In some people, this can reduce or prevent aspiration, but it is by no means appropriate for all people with dysphagia [22, 37, 38].

Taste and chemesthesis can facilitate swallow initiation. Chemesthesis is defined as the sense of oral irritation mediated by the trigeminal nerve and responsible for the perception of the hotness of chili pepper, coolness of menthol, and carbonation; it is distinctly different from taste and has different neural substrates [23, 24]. Sour taste promotes initiation of swallowing more effectively than the other tastes [25–27]. Chemesthetic stimuli, such as menthol and capsaicin, facilitate swallow initiation as well [28, 29].

Sequential straw or cup drinking, or drinking larger volume (20–50 mL) alters the location of the bolus at swallow initiation [30–35, 39]. In sequential or continuous swallowing of liquid, the bolus head typically reaches the valleculae or hypopharynx before swallow onset. Thus, the timing of swallow initiation for sequential drinking is relatively delayed in comparison to swallowing a single liquid bolus. Infants commonly collect milk in the hypopharynx and valleculae

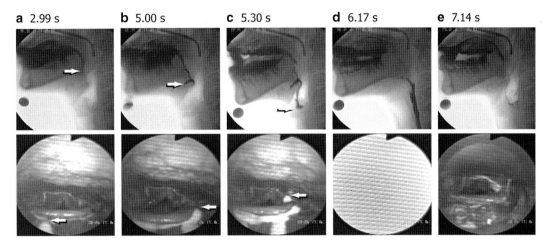

a 2.99 s   **b** 5.00 s   **c** 5.30 s   **d** 6.17 s   **e** 7.14 s

Fig. 8.4 Eating food with both liquid and soft solid phases (two-phase food). Selected images from concurrent videofluorographic and fiberoptic recordings of a healthy subject eating corned beef hash and liquid barium. *Arrows* on the images indicate the leading edge of the barium until swallowing. The liquid component enters (**a**) the valleculae, (**b**) hypopharynx, and (**c**) piriform sinus while chewing continues in the oral cavity prior to (**d**) swallow initiation. (**e**) There is no laryngeal penetration or aspiration

during one or more suckling cycles prior to swallowing [40].

The location of the leading edge of the barium at the time of swallow initiation is significantly different for eating food than swallowing liquid, especially single liquid swallows. Furthermore, when eating solid or semisolid food, the movement speed of the bolus in the pharynx and the amount and duration of food accumulating in the pharynx prior to swallow initiation are different among the initial food consistencies [2, 41]. Mastication modifies sold food, preparing a bolus with physical characteristics appropriate to initiate a swallow [42]. Prinz and Lucas hypothesize that cohesiveness of the food bolus is optimized for swallowing and that this depends on the size of food particles (a function of mastication) and mixing with the proper quantity of saliva [42]. The food particles processed by mastication and salivation, having reached optimal cohesiveness, are then transported to the pharynx (stage II transport) for bolus formation before swallowing. The optimized cohesive forces help to maintain bolus integrity in the pharynx both before and during swallowing, thus reducing the risk of aspiration. Prinz and Lucas further suggested that if swallowing is delayed, excessive saliva can flood the bolus, separating particles and reducing cohesion, increasing the risk of losing bolus integrity. This is similar to the situation that arises when eating a biphasic food that includes both soft solid and thin liquid components. As predicted by Prinz and Lucas, the low viscosity liquid component can flow rapidly down to the hypopharynx a few seconds before swallowing under the influence of gravity, while the solid component remains in the oral cavity for food processing [41]. As seen in Fig. 8.4, when liquid enters the hypopharynx during chewing, it approaches the laryngeal vestibule at a time when the larynx remains open. This may cause aspiration, especially in cases of dysphagia with impaired swallow initiation.

Mastication

Masticatory Function

The Process Model of Feeding describes the process of mastication and swallowing. This model has its origin in studies of mammalian feeding [43–48] and was later adapted to feeding in humans [12] (Fig. 8.5). When eating solid food,

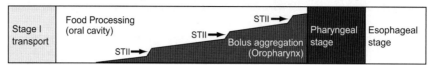

a Four sequence model: swallowing a liquid bolus

| Oral preparatory stage | Oral propulsive stage | Pharyngeal stage | Esophageal stage |

b Process model: eating food

Fig. 8.5 Models for consuming (**a**) liquids and (**b**) solids. (**a**) Drinking liquid, four-stage model. The bolus is placed in swallow-ready position (oral preparatory stage), propelled from the oral cavity to the pharynx (oral propulsive stage), through the pharynx and upper esophageal sphincter (pharyngeal stage), and finally down the esophagus and through the lower esophageal sphincter to the stomach (esophageal stage). Drinking liquids, there is minimal temporal overlap between stages. (**b**) When eating solid food, the food is chewed in the oral cavity (food processing). Chewing can continue while chewed food is propelled to the oropharynx (stage II transport, STII) and collected there (bolus aggregation) prior to the onset of the pharyngeal stage of swallowing. Thus, in the process model, food processing and stage II transport (with aggregation in the pharynx) can overlap substantially in time

the food is first transported to the occlusal surfaces of the postcanine dentition (stage I transport). Then, in chewing, the food is reduced in size and lubricated with saliva (food processing). Triturated food is transported to the oropharynx (stage II transport) and collects there (bolus aggregation) until swallow onset. Food processing often continues during stage II transport and bolus aggregation in the oropharynx. Thus, the oral preparatory phase (food processing) and oral propulsive phase (stage II transport and bolus aggregation) can overlap in time during feeding.

Stage I Transport

When food enters the mouth, it is positioned on the tongue surface. The mouth opens, then the tongue carries the food back to the postcanine region and rotates laterally, placing it on the occlusal surfaces of lower teeth for food processing (stage I transport, Fig. 8.6a). We call this process of carrying the food posteriorly on the surface of the tongue a "pullback" mechanism of intraoral food transport.

Food Processing

Food processing immediately follows stage I transport. During food processing, food particles are reduced in size by mastication and softened by saliva until the food consistency is appropriate

for swallowing. Rhythmic jaw movements for chewing continue until all of the food is prepared for swallowing, with only momentary pauses for each swallow. Cyclic movement of the jaw in processing is tightly coordinated with the movements of the tongue, cheek, soft palate, and hyoid bone. During food processing, the tongue and soft palate move cyclically in association with masticatory jaw movement. This keeps the fauces open so there is no seal between the oral cavity and pharynx [2, 3]. Jaw closing decreases the volume of the oral cavity and pumps air into the nasal cavity through the pharynx, delivering the food's aroma to chemoreceptors in the nasopharynx and nasal cavity [4–6].

Tongue movement during chewing is temporospatially linked with masticatory jaw movement during food processing [8, 11] (Fig. 8.7). Tongue movements during processing are large in both the anteroposterior and vertical dimensions; jaw movements are similarly large in the vertical dimension but smaller in the horizontal dimension. During jaw opening, the tongue generally moves forward as the jaw opens, and backward as it closes. The tongue also moves superoinferiorly and mediolaterally and rotates on its long (anteroposterior) axis during chewing [8]. These movements help keep the food on the occlusal surface of the lower teeth. As the teeth

a Stage I transport

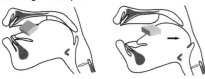

b Stage II transport

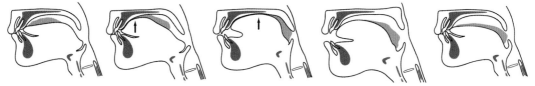

Fig. 8.6 Schematic images of stage I (**a**) and stage II transport (**b**). *Arrows* indicate the direction of tongue movement. (**a**) Ingested food is transported to the molar region by *pullback* and rotation of the tongue. The food does not push upward against the palate. Food processing begins immediately after stage I transport is completed.

(**b**) Chewed food is positioned on the center of the tongue and transported to the oropharyngeal tongue surface by *squeeze-back* of the food by the tongue pressing upward against the palate. Stage II transport occurs intermittently during food processing so a bolus can gradually accumulate in the oropharynx prior to swallow onset

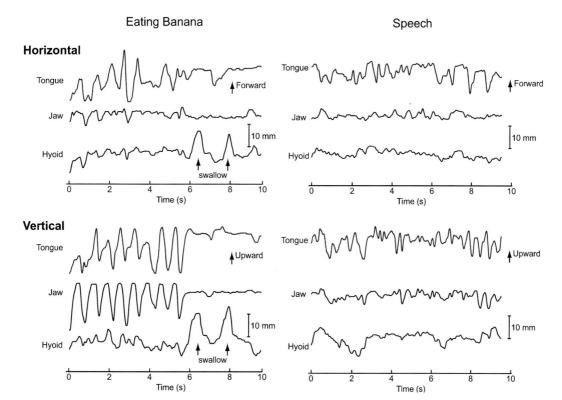

Fig. 8.7 Eating and Speaking: graph showing motions of an anterior tongue surface marker (tongue), the jaw, and the hyoid bone in the horizontal and vertical dimensions [7]. A complete sequence of a healthy subject eating banana is shown on the *left*; motion while the same subject reads a portion of the "Grandfather Passage" is shown on the *right*. *Upward* on the graphs represents motions

forward or upward. When eating banana, the tongue moves cyclically in horizontal and vertical dimensions. Tongue movement showed tight temporospatial linkage to jaw and hyoid movements during feeding, especially in the vertical dimension. In speech, the displacements were relatively small and irregular, and the temporospatial linkages among structures were weak

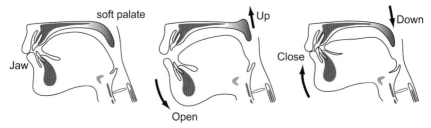

a soft plate motion associated with masticatory jaw movement

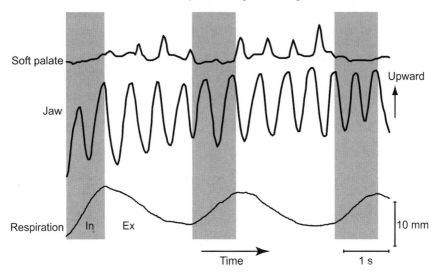

b vertical movement of the soft plate and jaw during mastication

Fig. 8.8 The soft palate in mastication. (**a**) Movements of the soft palate associated with masticatory jaw movement. The soft palate moves upward as the jaw opens, and moves downward as the jaw closes. (**b**) *Vertical positions* of the soft palate and jaw, and respiration (lower trace) over time during mastication. *Upward* on the figure represents movement upward or increasing tidal volume. Motion of the soft palate is temporally linked to jaw movement but not in every motion cycle. Soft palate motion is diminished during inspiration

approach occlusion during the closing stroke, the particle of the food is squeezed off the occlusal surfaces of the lower teeth. The tongue and cheek alternately push against the medial and lateral surfaces of the food, respectively, during jaw opening, pushing the food back onto the occlusal surfaces. After one or more cycles of the tongue pushing the food laterally, the food is shifted to lateral sulcus. The cheek then pushes it medially to replace it on the occlusal surfaces.

During mastication, active food reduction is generally performed on one side of the mouth at a time; this side is called the "working side," while the opposite side is known as the "balancing side."

Mastication can also be performed on both sides simultaneously but this "bilateral mastication" is less common. The tongue sometimes carries the whole piece or a portion of the food from the working side to the balancing side of the mouth for brief storage on the balancing side, for bilateral chewing, or to reverse the balancing and working sides [8].

The soft palate moves cyclically during chewing, and this movement is temporally (but not mechanically) linked to jaw movement [3] (Fig. 8.8a). The soft palate often elevates intermittently during processing and stage II transport. However, the temporospatial relationship between movements of the jaw and soft palate during food processing is totally different from their relationship during swallowing [49]. In chewing, the soft palate moves upward as the jaw opens and downward as the jaw closes. This masticatory soft palate elevation is less frequent during inspiration than expiration probably because soft palate elevation is suppressed to maintain retropalatal airway patency during inspiration [50] (Fig. 8.8b).

Stage II Transport

When a portion of the masticated solid food in the oral cavity is suitable for swallowing, the triturated food is segregated from the particles on the occlusal surface and gathered on the dorsal surface of the tongue. The food is propelled back through the fauces to the oropharynx by the tongue squeezing it back along the palate (stage II transport, Fig. 8.6b) [2, 51]. Stage II transport is primarily driven by the tongue, and does not require gravity, though it is assisted by gravity in the upright position [41, 52]. During stage II transport cycles, the tongue squeezes the food bolus back along the palate during jaw opening, and the soft palate elevates briefly after that squeeze-back action [3]. We call this mechanism of food transport by pressing back along the palate "squeeze back" to differentiate from the pullback mechanism of stage I transport, wherein the tongue remains in a lowered position so the food does not contact the palate. The mechanism for the oral propulsive phase when drinking liquids is similarly a squeeze-back mechanism. The neural mechanism underlying stage II transport is not known. It is possible that the same neural mechanism controls the oral squeeze-back action for liquid swallows and for stage II transport of masticated solid food.

Stage II transport occurs intermittently during food processing [3], but the frequency of stage II transport cycles increases over time from initial ingestion toward the swallow. The transported food accumulates on the oropharyngeal surface of the tongue and in the valleculae. Chewing continues, and the bolus in the oropharynx is increased incrementally by subsequent stage II transport cycles. The duration of bolus aggregation in the oropharynx ranges from a fraction of a second to about ten seconds, and has substantial interindividual variation [2]. The bolus aggregation in the pharynx ends when a swallow is initiated.

Factors Influencing Masticatory Performance

Masticatory performance is basically controlled by the central nervous system, but also influenced by internal factors such as dentition, bite force, saliva production, and external factors such as food texture, or other physical properties of the food (Table 8.3).

Dentition

Dentition has a significant impact on masticatory performance. Missing teeth, decrease in occlusal contact areas, use of removal prosthetic devices, and reduction in bite force can reduce masticatory performance [53, 54, 56–58]. Subjects with a decreased number of postcanine teeth or reduced functional occlusal contact areas need more chewing strokes compared to subjects with natural dentition [56, 57]. But the particle size of the swallowed bolus is larger for subjects with decreased dentition or denture wearer due to lower masticatory efficiency [57, 59]. The number of occlusal units has significant influence on the swallowing threshold, defined here as the number of chewing strokes used to prepare a given piece of food for swallowing [55, 56]. There is a small effect of gender or age on masticatory performance when eliminating the confounding effects of missing teeth or the other illness [53, 56, 60]. On the other hand, there is substantial variation in masticatory performance among subjects [2, 56]. The swallowing threshold depends on individual performance; there are slow and fast eaters.

Food Properties

The physical and sensory characteristics of food affect feeding behavior including food processing and pre-swallow food transport [2, 61]. The influence of food hardness on chewing behavior has been studied extensively using both natural foods and artificial test foods. The number of chewing cycles and chewing duration to prepare

Table 8.3 Internal and external factors affecting masticatory function

Influence factors	Outcome of masticatory functions
Internal factors	
Loss of post-canine teeth; reduced area of functional occlusal contacts; or use of dentures	Increased number chewing strokes [50, 51]
	Larger particle size of the swallowed bolus [51, 53]
Age, gender	A small effect on masticatory performance but significant interindividual difference [50, 52, 54]
External factors	
Hardness of food	Increased number of chewing strokes
	Longer duration of chewing and pharyngeal aggregation [2]
Dryness of food	Increased chewing duration, more saliva [55]

a food for swallowing increase with hardness of food. The duration that the masticated food is aggregated on the pharyngeal surface of the tongue is also extended with greater hardness of the food [2]. Dryness also influences masticatory performance. The duration of chewing cycles needed to reduce food particle sizes is longer with dry foods.

Salivary Production

Salivary flow has several protective functions for oral health; it prevents tooth decay, aids digestion by providing digestive enzymes, acts as a buffer to protect the mucosa from acids or alkali, moistens the oral mucosa, washes out dental plaques, and lubricates food during chewing to form an optimized bolus during mastication (Table 8.4). Healthy adults produce and swallow 1.0–1.5 L of saliva per day on the average. The autonomic nervous system controls saliva secretion including the balance of serous and mucous fluid. Dysphagic individuals can have difficulty dealing with the normal amount of salivary secretion and fail to swallow it, resulting in overflow aspiration or anterior loss of saliva (drooling from the mouth). On the other hand, xerostomia or dry mouth after radiotherapy can also worsen dysphagia.

Anatomy of Salivary Glands

Saliva is secreted from the major and minor salivary glands. The parotid, submandibular, and

Table 8.4 Salivary functions

Antimicrobial	Antimicrobial compounds and immunoglobulins control normal bacteria flora and protect the oral cavity from the pathogens
Buffering	Bicarbonate system neutralizes acids produced by bacteria or gastric secretions
Digestive	Digestive enzymes (e.g., amylase and lipase) decompose starch and lipids
Feeding	Saliva releases the taste and flavor of food during chewing, and lubricates the chewed food to facilitate bolus formation and swallowing
Protective	Mucin coats the oral mucosa
Remineralization	Calcium and phosphonate repair dental enamel

sublingual glands are the major salivary glands. Saliva secretion is controlled by both sympathetic and parasympathetic nervous systems, but mainly by the parasympathetic. The parotid is the largest salivary gland and is located antero-inferior to the auricle. The parotid gland mainly produces serous fluid. Preganglionic parasympathetic fibers originate in the inferior salivatory nucleus located in the medulla, and synapse in the otic ganglion. Postganglionic fibers travel to the parotid gland in the glossopharyngeal nerve. The submandibular glands are located in the digastric triangle on each side, bordered above by the lower border of the body of the mandible and inferiorly by the anterior and posterior bellies of the digastric muscle. The sublingual glands are above the mylohyoid muscle. The submandibular and sublingual glands produce both serous and mucous fluid. Pregangliotic parasympathetic fibers originate in the superior salivatory nucleus and synapse in the submandibular ganglion. Postganglionic fibers to the submandibular and sublingual glands travel in the facial nerve (corda tympani branch). Parasympathetic fibers promote serous saliva secretion, and a small amount of mucous saliva is secreted when the sympathetic innervation is stimulated. The minor salivary glands are located in the mucosa of the lips, cheeks, tongue, and palate. Saliva secretion is stimulated by gustatory and mechanical inputs from oral mucosa, and modified by the supratentorial region.

Table 8.5 Causes of dry mouth

Functional issues of salivary glands
Sjögren's syndrome
Sarcoidosis
Malignant lymphoma
Acquired immunodeficiency syndrome (AIDS)
Graft versus host disease (GVHD)
Iatrogenic issues
Radiation therapy for head–neck cancer treatment
Anticholinergic medications
Systemic issues
Metabolic: dehydration, diabetes mellitus, kidney failure, heart failure, hyperthyroidism, diarrhea, diabetes insipidus
Evaporative: open mouth, mouth breathing, hyperpnea

Function of Saliva

Saliva is a liquid containing various elements. Antimicrobial compounds and immunoglobulins control the normal bacteria flora and protect the oral cavity from pathogenic bacteria to protect teeth from dental caries. Saliva is a buffer to neutralize acid produced by bacteria or gastric acid that may reach the oral cavity via extraesophageal reflux or regurgitation. Oral digestive enzymes, such as amylase or lipase, decompose starch or lipid to help digestion.

Saliva also plays an important role in feeding. Saliva flow rates are increased by the presence of food in the mouth and further increased by mastication [62]. When masticating food, saliva lubricates the food to assist in bolus formation on tongue surface before swallowing. The characteristics of the food also affect the amount of saliva during mastication. Dry food facilitates secretion of more saliva than does moist food. Saliva is also important to perception of taste and flavor. When particles of food are mixed with saliva, we can perceive the taste and flavor released from the food matrix [63].

Factors Affecting Saliva Production

Salivary gland hypofunction and xerostomia (dry mouth) are produced by various factors such as Sjögren's syndrome, and radiation therapy

for cancer of the head or neck [64] (Table 8.5). The salivary changes are often permanent. Various medications with anticholinergic side effects hamper saliva flow. Salivary gland hypofunction and xerostomia, the subjective sensation of a dry mouth, lead to deterioration of oral health and health-related quality of life. Poor salivary flow causes dental caries and periodontal disease which can be severe. Patients with xerostomia have trouble in eating due to inability to lubricate masticated food with resulting difficulty forming a bolus. Perception of taste and flavor sensation can also be impaired, with resulting loss of the enjoyment of eating.

References

1. Rodenstein DO, Stanescu DC. The soft palate and breathing. Am Rev Respir Dis. 1986;134:311–25.
2. Hiiemae KM, Palmer JB. Food transport and bolus formation during complete feeding sequences on foods of different initial consistency. Dysphagia. 1999;14:31–42.
3. Matsuo K, Hiiemae KM, Palmer JB. Cyclic motion of the soft palate in feeding. J Dent Res. 2005;84:39–42.
4. Hodgson M, Linforth RS, Taylor AJ. Simultaneous real-time measurements of mastication, swallowing, nasal airflow, and aroma release. J Agric Food Chem. 2003;51:5052–7.
5. Palmer JB, Hiiemae KM. Eating and breathing: interactions between respiration and feeding on solid food. Dysphagia. 2003;18:169–78.
6. Buettner A, Beer A, Hannig C, Settles M. Observation of the swallowing process by application of videofluoroscopy and real-time magnetic resonance

imaging-consequences for retronasal aroma stimulation. Chem Senses. 2001;26:1211–9.

7. Matsuo K, Palmer JB. Kinematic linkage of the tongue, jaw, and hyoid during eating and speech. Arch Oral Biol. 2010;55:325–31.

8. Mioche L, Hiiemae KM, Palmer JB. A postero-anterior videofluorographic study of the intra-oral management of food in man. Arch Oral Biol. 2002;47:267–80.

9. Dodds WJ, Stewart ET, Logemann JA. Physiology and radiology of the normal oral and pharyngeal phases of swallowing [see comments]. AJR Am J Roentgenol. 1990;154:953–63.

10. Logemann JA. Evaluation and treatment of swallowing disorders. 2nd ed. Austin, TX: Pro-Ed; 1998.

11. Palmer JB, Hiiemae KM, Liu J. Tongue-jaw linkages in human feeding: a preliminary videofluorographic study. Arch Oral Biol. 1997;42:429–41.

12. Palmer JB, Rudin NJ, Lara G, Crompton AW. Coordination of mastication and swallowing. Dysphagia. 1992;7:187–200.

13. Sanguineti V, Laboissiere R, Ostry DJ. A dynamic biomechanical model for neural control of speech production. J Acoust Soc Am. 1998;103:1615–27.

14. Green JR, Wang YT. Tongue-surface movement patterns during speech and swallowing. J Acoust Soc Am. 2003;113:2820–33.

15. Hiiemae KM, Palmer JB, Medicis SW, Hegener J, Scott Jackson B, Lieberman DE. Hyoid and tongue surface movements in speaking and eating. Arch Oral Biol. 2002;47:11–27.

16. Thexton AJ, Crompton AW, German RZ. Transition from suckling to drinking at weaning: a kinematic and electromyographic study in miniature pigs. J Exp Zool. 1998;280:327–43.

17. Rodenstein DO, Stanescu DC. Soft palate and oronasal breathing in humans. J Appl Physiol. 1984;57:651–7.

18. Hairston LE, Sauerland EK. Electromyography of the human palate: discharge patterns of the levator and tensor veli palatini. Electromyogr Clin Neurophysiol. 1981;21:287–97.

19. Tangel DJ, Mezzanotte WS, White DP. Respiratory-related control of palatoglossus and levator palatini muscle activity. J Appl Physiol. 1995;78:680–8.

20. Tsuiki S, Ono T, Ishiwata Y, Kuroda T. Functional divergence of human genioglossus motor units with respiratory-related activity. Eur Respir J. 2000;15:906–10.

21. Hiss SG, Strauss M, Treole K, Stuart A, Boutilier S. Effects of age, gender, bolus volume, bolus viscosity, and gustation on swallowing apnea onset relative to lingual bolus propulsion onset in normal adults. J Speech Lang Hear Res. 2004;47:572–83.

22. Robbins J, Gensler G, Hind J, Logemann JA, Lindblad AS, Brandt D, Baum H, Lilienfeld D, Kosek S, Lundy D, Dikeman K, Kazandjian M, Gramigna GD, McGarvey-Toler S, Miller Gardner PJ. Comparison of 2 interventions for liquid aspiration on pneumonia incidence: a randomized trial. Ann Intern Med. 2008;148:509–18.

23. Dessirier JM, Simons CT, Carstens MI, O'Mahony M, Carstens E. Psychophysical and neurobiological evidence that the oral sensation elicited by carbonated water is of chemogenic origin. Chem Senses. 2000;25:277–84.

24. Green BG, Alvarez-Reeves M, George P, Akirav C. Chemesthesis and taste: evidence of independent processing of sensation intensity. Physiol Behav. 2005;86:526–37.

25. Logemann JA, Pauloski BR, Colangelo L, Lazarus C, Fujiu M, Kahrilas PJ. Effects of a sour bolus on oropharyngeal swallowing measures in patients with neurogenic dysphagia. J Speech Hear Res. 1995;38:556–63.

26. Pelletier CA, Lawless HT. Effect of citric acid and citric acid-sucrose mixtures on swallowing in neurogenic oropharyngeal dysphagia. Dysphagia. 2003;18:231–41.

27. Leow LP, Huckabee ML, Sharma S, Tooley TP. The influence of taste on swallowing apnea, oral preparation time, and duration and amplitude of submental muscle contraction. Chem Senses. 2007;32:119–28.

28. Ebihara T, Ebihara S, Watando A, Okazaki T, Asada M, Ohrui T, Yamaya M, Arai H. Effects of menthol on the triggering of the swallowing reflex in elderly patients with dysphagia. Br J Clin Pharmacol. 2006;62:369–71.

29. Yamasaki M, Ebihara S, Ebihara T, Yamanda S, Arai H, Kohzuki M. Effects of capsiate on the triggering of the swallowing reflex in elderly patients with aspiration pneumonia. Geriatr Gerontol Int. 2010;10:107–9.

30. Daniels SK, Foundas AL. Swallowing physiology of sequential straw drinking. Dysphagia. 2001;16:176–82.

31. Martin-Harris B, Brodsky MB, Michel Y, Lee FS, Walters B. Delayed initiation of the pharyngeal swallow: normal variability in adult swallows. J Speech Lang Hear Res. 2007;50:585–94.

32. Stephen JR, Taves DH, Smith RC, Martin RE. Bolus location at the initiation of the pharyngeal stage of swallowing in healthy older adults. Dysphagia. 2005;20:266–72.

33. Chi-Fishman G, Stone M, McCall GN. Lingual action in normal sequential swallowing. J Speech Lang Hear Res. 1998;41:771–85.

34. Chi-Fishman G, Sonies BC. Motor strategy in rapid sequential swallowing: new insights. J Speech Lang Hear Res. 2000;43:1481–92.

35. Chi-Fishman G, Sonies BC. Kinematic strategies for hyoid movement in rapid sequential swallowing. J Speech Lang Hear Res. 2002;45:457–68.

36. Dantas RO, Kern MK, Massey BT, Dodds WJ, Kahrilas PJ, Brasseur JG, Cook IJ, Lang IM. Effect of swallowed bolus variables on oral and pharyngeal phases of swallowing. Am J Physiol. 1990;258:G675–81.

37. Lazarus CL, Logemann JA, Rademaker AW, Kahrilas PJ, Pajak T, Lazar R, Halper A. Effects of bolus volume, viscosity, and repeated swallows in nonstroke subjects and stroke patients. Arch Phys Med Rehabil. 1993;74:1066–70.

38. Clave P, de Kraa M, Arreola V, Girvent M, Farre R, Palomera E, Serra-Prat M. The effect of bolus viscosity on swallowing function in neurogenic dysphagia. Aliment Pharmacol Ther. 2006;24:1385–94.

39. Daniels SK, Corey DM, Hadskey LD, Legendre C, Priestly DH, Rosenbek JC, Foundas AL. Mechanism of sequential swallowing during straw drinking in healthy young and older adults. J Speech Lang Hear Res. 2004;47:33–45.

40. Newman LA, Cleveland RH, Blickman JG, Hillman RE, Jaramillo D. Videofluoroscopic analysis of the infant swallow. Invest Radiol. 1991;26:870–3.

41. Saitoh E, Shibata S, Matsuo K, Baba M, Fujii W, Palmer JB. Chewing and food consistency: effects on bolus transport and swallow initiation. Dysphagia. 2007;22:100–7.

42. Prinz JF, Lucas PW. An optimization model for mastication and swallowing in mammals. Proc R Soc Lond B Biol Sci. 1997;264:1715–21.

43. German RZ, Saxe SA, Crompton AW, Hiiemae KM. Food transport through the anterior oral cavity in macaques. Am J Phys Anthropol. 1989;80:369–77.

44. Hiiemae KM. Feeding in mammals. In: Schwenk K, editor. Feeding: form, function, and evolution in tetrapod vertebrates. 1st ed. San Diego, CA: Academic; 2000. p. 411–48.

45. Franks HA, Crompton AW, German RZ. Mechanism of intraoral transport in macaques. Am J Phys Anthropol. 1984;65:275–82.

46. Franks HA, German RZ, Crompton AW, Hiiemae KM. Mechanism of intra-oral transport in a herbivore, the hyrax (Procavia syriacus). Arch Oral Biol. 1985;30:539–44.

47. Thexton A, Hiiemae KM. The effect of food consistency upon jaw movement in the macaque: a cineradiographic study. J Dent Res. 1997;76:552–60.

48. Hylander WL, Johnson KR, Crompton AW. Loading patterns and jaw movements during mastication in Macaca fascicularis: a bone-strain, electromyographic, and cineradiographic analysis. Am J Phys Anthropol. 1987;72:287–314.

49. Matsuo K, Metani H, Mays KA, Palmer JB. Tempospatial linkage of soft palate and jaw movements in feeding [Japanese]. Jpn J Dysphagia Rehabil. 2008;12:20–30.

50. Matsuo K, Metani H, Mays KA, Palmer JB. Effects of respiration on soft palate movement in feeding. J Dent Res. 2010;89:1401–6.

51. Matsuo K, Palmer JB. Anatomy and physiology of feeding and swallowing: normal and abnormal. Phys Med Rehabil Clin North Am. 2008;19:691–707.

52. Palmer JB. Bolus aggregation in the oropharynx does not depend on gravity. Arch Phys Med Rehabil. 1998;79:691–6.

53. Hatch JP, Shinkai RS, Sakai S, Rugh JD, Paunovich ED. Determinants of masticatory performance in dentate adults. Arch Oral Biol. 2001;46:641–8.

54. Carlsson GE. Masticatory efficiency: the effect of age, the loss of teeth and prosthetic rehabilitation. Int Dent J. 1984;34:93–7.

55. Bourdiol P, Mioche L. Correlations between functional and occlusal tooth-surface areas and food texture during natural chewing sequences in humans. Arch Oral Biol. 2000;45:691–9.

56. Fontijn-Tekamp FA, van der Bilt A, Abbink JH, Bosman F. Swallowing threshold and masticatory performance in dentate adults. Physiol Behav. 2004; 83:431–6.

57. van der Bilt A, Olthoff LW, Bosman F, Oosterhaven SP. The effect of missing postcanine teeth on chewing performance in man. Arch Oral Biol. 1993;38:423–9.

58. Wayler AH, Muench ME, Kapur KK, Chauncey HH. Masticatory performance and food acceptability in persons with removable partial dentures, full dentures and intact natural dentition. J Gerontol. 1984;39: 284–9.

59. Yven C, Bonnet L, Cormier D, Monier S, Mioche L. Impaired mastication modifies the dynamics of bolus formation. Eur J Oral Sci. 2006;114:184–90.

60. Karlsson S, Carlsson GE. Characteristics of mandibular masticatory movement in young and elderly dentate subjects. J Dent Res. 1990;69:473–6.

61. Hiiemae K, Heath MR, Heath G, Kazazoglu E, Murray J, Sapper D, Hamblett K. Natural bites, food consistency and feeding behaviour in man. Arch Oral Biol. 1996;41:175–89.

62. Watanabe S, Dawes C. A comparison of the effects of tasting and chewing foods on the flow rate of whole saliva in man. Arch Oral Biol. 1988;33:761–4.

63. Engelen L, van den Keybus PA, de Wijk RA, Veerman EC, Amerongen AV, Bosman F, Prinz JF, van der Bilt A. The effect of saliva composition on texture perception of semi-solids. Arch Oral Biol. 2007;52:518–25.

64. Ship JA, Pillemer SR, Baum BJ. Xerostomia and the geriatric patient. J Am Geriatr Soc. 2002;50: 535–43.

Deglutitive Oral Pressure Phenomena

9

Robert M. Siwiec and Reza Shaker

Abstract

Intra-oral deglutitive pressure phenomena has been the topic of fewer studies compared to the other members of swallowing apparatus. Available studies mostly focus on swallow-induced and non-swallow-induced pressures generated by the tongue. They also address the effect of gender and age but rarely the effect of disease on lingual pressure. Available studies, have described the existence of an infra- lingual pressure phenomenon generated by apposition of the muscles of the floor of the mouth and the inferior/ventral surface of the tongue, as well as the supra lingual pressure phenomenon developed by sequential contact of the dorsum of the tongue with the hard palate generating the deglutitive lingual peristalsis that propels the bolus into the pharynx. Deglutitive activities of the base of the tongue contribute to the swallow related pharyngeal pressure phenomenon and is covered elsewhere.

Keywords

Deglutitive oral pressure phenomena • Supralingual pressure • Infralingual pressure • Taltic lingual • Oral pressure complex

R.M. Siwiec, MD
Division of Gastroenterology & Hepatology,
Gastroenterology Fellow, Medical College of Wisconisn,
Milwaukee, WI, USA

R. Shaker, MD (✉)
Division of Gastroenterology and Hepatology,
Digestive Disease Center, Clinical and Translational
Science Institute, Medical College of Wisconsin,
9200 W. Wisconsin Ave, Milwaukee, WI 53226, USA
e-mail: rshaker@mcw.edu

Based on radiographic observations, a considerable amount of information exists about the oral phase of swallowing [1–4]. However, the regional pressure phenomenon within the oral cavity during swallowing has been more difficult to study. Pressure events during the oral phase of swallowing have a short duration (0.5–1.1 s) and fast rise rate. The oral phase of swallowing exhibits a wide range of intersubject as well as intrasubject pressure variations.

The oral cavity exhibits two distinct pressure compartments during swallowing: supralingual and infralingual [5, 6].

R. Shaker et al. (eds.), *Principles of Deglutition: A Multidisciplinary Text for Swallowing and its Disorders*,
DOI 10.1007/978-1-4614-3794-9_9, © Springer Science+Business Media New York 2013

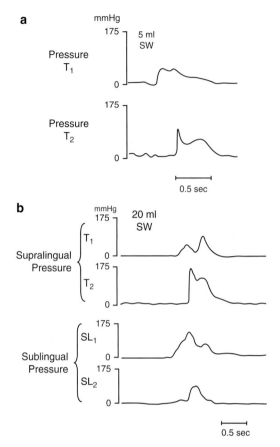

Fig. 9.1 (**a**). Supralingual pressures recorded during the oral phase of swallowing at the tip of the tongue (T1) and at the middle of the tongue (T2). The subject swallowed (SW) 5 ml of water. A peristaltic pressure wave is seen to propagate from T1 to T2. The wave at T1 is monophasic, whereas the wave at T2 has a spike and dome configuration, (**b**). Supralingual and sublingual pressures recorded during swallowing of a 20 ml bolus of water. Supralingual pressures were recorded at the tip of the tongue (T1) and at the middle of the tongue (T2). Sublingual pressure (SL) was recorded in the anterior mouth (SL1) and at the mid-mouth (SL2). With swallowing, a sequential peristaltic pressure wave is seen to propagate from T1 to T2. The wave at T1 is biphasic. From R. Shaker and I.M. Lang. Dysphagia 1994;9(4):221–8 with permission of Springer

The supralingual pressure complex is initiated in the anterior of the mouth when the tip of the tongue contacts in the front portion of the hard palate and begins to make sequential contact posteriorly toward the pharynx, thereby generating the peristaltic lingual/oral pressure complex (Fig. 9.1).

The amplitude, duration, and velocity of such oral peristaltic waves are not influenced

significantly by the volume of a swallowed water bolus, whereas the amplitude of such waves is significantly greater with a comparable volume of a semisolid such as mashed potato (Table 9.1). The increase in bolus consistency also seems to slow down the velocity of lingual peristalsis. During swallowing, the supralingual pressure complex demonstrates substantial radial asymmetry. The highest pressures are recorded when the manometric transducers face the tongue (Fig. 9.2).

The infralingual pressure complex also shows radial asymmetry. The highest pressures are recorded with the transducers facing the tongue. The infralingual peristaltic pressure waves have a longer duration than supralingual waves and generally are dome shaped. We propose that the sublingual pressure complex is produced by apposition of the inferior aspect of the tongue with the floor of the mouth, including the genioglossal, geniohyoid, and mylohyoid muscles, and at the onset of swallowing stabilizes the floor of the mouth [7, 8]. It is likely that contraction of these muscle groups explains the manometric phenomenon of the infralingual deglutitive pressure waves.

In the majority of subjects, water swallows, regardless of volume, are associated with a pressure wave that is recorded from the proximal part of the sublingual compartment and precedes the supralingual pressure wave. During dry swallows, the pressure waves that occur concurrently in the proximal and distal sublingual region coincide with the initiation of the pressure wave at the tip of the tongue. These findings suggest that the muscles of the floor of the mouth not only support the mouth floor, but also, by their early contraction, act in concert with extrinsic tongue muscles to provide a stable base upon which the tongue is able to push the bolus towards the pharynx. This notion is consistent with reported electromyographic data [7]. Analysis of the concurrent oral videoradiography and manometry clearly establishes that the point of glosso-palatal contact, immediately proximal to the tail of the bolus, corresponds to the upstroke onset of the peristaltic pressure wave recorded by manometry. Furthermore, the progression of the bolus tail, as seen on video recording, occurs at the same rate as

Table 9.1 Manometric features of supralingual peristaltic pressure waves: composite data from five normal subjects

Bolus	Tongue tips (T1)		Middle tongue (T2)		Transit time (s)
	Amplitude (mmHg)	Duration (s)	Amplitude (mmHg)	Duration (s)	T1–T2
DS (0 ml)	193±16	0.99±0.05	214±18	0.86±0.06	0.23±0.03
WS (2 ml)	158±12	1.01±0.05	192±20	0.87±0.05	0.21±0.03
WS (5 ml)	171±13	0.96±0.04	247±21	0.82±0.03	0.23±0.04
WS (10 ml)	166±10	0.99±0.04	225±16	0.71±0.04	0.25±0.03
WS (20 ml)	164±15	0.90±0.02	209±15	0.72±0.04	0.23±0.03
MP (5 ml)	383±30*	0.98±0.04	485±52*	0.77±0.03	0.33±0.03

Adapted from [6]
Values given as $x\pm$SE
DS dry swallow, *WS* west swallow, *MP* mashed potato
*Differed significantly ($p<0.05$) from WS (5 ml)

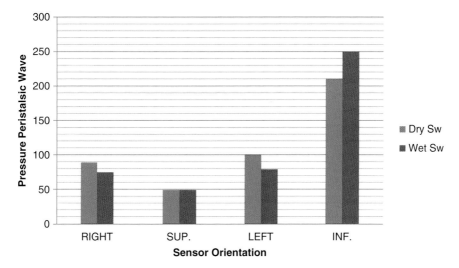

Fig. 9.2 Composite supralingual peristaltic pressure recorded from the mid-mouth in five normal subjects. Effect of radial orientation of the pressure transducer data is plotted as mean±1 SE for dry swallows and 5 ml wet swallow of water. Pressures recorded inferiorly (INF) with the transducer facing the tongue were substantially greater ($p<0.01$) than those recorded in any other radial orientation. From R. Shaker and I.M. Lang. Dysphagia 1994;9(4):221–8 with permission of Springer

the peristaltic pressure wave recorded manometrically. Sequential caudad contact of the tongue with the hard palate constitutes the major propulsive force during the oral phase of swallowing.

The increase in amplitude of the lingual pressure complexes for the mashed potato swallows suggests that feedback modulation related to bolus consistency exists between the mouth and the swallowing centers in the brainstem. On the other hand, the lack of correlation between liquid bolus volume and pressure complex amplitude or velocity suggests that feedback modification of intra-oral pressure activity is not volume dependent [5].

Earlier studies have documented significantly reduced isometric tongue pressure in the elderly compared to the young without an appreciable difference in maximal tongue pressure generated during swallowing between the two groups [9, 10].

Nondeglutitive and deglutitive lingual pressure measurements have been used to study the effect of age and gender and to determine the impact of various exercises and therapeutic approaches.

Using the Iowa Oral Performance Instrument with pressure transducers, tongue strength and endurance in 99 healthy volunteers ranging from

21 to 96 years of age were studied [11]. This study suggests that tongue strength is gender- and age-dependent and follows the same trends as hand function. Tongue strength is decreased in older individuals and females, while tongue endurance is gender- and age-independent.

Tongue-palate pressures recorded in healthy young adults performing water and nectar-thick juice swallows, effortful and noneffortful saliva swallows, as well as tongue-palate partial-pressure tasks have shown that there are pressure profile similarities between tongue resistance training tasks and liquid swallows [12].

Using lingual pressure recording devices, investigators have developed training strategies to improve tongue strength and pressure-generation precision in older individuals with dysphagia [13].

In conclusion, during the oral phase of swallowing lingual function produces a peristaltic pressure wave which propels the bolus into the pharynx. The upstroke of this peristaltic pressure wave is temporally associated with the tail of the propelled bolus. Preceding the lingual peristalsis is the development of sublingual pressure, reflecting contraction of the muscles of the floor of the mouth. Tongue strength is negatively affected by age and gender but can be modified by training exercises. Pressure signatures produced by lingual function can be used to objectively measure tongue strength and determine therapy outcomes.

References

1. Curtis DJ, et al. Timing in the normal pharyngeal swallow prospective selection and evaluation of 16 normal asymptomatic patients. Invest Radiol. 1984;19(6):523–9.
2. Donner MW. Swallowing mechanism and neuromuscular disorders. Semin Roentgenol. 1974;9(4):273–82.
3. Logemann J. Evaluation and treatment of swallowing disorders. San Diego, CA: College Hill Press; 1983.
4. Ramsey GH, et al. Cinefluorographic analysis of the mechanism of swallowing. Radiology. 1955;64(4): 498–518.
5. Shaker R, et al. Pressure-flow dynamics of the oral phase of swallowing. Dysphagia. 1988;3(2):79–84.
6. Shaker R, Lang IM. Effect of aging on the deglutitive oral, pharyngeal, and esophageal motor function. Dysphagia. 1994;9(4):221–8.
7. Doty RW. Neural organization of deglutition, in Handbook of Physiology. 1968. Publisher-American Physiology, Washington D.C.
8. Miller AJ. Neurophysiological basis of swallowing. Dysphagia. 1986;1:91–100.
9. Robbins J, et al. Oropharyngeal swallowing in normal adults of different ages. Gastroenterology. 1992;103(3):823–9.
10. Robbins J, et al. Age effects on lingual pressure generation as a risk factor for dysphagia. J Gerontol A Biol Sci Med Sci. 1995;50(5):M257–62.
11. Crow HC, Ship JA. Tongue strength and endurance in different aged individuals. J Gerontol A Biol Sci Med Sci. 1996;51(5):M247–50.
12. Steele CM, et al. Pressure profile similarities between tongue resistance training tasks and liquid swallows. J Rehabil Res Dev. 2010;47(7):651–60.
13. Yeates EM, Molfenter SM, Steele CM. Improvements in tongue strength and pressure-generation precision following a tongue-pressure training protocol in older individuals with dysphagia: three case reports. Clin Interv Aging. 2008;3(4):735–47.

Effects of Aging on the Oral Phase of Deglutition

10

Georgia A. Malandraki and JoAnne Robbins

Abstract

Swallowing is a highly complex activity that requires the sensorimotor integration and coordination of multiple anatomic structures, muscles, nerves and the brain. All of these functional components go through healthy chronologically-related anatomical and physiological changes as people age. The present chapter aims to focus on the aging changes that occur in primarily, but not solely, oral components of the swallowing process, highlighting the crucial role of the oral cavity in the initial stages of the swallowing mechanism and process. The oral components of normal deglutition are described in detail followed by a comprehensive summary of all the known motor, taste, sensory and neural changes affecting the oral swallow in healthy elders. Although these changes appear to be modest and to occur slowly and insidiously in most elders, at times they may signify reductions in the swallowing functional reserve capacity and endurance, increasing their vulnerability to dysphagia and airway invasion secondary to disease and environmental complications. Understanding these changes and their underlying peripheral and central mechanisms is necessary in finding solutions to treat and even prevent certain conditions.

Keywords

Effects of aging • Oral phase of deglutition • Oral cavity • Swallowing • Oral presbyphagia • Oropharyngeal swallow • Coupling and uncoupling • Neural implications

G.A. Malandraki, PhD, CCC-SLP
Program of Speech and Language Pathology,
Department of Biobehavioral Sciences,
Teachers College, Columbia University, 525 West 120th
Street, Thorndike Hall, Room 1052A, New York,
NY 10027, USA

J. Robbins, PhD, CCC-SLP, BRS-S (✉)
UW Department of Medicine, University of Wisconsin,
Wm. S. Middleton Memorial Veterans Hospital,
2500 Overlook Terrace, GRECC 11G, Madison,
WI 53705, USA
e-mail: jrobbin2@wisc.edu

R. Shaker et al. (eds.), *Principles of Deglutition: A Multidisciplinary Text for Swallowing and its Disorders*, 137
DOI 10.1007/978-1-4614-3794-9_10, © Springer Science+Business Media New York 2013

Introduction

Aging is a phenomenon with manifestations that depend on both environmental and genetic influences. The attempt to define aging and the concept of "elderly" can be challenging. Senescence (the preferred term by many scientists) is physiologically defined as the biological process that typically leads to a functional decline with age and ultimately to death [1, 2]. According to the World Health Organization [WHO], most developed world countries use the chronological age of 65 years as a definition of "elderly" [3], as the age at which individuals usually start receiving pension benefits, although no major specific change in physiological processes occur or start declining at that precise age.

With the time-delayed impact of high fertility rates after World War II, and the exciting improvements in healthcare and technology in recent years, life expectancy has significantly increased, while death rates at older ages have decreased pushing back death to "old old" age. According to the US Census bureau, the older US population (people aged 65 years and over) grew from 3 million in 1900 to 39 million in 2008, and in 2030 it is projected to be 72 million, representing nearly 20 % of the total US population. The oldest-old population (those aged 85 and over) grew from 100,000 in 1900 to 5.7 million in 2008, and could grow to 19 million by 2050. These increases are the result of great health and technological advancements, and bring many joys and satisfactions with them. At the same time, they raise concerns given the certain declines in many physiological and systemic functions seen in elders, and the need for effective prevention and rehabilitation of these declines.

The ability to swallow is not only one of the main processes that enables us to sustain life, but also is a significant part of the social everyday activities of all humans. As leisure time increases with the anticipated extended retirements of our increasing elderly population, and older adults look forward to more opportunities to participate in social activities that include eating and drinking, an ultimate irony is the anatomical and physiological changes that take place, increasing the risk for disordered swallowing with advancing age. Indeed, the loss of swallowing function can have devastating health implications, including nutrition and hydration declines, changes in health status, including pneumonia, and increased need for care provision, especially for older adults.

Swallowing is a highly complex activity that requires the sensorimotor integration and coordination of multiple anatomic structures, muscles, nerves, and the brain. All of these functional components, however, that are necessary for a complete and functional swallow to occur, go through "normal" or healthy chronologically related anatomical and physiological changes as people age.

The present chapter aims to focus on the aging changes that occur in primarily, but not solely, oral components of the swallowing process, highlighting the crucial role of the oral cavity in the initial stages of the swallowing mechanism and process. It has to be emphasized, however, that the division of swallowing into different stages is artificial, as swallowing is truly an integrated, dynamic and very rapid oropharyngeal process with downstream events, for instance, airway protection (e.g., vocal fold closing) occurring even simultaneously while food, liquid, and saliva are positioned on the anterior tongue initiating swallow activity [4].

Roles of Oral Cavity in Swallowing

The oral cavity serves multiple essential functions for human beings. Some of these include contributions in speaking, masticating, tasting, swallowing, laughing, smiling, and kissing [5]. For swallowing, the oral cavity is the location where the swallowing sequence is initiated. As already reported, the division of swallowing into different stages is artificial. Terms and concepts such as oral or pharyngeal stages or phases reflect the sequential course of bolus transit rather than the generally time-linked overlapping physiologic events in the oral cavity, pharynx, and larynx that affect healthy, safe swallowing. For the purposes of this chapter, however, this "stage or phase" traditional division will be utilized, with the reminder that this is merely organizational for our review purposes and is limited, representing the sequential morphologic pathway [lips to upper esophageal sphincter (UES)] through which bolus flows, not capturing the simultaneous or overlapping events up or down stream to ensure safe and effective swallowing.

Physiology of the Oral Stage of Swallowing

The oral stage of swallowing is reported to involve two functional phases, the oral preparatory and the oral transport phases [6].

Oral Preparatory Phase

In the oral preparatory phase, the material, which may comprise food, liquid, medication, or secretions referred to as the bolus, is prepared to be swallowed. This phase is under complete conscious control and the duration is variable and difficult to predict because it depends on bolus-related factors such as viscosity and volume, sensory factors including taste and temperature, and human status factors such as environment, age, hunger, motivation, and consciousness [7, 8]. For the oral preparatory phase to be initiated, sensory awareness of the food or liquid presence in the oral cavity, as well as taste input to the brainstem and the brain, is crucial before motor actions can be initiated. According to Blitzer, there are five motor actions that contribute to the success of the oral preparatory phase, once sensation and taste have been achieved: labial seal, buccal and facial tone, adequate and appropriate tongue movements, lowering of the velum, and, when necessary, mastication of the material, with lateral and rotary motion of the mandible [9].

Labial seal is achieved by the movements of the upper and lower lips after the material has entered the oral cavity and is intended to prevent anterior loss of the food or liquid from the mouth [10]. During labial seal, an open nasal airway is essential to maintenance of breathing [11]. This is accomplished with the lowering of the velum and

the elevation of the tongue base simultaneously also creating a barrier preventing the premature escape of the bolus into the pharynx [12].

Manipulation of the bolus during this phase requires movements of several structures that occur in temporal proximity. For liquid swallows the initial tongue tip motion for bolus manipulation is immediately followed by tongue base elevation, and subsequently by onset of superior hyoid bone movement and the initiation of the submental musculature activity [13]. These actions are usually completed in sequence and occur within approximately 200 milliseconds (ms) of one another [13].

When the food is to be masticated, the oral preparatory phase also can be subdivided into two components: an initial transport component, during which the tongue contributes to the placement of food between the molars and a reduction component which involves the segmentation of the food into smaller pieces and its mixture with saliva to become a bolus [14, 15]. Saliva production by the multiple salivary glands also is important, as it will maintain mucosa lubrication and will help with food manipulation, transport and digestion.

Oral Transport Phase

The oral transport phase of swallowing involves the transition of the bolus from the mouth to the oropharynx [16]. After the bolus has been formed, the tip of the tongue is elevated toward the superior alveolar ridge while the soft palate elevates and the posterior tongue depresses [17, 18]. The bolus is then propelled to the oropharynx as lingual muscles push the bolus superiorly and posteriorly [9, 17]. The onset of the oral transport phase is voluntary, but once the transport begins, conscious control of this phase is reduced. The oral transport phase generally takes 1–1.5 s to complete, but duration might be slightly longer with more viscous food [11]. It has been found that ~150 ms after the tongue starts its propelling movement, the hyoid bone initiates its anterior motion, immediately followed by epiglottic inversion and velar retraction and elevation [19]. In anticipation of bolus arrival, the UES starts to open

Table 10.1 Functional and anatomical components involved in the oral stage of swallowing

Swallowing phase	Function	Sensors/glands/muscles	Cranial nerves involved
Oral preparatory	Sensory awareness and taste	Mechanoreceptors, thermosensors, and chemoreceptors	V, VII and IX
	Saliva production	Salivary glands	VII and IX
	Labial seal	Facial muscles (orbicularis oris)	VII
	Buccal and labial tone	Facial muscles	VII
	Tongue movements	Lingual muscles	XII
	Linguavelar closure	Velar muscles	CN X and pharyngeal plexus
	Mastication	Muscles of mastication	V
	Initiation of pharyngeal events—hyoid movement and UES opening	Submental muscles and CP	V, IX, X, XI
Oral transport	Tongue movements—propelling	Lingual muscles	XII
	Buccal tone	Facial muscles	VII
	Velar elevation	Velar muscles	CN X and pharyngeal plexus

anytime between 400 and 750 ms subsequent to the initiation of the tongue propelling movement [13]. Bolus volume increases cause all these actions to occur earlier in time [13]. Events that are initiated during the oral transport phase also are considered to be critical to the successful implementation of laryngeal and pharyngeal physiological events. Anatomic and functional components of the oral preparatory and oral transport phases are included in Table 10.1.

Oral Presbyphagia

Aging affects swallowing just like it affects most other processes of the human body. Changes in both the functional and the anatomical components of the oral swallow have been reported in the literature. However, not all of these changes are statistically or functionally significant. Indeed, many healthy older adults can maintain and enjoy functional oral health and a completely functional oropharyngeal swallow until later in life [20, 21].

The age-related swallowing changes in healthy aging in the absence of disease are collectively termed presbyphagia [20, 22–24]. These include alterations in both the sensory and motor aspects of the oropharyngeal swallowing mechanism [20, 25–31].

Sensory Changes in Oral Swallowing

Taste, Smell, and Oral Sensation

Changes in taste perception, smell, and oral somatic sensation have been identified in healthy elders [32–35], and some of these changes may be responsible for several swallowing-related declines observed in the older population. Although, a direct correlation of reduced chemosensory abilities and oral sensation with aging swallowing has not been extensively investigated to date, these sensory losses are known to affect overall health, quality of life, pleasure levels during eating, nutritional choices, and status among elders [32, 34, 35]. Furthermore, chemosenses are important in preparing the body for digestion by eliciting secretions from the salivary glands, and the entire gastrointestinal system, therefore playing a significant role in the digestive tract [36, 37].

Specifically, regarding taste, older healthy adults are known to exhibit reduced sensitivity for all major tastes, including sour, sweet, bitter, salty, and amino acid tastes [38–40]. These reductions, however, are frequently reported only to be modest for older adults free of medical conditions and/or medication use [41]. Nevertheless, they can be significant for those who receive small or moderate amounts of medications even without a profound underlying medical condition, which is the case for the majority of older adults [34, 38]. Additionally, elders have been found to perceive a wide range of tastes as less intense than young adults [42, 43], and to have difficulty accurately correlating increases in concentration of tastant with increased perceptual intensity of the stimulus [41]. The cause(s) of these age-related taste changes are not known. In some studies anatomical alterations such as reduced number of taste buds or papillae have been reported [44], while other investigations hypothesize changes in the taste cell membranes [45]. In general, researchers agree that most taste changes seen in elders are secondary to medical conditions and medication use and are not primary aging consequences.

Taste is greatly associated with smell. Not infrequently, individuals will report reduced taste of a specific tastant, when in fact they may be unable to smell it. This is because food in the oral cavity is perceived through taste buds, but also through its odor which travels retronasally to the nasal cavity [34]. Indeed, changes in smell perception are more significant with aging than are taste changes. Odor recognition thresholds have been reported to be 2–15 times higher in healthy elders compared with younger counterparts [46, 47]. Discriminating different odors, as well as odor recall memory and odor recognition memory also become more challenging as people age [35, 48–50], with approximately 75 % of people over 80 years of age reported to have significant difficulty identifying odors [51]. These findings also were recently supported by neuroimaging research showing reduced neural orbitofrontal activations in elders during odor smelling functional Magnetic Resonance Imaging (fMRI) paradigms [52, 53].

Although taste and smell perceptions are decreased in older adults (smell more so than taste), oral somatic sensation is relatively retained [32, 33]. In a study by Fucci and colleagues, a statistically significant increase in the oral sensation detection threshold with an accompanying decrease in lingual sensation in elders was found [54]; however, increasing the

duration of the lingual stimulus improved their sensory responses [55]. In a more recent study of 60 healthy adults included in five different age groups, no age differences were found in thermal or somesthetic sensation and proprioception. Two point discrimination on the lips and cheeks seemed to reduce after the age of 80 [33], while tongue and palate sensation remained intact.

Motor Changes in the Oral Stage

Mastication

Masticatory performance is relatively maintained in old age [25, 56, 57]. Older adults have been observed to require an increased number of chewing strokes and increased time to prepare a bolus [25]. Additionally, breaking down a bolus into smaller pieces before swallowing is more frequent in healthy elders over 80 years of age compared with young healthy adults [58]. However, most reduced masticatory abilities seen in older individuals have been attributed to tooth loss, and/or artificial dentition [5]. Individuals wearing dentures are known to have less masticatory strength [56, 57], require even more time to masticate [56, 59], and have reduced masticatory efficiency by approximately 16–50 % [56]. When normal dentition is maintained until later in life, masticatory difficulties are usually not seen in healthy elders.

Saliva Production

Saliva serves multiple functions that are important for maintenance of oral health, normal swallowing, and digestive status. These include lubricating the oral tissues and providing moisture to help with food manipulation and swallowing, enhancing speech, helping with retention of dentures, cleansing effects of the oropharyngeal mucosa, and initiation of digestion of starches [60]. Histologically, salivary glands are structures including fat, fibrovascular tissue, and acini [60]. With age, the fat and fibrovascular tissues increase, while acini undergo reduction, thus leading to a decrease of the glands parenchymal component [61, 62]. Despite these anatomic alterations, there are contradictory findings in terms of the overall salivary flow rates of healthy elderly individuals. Some researchers report relatively constant salivary flow rates across age [63], while others found age-related reductions [64]. Specifically, when saliva flow is mildly stimulated and un-stimulated, salivary flow rates tend to be only mildly reduced in normal healthy elders; when stimulation is continuous for a short period of time, saliva flow rates are comparable to young adults; however, when stimulation is prolonged, these rates can be significantly decreased [60].

Overall indications, in general, show that saliva production in healthy elders is sufficient for most oropharyngeal functions associated with it. Despite this, approximately 25 % of elderly individuals complain of oral dryness or xerostomia [65]. It appears that the most frequent cause of this complaint is medication use, with research showing that there is a clear inverse relationship between number of medications received and reduction of salivary flow rates [66]. Other causes of xerostomia in elders include Sjogren's disease and radiotherapy exposure after diagnosis of head and neck cancer [67, 68].

The effects of xerostomia on the oral swallowing events of healthy individuals have received limited attention to date. A study of 15 young healthy adults who were exposed to artificial oral dryness (via an intramuscular injection of methylscopolamine) found increased number of chewing strokes for harder solid foods, but no difference for softer and chewy materials [69]. Logemann and colleagues also reported that chemoradiation-induced xerostomia in head and neck cancer patients (3 and 12 months post treatment) affects the sensory properties of eating and meal satisfaction, while the physiological bolus transport properties remain relatively unaffected [70, 71].

Facial, Lingual, and Oral Contributions

Aging is known to be accompanied by tissue sagging under the skin, wrinkling, increase in adipose tissue in the orofacial area, and bony prominences [72]. It is logical that facial muscles—like all muscles in the human body—undergo atrophy and reductions in muscle fibers and tone, which result in the aforementioned facial symptoms. These changes, however, are not known to affect speech or swallowing [73].

Lingual pressure generation is an important contributor to the swallowing process as it enables food manipulation and bolus propulsion from the oral cavity into the pharynx and into the esophagus. Although maximum lingual pressure generated during swallowing does not decline significantly with age, maximum isometric lingual pressure significantly decreases [28]. This suggests that young adults have a reserve capacity of tongue strength although not utilized during swallowing, and that older adults have a significant decline in this reserve capacity [28]. Therefore, older individuals have reduced access to such in the later years when most needed in response to age-related increase in risk factors for dysphagia. It has been further indicated that this decline results in increased (longer) time to generate peak lingual pressures [30] during isometric pressure generation and, perhaps more importantly, during liquid swallows. This increase in *time to reach peak swallowing pressure* was found to be significantly increased with age for liquids but not semisolids. This may, at least in part, explain findings that older individuals aspirate most commonly on liquids, which generally have rapid flow rates (particularly "thin" fluids), as opposed to other types of material [74] (Fig. 10.1). Additionally, healthy elders are, in general, slower eaters than their younger counterparts [20, 26]. Etiological explanation of these motor declines influencing swallowing, partially comes from the evidence that sarcopenia is present in the striated muscles of the upper aerodigestive tract in old age [75–77]. Sarcopenia is defined as the age-related reduction in muscle mass and cross-sectional area and in

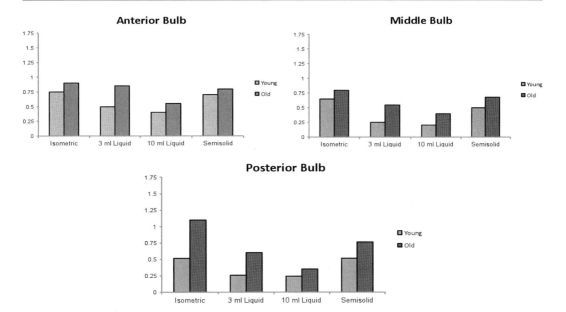

Fig. 10.1 Time to reach peak pressure was reduced with age for both the isometric task and liquid swallows, with no difference found for semisolids, at each bulb location. From M.A. Nicosia et al. J Gerontol A Biol Sci Med Sci 2000;55:M634–40 with permission from Oxford University Press

the number of selective muscle fibers. Strength and functional changes demonstrated in the motor components of the oropharyngeal swallow have been found to be associated with reduction in lingual muscle composition [78, 79], thus attributing some of the aging swallowing motor changes to the end organ, the muscle.

Although there is an abundance of literature on age-related changes in skeletal muscle strength (though little specific to the head and neck), surprisingly less information exists on the relationship between muscle endurance and aging. Muscle endurance is generally described as the ability to maintain a required or expected force and is operationally defined as "the time to task failure for a sustained isometric contraction performed at a submaximal intensity" [80]. Fatigue, an antonym of endurance, is described as the failure to maintain a prescribed force and often includes components such as "an acute impairment in performance" and "an increase in the perceived effort necessary to exert a force" [81]. Fatiguing effects of eating a meal (dining) on tongue and swallowing endurance have not been

extensively examined. To date, most studies have focused on a few swallows of controlled barium boluses as imaged with videofluoroscopy. Recently, Kays and colleagues examined the effects of consuming an entire meal on tongue endurance in healthy young and old adults, with respect to factors such as meal duration, meal-related perceptions of effort, and clinical signs of swallowing difficulty [82]. Results suggest that both young and old adults demonstrate reduced tongue strength and endurance post-meal. Young adults showed a larger difference between pre- and post-meal anterior tongue endurance than older adults and had significantly reduced anterior tongue endurance values post-meal, while older men exhibited reduced posterior tongue endurance. Interestingly, three subjects, all in the oldest age group, demonstrated clinical signs of aspiration during the meal. These results suggest that the daily act of dining decreases tongue strength and tongue endurance in both young and old adults, with potentially harmful effects (aspiration) in older individuals due to decreased swallowing reserve in the latter group.

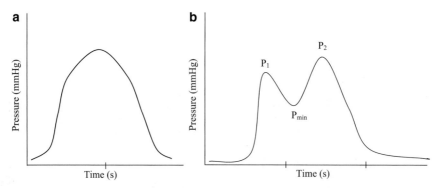

Fig. 10.2 Example waveforms of swallowing pressure versus time, illustrating the method used to determine whether a waveform has single (**a**) or multiple (**b**) peaks. Swallow (**b**) was considered to have two peaks if the ratios, Pmin/P1 and Pmin/P2, were both less than some value α. As the parameter α is arbitrary, values of $\alpha=0.25$, 0.5, and 0.75 were examined. From M.A. Nicosia et al. J Gerontol A Biol Sci Med Sci 2000;55:M634–40 with permission

Timing Events

Most studies investigating aging effects on the timing of swallowing events have focused on initiation, also referred to as the "triggering" of the pharyngeal swallow and on pharyngeal components. However, a few investigators have studied the timing of the oral phase in elderly participants. Specifically, oral transit time has been found to be slightly longer in older individuals by approximately 200–300 ms when compared with younger adults [26, 83]. Even in healthy elders over 80 years of age, this delay is usually ~250 ms [58].

Robbins and colleagues tested the hypothesis that older individuals may require more time to build the pressures necessary (and equivalent to young) for oropharyngeal bolus transport, thereby increasing oral duration [28]. Different patterns of pressure generation were found only in the elders, increasing time to reach peak pressure on multiple peaked waveforms generated during liquid swallows (Fig. 10.2). This different pattern (multiple peaked waveforms) than demonstrated by the younger cohort who were able to reach maximum pressure on their first peak led to increased time for the elders to reach peak pressure and is termed "pressure building" [30].

Oropharyngeal Swallow, Coupling, and Uncoupling: Neural Implications

The young, healthy adult oropharyngeal swallow is a rapid and well-coordinated series of oral and pharyngeal events that occur within milliseconds, may overlap and often appear as one very precisely controlled sequence of activity from start of bolus transit to its passage into the esophagus. In contrast, a delay in the initiation of the pharyngeal response has been reported to be relatively common in older healthy adults [20, 27]. This delay or lapse in time, during which the oral events have been completed and remaining pharyngeal events have not initiated, appears as an uncoupling of the typical (seen in young adults) single swift oropharyngeal swallow into two time-distinct groups of events, functionally separating the oral and the pharyngeal events [84] (Fig. 10.3). Essentially, as people age, the more voluntary—more cortically regulated—oral events of swallowing become neurologically "un-coupled" from the more automatic—brainstem regulated—pharyngeal response, suggesting a central neural component underlying these declines. The presence of increased periventricular white matter lesions has been associated with slower swallowing and appears to be at least one contributor to the "uncoupling" process with aging [85] (Fig. 10.4).

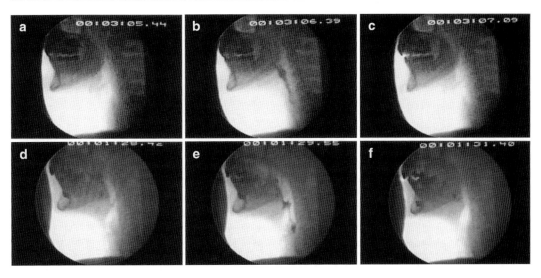

Fig. 10.3 Healthy young swallowing documented with videofluoroscopy. (**a**) Bolus in oral cavity, ready to be swallowed. (**b**) Bolus appears as a "column" of material swiftly moving through the pharynx. (**c**) Oropharynx cleared of material when the swallow is completed. Healthy old swallowing documented with videofluoroscopy. (**d**) Bolus in mouth ready for swallowing. (**e**) Bolus pooled in vallecula and pyriform sinus during delayed onset of pharyngeal response. (**f**) Bolus cleared of material when the swallow is completed. From J. Robbins. Semin Neurol 1996;16:309–17 with permission

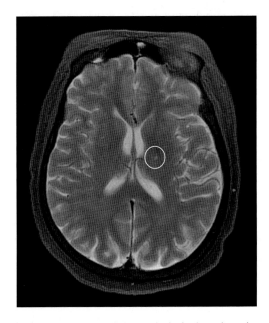

Fig. 10.4 Grade = 1, Lower cortical, single periventricular *white* matter lesion aka UBO with subcortical region (*white small*)

Further evidence for this uncoupling concept comes from recent functional neuroimaging research. In a recent fMRI study of healthy young and older adults, where participants completed one swallowing and three swallowing-related tasks, the latter group appeared to have significantly reduced activations in primary somatosensory areas and areas involved in sensorimotor integration (including subcortical areas), while primary motor areas remained relatively intact in the old group [86] (Fig. 10.5). Pharyngeal components of swallowing have been reported to rely more heavily on subcortical networks, whereas oral components are known to depend more on cortical sensorimotor cortex innervation [87]. These reduced activations seen in healthy elders may explain some of the sensory oropharyngeal age-related declines described earlier. Clinically, this is an important finding. If future research validates such a relationship, swallowing treatments aimed to improve the sensory components of the swallow will have to target the neurophysiological underpinnings of such sensory declines in order to be effective.

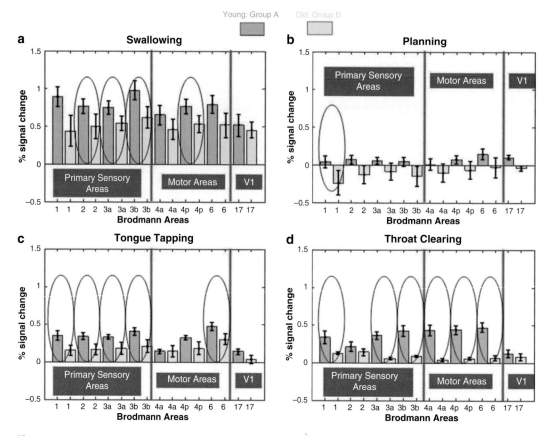

Fig. 10.5 Average % signal change in all regions of interest (ROIs) during (**a**) swallowing, (**b**) planning, (**c**) tongue tapping, and (**d**) throat clearing in both groups. *Green*: Young adults' activation (Group A); *Yellow*: Old adults' activation (Group B); circles indicate statistically significant amplitude differences between age groups ($p<0.05$). From G.A. Malandraki et al. Hum Brain Mapping 2011;32:730–43 with permission from Wiley and Sons

Conclusions

Oral anatomy, physiology, and neural integrity are intimately and dynamically integrated in the healthy oropharyngeal swallow and therefore critical to the safe and effective execution of multiple everyday functions, including eating and speech. Maintenance of oral health is crucial in old age in order to preserve chemosensory and motor function, nutritional health, and ultimately quality of life. Anatomic and functional sensorimotor components of oral physiology and the early initial events for swallowing, specifically, undergo gradual changes as people age. These changes appear to be modest enough or occur so slowly and insidiously that spontaneous compensation, occurring at a subconscious level, precludes their interference with swallowing functionality and safety in most healthy older adults. They may, however, signify reductions in the swallowing functional reserve capacity and endurance in elders, increasing their vulnerability to dysphagia and airway invasion secondary to disease and environmental complications. Understanding these changes and their underlying peripheral and central mechanisms is necessary in finding solutions to treat and even prevent certain conditions. Recent developments in imaging and electrophysiological methods now facilitate study of these changes relatively non-invasively and promise to provide breakthrough mechanistic information in order to improve our diagnostic methods, treatment, practice patterns, and prevention protocols.

References

1. Comfort A. Ageing: the biology of senescence. London: Routledge & Kegan Paul; 1964.
2. Finch CE. Senescence, longevity, and the genome. Chicago: The University of Chicago Press; 1990.
3. World Health Organization. Information needs for research policy and action on ageing and older adults: report of a workshop on creating a minimum data set (MDS) for research, policy and action on ageing and the aged in Africa (WHO/NMH/HPS/00.7). Harare, Zimbabwe; 2011.
4. Zamir Z, Ren J, Hogan WJ, Shaker R. Coordination of deglutitive vocal cord closure and oral-pharyngeal swallowing events in the elderly. Eur J Gastroenterol Hepatol. 1996;8:425–9.
5. Kossioni AE, Dontas AS. The stomatognathic system in the elderly. Useful information for the medical practitioner. Clin Interv Aging. 2007;2:591–7.
6. Perlman AL. Normal swallowing physiology and evaluation. Curr Opin Otolaryngol Head Neck Surg. 1994;2:226–32.
7. Ertekin C, Aydogdu I. Neurophysiology of swallowing. Clin Neurophysiol. 2003;114:2226–44.
8. Vaiman M, Eviatar E, Segal S. Surface electromyographic studies of swallowing in normal subjects: a review of 440 adults. Report 1. Quantitative data: timing measures. Otolaryngol Head Neck Surg. 2004;131:548–55.
9. Blitzer A. Approaches to the patient with aspiration and swallowing disabilities. Dysphagia. 1990;5:129–37.
10. Gay T, Rendell JK, Spiro J, Mosier K, Lurie AG. Coordination of oral cavity and laryngeal movements during swallowing. J Appl Physiol. 1994;77:357–65.
11. Logemann J. Evaluation and treatment of swallowing disorders. Austin, TX: Pro-Ed Inc.; 1998.
12. Perlman AL, Christenson J. Topography and functional anatomy of the swallowing structures. In: Perlman AL, Schulze-Delrieu KS, editors. Deglutition and its disorders. San Diego, CA: Singular Publication Group; 1997. p. 15–42.
13. Cook IJ, Dodds WJ, Dantas RO, Kern MK, Massey BT, Shaker R, Hogan WJ. Timing of videofluoroscopic, manometric events, and bolus transit during the oral and pharyngeal phases of swallowing. Dysphagia. 1989;4:8–15.
14. Hiiemae KM, Crompton AW. Mastication, food transport and swallowing. In: Hildebrand M, Bramble D, Liem K, Wale D, editors. Functional vertebrate morphology. Cambridge, MA: Belknap; 1985. p. 262.
15. Luschei ES, Goodwin GM. Patterns of mandibular movement and jaw muscle activity during mastication in the monkey. J Neurophysiol. 1974;37:954–66.
16. Kahrilas PJ, Lin S, Logemann JA, Ergun GA, Facchini F. Deglutitive tongue action: volume accommodation and bolus propulsion. Gastroenterology. 1993;104:152–62.
17. Dodds WJ, Stewart ET, Logemann JA. Physiology and radiology of the normal oral and pharyngeal phases of swallowing. AJR Am J Roentgenol. 1990;154:953–63.
18. Shaker R, Cook IJS, Dodds WJ, Hogan WJ. Pressure flow dynamics of the oral phase of swallowing. Dysphagia. 1988;3:79–84.
19. Yotsuya H, Saito Y, Ide Y. Studies on temporal correlations of the movements of the pharyngeal organs during deglutition by X-ray TV cinematography. Bull Tokyo Dent Coll. 1981;22:171–81.
20. Robbins J, Hamilton JW, Lof GL, Kempster GB. Oropharyngeal swallowing in normal adults of different ages. Gastroenterology. 1992;103:823–9.
21. Ship JA. The influence of aging on oral health and consequences for taste and smell. Physiol Behav. 1999;66:209–15.
22. Leslie P, Drinnan MJ, Ford GA, Wilson JA. Swallow respiratory patterns and aging: presbyphagia or dysphagia? J Gerontol A Biol Sci Med Sci. 2005;60:391–5.
23. Ney DM, Weiss JM, Kind AJ, Robbins J. Senescent swallowing: impact, strategies, and interventions. Nutr Clin Pract. 2009;24:395–413.
24. Wikipedia. Presbyphagia. http://en.wikipedia.org/wiki/Presbyphagia (2008). Accessed 20 May 2011.
25. Feldman RS, Kapur KK, Alman JE, Chauncey HH. Aging and mastication: changes in performance and in the swallowing threshold with natural dentition. J Am Geriatr Soc. 1980;28:97–103.
26. Cook IJ, Weltman MD, Wallace K, Shaw DW, McKay E, Smart RC, Butler SP. Influence of aging on oral-pharyngeal bolus transit and clearance during swallowing: scintigraphic study. Am J Physiol. 1994;266:G972–7.
27. Shaker R, Ren J, Zamir Z, Sarna A, Liu J, Sui Z. Effect of aging, position, and temperature on the threshold volume triggering pharyngeal swallows. Gastroenterology. 1994;107:396–402.
28. Robbins J, Levine R, Wood J, Roecker EB, Luschei E. Age effects on lingual pressure generation as a risk factor for dysphagia. J Gerontol A Biol Sci Med Sci. 1995;50:M257–62.
29. Logemann JA, Pauloski BR, Rademaker AW, Colangelo LA, Kahrilas PJ, Smith CH. Temporal and biomechanical characteristics of oropharyngeal swallow in younger and older men. J Speech Lang Hear Res. 2000;43:1264–74.
30. Nicosia MA, Hind JA, Roecker EB, Carnes M, Robbins JA. Age effects on the temporal evolution of isometric and swallowing pressure. J Gerontol A Biol Sci Med Sci. 2000;55:M634–40.
31. Daniels SK, Corey DM, Hadskey LD, Legendre C, Priestly DH, Rosenbek JC, Foundas AL. Mechanism of sequential swallowing during straw drinking in healthy young and older adults. J Speech Lang Hear Res. 2004;47:33–45.
32. Fukunaga A, Uematsu H, Sugimoto K. Influences of aging on taste perception and oral somatic sensation. J Gerontol A Biol Sci Med Sci. 2005;60:109–13.
33. Calhoun KH, Gibson B, Hartley L, Minton J, Hokanson JA. Age-related changes in oral sensation. Laryngoscope. 1992;102:109–16.

34. Schiffman SS. Taste and smell losses in normal aging and disease. J Am Med Assoc. 1997;278:1357–62.

35. Doty RL, Shaman P, Applebaum SL, Giberson R, Siksorski L, Rosenberg L. Smell identification ability: changes with age. Science. 1984;226:1441–3.

36. Schiffman SS, Warwick ZS. The biology of taste and food intake. In: Bray GA, Ryan DH, editors. The science of food regulation. Baton Rouge, LA: Louisiana State University Press; 1992.

37. Teff KL, Engelman K. Palatability and dietary restraint: effect on cephalic phase insulin release in women. Physiol Behav. 1996;60:567–73.

38. Stevens JC, Cruz LA, Hoffman JM, Patterson MQ. Taste sensitivity and aging: high incidence of decline revealed by repeated threshold measures. Chem Senses. 1995;20:451–9.

39. Bradley RM. Effects of aging on the anatomy and neurophysiology of taste. Gerodontics. 1988;4:244–8.

40. Schiffman SS, Clark 3rd TB. Magnitude estimates of amino acids for young and elderly subjects. Neurobiol Aging. 1980;1:81–91.

41. Murphy C. The chemical senses and nutrition in older adults. J Nutr Elder. 2008;27:247–65.

42. Nordin S, Razani LJ, Markison S, Murphy C. Age-associated increases in intensity discrimination for taste. Exp Aging Res. 2003;29:371–81.

43. Schiffman SS, Lindley MG, Clark TB, Makino C. Molecular mechanism of sweet taste: relationship of hydrogen bonding to taste sensitivity for both young and elderly. Neurobiol Aging. 1981;2:173–85.

44. Mistretta CM. Aging effects on anatomy and neurophysiology of taste and smell. Gerodontology. 1984;3:131–6.

45. Schiffman SS. Drugs influencing taste and smell perception. In: Getchell TV, Doty RL, Bartoshuk LM, Snow JB, editors. Smell and taste in health and disease. New York, NY: Raven; 1991. p. 845–50.

46. Cain WS, Stevens JC. Uniformity of olfactory loss in aging. Ann N Y Acad Sci. 1989;561:29–38.

47. Stevens JC, Cain WS. Age-related deficiency in the perceived strength of six odorants. Chem Senses. 1985;10:517–29.

48. Morgan CD, Covington JW, Geisler MW, Polich J, Murphy C. Olfactory event-related potentials: older males demonstrate the greatest deficits. Electroencephalogr Clin Neurophysiol. 1997;104:351–8.

49. Murphy C, Nordin S, Acosta L. Odor learning, recall, and recognition memory in young and elderly adults. Neuropsychology. 1997;11:126–37.

50. Larsson M, Backman L. Modality memory across the adult life span: evidence for selective age-related olfactory deficits. Exp Aging Res. 1998;24:63–82.

51. Doty RL. Olfactory capacities in aging and Alzheimer's disease. Psychophysical and anatomic considerations. Ann N Y Acad Sci. 1991;640:20–7.

52. Cerf-Ducastel B, Murphy C. FMRI brain activation in response to odors is reduced in primary olfactory areas of elderly subjects. Brain Res. 2003;986: 39–53.

53. Wang J, Eslinger PJ, Smith MB, Yang QX. Functional magnetic resonance imaging study of human olfaction and normal aging. J Gerontol A Biol Sci Med Sci. 2005;60:510–4.

54. Fucci D, Petrosino L, Robey RR. Auditory masking effects on lingual vibrotactile thresholds as a function of age. Percept Mot Skills. 1982;54:943–50.

55. Petrosino L, Fucci D, Robey RR. Changes in lingual sensitivity as a function of age and stimulus exposure time. Percept Mot Skills. 1982;55:1083–90.

56. Heath MR. The effect of maximum biting force and bone loss upon masticatory function and dietary selection of the elderly. Int Dent J. 1982;32:345–56.

57. Carlsson GE. Masticatory efficiency: the effect of age, the loss of teeth, and prosthetic rehabilitation. Int Dent J. 1984;34:93–7.

58. Yoshikawa M, Yoshida M, Nagasaki T, Tanimoto K, Tsuga K, Akagawa Y, Komatsu T. Aspects of swallowing in healthy dentate elderly persons older than 80 years. J Gerontol A Biol Sci Med Sci. 2005;60:506–9.

59. Helkimo E, Carlsson GE, Helkimo M. Chewing efficiency and state of dentition. A methodologic study. Acta Odontol Scand. 1978;36:33–41.

60. Vissink A, Spijkervet FK, Van Nieuw Amerongen A. Aging and saliva: a review of the literature. Spec Care Dentist. 1996;16:95–103.

61. Scott J. Quantitative age changes in the histological structure of human submandibular salivary glands. Arch Oral Biol. 1977;22:221–7.

62. Drummond JR, Chisholm DM. A qualitative and quantitative study of the ageing human labial salivary glands. Arch Oral Biol. 1984;29:151–5.

63. Shern RJ, Fox PC, Li SH. Influence of age on the secretory rates of the human minor salivary glands and whole saliva. Arch Oral Biol. 1993;38:755–61.

64. Percival RS, Challacombe SJ, Marsh PD. Flow rates of resting whole and stimulated parotid saliva in relation to age and gender. J Dent Res. 1994;73:1416–20.

65. Osterberg T, Carlsson GE. Symptoms and signs of mandibular dysfunction in 70-year-old men and women in Gothenburg, Sweden. Commun Dent Oral Epidemiol. 1979;7:315–21.

66. Narhi TO. Prevalence of subjective feelings of dry mouth in the elderly. J Dent Res. 1994;73:20–5.

67. Atkinson JC, Travis WD, Pillemer SR, Bermudez D, Wolff A, Fox PC. Major salivary gland function in primary Sjogren's syndrome and its relationship to clinical features. J Rheumatol. 1990;17:318–22.

68. Liu RP, Fleming TJ, Toth BB, Keene HJ. Salivary flow rates in patients with head and neck cancer 0.5 to 25 years after radiotherapy. Oral Surg Oral Med Oral Pathol. 1990;70:724–9.

69. Liedberg B, Owall B. Masticatory ability in experimentally induced xerostomia. Dysphagia. 1991;6:211–3.

70. Logemann JA, Smith CH, Pauloski BR, Rademaker AW, Lazarus CL, Colangelo LA, Mittal B, MacCracken E, Gaziano J, Stachowiak L, Newman LA. Effects of xerostomia on perception and performance of swallow function. Head Neck. 2001;23:317–21.

71. Logemann JA, Pauloski BR, Rademaker AW, Lazarus CL, Mittal B, Gaziano J, Stachowiak L, MacCracken E, Newman LA. Xerostomia: 12-month changes in saliva production and its relationship to perception and performance of swallow function, oral intake, and diet after chemoradiation. Head Neck. 2003;25:432–7.

72. Kahane JC. Anatomic and physiologic changes in the aging peripheral speech mechanism. In: Beasley DS, Davis GA, editors. Aging: communication processes and disorders. New York, NY: Grune & Stratton; 1981.

73. Sonies B, Stone M, Shawler T. Speech and swallowing in the elderly. Gerodontology. 1984;3:115–23.

74. Roos MR, Rice CL, Vandervoort AA. Age-related changes in motor unit function. Muscle Nerve. 1997;20:679–90.

75. Cartee GD. What insights into age-related changes in skeletal muscle are provided by animal models? J Gerontol A Biol Sci Med Sci. 1995;50:137–41. Spec No.

76. Evans WJ. What is sarcopenia? J Gerontol A Biol Sci Med Sci. 1995;50:5–8. Spec No.

77. Faulkner JA, Brooks SV, Zerba E. Muscle atrophy and weakness with aging: contraction-induced injury as an underlying mechanism. J Gerontol A Biol Sci Med Sci. 1995;50:124–9. Spec No.

78. Price PA, Darvell BS. Force and mobility in the aging human tongue. Med J Aust. 1982;1:75–8.

79. Newton JP, Abel EW, Robertson EM, Yemm R. Changes in human masseter and medial pterygoid muscles with age: a study by computed tomography. Gerodontics. 1987;3:151–4.

80. Hunter SK, Critchlow A, Enoka RM. Muscle endurance is greater for old men compared with strength-matched young men. J Appl Physiol. 2005;99:890–7.

81. Enoka RM, Stuart DG. Neurobiology of muscle fatigue. J Appl Physiol. 1992;72:1631–48.

82. Kays S, Hind J, Gangnon R, Robbins J. Effects of dining on tongue endurance and swallowing-related outcomes. J Speech Lang Hear Res. 2010;53:898–907.

83. Shaw D, Cook IJ, Gabb M, Holloway R, Simula M, Panagopoulos V, Dent J. Influence of normal aging on oral-pharyngeal and upper esophageal sphincter function during swallowing. Am J Physiol Gastrointest Liver Physiol. 1995;268:G389–96.

84. Robbins J. Normal swallowing and aging. Semin Neurol. 1996;16:309–17.

85. Levine R, Robbins JA, Maser A. Periventricular white matter changes and oropharyngeal swallowing in normal individuals. Dysphagia. 1992;7:142–7.

86. Malandraki GA, Sutton BP, Perlman AL, Karampinos DC. Reduced somatosensory activations in swallowing with age. Hum Brain Mapp. 2011;32:730–43.

87. Malandraki GA, Sutton BP, Perlman AL, Karampinos DC, Conway C. Neural activation of swallowing and swallowing-related tasks in healthy young adults: an attempt to separate the components of deglutition. Hum Brain Mapp. 2009;30:3209–26.

Nascent Oral Phase

11

Amy L. Delaney and Colin Rudolph

Abstract

The oral phase of swallowing is characterized by sucking in the newborn. Over the first years of life the anatomy alters from one adapted perfectly to sucking, to one more similar to adult anatomy, allowing mastication skills to emerge. Changes in anatomic structural relationships confound attempts to precisely quantify this developmental process such that our understanding of the exact developmental timing for mastery of various feeding skills is incomplete. Previous research has focused upon the development of sucking and chewing where some normative data is available. This chapter reviews the available knowledge about the normal emergence and mastery of the oral skills required for feeding. The implication of variation from these expected developmental patterns is also briefly discussed.

Keywords

Anatomic changes impacting feeding • Nascent oral phase • Prenatal development • Frequency of sucking • Periodicity of sucking • Amplitude of sucking pressure

Prenatal Development of Feeding and Swallowing Performance

Embryologic formation of the oropharyngeal cavity, esophagus, and trachea occurs during first 8 weeks of gestation [1–3]. Subsequent growth and remodeling of these structures continues throughout fetal development and the first 2 years of life [1–7]. Myelination of the cranial nerves required for sucking (glossopharyngeal, hypoglossal, and facial) occurs by 20–24 weeks gestation. Thus by about 24 weeks, the apparatus for sucking appears to be established.

Ultrasound technology has been used to evaluate the fetal development of the anatomic structures involved in feeding and to observe the timing of both emergence, and consistent performance of movements related to postnatal feeding and swallowing [6, 8–10] (Table 11.1). This normative data allows comparison with infants from

A.L. Delaney, PhD, CCC-SLP
Children's Hospital of Wisconsin,
Medical College of Wisconsin, Milwaukee, WI, USA
e-mail: adelaney@chw.org

C. Rudolph, MD, PhD (✉)
Mead Johnson Nutrition, Evansville, IN, USA
e-mail: colin.rudolph@mjn.com

Table 11.1 Gestational age of the earliest observation and age with consistent performance of skills associated with feeding

	Earliest	Consistent
Mouthing action	16 weeks	17 weeks defined jaw opening/closing
Tongue thrusting	15 weeks	After 21 weeks
Swallowing	15 weeks	22–24 weeks
Laryngeal contraction	15 weeks	26 weeks (decreasing by 38 weeks)
Tongue cupping	16 weeks	28 weeks
Tongue protrusion "suckling"	18 weeks	28 weeks
Licking, munching	n/a	31 weeks
Rapid, low-amplitude sucking	n/a	32 weeks
Irregular sucking	n/a	34 weeks

Reference: Miller et al. [6]

Table 11.2 Growth patterns of oral and pharyngeal structures

	% adult size	
Structure	18 months	6 years
Maxillary lip thickness	60	70
Mandibular length	55	75
Hard palate length	80	90
Mandibular depth	65	80
Soft palate length	65	80
Laryngeal descent	55	65
Tongue length	60	70
Vocal tract length	55	75

References: Vorperian et al. [11, 12]

high-risk groups such as infants of diabetic mothers and those with genetic disorders who are more likely to have feeding problems after birth.

Basic mouthing actions and tongue thrust movements evolve to complex actions between 28 and 34 weeks. Oral-lingual movements appear earlier in females [6, 7]. Irregular sucking evolves to rhythmic sucking similar to that seen in the newborn by term. This data provides a perspective on the feeding skills that can be expected in preterm infants.

Anatomic Changes Impacting Feeding in Infants and Children

Rapid growth of the oral and pharyngeal cavities occurs in the first several years of life with continued growth into adulthood. The oral structures reach adult proportions earlier than pharyngeal structures [11, 12] with rapid growth of the pharyngeal structures between 8 and 14 years as summarized in Table 11.2.

The differences in size of the oral cavity facilitate sucking in the infant. The small size and shape of the infant oral cavity are ideal for sucking. The buccal fat pads and palate stabilize the lateral and superior walls of the oral cavity. To suck, the lips close around the breast or nipple, and the tongue seals against the pharynx posteriorly forming a closed intraoral chamber. Depression of the tongue and mandible generates suction up to 150 mmHg in the oral cavity. As the infant matures, the oral cavity enlarges which allows manipulation of a pureed or solid food bolus. Subsequently, the alveolar ridges and teeth develop to facilitate biting and mastication. The anatomic relationships then no longer favor sucking but rather promote cup and spoon-feeding patterns. Similar changes occur in the pharynx with enlargement of the pharyngeal cavity and descent of the larynx. During the first 2 years of life the human larynx remains relatively high in the neck with the major descent occurring between 2 and 3 years of age as the upper border of the larynx descends to the level of cervical vertebra C3 and the lower border of the larynx to C5 [13]. The descent of the larynx prevents the epiglottis from approximating the soft palate. Thus, in the mature human, even during maximum laryngeal elevation a region of oropharynx is always located above the laryngeal inlet and the airway and digestive pathways cannot be entirely separated. Among mammals, this anatomic arrangement is unique to the adult human, probably evolving to allow the use of the larger tongue surface to form a broader range of sounds for communication. Unfortunately, the sophisticated neuromuscular protective mechanisms, which evolved to prevent aspiration, are less robust than the simpler mechanical protection provided by anatomic positioning of the larynx above the digestive pathway. Minor anatomic or neuromuscular disorders that are not problematic in an infant can compromise protective mechanisms when the larynx descends because the separation of air and digestive pathways becomes more challenging.

Factors Impacting Feeding Performance in Infants

Changes in feeding and swallowing physiology are measured by several different performance variables. The overall efficiency of feeding is dependent on the volume and/or rate of consumption within a specified time segment. More specifically, feeding efficiency is measured relative to the suck–swallow–breath sequence in an infant and by evaluation of chewing skills in a child. The general health and well-being of an infant impact their feeding experiences as related to the level of alertness, self-regulation, and strength [14] and any alterations during these developmental periods can have considerable impact on the prognosis for feeding and swallowing development.

Sucking

Two types of sucking are observed in infants. *Non-nutritive sucking* that comforts and soothes the infant and *nutritive sucking* that provides the sole source of nutrient ingestion for infants until they begin receiving complementary foods between 4 and 6 months of age. Because nutrient sucking is required for normal growth and development, it is the usual variable focused upon for evaluation of feeding during the neonatal period. Nutritive sucking consists of the rhythmic alteration of suction and expression [15] that extracts liquid from the breast or bottle for swallowing. Suction occurs during jaw depression [16] generating negative oral pressure [15] due to the coupling of the soft palate and epiglottis. In addition, to this negative pressure the expression of liquid occurs due to a positive pressure exerted around the nipple during stripping of the nipple between the hard palate and tongue [15].

Table 11.3 Quantitative parameters used to evaluate feeding and sucking

Feeding Efficiency During Nutritive Sucking (Volume/Duration)
Suck (Frequency and Periodicity)
Suck: # and duration Burst: # and duration Sucks per burst Pauses: # and duration Suck per time period (seconds, minute, entire feeding) Volume per suck Volume per time period Amplitude / Pressures
Swallow (Temporal Physiologic and Bolus Flow Measures)
Onset of oral movements and bolus transit SSR (suck:swallow ratio) Bolus size Onset of pharyngeal movements and bolus transit Cricopharyngeal elevation and opening/closing Muscle activation and duration
Breathe (Respiration)
Respiratory pattern O2 saturations Rest/pause duration

Measurement of nutritive sucking performance has been accomplished with several different methodologies including visual observation [17–19], volume measurement [17, 20–22], ultrasound [6, 8, 23], fluoroscopy [24, 25], pressure transducers [21, 22, 26–28], and electromyography [29]. A variety of parameters that may impact feeding efficiency during nutritive sucking (amount consumed within a specified period of time) are shown in Table 11.3. Most of the variables vary depending upon the age of the infant, rate of breast milk delivery from the mother or nipple, and physiologic state of the infant. While the parameters used to measure individual sucking motions are useful for understanding normal patterns of development, coordination of sucking with swallowing and breathing is likely more important for successful feeding. Three general areas are considered for evaluation of nutritive sucking: frequency and periodicity of sucking events; timing of swallowing events; and respiratory patterns (Table 11.3).

Table 11.4 Total oral intake per specified time

DOL/Age	Breast	Duration	Bottle	Duration
1 day	9.6 +/−10.3 ml	n/a	18.5+/−9 ml	n/a
	13+/−16 ml	n/a	n/a	n/a
2 days	13.0+/−11.3 ml	n/a	42.2+/−14.2 ml	n/a
	40+/−23 ml	n/a	n/a	n/a
1–4 days	n/a	n/a	44 ml	n/a
6 days	67+/−2 ml	25 min	75+/−6 ml	25+/−3 min
1 month	n/a	n/a	101 ml	n/a
	60+/−31.6 ml	(9.5 min) 575+/−168 s	68.1+/−15.1	(4.3 min) 259+/−81 s
3 months	81.3+/−39.0 ml	(7.7 min) 464+/−180 s	90+/−20 ml	(4.5 min) 270+/−57 s
6 months	108.8+/−42.6 ml	(5.8 min) 350+/−147 s	122.5+/−21.9 ml	(4.6 min) 276+/−103 s

References: Casey et al. [17]; Dollberg [18]; Lucas et al. [19]; Qureshi et al. [21]; Taki et al. [22] (n/a=no reported duration)

Volume and Length of Feeding in Infants

The feeding efficiency of infants is determined if the volume of feeding ingested is taken within a reasonable amount of time and is adequate to maintain growth and nutrition. If a child is not achieving normal growth, or is taking a prolonged amount of time to ingest adequate calories a feeding problem exists. Normal volumes ingested by infants at various ages from birth to age 6 months are shown in Table 11.4.

Dollberg and colleagues [18] found that bottle-fed neonates on day of life (DOL) 1 and 2 had greater intake and less weight loss. As well, infants with greater intake on DOL 1 had greater intake on DOL 2 when compared to breastfed infants. From DOL 1–4 to 1 month of age, volumes doubled [21]. On DOL 6, there was no difference in intake during the first 4 min of a feeding [19]. As the feeding progressed, bottle-fed infants demonstrated a linear pattern of intake taking 81% of total intake within the first 10 min and 93% by 15 min. Instead, breastfed infants demonstrated a biphasic pattern of intake taking 55% of total intake within the first 10 min of a feeding. However, when eliminating the pause in feeding for changing breasts, breastfed infants' intake increased to 83% of total volume in 8 min of active eating [19]. Intake was greater for infants 6 months of age than 1 month for both breast and bottle-feeding with a significantly shortened total duration [22]. Volume per suck was not significantly different for age or method but volume per minute systematically increased with age [22]. Overall, the total duration of feedings of those reported lasted no longer than 25 min and this duration has been used as a marker for efficient feeding in typically developing infants.

The nutritive sucking skills used by an infant vary and impact the intake during a feeding. For comparison of data, number of sucks, number of bursts and volume of intake are difficult to compare without reporting of the duration of time that these data were monitored since these rates can vary from the beginning to the end of a feeding. Duration data is not required when comparing findings for the number of sucks/burst (S/B), suck/swallow ratio, sucking rate and pressures. Table 11.5 summarizes data on term healthy infants from first day of life to 16 months of age. Missing data reflect differing methodologies.

Frequency and Periodicity of Sucking

The number of occurrences of sucking events over a specified time period is of interest. The frequency of these sucking events includes the number of sucks, groups of sequential sucks known as "bursts", pauses, and swallows. The specified time period may include the duration of the suck, burst, pause, swallow, and entire feeding. All of these measurements impact upon the total

Table 11.5 Nutritive sucking data for term healthy infants (bottle unless otherwise indicated)

DOL/age	Duration (minutes)	Sucks/burst (+/−SD or range)	# Sucks	# Bursts	Mean sucks/min	Mean suck rate (sucks/s) (+/−SD or range)	Pressure
1 day	5	10.27 (+/−14.56)	163.41 (+/−91.3)	19.26 (+/−10.26)	n/a	n/a	107.81 (+/−47.15)
2 days	5	13.04 (+/−13.72)	216.14 (+/−87.1)	21.69 (+/12.04)	n/a	n/a	117.9 (+/−41.57)
	5	13.6 (+/−8.7)	n/a	n/a	n/a	n/a	100.3 (+/−36)
	1	56 median (17.3–66.0)	56 median (52–66)	1	56	0.93	n/a
1–4 days	Full feed	10	n/a	n/a	55	1.10 (+/−0.145)	n/a
4–6 days	n/a	n/a	n/a	n/a	n/a	1.0 (0.8–1.2)	n/a
21–28 days	n/a	n/a	n/a	n/a	41–42	n/a	n/a
1 months	Full feed	21	n/a	n/a	68	0.87 (+/−0.145)	n/a
	Full feed 4.3[a]	37.7 (+/−12.2)	290 (+/−111)	8.3 (+/−4.3)	67[a]	1.1[a]	−126 (+/−24) mmHg
	Full feed 9.6[a] (Breast)	17.8 (+/−8.8)	585 (+/−288)	33.9 (+/−13.9)	60.9[a]	1.01[a]	−155 (+/−76) mmHg
0–7 weeks	8	77.1	349	10.4	43.6[a]	1.14 (+/−0.10)	−0.102
2 weeks to 2 months	n/a	n/a	n/a	n/a	n/a	1.3 (1.1–15)	n/a
3 months	Full feed 4.5[a]	43.3 (+/−7.4)	315 (+/−78)	7.3 (+/−1.4)	70	1.2[a]	−137 (+/−10) mmHg
	Full feed 7.7[a] (Breast)	23.8 (+/−8.3)	606 (+/−353)	28 (+/−18.2)	78.7[a]	1.3[a]	−122 (+/−50) mmHg
6 months	Full feed 4.6[a]	82.3 (+/−22.0)	372 (+/−131)	4.5 (+/−1.3)	80.9[a]	1.3[a]	−143 (+/−15) mmHg
	Full feed 5.8[a] (Breast)	32.4 (+/−15.3)	524 (+/−321)	18.6 (+/−12.8)	90.3[a]	1.5[a]	−131 (+/−60) mmHg
7–9 months	n/a	n/a	n/a	n/a	n/a	1.5 (1.3–1.6)	n/a
13–16 months	2	228 (+/−224)	480 (+/−128)	2.2 (+/−1.74) (segment 2–4 min)	60[a]	1.35 (+/−0.179)	−0.148 (+/−0.069)

References: Lang et al. [26]; Medoff-Cooper et al. [28]; Qureshi et al. [21]; Rocha et al. [30]; Taki et al. [22]

n/a not reported or not part of methodology

[a]Estimates calculated from data provided; actual findings not specifically provided within reference (raw data for duration of feeding measured found in Table 11.4)

volume consumed within the expected time period for adequate growth, nutrition, and development. While both volume and duration parameters allow for comparison across studies, often one of these factors is not reported.

Non-nutritive sucking patterns occur at twice the rate of nutritive sucking with sucks segmented into bursts and pauses [31]. Nutritive sucking occurs with a mean rate of 1 suck per second with equally spaced sucks.

An increase in sucking performance is evident from DOL 1–2 and throughout early infancy. Neonates from DOL 1 to DOL 2 demonstrated differences in the number of sucks as more sucks occurred on DOL 2 when behavioral state was held constant [28]. The total number of sucks per feeding was not significantly different for age or within method but there were a greater number of sucks during breast-feeding at 1 and 3 months of age than during bottle-feeding [22].

Sucking performance changes over the course of a feeding. The mean number of sucking movements per minute decreased from ~60 to ~35 over ten total minutes for infants 21–28 days of age [32]. Mean number of sucks decreased over each 2 min time segment from an average of 118 sucks in the first 2 min to an average of 58 sucks in the last 2 min of an 8 min feeding for infants at birth to 7 weeks [26]. Mean number of sucks per minute also decreased for infants 3–5 months of age from ~70 to ~30 sucking movements per minute over 15 total minutes [32].

Bursts are measured as the number of sucks produced within a burst (S/B). For a series of sucks to be considered a burst, it must contain at least one [33], two [30], or three [21, 22] sucks and the timing between each of the sucks must be 2 s or less [21, 30, 33]. Two [22, 27, 30] or three [26] or more seconds without a suck marks the end of the burst.

Increases in bursting performance are evident from DOL 1–2 and throughout early infancy. Neonates from DOL 1 to DOL 2 demonstrated differences in the number of bursts as more bursts occurred on DOL 2 when the behavioral state was held constant [28]. Generally, a greater number of sucks per burst occur [21, 22] with increased duration of bursts occurring as children age [22]. With age and efficiency, the number of bursts per feeding and the duration between bursts decrease [22]. Mean burst duration was 10.14 s (+/−8.61) for infants DOL 1–4 [21], 20.99 s (+/−22.65) for infants 1 month of age [21], and 66.2 (for full cohort of 91 infants) for infants 0–7 weeks of age [26]. More specifically, the duration of bursts significantly increased from 1 month to 6 months of age for both breast- and bottle-fed infants [22]. Duration of bursts

increased from 11.2 s (+/− 6.1) to 17.9 s (+/−8.8), respectively, from 1 to 6 months of age for breast-fed infants and from 27.5 s (+/−12.3) to 57.2 s (+/−13.5), respectively, from 1 to 6 months of age for bottle-fed infants [22] and continuing to increase with age to 166 s (+/− 154) for a subset of 15 infants when retested at 13–16 months of age [26]. Conversely, the total number of bursts per feeding significantly decreased from 1 to 6 months of age [22].

Bursting performance changes over the course of a feeding. The number of sucks per burst and duration of bursts decreased from the first 2 min to the last 2 min of a feeding for healthy term infants 0–7 weeks of age [26]. The average number of bursts fluctuated over a feeding, increasing from the first 2 min to the second 2 min and then declining over the last 4 min [26]. The duration of bursts significantly decreased from a mean of 107 s to a mean of 64 s over an 8-min feeding [26].

Amplitude of Sucking Pressure

The amplitude of the suck is measured by the pressure or force exerted during the suck. These measurements are made using pressure transducers placed in the oral cavity during sucking activity. The unit of pressure measurement is cmH_2O or mmHg. The expressed positive and negative pressure indicates the presence of sucking force between 0.27 and 1.35 cm H_2O and −3.39 to −21.75 cm H_2O [9, 30] (Table 11.5). Significant differences were reported in sucking pressures from DOL 1–2 [28] yet no differences in sucking pressures for age or method of feeding was found for healthy term infants 1–6 months of age [22]. However, a reduction in the mean sucking pressure occurred from the start to the end of the feeding [26] and infants adjust the magnitude of pressure to adjust to variable nipple flow [21, 34].

Suck and Swallowing Timing and Coordination

The suck–swallow ratio (SSR) is a key measure used to during the evaluation of infant sucking

Table 11.6 Mean oral transit time for liquids

Duration (seconds = s)	Age
0.7 s	Mean 2.2 months
0.88 s (0.26–4.67)	<6 months
0.6 s	Mean 10 months
0.8 s	Mean 3 years
0.64 s (+/−0.17 s)	6–12 years

References: Casas et al. [36]; Newman et al. [24]; Weckmueller et al. [25]

Table 11.7 Mean pharyngeal transit time for liquids

Duration (seconds = s)	Age
0.2 s	Mean 2.2 months
0.66 s (0.46–0.89)	<6 months
0.55 s	Mean 10 months
0.2 s	Mean 3 years
1.0 s (+/−0.58 s)	6–12 years

References: Casas et al. [36]; Newman et al. [24]; Weckmueller et al. [25]

performance [8, 31] described nutritive sucking as a steady rate of one suck per second. Qureshi and colleagues (2002) confirmed that a 1:1 SSR was utilized on nearly 79% (SD 20.1) of sucks for neonates (DOL 1–4). The percentage decreased to 57% (SD 25.8) with an increase in 2:1 and 3:1 SSR in the 1-month cohort. This may reflect the shift from purely reflexive feeding to commencement of more voluntary mediation, based on myelination and sensory-motor experience [8, 35]. Typically developing infants under 6 months of age continue to utilize a mean SSR of 1.74 (+/−1.45) even with growth and experience.

Data on typically developing infants without feeding or swallowing difficulties are limited. Temporal physiologic events and bolus flow measures for swallowing in children from the limited data available coincide with adult data based on fluoroscopy, ultrasound, and EMG.

Oral phase durations for liquids did not differ by age or method of intake for infants [25] (Table 11.6). Oral transit times lasted less than 1 s. Only Casas et al. [36] controlled bolus size. Data are presumed to occur during sequential swallowing. Higher standard deviations were reflective of variations in SSRs.

Pharyngeal transit time for liquids did not differ by age or method of intake for infants [25] (Table 11.7). Pharyngeal transit times lasted less than 1 s. Total swallow time was 1.48 s without age or gender-specific differences [24].

Newman and colleagues [24] studied infants under 6 months of age using fluoroscopy and noted that they collect the bolus equally between the midtongue and hard palate (35%) and over tongue base within the valleculae (40%) prior to swallow initiation. There was no collection or

hesitation of the bolus in the 20% of infants (four children) using a 1:1 SSR. Mild consistent residue in the valleculae was also reported. Laryngeal closure was not observed until the bolus head reached the valleculae in younger, bottle-fed infants, and until the entire bolus was contained within the valleculae for older, cup-fed children [25]. Isolated laryngeal penetration occurred for 97% (33 of 34) of typically developing children (mean 4 months; 7 days–16 months) without history or clinical suspicion for swallowing dysfunction undergoing an upper GI study [37]. More specifically, 47% (16 of 34) of children had laryngeal penetration on more than 50% of swallows [37]. Data were not age-specific.

Suck and Swallow Coordination with Respiration

The coordination and breathing patterns during nutritive sucking are distinct. Oxygen saturations are expected to remain at or above 90% during feedings to demonstrate respiratory stability and endurance. Healthy term infants on day of life 4 and 5 were monitored for saturation levels while bottle- or breast-feeding. Both groups remained at 93% or greater saturation levels throughout the majority of the feeding. Mean saturation levels were 96 +/−2% for breastfed infants and 95+/−3% for bottle-fed infants. Breastfed infants spent more than 50% of the feeding above 95% saturation levels and bottle-fed infants demonstrated rare drops to 87–89% saturation. Infants falling below 90% tended to drop within 5 min of completion of the feeding rather than occurring during a feeding.

The intricate coordination of breathing cessation for swallowing is crucial for safe feeding. This interruption in breathing during swallowing is called *swallowing apnea*. Infants with tachypnea due to underlying pulmonary or cardiac disease often are unable to cease respiration for a long enough period to permit swallowing. This results in poor feeding efficiency with inadequate nutrient ingestion. Respiration patterns during swallowing in healthy term infants changes rapidly over the first year of life. Neonates within the first 48 h of life predominately swallow mid-expiration [38]. Infants between 9 and 12 months of age predominately swallow after expiration matching adult-like patterns [38].

Drinking

Children transition from sucking from breast or bottle at variable ages. By 1 year of age most children can drink efficiently from a cup. The measurement variables used to evaluate drinking in adults are generally applied to describe liquid ingestion during this transition period. As in adults, it appears that children can accomodate to variable sizes of bolus. In adults, liquid bolus volume size ranges from 1 ml (saliva bolus) to 17–20+ ml during cup drinking. This variabilty is accomplished by accomodating the large bolus volume size in a deeper cavity formed within the tongue [39, 40].

Understanding the developmental progression needed to accommodate differing or increasing bolus size in children is an important consideration when assessing and treating children with feeding and swallowing difficulties. Measures include bolus volume per sip and number of swallows per measured bolus along with duration and magnitude of muscle activation as related to discrete and sequential swallowing, viscosity, and method.

Discrete Swallows in Children

Distinct differences in the volume of thin liquid consumed per swallow vary by age and method of study. On average, preschool-aged children

Table 11.8 Average bolus size per discrete sip of thin liquid in typically developing children

Age (years)	Method	Mean volume (ml)
2–5	Straw (2.8 cm)	4.9
2–5.5	Cup (6.5 cm)	5.4
3.5–5.5	Cup	7.34 check method as outlier[a]
4–5	Cup	5.5
6–8	Cup	6.5
9–12	Cup	7.2
Narrow diameter straw and cup		
2–5	Straw (0.7 cm)	3.3
2–5.5	Cup (1.5 cm diameter)	1.7

References: Lawless et al. [41]; Ruark et al. [44]; Steele et al. [43]; Vaiman et al. [45]; Watson et al. [46]

handle a 5 ml bolus of thin liquid during an individual swallow. The average volume per swallow increases with age for thin liquids (Table 11.8). Increasing resistance by drinking low viscosity liquids through a smaller diameter straw resulted in smaller volume swallows. However, when a high viscosity liquid was given, alterations in straw size had less of an effect on bolus size which was reduced compared with low viscosity bolus size.

Volume per swallow is also impacted by the amount given and between natural sips versus experimental tasks [47]. This likely correlates to the reduction in the average volume per swallow (0.85 ml, 2.14 ml, 4.06 ml, 6.13 ml) in 5-year-olds when given a measured bolus (i.e., 1, 3, 5, 10 ml) versus when instructed to take a sip from a larger presented volume [44].

Sequential Swallows in Children

Sequential swallowing is evaluated by determining the number of swallows used to ingest a known volume. Four to 8-years-old children average a volume of 4.8 ml per swallow while 9–12-year-old children average volumes of 7.2 ml per swallow [45]. Five-year-old children use an average of 1.63 swallows for 10 ml, 1.23 swallows for 5 ml, 1.4 swallows for 4 ml, and 1.17 swallows for 1 ml [44]. A significant difference was found for 1 and 5 ml bolus compared to the 10 ml bolus. The

Table 11.9 Duration of muscle activation during thin liquid swallow

Age (years)	Discrete swallow (s)	Sequential swallow (seconds/swallow)
4–6	4.9	1.75
6–8	4.5	1.64
Adult	3.37	1.51

Reference: Vaiman et al. [45]

average volume per swallow was calculated from these data (number of swallows divided by measure bolus) in order to compare to the discrete swallow data.

Muscle Activation Patterns

Electromyographic (EMG) studies of muscle activation pattern and duration, in 5–8-year-old children found systematically increased muscle duration activity as bolus viscosity was increased that is the lowest magnitude of muscle activity occurred with thin liquid swallows (1.0 s submental activity; 1.0 s laryngeal strap activity). The average duration of muscle activity was typically shorter in children than adults for all consistencies studied except for pudding, where an adult-type pattern of muscle activation was noted [44].

The duration of muscle activation was longer for both discrete and sequential swallowing in children. This increase was due to the highly variable oral stage duration (Table 11.9) [45]. Overall, in sequential swallowing the duration of muscle activation was shorter than in discrete swallows.

Development of Chewing Skills

As children develop over the first year of life, they are reliant on chewing and swallowing solids as an increasingly major portion of their nutritional intake. As with nutritive sucking, a variety of parameters may impact feeding efficiency during chewing. Most of the parameters vary depending upon the age of the child and type of food texture studied. Measurement of chewing performance has been accomplished with several different

methodologies including visual observation [45, 48, 49], timing [50, 51], pressure transducers [52, 53], kinematics [54–56], and electromyography [54, 57]. Current findings reveal age-related changes and expectations [1, 2].

Three general areas are considered for evaluation of chewing: frequency and periodicity of chewing events; timing of swallowing events; and respiratory patterns. The frequency and periodicity of chewing events will be discussed here.

Chewing requires coordinated muscle activation and movement patterns of the jaw and lips and lip closure. Measures of muscle coordination, lip strength, chewing efficiency and rate are typically used to evaluate chewing skills. Muscle activation patterns for chewing have been studied using both electromyography and kinematic approaches in both children and adults. Reciprocal activation of antagonist muscle groups, distinct from speech activation patterns, is found in both children and adults [54, 57]. This pattern is evident as early as 9 months of age [57]. Previous dogma based upon limited visual observation described the development of chewing patterns as a uniform predictable process for infants and children [8, 49]. However, these studies used less sensitive methods that were unable to capture age-related change and alterations in bolus viscosity such effecting jaw speed and movement patterns.

Recent studies using kinematic tracings and speed measures have shown continued refinements of chewing skills until at least age 3 years. As the child develops, the horizontal component of jaw motion, that is the jaw motion used in rotary chewing, and chewing speed are reduced with presentation of pureed foods suggesting refinement of motion. Nine to 18-month-old children are unable to modify jaw movements and force to adjust to the consistency of foods [56]. By 18 months of age children alter jaw movements and bite force for puree but the ability to adjust jaw movements during chewing of solid consistency (e.g., Cheerio) is not present even at 30 months of age, indicating that rotary chewing remains poorly developed at this age. These observations contrast with the previous established belief that children develop chewing as a primary vertical motion during infancy and progress to lateral and rotary chewing motions by the second year of life.

Chewing Efficiency

Gisel and colleagues performed landmark studies evaluating chewing efficiency changes as children age [50, 51]. Children use fewer chewing cycles (each cycle consists of one down and up movement of the jaw) this shortens the duration for ingestion of a solid as children progress through a transitional feeding period when pureed and solid foods are introduced [50]. Chewing patterns and efficiency stabilize sometime after 3 years of age based on a definition of stabilization, that is a consistent pattern is established across two age groups [50]. EMG measurements also show that there are shorter bursts of muscle activation during chewing by older children when compared to chewing activity in younger children [54]. Chewing cycles are defined as an upward and downward movement of the chin. Time/cycle ratios are defined as the total time, from the moment food is placed in the mouth until the final swallow occurs and is divided by the number of cycles counted for the period (Table 11.10).

Gisel also observed that the duration for chewing solids exceeds that of purees [51]. Time/cycle ratios were generally between 1.0 and 1.5 for all textures with no significant differences found in age group or texture tested [51]. The only gender difference observed was that girls took more time to chew solids than boys [51]. This finding may reflect more global eating behavioral differences between genders. With altered textures across genders the duration of chewing may be significantly different but the time/cycle ratio remained constant.

Chewing Rate

Gisel's [51] initial observations have been confirmed by others with demonstration of consistent chewing rates of approximately 1 Hz per second regardless of age or texture [54, 57, 58]. Since chewing duration and the number of cycles used to chew decrease with age, this suggests that

Table 11.10 Chewing duration in seconds for 6–24-month-old typically developing children by food texture

| Age | Time (seconds) (approximated) by texture | | | |
	Puree	Viscous-large	Viscous-small	Solid
6 months	8	11	11	41[a]
8 months	7	10	7	32[a]
10 months	6	8	8	26
12 months	6	9	8	25[b]
18 months	4	7	6	18[b]
24 months	5	7	6	17

| Age | Number of cycles (approximated) by texture | | | |
	Puree	Viscous-large	Viscous-small	Solid
6 months	5	10	10	30
8 months	4	9	6[a]	24
10 months	3.5	8	8[a]	22[a]
12 months	3[a]	6	5[b]	17[a, b]
18 months	2[a]	5	4[b]	13[b]
24 months	2	5	5	14

Number of cycles used to chew for 6–24-month-old typically developing children by food texture
Normative data were reported for chewing duration, number of cycles used to chew and time/cycle ratios for age and consistency. Times and cycles were approximated from the bar graphs provided in the article, as specific times were not reported
Adapted from Gisel [53]
[a]Notation indicates significant differences between two consecutive age groups
[b]Notation indicates significant difference between two consecutive age groups

even infants just learning to chew, do so at the same rate as adults across textures [55].

Delaney [48] recently revealed trends in the development of the movement patterns of individual oral-motor movements studied in 63 typically developing infants. The emergence and mastery of 52 oral skills was studied finding that infants 8–12 months of age similarly performed 21 of 52 skills regardless of age, texture, and experience. These findings demonstrated that skills emerge and plateau before 8 months of age, which refutes the conventional wisdom that oral skills for feeding develop in a step-wise process over the first year of life. Overall, there were fewer differences in performance than expected across the age groups [48].

Other aspects of chewing skill performance will not be addressed here. In brief, lip and tongue strength increase with age without significant gender differences [52, 53]. Midline lip pressure and tongue strength decreased in variability with age. Other observational studies detail changes in skill development and performance [48, 51, 59, 60].

Nutritive sucking and chewing performance are measured in different ways. Age and texture-related changes exist and should always be considered when evaluating and treating infants and young children. Continued research will help to further define normal developmental parameters and advance evidence-based practice.

References

1. Arvedson JC, Delaney AL. Development of oromotor functions for feeding, in Oromotor disorders in childhood, M.R.-Q.L. Pennington, editor, Viguera Editores, S.L.: Barcelona; 2011.
2. Delaney AL, Arvedson JC. Development of swallowing and feeding: prenatal through first year of life. Dev Disabil Res Rev. 2008;14(2):105–17.
3. Moore K, Persaud R. The developing human: clinically oriented embryology. 7th ed. Amsterdam: Elsevier—Health Sciences Division; 2003.
4. Cajal C. Description of human fetal laryngeal function: phonation. In: Early human development. 1996;45(1-2):63–2.
5. Humphrey T. Reflex activity in the oral and facial area of the human fetus. In: Bosma JF, editor Second Symposium on oral sensation and perception. 1967, Charles C. Thomas: Springfield.
6. Miller JL, Sonies BC, Macedonia C. Emergence of oropharyngeal, laryngeal and swallowing activity in the developing fetal upper aerodigestive tract: an ultrasound evaluation. Early Hum Dev. 2003;71(1):61–87.
7. Miller JL, Macedonia C, Sonies BC. Sex Differences in prenatal oral motor function and development. Dev Med Child Neurol. 2006;48:465–70.
8. Bosma JF. Development of feeding. Clin Nutr. 1986;5(5):210–8.
9. Hack M, Estabrook MM, Robertson SS. Development of sucking rhythm in preterm infants. Early Hum Dev. 1985;11(2):133–40.
10. Ianniruberto A, Tajani E. Ultrasonographic study of fetal movements. Semin Perinatol. 1981;5(2):175–81.
11. Vorperian H, et al. Anatomic development of the oral and pharyngeal portions of the vocal tracts: An imaging study. J Acoust Soc Am. 2009;1(3):1666–78.
12. Voerperian H, et al. Development of vocal tract length during early childhood: a magnetic resonance imaging study. J Acoust Soc Am. 2005;117(1): 338–50.
13. Lieberman DE, et al. Ontogeny of postnatal hyoid and larynx descent in humans. Arch Oral Biol. 2001;46(2): 117–28.
14. da Costa SP, van den Engel-Hoek L, Bos AF. Sucking and swallowing in infants and diagnostic tools. J Perinatol. 2008;28(4):247–57.
15. Lau C, Schanler RJ. Oral motor function in the neonate. Clin Perinatol. 1996;23(2):161–78.
16. Barlow SM. Central pattern generation involved in oral and respiratory control for feeding in the term infant. Curr Opin Otolaryngol Head Neck Surg. 2009;17(3):187–93.
17. Casey CE, et al. Nutrient intake by breast-fed infants during the first five days after birth. Am J Dis Child. 1986;140(9):933–6.
18. Dollberg S, Lahav S, Mimouni FB. A comparison of intakes of breast-fed and bottle-fed infants during the first two days of life. J Am Coll Nutr. 2001;20(3): 209–11.
19. Lucas A, Lucas PJ, Baum JD. Differences in the pattern of milk intake between breast and bottle fed infants. Early Hum Dev. 1981;5(2):195–9.
20. Hammerman C, Kaplan M. Oxygen saturation during and after feeding in healthy term infants. Biol Neonate. 1995;67(2):94–9.
21. Qureshi MA, et al. Changes in rhythmic suckle feeding patterns in term infants in the first month of life. Dev Med Child Neurol. 2002;44(1):34–9.
22. Taki M, et al. Maturational changes in the feeding behaviour of infants—a comparison between breast-feeding and bottle-feeding. Acta Paediatr. 2010;99(1): 61–7.
23. Geddes DT, et al. Ultrasound imaging of infant swallowing during breast-feeding. Dysphagia. 2010;25(3): 183–91.
24. Newman LA, et al. Videofluoroscopic analysis of the infant swallow. Invest Radiol. 1991;26(10):870–3.
25. Weckmueller J, Easterling C, Arvedson J. Preliminary temporal measurement analysis of normal oropharyngeal swallowing in infants and young children. Dysphagia. 2011;26(2):135–43.
26. Lang WC, et al. Quantification of intraoral pressures during nutritive sucking: methods with normal infants. Dysphagia. 2011;26(3):277–86.
27. Medoff-Cooper B. Nutritive sucking research: from clinical questions to research answers. J Perinat Neonatal Nurs. 2005;19(3):265–72.
28. Medoff-Cooper B, Bilker W, Kaplan JM. Sucking patterns and behavioral state in 1- and 2-day-old full-term infants. J Obstet Gynecol Neonatal Nurs. 2010;39(5):519–24.
29. Gomes CF, Thomson Z, Cardoso JR. Utilization of surface electromyography during the feeding of term and preterm infants: a literature review. Dev Med Child Neurol. 2009;51(12):936–42.
30. Rocha AD, et al. Development of a technique for evaluating temporal parameters of sucking in breastfeeding preterm newborns. Early Hum Dev. 2011;87(8):545–8.
31. Wolff PH. The serial organization of sucking in the young infant. Pediatrics. 1968;42(6):943–56.
32. Moral A, et al. Mechanics of sucking: comparison between bottle feeding and breastfeeding. BMC Pediatr. 2010;10(6):1–8.

33. Pickler RH, Chiaranai C, Reyna BA. Relationship of the first suck burst to feeding outcomes in preterm infants. J Perinat Neonatal Nurs. 2006;20(2):157–62.

34. Mathew OP, Belan M, Thoppil CK. Sucking patterns of neonates during bottle feeding: comparison of different nipple units. Am J Perinatol. 1992;9(4):265–9.

35. Stevenson RD, Allaire JH. The development of normal feeding and swallowing. Pediatr Clin North Am. 1991;38(6):1439–53.

36. Casas MJ, McPherson KA, Kenny DJ. Durational aspects of oral swallow in neurologically normal children and children with cerebral palsy: an ultrasound investigation. Dysphagia. 1995;10(3):155–9.

37. Delzell PB, et al. Laryngeal penetration: a predictor of aspiration in infants? Pediatr Radiol. 1999;29(10):762–5.

38. Kelly BN, et al. The first year of human life: coordinating respiration and nutritive swallowing. Dysphagia. 2007;22(1):37–43.

39. Hiiemae KM, Palmer JB. Tongue movements in feeding and speech. Crit Rev Oral Biol Med. 2003;14(6):413–29.

40. Kahrilas PJ, et al. Deglutitive tongue action: volume accommodation and bolus propulsion. Gastroenterology. 1993;104(1):152–62.

41. Lawless HT, et al. Gender, age, vessel size, cup vs. straw sipping, and sequence effects on sip volume. Dysphagia. 2003;18(3):196–202.

42. Saylor JH. Volume of a swallow: role of orifice size and viscosity. Vet Hum Toxicol. 1987;29(1):79–83.

43. Steele CM, Van Lieshout PH. Influence of bolus consistency on lingual behaviors in sequential swallowing. Dysphagia. 2004;19(3):192–206.

44. Ruark J, Mills C, Muenchen R. Effects of bolus volume and consistency on multiple swallow behavior in children and adults. J Med Speech Lang Pathol. 2003;11(4):79–83.

45. Vaiman M, Segal S, Eviatar E. Surface electromyographic studies of swallowing in normal children, age 4–12 years. Int J Pediatr Otorhinolaryngol. 2004;68(1):65–73.

46. Watson WA, Bradford DC, Veltri JC. The volume of a swallow: correlation of deglutition with patient and container parameters. Am J Emerg Med. 1983;1(3):278–81.

47. Bennett JW, et al. Sip-sizing behaviors in natural drinking conditions compared to instructed experimental conditions. Dysphagia. 2009;24(2):152–8.

48. Delaney A. Oral-motor movement patterns in feeding development. Madison, WI: University of Wisconsin; 2010.

49. Morris SE. Pre-speech assessment scale. Clifton: J.A. Preston Corporation; 1982.

50. Gisel EG. Chewing cycles in 2- to 8-year-old normal children: a developmental profile. Am J Occup Ther. 1988;42(1):40–6.

51. Gisel EG. Effect of food texture on the development of chewing of children between six months and two years of age. Dev Med Child Neurol. 1991;33(1):69–79.

52. Chigira A, et al. Lip closing pressure in disabled children: a comparison with normal children. Dysphagia. 1994;9(3):193–8.

53. Potter NL, Short R. Maximal tongue strength in typically developing children and adolescents. Dysphagia. 2009;24(4):391–7.

54. Green JR, et al. Development of chewing in children from 12 to 48 months: longitudinal study of EMG patterns. J Neurophysiol. 1997;77(5):2704–16.

55. Wilson EM. Kinematic description of chewing development. Madison, WI: University of Wisconsin; 2005.

56. Wilson EM, Green JR. The development of jaw motion for mastication. Early Hum Dev. 2009;85(5):303–11.

57. Steeve RW, et al. Babbling, chewing, and sucking: oromandibular coordination at 9 months. J Speech Lang Hear Res. 2008;51(6):1390–404.

58. Schwaab LW, Niman CW, Gisel EG. Comparison of chewing cycles in 2-, 3-, 4-, and 5-year-old normal children. Am J Occup Ther. 1986;40(1):40–3.

59. Carruth BR, Skinner JD. Feeding behaviors and other motor development in healthy children (2–24 months). J Am Coll Nutr. 2002;21(2):88–96.

60. Stolovitz P, Gisel EG. Circumoral movements in response to three different food textures in children 6 months to 2 years of age. Dysphagia. 1991;6(1):17–25.

Part IV

Pharyngeal Phase of Deglutition

Development, Anatomy, and Physiology of the Pharynx

12

Peter C. Belafsky and Catherine Rees Lintzenich

Abstract

The pharynx plays an essential role in deglutition. It is a highly complex common cavity for swallowing and respiration and serves a vital function in the fundamental separation of food passage and air exchange. A thorough understanding of pharyngeal anatomy and physiology is essential to understand swallowing.

Keywords

Pharynx • Nasopharynx • Oropharynx • Hypopharynx • Anatomy • Physiology • Embryology

Development

The pharyngeal apparatus begins embryologic development from the foregut at week four of gestation. It consists of a paired network of five arches, clefts, and pouches that develop as a series of mesodermal outpouchings on the sides of the pharynx. The fifth arch is vestigial and is nonexistent in humans. The structures, therefore, are named the first, second, third, fourth, and sixth pharyngeal arches. Each arch contains a cartilaginous bar, a cranial nerve, muscle, and

P.C. Belafsky, MD, MPH, PhD (✉)
Department of Otolaryngology/Head and Neck Surgery,
University of California, Davis Medical Center
Sacramento, CA, USA
e-mail: pbelafsky@sbcglobal.net

C.R. Lintzenich, MD
Department of Otolaryngology, Wake Forest School of
Medicine, Winston Salem, NC, USA

artery. The arches are separated by endodermally lined pouches and ectodermally lined clefts (Fig. 12.1). The first arch develops into the maxillary and common carotid arteries, the mandible and maxilla, the muscles of mastication, the mandibular division of the trigeminal nerve, the mylohyoid, the anterior belly of the digastric, the tensor tympani, and the tensor veli palatini muscles. The second arch develops into the stapedial artery, the facial nerve, and part of the stapes, incus, malleus, styloid, and stylohyoid ligament, and lesser cornu of the hyoid bone. Muscular derivatives of the second arch include the muscles of facial expression, the posterior belly of the digastric, the stylohyoid, and the stapedius muscles. The third pharyngeal arch develops into the common and internal carotid arteries, the greater cornu of the hyoid bone, the glossopharyngeal nerve, and the stylopharyngeus muscle. The fourth arch develops into the aortic arch and right subclavian artery, the epiglottis and thyroid

R. Shaker et al. (eds.), *Principles of Deglutition: A Multidisciplinary Text for Swallowing and its Disorders*,
DOI 10.1007/978-1-4614-3794-9_12, © Springer Science+Business Media New York 2013

1st Arch	Derivatives
Artery	Maxillary, external carotid
Cartilage	Mandible, maxilla, zygoma, squamous portion temporal bone, part of ossicles
Nerve	Trigeminal nerve
Muscles	Muscles of mastication, mylohyoid, anterior belly of digastric, tensor tympani, tensor veli palatini

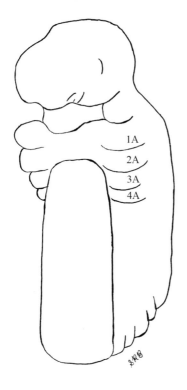

2nd Arch	Derivatives
Artery	Stapedial artery
Cartilage	Part of ossicles, lesser cornu of hyoid bone, styloid, stylohyoid ligament
Nerve	Facial nerve
Muscles	Muscles of facial expression, posterior belly of the digastric, stylohyoid, stapedius

3rd Arch	Derivatives
Artery	Common carotid, internal carotid
Cartilage	Greater cornu of hyoid
Nerve	Glossopharyngeal
Muscles	Stylopharyngeus

4th Arch	Derivatives
Artery	Arch of aorta, right subclavian
Cartilage	Epiglottis, thyroid, cuneiform
Nerve	Superior laryngeal nerve
Muscles	Pharyngeal constrictors, cricothyroid, levator veli palatini

6th Arch	Derivatives
Artery	Pulmonary, ductus arteriosus
Cartilage	Arytenoid, corniculate, cricoid
Nerve	Recurrent laryngeal nerve
Muscles	Intrinsic laryngeal muscles

*The 6th arch is buried and is not visible on the surface of the embryo.

Fig. 12.1 Human embryo at 4 weeks gestation showing the branchial arches and their derivatives. 1A = first branchial arch, 2A = second branchial arch, 3A = third branchial arch, 4A = fourth branchial arch

cartilage, the superior laryngeal nerve, the pharyngeal constrictors, cricothyroid, and levator veli palatini muscles. The sixth arch develops into the pulmonary arteries, the cricoid and arytenoid cartilages, the recurrent laryngeal nerve, and the intrinsic muscles of the larynx.

The pharyngeal pouches develop between the arches. The first pouch develops into the eustachian tube and middle ear, the second pouch into the palatine tonsil, the third pouch into the inferior parathyroid and thymus glands, and the fourth pouch develops into the superior parathyroids and the parafollicular cells of the thyroid gland.

Anatomy

The pharynx extends from the skull base to the inferior aspect of the cricoid cartilage. It is divided into the nasopharynx, oropharynx, and hypopharynx (Fig. 12.2). The mucosa of the nasopharynx is ciliated pseudostratified columnar epithelium and resembles that of the nose. The mucosa of the lower pharynx is stratified squamous epithelium similar to that of the mouth. The muscular tube of the pharynx is made up of a set of three pharyngeal constrictors covered by a layer of buccopharyngeal

fascia. The space between the buccopharyngeal fascia and the alar fascia is called the retropharyngeal space. The space between the alar fascia and the prevertebral fascia is called the danger space. Unlike the retropharyngeal space, the danger space lacks a midline raphe and infection can spread easily to the mediastinum. All of the muscles of the pharynx except the stylopharyngeus (CN IX) are innervated by the pharyngeal plexus of the vagus nerve.

Nasopharynx

The nasopharynx extends superiorly from the occipital bone of the skull base to the superior surface of the soft palate inferiorly. It is bound anteriorly by the choanae of the nasal cavity, superiorly by the skull base, inferiorly by the junction of the hard and soft palate, and posteriorly

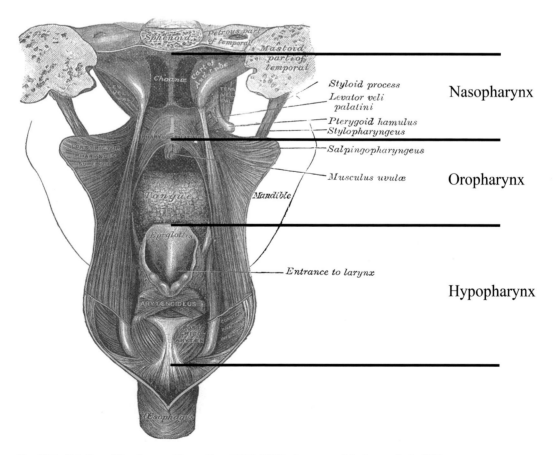

Fig. 12.2 Subsites of the pharynx. Henry Gray (1825–1861). Anatomy of the human body 1918

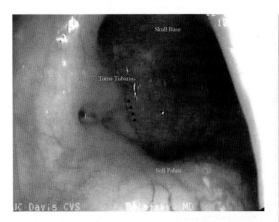

Fig. 12.3 The boundaries of the nasopharynx seen on flexible endoscopic view though the right posterior nasal aperture (choanae). The boundaries are the base of skull superiorly, the torus tubarius, eustachian tube orifice (E), and the salpingopharyngeal fold (*arrowheads*) laterally, the superior pharyngeal constrictor posteriorly, and the choanae anteriorly

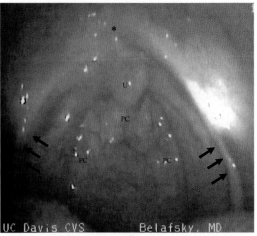

Fig. 12.4 The boundaries of the oropharynx seen on flexible endoscopic view through the mouth. The anterior border is the palatoglossal fold (anterior tonsillar pillar— *black arrows*). The posterior and lateral boundary is the superior and middle pharyngeal constrictors (PC). The inferior border is the foramen cecum (not seen on this image) and the superior border is the junction of the hard and soft palate (*asterisks*) just above the uvula (U)

and laterally by the superior pharyngeal constrictor, levator veli palatini, tensor veli palatini, and salpingopharyngeus muscles (Fig. 12.3).

The contents of the nasopharynx include the pharyngeal tonsil (adenoid) and the eustachian tube. The pharyngeal tonsil forms the posterior superior aspect of an incomplete ring of lymphoid tissue called Waldeyer's ring. This ring is made up of the palatine tonsils laterally, the lingual tonsils anteriorly, and the pharyngeal tonsil (adenoid) posterosuperiorly. Enlargement of the pharyngeal tonsil can lead to chronic nasal obstruction, otitis media, and speech disturbance. The eustachian tube is approximately 3.5 cm in length. It connects the nasopharynx to the middle ear cavity and consists of an anterior cartilaginous and a posterior osseous component.

Oropharynx

The oropharynx extends from the soft palate to the hyoid bone (Fig. 12.2). The anterior borders of the oropharynx include the anterior tonsillar pillars laterally, the foramen cecum inferiorly (dividing the anterior 2/3 of the tongue from the posterior 1/3 of the base), and the junction

between the hard and soft palate superiorly (Fig. 12.4). The posterior and lateral boundary of the oropharynx is the superior and middle pharyngeal constrictors, innervated by the pharyngeal plexus of the vagus nerve (CN X). The superior, middle, and inferior constrictor muscles create the tubular pharynx and join in a posterior midline raphe. The superior pharyngeal constrictor muscle has complex attachments to the buccinator muscle, the mandible, and the tongue base. From the pharyngeal wall, the stylopharyngeus muscle extends up to the styloid process of the temporal bone. This muscle, along with the palatopharyngeus muscle, assists in vertical shortening of the pharynx during deglutition. The human constrictor muscles are comprised of a slow inner layer of muscle fibers, innervated by the glossopharyngeal nerve (CN IX), and a fast outer layer of fibers, innervated by the vagus nerve (CN X) [1]. This fast outer layer is felt to be more important in deglutition, while the slow inner layer likely plays a more prominent role in respiration and speech. The inferior border of the oropharynx is demarcated by the tip of the epiglottis. The epiglottis is connected to the

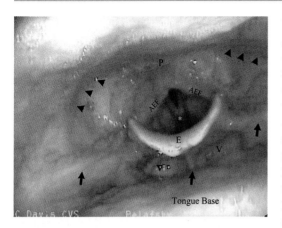

Fig. 12.5 The boundaries of the hypopharynx seen on flexible endoscopic view through the nasal cavity. The boundaries are the tip of the epiglottis (E) superiorly, the hypopharyngeal walls (*black arrowheads*) posterolaterally, and the posterior cricoid region inferiorly (P). The aryepiglottic folds (AEF) separate the hypopharynx from the endolarynx (*asterisk*). Also seen on this image is the median and lateral glossoepiglottic ligaments (*black arrows*), the tongue base, and vallecula (V)

tongue by the median glossoepiglottic ligament and the paired lateral glossoepiglottic ligaments (Fig. 12.5). The space between lateral glossoepiglottic ligaments is the vallecula. The sensory input to the oropharynx and hypopharynx is from the glossopharyngeal nerve (CN IX) and the vagus nerve (CN X). Blood supply to the pharynx is from the external carotid artery.

The contents of the oropharynx include the palatine tonsils, the lingual tonsils, and vallecula. The palatopharyngeus muscle forms the posterior tonsillar pillar, and the palatoglossus muscle makes up the anterior tonsillar pillar. The paired palatine tonsils reside between the anterior and posterior pillars. The palatal arches meet in the midline at the uvula, a pendulous projection comprised of the uvulus muscle.

The base of the tongue (posterior 1/3) is relatively fixed compared to the freely mobile oral tongue. The intrinsic tongue musculature includes longitudinal, vertical, and transverse muscle fibers innervated by the hypoglossal nerve (CN XII). The intrinsic muscles do not have bony attachments. The longitudinal fibers shorten the tongue, the vertical fibers flatten and widen the tongue, and the transverse fibers narrow and elongate the

tongue. The extrinsic tongue muscles include the genioglossus, the hyoglossus, the styloglossus, and the palatoglossus. All of the extrinsic tongue muscles are innervated by the hypoglossal nerve (CN XII), except the palatoglossus, which is innervated by the vagus nerve (CN X). The hyoglossus and styloglossus muscles attach to the hyoid bone and styloid process, respectively. The hyoglossus muscle depresses and flattens the tongue. The styloglossus muscle retracts the tongue and makes the surface concave. The genioglossus muscle is a large fan-shaped muscle arising from the mental spine on the posterior surface of the mandible and inserting on the tongue dorsum and hyoid bone. This muscle is primarily responsible for extruding and depressing the tongue.

The suprahyoid muscles assist in movement of the tongue as well as elevation of the larynx. The geniohyoid muscle, innervated by C1 hitchhiking along the hypoglossal nerve, arises from the inferior mental spine of the mandible and attaches to the anterior hyoid. The anterior belly of the digastric muscle and the mylohyoid muscle, innervated by the mandibular branch of the trigeminal nerve (CN V3) also assist in elevating the hyoid and pulling the tongue forward.

Sensory innervation to the tongue base is supplied by the glossopharyngeal nerve (CN 9), as opposed to the anterior oral tongue that is supplied by the trigeminal nerve (CN V). The special sensory innervation taste is delivered via the branches of the glossopharyngeal nerve (CN IX) and the internal laryngeal nerve (CN X) in the tongue base. Anterior tongue taste occurs via the chorda tympani nerve (CN VII). The large circumvallate papillae can be visualized on the posterior tongue. Beyond this, the lingual tonsil covers the posterior portion of the tongue.

Hypopharynx

The hypopharynx is part of the laryngopharynx, which includes both the larynx and the hypopharynx (Fig. 12.5). The superior margin of the hypopharynx is the tip of the epiglottis and the inferior border is the lower edge of the cricoid cartilage (Fig. 12.2). The hypopharyngeal walls make up the posterolateral boundary and the aryepiglottic folds separate the hypopharynx from the endolarynx. The hypopharynx can be divided into the pharyngeal walls, the piriform sinuses, and the postcricoid region.

The pharyngeal walls are covered in mucosa and formed by the pharyngeal constrictor muscles. The superior, middle, and inferior constrictor muscles create the tubular pharynx and join in a posterior midline raphe. From the pharyngeal wall, the stylopharyngeus muscle, innervated by the glossopharyngeal nerve (CN IX) extends to the styloid process of the temporal bone, and the palatopharyngeus muscle extends to the soft palate.

The piriform sinuses are lateral to the larynx and extend inferior to the larynx. These recesses act as gutters during swallowing. If lingual and pharyngeal peristalsis do not effectively transport a bolus into the esophagus, these reservoirs serve to retain food, liquid, and secretions and keep them out of the airway. The borders of the piriform sinus are the aryepiglottic folds medially, the thyrohyoid membrane anteriorly, and the thyroid ala or cartilage laterally.

Because of its location, the region between the hypopharynx and esophagus has been referred to as the pharyngoesophageal segment or PES. The upper esophageal sphincter (UES) specifically refers to the intra-luminal high-pressure zone visualized on manometry. The PES refers to the anatomic components that make up the high-pressure zone. The UES and PES are synonymous and may be used interchangeably. The cricopharyngeus muscle (CPM) makes up only one component of the PES. The anatomy and physiology of this region will be addressed in a subsequent chapter.

The postcricoid region is the mucosal area posterior to the larynx, bordered anteriorly by the arytenoid cartilages and the posterior commissure of the larynx (Fig. 12.6). This area is difficult to visualize in the awake patient because the pharyngoesophageal segment is closed, obliterating the postcricoid region. Occasionally the mucosa of

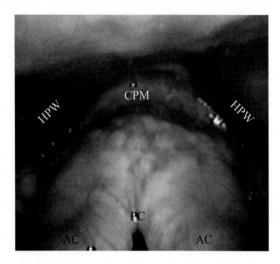

Fig. 12.6 The posterior cricoid region seen on flexible endoscopic view. The anterior boundaries are the arytenoid cartilages (AC) and posterior commissure of the glottis (PC). The posterolateral boundary is the hypopharyngeal wall (HPW), and the inferior boundary is the cricopharyngeus muscle (CPM)

this region can be inspected during a swallow or a belch, but usually general anesthesia with rigid endoscopy is required for adequate exposure of the postcricoid region. Because of the limitations of examination in this area, malignancies of the postcricoid region may be missed. Postcricoid tumors should always be considered in a patient with unexplained postcricoid and/or pyriform sinus residue and in patients with painful swallowing (odynophagia).

Physiology of the Pharyngeal Phase of Deglutition

Because of the principal requirement to separate food and air movement through the upper aerodigestive tract, coordination between respiration and deglutition during the pharyngeal phase is fundamental and largely involuntary. After preparation of the food bolus in the oral cavity (Fig. 12.7a), the bolus is moved to the posterior

Fig. 12.7 (continued) Passive compression of the epiglottis by the advancing bolus and contraction of the pharyngeal constrictors, thyroepiglottic and aryepiglottic muscles rotate the epiglottis from a horizontal to a transverse orientation facing the esophageal inlet (*black arrow*).

Note the cricopharyngeus muscle bar at the distal aspect of pharyngoesophageal segment (*asterisks*). (**f**) The elastic pharyngoesophageal segment closes behind the tale of the bolus and the pharyngeal phase of the swallow is complete

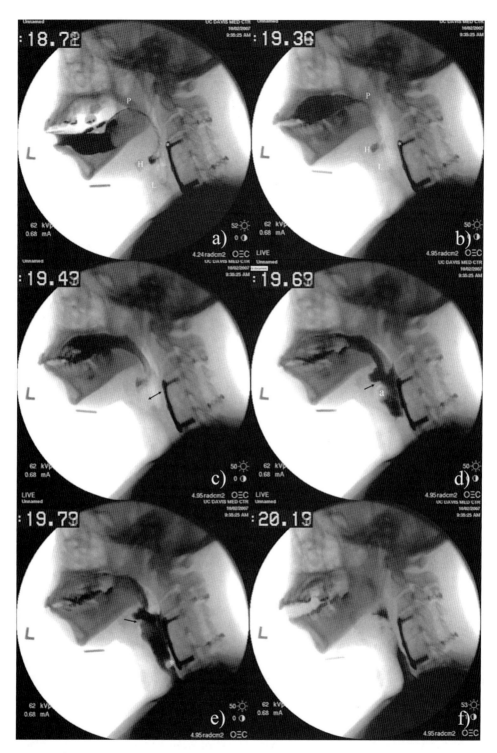

Fig. 12.7 Lateral fluoroscopic view during deglutition. (**a**) The bolus is held in the anterior oral cavity and the hyoid (H), larynx (L), and palate (P) are at their resting position. Note the relationship of the hyoid and larynx to the position of the anterior C4–C6 cervical hardware. The hyoid sits below the rostral margin of the plate (*asterisk*). (**b**) The bolus is prepared in the oral cavity and transferred to the posterior tongue. The palate (P) begins to close off the nasopharynx and the hyoid (H) and larynx (L) begin their ascent. The hyoid is now above the rostral margin of the plate (*asterisk*).

(**c**) The bolus is transported past the anterior tonsillar pillars and the pharyngeal phase of deglutition is initiated. The larynx and hyoid remain elevated off of the spine and the pharyngeal area is enlarged (*black double arrow*). (**d**) The arytenoids (**a**) are pulled toward the laryngeal surface of the epiglottis and the epiglottis is passively rotated into a horizontal position to protect the endolarynx (*black arrow*). (**e**) Lingual and pharyngeal driving pressure in addition to negative hypopharyngeal pressure work in concert to transport the bolus through the pharynx and into the cervical esophagus.

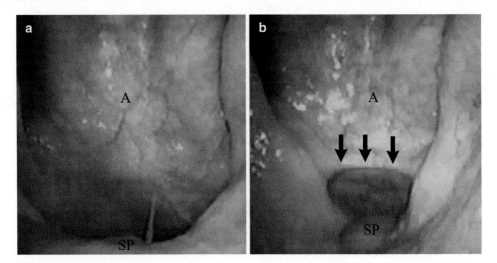

Fig. 12.8 Flexible endoscopic view of Passavant's ridge through the left nasal cavity. (**a**) The nasopharynx and soft palate (SP) are at rest. The regressed adenoid (**a**) is seen posteriorly. (**b**) The nasopharynx and soft palate (SP) contract bringing Pasavant's ridge into view (*black arrows*)

tongue (Fig. 12.7b). The bolus is stripped by the piston-like action of the tongue against the hard and then soft palate. As the bolus crosses the anterior tonsillar pillars, the pharyngeal phase of deglutition is initiated (Fig. 12.7c). The palatopharyngeal folds approximate toward the midline to form a funnel that guides the bolus through the upper pharynx. The soft palate moves superiorly to isolate the nasopharynx from the oropharynx. Successful closure of both the nasopharynx and oropharynx is essential in bolus propagation through the lower pharynx. During the swallow, the levator veli palatini, innervated by the pharyngeal branch of the vagus nerve (CN10), and the tensor veli palatini, innervated by the mandibular branch of the trigeminal nerve (CN, V3) elevate the soft palate to close off the nasopharyx. The salpingopharyngeus muscle, innervated by the pharyngeal plexus of the vagus nerve, serves two primary purposes. It elevates the pharynx and larynx to assist with deglutition and, in conjunction with the tensor veli palatini, opens the eustachian tube to equalize air pressure between the middle ear and nasopharynx during swallowing and yawning. Contraction of the lateral and posterior nasopharyngeal walls helps create a muscular barricade

to nasal regurgitation called Passavant's ridge (Fig. 12.8). Posterior movement of the tongue and closure of the naso- and oropharynx creates a pressure differential that forces the bolus inferiorly (Fig. 12.7d). As the bolus traverses the lower pharynx, three events are responsible for airway protection:

1. *Movement of the hyoid and larynx superiorly and anteriorly.* This motion protects the larynx underneath the base of tongue and elevates the laryngeal framework off of the spine. Elevation shortens and enlarges the pharynx, assists with UES opening, and creates negative hypopharyngeal pressure to assist with bolus propagation. The negative hypopharyngeal pressure ahead of the advancing bolus, coupled with the tongue and pharyngeal driving pressure behind the tail of the bolus, creates a pressure gradient that favors bolus movement into the esophagus.

2. *Glottic closure.* Airway protection is provided by a three-tiered protective mechanism. Glottic closure occurs at the level of the true, false, and aryepiglottic folds and proceeds in a rostral to caudal direction. Closure of the true vocal folds is thought to be the most important of the three protective mechanisms. Since the

vocal folds must close during deglutition, a period of apnea occurs during every swallow. Depending on the bolus size, this apneic period may last as long as 3.5 s [2–5].

3. *Epiglottis retroversion.* Closure of the epiglottis over the laryngeal vestibule has been described as a two-step procedure [6]. Fibroelastic ligaments fix the epiglottis to the surrounding hyoid bone, thyroid cartilage, and quadrangular membrane. Laryngopharyngeal elevation by the suprahyoid musculature (mylohyoid, stylohyoid, geniohyoid, thyrohyoid, and digastric) results in passive movement of the suspended epiglottis from a vertical to a horizontal orientation. Passive compression of the epiglottis by the advancing bolus and active contraction of the pharyngeal constrictors, along with the thyroepiglottic and aryepiglottic muscles then assist the epiglottis in progressing from its transverse orientation to its ultimate inverted position facing the esophageal inlet. Airway protection is now complete.

Four factors are thought responsible for bolus propagation past the protected larynx. Tongue driving pressure, contraction of the pharyngeal constrictors, negative hypopharyngeal pressure, and gravity. McConnel referred to these mechanisms as the oropharyngeal propulsion pump (OPP) and the hypopharyngeal suction pump (HSP) [7]. The OPP is driven by the pressure generated from the anterior two-thirds of the tongue and contraction of the pharyngeal constrictor muscles. The negative pressure of the HSP is generated from enlargement of the pharynx and elevation of the hyoid and larynx (Fig. 12.7d). These mechanisms work in concert to drive a bolus through the pharynx at a rate of 9–25 cm/s [8, 9]. The upper esophageal sphincter opens by muscle relaxation, traction force through anterior hyolaryngeal excursion, intrabolus pressure, and UES muscle compliance. The opening of the UES is triggered at the initiation of the pharyngeal phase of swallowing. The UES remains open until the bolus has traversed the relaxed cricopharyngeous muscle and entered the esophagus, indicating the end of the pharyngeal phase of deglutition.

References

1. Mu L, Sanders I. Neuromuscular specializations within human pharyngeal constrictor muscles. Ann Otol Rhinol Laryngol. 2007;116(8):604–17.
2. Martin-Harris B, Brodsky MB, Price CC, Michel Y, Walters B. Temporal coordination of pharyngeal and laryngeal dynamics with breathing during swallowing: single liquid swallows. J Appl Physiol. 2003;94(5):1735–43.
3. Martin-Harris B, Brodsky MB, Michel Y, Ford CL, Walters B, Heffner J. Breathing and swallowing dynamics across the adult lifespan. Arch Otolaryngol Head Neck Surg. 2005;131:762–70.
4. Perlman AL, Ettema SL, Barkmeier J. Respiratory and acoustic signals associated with bolus passage during swallowing. Dysphagia. 2000;15(2):89–94.
5. Hårdemark Cedborg AI, Bodén K, Witt Hedström H, Kuylenstierna R, Ekberg O, Eriksson LI, Sundman E. Breathing and swallowing in normal man--effects of changes in body position, bolus types, and respiratory drive. Neurogastroenterol Motil. 2010;22(11): 1201–8. e316.
6. Ekberg O, Sigurjónsson SV. Movement of the epiglottis during deglutition. A cineradiographic study. Gastrointest Radiol. 1982;7(2):101–7.
7. McConnel FMS, Cerenko D, Mendelsohn MS. Manofluorographic analysis of swallowing. Oto Clin North Am. 1988;21:625–35.
8. Dodds WJ, Stewart ET, Logemann JA. Physiology and radiology of the normal oral and pharyngeal phases of swallowing. AJR Am J Roentgenol. 1990; 154(5):953–63.
9. Dodds WJ. The physiology of swallowing. Dysphagia. 1989;3:171–8.

Development, Anatomy, and Physiology of the Larynx

13

Mikhail Wadie, Stewart I. Adam,
and Clarence T. Sasaki

Abstract

The human larynx, located at the crossroads of the upper digestive tract and tracheobronchial tree, has evolved structural and functional components to safely facilitate respiration, swallowing, airway protection, and vocalization. The larynx, trachea, and lungs begin formation at 28 days of life. Development continues into the neonatal period and through puberty, with cartilage maturation and larynx and hyoid decent. Detailed knowledge of the laryngeal cartilage skeleton and neurovascular structures is vital for both the head and neck surgeon and speech pathologist. A complex set of afferent and efferent pathways govern neuromuscular physiology, which dictate basic laryngeal functions through a delicate coordination of precisely organized brainstem reflexes. Significant work has been invested into understanding the unique and phylogenetically advanced protective, respiratory, and phonatory reflexes of the human larynx.

Keywords

Development • Anatomy • Physiology • Larynx • Airway protection • Respiration • Phonation

The human larynx is a multitask organ that balances respiration, swallowing, airway protection, and vocalization. These functions are intrinsically related to the structure and location of the larynx, which is a valve at the crossroads of the upper digestive tract and tracheobronchial tree. Complex neural control, coupled with specialized tissue adaptations, govern the vitality of laryngeal function. Understanding how laryngeal evolution and development relate to specialized anatomy paves the way for an appreciation of its complex functional behaviors.

M. Wadie, MD • S.I. Adam, MD
Department of Otolaryngology, Yale New Haven
Hospital, New Haven, CT, USA

C.T. Sasaki, MD (✉)
Department of Surgery-Otolaryngology, Yale
Comprehensive Cancer Center, Yale New Haven
Hospital, New Haven, CT, USA
e-mail: clarence.sasaki@yale.edu

Development

Negus classically articulated the functioning priorities of the larynx in his evolutionary studies, which demonstrated (1) airway protection,

(2) respiration, (3) and phonation to be the order [1]. Bichir lungfish, with the most primitive larynx, developed a simple sphincter for lower airway protection. African lungfish evolved musculature to open and close its laryngeal sphincter, creating a primitive respiratory system. Vertebrates, with the aid of their thoracoabdominal diaphragm, can use the larynx as a flutter valve for sound production by varying airflow during respiration [2].

According to the Carnegie staging system for human embryologic development, there are two periods of development. The first period, the embryonic period, comprises the first 8 weeks of gestation and is subdivided into 23 stages. The second period, the fetal period, spans the remaining

32 weeks of gestation. The larynx begins to develop during stage 11 of the embryonic period at 25–28 days (Fig. 13.1).

At 28 days of intrauterine life, the larynx, trachea, and lungs begin to form as the laryngotracheal diverticulum (respiratory diverticulum). These structures commence as an endodermal outgrowth in the ventral wall of the foregut just caudal to the fourth pair of pharyngeal pouches [4]. The epithelial lining and glands for the larynx, trachea, and lungs arise from the foregut endodermal lining of the diverticulum. Splanchnic mesenchyme forms an investing layer around the lengthening diverticulum, which gives rise to smooth muscle, cartilage, connective tissue, and

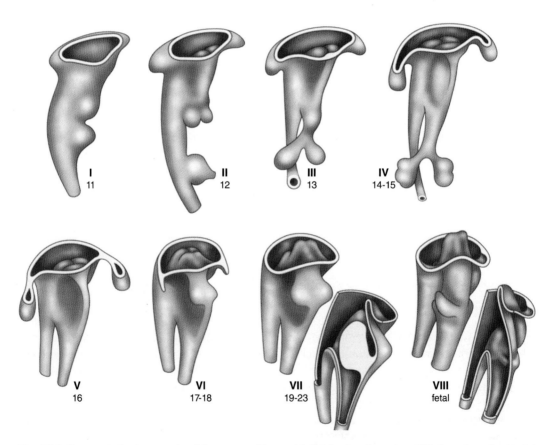

Fig. 13.1 Laryngeal development in eight stages with Carnegie Institute embryologic stages (11–23), as illustrated in Holinger et al. Pertinent ideas: I- ventral foregut produces respiratory diverticulum; II- bronchopulmonary bud formation; III-development of tracheobronchial tree; IV- arytenoids swellings, developing epiglottis, and epithelial lamina formation; VII- inception of epithelial lamina recanalization; VIII-formation of laryngeal ventricles. From D.H. Henick and L.D. Holinger. Pediatric laryngology and bronchoesophagology. Philadelphia: Lippincott-Raven; 1997:1–17 with permission

the primordial lung bud by the end of the fourth week. Zaw-Tun and Burdi demonstrated that the separation of the trachea and esophagus results from the continued ventrocaudal lengthening of the respiratory diverticulum as an outgrowth of foregut lumen, which replaced the century old His paradigm of an ascending tracheoesophageal septum. The developing respiratory system, including the larynx and the foregut, continue their separate development in a cranial to caudal direction [3, 5, 6].

The primitive pharyngeal floor, equivalent to the level of the fourth pouch and site of origin of the respiratory diverticulum, develops into the glottic region. A segment of foregut consisting of the primitive laryngopharynx becomes the supraglottic larynx; it separates the primitive pharyngeal floor from the pharyngeal floor formed by the fourth branchial pouches. As the bronchopulmonary buds migrate caudally, the two main bronchi and carina take form, and the infraglottis develops from the cephalic portion of respiratory diverticulum. The infraglottis becomes separated from the carina by the developing trachea. With continued elongation of the foregut and respiratory diverticulum, the esophagus lengthens in the coming weeks.

Mesenchyme in the ventral portion of the developing larynx proliferates rapidly in the sixth week, gradually obliterating the lumen and giving rise to the epithelial lamina. Arytenoid swellings develop from the pharyngeal floor, causing the laryngeal inlet to be seen as a T-shape between the developing arytenoids and central epiglottic swelling. The epithelial lamina continues to obliterate the primitive laryngopharyx in a ventral to dorsal direction almost completely, aside from a narrow communication between the hypopharynx and infraglottis called the pharyngoglottic duct. The laryngeal cecum, a depression that develops between the arytenoid swellings and epiglottis, descends ventrally along the epithelial lamina toward the glottis [7].

The epithelial lamina begins to recanalize from a dorsocephalic to ventrocaudal direction during the tenth week of development. This process establishes a communication between the laryngeal cecum and dorsal phayrngoglottic duct, connecting the supraglottis and infraglottis. The laryngeal ventricle is one of the last structures to develop during the recanalization period, as ventricular outgrowths from lateral aspects of the laryngeal cecum. The upper and lower lips of this lateral outgrowth form the false and true vocal folds, respectively. Failure of the recanalization process is the source of congenital laryngeal webs and atresias [8].

The epithelial lining of the larynx is derived from endoderm, as described above. During the fifth to eighth week of development, the laryngeal cartilages take form and musculature is clearly delineated. The hyaline cartilages—thyroid, cricoid, and arytenoid—are formed by fusion of mesenchymal neural crest in the fourth and sixth branchial arches. The elastic cartilages—epiglottic, cuneiform, and corniculate—are formed from mesenchyme in the pharyngeal floor. The cricoid and arytenoids chondrify bilaterally from a single center in the ventral arch. The thyroid alae chondrify at two centers. The epiglottis forms last from the hypobronchial eminence, a proliferation of mesenchyme in the ventral ends of the third and fourth arches.

At the same time, laryngeal musculature develops from mesenchymal condensation within the larynx. The cricothyroid, stemming from the ventral portion of the inferior pharyngeal constrictor, is a fourth arch derivative and innervated by the superior laryngeal nerve. The other intrinsic muscles are derived from the sixth arch, innervated by the recurrent laryngeal nerve [9, 10].

The laryngeal cartilages continue to mature during the ensuing fetal period. The larynx is at the body of the second cervical vertebra in the newborn, whereas the adult larynx may be as low as the sixth cervical vertebra. The larynx continues to rapidly develop during the first few years of life, giving all cartilages their mature shape and form. During puberty, there is a brisk lowering of the larynx and hyoid bone relative to the base of tongue. This process corresponds to voice changes, which garners unique human function.

Anatomy

Skeletal Structure (Figs. 13.2 and 13.3) [11]

Thyroid Cartilage

The thyroid cartilage is the largest laryngeal cartilage. It forms a shield over the anterior portion of the larynx, protecting the internal laryngeal structures. It is a wedge-shaped structure, with two lateral wings called laminae or alae. The midline fusion of the alae at the apex of the wedge occurs at approximately 90° in men, accounting for the laryngeal prominence ("Adams's apple"). The prominence is less prominent in females because the alae fuse more obliquely at 120°. A superior tissue deficiency at the juncture point creates the thyroid notch. Laterally, at the posterior edges of the alae are a superior greater and inferior lesser cornu or horn. Thyroid cartilage articulates with a facet on the cricoid cartilage at the inferior bilateral cornu to form the cricothyroid joint. This synovial joint allows rotation of the cricoid cartilage, which varies tension on the vocal folds. Thyroid cartilage is attached to the hyoid bone by the thryohyoid membrane. The thickened middle and edges of the membrane are called the median and lateral thryohyoid ligaments (often containing small triticeal cartilages), where the superior cornu attaches to the greater cornu of the hyoid bone [12–16].

The superior tubercle is a protuberance at the attachment of the superior cornu to the thyroid alae. The superior laryngeal artery and the internal branch of the superior laryngeal nerve pierce the thyrohyoid membrane about 1 cm anterior and superior to the tubercle, supplying the supraglottic portion of the larynx. The tubercle is a landmark for transcutaneous anesthesia of the internal branch. The oblique line runs from the anterior commissure to the posterior edge of the ala, affording attachment for the thyrohyoid, sternohyoid, and inferior constrictor muscles.

A thick layer of perichondrium lines the thyroid cartilage on all surfaces sans the inner portion at the anterior commissure. Five ligaments attach at the anterior commissure providing support to the laryngeal folds. The median thyroepiglottic ligament (median thyrohyoid fold), bilateral vestibular ligaments (false folds), and bilateral vocal ligaments (vocal folds) run from superior to inferior. Broyles' ligament is formed through the fibrous attachments of these ligaments penetrating the inner perichondrium, providing a barrier to the spread of laryngeal neoplasms.

An understanding of the relation of surface anatomy to internal laryngeal anatomy is vital for surgical approaches such as a supraglottic laryngectomy or thyroplasty procedures, where the level of the true vocal cords in relation to the thyroid cartilage is most important. The midline vertical distance from the thyroid notch to the inferior border of the thyroid cartilage ranges from 20 to 47 mm in men and from 15.5 to 38 mm in women [10]. The midpoint between these two landmarks houses the anterior commissure with the vocal folds lying below the vertical midline of the thyroid cartilage. The posterior portion of the folds is anterior to and in the middle third of the oblique line [17].

Cricoid Cartilage

The tracheal entrance and lower portion of the laryngeal wall are buttressed by cricoid cartilage, which is a complete ring and the only supporting structure of the larynx and trachea extending completely around the airway. Described as a signet ring, its narrow anterior arch and expanded posterior lamina are 0.5–1 cm and 2–3 cm in vertical height, respectively. The horizontal inferior border is attached to first tracheal cartilage by the cricotracheal ligament [11, 12].

The posterior cricoarytenoid muscles, the only abductor of the vocal fold, attach in depressions separated by a midline vertical ridge on the posterior cricoid surface. Two fasciculi of esophageal longitudinal fibers are attached to the midline ridge. The lateral cricoarytenoid muscles are attached anteriorly. Laterally, the cricoid cartilage receives the lowermost fibers of the inferior constrictor muscle and the semicircular fibers of the cricopharyngeus muscle of the upper esophageal sphincter.

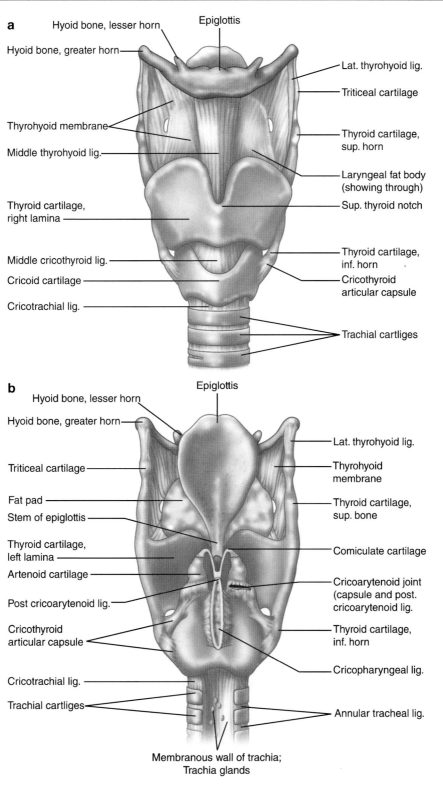

Fig. 13.2 Anterior view of the laryngeal framework—cartilages and ligaments—and hyoid bone (*top*). Posterior view of the laryngeal cartilages, ligaments, and infrastructure (*bottom*). From C.T. Sasaki et al. Ballenger's Otorhinolaryngology head and neck surgery, 17th ed. Shelton, CT: Decker; 2009:849 with permission

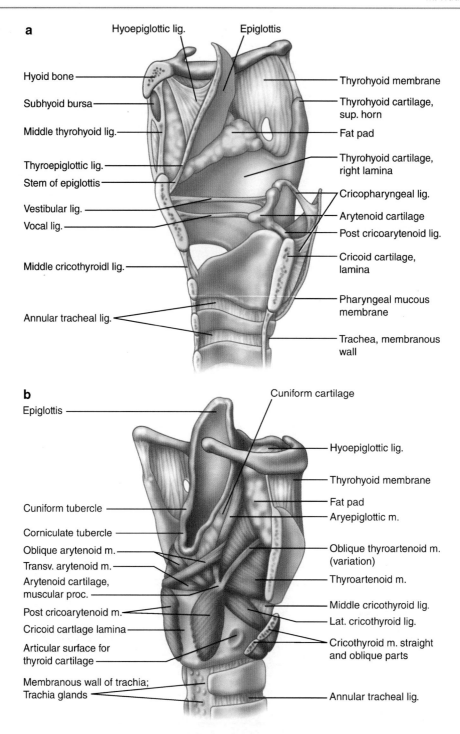

Fig. 13.3 *Sagital view* of laryngeal ligaments and infrastructure (*top*). *Posterior lateral* view of laryngeal intrinsic musculature (*bottom*). From C.T. Sasaki et al. Ballenger's Otorhinolaryngology head and neck surgery, 17th ed. Shelton, CT: Decker; 2009:849 with permission

The paired arytenoid cartilages are on the superior surface of the posterior lamina. The cricoid lamina slopes downward, posterior to anterior to the cricoid arch, the superior portion of which attaches to the inferior border of thyroid cartilages by the midline cricothyroid membrane. The anterolateral portion of this membrane is subcutaneous and is incised when performing an emergency cricothyrotomy.

Arytenoid Cartilages

The paired arytenoid cartilages attach to the posterior ends of the vocal ligament and sit on the posterosuperior portion of the cricoid cartilage. The arytenoids are pyramidal, each with a triangular base. The base provides a lateral muscular process, anterior vocal process, and an inferior articular facet. The synovial cricoarytenoid joint provides movements for the complex laryngeal functions. The most important movement of the joint is a downward and lateral or upward and medial sliding of arytenoid on cricoid, accompanied by a rocking and twisting motion of the cartilage around the long axis of its facet. The vestibular ligament, along with the thyroarytenoid muscle and vocalis as its medial belly, attaches to the anterolateral surface. The posterior surface contains muscular attachments, and the posterior cricoarytenoid ligament is attached to the medial surface. The corniculate cartilage sits at the apex of the arytenoid [12, 14–16].

Corniculate and Cuneiform Cartilages

The corniculate cartilage (of Santorini) and cuneiform cartilage (of Wrisberg) are small fibroelastic cartilages. The corniculates are surmounted on the arytenoid apex, and the cuneiforms, when present, are lateral to the corniculate in the aryepiglottic folds. Regarded as rudimentary and vestigial, the cuneiforms add rigidity to the aeryepiglottic folds, driving swallowed material laterally into the pyriform sinuses away from the larynx [12–16].

Epiglottis

The leaf-shaped elastic fibrocartilage of the epiglottis serves as a safety-net, preventing swallowed matter from entering the laryngeal aditus.

The epiglottis is displaced posteriorly over the laryngeal aditus by the tongue base during the swallow reflex, as the larynx is raised anterosuperiorly. The epiglottis is anchored anterosuperiorly by the hyoepiglottic ligament. It is anchored anteroinferiorly by the attachment of the thyroepiglottic ligament at the inner surface of the thyroid cartilage to its pointed inferior pole (petiolus). Numerous pits and mucous glands cover the surface of the epiglottic cartilage; the pits serve as sites for the potential spread of cancer [15, 16].

The epiglottis can be divided into a suprahyoid and infrahyoid portion. The laryngeal and lingual surfaces of the suprahyoid portion are both free. Laryngeal mucosa is more adherent than lingual. Two lateral glossoepiglottic folds and one median glossoepiglottic fold stem from the reflection of laryngeal mucosa onto the base of tongue. The valleculae (*little depression* in Latin) are formed by the two depressions from these folds. Only the laryngeal surface of the infrahyoid portion is free. The potential space between the anterior surface of the epiglottis and the inner surface of the thyrohyoid membrane and thyroid cartilage is the preepiglottic space. Carcinoma of the larynx may invade this space, requiring removal with the epiglottis. The aryepiglottic fold attaches laterally on each side of the epiglottis as a quadrangular membrane, extending to the arytenoid and corniculate cartilages [12–16].

Ossification of Laryngeal Cartilages

An awareness of the normal pattern and variation in the ossification of laryngeal cartilages has been of clinical importance since the advent of radiographs, in which incomplete ossification may be mistaken for a foreign body. Only structures composed of hyaline cartilage will undergo ossification (thyroid, cricoid, and arytenoid). The hyoid bone is usually not a point of radiologic confusion, as it is completely ossified by 2 years of age [18, 19].

The thyroid cartilage begins ossification around the age of 20 years in the male and 22 years in the female. The process begins posteroinferiorly on the lamina, extending anteriorly and superiorly on the inferior and posterior borders, respectively. The inferior and superior cornua have centers of ossification at this time. Ossification of the cricoid and arytenoid begin after that of the thyroid cartilage, commencing at the inferior border of the cricoid. Invasion of the thyroid cartilages by a neoplastic process takes place in the ossified portions; incomplete ossification increases difficulty in differentiating small areas of invasion [15, 16].

Elastic Tissues (Fig. 13.4) [20]

The two portions of elastic tissue in the adult larynx are the quadrangular membrane of the supraglottic larynx and the conus elasticus and vocal ligaments of the glottic and infraglottic larynx. The quadrangular membrane extends from the sides of the epiglottic cartilage to the corniculate and arytenoid cartilages. It forms the aryepiglottic fold with the mucous membrane covering it. The fold forms both parts of

the medial walls of the pyriform sinus. Inferiorly, the quadrangular membrane forms the vestibular ligaments that help produce the false vocal folds.

The conus elasticus is a more strongly developed layer of elastic tissue than the quadrangular membrane. Its inferior attachment is at the superior border of the cricoid cartilage. With superior and medial projection of the conus, the anterior commissure of the thyroid cartilage and the vocal processes of the arytenoid serve as the superior attachments. The conus thickens to form a vocal ligament between these superior attachments. The cricothyroid membrane, with its midline thickening into the cricothyroid ligament, is formed by the conus anteriorly. The thyroglottic membrane, which parallels the superior surface of the true vocal fold, is the superior extension of the conus. The thyroglottic membrane forms an incomplete barrier to the extension of transglottic cancer due to normal dehiscence in the membrane [12, 15, 16].

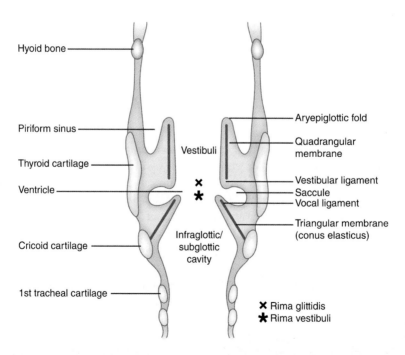

Fig. 13.4 Internal cavity and subdivisions of larynx in coronal view. From C.T. Sasaki et al. Ballenger's otorhinolaryngology head and neck surgery, 17th ed. Shelton, CT: Decker; 2009:852 with permission

Internal Anatomy

The laryngeal aditus, or entrance into the larynx, is triangular shaped in the anterior wall of the pharynx. The internal anatomy has three portions—the vestibule, ventricle, and infraglottic cavity—demarcated by the false and true vocal cords [11–16].

Vestibule

As seen through the laryngoscope, the vestibule extends from the tip of the epiglottis to the false vocal (vestibular) folds. The epiglottis, aryepiglottic folds, arytenoid, and corniculate cartilages are its anterior, lateral, and posterior borders, respectively. The anterior commissure is frequently hidden by the epiglottic tubercle during laryngoscopy. The inferior border of the quadrangular membrane provides mucosa to overlay the vestibular ligament, forming the vestibular folds. Numerous seromucinous glands are within the submucosa, aiding in mechanical and immune protection.

Ventricle

The false vocal folds hide much of the true vocal folds during laryngoscopy. The ventricle of the larynx (sinus of Morgani) extends between the false and true vocal folds. A diverticulum known as the laryngeal saccule is at the anterior end of the ventricle, extending between the vestibular fold and inner surface of thyroid cartilage. A number of mucous glands line the saccule, along with fibers of thyroarytenoid muscle, whose contractions express mucous and lubricate the vocal fold. Laryngocele occurs with abnormal enlargement of the saccule with air.

Vocal Folds (Fig. 13.5)

The true vocal folds, extending from the anterior commissure to the vocal process of the arytenoid, are inferior to the ventricle. The glottis is defined as the vocal folds and the slit between them (rima glottidis) and is normally the narrowest portion of the larynx. The intermembranous portion of

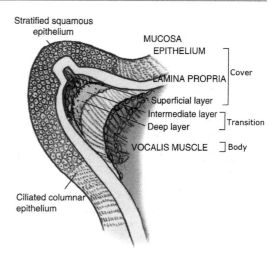

Fig. 13.5 Microanatomy of the adult vocal fold illustrating the body-cover concept elucidated by Hirano. From M. Suzuki and J.A. Kirchner. Ann Otol Rhinol Laryngol 1968;77:1059 with permission

the rima (rima glottidis vocalis) is the space between the edges of the anterior three-fifths of the vocal folds, formed by the vocal folds with its ligament and covering epithelium. The intercartilaginous part of the rima (respiratory portion) is the posterior two-fifths of the vocal folds, formed by the vocal process of the arytenoid cartilages.

The membranous (vibratory) portion has three structural layers, the epithelium, lamina propria, and vocalis muscle, from superficial to deep. Hirano developed the cover-body concept in describing this microanatomy [22–24]. The cover consists of the stratified squamous epithelium overlying the gelatinous layer of superficial lamina propria. The vocalis muscle is the rubber-band like body. A transition zone of deep lamina propria (intermediate elastic and deep collagenous) separates the cover and body. The body provides the rigid base on which the cover vibrates. The anterior and posterior macula flava, at the anterior and posterior ends of the vocal folds, are a thickening of the intermediate elastic layer. They are believed to protect the ends of the vocal folds from vibratory damage. The pediatric larynx lacks this protective cushion, as well as the cover-body microanatomy, due to a single-layered lamina propria, which does not approximate adult form until the age of 10 years [22]. The geriatric larynx develops a thickened and edematous cover with age-related changes in the superficial lamina propria, while the vocalis muscle atrophies.

Infraglottic Cavity

The infraglottic cavity is the space from the glottis to the inferior border of the cricoid cartilage. The conus elasticus and cricoid cartilage laterally bound this space.

Mucosa

The laryngeal mucosa is largely of the respiratory type (pseudostratified ciliated columnar), with a portion covered by stratified squamous epithelium. The squamous epithelium is limited to the upper half of the posterior surface of epiglottis, the upper part of the aryepiglottic folds, and the vocal folds themselves. Beneath the epithelial covering is a variable basement membrane, separated by a layer of loose tissue stroma. This stromal layer is absent on the true vocal folds and on the posterior surface of the epiglottis, accounting for the more intense swelling of the anterior surface of the epiglottis during inflammatory conditions of the larynx.

Preepiglottic Space

The epiglottis is the posterior boundary of the preepiglottic space, which lies anterior to the epiglottis. The thyrohyoid membrane and inner surface of the thyroid lamina are the anterior borders. The hyoepiglottic ligament and mucosa of the vallecula and thyroepiglottic ligament are the superior and inferior boundaries, respectively. The preepiglottic space opens into the paraglottic space laterally. The preepiglottic space is an important barrier for the spread of cancer, which can access the space via the infrahyoid portion of the epiglottis.

Paraglottic Space

The paraglottic space plays an important role in the extralaryngeal spread of laryngeal cancer. This space is superior and inferior to the true and false vocal folds on both sides of the glottis.

The cricothyroid membrane and perichondrium of the thyroid lamina define the space laterally, while the quadrangular membrane, ventricle, and conus elasticus serve as the medial borders. The space opens into the posterior preepiglottic space anterosuperiorly. Pyriform sinus mucosa forms the posterior boundary. Supraglottic cancer penetrating this space may be marked by rapid extralaryngeal spread [16].

Pyriform Sinus

The pyriform sinus is part of the hypopharyx and it has important anatomic relationships to the larynx. Superiorly, the pyriform sinus begins as the lateral glossoepiglottic fold. The apex of the sinus meshes with the esophageal inlet inferiorly at the superior border of the cricoid. It is essentially a gutter, medially formed by the aryepiglottic fold, arytenoid cartilage, and superior cricoid cartilage. Its lateral borders are the thyrohyoid membrane and internal surface of the thyroid lamina. The superior laryngeal nerve marks its course anteriorly in the sinus floor. The nerve's submucosal plane makes it amendable to topical anesthesia in this space. Additionally, the superior cornu of the thyroid cartilage may protrude into the pyriform sinus and should not be confused with a neoplastic process.

Vessels

Arteries and Veins

The paired superior and inferior laryngeal arteries are the main arterial supply to the larynx. The superior thyroid artery is the first branch off the external carotid artery, and after coursing lateral to the laryngohyoid complex, the superior laryngeal artery branches off at about the hyoid level. The superior laryngeal artery runs horizontally across the posterior portion of the thyroid membrane, along with the internal branch of the superior laryngeal nerve. The artery penetrates the thyrohyoid membrane inferior to the nerve, entering the submucosa of the pyriform sinus, where it supplies the mucosa and musculature of the larynx. At the level of the cricothyroid membrane, the superior thyroid artery gives off a small cricothyroid artery, which passes horizontally below the cricoid cartilage. The inferior laryngeal artery, a branch of the inferior thyroid artery that emanates from the subclavian artery via the thyrocervical trunk, takes a course posterior to the cricothyroid joint with the recurrent laryngeal nerve. The inferior thyroid artery accesses the larynx through a gap in the inferior constrictor muscle known as the Killian-Jamieson area. Within the larynx the artery branches and supplies mucosa and musculature, anastomosing with the superior laryngeal artery.

Superior and inferior laryngeal veins parallel the arteries, joining the superior and inferior veins, respectively.

Lymphatics

The lymphatics of the larynx have numerous divisions, an understanding of which is essential in contemplating the spread of laryngeal cancer and its treatment modalities. The divisions start with superficial (intramucosal) and deep (submucosal) groups, which are further divided into right and left halves, broken down into supraglottic, glottic, and subglottic. The deep portion is more important in the spread of cancer. The supraglottic region (false cords and aryepiglottic folds) flows to the deep jugular chain near the carotid bifurcation, as the lymphatic channels follow the superior laryngeal and superior thyroid vessels from the pyriform sinus through the thyrohyoid membrane. The epiglottis, as a midline structure, has bilateral drainage. The ventricle is drained through the cricothyroid membrane and ipsilateral thyroid lobe. There are two systems in the lymphatic drainage of the subglottic larynx. The first system ends in the subclavian, paratracheal, and tracheoesophageal chains, as well as the lower portion of the deep jugular chain by following the inferior thyroid vessels. The other system drains bilaterally to the middle deep cervical nodes and prelaryngeal (Delphian) nodes by piercing the cricothyroid membrane. Cancer localized to the true vocal folds has a high curability rate because there is no lymphatic drainage of this structure [12–16, 23].

Muscles (Fig. 13.6) [24]

Extrinsic Muscles

The extrinsic muscles of the larynx, also referred to as the strap muscles, function to raise, lower, or stabilize the larynx. The infrahyoid group includes the omohyoid, sternothyroid, thyrohyoid, and sternohyoid muscles, which are innervated by the ansa cervacalis. These muscles depress the larynx, displacing it downward during inspiration. The suprahyoid group of muscles includes the digastrics, stylohyoid, geniohyoid, mylohyoid, and stylopharyngeus. These muscles elevate and anteriorly displace the larynx during swallowing and help suspend the larynx from the skull base and mandible via the hyoid bone. The middle and inferior constrictors, as well as the cricopharyngeus muscles, are also extrinsic muscles that play an imperative role in the precisely timed act of deglutition [12–16].

Intrinsic Muscles

The intrinsic laryngeal muscles act in synchrony to modify the size of the glottic opening, as well as both the length and tension of the vocal folds (Fig. 13.6). These muscles are restricted to the internal larynx and they consist of numerous adductors and a single abductor. The intrinsic muscles are paired, with the exception of the interarytenoid [25].

Cricothyroid Muscle

The cricothyroid muscle arises from the external surface of the anterior cricoid arch and it is divided into two bellies. An anterior-superior pars recta runs upward and laterally from the cricoid arch toward the inferior border of thyroid cartilage. The posterior and inferior pars obliqua runs obliquely upward from the anterolateral border of the cricoid arch to the anterior portion of the inferior cornu. Contraction of the cricothyroid tilts the cricoid at the cricothyroid joint. During contraction, the posterior cricoid lamina and arytenoid cartilages are displaced inferiorly, while the anterior cricoid arch is brought superiorly toward the inferior border of the thyroid alae. The inferior displacement of the posterior cricoid

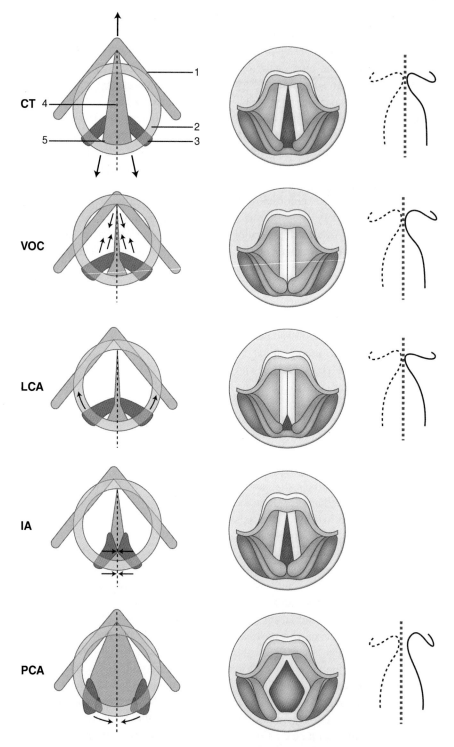

Fig. 13.6 Illustration of laryngeal muscle action. *Left column* shows vocal fold edges and cartilage location at laryngeal muscle activation. *Arrows show* vector of force. *CT* cricothyroid muscle; *IA* interarytenoid muscle; *LCA* lateral cricoarytenoid muscle; *PCA* posterior cricoarytenoid; *VOC* vocalis; *1* thyroid cartilage; *2* cricoids cartilage; *3* arytenoids; *4* vocal ligament; *5* posterior cricoarytenoid ligament. *The middle column* shows laryngoscopic view. *The right column* shows the middle membranous portion of the vocal fold. The dotted line demonstrates a neutral position with no muscle activated. From C.T. Sasaki and G. Isaacson. Probs Anesth 1988;2(2):163–74 with permission

lamina increases the distance between the anterior commissure and the vocal processes. This process stretches, elongates, and thins the vocal folds, adducting them into a paramedian position. Contraction of the cricothyroid during inspiration increases the antero-posterior glottis dimension, while during phonation it results in a higher fundamental frequency produced by the vocal folds.

Lateral Cricoarytenoid Muscle

Arising from the upper border of the cricoid arch, the lateral cricoarytenoid extends posterosuperiorly to insert at the arytenoid muscular process. During contraction, it slides the arytenoid cartilage superiorly and medially on the cricoid with an anterolateral pull, adducting and lowering the tip of vocal process, both elongating and thinning it. The lateral cricoarytenoid thus acts as the antagonist to the posterior cricoarytenoid.

Posterior Cricoarytenoid Muscle

It is the sole abductor of the vocal folds. From its origin on posterior surface of the cricoid cartilage lamina, the posterior cricoarytenoid fibers insert into the arytenoid muscular process after taking an oblique, lateral, and superior course. Contraction slides the arytenoid cartilage inferiorly and laterally on the cricoid with a posteromedial pull. It therefore abducts and elevates the tip of the vocal process, elongating and thinning the vocal fold, causing its edge to be rounded. All layers of the vocal fold are passively stiffened.

Interarytenoid/Aryepiglottic Muscle

The unpaired interarytenoid muscle has two types of muscle fibers. Transverse muscle fibers stretch between the posterior surfaces of the two arytenoid cartilages, which are approximated upon contraction of the fibers. This process assists in the closure of the posterior glottic portion with little affect on the mechanical property of the vocal fold. The oblique fibers cross in the midline as they pass from the posterior arytenoid portion on one side to the arytenoid apex on the other side. Some fibers insert at the apex, while others fan out along the quadrangular membrane (aryepiglottic muscle). The oblique fibers narrow the laryngeal aditus.

Thyroarytenoid Muscle

The thyroarytenoid has an internal and external component, both with the same attachments. The internus lies deep to the externus and is more well developed. Arising from the inner surface of thyroid cartilage at the commissure, the externus inserts at the lateral surface of arytenoid cartilage. It brings the arytenoid cartilage anteromedially during contraction, thus adducting the vocal folds. The externus also adducts the false folds and, with the transverse arytenoid, acts as the sphincter mechanism at the false fold level. The thyroarytenoid internus, or vocalis muscle, extends from the anterior commissure to the vocal process, with a few fibers attaching to the outer surface of the conus elasticus inferior to the vocal ligament. Contraction adducts, shortens, and thickens the vocal fold, as the body (muscular layer) is actively stiffened and the cover is passively slackened.

Physiology

Structural Considerations

The upper airway in the adult human traverses the digestive tract in the region of the pharynx, providing sphincteric protection while complicating the respiratory function of the lower airway. Two important organic modifications developed during evolution to resolve this functional difficulty: structural adaptation and delicate coordination among the three basic laryngeal functions as dictated by precisely organized brainstem reflexes.

Many mammalian species are provided with a relatively high-riding larynx, affording its close approximation with structures of the posterior nasal cavities. The intracranial position of the larynx, which secures a continuous airway from the nose to the bronchi, decreases the risk of pulmonary contamination by swallowed matter.

The human newborn exhibits similar nasolaryngeal connection by the approximation of its epiglottis with the posterior surface of its palate, thus ensuring against aspiration.

In the adult, the characteristic flat, shield-like configuration of the epiglottis serves to direct swallowed food laterally into the pyriform sinuses, away from the midline laryngeal aperture. Furthermore, in adult humans, elevation of the larynx toward the nasal cavity during the height of deglutition exaggerates this protective function. The aryepiglottic folds act as ramparts to the larynx, allowing food to pass on either side of the epiglottis along the gutter produced between each fold and the lateral pharyngeal wall. It appears that the primary function of the supraglottic larynx lies in its protection of the lower airway.

The ability of the larynx to perform as an effective valve depends on the unique shelf-like configuration of its bilateral superior and inferior folds. The ventricular folds, which are located superiorly, act as an exit valve, preventing the escape of air from the lower respiratory tract. When medialized by muscular contraction, these false cords seal even more tightly as tracheal pressure is increased below. This feature of adducted false cords is attributable to their unique shape, characterized by the down-turned direction of their free margins.

Conversely, the true cords behave as a one-way valve in the opposite direction, obstructing the ingress of air or fluid. The false cords prevent the egress of air from the lungs, and the true cords with their upturned margins are capable of arresting its ingress. The structural adaptation of the larynx in man aids in maintaining the functional diversity of this organ.

Neuromuscular Physiology

Afferent System

Sensory nerve fibers to the larynx are derived from the internal branch of the superior laryngeal nerve. Each nerve innervates the ipsilateral upper half of the larynx to the level of the true vocal cord, Likewise, below the true cords ipsilateral sensation is mediated by each recurrent laryngeal nerve. Suzuki and Kirchner [21] however, demonstrated that a diamond-shaped area in the anterior midline of the subglottic space in the cat is innervated by both external branches *of* the superior laryngeal nerve. Afferent impulses from deep muscle receptors and cricothyroid joints also travel cephalad in this nerve branch (Table 13.1) [24]. The density of sensory innervation appears

Table 13.1 Sensory innervation

Nerve	Distribution
Superior laryngeal (internal division)	Supraglottic mucosa
	Thyroepiglottic joint
	Cricothyroid joint
Superior laryngeal (external division)	Anterior subglottic mucosa
Recurrent laryngeal	Subglottic mucosa
	Muscle spindles
Nerve of Galen (communicating branch between superior and recurrent nerves)	Aortic arch

greatest in the laryngeal inlet. This is logical since the entrance to the larynx is thought to serve as a protective zone for more distal parts of the respiratory system. When nerve staining techniques are used, the laryngeal surface of the epiglottis appears to contain the most compact innervation, whereas the true cords exhibit lesser degrees of sensory density [26, 27]. Further, the posterior half of the true cord is more heavily furnished with touch receptors than its anterior portion. The distribution of chemical and thermal sensors is different. These appear limited to the supraglottic larynx and are sensitive to a variety of noxious substances. Measurement of single nerve fiber potentials from the superior laryngeal nerve in sheep shows chemosensitivity to KCl, NH_4Cl, $NaCl$, $LiCl$, distilled water, citric acid, and dilute hydrochloric acid, in order of decreasing sensitivity [28, 29].

Water chemoreceptors on the epiglottis have been implicated experimentally in the production of prolonged apnea. Furthermore, it has been demonstrated that the respiratory response to water-aerosol inhalation for treatment of croup and other upper airway obstruction may be related to the exquisite water sensitivity of these epiglottic receptors. The effect produced consists of respiratory slowing with a concomitant increase in tidal volume—certainly an effect beneficial in partial airway obstruction. In addition, this centrally mediated respiratory response appears to be greater in early life than in adulthood [30].

It is generally agreed that sensory components of the superior laryngeal nerve include representation from mucosal touch receptors, epiglottic chemoreceptors, joint receptors, aortic baroreceptors, and stretch receptors from the intrinsic laryngeal muscles [31]. Afferent impulses are delivered through the ganglion nodosum to the brainstem tractus solitarius.

Efferent System

Motor innervation of the larynx is no less complex (Table 13.2) [27]. It is generally agreed that the motor distribution of the intrinsic laryngeal musculature originates in the medullary nucleus ambiguus. This motor nucleus is topographically divided into abductor and adductor zones. Each recurrent laryngeal nerve ipsilaterally innervates all muscles except the cricothyroid muscle, which receives its motor impulses from the external division of its ipsilateral superior laryngeal nerve. The interarytenoid muscles, however, receive bilateral innervation from both recurrent laryngeal nerves. The muscle that widens the glottic chink, as takes place in respiration, is solely the posterior cricoarytenoid muscle (laryngeal abductor). It extends from the posterior aspect of the cricoid plate to the muscular process of the arytenoid (Fig. 13.7a) [27]. Exerting a posterolateral pull on the arytenoid body will rotate the vocal fold outward, effecting cord abduction on inspiration. On the other hand, vocal fold adduction results from *contraction* of all other intrinsic musculature, major contributions arising from the action of thyroarytenoid and lateral cricoarytenoid muscles (Fig. 13.7b, c)

[27]. The interarytenoid muscles serve to close the posterior gap in the glottis (Fig. 13.7d) [27], while the cricothyroid muscle adducts and tenses the vocal cord, passively lengthening it by 30 %. This is accomplished by shortening the anterior distance between the cricoid and thyroid cartilages, resulting in dorsal and posterior displacement of the posterior cricoid plate. The vocal cord therefore undergoes a mechanical stretch displacement, resulting in an increase in the anteroposterior diameter of the laryngeal aperture (Fig. 13.7e) [27].

Briefly, when one cricothyroid muscle is denervated by sectioning the superior laryngeal nerve, the unopposed contraction of the contralateral cricothyroid muscle results in rotation of the posterior commissure toward the inactive side, with foreshortening of the cord on the side of denervation. On the other hand, it is agreed that unilateral recurrent laryngeal nerve injury results in the paramedian position of that cord because the unopposed action of the ipsilateral cricothyroid muscles, innervated by an intact superior laryngeal nerve, produces cord adduction on the side of recurrent laryngeal nerve injury.

Since the recurrent laryngeal nerve contains mixed adductor and abductor fibers, repair of this nerve following section offers little hope of orderly re-innervation and laryngeal function. Still, experiments with electrical stimulation of the larynx may lead someday to laryngeal reanimation. It has been demonstrated in dogs that the abductor and adductor muscles respond to different frequencies of stimulation. At stimulation rates less than 30 Hz, vocal abduction is observed.

Table 13.2 Motor innervation

Nerve	Distribution	Action
Superior laryngeal (external division)	Cricothyroid joint	Adductor, isotonic tensor
Recurrent laryngeal	Thyroarytenoid muscle	Adductor, isometric tensor
	Lateral cricoarytenoid muscle	Adductor
	Interarytenoid muscle	Adductor
	Posterior cricoarytenoid muscle	Abductor
Nerve of Galen (communicating branch between superior and recurrent nerves)	Tracheoesophageal mucosa	Autonomic (secretory)
	Tracheal smooth muscle	Autonomic

Actions of intrinsic laryngeal muscles

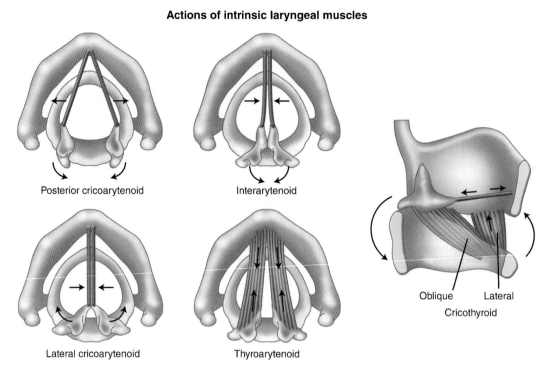

Fig. 13.7 The intrinsic muscles responsible *for* vocal cord position

At greater rates, adduction occurs [32]. This experimental finding and related experiments with direct posterior cricoarytenoid electrical stimulation in synchrony with phrenic activity may someday lead to practical laryngeal pacing in the setting of vocal cord paralysis. More immediately, transmucosal stimulation of laryngeal musculature by electrode arrays placed in the pyriform sinuses of dogs have been used to open and close the laryngeal aperture. Similar devices may prove useful to the anesthesiologist in overcoming laryngospasm and as an aid to intubation in humans [33].

Laryngeal Reflexes

Basic functions of the larynx (protective, respiratory, and phonatory) are derived from a complex interrelationship of diverse polysynaptic brainstem reflexes. Protective function is entirely reflexive and involuntary, constituting one end of a spectrum that is balanced by voluntary respiratory and phonatory performances regulated involuntarily through an array of feedback reflexes.

Protective Reflexes

Stimulation of the upper respiratory tract, especially the larynx, evokes a strong glottic closure reflex (GCR). The afferent sensory impulses via the internal branch of SLN project to the ipsilateral nucleus ambiguus after synapsing in the nucleus tractus solitarius. The motor neurons within the nucleus ambiguus then project through the RLN, completing the efferent limb of the ipsilateral GCR (Fig. 13.8) [34].

The functional analog of this reflex is reproduced as protective glottic closure during deglutition. Touch and chemical and thermal stimulation of the laryngeal aditus produce the same response as seen experimentally with electrostimulation of the SLN. In an experimental setup, it has been observed that stimulation of ipsilateral internal SLN elicits three categories of brainstem laryngeal

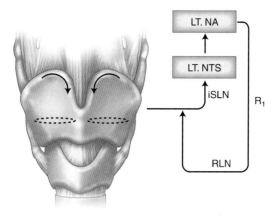

Fig. 13.8 Organizational model of the ipsilateral GCR

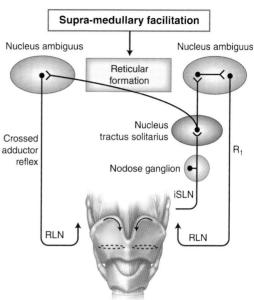

Fig. 13.9 Organizational model of the ipsilateral and crossed adductor reflex pathway in man

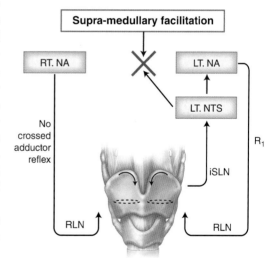

Fig. 13.10 Organizational model demonstrating the loss of contralateral R1 under deep anesthesia

responses. First, an early response involves adduction of the ipsilateral vocal cord with a latency of approximately 10–18 ms in anesthetized cat, dog, and pig. This short latency R1 evoked response has been consistently noted in anesthetized humans [30, 35]. A second category of short latency R1 response involves simultaneous contralateral adduction also known as the crossed adductor reflex. The existence of crossed GCR pathway (Fig. 13.9) [36] has been hypothesized in a human study [35]. In the same study, it was also demonstrated that as depths of anesthesia increased, the crossed reflex is suppressed. Still, a third category of adductor response involving a longer latency reflex, termed R2, has been observed to produce bilateral vocal *fold* responses, but its presence appears to be most readily noted in awake human subjects; it has a latency of 50–80 ms. [36]

From these observations it is seen that the crossed GCR is centrally mediated and is suppressed with increasing depths of anesthesia converting GCR into a unilateral one (Fig. 13.10) [36], weakening the glottic closing force and making one prone to aspiration under anesthesia and deep sedation [37].

Interestingly, in another experimental study, Sasaki et al. demonstrated that selective denervation of larynx has a profound biomechanical effect on glottic closing force [38]. They showed that unilateral SLN and RLN sectioning reduced GCF by 46 % and 76 %, respectively. However, combined SLN and RLN sectioning on the ipsilateral side further reduced it to only 77 %, thereby suggesting an organizational configuration in which motor neurons functionally involved ipsilaterally likely outnumber those contralaterally (Fig. 13.11) [36].

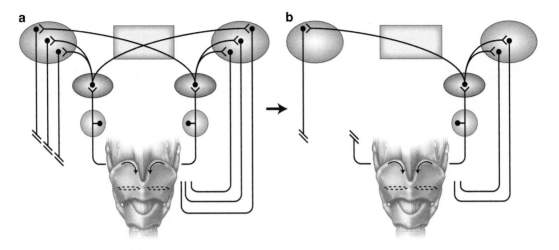

Fig. 13.11 Organizational model demonstrating the effect of converting a unilateral RLN section (**a**) to a combined unilateral RLN-SLN section (**b**) when motor neurons functionally involved ipsilaterally outnumber those contralaterally

Bilateral SLN stimulation results in sphincteric closure of the upper airway of its three muscular tiers within the laryngeal framework. The highest occurs at the level of the aryepiglottic folds, which contain the superior-most divisions of the thyroarytenoid muscle. The contraction of these fibers approximates the aryepiglottic folds to cover the superior inlet of the larynx, and with the arytenoid cartilages in the posterior gap, completes the first of the three sphincteric tiers of protection. The second tier of protection occurs at the level of the false cords, consisting of bilateral folds forming the roof of each laryngeal ventricle. The third tier of protection occurs at the level of the true vocal cords, which in man are shelf like with a slightly upturned free border. The inferior division of the thyroarytenoid muscle forms the bulk of this shelf, and with the passive valvular effect of the upturned border or the true cord margin, the true vocal folds are perhaps the most significant of the three barriers to aspiration.

Mechanical stimulation applied to the upper respiratory tract, which is innervated by the trigeminal and glossopharyngeal nerves or the electrical stimulation of all major cranial afferent nerves produces strong laryngeal adductor responses. In the cat, reflex action potentials in the adductor branch of RLN can he elicited by electrostimulation of the optic, acoustic, chorda tympani, trigeminal, splanchnic, vagus, radial, and intercostals nerves [39]. The susceptibility of this reflex response to such diverse sensory stimulation is unique and emphasizes its primitive role in respiratory protection of the organism from a wide variety of potentially noxious influences.

Physiologic exaggeration of the GCR is called laryngospasm, which is clinically observed as a strong prolonged closure of the glottis when the adductor muscle is tonically contracted and maintained well beyond the cessation of mucosal irritation. From neurophysiologic analysis, laryngeal spasm consists of prolonged tonic adductor spike activity in the RLN that bears no precisely reproducible temporal relationship or latency, to its initiating stimulus. This observation is based on the fact that laryngeal spasm is solely mediated by stimulation of the SLN. In fact high frequency stimulation of other afferent nerves, capable of eliciting simple glottic closure, produces little adductor after discharge activity that is characteristic of laryngospasm.

Adductor motor depression caused by hypoventilation is supported by other experimental data indicating preferential abolition of postsynaptic potentials by hypoxia [40]. This experimental evidence further indicates that, in hypoxic states, postsynaptic recovery lags behind the presynaptic recovery producing a net depressive effect on all reflex neural activity, Hypoventilation, therefore, understandably impairs the output capability of the brainstem adductor motor aggregate to repetitive SLN stimulation. Such experimental data seem to support the clinical observation that laryngeal spasm occurs more often in well-ventilated rather than cyanotic patients. Aside from the variety of excitatory adductor responses it produces, SLN stimulation also exerts an inhibitory effect on the medullary inspiratory motor neurons. Not only does laryngeal abductor activity cease but phrenic activity is also inhibited, resulting in various degrees of reflex apnea.

Respiratory Reflex

The inputs of central and peripheral chemoreceptors and of vagally mediated thoracic stretch receptors in the regulation of breathing were among the great conceptual strides of the nineteenth century. The respiratory contribution of the larynx, however, was not appreciated until 1949 when Negus noted that the glottis opened a fraction of a second before air was drawn in by the descent of the diaphragm [1]. The neurophysiology behind this observation was clarified by Suzuki and Kirchner, who established this activity as a direct effect of the medullary respiratory center. Having shown that widening of the glottis occurred with rhythmic bursts of activity in the recurrent laryngeal nerve, Suzuki and Kirchner then demonstrated that, like phrenic activity, this rhythmicity was accentuated by hypercapnia and ventilatory obstruction and depressed by hyperventilation and resultant hypocapnia [41].

Likewise, as phrenic activity is modified by ventilatory resistance, it would seem reasonable that glottic widening, influenced by the respiratory center, would be similarly modified.

From a purely structural perspective, the true vocal folds passively act to obstruct the ingress of air to the lungs. Thus, to relieve this obstruction active inspiratory abduction, the product of phasic muscular contraction by the posterior cricoarytenoid muscle must take place. Further, this activity has been demonstrated to be synchronous with inspiration [42]. The degree of abductor activity appears to vary directly with ventilatory resistance, disappearing entirely when inspiratory resistance is removed and returning when resistance to ventilation is reestablished. Because vagotomy abolishes this response, it is thought that the afferent limb for the reflex regulation of phasic inspiratory abduction lies within the ascending vagus nerve [43]. End organ receptors contributing to this reflex presumably lie within the thorax, although their exact nature and location remain unknown.

The cricothyroid muscle behaves in an unusual way as a respiratory muscle. It is known to be a vocal cord adductor and isotonic tensor. It is odd then that it is seen to contract during inspiration when adduction would seem counterproductive [44]. In fact, its role in cord lengthening actually enhances the cross-sectional diameter of the glottis by increasing its anteroposterior dimension. Thus, the posterior cricoarytenoid and cricothyroid muscles act together to widen and lengthen the glottic chink.

One must also consider the role of the larynx in controlling expiration. In eupneic states, expiratory flow and duration are principal determinants of respiratory frequency. As others have demonstrated in both animal and human investigations, variations in respiratory rate result primarily from changing the duration of the expiratory phase rather than the inspiratory phase of the respiratory cycle [45, 46]. In this regard the larynx exerts a major valvular effect on ventilatory resistance, significantly influencing the expiratory phase of respiration.

The cricothyroid muscle is closely linked to this expiratory control, Cricothyroid activity is evoked by positive intratracheal pressure independent of respiratory rate. Cricothyroid activity continues as long as positive pressure is maintained and ceases with the loss of this pressure. In addition, the rate of change of intratracheal pressure appears important in triggering cricothyroid activity with a critical level at approximately 30 cm H_2O/s.

There is evidence that the expiratory activity of the cricothyroid muscle is solely mediated peripherally, lacking the medullary control exerted during the inspiratory phase. Cricothyroid tracking of intratracheal pressure changes is abolished by bilateral vagotomy, although medullary and efferent components are left intact.

Phonatory Reflex System

The phonatory function of the larynx is probably least well understood of its three basic functions. With advances in investigative technique, many established hypotheses based on animal models have been challenged, a result in large measure to the advent of more specialized technology based on human study. High-speed cinematography, electro- *and* photoglottography, improved endoscopic techniques using the video stroboscope, and direct human electromyographic measurements made possible by hooked-wire electrodes combined with advanced aerodynamic measurements are largely responsible for these newer additions.

It is generally agreed that speech results from the production of a fundamental tone at the larynx and is modified by resonating chambers of the upper aerodigestive tract. Intelligible speech, therefore, represents the combined effect of the larynx, tongue, palate, and related structures of the oral vestibule. The fundamental tone is produced by vibration of the vocal folds against each other, powered by the passage of air between them. The passive nature of vocal cord vibration forms the basis of the aerodynamic theory of sound generation. Such a theory is supported by the observation that a completely paralyzed larynx is capable of producing sound, as is the cadaver larynx when air is blown through it. Furthermore, vocal cord vibration ceases when a tracheostomy is performed for diversionary purposes. The aerodynamic theory of sound production replaces the neurochronaxic theory proposed by Husson, who postulated that the central generation of RLN impulses produces cord vibrations by active contraction of the thyroarytenoid

muscles [47]. According to this theory, each vibration represented the result of beat-by-beat impulses through the RLN. This concept is no longer accepted as tenable on acoustic or neurophysiological grounds.

Although sound production may be considered a passive function, the regulation of its acoustic quality is not. Rather vocal cord shaping and positioning are under active neurophysiological regulation. During phonation the vocal folds are positioned near the midline by isotonic tensing provided by the cricothyroid muscles. Additionally, the thyroarytenoid muscles provide finer shaping of the vocal folds. The effect of shaping may be appreciated when the vocal folds are viewed in the frontal plane during phonation. During the production of high-pitched notes, the folds seen on cross section appear thin, but during low pitches the folds appear thickened considerably. Thus, the frequency of vibration depends on the vibratory mass of both cords, their anteroposterior tension, functional damping at high pitches, and subglottic pressure. As pitch increases, the true cords lengthen and tense isotonically through the action of the cricothyroid muscles. Although cord lengthening alone might serve to lower pitch, cord thinning produced by thyroarytenoid action, which also increases the internal tension of the true cord, offsets this effect. It must also be recognized that the activity of the extrinsic laryngeal muscles affects pitch by altering the spatial relationship between the cricoid and the thyroid cartilages. The sternothyroid muscle is felt to influence pitch in this way. Table 13.3 [24] summarizes the influence of each of the intrinsic and extrinsic muscles on the shape and tension of the glottis during phonation.

In considering the phonatory process, a variety of factors necessarily contribute to the acoustic product as defined in Table 13.4 [22].

A variety of feedback mechanisms aid in the fine-tuning of the voice. The contribution of auditory input is demonstrated by observing a nonprofessional singer's ability to hit a desired note when hearing is masked by white noise. Mucosal receptors in the pharynx and larynx also supply

Table 13.3   Characteristic functions of the laryngeal muscles in the vocal fold adjustments

	CT	VOC	LCA	IA	PCA
Position	Paramed	*Adduct*	*Adduct*	*Adduct*	*Adduct*
Level	Lower	Lower	*Lower*	0	*Elevate*
Length	*Elongate*	*Shorten*	Elongate	(Shorten)	*Elongate*
Thickness	*Thin*	*Thicken*	Thin	(Thicken)	Thin
Edge	*Sharpen*	*Round*	Sharpen	0	Round
Muscle (body)	*Stiffen*	*Stiffen*	Stiffen	(Slacken)	Stiffen
Mucosa (cover and transition)	*Stiffen*	Slacken	Stiffen	(Slacken)	Stiffen

0 no effect; *()* slightly; *italics* markedly; *CT* cricothyroid muscle; *VOC* vocalis muscle; *LCA* lateral cricoarytenoid muscle; *IA* interarytenoid muscle; *PCA* posterior cricoarytenoid muscle. Adapted from Hirano M. Clinical examination of voice. New York: Springer: 1981

Table 13.4   Parameters in the peripheral process of the production and perception of voice.

	Parameters that regulate vibratory pattern of vocal fold		Parameters that specify vibratory pattern	Parameters that specify sound generated	
Level	*Physiologic*	*Physical*	*Physical*	*Acoustic*	*Psychoacoustic*
Parameters	Neuromuscular control	(Primary)	Fundamental period	Fundamental frequency	Pitch
	Respiratory muscles	Expiratory force	Symmetry	Amplitude (intensity)	Loudness
			Periodicity		
	Laryngeal muscles	Vocal fold	Uniformity	Waveform	
		Position	Glottal closure	Acoustic spectrum	Quality
		Shape and size	Amplitude		
		Elasticity	Mucosal wave	Fluctuations	Fluctuations
		Viscosity	Speed of excursion		
	Articulatory muscles	State of vocal tract (Secondary)	Glottal area waveform		
		Pressure drop across glottis			
		Volume velocity			
		Glottal impedance			

important information, the transmission of which can be blocked by topical anesthetics. Finally, stretch receptors in the laryngeal joint capsules give critical proprioceptive information [27, 32, 48].

Despite recent advances in our understanding of the mechanisms of the larynx, the precise mechanism of voice regulation remains a matter of continued fascination.

References

1. Negus VE. The comparative anatomy and physiology of the larynx. London: Heinemann; 1949.
2. Sasaki CT, Weaver EM. Physiology of the larynx. J Am Med. 1997;103:9–18.
3. Henick DH, Holinger LD. Laryngeal development. In: Holinger LD, Lusk RP, Green CG, editors. Pediatric laryngology and bronchoesophagology. Philadelphia: Lippincott-Raven; 1997. p. 1–17.

4. Sanudo JR, Domenech-Mateu JM. The laryngeal primordium and epithelial lamina: a new interpretation. J Anat. 1990;171:207–22.

5. Moore KL, Persaud TVN. The pharyngeal apparatus. In: Moore KL, Persaud TVN, editors. The developing human: clinically orientated embryology. 8th ed. Philadelphia: W.B. Saunders; 2008. p. 159–96.

6. Milczuk HA, Smith JD, Everts EC. Congenital laryngeal webs: Surgical management and clinical embryology. Int J Pediatr Otorhinolaryngol. 2000;52:1–9.

7. Pohunek P. Development, structure, and function of the upper airways. Paediatr Respir Rev. 2004;5:2–8.

8. Hartnick CJ, Cotton RT. Congenital laryngeal anomalies. Laryngeal atresia, stenosis, webs, and clefts. Otolaryngol Clin North Am. 2000;33:1293–308.

9. Spector GJ. Developmental anatomy of the larynx. In: Ballenger JJ, editor. Diseases of the nose, throat, ear, head and neck. 13th ed. Philadelphia, PA: Lea & Febiger; 1985. p. 369–75.

10. Zaw-Tun HA, Burdi AR. Reexamination of the origin and early development of the human larynx. Acta Anat. 1985;122:163–84.

11. Sasaki CT, Young-Ho K, LeVay AJ. Development, anatomy, physiology of the larynx. In: Snow JB, Wackym PA, eds. Ballenger's Otorhinolaryngology head and neck surgery 17th edition. Shelton, CT:BC Decker;2009:849.

12. Maue WM, Dickinson DR. Cartilages and ligaments of the adult larynx. Arch Otolaryngol. 1971;92: 432–9.

13. Hollinshead WH. The pharynx and larynx. In: Hollinshead WH, editor. Anatomy for surgeons, volume 1: the head and neck. 3rd ed. Philadelphia: JB Lippincott; 1982. p. 389–441.

14. Hanafee WN, Ward PH. Anatomy and physiology. In: Hanafee WN, Ward PH, editors. Clinical correlations in the head and neck, volume 1: the larynx. New York: Thieme Medical Publishers; 1990. p. 1–7.

15. Tucker HM. Anatomy of the Larynx. In: Tucker HM, editor. The Larynx. 2nd ed. New York: Thieme Medical Publishers; 1993.

16. Spector GJ. Anatomy of the larynx. In: Ballenger JJ, editor. Diseases of the nose, throat, ear, head and neck. 13th ed. Philadelphia, PA: Lea & Febiger; 1985. p. 376–85.

17. Sasaki CT, Young-Ho K, LeVay AJ. Development, anatomy, physiology of the larynx. In: Snow JB, Wackym PA, editors. Ballenger's otorhinolaryngology head and neck surgery. 17th ed. Shelton, CT: BC Decker; 2009. p. 852.

18. Chamberlain WE, Young B. Ossification (so-called "calcification") of normal laryngeal cartilages mistaken for foreign body. Am J Roentgen Rad Ther. 1935;33:441–50.

19. Hately W, Evison E, Samuel E. The pattern of ossification in the laryngeal cartilages: A radiological study. Br J Radiol. 1965;38:585–91.

20. Cooper MH. Anatomy of the larynx. In: Blitzer A, Brin MF, Sasaki CT, Fahn S, Harris K, editors. Neurologic disorders of the larynx. New York: Thieme Medical Publishers; 1992. p. 3–11.

21. Suzuki M, Kirchner JA. Afferent nerve fibers in the external branch of the superior laryngeal nerve in cat. Ann Otol Rhinol Laryngol. 1968;77:1059.

22. Bosely ME, Hartnick CJ. Development of the human true vocal fold: depth of cell layers and quantifying cell types within the lamina propria. Ann Otol Rhinol Laryngol. 2006;115:784–8.

23. Johner CH. The lymphatics of the larynx. Otolaryngol Clin North Am. 1970;3:439–51.

24. Sasaki CT, Isaacson G. Dynamic anatomy of the larynx. Probs Anesth. 1988;2(2):163–74.

25. Hirano M. Outline of voice production and its examination. In: Hirano M, editor. Clinical examination of voice. New York: Springer; 1981. p. 1–100.

26. Koizumi H. On sensory innervation of the larynx in dog. J Exp Med. 1953;58:199.

27. Shin T, Wantanbe S, Wada S, et al. Sensory nerve endings in the mucosa of the epiglottis—Morphologic investigations with silver impregnation, immunohistochemistry, and electron microscopy. Otolaryngol Head Neck Surg. 1987;96:55.

28. Bradley RM, Stedman HM, Mistretta CM. Superior laryngeal nerve response patterns to chemical stimulation of sheep epiglottis. Brain Res. 1983;275:81.

29. Goding GS, Richardson MA, Trachy RE. Laryngeal chemoreflex: Anatomic and physiologic study by use of the superior laryngeal nerve in the piglet. Otolaryngol Head Neck Surg. 1987;97:28.

30. Sasaki CT, Suzuki M. The respiratory mechanism of aerosol inhalation in treatment of partial airway obstruction. Pediatrics. 1977;59:689.

31. Bowden REM. Innervation of intrinsic laryngeal muscles. Ventilatory and phonatory control systems. Woke B (editor) Oxford University Press; London 1974.

32. Sanders I, Aviv J, Biller HF. Transcutaneous electrical stimulation of the recurrent laryngeal nerve: A method of controlling vocal cord position. Otolaryngol Head Neck Surg. 1986;95:152.

33. Kraus WM, Sanders I, Aviv JE, et al. The laryngeal electrode platform: An indwelling device for mobilization of the vocal cords. Ann Otol Rhinol Laryngol. 1987;96:674.

34. Sasaki CT, Hundal J, Ross DA. Laryngeal physiology. In: Fried MP, Ferlito A, Rinaldo A, Smith R, editors. The Larynx. 3rd ed. San Diego, CA: Plural Publishing Inc; 2009. p. 101–12.

35. Sasaki CT, Suzuki M. Laryngeal reflexes in cat, dogs and man. Arch Otolarvitgol. 1976;102:400–2.

36. Ludlow CL, Van Pelt F, Koda J. Characteristics of late responses to superior laryngeal nerve stimulation in humans. Ann Otol Rhinol Laryngol. 1992;101: 127–34.

37. Sasaki CT, Jassin B, Kim YH, et al. Central facilitation of the glottic closure reflex in humans. Ann Otol Rhinol laryngol. 2003;112:293–7.

38. Sasaki CT, Hundal JS, Kim YH. Protective glottic closure:biomechanical effects of selective laryngeal

denervation. Ann Otol Rhinol Laryngol. 2005;114:
271–5.

39. Suzuki M, Sasaki CT. Effect of various sensory stimuli on reflex laryngeal adduction. Ann Otol. 1977;86:
30–6.

40. Chang HT. Activation of internuncial neurons through
collaterals of pyramidal fibers at cortical level. J
Neurophysiol. 1955;18:452–71.

41. Suzuki M, Kirchner JA. The posterior cricoarytenoid
as an inspiratory muscle. Ann Otol Rhinol Larvngol.
1969;78:849.

42. Sasaki CT, Fukuda H, Kirchner JA. Laryngeal abductor activity in response to varying ventilatory resistance. Trans Am Acad Ophthalmol Otolaryngol.
1973;77:403.

43. Fukuda H, Sasaki CT, Kirchner JA. Vagal afferent
influences on the phasic activity of the posterior

cricoarytenoid muscle. Acta Otolaryngol. 1973;
75:112.

44. Suzuki M, Kirchner JA, Murakami Y. The cricothyroid as a respiratory muscle. Ann Otol Rhinol Laryngol.
1970;79:1.

45. Bendixen HH, Smith GM, Mead J. Pattern of ventilation in young adults. J Appl Physiol. 1964;
19:195.

46. Remmers JE, Bartlett Jr D. Reflex control *of* expiratory airflow and duration. J Appl Physiol. 1977;
42:80.

47. Husson R. Etude des phénomènes physiologiques et
Acoustiques Fondamentaux de la Voix Chantée. Paris,
France: These Fac Sc; 1950.

48. Gracheva MS. On sensory innervations of the framework of the motor apparatus of the larynx[in Russian].
Arkh Anat Gistol Embriol. 1963;44:77–80.

Development, Anatomy, and Physiology of the Lungs

14

Rade Tomic, Andreea Antonescu-Turcu, and Elizabeth R. Jacobs

Abstract

Because of the anatomic proximity of the upper airway and gastrointestinal (GI) tracts, there is a risk of lung injury through aspiration. A number of lines of defense counter penetration of gastric acid or meals into the airways, including laryngeal closure, swallowing apnea and cough. Nonetheless, the prevalence of aspiration is greatly increased in a number of chronic diseases including chronic cough, asthma, interstitial lung diseases, lung transplantation and others. A causal relationship between these disorders and aspiration is not established, neither is there a clear benefit to treating aspiration. In part, this relationship may be difficult to prove due to limitations in detection of aspiration. This chapter focuses on systems of protection against aspiration, methods to detect aspirations of meals into the upper and lower airways, common pulmonary disorders associated with increased risk of aspiration and responses of normal lung tissue to acidification of the distal esophagus.

Keywords

Dysphagia • Pulmonary • Aspiration • Asthma • Idiopathic pulmonary fibrosis • Lung transplantation

R. Tomic, MD
Division of Pulmonary and Critical Care,
Department of Medicine, Froedtert Hospital, Medical College of Wisconsin, 9200 W. Wisconsin Ave, Milwaukee, WI 53226, USA

A. Antonescu-Turcu, MD
Medical College of Wisconsin, 9200 W Wisconsin Ave, Suite 5200, Milwaukee, WI 53226, USA

E.R. Jacobs, MD, MBA (✉)
Pulmonary and Critical Care Medicine, Medical College of Wisconsin, 8701 Watertown Plank Road, Milwaukee, WI 53226, USA

Clement J. Zablocki VA Medical Center,
5000 W. National Ave, Milwaukee, WI 53295, USA
e-mail: ejacobs@mcw.edu

Introduction

Breathing and swallowing are both essential functions for survival and normally occur in mammals at different frequencies. The close anatomic relationship of the esophagus and trachea confers a substantial risk for deleterious respiratory consequences in case of oral-pharyngeal dysfunction. Accordingly, redundant mechanisms to protect the airways from aspiration evolved. Despite the barriers to aspiration of meals, complications of oral contents reaching the upper and lower airways are common. For example, in excess of

10 % of healthy patients over 70 years of age and ~70 % of individuals poststroke are reported to have dysphagia and aspiration [1–3]. The risk of dysphagia is greatly increased by chronic diseases such as COPD or congestive heart failure (CHF), and the presence of dysphagia extends hospitalization costs [3]. Therefore, pulmonary complications of aspiration are of some importance to clinicians. The focuses of this review are (1) developmental aspects of esophageal and pulmonary growth; (2) anatomic and physiologic mechanisms of airway protection, including signaling pathways which control breathing and swallowing; (3) methods to detect aspiration; (4) implications of disorders of swallowing in specific respiratory disorders; and (5) summary and future directions.

Implications of Pulmonary and Esophageal Development

The mammalian lung first develops as an outpouching from the foregut endoderm into the adjacent splanchnic mesenchyme [4, 5]. Separate regions of the foregut differentiate into distinct thoracic and visceral organs. Lung-buds elongate and branch, the foregut longitudinally separates into the esophagus and trachea. This process begins by 3–4 weeks of embryonic development in humans. Many generations of

dichotomous branching are completed prior to parturition; secularization and alveolarization occur both pre- and postnatally.

Congenital Abnormalities

The most frequent congenital disorder affecting breathing and swallowing is a tracheoesophageal fistula (TEF), which consists of a communication between the trachea and esophagus [5]. Because TEFs render ineffective most defenses against aspiration, they lead to severe and sometimes fatal pulmonary complications. The incidence of congenital TEFs is estimated to be one case in 2,000–4,000 live births, and most patients with congenital TEFs are diagnosed immediately following birth or during infancy. However, in rare cases, congenital TEFs are not detected until adulthood [6]. In excess of 50 % of children with TEFs have associated developmental anomalies including Down syndrome, duodenal atresia, and cardiovascular defects (patent ductus arteriosus, atrial septal defect, ventricular septal defect, or Tetralogy of Fallot) [5]. Congenital TEFs are classified into one of five groups (see Fig. 14.1; [5]) based upon their anatomy. Proximal esophageal atresia and distal fistulous connection to the esophagus to the trachea are far the most common of these abnormalities.

Acquired TEFs occur secondary to malignant disease, infection, ruptured diverticula and trauma.

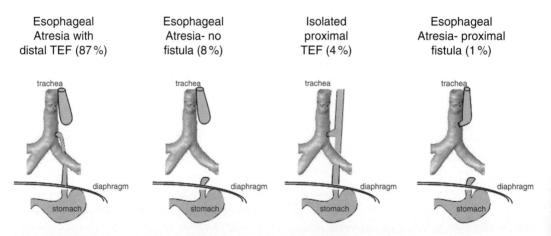

Fig. 14.1 Five variations of tracheoesophageal fistulas based upon anatomy and frequency of presentation

TEFs may also develop following prolonged mechanical ventilation with either an endotracheal or tracheostomy tube [5]. Diagnosis of this condition is often delayed or missed since signs and symptoms are indistinguishable from ventilator-associated pneumonia, e.g., cough, aspiration, fever and infiltrates on roentgenographic studies of the chest. Instillation of contrast media into the esophagus or by direct visualization by flexible esophagoscopy or bronchoscopy can be diagnostic. However, because communication tracts between the trachea and esophagus are generally small and movement of fluid between these structures is intermittent, persistence and a high index of suspicion may be required to make the diagnosis [5].

Anatomy and Physiology of Deglutition

Deglutition is traditionally divided into three neuro-anatomical phases: oral, pharyngeal and esophageal [7]. When food enters the mouth, the oral phase begins with manipulation of the bolus. The orbicularis oris and buccinators muscles provide support to maintain the bolus in the oral cavity, while the teeth accomplish mastication. Food is reduced to small particles using primarily temporalis, masseter, medial and lateral pterygoid muscles. Mechanoreceptor cells concentrated on the tip of the tongue and soft palate provide information about the position and size of food bolus via trigeminal nerve. The oral transport phase starts with peristaltic movements of the tongue that stimulates mechanoreceptors in the hard palate. This phase is voluntary and is controlled by the cerebral cortex and the corticobulbar tracts.

When the bolus is transferred to the oropharynx, the pharyngeal phase of swallowing is initiated [8]. From this point forward, swallowing is involuntary. Mediated largely by vagus and glossopharyngeal nerves, pharyngeal swallowing involves synergized contractions of genioglossus and mylohyoid muscles and cooperative actions of suprahyoid musculature [7]. In this phase of swallowing, the primary risk to aspiration during eating and drinking occurs. Coordinated contraction of more than 29 pairs of muscles contribute to tongue retraction, velopharyngeal closure, pharyngeal contraction, closing of the larynx at the level of the true vocal cords, false vocal folds and epiglottis-aryepiglottic folds. Key to protection of the airway is descent of the epiglottis and elevation of the arytenoid processes to provide an anatomic barrier to entry of liquids or solids into the airway. Also serving as a barrier to aspiration, the vocal cords are maximally adducted and do not reopen until the pharyngeal phase of swallowing is complete [9]. Interestingly, vocal cord closure may be neurally controlled via pathways that are independent from swallow apnea [10]. The pharyngeal phase ends with elevation of the larynx, relaxation of the cricopharyngeal muscle [8], and by-passage of food bolus through the upper esophageal sphincter (UES). These complex interactions take place in less than 1 s.

The *esophageal phase* is the last facet of swallowing, which involves the movement of the bolus from the cervical esophagus to the stomach by a peristaltic wave coordinated by the brain stem and the intrinsic myenteric plexus. The lower esophageal sphincter (LES) is located near gastroesophageal junction [7, 8]. Stimulation of the vagus nerve by food passage through the esophagus causes inhibition of LES activity and a decrease in tonic myotonic activity.

Swallowing Apnea

Beyond the anatomical barriers to aspiration defined above, a fundamental protective mechanism of the lungs is a cessation of breathing during swallowing, or "swallowing apnea" [10, 11]. Mechanisms to coordinate swallowing with breathing include neural and physiological interconnections (signaling pathways), the exact nature of which remains uncertain despite intense interest in this area for more than 30 years. However, several characteristics of swallowing apnea are well established. The breathing cycle is not simply paused during swallowing. Rather a different pattern of breathing during swallowing emerges

[12]. In normal subjects, swallowing apnea most often interrupts the exhalation phase of respiration, with completion of exhalation after swallowing and before initiation of a new breath. However, conscious humans are able to swallow and stop in any phase of a breathing cycle. Apnea begins just before the pharyngeal phase of swallowing and prior to the onset of laryngeal elevation and continues through all pharyngeal phases of deglutition.

Phase Effects of Swallowing

Swallowing during either inspiration or expiration is reported to increase the phase of respiration in which it occurs, but the effects of swallowing on breathing appear more complex than that [13]. In unanesthetized goats, Feroah et al. observed multiple, within-cycle effects on respiratory timing and output. During inspiration, the later the onset of swallowing, the greater the increases in inspiratory time and tidal volumes. Swallows which occur later in the expiratory phase increase expiratory time, and cause increases in inspiratory time and tidal volumes in the subsequent breath [13]. Costa and Leme [10] confirmed a similar coordination in human subjects and noted that cessation of breathing occurred just under 90 % of the time in periods of lowest elastic resistance of the lung (end expiration or early inspiration). They concluded that neural mechanisms responsible for the interruption of the breathing cycle during swallowing may be linked to the elastic resistance of the lungs.

If anatomic barriers and swallow apnea are insufficient to prevent aspiration, the last line of defense is a cough. Involuntary or reflexive cough can be activated by mechanical or chemical stimulation of irritant receptors in either the larynx or trachea [14] which then carry afferent signals through the vagus to initiate a cough. The central nervous system (CNS) coordinates closure of the epiglottis and larynx and simultaneously, contraction of abdominal and intercostal muscles, thereby increasing the subglottic pressure. When the vocal cords open, air is expelled past the upper airway at speeds in excess of 100 miles per hour. In addition to clearing airway secretions, coughing evicts aspirated food and liquid from the lower respiratory tract. Thus, reflexive cough forms one more line of protection against tracheobronchial aspiration.

Central Neuronal Mechanisms That Facilitate Coordination of Swallowing and Breathing

Central pattern generators (CPGs) for breathing are located in the dorsomedial and ventrolateral brain stem (see Fig. 14.2). The best recognized respiratory centers consist of the dorsal respiratory group and the ventral respiratory column in the medulla and pneumotactic centers in the pons [13, 15]. Swallowing CPGs are largely located in the medulla oblongata and include a dorsal swallowing group (DSG) in the nucleus tractus solitarius and a ventral swallowing group (VSG) within the ventrolateral medulla above the nucleus ambiguus. Both respiratory and swallowing centers receive afferent sensory input from the laryngeal via the vagal nerves, as well as modulating signals from cortical centers and several other CNS sites such as the cerebellum [11].

There is a great deal of cross-talk between swallowing and respiratory CPGs. For example, about one half of the VSG inspiratory augmenting and decrementing neurons exhibit discharge during swallowing. This neural exchange and synaptic inhibition facilitates coordination of swallowing and breathing, including inhibition of diaphragmatic contraction during swallowing [11]. Input to the respiratory CPG triggers protective and expulsive reflexes, first through efferents to pre-motoneurons, then to motor neurons including the cranial nerves VI, IX, X, and XII (which control pharyngeal and genioglossus muscles), diaphragmatic, abdominal and intercostals muscles [11]. Loss of swallow apnea due to central or motor dysfunction is associated with dysphagia, coughing, aspiration and weight loss [16].

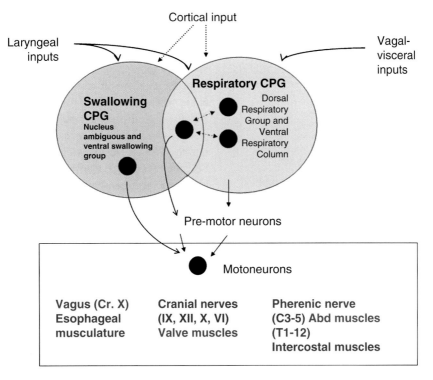

Fig. 14.2 Sensory input from the laryngeal and vagal nerves as well as higher cortical sites feed input to the respiratory central pattern generators (CPGs) for breathing located in the dorsomedial and ventrolateral brain stem and swallowing CPG located in the medulla oblongata. Respiratory centers consist of the dorsal respiratory group and the ventral respiratory column in the medulla and pneumotactic centers in the pons.

Swallowing centers include the dorsal swallowing group (DSG) in the nucleus tractus solitarius and a ventral swallowing group (VSG). There is overlap and cross-talk between swallowing and respiratory CPGs. Efferents to pre-motoneurons, then to motor neurons including the cranial nerves VI, IX, X, and XII control pharyngeal and genioglossus muscles, diaphragmatic, abdominal and intercostals muscles

Signaling Pathways Through Which Esophageal Disorders Affect Breathing

There are excellent data in experimental animals that acidification of the distal esophagus with physiological concentrations of hydrochloric acid (HCl, 0.1 N) results in not only modest decreases in the diameter of small airways, but also substantial increases in mucous secretion or airway microvascular leakage and decreased tracheomucociliary transport [17, 18]. Signaling mechanisms through which esophageal acidification stimulate the airways are incompletely understood. Broadly, these signaling mechanisms may consist of neural or humoral pathways. Below, we summarize signaling pathways which have been reported to link esophageal acidification to

bronchoconstriction or stimulated mucous secretion (see Table 14.1).

Neural (reflex). Bronchoconstriction in persons or experimental animals with acid reflux and mild asthma is decreased by treatment with atropine or vagotomy, suggesting mediation by the vagus nerve and cholinergic release [19, 20]. Most investigators now accept this signaling pathway and involvement of some of the below intermediates as a good explanation of most gastroesophageal reflux disease (GERD)-induced bronchospasm.

Tachykinins. In the airways, the activation of C-fiber afferent nerves leads to local release of tachykinins, a group of neuropeptides including substance P (SP), neurokinin A (NKA), neurokinin

Table 14.1 Signaling of bronchoconstriction, extravasation of fluids

Signaling Pathway	Mechanism of action	References
Reflex theory	Vagus nerve and cholinergic stimulation of airway	[19, 20]
Tachykinins	tachykinins act on NK1 and NK2 receptors in the airways to evoke bronchoconstriction plasma extravasation	[21–23]
Nitrogen oxides	NO release from smooth muscle increases nitrotyrosine and activation of vanilloid receptors	[24]
Vanilloid receptors	TRYPV1 receptors are increased by esophagitis and mediate vagally effected pulmonary inflammation	[23, 25]
Opiod receptors	Plasma extravasation induced by esophageal HCl is mediated by pre-junctional opiod receptors	[18, 26]

B (NKB). Tachykinins are present in several types of peripheral tissues, including the gastrointestinal tract, they induce bronchospasm, increase in microvascular permeability, vasodilatation, stimulation of glandular secretions, facilitation of cholinergic neurotrans-mission and the recruitment and activation of neutrophils [21]. HCl-induced sensory nerve stimulation in the esophagus evokes release of tachykinins probably through para-sympathetic ganglions, which act on neurokinin (NK)1 and NK2 receptors in the airways to evoke bronchoconstriction [22, 27].

Vanilloid receptors. Transient Receptor Potential Vanilloid (TRPV) 1 receptors are present on intrinsic neurons in the esophageal submucosa and esophageal epithelial cells [23]. HCl-induced activation of TRPV1 receptors in the esophageal mucosa causes release of substance P and calcitonin gene receptor peptide (CGRP) from neurons as well as release of PAF substance P, which are hypothesized to cause a subsequent cascade of inflammatory mediators in the lung [25].

Nitrogen oxides. Release of tachykinins or other proinflammatory mediators from airway branches of the vagus nerve (so-called neurogenic inflammation) enhances acid production and release in the airways, through recruitment of neutrophils and other such cells [24]. Acids stimulate release of nitric oxide (NO) from any other three major nitric oxide synthase isoforms in the airway. Excess NO promotes the formation of injurious nitrospecies including peroxynitrite, pernitrous acid, and other reactive species which nitrate tyrosine residues. It is postulated that tyrosine residues have adverse effects on both the innate and acquired immune systems [24].

Opioid receptors. Activation of opiod receptor-like 1 receptors (NOP) inhibits airway microvascular leakage induced by HCl in guinea pigs [18, 26]. It is postulated that opioid receptors play a role in regulating tachykinin transmission in the airways, acting on sensory nerves at the presynaptic level.

Methods to Detect Aspiration

A problem common to all studies addressing the importance of aspiration in lung function is substantial limitations to the methods presently available to detect this condition. Below (and summarized in Table 14.2), we review the advantages and challenges of tests to detect aspiration.

Videofluoroscopic swallow studies are widely available, noninvasive and remain the standard against which other methods to detect aspiration are measured. When fluoroscopic aspiration is observed, there is a correlation to pulmonary complications including pneumonias (e.g., [28, 29]). Alternatively, direct visualization of meal penetration into the trachea can be achieved by flexible endoscopic evaluation during swallowing [30]. While potentially useful, these examinations miss intermittent aspiration. In addition, penetration of particularly liquid meals past the vocal cords, though not to lower airways, has been reported in 11 % of normal individuals [29].

Aspiration has also been detected by labeling meals with radionucleotide tracers such as technetium and then assessing pulmonary signals. This technique appears to be plagued with false negatives (low sensitivity) and frequent positive results in apparently normal subjects [31–33].

Table 14.2 Detection of aspiration

Method of detection	Challenges	References
Videofluoroscopic or direct visualization of aspiration of meal into trachea	Gold standard, but misses intermittent and/or small volume aspiration	[28–30]
Radionucleotide tracers	High rate of false positive	[31–33]
pH detection in trachea	Invasive and does not correlate well to clinical disorders	[34]
Measurement of glucose in respiratory secretions or lavage	False positive with blood in the airway, less useful in the absence of enteral feedings	[35]
Lipid-laden macrophages	Limited sensitivity and specificity	[36–38]
Dyes (methylene blue)	Mitochondrial toxicity	[39, 40]
Detection of GI-specific proteins, solutes, or pH in exhaled breath condensates	Difficulty in determining dilution of respiratory droplets; sensitivity of assays inadequate	[41–43]

pH monitoring of the distal and proximal esophagus has been proposed as a means to detect reflux and aspiration of acid gastric contents, particularly that contributing pathophysiologically to asthma [34]. However, the strongest correlation between acidification and bronchoconstriction derives from pH probes inserted into the trachea through the cricothyroid membrane, thereby documenting acidification of the upper airway [44]. If true, noninvasive monitoring of airway pH in asthmatic individuals attains clinical significance [24], but accurate measurements of this endpoint remain elusive [41]. The invasive nature of placing transcricothyroid pH probes limits this approach.

Winterbauer et al. [35] first suggested measurements of glucose via glucose oxidase test strips in respiratory secretions to detect acid reflux. The basis for this test is the fact that glucose concentrations in respiratory secretions in normal subjects are normally less than 5 mg/dL, whereas enteral feedings have glucose concentrations in excess of 300 mg/dL. Contamination of specimens by even relatively small amounts of blood can raise glucose concentrations in the absence of aspiration. In addition, the likelihood of detecting elevated glucose concentrations in respiratory secretions from individuals not receiving enteral foods decreases greatly.

Identification of lipid-laden macrophages in respiratory secretions obtained by bronchoalveolar lavage (BAL) is frequently cited as evidence of aspiration [36]. However, the presence of lipid-laden macrophages in airway fluids lacks sensitivity and specificity, and the samples cannot be obtained easily in an unanesthetized subject [37, 38].

Addition of dyes such as methylene blue to enteral feedings to detect aspiration in suctioned secretions has been used historically [39]. Not only does this additive stain skin, urine and stool green, but it can also be absorbed across intestinal mucosa resulting in mitochondrial poisoning [40]. Therefore, use of this method to identify aspiration has fallen out of favor.

Finally, detection of proteins unique to the digestive tract (e.g., pepsin) or acid pH in exhaled breath condensates or secretions has theoretical potential to identify aspiration [41–43]. Accurate measurements of solute dilution by water vapor or BAL and sufficient sensitivity of assays limit the utility of this method at this writing [41].

Lung Diseases and Aspiration

Many lung diseases are associated with aspiration, but the nature and scope of this relationship are debated. There are two mechanisms by which micro-aspirations produce lung disease: (1) neural mechanisms occurring during reflux events limited to the lower esophagus (distal gastroesophageal reflux) and (2) direct effect from gastric contents refluxed above the UES (proximal gastro esophageal reflux) producing upper airway injury and, if aspirated into the tracheobronchial tree, lung disease (e.g., [45]). Below (and in Table 14.3), we review the data implicating aspiration in pulmonary disorders including cough, asthma or COPD, lung transplant and fibrosing lung diseases.

Table 14.3 Respiratory disorders related to GERD or aspiration

Disorder	Factors linking this disorder to GERD	Limitations to pathophysiologic relation to GERD	References
Cough	Roughly 40 % patients with chronic cough respond to anti-reflux therapy	Randomized controlled trials do not support improvement in cough with acid-suppressive therapy	[14, 16, 46]
Asthma and COPD	Treatment of GERD improves asthma control in some trials; experimental studies support bronchoconstriction by esophageal acidification	Treatment of GERD does not consistently improve objective or subjective symptoms of asthma	[44, 47–53]
Lung transplant	Correlation between severity of reflux and bile acid presence in BAL with bronchiolitis obliterans	Treatment of GERD alone does not prevent deterioration of lung function after lung transplantation	[54–58]
Scleroderma	Esophageal reflux is increased in patients with scleroderma correlated with the severity of disease	Association severity of GERD and scleroderma may represent disease severity	[59–62]
Interstitial pulmonary fibrosis	Aspiration may cause acute exacerbations and prevalence is increased	A minority of patients with IPF have proximal reflux aspiration	[63, 64]

Cough and Aspiration

Reflux-associated cough has been recognized for many years, with primary care and pulmonary physicians consistently reporting up to 40 % of patients with chronic cough responding to anti-reflux therapy [14]. Despite these impressive numbers, randomized placebo-controlled trials linking acid suppression therapy and cough are inconclusive. Reflexive cough while eating and drinking in adult patients with an abnormal pharyngeal swallow phase supports cough secondary to aspiration [16]. Symptoms and findings that suggest that the cough is associated with penetration or aspiration include increased cough with thin—as opposed to thick—liquids, a history of stroke or progressive neurologic disease, a history of oropharyngeal dysphagia, a history of head and neck cancer or head and neck surgery, the presence of a wet vocal quality, hoarseness and coughing with meals as opposed to after meals [46]. Some patients with a hypersensitive larynx also report coughing with meals. Hence it is important to differentiate persons with a hypersensitive larynx from persons with oropharyngeal dysphagia who are at risk for aspiration.

Cough Response to Tussigenic Challenges

Impaired cough reflex sensitivity in response to tussigenic challenges has been reported to predict the development of pneumonia in the elderly [65]. Cough sensitivity to inhaled capsaicin was measured in a small consecutive group of patients ($n=7$) with recurrent pneumonia (2–6 episodes each), all of whom had chest radiographic findings consistent with aspiration. The concentration of capsaicin needed to induce reflex coughs was higher ($p < 0.0001$) in pneumonia patients than in age- and gender-matched control subjects, implying that patients with recurrent pneumonia had reduced sensitivity to stimulation of irritant receptors in the laryngeal area [66]. Not all investigators have found a tight correlation between pneumonia and positive tussigenic challenges [67]. For example, cough thresholds to inhaled capsaicin in patients ($n=28$) with a variety of neurologic impairments were not different based upon normal or abnormal swallow studies ($n=28$) [68].

Asthma and COPD

Asthma affects roughly 9 % of the population, while GERD symptoms occur daily in approximately 7–20 % of the US adult population [47]. Therefore, many asthmatic patients should also have GERD purely based on the probability of having two common diseases. However, asthmatic patients have a greater prevalence of GERD (up to 80 % in some studies) than the general population, which has led to consideration of a pathologic link between the two disease states. Although many asthmatic patients with positive pH probe findings have typical GERD symptoms such as heartburn, approximately 40 % are asymptomatic [48].

Because acidification of the distal esophagus induces bronchospasm and micro-aspiration induces chronic inflammatory changes [17, 69], it is postulated that GERD and asthma are pathophysiologically linked. In addition, descent of the diaphragm in the setting of lung hyperinflation increases the pressure gradient between the abdomen and chest and may cause the LES to herniate into the chest where its barrier function is impaired [70]. Compounding matters, asthma medications may promote acid reflux; beta agonists and methylxanthine bronchodilators decrease LES tone, which may foster acid reflux. Several studies suggesting that treatment of GERD improved asthma control prompted recommendations for such treatment in all poorly controlled asthmatic patients, irrespective of GERD symptoms (Table 14.3) [44, 49]. Improvement of asthma control in more than 80 % of patients in some studies who undergo laparoscopic fundoplication further supports the notion that esophageal reflux plays a role in asthma [71].

However, clinical trials are inconsistent in demonstrating positive effects of acid suppression on lung function, asthma symptoms, or asthma-related quality of life [50, 72]. A meta-analysis concluded that treatment of GERD with the goal of improving asthma control cannot be supported by the literature [73]. Littner et al. [51] conducted a 6-month placebo-controlled trial involving 207 patients with moderate-to-severe asthma with symptomatic GERD treated with lanzoprazole twice daily. Treatment of symptomatic GERD resulted in a reduction in exacerbations and an improvement in asthma-related quality of life, but did not improve the primary outcome of daily asthma symptoms [51]. Kiljander et al. [49] conducted a similar trial involving patients with mild-to-moderate asthma and patient reported symptoms of gastroesophageal reflux treated with proton pump inhibitors. Overall, there were no improvements in daily peak expiratory flow rate, exacerbations, or asthma symptoms in patients treated for GERD. A subsequent study [52] reported that patients with moderate to severe GERD experienced modest improvement in asthma control with anti-reflux therapy.

To evaluate the potential effect of *silent* GERD on asthma control, the Asthma Clinical Research Centers (ACRC) conducted a trial of patients with poorly controlled asthma without symptoms of GERD on a stable dose of inhaled corticosteroids. Participants were randomized to proton pump inhibitor esomeprazole (40 mg twice daily) or placebo and followed for 6 months [48]. Patients treated with esomeprazole did not experience any benefit with respect to the rate of asthma attacks, asthma symptoms, nocturnal awakening, quality of life, or lung function. In addition, nearly half of the participants had silent GERD based upon ambulatory pH probe measurements. No subgroup likely to benefit from therapy with proton pump inhibitors was identified [48].

Acid reflux may not correlate with asthma even if there is a pathophysiologic relationship. Ambulatory 24-h esophageal pH monitoring is the reference standard for the diagnosis of gastroesophageal reflux. Acid reflux is diagnosed when distal esophageal pH is less than 4 for ≥5 % of the total study time, a definition which correlates well with endoscopically diagnosed erosive esophagitis [74]. Poor correlation between asthma and reflux may be because 24-h pH studies do not evaluate the volume or proximal extent of reflux, factors that may be important for the development of pulmonary symptoms. In fact, Tomonaga et al. [75] reported that patients with acid reflux detected at both a proximal and distal pH probe had a higher incidence of nocturnal cough than those in whom acid reflux was detected only at the distal probe. On the other hand, the ALA–ACRC Study of Acid Reflux and Asthma (SARA) trial demonstrated no effect on asthma control with acid suppression targeted to neutralization of proximal versus distal GERD or both proximal and distal GERD [76]. There is also some evidence that nonacid reflux may impact asthma control [53]. Reflux of pepsin, bile acids, or pancreatic enzymes, or mechanical distention of the esophagus could elicit symptoms in patients with asthma that are resistant to proton-pump inhibitors. Based upon available data, we conclude that (a) there is no clear benefit of treatment with a proton pump inhibitor in patients with poorly controlled asthma and (b) pH probe monitoring does not identify asthmatic patients likely to benefit from GERD treatment.

Lung Transplant and GERD

Lung transplantation has become a life-saving therapy for patients with end-stage lung disease, but a major limitation to the long-term success of this therapy is the development of posttransplant bronchiolitis obliterans, a process of fibrous obliteration of the small airways with progressive airflow obstruction. Bronchiolitis obliterans usually develops between 6 months and 2 years after transplant and affects 50–60 % of patients within 5 years after transplant [54]. It is increasingly clear that bronchiolitis obliterans (BO) represents the response of the lung to multiple injurious processes, possibly including GERD and/or aspiration.

Immunosuppressive drugs prolong gastric emptying. Combined with potential for iatrogenic vagal nerve injury during lung implantation, GERD may be exacerbated after lung transplantation [55, 77]. Lung defense mechanisms such as cough reflex and mucociliary clearance of foreign bodies are significantly impaired in lung transplant patients [78]. It is postulated that a prolonged contact time of aspirated gastric contents may lead to greater lung injury. Aspirated material can act as detergents in

disrupting the lipid layers of pulmonary surfactant. Alternatively, bile acids may cause direct injury to type-II pneumocytes responsible for the surfactant protein, phospholipid production and homeostasis [79]. Furthermore, bile acids appear to downregulate the innate immunity via specific receptors (TGR5) abundantly expressed in monocytes and macrophages [80]. Rabbit alveolar macrophage phagocytosis and lipopolysaccharide-stimulated cytokine production are impaired by bile acid. By disrupting loco-regional innate immunity, GERD aspirate may promote infections and/or maintain chronic infections and this could secondarily be responsible for upregulation of the adaptive immune response [81]. Recent evidence suggests that BO is associated with impaired innate defenses within the lungs. Some combination of these defects may account for accelerated aspiration-induced lung injury in persons with transplanted lungs.

Hartwig et al. [56] documented that chronic aspiration of acid gastric material accelerates the pulmonary allograft dysfunction in a rat model of lung transplantation. It is not clear if the injurious agent is gastric acid or other gastro-duodenal components such as pepsin, trypsin, or bile acids. D'Ovidio et al. [82] reported abnormal esophageal pH measurements in 30 % of lung transplant patients 3 months after transplantation and in 50 % of lung transplant patients 1 year after lung transplantation. Seventy percent of patients with high levels of bile acids in bronchoalveolar lavage fluid (BALF) will develop bronchiolitis obliterans 1 year after lung transplant, and nearly one-third of patients posttransplant will have only nonacid reflux [57]. Atkins et al. [83] reported that 64 % of lung transplant patients aspirate during swallowing and 78 % of these were asymptomatic. These patients have increased frequency of BO. Young et al. [84] documented increased GERD and increased acid contact time after lung transplantation. GERD correlates with worse results in pulmonary function tests (PFTs) in posttransplant population [58] and retrospective analyses suggest that anti-reflux procedures could improve pulmonary function in patients with BOS and GERD [85]. Complicating interpretation of these data are the facts that GERD symptoms are frequently absent posttransplantation due to esophageal denervation and do not correlate with objective measurements of esophageal pH.

Conservative therapy for GERD including proton pump inhibitors is usually insufficient to prevent BO after lung transplant, possibly because it does not prevent nonacid reflux and aspiration. Besides prednisone, azithromycin is now advocated in patients with BO because of its anti-inflammatory, antibacterial and pro-motile effect; esophageal motility; or promotion of ciliary motion [86]. Other experimental therapies including endoscopic reflux therapy with endoluminal gastroplication, suturing, radiofrequency ablation, or injecting the gastroesophageal junction to decrease GER have been advocated [55, 87].

When conservative therapies for reflux fail in transplant patients, surgical interventions have been advocated. Balsara et al. [88] suggest that anti-reflux surgery in this population may increase survival and improved lung function. Limited data support early fundoplication (within 90 days after lung transplant) as yielding better outcomes than late fundoplication, possibly because patients with more advanced BO have irreversible fibrotic changes [55, 88]. Published reports favor laparoscopic over open anti-reflux procedures in lung transplant patients [55]. Although these results are intriguing, prospective randomized clinical trials are needed to determine the relationship between aspiration and BO as well as the role of interventions in prevention of this disorder.

Fibrosing Lung Diseases

The classic fibrosing lung disease, interstitial pulmonary fibrosis (IPF) progresses to death within 3–5 years in most patients. Recurrent micro-aspiration has been identified as a potential risk factor for IPF and is postulated as pathophysiologically important [45]. Esophageal dysfunction occurring in a variety of interstitial lung diseases has been reported [89], suggesting that GERD in fibrotic lung diseases results from other than disease-specific changes in pulmonary mechanics and trans-diaphragmatic pressure gradient. Bile acids, identified in increased levels in the sputum of patients with GERD [79], induce

in vitro production of transforming growth factor (TGF)-$\beta 1$ by human epithelial cells. As TGF-β is an important mediator of the fibro-proliferative processes in IPF [90], this mechanism is postulated to contribute to development and progression of this disease. Below, we review data related to specific fibrotic diseases and aspiration.

Scleroderma-Associated Lung Fibrosis

Studies evaluating the role of esophageal reflux in the development of scleroderma-associated pulmonary fibrosis are limited to small case series employing a variety of indices of esophageal function. Johnson et al. [91] studied 13 patients with scleroderma, all of whom had abnormal LES function and biopsy evidence of GERD. Ten of these patients had a reduced diffusing capacity for carbon monoxide ($D_{L,CO}$), a proxy for capillary surface area, which was inversely correlated with GERD severity. Two patients had aspiration as demonstrated by scintigraphic study. Another series of 43 patients demonstrated a correlation between abnormal esophageal motility and poor lung function [59]. Kinuya et al. [92] evaluated 47 scleroderma patients and found that higher esophageal retention of a nuclear tracer (a marker of impaired peristalsis) correlated with impairment in both $D_{L,CO}$ and forced vital capacity. Marie et al. [60] studied 43 scleroderma patients with esophageal manometry showing that although the patients did not differ with respect to disease duration, systemic disease manifestations, or inflammatory markers, more severe esophageal dysfunction was correlated with interstitial changes as shown by high-resolution computed tomography (HRCT) and reduced $D_{L,CO}$, with a trend toward lower lung volumes. Savarino et al. [61] studied 40 consecutive scleroderma patients with combined esophageal pH and impedance testing. HRCT evidence of pulmonary fibrosis was found in 18 out of 40 patients, and this group had significantly lower LES pressure, more esophageal acid exposure and more total and proximal reflux events. They also had a higher percentage of proximal reflux episodes compared to those without fibrosis. In contrast, another study of 47 patients found that the presence of proximal reflux was not correlated with lung function, although $D_{L,CO}$ was reduced in patients both with and without reflux [62]. These studies may support the premise that recurrent aspiration could play a role in the progression of scleroderma-associated lung fibrosis. It is equally possible that the association of pulmonary and esophageal dysfunction simply reflects a more advanced stage of disease.

Interstitial Pulmonary Fibrosis

Similar to scleroderma, patients with IPF have a high prevalence of GERD, supporting the hypothesis that recurrent occult micro-aspiration may drive ongoing fibrosis. There is some evidence that micro-aspiration can cause acute exacerbations in addition to being a primary cause of IPF. Mays et al. [63] reported 131 patients with radiographic pulmonary fibrosis; six of these patients had recurrent aspiration as their primary diagnosis. Another 63 were ultimately diagnosed as "idiopathic" fibrosis, and 79 % of this group had symptoms of GERD.

Recognition of GERD as a potential etiological factor in IPF has important treatment implications. Trials of therapy for GERD in patients with established IPF are limited to one retrospective case series of four patients with IPF and documented GERD who were treated with only proton pumps inhibitors (PPI) [64]. With treatment, these patients stabilized or improved over a 2–3-year period. While micro-aspiration is inferred as a contributor to IPF, scintigraphic studies in patients with upper airway complaints suggest that this may be a false assumption as only a minority of patients with IPF have proximal reflux aspiration [93]. The question of whether GERD initiates the fibrotic process, participates in driving already established fibrosis, or is an irrelevant bystander remains unresolved.

Treatment of Oralpharyngeal Dysphagia

Therapy for oralpharyngeal dysphagia has been reported to result in a reduction of swallowing-related medical complications, chest infection, and death or institutionalization and an increase in the proportion of patients regaining swallowing function [94]. Treatment methods including muscle strengthening, compensatory maneuvers and neuromuscular stimulation are now proposed to improve oralpharyngeal swallow function. These treatment approaches are in the exploratory stage, i.e., they are under development and are considered to show promise and efficacy in certain patient groups. An evidence-based systematic review of treatments for oralpharyngeal dysphagia is underway by the American Speech Language and Hearing Association and results will be available online at http://www.asha.org in the near future.

Pharmacologic agents that modulate dopamine metabolisms are also being investigated to improve swallowing and the cough reflex in the elderly. These investigations are focused on the decrease of substance P in patients with CVAs who are at increased risk of subclinical aspiration and an increased incidence of pneumonia [95]. Treatment for patients with dysphagia including pharmacologic measures, electrical stimulation of oralpharyngeal musculature and muscle strengthening are reported to result in a decrease in morbidity and mortality [95, 96].

Summary and Future Directions

Despite intense interest and study, we have yet to really identify the extent of aspiration injury on lung function. We need an equivalent of hemoglobin A1C to measure the cumulative effects of micro-aspiration over time on lung function. Reliable biomarkers of aspiration in sputum or BAL samples are similarly lacking. Until such barometers are developed, the pathophysiological association of GERD with lung diseases will remain speculative.

We do not fully understand how acid or gastric contents in the esophagus mediate altered lung function, including endpoints such as bronchospasm, increased vascular permeability and enhanced mucous secretion. There is evidence of both humoral and neural connections between the esophagus and lung, as well as studies to implicate specific receptors. Nevertheless, the tools to identify these signaling pathways are crude. If these pathways were defined, then therapeutic implications (e.g., inhibition of NK1 or NK2 receptors) should emerge. The association of GERD with a variety of lung diseases ranging from cough, asthma, to transplanted lung and idiopathic IPF cannot be causally related, neither can therapies for GERD be clearly related to better outcomes in individuals with these disorders. Better therapies to treat individuals with oralpharyngeal aspiration are sorely needed.

Key points

- Proximity of the upper respiratory and gastrointestinal (GI) tracts confers substantial risk for aspiration.
- Tests for aspiration do not have high sensitivity and specificity.
- GERD and aspiration are common in the general population and are increased by factors including advanced age and chronic diseases.
- It is difficult to establish a causal relationship between pulmonary diseases including cough, asthma, lung transplant, or idiopathic pulmonary fibrosis (IPF) and others to GERD or aspiration, though the incidence of GERD is substantially increased in these populations.
- There are very limited data to support the concept that treatment of GERD may improve objective outcomes in patients with the above diseases, leaving room for future studies.

References

1. Nakagawa T, Sekizawa K, Nakajoh K, Tanji H, Arai H, Sasaki H. Silent cerebral infarction: a potential risk for pneumonia in the elderly. J Intern Med. 2000;247(2):255–9.
2. Martino R, Foley N, Bhogal S, Diamant N, Speechley M, Teasell R. Dysphagia after stroke: incidence, diagnosis, and pulmonary complications. Stroke. 2005;36(12):2756–63.
3. Altman KW, Yu GP, Schaefer SD. Consequence of dysphagia in the hospitalized patient: impact on prognosis and hospital resources. Arch Otolaryngol Head Neck Surg. 2010;136(8):784–9.
4. Chinoy MR. Lung growth and development. Front Biosci. 2003;8:d392–415.
5. Sharma S DD. Tracheoesophageal fistula. http://emedicine medscape com/article/186735-overview. 2010; eMedicine/Gastroenterology/Esophagus(January 10, 2010).
6. Acosta JL, Battersby JS. Congenital tracheoesophageal fistula in the adult. Ann Thorac Surg. 1974; 17(1):51–7.
7. Plant RL. Anatomy and physiology of swallowing in adults and geriatrics. Otolaryngol Clin North Am. 1998;31(3):477–88.
8. Kahrilas PJ. Pharyngeal structure and function. Dysphagia. 1993;8(4):303–7.
9. Martin BJ, Logemann JA, Shaker R, Dodds WJ. Coordination between respiration and swallowing: respiratory phase relationships and temporal integration. J Appl Physiol. 1994;76(2):714–23.
10. Costa MM, Lemme EM. Coordination of respiration and swallowing: functional pattern and relevance of vocal folds closure. Arq Gastroenterol. 2010;47(1):42–8.
11. Bianchi AL, Gestreau C. The brainstem respiratory network: an overview of a half century of research. Respir Physiol Neurobiol. 2009;168(1–2):4–12.
12. Shaker R, Dua KS, Ren J, Xie P, Funahashi A, Schapira RM. Vocal cord closure pressure during volitional swallow and other voluntary tasks. Dysphagia. 2002;17(1):13–8.
13. Feroah TR, Forster HV, Fuentes CG, et al. Effects of spontaneous swallows on breathing in awake goats. J Appl Physiol. 2002;92(5):1923–35.
14. Smith J, Woodcock A, Houghton L. New developments in reflux-associated cough. Lung. 2010;188 Suppl 1:S81–6.
15. Bonis JM, Neumueller SE, Marshall BD, et al. The effects of lesions in the dorsolateral pons on the coordination of swallowing and breathing in awake goats. Respir Physiol Neurobiol. 2011;175(2):272–82.
16. Smith Hammond CA, Goldstein LB. Cough and aspiration of food and liquids due to oral-pharyngeal dysphagia: ACCP evidence-based clinical practice guidelines. Chest. 2006;129 Suppl 1:154S–68.
17. Lang IM, Haworth ST, Medda BK, Roerig DL, Forster HV, Shaker R. Airway responses to esophageal acidification. Am J Physiol Regul Integr Comp Physiol. 2008;294(1):R211–9.
18. Rouget C, Cui YY, D'Agostino B, et al. Nociceptin inhibits airway microvascular leakage induced by HCl intra-oesophageal instillation. Br J Pharmacol. 2004; 141(6):1077–83.
19. Colson DJ, Campbell CA, Wright VA, Watson BW. Predictive value of oesophageal pH variables in children with gastro-oesophageal reflux. Gut. 1990;31(4):370–3.
20. Andersen LI, Schmidt A, Bundgaard A. Pulmonary function and acid application in the esophagus. Chest. 1986;90(3):358–63.
21. Hamamoto J, Kohrogi H, Kawano O, et al. Esophageal stimulation by hydrochloric acid causes neurogenic inflammation in the airways in guinea pigs. J Appl Physiol. 1997;82(3):738–45.

22. Daoui S, D'Agostino B, Gallelli L, Alt XE, Rossi F, Advenier C. Tachykinins and airway microvascular leakage induced by HCl intra-oesophageal instillation. Eur Respir J. 2002;20(2):268–73.

23. Cheng L, de la Monte S, Ma J, et al. HCl-activated neural and epithelial vanilloid receptors (TRPV1) in cat esophageal mucosa. Am J Physiol Gastrointest Liver Physiol. 2009;297(1):G135–43.

24. Hunt J. Airway acidification: interactions with nitrogen oxides and airway inflammation. Curr Allerg Asthma Rep. 2006;6(1):47–52.

25. Peles S, Medda BK, Zhang Z, et al. Differential effects of transient receptor vanilloid one (TRPV1) antagonists in acid-induced excitation of esophageal vagal afferent fibers of rats. Neuroscience. 2009;161(2): 515–25.

26. Banerjee B, Medda BK, Zheng Y, et al. Alterations in N-methyl-D-aspartate receptor subunits in primary sensory neurons following acid-induced esophagitis in cats. Am J Physiol Gastrointest Liver Physiol. 2009;296(1):G66–77.

27. Gallelli L, D'Agostino B, Marrocco G, et al. Role of tachykinins in the bronchoconstriction induced by HCl intraesophageal instillation in the rabbit. Life Sci. 2003;72(10):1135–42.

28. Pikus L, Levine MS, Yang YX, et al. Videofluoroscopic studies of swallowing dysfunction and the relative risk of pneumonia. AJR Am J Roentgenol. 2003;180(6):1613–6.

29. Allen JE, White CJ, Leonard RJ, Belafsky PC. Prevalence of penetration and aspiration on videofluoroscopy in normal individuals without dysphagia. Otolaryngol Head Neck Surg. 2010;142(2): 208–13.

30. Langmore SE, Schatz K, Olsen N. Fiberoptic endoscopic examination of swallowing safety: a new procedure. Dysphagia. 1988;2:216–9.

31. Ghaed N, Stein MR. Assessment of a technique for scintigraphic monitoring of pulmonary aspiration of gastric contents in asthmatics with gastroesophageal reflux. Ann Allerg. 1979;42(5):306–8.

32. Ruth M, Carlsson S, Mansson I, Bengtsson U, Sandberg N. Scintigraphic detection of gastro-pulmonary aspiration in patients with respiratory disorders. Clin Physiol. 1993;13(1):19–33.

33. Ravelli AM, Panarotto MB, Verdoni L, Consolati V, Bolognini S. Pulmonary aspiration shown by scintigraphy in gastroesophageal reflux-related respiratory disease. Chest. 2006;130(5):1520–6.

34. Gastal OL, Castell JA, Castell DO. Frequency and site of gastroesophageal reflux in patients with chest symptoms. studies using proximal and distal pH monitoring. Chest. 1994;106(6):1793–6.

35. Winterbauer RH, Durning Jr RB, Barron E, McFadden MC. Aspirated nasogastric feeding solution detected by glucose strips. Ann Intern Med. 1981;95(1):67–8.

36. Corwin RW, Irwin RS. The lipid-laden alveolar macrophage as a marker of aspiration in parenchymal lung disease. Am Rev Respir Dis. 1985;132(3): 576–81.

37. Furuya ME, Moreno-Cordova V, Ramirez-Figueroa JL, Vargas MH, Ramon-Garcia G, Ramirez-San Juan DH. Cutoff value of lipid-laden alveolar macrophages for diagnosing aspiration in infants and children. Pediatr Pulmonol. 2007;42(5):452–7.

38. Parameswaran K, Anvari M, Efthimiadis A, Kamada D, Hargreave FE, Allen CJ. Lipid-laden macrophages in induced sputum are a marker of oropharyngeal reflux and possible gastric aspiration. Eur Respir J. 2000;16(6):1119–22.

39. Potts RG, Zaroukian MH, Guerrero PA, Baker CD. Comparison of blue dye visualization and glucose oxidase test strip methods for detecting pulmonary aspiration of enteral feedings in intubated adults. Chest. 1993;103(1):117–21.

40. Maloney JP, Ryan TA, Brasel KJ, et al. Food dye use in enteral feedings: a review and a call for a moratorium. Nutr Clin Pract. 2002;17(3):169–81.

41. Effros RM. Exhaled breath condensate: delusion or dilution? Chest. 2010;138(3):471–2.

42. Metheny NA, Chang YH, Ye JS, et al. Pepsin as a marker for pulmonary aspiration. Am J Crit Care. 2002;11(2):150–4.

43. Ward C, Forrest IA, Brownlee IA, et al. Pepsin like activity in bronchoalveolar lavage fluid is suggestive of gastric aspiration in lung allografts. Thorax. 2005;60(10):872–4.

44. Harding SM, Richter JE, Guzzo MR, Schan CA, Alexander RW, Bradley LA. Asthma and gastroesophageal reflux: acid suppressive therapy improves asthma outcome. Am J Med. 1996;100(4):395–405.

45. American Thoracic Society (ATS) and European Respiratory Society (ERS). Idiopathic pulmonary fibrosis: diagnosis and treatment. International consensus statement. American Thoracic Society (ATS) and the European Respiratory Society (ERS). Am J Respir Crit Care Med. 2000;161(2):646–64.

46. Amin MR, Belafsky PC. Cough and swallowing dysfunction. Otolaryngol Clin North Am. 2010;43(1): 35–42. viii.

47. Locke 3rd GR, Talley NJ, Fett SL, Zinsmeister AR, Melton 3rd LJ. Prevalence and clinical spectrum of gastroesophageal reflux: a population-based study in olmsted county, minnesota. Gastroenterology. 1997;112(5):1448–56.

48. American Lung Association Asthma Clinical Research Centers, Mastronarde JG, Anthonisen NR, et al. Efficacy of esomeprazole for treatment of poorly controlled asthma. N Engl J Med. 2009;360(15):1487–99.

49. Kiljander TO, Salomaa ER, Hietanen EK, Terho EO. Gastroesophageal reflux in asthmatics: a double-blind, placebo-controlled crossover study with omeprazole. Chest. 1999;116(5):1257–64.

50. Boeree MJ, Peters FT, Postma DS, Kleibeuker JH. No effects of high-dose omeprazole in patients with severe airway hyperresponsiveness and (a) symptomatic gastro-oesophageal reflux. Eur Respir J. 1998;11(5):1070–4.

51. Littner MR, Leung FW, Ballard 2nd ED, Huang B, Samra NK, Lansoprazole Asthma Study Group.

Effects of 24 weeks of lansoprazole therapy on asthma symptoms, exacerbations, quality of life, and pulmonary function in adult asthmatic patients with acid reflux symptoms. Chest. 2005;128(3):1128–35.

52. Kiljander TO, Junghard O, Beckman O, Lind T. Effect of esomeprazole 40 mg once or twice daily on asthma: a randomized, placebo-controlled study. Am J Respir Crit Care Med. 2010;181(10):1042–8.

53. Asano K, Suzuki H. Silent acid reflux and asthma control. N Engl J Med. 2009;360(15):1551–3.

54. Boehler A, Kesten S, Weder W, Speich R. Bronchiolitis obliterans after lung transplantation: a review. Chest. 1998;114(5):1411–26.

55. Cantu 3rd E, Appel 3rd JZ, Hartwig MG, et al. J. Maxwell Chamberlain Memorial Paper. Early fundoplication prevents chronic allograft dysfunction in patients with gastroesophageal reflux disease. Ann Thorac Surg. 2004;78(4):1142–51. discussion 1142–51.

56. Hartwig MG, Appel JZ, Li B, et al. Chronic aspiration of gastric fluid accelerates pulmonary allograft dysfunction in a rat model of lung transplantation. J Thorac Cardiovasc Surg. 2006;131(1):209–17.

57. Blondeau K, Mertens V, Vanaudenaerde BA, et al. Gastro-oesophageal reflux and gastric aspiration in lung transplant patients with or without chronic rejection. Eur Respir J. 2008;31(4):707 13.

58. Hadjiliadis D, Duane Davis R, Steele MP. Gastroesophageal reflux disease in lung transplant recipients. Clin Transplant. 2003;17(4):363–8.

59. Lock G, Pfeifer M, Straub RH, et al. Association of esophageal dysfunction and pulmonary function impairment in systemic sclerosis. Am J Gastroenterol. 1998;93(3):341–5.

60. Marie I, Dominique S, Levesque H, et al. Esophageal involvement and pulmonary manifestations in systemic sclerosis. Arthritis Rheum. 2001;45(4):346–54.

61. Savarino E, Bazzica M, Zentilin P, et al. Gastroesophageal reflux and pulmonary fibrosis in scleroderma: a study using pH-impedance monitoring. Am J Respir Crit Care Med. 2009;179(5):408–13.

62. Troshinsky MB, Kane GC, Varga J, et al. Pulmonary function and gastroesophageal reflux in systemic sclerosis. Ann Intern Med. 1994;121(1):6–10.

63. Mays EE, Dubois JJ, Hamilton GB. Pulmonary fibrosis associated with tracheobronchial aspiration. A study of the frequency of hiatal hernia and gastroesophageal reflux in interstitial pulmonary fibrosis of obscure etiology. Chest. 1976;69(4):512–5.

64. Raghu G, Yang ST, Spada C, Hayes J, Pellegrini CA. Sole treatment of acid gastroesophageal reflux in idiopathic pulmonary fibrosis: a case series. Chest. 2006;129(3):794–800.

65. Vergis EN, Brennen C, Wagener M, Muder RR. Pneumonia in long-term care: a prospective case-control study of risk factors and impact on survival. Arch Intern Med. 2001;161(19):2378–81.

66. Niimi A, Matsumoto H, Ueda T, et al. Impaired cough reflex in patients with recurrent pneumonia. Thorax. 2003;58(2):152–3.

67. Nakajoh K, Nakagawa T, Sekizawa K, Matsui T, Arai H, Sasaki H. Relation between incidence of pneumonia and protective reflexes in post-stroke patients with oral or tube feeding. J Intern Med. 2000;247(1):39–42.

68. Smith PE, Wiles CM. Cough responsiveness in neurogenic dysphagia. J Neurol Neurosurg Psychiatry. 1998;64(3):385–8.

69. Jack CI, Calverley PM, Donnelly RJ, et al. Simultaneous tracheal and oesophageal pH measurements in asthmatic patients with gastro-oesophageal reflux. Thorax. 1995;50(2):201–4.

70. Zerbib F, Guisset O, Lamouliatte H, Quinton A, Galmiche JP, Tunon-De-Lara JM. Effects of bronchial obstruction on lower esophageal sphincter motility and gastroesophageal reflux in patients with asthma. Am J Respir Crit Care Med. 2002;166(9):1206–11.

71. Rakita S, Villadolid D, Thomas A, et al. Laparoscopic nissen fundoplication offers high patient satisfaction with relief of extraesophageal symptoms of gastroesophageal reflux disease. Am Surg. 2006;72(3):207–12.

72. Levin TR, Sperling RM, McQuaid KR. Omeprazole improves peak expiratory flow rate and quality of life in asthmatics with gastroesophageal reflux. Am J Gastroenterol. 1998;93(7):1060–3.

73. Gibson PG, Henry RL, Coughlan JL. Gastro-oesophageal reflux treatment for asthma in adults and children. http://www.ncbi.nlm.nih.gov/pubmed/12804410. Cochrane Database Syst Rev. 2003;(2): CD001496. Review. PMID: 12804410.

74. Koufman JA. The otolaryngologic manifestations of gastroesophageal reflux disease (GERD): a clinical investigation of 225 patients using ambulatory 24-hour pH monitoring and an experimental investigation of the role of acid and pepsin in the development of laryngeal injury. Laryngoscope. 1991;101(4 Pt 2 Suppl 53):1–78.

75. Tomonaga T, Awad ZT, Filipi CJ, et al. Symptom predictability of reflux-induced respiratory disease. Dig Dis Sci. 2002;47(1):9–14.

76. DiMango E, Holbrook JT, Simpson E, et al. Effects of asymptomatic proximal and distal gastroesophageal reflux on asthma severity. Am J Respir Crit Care Med. 2009;180(9):809–16.

77. Lubetkin EI, Lipson DA, Palevsky HI, et al. GI complications after orthotopic lung transplantation. Am J Gastroenterol. 1996;91(11):2382–90.

78. Reid KR, McKenzie FN, Menkis AH, et al. Importance of chronic aspiration in recipients of heart-lung transplants. Lancet. 1990;336(8709):206–8.

79. Perng DW, Chang KT, Su KC, et al. Exposure of airway epithelium to bile acids associated with gastroesophageal reflux symptoms: a relation to transforming growth factor-beta1 production and fibroblast proliferation. Chest. 2007;132(5):1548–56.

80. Chang KO, Sosnovtsev SV, Belliot G, Kim Y, Saif LJ, Green KY. Bile acids are essential for porcine enteric calicivirus replication in association with downregulation of signal transducer and activator of transcription 1. Proc Natl Acad Sci USA. 2004;101(23): 8733–8.

81. Wright JR, Borron P, Brinker KG, Folz RJ. Surfactant protein A: regulation of innate and adaptive immune responses in lung inflammation. Am J Respir Cell Mol Biol. 2001;24(5):513–7.

82. D'Ovidio F, Mura M, Ridsdale R, et al. The effect of reflux and bile acid aspiration on the lung allograft and its surfactant and innate immunity molecules SP-A and SP-D. Am J Transplant. 2006;6(8):1930–8.

83. Atkins BZ, Trachtenberg MS, Prince-Petersen R, et al. Assessing oropharyngeal dysphagia after lung transplantation: altered swallowing mechanisms and increased morbidity. J Heart Lung Transplant. 2007;26(11):1144–8.

84. Young LR, Hadjiliadis D, Davis RD, Palmer SM. Lung transplantation exacerbates gastroesophageal reflux disease. Chest. 2003;124(5):1689–93.

85. Davis Jr RD, Lau CL, Eubanks S, et al. Improved lung allograft function after fundoplication in patients with gastroesophageal reflux disease undergoing lung transplantation. J Thorac Cardiovasc Surg. 2003;125(3):533–42.

86. Yates B, Murphy DM, Forrest IA, et al. Azithromycin reverses airflow obstruction in established bronchiolitis obliterans syndrome. Am J Respir Crit Care Med. 2005;172(6):772–5.

87. Chen D, Barber C, McLoughlin P, Thavaneswaran P, Jamieson GG, Maddern GJ. Systematic review of endoscopic treatments for gastro-oesophageal reflux disease. Br J Surg. 2009;96(2):128–36.

88. Balsara KP, Shah CR, Hussain M. Laparoscopic fundoplication for gastro-esophageal reflux disease: an 8 year experience. J Minim Access Surg. 2008;4(4): 99–103.

89. Tobin RW, Pope 2nd CE, Pellegrini CA, Emond MJ, Sillery J, Raghu G. Increased prevalence of gastroesophageal reflux in patients with idiopathic pulmonary fibrosis. Am J Respir Crit Care Med. 1998; 158(6):1804–8.

90. Krein PM, Winston BW. Roles for insulin-like growth factor I and transforming growth factor-beta in fibrotic lung disease. Chest. 2002;122 Suppl 6:289S–93.

91. Johnson DA, Drane WE, Curran J, et al. Pulmonary disease in progressive systemic sclerosis. A complication of gastroesophageal reflux and occult aspiration? Arch Intern Med. 1989;149(3):589–93.

92. Kinuya K, Nakajima K, Kinuya S, Michigishi T, Tonami N, Takehara K. Esophageal hypomotility in systemic sclerosis: close relationship with pulmonary involvement. Ann Nucl Med. 2001;15(2):97–101.

93. Songur N, Songur Y, Cerci SS, et al. Gastroesophageal scintigraphy in the evaluation of adult patients with chronic cough due to gastroesophageal reflux disease. Nucl Med Commun. 2008;29(12):1066–72.

94. Carnaby G, Hankey GJ, Pizzi J. Behavioural intervention for dysphagia in acute stroke: a randomised controlled trial. Lancet Neurol. 2006;5(1):31–7.

95. Teramoto S. Novel preventive and therapuetic strategy for post-stroke pneumonia. Expert Rev Neurother. 2009;9(8):1187–200.

96. White GN, O'Rourke F, Ong BS, Cordato DJ, Chan DK. Dysphagia: causes, assessment, treatment, and management. Geriatrics. 2008;63(5):15–20.

Effect of Aging of the Pharynx and the UES

15

Rebecca J. Leonard and Reza Shaker

Abstract

Oral-pharyngeal dysphagia is increasingly recognized as a health risk in generally healthy, but elderly, adults. The focus of this chapter is to review evidence of aging effects on the pharynx that may contribute to this difficulty. Information reflecting multiple focus areas and investigative techniques is considered. Collectively, the evidence suggests declining efficiency and an increased need for adaptation to offset structural and functional changes in the pharynx associated with aging.

Keywords

Effect of aging of the pharynx • Effect of aging of the UES • The aging pharynx • Implications for swallowing • Temporal characteristics • Displacement characteristics

Structures of the head and neck critical to deglutition can be described simply as a series of chambers and valves [1]. Chambers, including the oral cavity and pharynx, expand and compress. Expansion permits accommodation of bolus material, while peristaltic compression is necessary to direct and clear bolus material through and from each chamber, respectively. Valves are structures that open or close to permit or prevent bolus flow from one chamber to another. For example, the tongue-palate valve contains material in the oral cavity and then permits its entry into the pharynx; the velopharyngeal valve prevents bolus entry into the nose. The laryngeal valves, including the aryepiglottic, true and false vocal folds, prevent bolus material from entering the laryngeal vestibule and tracheal airway. Finally, valving action of the upper esophageal sphincter permits bolus entry into the esophagus, and strives to prevent it from reentry into the pharynx. In normal swallowing, valves and chambers act in a highly integrated manner to ensure safe and efficient food transport from the mouth

R.J. Leonard, AB, MS, PhD
Department of Otolaryngology/HNS, University of California, Davis, Medical Center/Health System, 2521 Stockton Blvd., Ste. 7200, Sacramento, CA 95817, USA

R. Shaker, MD (✉)
Division of Gastroenterology and Hepatology, Digestive Disease Center, Clinical and Translational Science Institute, Medical College of Wisconsin, 9200 W. Wisconsin Ave, Milwaukee, WI 53226, USA
e-mail: rshaker@mcw.edu

R. Shaker et al. (eds.), *Principles of Deglutition: A Multidisciplinary Text for Swallowing and its Disorders*, DOI 10.1007/978-1-4614-3794-9_15, © Springer Science+Business Media New York 2013

to the esophagus. Dysfunction of a chamber may lead to insufficient compression to propel and clear bolus material. Failure of valves may result in inappropriate bolus entry to, or exit from, a chamber.

Effects of aging on pharyngeal chambers and valves, as well as on other swallowing-related mechanisms, are important to understand. Epidemiological studies suggest dysphagia affects 22% of adults over the age of 50 years [2]. Individuals over the age of 65 years comprised 12.9% of the U.S. population in 2009, and are expected to represent 19% of the population by 2030 [3]. If we can differentiate expected changes in swallow function from those that are atypical, our ability to diagnose dysphagia, and target specific therapies for it, is improved. Furthermore, if we understand typical changes in swallowing function with aging that are also aversive, we may be able to prevent or minimize swallowing difficulty in elderly individuals. The intent of this chapter is to review our current understanding of pharyngeal changes associated with aging, and the impact of these on deglutition in the elderly. Defining the "normal" aged pharynx is complicated by many factors, e.g., isolating aging effects from those related to diseases that are prevalent with aging, or treatments for these diseases, or from aging effects on related organs and systems. In other cases, available evidence has been documented for a nonmammalian species, or only for a particular system, e.g., cranial muscles, as opposed to spinal. These confounding issues notwithstanding, a growing literature suggests both structural and functional changes in the pharynx likely to impact deglutition in elderly individuals.

Evidence of Pharyngeal Changes with Aging

Evidence of pharyngeal change with aging comes from many sources and reflects a variety of investigative tools. Leonard recently summarized a number of fluoroscopic measurements from two large groups of normal, nondysphagic subjects, reported over several studies [4]. Sixty-three subjects were under the age of 65 years, and 74 were over 65 years. Median ages were 37 and 72 years, respectively. All subjects underwent fluoroscopic swallow studies from which both timing and displacement measures for several bolus types were extracted [5]. Subjective assessments of other variables were also described. These data are described below. For each finding, as available, pertinent data from related studies will also be presented.

Physical Characteristics

Most objective measures providing insights into size differences between young and elderly subjects were made from lateral view fluoroscopic images while subjects were holding a 1 cc bolus in the oral cavity. The position of structures at this point ("Hold" position) is used as the baseline referent for maximum displacements of structures. Findings are presented in Table 15.1 and Fig. 15.1:

(a) The distance between the mandible and hyoid was uniform across groups. However, the distance between the hyoid and larynx was greater in the elderly ($p=0.000$), a

Table 15.1 Total pharyngeal transit time for normal subjects under and over 65 years of age

	Age (years)	Total pharyngeal transit time (s)	Significance (p)	Standard deviation	Confidence interval (95%)
1 cc	<65	0.908	0.000	0.297	0.775–1.040
	>65	1.374		0.672	1.250–1.497
3 cc	<65	0.866	0.000	0.270	0.731–1.001
	>65	1.308		0.70	1.183–1.434
Paste	<65	0.897	0.000	0.368	0.714–1.081
	>65	1.420		0.945	1.250–1.590
20–30 cc	<65	0.917	0.000	0.288	0.777–1.057
	>65	1.378		0.718	1.248–1.508

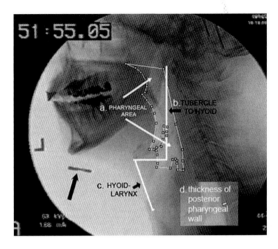

Fig. 15.1 Positions of structures with 1 cc bolus held in oral cavity. (**a**) Pharyngeal area outlined in lateral view; (**b**) distance from tubercle of atlas to hyoid; (**c**) distance from hyoid to larynx; and (**d**) thickness of posterior pharyngeal wall

Implications

Evidence suggests that the pharynx becomes larger, more dilated, with aging, and possibly, more vulnerable to collapse in some situations, i.e., supine position. Tissue changes identified are consistent with sarcopenia. Gravity may play an increasingly important role in clearing the pharyngeal chambers, and strategies that optimize flow direction (away from airway and towards esophagus) and speed may be practical and useful in some individuals.

Displacement Characteristics

Displacement differences between the two groups (Table 15.2; Fig. 15.2) were also noted during swallowing [11]. Findings presented here are for the largest bolus swallowed, i.e., 20–30 cc liquid, and corrected for gender:

nonsignificant trend previously reported by Logemann et al. for elderly males [6]. The distance between the tubercle of the atlas and the hyoid was also significantly greater in elderly controls ($p=0.000$), as was a measure of the two-dimensional pharyngeal area in the hold position ($p=0.000$).

Increased distance between the posterior nasal spine and superior epiglottis in elderly subjects, as compared to younger, has also been reported by Shigeta et al. [7]. Interestingly, acoustic studies used to investigate sleep apnea in older adults have identified reduced cross-sectional areas at selected points in the pharyngeal airway in supine position (not upright), suggesting increased potential for pharyngeal collapse in this population [8].

(b) Thickness of the posterior pharyngeal wall, measured at the midpoint of cervical vertebra 3, was significantly reduced in the elderly group ($p<0.01$).

Evidence of sarcopenia-like changes, i.e., reduced muscle mass and fiber diameter, loss of specific fiber types, have been previously demonstrated for the pharynx, as well as for the tongue and larynx [9, 10]. Leese and Hopwood described both atrophy and hypertrophy leading to increased variability of fiber size in pharynges of aged human cadavers [9].

(a) Hyoid displacement did not significantly differ, but hyoid to larynx approximation was significantly greater in the elderly ($p=0.037$), possibly representing an adaptation to the greater distance between hyoid and larynx in the "Hold" position. Gender differences were noted for hyoid displacements (young) and hyoid to larynx approximation (young and elderly).

(b) Thirty-two percent of elderly control subjects demonstrated a cricopharyngeal bar that could be described as mild, moderate, or marked [12]. No nontransient bars were identified in younger control subjects. Evidence for bars in this group of elderly subjects is consistent with findings on cadaver studies of elderly subjects [13].

(c) UES opening did not significantly differ between younger subjects and elderly subjects without bars, but was significantly reduced in the group of elderly subjects with bars. Gender differences were not identified for UES opening; however, bars were identified more frequently in males than in females. These fluoroscopic observations of reduced UES opening size and increased prevalence of cricopharyngeal bars in the elderly would appear to be consistent with previous manometric reports of increased obstruction to flow at the UES in elderly subjects.

Table 15.2 Distances, pharyngeal area, and thickness of posterior pharyngeal wall at cervical vertebra 3 with 1 cc bolus held in oral cavity

	Age	Mean (cm)	Significance (p)	Standard deviation	Confidence interval (95%)	N
Hyoid–larynx (cm)	<65	3.3486	0.024	0.70043	3.159–3.538	59
	>65	3.6425		0.75584	3.472–3.813	73
Tubercle–hyoid (cm)	<65	5.0102	0.000	0.77933	4.775–5.256	62
	>65	5.7205		1.03896	5.500–5.933	73
Pharyngeal area (hold) (cm²)	<65	7.2463	0.000	2.02260	6.541–7.903	61
	>65	9.5392		3.07255	8.947–10.171	73
Posterior pharyngeal wall (cm)	<65	0.3479	0.000	0.08024	0.297–353	59
	>65	0.2953		0.08086	0.282–335	73

Data for normal subjects under and over 65 years of age

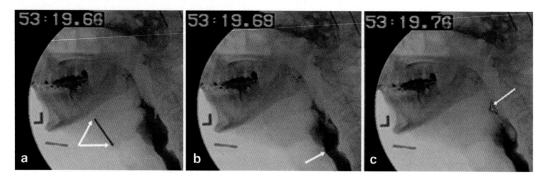

Fig. 15.2 Structures maximally displaced during swallow. (**a**) Hyoid and larynx; (**b**) UES opening; (**c**) pharynx maximally constricted (residual air and bolus are outlined)

For example, Bardan et al. described a significant increase in trans-UES sphincter pressure gradient with aging [14]. In earlier work, these investigators noted increased intrabolus pressure and elevated pharyngeal outflow resistance in elderly nondysphagic subjects. Impaired opening of the UES and reduced UES resting tone have been reported by numerous groups, including McKee et al., Shaw et al., Shaker et al., and Shaker et al. [15–19]. The latter authors suggested that an increase in both amplitude and duration of the hypopharyngeal pressure wave identified in their elderly subjects may represent a necessary adaptation to the associated increase in pharyngeal outflow resistance. Similar findings of elevated pharyngeal contraction pressures with aging have been reported by Wilson et al. [20]. Increased pharyngeal peri-staltic waves and increased peak pressure durations were reported by Yokoyama et al. [21]. In some contrast to these findings, Tracy et al. described decreases in pharyngeal peristaltic amplitude, velocity and pressure, as well as a decrease in the duration of cricopharyngeal opening, in their elderly subjects [22]. Interestingly, in the Tracy et al. study, UES opening duration was decreased even though pharyngeal swallow duration was increased [22].

(d) Thickness of the posterior pharyngeal wall at its point of maximum constriction during the large liquid bolus swallow, measured again at C3, was significantly reduced in the elderly ($p=0.001$).

(e) A measure of pharyngeal constriction, referred to as the pharyngeal constriction ratio (PCR), is determined by dividing the two-dimensional area of the pharynx at the point of maximum constriction by the area with the 1 cc bolus held in the oral cavity (Figs. 15.1 and 15.2). The ratio was significantly elevated in the elderly, indicating reduced ability to constrict the pharynx during swallow [23]. In the anterior–posterior view, a measure of pharyngeal width at the point of maximum pharyngeal expansion was also elevated in the elderly, again suggesting increased dilation of the pharynx with aging [23].

Implications

Evidence suggests that some structural displacements associated with swallowing are diminished with aging. Hyoid displacement may be unchanged, but hyoid to larynx approximation is increased, possibly reflecting an adaptation to the increased resting distance between hyoid and larynx. Pharyngeal constriction is reduced. The combination of enlarged, dilated pharyngeal chambers and reduced potential to compress, shorten, and clear them likely contributes to increased effort needed for swallowing. Obstruction at the UES valve, related to the presence of a cricopharyngeal bar, further hinders bolus passage and may affect 30% or more of the elderly population.

Temporal Characteristics

Timing of bolus transit, and of the coordination between bolus transit and swallow gesture times, was also investigated in the young and elderly subjects described [11]. Results are summarized

below and, again, are presented with results from related studies:

1. Total pharyngeal transit time was significantly prolonged in the elderly subjects, as compared to younger subjects, for a 1 cc, 3 cc, 20 cc, and paste bolus (Tables 15.1 and 15.3; Fig. 15.3). No gender differences were identified for any timing measure. Prolonged pharyngeal transit times in elderly individuals have been reported by several investigators [18, 21, 22, 24–29]. Bardan et al. further described differences in hypopharyngeal bolus acceleration between young and older subjects [14]. In particular, acceleration through the hypopharynx typical of younger individuals was not identified in elderly subjects.

2. A comparison of non-dysphagic elderly individuals with no chronic medical condition to nondysphagic elderly individuals with either hypertension or osteoarthritis, respectively, revealed that both chronic condition groups tended to have longer oropharyngeal and hypopharyngeal transit times than controls, but differences were significant only for a 1 cc bolus, and only for oropharyngeal transit (bolus transit from posterior nasal spine to valleculae). No significant differences were identified for a 20 cc bolus [12].

3. Bolus transit times provide, primarily, insights into flow or transport efficiency. Timing measures that consider both *bolus transit* and *swallowing gesture* times, however, are of further value because they reflect coordination between bolus material and the structural movements responsible for transporting it. For example, we would expect protective

Table 15.3 Displacements and pharyngeal constriction ratio (PCR) for 20–30 cc bolus

	Age	Significance (*p*)	Mean (cm)	Standard deviation	*N*
Max. hyoid displacement (cm)	<65		2.15758	0.852677	62
	>65	ns	2.05662	0.643690	71
Max hyoid–larynx approximation (cm)	<65		1.14177	0.497045	62
	>65	*p* = 0.04	1.37141	0.656221	71
Max. PES opening (cm) (exclude ss with CP bars)	<65		0.88661	0.273573	62
	>65	ns	0.83676	0.241961	48
Pharyngeal constriction ratio (PCR)	<65		0.03252	0.028289	62
	>65	*p* = 0.000	0.11244	0.113100	71

Data presented for normal subjects under and over 65 years of age. Data are combined across gender

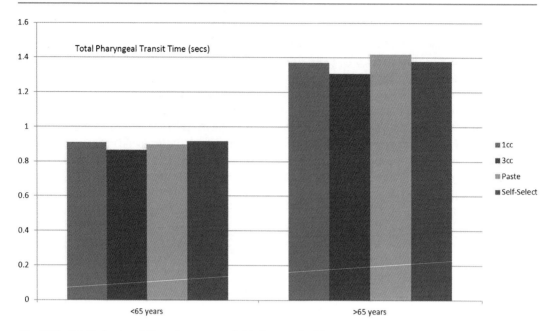

Fig. 15.3 Total bolus transit times for young and elderly normal subjects

mechanisms of the airway to close prior to the bolus head entering the esophagus. If not, the airway is vulnerable to penetration or aspiration. In most normal subjects investigated here [23], young and elderly, this observation was true, that is, the laryngeal vestibule closed prior to bolus entering the UES. But in some normal subjects in both groups, the airway remained open *after* the bolus entered the UES. The delay was never more than 0.1 s in any subject, for any bolus. Elderly subjects closed the airway significantly earlier prior to UES opening than younger subjects for the largest bolus ($p < 0.001$). No significant difference was noted for a 1 cc bolus.

Interestingly, Ren et al. [30], using simultaneous endoscopy, manometry, respirography and submental surface electromyography, found that the onset of vocal fold closure always preceded the onset of UES relaxation, in both young and elderly healthy subjects. How these data relate to the previous fluoroscopic evidence of airway closing sometimes occurring after UES opening, in both young and older subjects, is not completely clear, but may reflect different investigative techniques. That is, in the Kendall et al.

fluoroscopic study, airway closure was indicated by approximation of the arytenoids and epiglottis closing the laryngeal vestibule, not by vocal fold adduction, which was observed by Ren et al. [30]. Further, in the Kendall et al. study, UES opening in the lateral view was observed; in Ren et al., UES relaxation, not opening, was monitored [30].

Zamir et al. [31] described subtle age differences in the coordination of glottic closure and the onset of bolus movement from the mouth into the pharynx. In young subjects, bolus movement always occurred after maximal vocal fold adduction was observed; in the elderly, bolus movement sometimes followed, and sometimes preceded, maximal vocal fold adduction [31]. The authors further concluded that, subtle differences notwithstanding, the coordination between oropharyngeal bolus transit and airway protection appears preserved with aging.

4. Other differences between groups were found for the latency between onset of hyoid displacement leading to a swallow and various points of bolus transit [32]. Bolus movement past the posterior nasal spine typically preceded hyoid onset in both younger and older subjects, but

the interval was significantly longer in elderly controls ($p<0.002$). Latency between hyoid onset and bolus transit past the mandibular ramus did not differ between groups, but latency between hyoid onset and bolus entrance to the UES was again significantly prolonged in the elderly ($p<0.001$). This timing evidence is consistent with the previous findings of structural similarities and differences between the young and elderly normal subjects with a 1 cc bolus held in the oral cavity, i.e., "Hold." That is, there was no difference between groups in the distance between hyoid and mandible, but significant differences for distances between the tubercle of atlas and hyoid, and between the hyoid and larynx.

Mendell and Logemann [33] investigated temporal relationships between various bolus arrival points and structural movements, each referenced to UES opening, in young and elderly normal subjects. The authors found that temporal relationships were generally longer in the elderly group, and, in both groups, affected by size and consistency of the bolus.

Implications

Evidence from numerous studies, based on both fluoroscopic and manometric data, demonstrates that bolus transport is prolonged with aging. How these findings relate to associated findings of alterations in pharyngeal size and compression capabilities, bolus acceleration and velocity, as well as sensory integrity of tissues, is not completely clear. Prolonged times render the airway more at risk, but may also reflect increased effort and, in some individuals, may offer an advantage to bolus control. Timing differences for small bolus sizes may be particularly sensitive to the effects of intercurrent disease, or to declining sensory function. It also appears to be the case that some latencies between individual swallow events may be more sensitive to age-related timing differences than others.

Subjective Observations

1. A review of all swallows (596) in 136 individuals for evidence of aspiration and penetration revealed only one instance of aspiration (0.6%) and 17 instances of penetration (2.9%). Differences according to age were not significant, but significantly more penetration occurred on larger boluses, and on liquid, as compared to paste [34]. These data are similar to findings reported by Robbins et al., also based on fluoroscopy [29]. Butler et al., based on endoscopic evaluations of 20 normal individuals, mean age 79 years, identified aspiration on 3% of a total of 560 swallows, and penetration on 15% of swallows [35]. Seventy-five percent of the subjects demonstrated penetration, and 30% demonstrated aspiration, across all swallows, but in particular, on thin liquid boluses.

   Differences in findings across these and other studies [36] may in part be related to the method of investigation, i.e., endoscopy vs. fluoroscopy. For example, on endoscopy (and perhaps on fluoro by some judges), bolus material on any portion of the laryngeal surface of the epiglottis is often considered penetration; on our fluoroscopic studies, it is bolus advance beyond the contact point (or presumed point) of arytenoid and epiglottis that is defined as penetration. Viscosity and bolus size also appear to influence results. In any event, our own data suggest that aspiration on fluoroscopy is very rare in normal individuals, and that penetration occurs, but in fewer than 10% of our normal, aged subjects.

2. Epiglottic inversion was judged as complete, incomplete or absent on all swallows. If inversion is absent or incomplete, both airway protection and pharyngeal clearing can be affected. Interestingly, our young and elderly normal subjects did not appear to differ significantly on this variable. Incomplete inversion was identified on 5% of all swallows in the elderly; 3% in the younger subjects. Absent inversion was not noted on any swallow in the young group, and on 3 of 344 swallows (0.008%) in the elderly, and always on a 1 cc or 3 cc bolus [4].

3. Our normal elderly subjects did not describe eating or swallowing difficulties. When carefully questioned, however, several acknowledged greater care taken with swallowing, i.e., thorough chewing, smaller pieces of solids,

repeat swallows, liquid flushes, avoidance of some foods. This is consistent with fluoroscopic observations, i.e., poorer pharyngeal clearing, greater likelihood of obstruction at the UES. These adaptations appear to have occurred so gradually, and were sufficiently effective, that they were not perceived as a problem in this group of subjects. Obviously, such strategies may also be helpful to patients seen clinically.

In an investigation of normal aging subjects living in a retirement village, Wilkinson and de Picciotto [37] reported subjective swallowing difficulty significant enough to interfere with daily function in 44% of 25 subjects interviewed. Most of the interviewees appeared to experience difficulty related to both pharyngeal and esophageal stages of deglutition. More recently, Chen et al. [38] described perceived dysphagia in 107 individuals residing in an independent living facility. According to the authors, 15% of the population reported difficulty with swallowing. Interestingly, 25% of this group described difficulty with swallowing (and voice) as a natural part of aging.

Implications

Though reports vary regarding the number of healthy, elderly individuals who experience alterations in swallow function, evidence suggests that perceived swallow difficulty is associated with aging, and that possibly many elderly individuals make ongoing adaptations to accommodate these "typical" changes.

Evidence of Neural Changes Affecting the Pharynx with Aging

Few studies have considered sensorimotor changes with aging that are specific to the pharynx. Teismann et al. [39] recently reported increased somatosensory cortical activation during swallow in elderly individuals and suggested it may represent a cerebral adaptation to aging. Similar evidence indicates a loss of laterality in cortical function, and increased bilateral activation, in both motor and verbal task performance with aging [40]. The implication is that bilateral

activation reflects recruitment of alternate brain regions to counteract declining cognitive function. Similar evidence was reported by Humbert et al. [26] using combined fMRI and fluoroscopic examinations of swallowing in young and older adults. Of particular note, swallows of older individuals demonstrated greater cortical activity, involving more cortical regions, than younger individuals. Evidence of increased activity was noted in pericentral gyri and inferior frontal gyrus pars opercularis and pars triangularis, and was most apparent on saliva swallows, as opposed to water and barium swallows. An associated increase in swallow times, filmed fluoroscopically with subjects in a supine position, was also identified.

Other evidence indicates increased pharyngeal stimulation required to elicit vocal fold adduction and swallow during rapid pulse injection of water into the pharynx [41]. The authors note this may have particular implications for the management of small bolus sizes with aging. Similar evidence of reduced sensitivity in the elderly has been reported by Aviv et al. [42] and Aviv [43]. These investigators applied air pulses of varying intensities to subjects' pyriform sinuses in an attempt to determine the threshold stimulation required to elicit vocal fold adduction. Sensitivity progressively deteriorated with age. Reduced UES response to both pharyngeal and laryngeal stimulation has also been noted [44, 45]. Ren et al. reported that the volume of water required to elicit the pharyngo-UES contractile reflex, or contraction of the UES, was increased in the elderly [45]. In addition, in the presence of continuous water infusion of the pharynx, elderly subjects, in contrast to young, did not demonstrate an increase in UES resting pressure. Theurere et al. recently reported an increase in the rate of saliva swallows in response to bilateral oropharyngeal air pulses in both young and elderly subjects [46]. However, younger subjects reported a strong urge to swallow in the presence of stimulation, an experience not reported by the older individuals. Smith et al. reported differences in oral and oropharyngeal perceptions of fluid viscosity in younger and older normal subjects [47]. In particular, elderly subjects demonstrated poorer sensitivity than younger subjects, with older men demonstrating greater deterioration than women.

Evidence of age-related alterations in sensitivity in tissues of the pharynx and larynx suggests possible alterations in the superior laryngeal nerve with aging. Tiago et al. recently investigated age-related changes in human superior and recurrent laryngeal nerves [48]. Cadaver tissues from individuals under and over 65 years of age were studied. The authors reported no differences in the number of myelinated fibers between groups for the superior laryngeal nerve. The younger group, however, demonstrated a larger number of myelinated fibers in the recurrent laryngeal nerve, and a greater number of total myelinated fibers, as compared to older individuals. Significant age-related loss of myelinated nerve fibers in the superior laryngeal nerve with aging has been reported by Mortelliti et al. [49]. These investigators compared specimens from individuals 20–30 years of age, and 60 years or older, and found 31% fewer myelinated fibers in the older individuals. In particular, small myelinated fibers (1–2 μm) were affected. Axonal diameter of myelinated fibers was also decreased in the older group. Differences between the Tiago et al. and Mortelliti et al. studies may reflect differences in the particular age groups investigated. In general, there appears to be agreement that aging in the laryngeal nerves affects both number and size of myelinated fibers.

Implications

Evidence for changes in sensory and motor functions with aging have been identified in the pharynx, and are well-documented for many specific mechanisms, i.e., taste and smell. Sensory changes are likely to affect, in particular, timing characteristics of swallowing, and may be mediated by specific bolus characteristics. Other changes are likely to impact critical features of chamber and valve functions, e.g., completeness of compression, and possibly, both the speed and completeness of valve opening and closing.

The Aging Pharynx and Deglutition: Implications for Clinical Practice

It is clear that pharyngeal changes associated with aging can impact swallowing. Increased pharyngeal dilation and reduced pharyngeal constriction and shortening, as well as the increased incidence of cricopharyngeal bar, support a hypothesis of added work required for effective swallow. Prolonged pharyngeal transit times associated with aging pose additional risk for airway safety, but may also offer an advantage to bolus control in some individuals. Measures of pharyngeal wall thickness, added to available histological investigations, suggest sarcopenia-like changes, findings not inconsistent with evidence of increased dilation and diminished contractility in the aged pharynx. Declining sensory capability in the pharynx is consistent with system-wide evidence of alterations in aged sensory end-organs and cortical function. Evidence for aging and swallowing is incomplete; however, the picture currently available is one of declining integrity in swallowing efficiency and an increasing need for adaptation in order to maintain swallow effectiveness.

Implications of the available evidence for clinical practice are several. Fluoroscopic examinations in the elderly should, e.g., focus on obstructive processes, i.e., cricopharyngeal bars, osteophytes, as well as on the integrity of airway protection and pharyngeal clearing mechanisms. The possible impact of intercurrent diseases and their treatments needs to be considered in many elderly patients. It is also important to recognize that even "typical" changes associated with pharyngeal aging may represent dysphagia risks in some individuals. Clinicians need to understand these changes in order to differentiate them from other etiologies for dysphagia, and to develop tools to prevent or minimize swallowing difficulty related *primarily* to aging. This suggests that enhancing sensory properties of foods, and maximizing nutrition per quantity, should receive increasing attention from food science investigators. Emphasis on eating as a social activity, as well as preventive measures related to dentition and oral hygiene, should be standard inclusions in counseling the elderly. Insufficient evidence is available regarding the role of exercise in maintaining swallow health, but promising findings in nondysphagic elderly subjects have been reported for improving lingual pressures [50–53], UES opening, and respiratory strength [54]. Precautionary measures such as early airway closure and repeat swallows are relatively easy to implement in many individuals. As our knowledge of aging and "normal" anatomy and physiology advances, our ability to recognize and understand both swallowing potential and dysphagia risk in this population will also improve. For the dysphagia clinician working with elderly patients, the need for such information, and the ability to implement it thoughtfully and appropriately in clinical practice, is critical.

References

1. Anatomy: Head and Neck, In: The New Werner Twentieth Century Edition of the Encyclopedia Britannica. 1907.
2. Howden CW. Management of acid-related disorders in patients with dysphagia. Am J Med. 2004;117(Suppl 5A):44S–8.
3. Administration on Aging, U.S.D.o.H.a.H.R., A Profile of Older Americans: 2010.
4. Leonard R. Swallowing in the elderly: evidence from fluoroscopy. Perspect Swallowing Disorders. 2010;19(3):103–14.
5. Leonard R, McKenzie S. Dynamic swallow studies: measurement techniques. In: Leonard R, Kendall K, editors. Dysphagia assessment and treatment planning: a team approach. San Diego: Plural Publishing Co; 2008. p. 265–94.
6. Logemann JA, et al. Temporal and biomechanical characteristics of oropharyngeal swallow in younger and older men. J Speech Lang Hear Res. 2000;43(5): 1264–74.
7. Shigeta Y, et al. Gender- and age-based differences in computerized tomographic measurements of the orophaynx. Oral Surg Oral Med Oral Pathol Oral Radiol Endod. 2008;106(4):563–70.
8. Eikermann M, et al. The influence of aging on pharyngeal collapsibility during sleep. Chest. 2007;131(6): 1702–9.
9. Leese G, Hopwood D. Muscle fibre typing in the human pharyngeal constrictors and oesophagus: the effect of ageing. Acta Anat (Basel). 1986;127(1):77–80.
10. Rodeno MT, Sanchez-Fernandez JM, Rivera-Pomar JM. Histochemical and morphometrical ageing changes in human vocal cord muscles. Acta Otolaryngol. 1993;113(3):445–9.
11. Leonard RJ, et al. Structural displacements in normal swallowing: a videofluoroscopic study. Dysphagia. 2000;15(3):146–52.
12. Leonard R, Kendall K, McKenzie S. UES opening and cricopharyngeal bar in nondysphagic elderly and nonelderly adults. Dysphagia. 2004;19(3): 182–91.
13. Xu S, et al. Is the anatomical protrusion on the posterior hypopharyngeal wall associated with cadavers of only the elderly? Dysphagia. 2006;21(3): 163–6.
14. Bardan E, et al. Effect of aging on bolus kinematics during the pharyngeal phase of swallowing. Am J Physiol Gastrointest Liver Physiol. 2006;290(3): G458–65.
15. Fulp SR, et al. Aging-related alterations in human upper esophageal sphincter function. Am J Gastroenterol. 1990;85(12):1569–72.
16. McKee GJ, et al. Does age or sex affect pharyngeal swallowing? Clin Otolaryngol Allied Sci. 1998;23(2):100–6.
17. Shaker R, Lang IM. Effect of aging on the deglutitive oral, pharyngeal, and esophageal motor function. Dysphagia. 1994;9(4):221–8.
18. Shaw DW, et al. Influence of normal aging on oral-pharyngeal and upper esophageal sphincter function during swallowing. Am J Physiol. 1995;268(3 Pt 1):G389–96.
19. Shaker R, et al. Effect of aging and bolus variables on pharyngeal and upper esophageal sphincter motor function. Am J Physiol. 1993;264(3 Pt 1):G427–32.
20. Wilson JA, et al. The effects of age, sex, and smoking on normal pharyngoesophageal motility. Am J Gastroenterol. 1990;85(6):686–91.
21. Yokoyama M, et al. Role of laryngeal movement and effect of aging on swallowing pressure in the pharynx and upper esophageal sphincter. Laryngoscope. 2000;110(3 Pt 1):434–9.
22. Tracy JF, et al. Preliminary observations on the effects of age on oropharyngeal deglutition. Dysphagia. 1989;4(2):90–4.
23. Leonard R, Kendall KA, McKenzie S. Structural displacements affecting pharyngeal constriction in nondysphagic elderly and nonelderly adults. Dysphagia. 2004;19(2):133–41.
24. Cook IJ, et al. Influence of aging on oral-pharyngeal bolus transit and clearance during swallowing: scintigraphic study. Am J Physiol. 1994;266(6 Pt 1): G972–7.
25. Dejaeger E, et al. Manofluorographic analysis of swallowing in the elderly. Dysphagia. 1994;9(3): 156–61.
26. Humbert IA, et al. Neurophysiology of swallowing: effects of age and bolus type. Neuroimage. 2009; 44(3):982–91.

27. Steele CM, van Lieshout PH. Does barium influence tongue behaviors during swallowing? Am J Speech Lang Pathol. 2005;14(1):27–39.
28. Yoshikawa M, et al. Aspects of swallowing in healthy dentate elderly persons older than 80 years. J Gerontol A Biol Sci Med Sci. 2005;60(4):506–9.
29. Robbins J, et al. Oropharyngeal swallowing in normal adults of different ages. Gastroenterology. 1992; 103(3):823–9.
30. Ren J, et al. Effect of age and bolus variables on the coordination of the glottis and upper esophageal sphincter during swallowing. Am J Gastroenterol. 1993;88(5):665–9.
31. Zamir Z, et al. Coordination of deglutitive vocal cord closure and oral-pharyngeal swallowing events in the elderly. Eur J Gastroenterol Hepatol. 1996;8(5): 425–9.
32. Leonard R, McKenzie S. Hyoid-bolus transit latencies in normal swallow. Dysphagia. 2006;21(3):183–90.
33. Mendell DA, Logemann JA. Temporal sequence of swallow events during the oropharyngeal swallow. J Speech Lang Hear Res. 2007;50(5):1256–71.
34. Allen JE, et al. Prevalence of penetration and aspiration on videofluoroscopy in normal individuals without dysphagia. Otolaryngol Head Neck Surg. 2010; 142(2):208–13.
35. Butler SG, et al. Penetration and aspiration in healthy older adults as assessed during endoscopic evaluation of swallowing. Ann Otol Rhinol Laryngol. 2009; 118(3):190–8.
36. Daggett A, et al. Laryngeal penetration during deglutition in normal subjects of various ages. Dysphagia. 2006;21(4):270–4.
37. Wilkinson T, de Picciotto J. Swallowing problems in the normal ageing population. S Afr J Commun Disord. 1999;46:55–64.
38. Chen PH, et al. Prevalence of perceived dysphagia and quality-of-life impairment in a geriatric population. Dysphagia. 2009;24(1):1–6.
39. Teismann IK, et al. Age-related changes in cortical swallowing processing. Neurobiol Aging. 2010; 31(6):1044–50.
40. Drag LL, Bieliauskas LA. Contemporary review 2009: cognitive aging. J Geriatr Psychiatry Neurol. 2010;23(2):75–93.
41. Shaker R, et al. Pharyngoglottal closure reflex: characterization in healthy young, elderly and dysphagic patients with predeglutitive aspiration. Gerontology. 2003;49(1):12–20.
42. Aviv JE, et al. Age-related changes in pharyngeal and supraglottic sensation. Ann Otol Rhinol Laryngol. 1994;103(10):749–52.
43. Aviv JE. Effects of aging on sensitivity of the pharyngeal and supraglottic areas. Am J Med. 1997;103(Suppl 5A):74S–6.
44. Kawamura O, et al. Laryngo-upper esophageal sphincter contractile reflex in humans deteriorates with age. Gastroenterology. 2004;127(1):57–64.
45. Ren J, et al. Deterioration of the pharyngo-UES contractile reflex in the elderly. Laryngoscope. 2000; 110(9):1563–6.
46. Theurer JA, et al. Effects of oropharyngeal air-pulse stimulation on swallowing in healthy older adults. Dysphagia. 2009;24(3):302–13.
47. Smith CH, et al. Oral and oropharyngeal perceptions of fluid viscosity across the age span. Dysphagia. 2006;21(4):209–17.
48. Tiago R, Pontes P, do Brasil OC. Age-related changes in human laryngeal nerves. Otolaryngol Head Neck Surg. 2007;136(5):747–51.
49. Mortelliti AJ, Malmgren LT, Gacek RR. Ultrastructural changes with age in the human superior laryngeal nerve. Arch Otolaryngol Head Neck Surg. 1990; 116(9):1062–9.
50. Robbins J, et al. The effects of lingual exercise in stroke patients with dysphagia. Arch Phys Med Rehabil. 2007;88(2):150–8.
51. Robbins J, et al. Oral, pharyngeal and esophageal motor function in aging, in GI Motility Online. 2006.
52. Ibayashi H, et al. Intervention study of exercise program for oral function in healthy elderly people. Tohoku J Exp Med. 2008;215(3):237–45.
53. Lazarus C. Tongue strength and exercise in healthy individuals and in head and neck cancer patients. Semin Speech Lang. 2006;27(4):260–7.
54. Shaker R, et al. Augmentation of deglutitive upper esophageal sphincter opening in the elderly by exercise. Am J Physiol. 1997;272(6 Pt 1): G1518–22.

Nascent Pharynx, Physiology, Reflexes

16

Sudarshan R. Jadcherla

Abstract

The pharynx must maintain and coordinate the safety of airway and digestive functions regardless of maturational state or aging, activity or sleep state, postural variability, health, or illness. Life-threatening events are frequent in early stages of life, varying from apnea to laryngospasm to airway aspiration and may be the result of malfunction of pharyngeal–airway communications. Similarly, feeding and swallowing problems are also frequent in neonatal period, and dysphagia may result from malfunction of pharyngeal–esophageal communications. Hence, understanding the developmental physiology of deglutition and pharyngeal phase of swallowing is vital to the study of dysphagia in young infants. Unfortunately, not much is known about nascent human pharynx either during fetal life or in those born prematurely. Much of the knowledge is gleaned from animal studies or adult human studies. In this chapter, we attempt to elucidate what is known and relevant to the nascent pharyngeal anatomy and functions.

Keywords

Nascent pharynx • Physiology • Reflexes • Pharyngeal phase of deglutition • Pharyngeal–glottal reflexes • Aerodigestive safety •

Introduction

The pharynx must maintain and coordinate the safety of airway and digestive functions regardless of maturational state or aging, activity or sleep state, postural variability, health, or illness. Life-threatening events are frequent in early stages of life, varying from apnea to laryngospasm to airway aspiration and may be the result of malfunction of pharyngeal–airway communications. Similarly, feeding and swallowing problems are also frequent in neonatal period, and

S.R. Jadcherla, MD, FRCP (Irel), DCH, AGAF (✉)
Sections of Neonatology, Pediatric Gastroenterology and Nutrition, The Neonatal and Infant Feeding Disorders Program, Neonatal Nutrition Program, Neonatal Occupational and Physical Therapy Program, Nationwide Children's Hospital, 700 Childrens Drive, Columbus, OH 43205, USA
e-mail: Sudarshan.Jadcherla@nationwidechildrens.org

R. Shaker et al. (eds.), *Principles of Deglutition: A Multidisciplinary Text for Swallowing and its Disorders*, DOI 10.1007/978-1-4614-3794-9_16, © Springer Science+Business Media New York 2013

dysphagia may result from malfunction of pharyngeal–esophageal communications. Hence, understanding the developmental physiology of deglutition and pharyngeal phase of swallowing is vital to the study of dysphagia in young infants. Unfortunately, not much is known about nascent human pharynx either during fetal life or in those born prematurely. Much of the knowledge is gleaned from animal studies or adult human studies. In this chapter, we attempt to elucidate what is known and relevant to the nascent pharyngeal anatomy and functions.

The pharynx as an organ communicates with exterior via oral cavity and nasal cavity, with middle ear via eustachian tubes, with the rest of the foregut via the upper esophageal sphincter (UES) and esophagus, and with the airway via the hypopharynx and larynx. Thus the pharynx is a junction to five tubular pathways, the control and regulation of each of these subsystems maintains aerodigestive homeostasis and vital functions. In the developmentally immature infant, these functions are evolving along with somatic growth and neuronal maturation. The neonate has a nasopharynx and hypo-pharynx only at birth; subsequently the oro-pharynx develops during infancy as the growth triples that of birth weight concurrent with changes in somatic growth.

The functions of the pharynx can be several; however, in this chapter, we specifically illuminate the deglutition aspects of the pharyngeal phase of normal deglutition during maturation. Specifically, we elucidate development of the nascent pharynx and esophagus, neuro-anatomical relationships, pharyngeal reflexes that facilitate deglutition, and the pharyngeal and airway defense reflexes that facilitate safe swallowing.

Developmental Aspects of Aerodigestive Relationships

An intricate relationship between the foregut and the airway begins in embryonic life. The airway and the lung buds, the pharynx, the esophagus, the stomach, and the diaphragm are all derived from the primitive foregut and or its mesenchyme, and share similar control systems [1–4]. By 4 weeks of embryological life, tracheo-bronchial diverticulum appears at the ventral wall of the foregut, with left vagus being anterior and right vagus posterior in position. At this stage of development, the stomach is a fusiform tube with the dorsal side growth rate greater than the ventral side, creating greater and lesser curvatures. At 7 weeks of embryonic life, the stomach also rotates 90° clockwise, and the greater curvature is now displaced to the left. The left vagus innervates the stomach anteriorly and the right vagus innervates the posterior aspect of the stomach. At 10 weeks, the esophagus and the stomach are in the proper position, with the circular and longitudinal muscle layers and the ganglion cells are in place. As seen in fetal ultrasound studies, by 11 weeks, pharyngeal phase of swallowing activity is seen; by 18–20 weeks sucking movements appear. By full-term gestation the fetus can swallow and circulate nearly 500 ml of amniotic fluid. Thus, swallow-induced peristaltic activity begins in fetal life as evidenced by ultrasound studies [5, 6].

Between 6 and 7 weeks of gestation, supraglottal structures evolve to protect the vocal cords and lower airway. These structures consist of the epiglottis, ary-epiglottic folds, false vocal cords, and the laryngeal ventricles. The epiglottis begins as a hypobranchial eminence behind the future tongue, and by 7 weeks it is completely separated from the tongue. At the same time, two lateral folds connect to the base of the epiglottis, at the distal end of which develops the arytenoids cartilages. The larynx begins as a groove in the primitive foregut, which folds upon itself to become the laryngo-tracheal bud; from this phase, 20 generations of conducting airways form. The first 8 generations constitute bronchi and acquire cartilaginous walls. The next 9–20 generations comprise the non-respiratory bronchioles that are not cartilaginous and contain smooth muscle, and the subsequent divisions form the bronchopulmonary segments [7].

Innervation of Pharynx

The foregut originates as a tubular organ comprised of inner circular and outer longitudinal muscle layers with the myenteric plexus located between the muscle layers. The proximal part of the foregut is exclusively comprised of fast-acting striated muscle; this segment includes the pharynx, UES, and the proximal third of the esophagus. The UES underlies between the pharynx and the proximal esophagus and is characterized by a high-pressure zone generated by the cricopharyngeus (the principal muscle), proximal cervical esophagus, and inferior pharyngeal constrictor. The UES is innervated by (1) the vagus via the pharyngo-esophageal, superior laryngeal, and recurrent laryngeal branches; (2) the glossopharyngeal nerve; and (3) the sympathetics via the cranial cervical ganglion. The lower esophageal sphincter (LES) comprises the distal end of the esophagus, which consists of the specialized smooth muscle with its unique innervation from both excitatory and inhibitory components of vagal neurons [8]. The LES is an autonomous contractile apparatus that is tonically active to prevent gastro-esophageal reflux and relaxes periodically to facilitate bolus transit clearance.

The airways and the foregut share common innervations [9–11]. The afferent neurons from the foregut are derived from both vagal and dorsal root ganglions with cell bodies in the nodose ganglion. This afferent apparatus conveys signals to the neurons in the nucleus tractus solitarius, located in the dorsomedial medulla oblongata. These signals are integrated in a specific terminal site of the nucleus tractus solitarius, the subnucleus centralis, which is the sole point of termination of esophageal afferents. After sensory integration in the nucleus tractus solitarius, the signals in turn activate airway motor neurons in the nucleus ambiguous and the dorsal motor nucleus of the vagus, producing cholinergic somatic responses involved with striated muscles of larynx and UES.

In summary, the innervations of the aerodigestive tract are as follows: (a) the supraglottal mucosal areas from IX and X cranial nerves and muscular areas from X cranial nerve; (b) the infra-glottal mucosal and muscular areas from X cranial nerve; and (c) the pharynx and esophagus from IX and X cranial nerves.

Pharyngeal Reflexes Facilitating Deglutition

Deglutition is defined as the act of swallowing. Swallowing has three phases: oral phase, pharyngeal–upper esophageal sphincter phase, and esophageal phase. In this chapter, the reflexes involved with pharyngeal phase of swallowing in relation to UES are discussed. Pharyngeal swallowing reflexes can occur spontaneously as dry swallows and is considered as primary peristalsis. In contrast, this sequence can be induced upon pharyngeal provocation and is considered as pharyngeal reflexive swallow. Both types of swallows are associated with pharyngeal contraction, UES relaxation, and anterograde propagation (Fig. 16.1a, b). Unique to neonates and infants is the fact that pharyngeal phase of swallowing usually precedes mouthing and jaw movements or sucking bursts during feeding. Pharyngeal phase of swallowing is associated with deglutition apnea.

We evaluated consecutive spontaneous solitary swallows during longitudinal maturation in preterm infants by studying preterm at 33 weeks postmenstrual age and the same preterm infants studied again at 36 weeks postmenstrual age [12]. We also assessed the effect of gestational maturation and growth by comparing preterm-born with full-term-born infants. We confirmed significant ($p<0.05$) differences during longitudinal maturation and gestational maturation with regard to (1) the basal UES resting pressure; (2) UES relaxation parameters; (3) proximal and distal esophageal body amplitude and duration; (4) magnitude of esophageal waveform propagation; and (5) segmental peristaltic velocity. Specifically, the characteristics of UES and primary esophageal peristalsis exist by 33 weeks PMA; however, they undergo further maturation and differentiation during the postnatal growth, and are significantly different from that of adults [12].

The esophagus is the frequent target for the anterograde bolus from the oro-pharynx as in swallowing, and also for the retrograde bolus from the stomach as in gastro-esophageal reflux events. During either event, the bolus comes in close proximity to the airway, and evolving postnatal mechanisms facilitate pharyngeal and

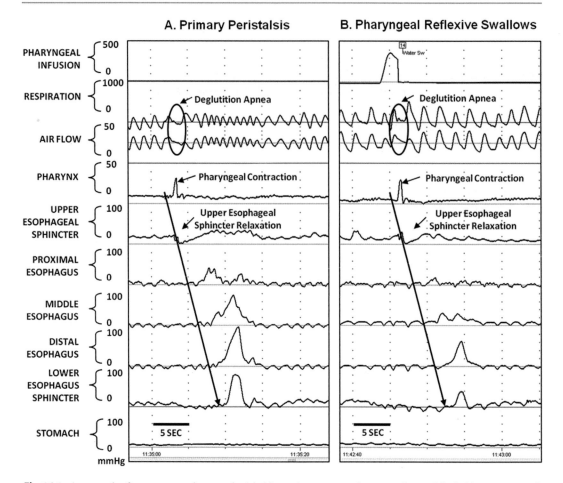

Fig. 16.1 An example of spontaneous primary peristalsis (**a**) and pharyngeal reflexive swallow evoked upon pharyngeal stimulation (**b**). Note the pharyngeal contraction, UES relaxation, anterograde propagation, and deglutition apnea associated with both these events. Note the changes in respiratory phase and air flow during pharyngeal contractile waveform

airway protection. For example, during primary esophageal peristalsis, there is a respiratory pause called deglutition apnea that occurs during the pharyngeal phase of swallow (Fig. 16.1b). This brief inhibition in respiration is due to a pause in the respiratory cycle (inspiratory or expiratory), and is a normal phenomenon [13, 14].

In contrast to spontaneous swallows, pharyngeal reflexive swallowing can be induced upon pharyngeal provocation with minute amounts of stimuli. Liquid stimuli are more potent modes of stimuli than air, in inducing pharyngeal reflexive swallowing, and the threshold volumes can be as low as 0.1 ml. However, there is a stimulus, volume–response relationship, in that the recruitment of pharyngeal reflexive swallows increases with

increments in provoking volumes. As a result, increased frequency of pharyngeal reflexive swallow sequences and longer deglutition apneas are noted (Fig. 16.2). In neonates, pharyngeal reflexive swallowing is the most frequent response. In adults, upon pharyngeal stimulation, pharyngo-upper esophageal sphincter contractile reflex (PUCR) is the most frequent response [15, 16].

Pharyngeal–Glottal Reflexes Maintaining Aerodigestive Safety

Upon birth, with the first breath, the glottal airway and pharyngo-esophageal functions are in parallel and assume different roles. Immediately

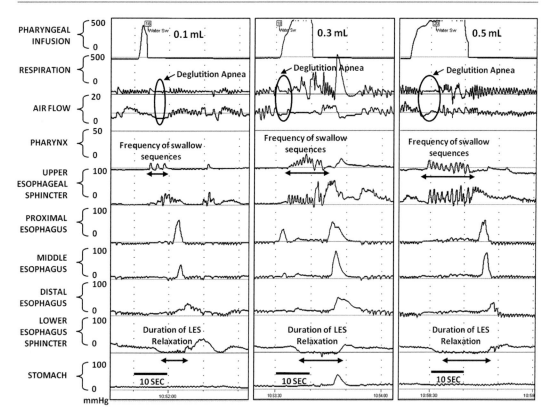

Fig. 16.2 An example of pharyngeal reflexive swallow and pharyngo-upper esophageal sphincter contractile reflex. Note the increases in the frequency recruitment of pharyngeal reflexive swallow sequences, duration of LES relaxation, and duration of deglutition apnea with increment in the volume of sterile water infusion stimulating the pharynx

after birth, pharyngo-esophageal functions continue to be responsible for swallowing, whereas the purpose of glottal opening and closure is to regulate the entry of air into and out of the lungs. Glottal motion occurs during normal inspiration and expiration to regulate air flow. However, complete glottal adduction can occur during the complex laryngeal chemoreflex, wherein the following phenomena can occur: laryngeal adduction, apnea, repetitive swallowing, startle, hypertension and bradycardia, and hypoxia [14]. In fetal and neonatal life, laryngeal chemoreflex and glottal closure can be observed and function to protect the airway from potential hazard such as aspiration. Also noted is repetitive swallowing performed to clear the pharyngeal airway of any material. In premature and full-term-born neonates apnea contributes in part to the important

airway protection mechanism, although the consequences of exaggerated apnea and laryngospasm can be deleterious as an absence of air flow and a lack of ventilation result in hypoxia. Subsequently, during infancy through adulthood, prolonged exhalations against a partially closed glottis occur in the form of cough reflex to clear the irritant away from the airway.

In summary, this chapter has described the developmental anatomy and neurophysiology of the pharynx and its aerodigestive relationships that facilitate swallowing, airway protection, and aspiration-preventing mechanisms. Mal-development and mal-adaptation of these functions in high-risk infants pose continued threats to pharyngeal function with the potential consequence being dysphagia, chronic airway problems, and impaired quality of life.

Acknowledgments This work is supported in part by NIH grant R01 DK 068158 (Jadcherla) and P01 DK 068051 (Jadcherla/Shaker). The author is grateful to Ms. Chin Yee Chan, MS, for assistance with this chapter.

References

1. Mansfield LE. Embryonic origins of the relation of gastroesophageal reflux disease and airway disease. Am J Med. 2001;111(Suppl 8A):3S–7.
2. Miller JL, Sonies BC, Macedonia C. Emergence of oropharyngeal, laryngeal and swallowing activity in the developing fetal upper aerodigestive tract: an ultrasound evaluation. Early Hum Dev. 2003;71:61–87.
3. Sadler TW. Respiratory system, Langman's medical embryology. 7th ed. Baltimore, MD: Williams and Wilkins; 1995.
4. Sadler TW. Digestive system, Langman's medical embryology. 7th ed. Baltimore, MD: Williams and Wilkins; 1995.
5. Sase M, Lee JJ, Park JY, et al. Ontogeny of fetal rabbit upper gastrointestinal motility. J Surg Res. 2001;101:68–72.
6. Sase M, Lee JJ, Ross MG, et al. Effect of hypoxia on fetal rabbit gastrointestinal motility. J Surg Res. 2001;99:347–51.
7. Langston C, Kida K, Reed M, et al. Human lung growth in late gestation and in the neonate. Am Rev Respir Dis. 1984;129:607–13.
8. Mittal RK, Balaban DH. The esophagogastric junction. N Engl J Med. 1997;336:924–32.
9. Goyal RK, Hirano I. The enteric nervous system. N Engl J Med. 1996;334:1106–15.
10. Goyal RK, Padmanabhan R, Sang Q. Neural circuits in swallowing and abdominal vagal afferent-mediated lower esophageal sphincter relaxation. Am J Med. 2001;111(Suppl 8A):95S–105.
11. Lang IM, Shaker R. Anatomy and physiology of the upper esophageal sphincter. Am J Med. 1997;103:50S–5.
12. Jadcherla SR, Duong HQ, Hofmann C, et al. Characteristics of upper oesophageal sphincter and oesophageal body during maturation in healthy human neonates compared with adults. Neurogastroenterol Motil. 2005;17:663–70.
13. Ren J, Shaker R, Zamir Z, et al. Effect of age and bolus variables on the coordination of the glottis and upper esophageal sphincter during swallowing. Am J Gastroenterol. 1993;88:665–9.
14. Thach BT. Maturation and transformation of reflexes that protect the laryngeal airway from liquid aspiration from fetal to adult life. Am J Med. 2001;111 (Suppl 8A):69S–77.
15. Jadcherla SR, Gupta A, Stoner E, et al. Pharyngeal swallowing: defining pharyngeal and upper esophageal sphincter relationships in human neonates. J Pediatr. 2007;151:597–603.
16. Ren J, Xie P, Lang IM, et al. Deterioration of the pharyngo-UES contractile reflex in the elderly. Laryngoscope. 2000;110:1563–6.

Part V

UES and Its Deglutitive Function

Development, Anatomy, and Physiology of the Upper Esophageal Sphincter and Pharyngoesophageal Junction

Ivan M. Lang

Abstract

The upper esophageal sphincter (UES) functions to close or to open the esophago-pharyngeal junction as needed. The UES closing muscles include the cervical esophagus, cricopharyngeus (CP), and inferior pharyngeal constrictor, but the primary functional muscle of the UES is the CP. The UES opening muscles include anteriorly the superior and inferior hyoid muscles and posteriorly the stylopharyngeus, palatopharyngeus, and pteropharyngeus. The UES is opened intermittently during various functions by relaxation of its closing muscles, contraction of its opening muscles, and bolus pulsion. The UES closing muscles contain two sets of muscle fibers: an inner layer of slow-twitch fibers and outer layer of fast-twitch fibers. It is hypothesized that these two fiber types serve the two basic functions of the UES closing muscles: slow tone generation and rapid reflex responsiveness. The UES motor and sensory functions are controlled by branches of the glossopharyngeal and vagus nerves. The motor nerve of the CP in animals is the pharyngoesophageal branch of the vagus nerve and may be the recurrent laryngeal nerve in humans. The nucleus ambiguus is the primary motor nucleus of the UES, and the nucleus tractus solitarius is the primary termination site of UES afferents. The UES opens and closes in complex patterns well coordinated with laryngeal movement to prevent aspiration during swallowing, belching, and vomiting. The UES tone increases during various digestive or respiratory tract reflexes to prevent the insufflation of air into the esophagus or the pharyngeal reflux of esophageal contents with possible aspiration. The specific actions of individual muscles of the UES differ among its various functions. The UES is fully functional as early as 33 weeks postmenstrual age although the specific parameters may differ.

I.M. Lang, DVM, PhD (✉)
Division of Gastroenterology and Hepatology,
Department of Medicine, Medical College of Wisconsin,
8701 Watertown Plank Road, Milwaukee, WI 53226, USA
e-mail: imlang@mcw.edu

R. Shaker et al. (eds.), *Principles of Deglutition: A Multidisciplinary Text for Swallowing and its Disorders*, DOI 10.1007/978-1-4614-3794-9_17, © Springer Science+Business Media New York 2013

Keywords

Upper esophageal sphincter • Cricopharyngeus • Swallowing • Belching • Vomiting

Introduction

The upper esophageal sphincter (UES) has two basic functions: opening and closing, and each is governed by a different set of muscles. The closing muscles consist of the cricopharyngeus (CP), inferior pharyngeal constrictor (IPC), and the cervical esophagus. The opening muscles consist of sets muscles anterior and posterior to the pharynx. The CP is the primary closing muscle of the UES. The CP is not only the major contributor to basal pressure of the UES, but it is the primary UES muscle that responds during various functions. The other UES closing muscles primarily contribute to the basal pressure of the UES.

Anatomy

Muscle Composition

UES Closing Muscles
Cricopharyngeus

The CP muscle attaches to the cricoid cartilage forming a muscular band at the junction of the esophagus and pharynx (Fig. 17.1). The CP is formed by two sets of muscle fibers. The obliquely oriented fibers, pars oblique (CPo), that are adjacent to the IPC extend from the cricoid cartilage to a median raphe [1]. The horizontally oriented fibers, i.e., pars fundiformis (CPh), are adjacent to the esophagus and extend between the lateral aspects of the lower portion of the cricoid cartilage without forming a median raphe [1]. The CP is a striated muscle composed of fibers 25–35 μm in diameter [1, 2] which forms a fiber network that inserts onto connective tissue [3]. The CP is composed of both slow- (type I, oxidative) and fast-twitch (type II, glycolytic) muscle fibers, but the type I fibers predominate [1–5]. The horizontal

fibers are composed of 76 % type I fibers whereas the oblique fibers contain 69 % type I fibers [5]. Both portions of the CP contain two layers and the inner layer is composed of significantly more type I fibers than the outer layer [5]. The layers not only differ in the amount of major myosin heavy chain (MHC) composition, but also in their unusual MHC isoform composition [6, 7]. The inner layer is composed of slow tonic and embryonic MHC isoforms, whereas the outer layer is composed of neonatal and alpha-cardiac MHC isoforms [7]. It is hypothesized that the isoform composition of the CP muscle layers, e.g., slow- vs. fast-twitch, is related to the function of the CP, e.g., tone generation vs. rapid responsiveness during swallowing, respectively [6, 7], but this hypothesis has not been tested. The role of the more unusual MHC isoforms in CP function is unknown.

The optimum length at which the CP reaches maximum active tension is about 1.7 times resting length [8], whereas this maximal tension in most striated muscles occurs at resting length. The source of this elasticity may be attributed to the connective tissue, i.e., collagen, elastin, sarcolemma, or the contractile proteins, actin and myosin [9]. The CP contains more elastic connective tissue and sarcolemma than most other striated muscles [2, 3]. This high degree of elasticity as well as the network arrangement of muscle fibers contributes to some important and distinctive characteristics of the UES. The UES is capable of maintaining a basal tone without active muscular contraction. The active tension of the UES increases throughout the range of distention [8] similar to Starling's law of the heart, allowing a greater force to be exerted by the UES behind a passing bolus. This characteristic would be important to propel larger boluses and to prevent reflux. In addition, the optimum length of

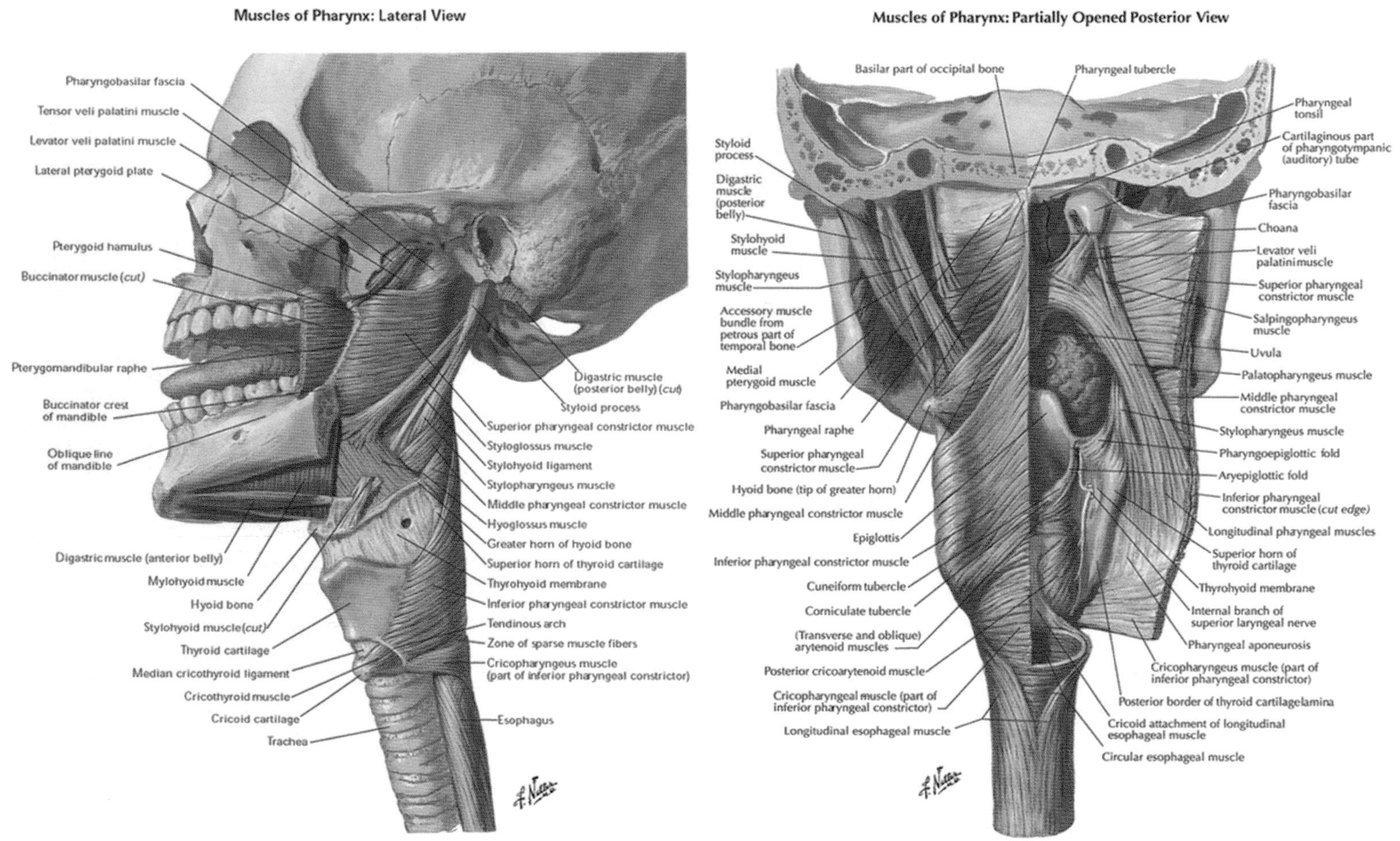

Muscles of Pharynx: Partially Opened Posterior View

Pharyngeal tonsil
Cartilaginous part of pharyngotympanic (auditory) tube
Pharyngobasilar fascia
Choana
Levator veli palatini muscle
Superior pharyngeal constrictor muscle
Salpingopharyngeus muscle
Uvula
Palatopharyngeus muscle
Middle pharyngeal constrictor muscle
Stylopharyngeus muscle
Pharyngoepiglotic fold
Aryepiglottic fold
Inferior pharyngeal constrictor muscle (cut edge)
Longitudinal pharyngeal muscles
Superior horn of thyroid cartilage
Thyrohyoid membrane
Internal branch of superior laryngeal nerve
Pharyngeal aponeurosis
Cricopharyngeus muscle (part of inferior pharyngeal constrictor)
Posterior border of thyroid cartilage lamina
Cricoid attachment of longitudinal esophageal muscle
Circular esophageal muscle

Pharyngeal tubercle
Basilar part of occipital bone
Styloid process
Digastric muscle (posterior belly)
Stylohyoid muscle
Stylopharyngeus muscle
Accessory muscle bundle from petrous part of temporal bone
Medial pterygoid muscle
Pharyngobasilar fascia
Pharyngeal raphe
Superior pharyngeal constrictor muscle
Hyoid bone (tip of greater horn)
Middle pharyngeal constrictor muscle
Epiglottis
Inferior pharyngeal constrictor muscle
Cuneiform tubercle
Corniculate tubercle
(Transverse and oblique) arytenoid muscles
Posterior cricoarytenoid muscle
Cricopharyngeus muscle (part of inferior pharyngeal constrictor)
Longitudinal esophageal muscle
Esophagus

Muscles of Pharynx: Lateral View

Pharyngobasilar fascia
Tensor veli palatini muscle
Levator veli palatini muscle
Lateral pterygoid plate
Pterygoid hamulus
Buccinator crest of mandible
Oblique line of mandible
Pterygomandibular raphe
Buccinator muscle (cut)

Digastric muscle (posterior belly)(cut)
Styloid process
Superior pharyngeal constrictor muscle
Styloglossus muscle
Stylohyoid ligament
Stylopharyngeus muscle
Middle pharyngeal constrictor muscle
Hyoglossus muscle
Greater horn of hyoid bone
Superior horn of thyroid cartilage
Inferior pharyngeal constrictor muscle
Thyrohyoid membrane
Tendinous arch
Zone of sparse muscle fibers
Cricopharyngeus muscle (part of inferior pharyngeal constrictor)
Esophagus
Trachea
Cricoid cartilage
Cricothyroid muscle
Median cricothyroid ligament
Thyroid cartilage
Stylohyoid muscle (cut)
Hyoid bone
Mylohyoid muscle
Digastric muscle (anterior belly)

Fig. 17.1 Anatomy of the closing and some opening muscles of the upper esophageal sphincter (UES). From I.M. Lang. GI motility online; 2006; doi:10.1038/gimo12

the CP is larger than the maximum bolus volume likely to occur [8], ensuring that the UES tension always accommodates the bolus. Finally the high degree of elasticity of the CP allows the UES to be opened by a bolus or distraction forces without relaxation of the CP [10].

Inferior Pharyngeal Constrictor

The fibers of the IPC insert onto the sides of the cricoid and thyroid cartilages (Fig. 17.1), run dorsally and medially, and meet at a fibrous raphe at the median line of the posterior pharynx [11]. The IPC, like the CP, differs anatomically in a rostrocaudal direction. The rostral fibers of the IPC [11] contain more (61 %) fast-twitch fibers than the caudal fibers (30 %). Similar to the CP, the IPC, both rostrally and caudally, is composed of two layers: an inner layer of slow-twitch muscle fibers and an outer layer of fast-twitch muscle fibers [12]. The inner layer of slow-twitch fibers of the caudal IPC is twice as thick as the outer layer of fast-twitch fibers, and this organization is reversed for the rostral IPC. The muscle fibers of the most caudal portion of the IPC are most similar to those of the most rostral portion of the CP. They have similar distribution of slow- and fast-twitch fibers (84 vs. 16 %) and both have similar proportional thicknesses of inner and outer layers (2:1 ratio). The IPC also has the similar composition of MHC isoforms as the CP as described earlier [5]. The IPC contains both collagen and elastin, but elastin content of the IPC is less than that of the CP.

Cervical Esophagus

The muscle fibers of the cervical esophagus (Fig. 17.1) are exclusively striated muscle for the first 1–5 cm and they are arranged in a strictly horizontal fashion [13]. The muscle fibers of the cervical esophagus are about the same size as the adjacent CP muscle fibers [14], and some have found that the CP contributes fibers to the cranial portion of the esophagus [15]. The predominant muscle fiber type of the cervical striated muscle esophagus in animals is fast twitch [15, 16], but this issue is unclear in humans because of significant differences among studies in handling of human tissues [13–16]. Unlike the IPC and CP,

no regional differences in fiber type have been found in the human esophagus [14]. The most proximal portion of the cervical esophagus has similar composition of MHC isoforms as the CP as described earlier [7]. The connective tissue composition of the cervical esophageal striated muscles is similar to other striated non-CP muscles.

UES Opening Muscles
Anatomy of the Anterior UES Opening Muscles

The anterior muscles include the superior and inferior hyoid muscles (Fig. 17.1). The superior hyoid muscles include the geniohyoideus, mylohyoideus, stylohyoideus, hyogolossus, and anterior belly of the digastricus. These muscles arise from various structures superior to the hyoid bone and insert onto the superior aspect of the hyoid bone so that their contraction acts to move the layngohyoid complex superiorly and anteriorly [17]. The inferior muscles include the thyrohyoideus, sternohyoideus, sternothyroideus, and omohyoideus. The thyrohyoideus arises from the thyroid cartilage, the strenohyoideus arises from the clavicle and manubrium, the sternothyroideus arises from the manubrium and upper vertebrae, and the omohyoideus arises from the scapula. All four muscles insert onto the inferior aspect of the hyoid bone [17]. The action of these muscles is to pull the hyoid bone and thyroid cartilage inferior and anterior. Most of the action of these anterior UES opening muscles is on the hyoid bone with the thyrohyoideus forming the connection between the hyoid and larynx. The simultaneous contraction of the anterior muscles, thus, acts to move the hyoid bone and larynx anteriorly. The relative contribution of these anterior muscles to opening of the UES depends on the function of the UES, and the stronger and wider the opening needed the more of these muscles are recruited.

Anatomy of the Posterior UES Opening Muscles

The posterior muscles (Fig. 17.1) include the stylopharyngeus, palatopharyngeus, pterygopharyngeus, and perhaps other superiorly directed posterior pharyngeal muscles [17]. The actions of these muscles are to elevate the pharynx and to stabilize the posterior wall of the pharynx by providing tension posteriorly.

Histology of the UES Opening Muscles

The UES opening muscles are histologically and histochemically similar to limb muscles and similar to each other [18–20]. The muscle fibers are oriented in parallel fashion, the fibers are uniform size, and there is little connective tissue. Most of the fibers, about 60–85 %, are composed of fast-twitch (type II) fibers and have a diameter of 20 to 40 μm. The only opening muscle that differs to a significant degree is the thyrohyoid which has more type I (40 %) and highly oxidative muscle fibers [20] than the other UES opening muscles. The increased fatigue resistance that results from these types of muscle fibers may contribute to the tonic functions of the thyrohyoid. The thyrohyoid maintains a constant distance between the thyroid and hyoid cartilages during many activities and tonically contracts to provide the main link between the suprahyoid muscles and the larynx.

Motor Innervation

UES Closing Muscles
Cricopharyngeus

The CP receives innervation from the pharyngeal plexus which is supplied by three nerves: vagus nerve branches, glossopharyngeal nerve (GPN), and sympathetic nerve fibers [17]. The vagal input to the pharyngeal plexus consists of three separate branches: the pharyngoesophageal nerve (PEN), the superior laryngeal nerve (SLN), and the recurrent laryngeal nerve (RLN). Although there is no prominent raphe of the CP, the CP is bilaterally innervated [21] with each half of the CP acting as a distinct motor unit [8]. The motor endplates of the CP form distinctive bands in each half of the CPh, but both CPo and CPh have endplates scattered throughout the muscle [4]. The sympathetic nerves probably innervate the blood vessels and epithelial mucous glands, but they have no role in motor control of the CP [22].

The motor innervation of the CP is species dependent. The PEN provides the motor innervation of the CP in most animal species. Electrical stimulation of the PEN in dogs and cats contracts the CP and transection of the PEN chronically paralyzes the CP [23]. The effects of electrical stimulation of three of the nerves supplying the pharyngeal plexus on glycogen depletion of the CP in rats were determined [24]. Glycogen depletion is an index of the amount of muscle contraction. It was found that the PEN had the greatest effect on glycogen depletion, followed by the SLN stimulation, whereas the RLN stimulation had no effect [24]. Studies of the effects of electrical stimulation of the GPN and all three branches of the vagus nerve on EMG and contractile activities in cats found similar results to the glycogen depletion studies in rats. Electrical stimulation of the PEN [8, 25] had the greatest effect on CP EMG and contractile activities, much less activation by SLN [8, 25] or GPN [25, 26] stimulation, and no effect of RLN [8, 25, 27] stimulation. In addition, in chronically instrumented dogs, transection of the PEN rather than the GPN or SLN had profound long-term deficits on swallowing and resting pharyngeal pressure, and produced denervation potentials in the CP [26, 28]. On the other hand, transection of the RLN unilaterally had no effect on resting UES pressure [29]. Furthermore in cats, transection of the PEN, but not SLN and RLN, bilaterally blocked the CP EMG responses during swallowing [8, 25].

The motor innervation of the CP in humans is unclear. A PEN has not been observed in humans [30] and data on the role of the RLN is contradictory. Some have suggested that the RLN innervates the CP based on visually tracing nerve fibers [4] or examining the effects of electrical stimulation of the RLN on electrical responses recorded from the CP [22, 31, 32]. On the other hand, CP of humans does not appear to be functionally innervated by the RLN as laryngeal paralysis due to RLN damage is not associated with UES contractile dysfunction [33].

Investigators found that electrical stimulation of the RLN caused electrical responses recorded from electrodes on the CP [31], but the source of these responses was not determined. It is possible that these CP electrical responses to RLN stimulation were due to the spread of current from the underlying laryngeal muscles, because transection of all of the nerves innervating the CP did not eliminate these responses [32]. In addition, the very same RLN stimulation caused electrical responses on the IPC as well as the CP [32], even though prior evidence found no innervation of the IPC by the RLN [4, 11]. Furthermore, the spread of current from underlying muscles can also explain the results of the other electrical recording studies. That is, the current needed to cause CP electrical responses to RLN stimulation [31] was much greater than that for PEN stimulation [8], and the magnitude of the electrical responses recorded from the CP during RLN stimulation [31] was much smaller than those activated by PEN stimulation [8]. In none of these electrical recording studies [22, 31, 32] of the CP were experiments performed to control for the possibility of spread of current from the underlying laryngeal muscles yet the RLN is the primary nerve innervating these laryngeal muscles.

Moreover, the ability of current spread from laryngeal muscles to electrodes on the CP has been observed in prior studies. That is, the electrical stimulation of the PEN or RLN caused electrical responses on the CP, but the electrical response to PEN stimulation was far greater (more than tenfold) and only PEN stimulation caused contraction of the CP [25]. One source of this current spread may be the posterior cricoarytenoideus (PCA) as the PCA lies just below the anterior border of the CP and the RLN innervates the PCA. Interestingly, the peak electrical response on the CP to RLN stimulation was at the anterior portion of the CP [22], which is the closest part of the CP to the underlying PCA. Therefore, the evidence supporting a role for the RLN in the motor innervation of the CP is weak.

In a retrospective review of clinical cases with nerve damage, investigators correlated dysfunction of various UES related muscles [34]. They found that CP dysfunction was very closely related to IPC dysfunction and minimally associated with laryngeal muscle dysfunction, suggesting that CP and IPC had common innervation and that CP and laryngeal muscles did not. Since the

RLN innervates the larynx and the pharyngeal plexus innervates the IPC, it was concluded that the major innervation of the CP was through the pharyngeal plexus and not RLN.

In summary, while the motor innervation of the CP of animals is clear from both anatomical and physiological studies, the innervation of the human CP is still unknown. It is suggested that the motor innervation of the human CP will not be defined until techniques that measure actual muscle contraction are employed.

Inferior Pharyngeal Constrictor

The motor innervation of the IPC is supplied primarily by the pharyngeal branch of the vagus nerve through the pharyngeal plexus [4, 11]; however, no physiological studies have been reported that have investigated this issue directly. Many studies have attempted to trace nerve fibers through the pharyngeal plexus to the IPC, but because this innervation is through a plexus of interconnecting nerves it is not possible to definitively determine which branch supplies the IPC using these techniques. The inferior IPC (iIPC) is supplied by the same branch of the pharyngeal branch of the vagus nerve that supplies the CP [11]. This implies similar control mechanisms, but no physiological studies have been reported to confirm this conjecture. The entire IPC muscle has a single vertical band of motor end plates that corresponds to the location of the pharyngeal plexus [4].

Cervical Esophagus

The motor innervation of the cervical esophagus is supplied by the RLN [4, 21, 23]. The terminal branches travel around the esophagus in a circular fashion and cross the midline both anteriorly and posteriorly [4].

UES Opening Muscles
Anterior Muscles

The individual anterior muscles have different motor innervations [17]. The motor nerves of the superior set of anterior muscles include the hypoglossal nerve for hypogolossal muscles, the facial nerve for the stylohyoideus, the first cervical nerve for the geniohyoideus, and the trigeminal nerve for both the mylohyoideus and the anterior belly of the digastricus. The inferior set of anterior muscles, thyrohyoideus, sternohyoideus, and sternothyroideus, all have the same motor nerves, the ansa cervicalis containing the first to third cervical nerves.

Posterior Muscles

The posterior opening muscles are innervated by different motor nerves. The GPN innervates the stylopharyngeus, and the accessory nerve innervates the palatopharyngeus.

Sensory Innervation

UES Closing Muscles

The epithelium and muscle fibers of the UES receive sensory innervation. The pharyngeal epithelium is innervated by branches of the GPN, SLN, and vagus nerves [35–39], and the esophageal epithelium is innervated by the vagus nerves, and the SLN [39] or RLN [32] depending on the species. The SLN mediates various reflexes from the pharynx and esophagus including swallowing and the esophago-UES contractile reflex from the most proximal portion of the esophagus [40]. The RLN mediates the afferent limb of esophago-UES contractile reflex from the distal portion of the cervical esophagus [23]. The vagus nerves mediate the afferent limb of the esophago-UES contractile reflex from the thoracic esophagus [41]. The GPN [42] mediates the afferent limb of the pharyngo-UES contractile reflex. The loss of sensory function of the UES may explain some of the swallowing deficits observed after transection of the GPN in dogs [26, 28]. The CP is devoid of muscle spindles [3, 4], but a Golgi tendon organ-like structure has been found in the human CP that may be involved in proprioception [43].

UES Opening Muscles

The UES opening muscles are all striated muscles and like most striated muscles they contain proprioceptors and the sensory nerves for these proprioceptors are the same as the motor nerves described earlier [44–47]. The UES opening muscles that do not have muscle spindles include the digastric [46] muscle, stylohyoideus [44], and stylopharyngeus [44].

Neurochemical Control

UES Opening and Closing Muscles

The only neurotransmitter of any of the UES opening or closing muscles found to mediate contraction is acetylcholine acting through nicotinic cholinergic receptors. However, the following neuropeptides have been found in the CP: neuropeptide Y, calcitonin gene related peptide (CGRP), tyrosine hydroxylase, substance P, vasoactive intestinal polypeptide (VIP), and galanin [48]. CGRP has also been found in the thyropharyngeus (TP, i.e., the inferior constrictor in animals) as well as the striated muscle esophagus, but there is less CGRP in the CP than TP [49, 50]. The functional significance of these neuropeptides in the UES muscles is unknown, but they may represent the autonomic innervation of the muscle because substance P, VIP, and galanin are found in parasympathetic nerves and CGRP, neuropeptide Y, and tyrosine hydroxylase are found in sympathetic nerves. In general, within the CP the sympathetic neuropeptides were more abundant than the parasympathetic neuropeptides. Parasympathetic ganglia have been found in the CP, but not the TP. The roles of the sympathetic or parasympathetic innervation and the neuropeptides in control of the UES are unknown, but they probably function to control blood flow to the UES and some aspects of epithelial function.

CNS Control

Motor neurons
UES Closing Muscles

Most of the motoneurons of the closing muscles of the UES, i.e., CP, IPC, and cervical esophagus, are located in the nucleus ambiguus (NA). The NA is topographically organized such that the more rostral portions of the NA contain the motoneurons to the more caudally located muscles [51–56]. The innervation of the IPC and the CP in those species in which the CP has a median raphe is mostly unilateral [52, 55], and this unilateral arrangement has been confirmed in physiological studies of swallowing [57]. In contrast, the reflex activation of the CP requires both halves of the brain stem and electrical stimulation of the nucleus tractus solitarius (NTS), the primary termination site of vagal afferents, causes bilateral activation of the CP [58]. These results suggest that control of the UES differs with different functions.

The neurons of the nucleus ambiguus have extensive dendritic arborization to the adjacent reticular formation [59], and ultrastructural studies indicate that the synapses on these neurons are both excitatory and inhibitory [60]. These findings provide an anatomical basis for the numerous excitatory and inhibitory responses of the UES and CP. Many pharyngeal motor neurons exhibit respiratory rhythm, but none of them have a spontaneous background discharge suggesting that the pharyngeal motor neurons are not the source of UES tone [61].

The NA is strongly activated during functions which involved significant changes in UES contractility including swallowing [62], secondary peristalsis [62, 63], and belching [63].

UES Opening Muscles

The motor nuclei of the UES opening muscles mirror the motor nerves [17]. The motor nuclei of the anterior suprahyoid muscles include the hypoglossal nucleus for hypogolossal muscles, the facial nucleus for the stylohyoideus, the first cervical division of the spinal cord for the geniohyoideus, and the trigeminal nucleus for both the mylohyoideus and the digastricus. The anterior infrahyoid muscles, thyrohyoideus, sternohyoideus, and sternothyroideus, all have motor nuclei in the first to third cervical divisions of the spinal cord. The motor nucleus of the posterior opening muscles is the nucleus ambiguus.

Sensory and Premotor Neurons
UES Closing Muscles

Pharyngeal vagal afferents have their cell bodies in the nodose ganglion [53] and terminate on premotor neurons found in the interstitial and intermediate subnuclei of the NTS [64–67]. However

stimulation of the pharynx using a physiological stimulus [62], i.e., water injection, activated neurons in the interstitial, intermediate, as well as the ventromedial subnucleus of the NTS. The specific premotor neurons participating in each reflex response initiated by stimulation of the pharynx are unknown.

Esophageal afferents have their cell bodies in the nodose ganglion [68, 69] and cervical and thoracic dorsal root ganglia of the spinal cord [68, 70]; the nodose fibers [68] terminate in premotor neurons [64, 67, 71] in the central subnucleus of the NTS. No studies have been conducted to specifically examine the most rostral portion of the cervical esophagus that forms part of the UES. It is possible that this area of the esophagus has similar distribution of premotor neurons as the pharynx. However, stimulation of specific esophageal mechanoreceptors [62, 63] and chemoreceptors [72], which activate different sets of physiological responses, activated different sets of subnuclei within the NTS. Therefore, different sets of premotor nuclei, activated by different types of esophageal stimuli, result in the activation of different responses.

UES Opening Muscles

The central nuclei mediating proprioception of the UES opening muscles include portions of the spinal cord and brainstem [17]. The sensory nuclei of the inferior set of anterior UES opening muscles as well as the geniohyoideus include the first three divisions of the cervical spinal cord. The sensory nucleus of the palatopharyngeus and hyoglossus is the medullary nucleus of the spinal tract of the trigeminal nerve, and the sensory nucleus of the mylohyodeus is the mesencephalic nucleus of the trigeminal nerve.

Physiology

UES Tone Generation

Tone is the constant force within the sphincter generated by both passive and active mechanical properties of the UES closing muscles which may be recorded intraluminally by pressure transducers.

Electromyographic (EMG) activity can also be used as an index of UES tone. Manometry, however, is subject to two limitations: (1) manometry cannot distinguish between passive and active tension and (2) pressure transducers create passive tension themselves by distending the elastic components of the UES muscles. The main limitation of EMG activity is that it can provide an index of active, but not passive tension. Another important consideration is that the UES is composed of striated muscles that unlike smooth muscles have no intrinsic tone generating mechanisms. All tone of the UES must arise from activation of the motor neurons.

Manometric studies have found a wide range, 35–200 mmHg, of resting UES pressure [73], which falls to very low levels during sleep [74] or anesthesia [75]. Chronic animal studies have found that CP EMG activity falls to very low levels when the animal is relaxed and its head supported (Fig. 17.2). In addition, pharyngeal motoneurons of decerebrate and paralyzed cats do not exhibit a spontaneous discharge [61]. Therefore, evidence suggests that the UES has no active basal tone, although a residual intraluminal pressure may be recorded manometrically due to the passive elastic properties of the UES closing muscles.

Although there is no basal tone of the UES, the tone of the UES is highly variable and can increase to very high levels. High UES pressures (Fig. 17.3) have been recorded during acute stress [76, 77] and other emotional states [78], and sharp increases in UES pressure have been recorded during waking [79]. In addition, large increases in ongoing EMG activity of the CP in animals [78] have been recorded during changes in posture and in response to stress or excitation. Therefore, while the UES has no basal tone, many reflexes function to alter UES tone.

The specific muscles involved in active UES tone generation have been investigated by recording EMG from the TP, CP, and proximal esophagus in conscious nonsedated and nonrestrained animals. Under these conditions, it was observed [78] that the TP EMG changed little regardless of excitability, arousal, and head position, whereas the CP EMG changed greatly (Fig. 17.4).

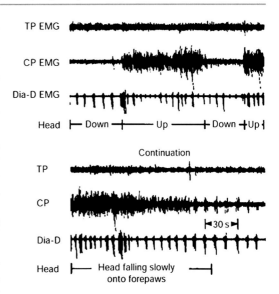

Fig. 17.2 High variability of CP but not TP EMG. This figure depicts the EMG responses of the TP, CP, and diaphragm in a minimally restrained awake chronically instrumented dog. Throughout this recording the dog is lying prone with its head upright or resting down on its paws. Note that the CP but not TP EMG varies with head position, and when the dog is relaxed at rest with its head down the TP EMG exceeds the CP EMG. *TP* thyropharyngeus, *CP* cricopharyngeus, *Dia-D* diaphragmatic dome fibers. From I.M. Lang. GI motility online; 2006; doi:10.1038/gimo12 with permission from Nature Publishing Group

In addition, correlation of basal TP and CP EMG with UES pressure during changes in excitability [78] revealed that CP but not TP EMG was related to UES pressure. Yet, even in these studies [78] it was found that peak pressure of the upper esophageal high pressure zone (UEHPZ) was observed at the distal end of the TP or proximal end of the CP (Fig. 17.5). However, as with similar human studies [79] these measurements were made with the animal relaxed and its head supported. Only under these conditions is the TP tone more active than the CP tone. Therefore, while peak UEHPZ may occur in or close to the TP, this finding only applies to the unusual conditions of the recording session and probably does not reflect the situation in a freely active individual. The UEHPZ may be higher in the vicinity of the TP under very low states of CP activation, because the TP is less compliant than the CP due to the high content of elastic tissue in the CP.

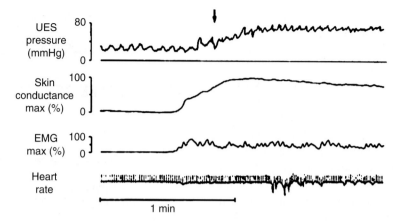

Fig. 17.3 Effect of stress on UES pressure. This figure depicts the tracings of UES pressure, skin conductance, integrated frontalis EMG, and heart rate before and during a stressful listening task (at *arrow*). Note the anticipatory rise in UES pressure about 15 s before the stress begins. From I.M. Lang. GI motility online; 2006; doi:10.1038/gimo12 with permission from Nature Publishing Group

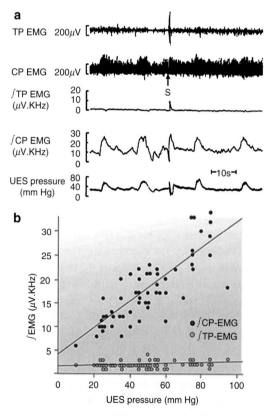

Fig. 17.4 Relationship of CP and TP EMG activities to UES pressure during rest and excitation. (**a**) Actual responses. (**b**) Graph of the relationship between EMG and UES pressure. The UES pressure changed five times: one swallow (S) preceded and followed by two rises in UES pressure induced by whistling in an awake dog lying on its side. Note that UES pressure changes correlated well ($p < 0.05$) with integrated CP-EMG but not integrated TP-EMG. *TP* thyropharyngeus, *CP* cricopharyngeus. From I.M. Lang. GI motility online; 2006; doi:10.1038/gimo12 with permission from Nature Publishing Group

The above studies recorded TP EMG 1–2 cm above the CP in dogs, but recent evidence suggests that the (iIPC) of humans has similar histochemical properties and innervation patterns as the CP [11], and therefore may also participate in the UEHPZ and tone generation. However, no physiological studies have been reported to date to confirm this conjecture.

UES Opening and Closing

The UES opens during various physiological states, e.g., swallowing, vomiting, and belching, to allow the passage of luminal contents, but the specific manner of the opening and the specific muscles involved differ with the physiological state. In all states, UES opening begins with UES relaxation followed briefly by contraction of UES distracting muscles, but the specific responses differ.

Swallowing

Opening of the UES during swallowing is a very complex maneuver. Simultaneous recordings of UES pressure and opening with EMG recording of UES muscles in awake and unanesthetized dogs found the following sequence of events during swallowing [78]. Firstly the CP muscle relaxed, about 100 ms later the UES pressure began to fall, i.e., UES relaxation, and this was followed about

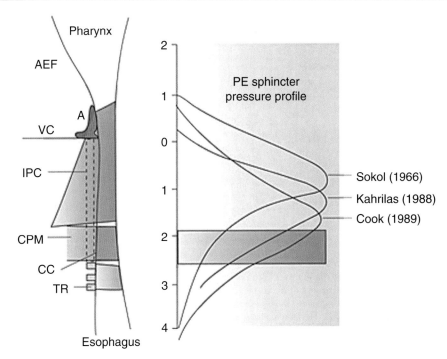

Fig. 17.5 Relationship of upper esophageal high-pressure zone (UEHPZ) to the pharyngoesophageal muscles. Data compiled from three different studies of the position of the UEHPZ with respect to individual pharyngeal muscles based on combined manometric and videofluoroscopic studies. Note that the peak pressures of the UEHPZ in humans at rest with the head fixed in all three studies coincide with the lower border of the IPC. *A* arytenoid, *AEF* aryepiglottic fold, *CC* cricoid cartilage, *ESO* esophagus, *IPC* inferior pharyngeal constrictor, *PE* pharyngoesophageal, *TR* tracheal ring, *VC* vocal cord. From I.M. Lang. GI motility online; 2006; doi:10.1038/gimo12 with permission from Nature Publishing Group

100 ms (150 ms in humans [80]) later by UES opening (Fig. 17.6). Videofluoroscopic studies [78, 80] found that UES opening was associated with superior and anterior movement of the hyoid and larynx (Fig. 17.7). The onset of the superior movement of the hyoid and larynx coincided with the beginning of UES relaxation and preceded anterior movement of the larynx and hyoid by about 100 ms in dogs [78] and over 200 ms in humans [74]. The anterior movement just preceded (humans [80]) or was concomitant (dogs [78]) with UES opening. The sequential movement of hyoid superiorly and anteriorly (Fig. 17.8) probably accounts for the elliptical pattern of movement of the hyoid bone observed during swallowing [80, 81].

The CP is the primary muscle that relaxes to permit UES opening [10, 78, 80, 81], while the TP muscle contracts during this time [78, 82, 83].

During swallowing the CP relaxes for about 0.5 s in humans [79, 81] and about 0.3 s in dogs [78, 82, 83]. Superior movement of the larynx and hyoid is probably caused by contraction of the superior hyoid muscles as all of these muscles begin to be activated (Fig. 17.9) concomitant with CP relaxation and this activation continues throughout CP relaxation [80, 83]. The inferior hyoid muscles completely relax during this time (Fig. 17.10) allowing maximum superior movement of the hyoid, larynx, and UES [78, 83]. Anterior movement of the hyoid and larynx corresponds with maximal activation of the geniohyoideus which suggests that the geniohyoideus is one of the primary suprahyoid muscles responsible for UES opening [78, 83]. The stylopharyngeus is activated concomitant with the geniohyoideus; therefore, it is likely that maximum opening of the UES is due not only to

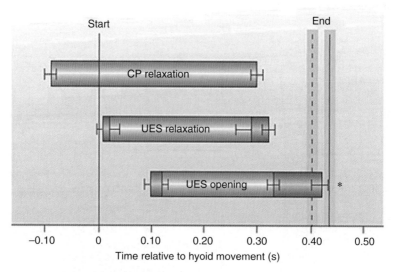

Fig. 17.6 Temporal relationship of UES pressure, opening, and CP EMG during 4-mL barium swallow relative to hyoid movement. The start and end of hyoid movement are indicated by *vertical lines* where the *shaded areas* indicate standard error (SE). Horizontal bars depict mean + SE onset and offset of measured variables relative to start of hyoid movement. *Green bars* depict data from noninstrumented dogs (*n*=8), and *blue bars* depict data from instrumented dogs (*n*=6). Note the electrode implantation significantly delayed time of UES closure. There is approximately a 100-ms difference between CP relaxation, UES relaxation, and UES opening. From I.M. Lang. GI motility online; 2006; doi:10.1038/gimo12 with permission from Nature Publishing Group

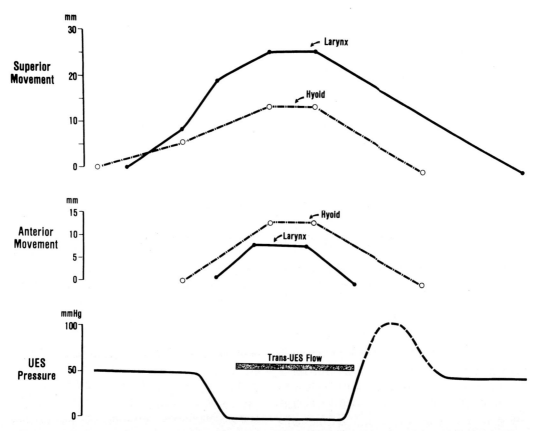

Fig. 17.7 Relationship among hyoid and laryngeal movement, UES relaxation, and UES opening for a 5 mL barium swallow. Note that superior relocation of the larynx precedes UES penetration by the bolus. Anterior movement of the hyoid and larynx precedes UES opening From I.J. Cook et al. Am JPhysiol 1989;257:G748–59 used with permission of the American Physiological Society

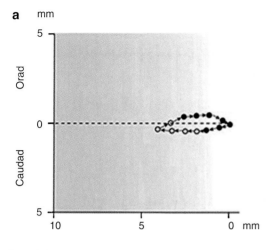

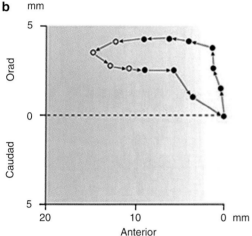

Fig. 17.8 Movement of the hyoid bone during belching (**a**) and swallowing (**b**). *Open circles* indicate UES opening observed by videofluoroscopy. Although hyoid bone movement during swallowing was invariably upward, forward, and counterclockwise, its movement during belching was mainly anterior and clockwise. The magnitude of hyoid bone movement during belching was significantly less than its movement during swallowing. Hyoid bone movement is an indication of the magnitude of the distraction forces that open the UES ($p < 0.02$). From I.M. Lang. GI motility online; 2006; doi:10.1038/gimo12 with permission from Nature Publishing Group

anterior movement of the pharynx caused by activation of the geniohyoideus, but also by posterior stabilization of the pharynx caused by activation of the stylopharyngeus and other posterior pharyngeal muscles.

Belching

Belching is characterized by a prolonged, over 1 s, drop in UES tone [84, 85], opening of the UES [84, 85], and relaxation of the UES muscles [65]. Unlike swallowing both the TP and CP relax during belching and the UES pressure drop during belching coincides with, rather than precedes, UES muscle relaxation [86]. In addition, during belching most of the distracting muscles are not active and the one active distracting muscle, the thyrohyoideus (Fig. 17.11), is activated at a low but constant level [88]. These small changes in UES distracting muscles probably account for the rather short anterior movement and lack of superior movement of the hyoid bone observed during belching [84, 85]. The role of infrahyoid and posterior pharyngeal muscles during belching remains to be studied, but given the small response of the anterior distracting muscles and small anterior movement of the hyoid [84, 85] it is suggested that UES opening during belching may be related more to the distracting effects of the bolus than occurs during other functions like swallowing. This effect may account for the observation that the delay from UES pressure drop to UES opening is longer during belching [85] than during swallowing [80].

Retching and Vomiting

The UES is involved in numerous functions during retching and vomiting and all three UES closing muscles participate in one or more of these responses (Fig. 17.12).

Preretch Tone Increase

Just prior to retching the tone of the UES increases greatly in phase with the diaphragm, and this increase in tone involves the CP and cervical esophagus, but not the TP [83]. The function of this increase in tone is to prevent air insufflation of the esophagus during the large negative thoracic pressure that is subsequently generated during the first very large inspiration of the first retch. This closing of the UES allows the lungs to fully inflate without allowing air into the esophagus or stomach. The LES is relaxed at this time so without UES closure the stomach would fill with air.

Dry   Food

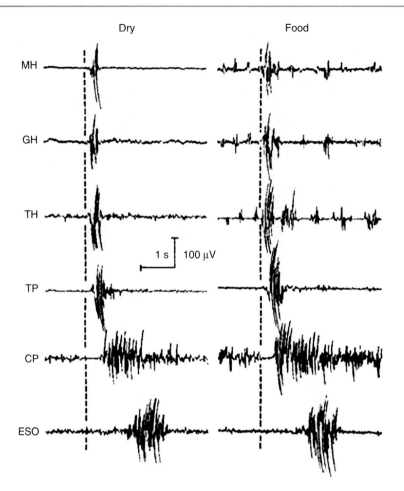

Fig. 17.9 Response of UES muscles during swallowing. This figure illustrates the EMG responses of the three UES closure muscles and many of the superior hyoid UES opening muscles during a dry swallow ad lib feeding of canned food in a chronically instrumented dog. Note that the three UES closing muscles respond quite differently during swallowing, but the superior opening muscles activate almost simultaneously. *MH* mylohyoideus, *GH* geniohyoideus, *TH* thyrohyoideus, *TP* thyropharyngeus, *CP* cricopharyngeus, *ESO* esophagus 2 cm below CP. From I.M. Lang. GI motility online; 2006; doi:10.1038/gimo12 with permission from Nature Publishing Group

Phasic Changes in UES Tone During Retching

After the first very large retch, the diaphragm and glottis then shift phase so that the diaphragm contracts during glottal closure instead of glottal opening [83]. This phase shift allows the diaphragm to be used as a pump to expel gastric contents and the external intercostal muscles then become the sole generator of inspiration. Thus, at the end of the inspiratory phase of the first retch, the glottis closes as the UES opens shifting the force of the diaphragmatic contraction to the stomach. The diaphragm then relaxes, glottis opens, and UES closes very strongly [83]. The function of this closure of the UES during this phase of retching is to prevent aspiration as this occurs during inspiration and gastric contents may be in the upper esophagus at this time [89]. Prior studies have found that gastric contents can be expelled to just below the UES during retching. This cycle continues until the end of retching.

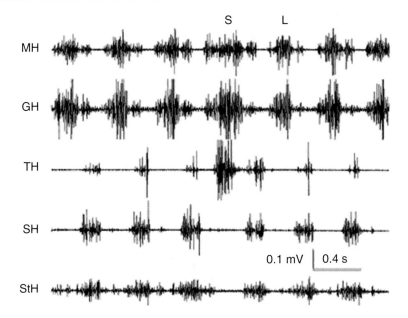

Fig. 17.10 Responses of superior and inferior hyoid muscles during swallowing. This figure illustrates the EMG responses of the superior (MH, GH) and inferior (TH, SH, StH) hyoid muscles during swallowing in a chronically instrumented dog. These muscles are capable of putting anterior traction on the larynx, thereby opening the UES. Note that during swallowing only the superior hyoid muscles are activated. *S* swallowing, *L* licking, *MH* mylohyoideus, *GH* geniohyoideus, *TH* thyrohyoideus, *SH* sternohyoideus, *StH* sternothyroideus. From I.M. Lang. GI motility online; 2006; doi:10.1038/gimo12 with permission from Nature Publishing Group

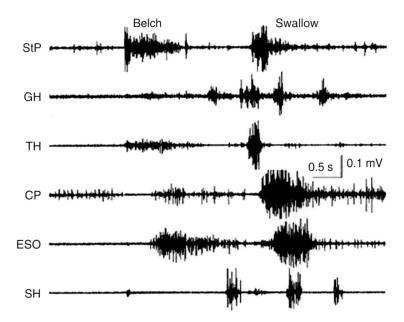

Fig. 17.11 Electromyography (EMG) responses of the opening and closing muscles of the UES during belching and swallowing activated by injection of 100 mL of air into the stomach of an awake and unanesthetized dog. Note that the only anteriorly directed UES opening muscle activated during belching is the TH and the main UES opening muscle activated is the posteriorly directed StP. These muscle responses are consistent with the movement of the hyoid during belching [87]. *StP* stylopharyngeus, *GH* geniohyoideus, *TH* thyrohyoideus, *CP* cricopharyngeus, *ESO* esophagus 1 cm below the CP, *SH* sternohyoideus. From I.M. Lang. GI motility online; 2006; doi:10.1038/gimo12 with permission from Nature Publishing Group

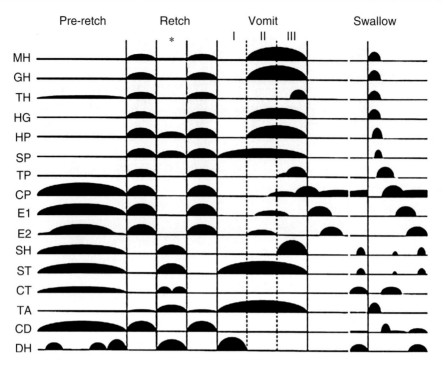

Fig. 17.12 Role of UES closure and opening muscles during the three phases of vomiting. Schematic illustration of typical pattern of activation of most pharyngeal, hyoid, and laryngeal muscles during vomiting derived from EMG data of chronically instrumented dogs stimulated to vomit by apomorphine. Note that during the preretch phase the tone of the CP and esophagus increase, significantly closing the UES. During retching the muscles pulling the UES open in a superior direction (superior hyoid muscles, HP and SP) are all activated in concert 180° out of phase with the UES opening muscles that open the UES in an inferior direction (inferior hyoid muscles). However, the UES does not open during superior movement because all of the UES closure muscles are activated as well. During vomiting, the superior and inferior hyoid and pharyngeal UES opening muscles are activated concomitantly with relaxation of all of the UES closure muscles, thereby causing maximum opening of the UES. *MH* mylohyoideus, *GH* geniohyoideus, *TH* thyrohyoideus, *HG* hyoglossus, *HP* hyopharyngeus, *SP* stylopharyngeus, *TP* thyropharyngeus, *CP* cricopharyngeus, *E#* esophagus number of centimeters from UES, *SH* stenohyoideus, *ST* sternothyroideus, *CT* cricothyroideus, *TA* thyroarytenoideus, *CD* cricoarytenoideus dorsalis, *DH* diaphragm hiatus. From I.M. Lang. GI motility online; 2006; doi:10.1038/gimo12 with permission from Nature Publishing Group

The UES during this phase of retching involves all three UES muscles, i.e., cervical esophagus, CP, and TP.

Vomitus Expulsion

During vomitus expulsion all of the UES closing muscles relax, and the UES is pulled open by contraction of the UES opening muscle. Not only are both the superior, i.e., suprahyoid muscles, and inferior, i.e., infrahyoid muscles, anterior UES opening muscles activated, but also the posterior UES opening muscles, e.g., stylopharyngeus [83]. The resultant force vector of simultaneous contraction of these muscles is a maximum anteriorly directed force which causes maximum opening of the UES. The primary UES opening muscles activated during vomitus expulsion are the mylohyoideus, geniohyoideus, sternohyoideus, and stylopharyngeus [83]. While the trajectory of the hyoid bone has not been determined during vomitus expulsion, based on the pattern of muscle activation the hyoid bone probably forms an elliptical path moving in the following sequence: posteriorly, superiorly, anteriorly, inferiorly, back to rest position. This movement pattern would be very different from that occurring during swallowing or belching.

UES Reflexes

Pharyngo-UES Contractile Reflex

Stimulation of the pharynx with light touch increases tone in the UES [90], and this response is due to activation of the TP and CP but primarily the CP [42]. It is unknown whether the cervical esophagus is involved in this reflex response. The most sensitive area of the pharynx was the hypopharynx and nasopharynx [42]. The afferent limb of this reflex is the GPN and the efferent limb is the pharyngeal branch of the vagus nerve [42]. This reflex may function to prevent air insufflation of the esophagus during strong inspiration as this reflex can be activated by air puffs and is strongest closest to the nasopharynx [90].

Esophago-UES Contractile Reflex

The slow distension of the esophagus causes an increase in tone of the UES or CP [41, 87, 91, 92], and this reflex involves all three UES muscles: CP, TP, and cervical esophagus, but primarily the CP. This reflex can be activated at all levels of the esophagus but is most sensitive near the UES [91], and the receptors for this reflex are probably slowly adapting muscular mechanoreceptors [41]. This reflex is stimulated not only by distension, but also by contraction of the esophageal wall and it is strongly activated by the propagating esophageal peristalsis [41]. The role of intraluminal acid in activating this reflex is equivocal as results have been contradictory [91, 93, 94]. The afferent limb of this reflex is complex. The afferent route from the thoracic esophagus are the vagus nerves [41, 68, 70], from the distal cervical esophagus are the caudally directed fibers of the RLNs [87], and from the proximal portion of the cervical esophagus are the rostrally directed fibers of the RLNs [29, 87]. It has been hypothesized [87] that these rostrally directed fibers connect to the nodose ganglia via the SLNs. The efferent limb of this reflex is the motor nerve of the cricopharyngeus which is the pharyngoesophageal branch of the vagus nerve in most animals [41] and possibly the RLN in humans. This reflex probably functions to prevent reflux of a bolus during its abroad propagation during esophageal peristalsis.

Esophago-UES Relaxation Reflex

The rapid distension of the esophagus causes relaxation of the UES [41, 84–86, 91] that involves the relaxation of the CP [41, 63, 86] and also probably the TP [41, 86]. This reflex is probably part of the belch response as it is activated by the same stimuli, and the pharyngeal and laryngeal motor responses that accompany this reflex are identical to those activated during belching as discussed previously [41]. In addition, spontaneous gastro-esophageal reflux episodes that cause esophageal common cavity or rapid increases in esophageal pressure are often associated with relaxation of the UES in what has been termed "microburps" [95]. The receptors for this reflex are probably rapidly adapting mucosal mechanoreceptors and the afferent limb of this reflex is the vagus nerve [41].

Vestibulo-UES Contractile Reflex

The UES tone changes greatly with change in head position and this tone change is due to activation of both the TP and CP, but primarily the CP [75, 78]. It is likely that this reflex is due to activation of the vestibular apparatus and may function to prevent pharyngeal reflux of esophageal contents when gravity is against the direction of peristalsis.

Lung-UES Contractile Reflex

The distension of the lungs above tidal volume or the rapid deflation of the lungs causes an increase in tone of the UES that is probably mediated by contraction of the TP and CP but primarily the CP [88]. The receptors for this reflex are probably rapidly adapting lung inflation receptors and the afferent limb of this reflex is the vagus nerve [96]. This reflex may be partly responsible for the respiratory rhythm that is often found on the UES [75, 78], and this reflex may function to prevent esophageal insufflation during deep inspirations. This reflex may also be partly responsible for the increase in UES pressure observed during phonation [97].

Development

The development of the UES and its functions has only recently been studied in humans, but the earliest age of development examined was 33 weeks postmenstrual age (PMA). The UES at 33 weeks PMA functions as in adulthood except that the specific parameters differ [98]. At 33 weeks PMA the UES of humans has a basal tone of 17 ± 7 mmHg which increases to 26 ± 14 at full term which is about one-half the adult level [98, 99]. On the other hand, the duration of the relaxation is about 2 s at 33 weeks PMA and at full term and this is about twice that of the adult [98]. In addition, the 33 weeks PMA infant has a functioning esophago-UES contractile reflex [98–101] as well as a pharyngo-UES contractile reflex [100]. The sensitivity of the esophago-UES contractile reflex increases from 33 to 36 weeks PMA [101]. Other UES functions have not been examined to date; however, the UES seems to be fully developed by at least 33 weeks PMA.

References

1. Brownlow H, Whitmore I, Willan P. A quantitative study of the histochemical and morphometric characteristics of the human cricopharyngeus muscle. J Anat. 1989;166:67–75.
2. Kristamundsdottir F, Mahon M, Froes MM, Cumming WJ. Histomorphometric and histological study of the human cricopharyngeus in health and in motor neuron disease. Neuropathol Appl Neurobiol. 1990;26:461–75.
3. Bonington A, Mahon M, Whitemore I. A histological and histochemical study of the cricopharyngeus muscle in man. J Anat. 1988;156:27–37.
4. Mu L, Sanders I. Neuromuscular organization of the human upper esophageal sphincter. Ann Otol Rhinol Laryngol. 2001;107:370–7.
5. Mu L, Sanders I. Muscle fiber-type distribution pattern in the human cricopharyngeus muscle. Dysphagia. 2002;17:87–96.
6. Mu L, Su H, Wang J, Sanders I. Myosin heavy chain-based fiber types in the adult human cricopharyngeus muscle. Muscle Nerve. 2007;35:637–48.
7. Mu L, Wang J, Su H, Sanders I. Adult human upper esophageal sphincter contains specialized muscle fibers expressing unusual myosin heavy chain isoforms. J Histochem Cytochem. 2007;55:199–207.
8. Medda BK, Lang IM, Dodds WJ, Christl M, Kern M, Hogan WJ, Shaker R. Correlation of electrical

and contractile activities of the cricopharyngeus muscle in the cat. Am J Physiol. 1997;273:G470–9.
9. Spiro D, Sonenblick EH. Comparison of the structural basis of the contractile process in heart and skeletal muscle. Circ Res. 1964;15 Suppl 11:14–7.
10. Asoh R, Goyal RK. Manometry and electromyography of the upper esophageal sphincter in the opossum. Gastroenterology. 1978;74:514–20.
11. Mu L, Sanders I. Neuromuscular compartments and fiber-type regionalization in the human inferior pharyngeal constrictor muscle. Anat Rec. 2001;264:367–77.
12. Mu L, Sanders I. Neuromuscular specializations within human pharyngeal constrictor muscles. Ann Otol Rhinol Laryngol. 2007;116:604–17.
13. Meyer GW, Austin RM, Brady CE, Castell DO. Muscle anatomy of the human esophagus. J Clin Gastroenterol. 1986;8:131–4.
14. Leese G, Hopwood D. Muscle fibre typing in the human pharyngeal constrictors and esophagus: effect of aging. J Anat. 1986;127:77–80.
15. Shedlofsky-Deschamps G, Krause WJ, Cutts JH, Hanson S. Histochemistry of the striated musculature in the opossum and human esophagus. J Anat. 1982;134:407–14.
16. Mascarello F, Rowlerson A, Scapolo PA. The fibre type composition of the striated muscle of the esophagus in ruminants and carnivores. Histochemistry. 1984;80:277–88.
17. Gray H, Goss CM. Anatomy of the human body. Philadelphia, PA: Lea & Febiger; 1968.
18. Bubb WJ, Sims MH. Fiber type composition of rostral and caudal portions of the digastric muscle in the dog. Am J Vet Res. 1986;47:1834–41.
19. Dick TE, Van Lunteren E. Fiber subtype distribution of pharyngeal dilator muscles and diaphragm in the cat. J Appl Physiol. 1990;687:2237–40.
20. Hisa Y, Malmgren LT, Lyon MJ. Quantitative histochemical studies on the cat infrahyoid muscles. Otolaryngol Head Neck Surg. 1990;103:723–32.
21. Mu L, Sanders I. The innervation of the human upper esophageal sphincter. Dysphagia. 1996;11:234–8.
22. Sasaki CT, Sims H, Kim Y-H, Czibulka A. Motor innervation of the human cricopharyngeus muscle. Ann Otol Rhinol Laryngol. 1999;108:1132–9.
23. Hwang K, Grossman MI, Ivy AC. Nervous control of the cervical portion of the esophagus. Am J Physiol. 1948;154:343–57.
24. Kobler JB, Datta S, Goyal RK, et al. Innervation of the larynx, pharynx, and upper esophageal sphincter of the rat. J Comp Neurol. 1994;349:129–47.
25. Lang IM, Medda BK, Shaker R. Functional studies of the innervation of the upper esophageal sphincter. Gastroenterology. 1998;114:A783.
26. Venker-van Haagen AJ, Hartman W, Wolvekamp WTC. Contributions of the glossopharyngeal nerve and the pharyngeal branch of the vagus nerve to the swallowing process. Am J Vet Res. 1986;47:1300–7.
27. Levitt MN, Dedo HH, Ogura JH. The cricopharyngeus muscle, an electromyographic study in the dog. Laryngoscope. 1965;75:122–36.

28. Venker-van Haagen AJ, Hartman W, Van den Brom WE, Wolvekamp WTC. Continuous electromyographic recordings of pharyngeal muscle activity in normal and previously denervated muscles in dogs. Am J Vet Res. 1989;50:1725–8.

29. Fukunaga Y, Higashino M, Osugi H, Tokuhara T, Kinoshita H. Function of the upper esophageal sphincter after denervation of recurrent laryngeal nerves and intramural nerves of the cervical esophagus in dogs. J Jap Surg Soc. 1994;95: 643–54.

30. Hwang K, Grossman MI. A note on the innervation of the cervical portion of the human esophagus. Gastroenterology. 1953;25:375–7.

31. Hammond CS, Davenport PW, Hutchison A, Otto RA. Motor innervation of the cricopharyngeus muscle by the recurrent laryngeal nerve. J Appl Physiol. 1997;83:89–94.

32. Brok HAJ, Copper MP, Stroeve RJ, Ongerboer BW, Venker-van Haagen AJ, Schouwenburg PF. Evidence for recurrent laryngeal nerve contribution in motor innervation of the human cricopharyngeal muscle. Laryngoscope. 1999;109:705–8.

33. Wilson JA, Pryde A, White A, Maran AGD. Swallowing performance in patients with vocal fold motion impairment. Dysphagia. 1995;10:149–54.

34. Halum SL, Shemirani N, Merati AL, Jaradeh S, Toothill RJ. Electromyography findings of the cricopharyngeus in association with ipsilateral pharyngeal and laryngeal muscles. Ann Otol Rhinol Laryngol. 2006;115:312–6.

35. Miyazaki J, Shin T, Murata Y, Masuko S. Pharyngeal branch of the vagus nerve carries intraepithelial afferent fibers in the cat pharynx: an elucidation of the origin and central and peripheral distribution of these components. Otolaryngol Head Neck Surg. 1999;120:905–13.

36. Maeyama T, Miyazaki J, Tsuda K, Shin T. Distribution and origin of the intraepithelial nerve fibers in the feline pharyngeal mucosa. Acta Otolaryngol Suppl. 1998;539:87–90.

37. Tanaka Y, Yoshida Y, Hirano M, Morimoto M, Kanaseki T. Intramucosal distribution of the glossopharyngeal sensory fibers of cats. Brain Res Bull. 1987;19:115–27.

38. Yoshida Y, Tanaka Y, Hirano M, Nakashima T. Sensory innervation of the pharynx and larynx. Am J Med. 2000;108(Suppl):51S–61.

39. Wank M, Neuhuber WL. Local differences in vagal afferent innervation of the rat esophagus are reflected by neurochemical differences at the level of the sensory ganglia and by different brainstem projections. J Comp Neurol. 2001;435:41–59.

40. Lang IM, Medda BK, Lamba R, Shaker R. Characterization and quantification of new aspects of the esophago-LES and -UES reflexes. Gastroenterology. 2011;140:T345.

41. Lang IM, Medda BK, Shaker R. Mechanisms of reflexes induced by esophageal distension. Am J Physiol. 2001;281:G1246–63.

42. Medda BK, Lang IM, Layman R, Dodds WJ, Hogan WJ, Shaker R. Characterization and quantification of a pharyngo-UES contractile reflex in cats. Am J Physiol. 1993;265:G963–72.

43. Nagai T. The occurrence and ultrastructure of a mechanoreceptor in the human cricopharyngeus muscle. Eur Arch Otorhinolaryngol. 1991;248:144–6.

44. Muntener M, Gottschall J, Neuhuber W, Mysicka A, Zenker W. The ansa cervicalis and the infrahyoid muscles of the rat. I. Anatomy; distribution, number and diameter of fiber types; motor units. Anat Embryol. 1980;159:49–57.

45. Maier A. Occurrence and distribution of muscle spindles in masticatory and suprahyoid muscles of the rat. Am J Anat. 1979;155:483–505.

46. Van Willigen JD, Morimoto T, Broekhuijsen ML, Bijl GK, Inoue T. An electromyographic study of whether the digastric muscles are controlled by jaw-closing proprioceptors in man. Arch Oral Biol. 1993;38:497–505.

47. Liss M. Muscle spindles in human levator veli palatini and palatoglossus muscles. J Speech Hear Res. 1990;33:736–46.

48. Tadaki N, Hisa Y, Uno T, Koike S, Okamura H, Ibata Y. Neurotransmitters for the canine inferior pharyngeal constrictor muscle. Otolaryngol Head Neck Surg. 1995;113:755–9.

49. Terenghi G, Polak JM, Rodrigo J, Mulderry PL, Bloom SR. Calcitonin gene-related peptide-immunoreactive nerves in the tongue, epiglottis and pharynx of the rat: occurrence, distribution and origin. Brain Res. 1986;365:1–14.

50. Rodrigo J, Polak JM, Fernandez L, Ghatei MP, Mulderry P, Bloom SR. Calcotinin gene-related peptide immunoreactive sensory and motor nerves of the rat, cat, and monkey esophagus. Gastroenterology. 1985;88:444–51.

51. Lawn AM. The localization in the nucleus ambiguus of the rabbit of the cells of origin of motor nerve fibers in the glossopharyngeal nerve and various branches of the vagus nerve by means of retrograde degeneration. J Comp Neurol. 1966;127:293–306.

52. Kitamura S, Ogata K, Nishiguchi T, Nagase Y, Shigenaga Y. Localization of the motoneurons supplying the rabbit pharyngeal constrictor muscles and the peripheral course of their axons: a study using retrograde HRP or fluorescent labeling technique. Anat Rec. 1989;229:399–406.

53. Bieger D, Hopkins DA. Viscerotopic representation of the upper alimentary tract in the medulla oblongata in the rat: the nucleus ambiguus. J Comp Neurol. 1987;262:546–62.

54. Holstege G, Graveland G, Bijker-Biemond C, Schuddeboom I. Location of motoneurons innervating soft palate, pharynx and upper esophagus. Anatomical evidence for a possible swallowing center in the pontine reticular formation. An HRP autoradiographic tracing study. Brain Behav Evol. 1983;23:47–62.

55. Collman PI, Tremblay L, Diamant N. The central efferent supply to the esophagus and lower esophageal

sphincter of the cat. Gastroenterology. 1993;104: 1430–8.

56. Lawn AM. The localization by means of electrical stimulation of the origin and path in the medulla oblongata of the motor nerve fibers of the rabbit esophagus. J Physiol. 1964;174:232–44.

57. Doty RW, Bosma JF. An electromyographic analysis of reflex deglutition. J Neurophysiol. 1956;19: 44–60.

58. Lang IM, Medda BK, Layman RD, Hogan WJ, Shaker R. Control of upper esophageal sphincter by the nucleus ambiguus. Gastroenterology. 1994;106: A529.

59. Altschuler SM, Bao X, Miselis RR. Dendritic architecture of nucleus ambiguus motoneurons projecting to the upper alimentary tract in the rat. J Comp Neurol. 1991;309:402–14.

60. Hayakawa T, Yajima T, Zyo K. Ultrastructural characterization of pharyngeal and esophageal motoneurons in the nucleus ambiguus of the rat. J Comp Neurol. 1996;370:135–46.

61. Grelot L, Barillot JC, Bianchi AL. Pharyngeal motoneurons: respiratory-related activity and response to laryngeal afferents in the decerebrate cat. Exp Brain Res. 1989;78:336–44.

62. Lang IM, Dean C, Medda BK, Aslam M, Shaker R. Differential activation of medullary vagal nuclei during different phases of swallowing in the cat. Brain Res. 2004;1014:145–63.

63. Lang IM, Medda BK, Shaker R. Differential activation of medullary vagal nuclei caused by stimulation of different esophageal mechanoreceptors. Brain Res. 2011;1368:119–33.

64. Altschuler SM, Bao X, Bieger D, Hopkins DA, Miselis RR. Visecerotopic representation of the upper alimentary tract in the rat: sensory ganglia and nuclei of the solitary tract and spinal trigeminal tracts. J Comp Neurol. 1989;283:248–68.

65. Brousard DL, Lyon RB, Wiedner EB, Altschuler SM. Solitarial premotor neuron projections to the rat esophagus and pharynx: implications for control of swallowing. Gastroenterology. 1998;114:1268–75.

66. Boa X, Wiedner EB, Altschuler SM. Transynaptic localization of pharyngeal premotor neurons in rat. Brain Res. 1995;696:246–9.

67. Hayakawa T, Takanaga A, Maeda S, Seki M, Yajima Y. Subnuclear distribution of afferents from the oral, pharyngeal, and laryngeal regions in the nucleus tractus solitarii of the rat: a study using transganglionic transport of cholera toxin. Neurosci Res. 2001; 39:221–32.

68. Collman PI, Tremblay L, Diamant NE. The distribution of spinal and vagal sensory n neurons that innervate the esophagus of the cat. Gastroenterology. 1992;103:817–22.

69. Neuhuber WL, Kressel M, Stark A, Berthoud HR. Vagal efferent and afferent innervation of the rat esophagus as demonstrated by anterograde DiI and DiA tracing: focus on myenteric ganglia. (J Auton Nerv Syst) JANS. 1998;70:92–102.

70. Qin C, Chandler MJ, Jou CI, Foreman RD. Responses and afferent pathways of C1-C2 spinal neurons to cervical and thoracic esophageal stimulation in rats. J Neurophysiol. 2004;91:2227–35.

71. Barrett RT, Bao X, Miselis RR, Altschuler SM. Brain stem localization of rodent esophageal premotor neurons revealed by transneuronal passage of pseudorabies virus. Gastroenterology. 1994;107: 728–37.

72. Lang IM, Medda BK, Shaker R. Differential activation of pontomedullary nuclei by acid perfusion of different regions of the esophagus. Brain Res. 2010;1352:94–107.

73. Castell JA, Dalton CB, Castell DO. Pharyngeal and upper esophageal sphincter manometry in humans. Am J Physiol. 1990;258:G173–8.

74. Kahrilas PJ, Dodds WJ, Dent J, Haebrle B, Hogan WJ, Arndorfer RC. Effect of sleep, spontaneous gastroesophageal reflux, and a meal on upper esophageal sphincter pressure in normal human volunteers. Gastroenterology. 1987;92:466–71.

75. Jacob P, Kahrilas PJ, Herzon G, McLaughlin B. Determinants of upper esophageal sphincter pressure in dogs. Am J Physiol. 1990;259:G245–51.

76. Cook IJ, Dent J, Shannon S, Collins SM. Measurement of upper esophageal sphincter pressure. Effect of acute emotional stress. Gastroenterology. 1987;93:526–32.

77. Cook IJ, Dent J, Collins SM. Upper esophageal sphincter tone and reactivity to stress in patients with a history of globus sensation. Dig Dis Sci. 1989;34: 672–6.

78. Lang IM, Dantas RO, Cook IJ, Dodds WJ. Videoradiographic, manometric and electromyographic assessment of upper esophageal sphincter. Am J Physiol. 1991;260:G911–9.

79. Goyal RK, Martin SB, Shapiro J, Spechler SJ. The role of cricopharyngeus muscle in pharyngoesophageal disorders. Dysphagia. 1993;8:253–8.

80. Cook IJ, Dodds WJ, Dantas RO, Massey B, Kern M, Lang IM, Brasseur J, Hogan WJ. Opening mechanisms of the upper esophageal sphincter. Am J Physiol. 1989;257:G748–59.

81. Kahrilas PJ, Dodds WJ, Dent J, Logemann JA, Shaker R. Upper esophageal sphincter function during deglutition. Gastroenterology. 1988;95: 52–62.

82. Lang IM, Sarna SK, Dodds WJ. The pharyngeal, esophageal, and gastric responses associated with vomiting. Am J Physiol. 1993;265:G963–72.

83. Lang IM, Dana N, Medda BK, Shaker R. Mechanisms of airway protection during retching, vomiting, and swallowing. Am J Physiol. 2002;283:G529–36.

84. Kahrilas PJ, Dodds WJ, Dent J, Wyman JB, Hogan WJ, Arndorfer RC. Upper esophageal function during belching. Gastroenterology. 1986;91:133–40.

85. Shaker R, Ren J, Kern M, Dodds WJ, Hogan WJ, Li Q. Mechanisms of airway protection and upper esophageal sphincter opening during belching. Am J Physiol. 1992;262:G621–8.

86. Lang IM, Dana N, Shaker R. The laryngeal, pharyngeal, and hyoid responses during swallowing, belching and vomiting. Gastroenterology. 2001;120:A122.

87. Freiman JM, El-Sharkaway TY, Diamant NE. Effect of bilateral vagosympathetic nerve blockade on response of the dog upper esophageal sphincter (UES) to intraesophageal distention and acid. Gastroenterology. 1981;81:78–84.

88. Monges H, Salducci J, Naudy B. The upper esophageal sphincter during vomiting, eructation, and distension of the cardia: an electromyographic study in the unanesthetized dog. In: Duthie HL, editor. Gastrointestinal motility in health and disease. Lancaster: MTP Press; 1978. p. 575–83.

89. Hesse O. Zur Kenntnes des Brechaktes. Nach Roentgenversuchen an Hunden. Pflugers Arch Gesamte Physiol. 1913;152:1–22.

90. Shaker R, Ren J, Xie P, Lang IM, bardan E, Sui Z. Characterization of the pharyngo-UES contractile reflex in humans. Am J Physiol. 1997;273:G854–8.

91. Szczesniak MM, Fuentealba SE, Burnett A, Cook IJ. Differential relaxation and contractile responses of the human upper esophageal sphincter mediated by interplay of mucosal and deep mechanorecptor activation. Am J Physiol. 2008;294:G982–8.

92. Enzmann DR, Harell GS, Zboralske FF. Upper esophageal responses to intraluminal distension in man. Gastroenterology. 1977;72:1292–8.

93. Vakil NB, Kahrilas PJ, Dodds WJ, Vanagunas A. Absence of an upper esophageal sphincter response to acid reflux. Am J Gastroenterol. 1989;84:606–10.

94. Gerhardt DC, Shuck TJ, Bordeaux RA, Winship DH. Human upper esophageal sphincter response to volume, osmotic and acid stimuli. Gastroenterology. 1978;75:268–74.

95. Pandolfino JE, Ghosh SK, Zhang Q, Han A, Kahrilas PJ. Upper sphincter function during transient lower oesophageal sphincter relaxation (tLOSR); it is mainly about microburps. Neurogastroenterol Motil. 2007;19(3):203–10.

96. Lang IM, Medda BK, Shaker R. Mechanism of the ventilatory cycle fluctuations in UES tone. Gastroenterology. 2000;118:A133.

97. Perera L, Kern M, Hofmann C, Tatro L, Chai K, Kuribayashi S, Lawal A, Shaker R. Manometric evidence for a phonation-induced UES contractile reflex. Am J Physiol. 2008;294:G885–91.

98. Jadcherla SR, Duong HQ, Hofmann C, Hofmann R, Shaker R. Characteristics of upper esophageal sphincter and oesophageal body during maturation in healthy human neonates compared with adults. Neurogastroenterol Motil. 2005;17:663–70.

99. Jadcherla SR, Duong HQ, Hoffman RG, Shaker R. Esophageal body and upper esophageal sphincter motor responses to esophageal provocation during maturation in preterm newborns. J Pediatr. 2003; 143:31–8.

100. Jadcherla SR, Gupta A, Stoner E, Fermande S, Shaker R. Pharyngeal swallowing: defining pharyngeal and upper esophageal sphincter relationships in human neonates. J Pediatr. 2007;151: 597–603.

101. Jadcherla SR, Hoffan RG, Shaker R. Effect of maturation of the magnitude of mechanosensitive and chemosensitive reflexes in the premature human esophagus. J Pediatr. 2006;147:77–82.

Deglutitive Pharyngeal and UES Pressure Phenomena

Erica A. Samuel and Reza Shaker

Abstract

Deglutitive pressure phenomena within the pharynx is generated by the contraction of pharyngeal constrictors, velum and posterior thrust of the tongue base. Due to axial as well as radial asymmetry, swallow induced pharyngeal pressure at any location varies depending on the radial directions and distance relative to the upper esophageal sphincter. With the recent availability of circumferential recording devices such those used in high resolution manometry, it is now possible to record average pressure at any location within the pharynx and overcome the radial asymmetry. The inherent shortening of the pharynx and the associated oral movement of the upper esophageal sphincter during swallowing poses a significant technical challenge in recognizing manometrically where the pharynx ends and where the UES begins. From a clinical perspective, however concurrent high resolution pharyngo-UES manometry can help ascertain pharyngeal peristalsis and its coordination with the UES relaxation, duration of UES relaxation and its coordination with pharyngeal peristalsis, hypopharyngeal intrabolus pressure.

Both UES resting pressure and its deglutitive manometric relaxation are multifactorial. UES resting high pressure zone is induced by coricopharyngeous muscle (main component), distal inferior pharyngeal

E.A. Samuel, MD
Division of Gastroenterology and Hepatology,
Medical College of Wisconsin, 9200 W. Wisconsin Ave,
Milwaukee, WI 53226, USA

R. Shaker, MD (✉)
Division of Gastroenterology and Hepatology, Digestive
Disease Center, Clinical and Translational Science
Institute, Medical College of Wisconsin, 9200 W.
Wisconsin Ave, Milwaukee, WI 53226, USA
e-mail: rshaker@mcw.edu

R. Shaker et al. (eds.), *Principles of Deglutition: A Multidisciplinary Text for Swallowing and its Disorders*, 257
DOI 10.1007/978-1-4614-3794-9_18, © Springer Science+Business Media New York 2013

constrictor and the most proximal part of the striated esophagus. Manometric UES relaxation observed during swallowing is induced by a) loss of tone of the UES muscles mainly cricopharyngeous and b) opening of the UES by the traction forces generated by the contraction of suprahyoid UES opening muscles. Distinguishing between these two effects based on manometric recording is virtually impossible, but based on earlier concurrent manometric, electromyographic and fluoroscopic recordings it seems that the sharp pressure decline reaching subatmospheric pressure is due to UES opening. Recent advances in reliable pharyngeal pressure recording, promises better defined clinical applications which await confirmation by adequate clinical trials.

Keywords

Deglutitive pharyngeal pressure phenomena • UES pressure phenomena • UES high pressure zone • Inter-cordal pressure • Intra-tracheal pressure • Straining • Swallowing • Coughing • Phonation

With the availability of reliable recording devices, an increased clinical and research interest has developed in the evaluation of pharyngeal and upper esophageal sphincter (UES) deglutitive pressure phenomena. Intraluminal manometry is now recognized to have the potential to provide important information about the physiology and pathophysiology of pharyngeal and UES motor function.

Three pressure events involving the oral cavity, glottis, and the UES occur temporally related to the pharyngeal pressure event during swallowing. Pressure events in the oral phase of swallowing are presented in earlier chapters. This review will provide basic information about intra-pharyngeal and UES pressure phenomena during swallowing and its relationship with the kinematics of solid and liquid boluses. In addition, the vocal cord closing pressure generated during swallowing as it counteracts and resists intra-bolus pressure, along with other known mechanisms to prevent aspiration, will be discussed.

Because of the axial asymmetry of the pharynx [1], the evaluation of pharyngeal peristaltic activity should reference recording sites to the UES high pressure zone (HPZ). This arrangement makes it possible to measure the parameters of pharyngeal peristalsis at sites with similar distances from the UES and to study the effect of bolus variables

such as volume, consistency, and temperature on pharyngeal peristalsis at comparable distances from the UES. Studying comparable sites in regard to their distance from the UES is also essential for reliable inter-group and inter-study comparisons.

The major finding of studies recording pharyngeal pressure phenomena is that in healthy young individuals the amplitude of the pharyngeal pressure wave increases precipitously while its duration decreases progressively as the wave travels from the proximal to the distal pharynx reaching maximum amplitude with the shortest duration in the hypopharynx [2]. These studies also show that the entire pharynx remains contracted until the hypo-pharyngeal pressure wave progresses into the UES. Among factors that may influence pharyngeal peristalsis, the effects of aging, bolus variables, and subject position have been well studied.

The major differences found between young and elderly, over the age of 70, were in the hypopharynx. The peristaltic pressure wave amplitude and duration were significantly greater in elderly compared with young healthy volunteers (Fig. 18.1) (Table 18.1, $p<0.05$) [2]. In addition, with regard to the duration of the pharyngeal peristaltic pressure wave, the pattern of precipitous aboral decrease in duration (seen in the

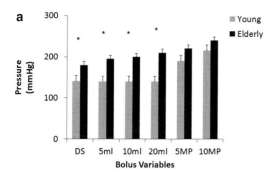

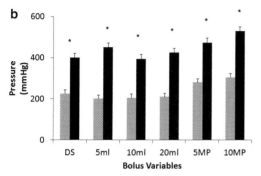

Fig. 18.1 Comparison of hypopharyngeal pressure wave amplitude (**a**) and duration (**b**) between young and elderly volunteers. For all tested boluses, hypopharyngeal pressure wave duration in the elderly was significantly longer than that of the young ($*p<0.01$). However, whereas hypopharyngeal pressure wave amplitude in the elderly during swallowing of 0–20 ml of water was significantly greater than that of the young ($*p<0.01$), these differences did not reach statistical significance for mashed potato swallows. From R. Shaker et al. Am J Physiol 1993;264:G427–32 with permission

young) is reported to be altered in the elderly, and the duration of the peristaltic pressure wave in the elderly at the hypopharynx is longer compared to more proximal sites (Fig. 18.2).

It is speculated that these changes in duration and amplitude of hypopharyngeal peristalsis with age are compensatory responses to the reduced cross-sectional area of the deglutitive UES opening [2, 3], causing an increase in outflow resistance. This is supported by the finding of increased intra-bolus pressure, a reliable indicator of resistance to the flow, in the hypo-pharynx of elderly subjects. In addition, in both young and elderly, the intra-bolus pressure in the supine position has been reported to be significantly higher compared with the upright position ($p<0.05$), which benefits from the effect of

gravity. These studies also show that although in both the young and elderly, bolus volume and temperature do not alter the parameters of the peristaltic pressure wave, swallowing of materials with higher consistency such as mashed potato significantly increases its amplitude and duration.

These findings suggest the existence of a consistency, but not volume, responsive modulatory mechanism between the pharynx and the brainstem. This is consistent with the effect of mashed potato on lingual peristalsis, reported earlier [4]. An interesting finding is that the amplitude of the hypopharyngeal peristaltic pressure wave during swallowing of mashed potato was found to be similar between the young and the elderly, whereas for dry and water swallows, it was significantly greater in the elderly. An explanation for this phenomenon could be that in the elderly, the peristaltic amplitude had already approached its maximum physiological limit for water swallows, and further increase with mashed potato swallows was not possible.

Correlation of the pharyngeal and UES pressure phenomena with the kinematics of a barium pellet as well as liquid barium has revealed interesting findings in healthy young individuals [5]. During each swallow, the velocity of the pellets varied as they traversed the pharynx, UES, and proximal esophagus. The velocity variability was location-dependent. There were two distinct zones of increasing velocity: over the tongue base and at the pharyngo-UES. These studies also have shown an influence of age on this relationship [6]. The average velocity of the pellet traversing the dorsum of the tongue averaged 18.4 (±1.3) and 17.2 (±3.1) cm/s for the young and elderly subjects, respectively. This velocity increased to 39.5 (±3.1) and 32.1 (±3.1) cm/s in the young and elderly subjects, respectively, while the pellet traversed the base of the tongue to the level of the inverted epiglottis (supraglottic region). During this time, the larynx had reached its maximum elevation and the epiglottis had assumed its horizontal orientation. The pellet velocity decreased significantly to 8.9 (±3.1) and 13.2 (±3.7) cm/s in the young and elderly subjects, respectively, while it traversed the area between the tip of the horizontal epiglottis and

Table 18.1 Effect of Aging and position on intrabolus pressure (mmHg) in hypopharynx

Bolus variables	WS$_5$		WS$_{10}$		WS$_{20}$		MP$_5$		MP$_{10}$	
	Young	Elderly	Young	Elderly	Young	Elderly	Young	Elderly	Young	Elderly
Upright	4.8±1.4	8.5±5*	5.7±1.3	11.2±3.2*	7.7±1.3	14.4±3.9*	10.4±2.4	18.8± 2.9	16.8± 3.1	34.5± 6.7*
Supine	13.3±2.1†	19.7± 1.5*,†	17.6± 1.7*,†	21.2±3.3*,†	Not tested		17.0±3.0†	29.0± 4.2*,†	23.6± 3.8†	42.8± 7.6*,†

Values are means ± SE; n = 14young and 12 elderly volunteers. P < 0.05 in *elderly volunteers compared with young and in †supine position compared to upright. WS$_5$: 5 mL water swallow, WS$_{10}$: 10 mL water swallow, WS$_{20}$: 20 mL water swallow, MP$_5$: 5 mL mash potato swallow, MP$_{10}$: 10 mL mash potato swallow. From R. Shaker, et al. Am J Physiol. 1993;264:G427–32 with permission

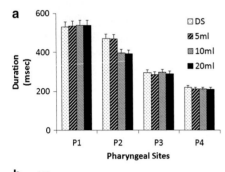

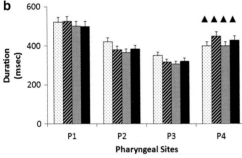

Fig. 18.2 Effect of volume and age on duration of pharyngeal peristaltic pressure wave. Although in the young (**a**) duration of peristaltic pressure wave showed precipitous aboral decrease from sites PI to P4 (p<0.01), in the elderly (**b**) this aboral decrease was interrupted at site P4, at which duration increased significantly instead of further decrease and became similar to site P2. Between-group comparison showed that in the elderly, duration of pharyngeal peristaltic for tested volumes at site P4 was significantly greater than that of the young (p<0.01). From R. Shaker et al. Am J Physiol 1993;264:G427–32 with permission

the posterior pharyngeal wall (pharyngo-epiglottic space). After the pellet passed this area, its velocity increased to an average of 31.8 (±2.4) cm/s in the young subjects (p<0.05) but remained at 13.2 (±1.7) cm/s in the elderly subjects while it passed through the pharyngo-UES

area to enter the proximal esophagus. After the pellet entered the esophagus, its velocity decreased to 11.8 (±1.2) and 10.7 (±3.0) cm/s in the young and elderly subjects, respectively (p<0.05 and p=not significant, respectively).

In these studies analysis of the concurrent manometric and videofluoroscopic recordings showed that, in both young and elderly groups, the pellet traveled ahead of the peristaltic pressure wave and the acceleration of the barium pellet was associated with incrementally decreasing pressure distal to the location of the pellet in the hypopharynx and across the UES. As the pellet passed each manometric recording site, the concurrent pressure at each site distal to it showed a progressive decline (Fig. 18.3).

For liquid boluses, the kinematic and dynamic characteristics of the bolus head were significantly different from those of the bolus tail. As with the pellet swallows, there was an incrementally decreasing pressure distribution distal to the bolus head. The temporal and spatial pressure distributions in the regions distal to the head of the barium bolus were similar to those for pellet swallows. The forces related to bolus tail kinematics were associated with the peristaltic pressure wave. Comparison of peristaltic pressure wave velocity, measured manometrically, and bolus tail speed, measured fluoroscopically, showed that the two phenomena were virtually identical: 11.0 (±0.3) and 10.9 (±0.3) cm/s, respectively, in the elderly subjects and 10.5 (±0.5) and 10.6 (±0.5) cm/s, respectively, in the young subjects.

Furthermore, analysis of the concurrent manometric and fluoroscopic recordings showed that the upstroke of the peristaltic pressure wave was

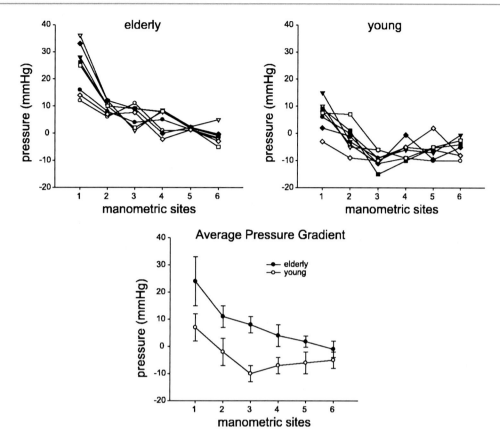

Fig. 18.3 Trans-sphincteric pressure gradient during pellet swallows in elderly and young subjects and average pressure gradient for each subject and grand average for each age group. Pressure values were evaluated at each manometric site at the instant the pellet was just above the most proximal pressure recording site. Nadir pressure and overall pressure gradient are higher in elderly than in young subjects. From E. Bardan et al. Am J Physiol Gastrointest Liver Physiol 2006;290:G458–465 with permission

always associated, both temporally and spatially, with the tail of the barium bolus. In addition, analysis of concurrent manometric and fluoroscopic recordings identified three different zones in relation to the position of the bolus: (1) the peristaltic zone, located behind the bolus, (2) the bolus zone, occupied by the bolus, and (3) the pre-bolus zone, located ahead of the bolus. In the peristaltic zone, the lumen is occluded by muscular contraction and exhibited positive maximum pressure averaging 178 (±16) and 133 (±11) mmHg in the elderly and young subjects, respectively. The bolus zone is the unclosed luminal region that is occupied by the bolus and reflects the intra-bolus pressure. The pre-bolus zone, i.e., the region immediately distal to the position of the bolus, exhibited a progressive decline in pressure across the pharyngo-esophageal junction, for which

sub-atmospheric pressures were commonly recorded as described above (Fig. 18.4).

Two significant differences between the elderly and young subjects have been revealed in regard to solid and liquid bolus kinematics and dynamics: (1) Young individuals have two zones of bolus acceleration in the pharynx, where in elderly the distal acceleration zone just above the UES is absent. (2) The downhill trans-sphincteric pressure gradient had a significantly higher nadir level in the elderly than in the young subjects. The presence of a decreasing pressure gradient throughout the pharyngo-esophageal segment ahead of the swallowed bolus has been previously reported in young healthy individuals [5]. Subsequent studies demonstrated the presence of similar gradients in intra-bolus pressure as liquid boluses traverse this segment [7].

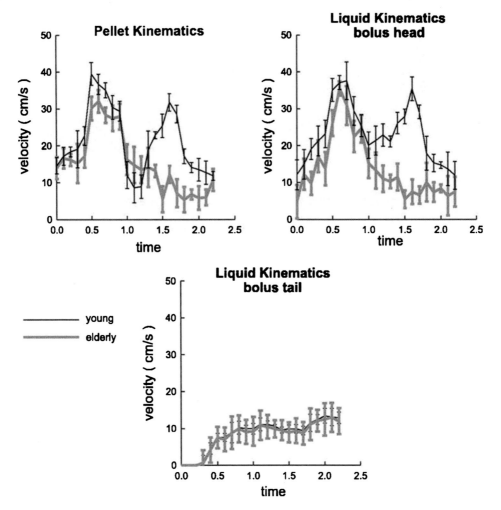

Fig. 18.4 Composite time history of average solid and liquid bolus head and tail kinematics in elderly and young subjects. Primary kinematic difference between the two age groups is the latter period of pellet and bolus head acceleration (at ~1.5 s), when young swallows are characterized by a substantial period of acceleration, but elderly swallows do not show the same pronounced increase in the velocity. From E. Bardan et al. Am J Physiol Gastrointest Liver Physiol 2006;290:G458–465 with permission

UES High Pressure Zone

The length of the UES HPZ in young health volunteers has been reported to average 3 cm (2.9±0.1 cm posterior; 3.1±0.2 cm anterior). This length is significantly longer than that of the elderly (2.1±0.7 cm posterior; 1.9±0.1 cm anterior) ($p < 0.01$). Resting UES pressure in the young (62±7 mmHg) is also significantly higher than that of the elderly (42±5 mmHg) ($p < 0.05$). Interestingly, the length of the lower esophageal sphincter HPZ is similar in the young (21±0.4 cm)

and elderly (21±0.2 cm) [8]. (For detailed discussion of UES relaxation and opening during swallowing refer to Chap. 37.)

It is noteworthy that aging affects the UES and LES differently, with regard to resting pressure and length. These findings suggest aging weakens the UES, but has no significant effect on the LES. The differences observed in these studies add to the list of previously reported significant reduction in biomechanical events with aging, such as anterior laryngeal excursion and UES opening.

Radial asymmetry of the UES HPZ is an accepted notion based on manometric studies profiling the resting pressure phenomenon within the UES [9–11]. Pressures are found to be lower in the lateral orientation compared with antero-posterior pressures due to differences in anatomy of the UES [11]. This finding however has been reevaluated recently and the influence of diameter and shape of recording device has been documented [12].

UES pressure measurement historically has been modeled after that of the lower esophageal sphincter [12] and as such, a cylindrical catheter has been used for defining its radial and axial pressure profile. However, UES anatomical configuration is quite different from that of the LES. Different configurations of pressure measurement influence the pressures measured due to the elliptical configuration of the UES.

The effect of catheter diameter and configuration on the measured pressures within the UES has been determined by comparing the pressure profile of the UES obtained using a round catheter assembly with an outer diameter of 4.8 mm, commonly used for manometric studies, to those obtained using a flat ribbon-shaped catheter assembly (4.8×1.2 mm) that conformed to the anatomy of the UES. In addition, comparisons have been made between the UES pressure profile in healthy elderly and young subjects. The round catheter assembly measured pressures that were significantly greater anteriorly and posteriorly compared with pressures recorded from lateral directions. This radial asymmetry was not found in the UES pressure profile when the smaller diameter conforming catheter assembly was used for measurement. The absence of radial asymmetry was due to a significant decrease in the anteriorly and posteriorly recorded pressures within the UES resulting in similarity of anteriorly, posteriorly, and laterally oriented pressures [12].

The effect of catheter diameter on UES pressure has been investigated previously [13–15] and has shown a direct relationship between the diameter of the recording catheter and the magnitude of UES pressure, a phenomenon attributed to the length–tension characteristic of the UES muscles. These findings lead to the following conclusions in regard to UES pressure asymmetry: (1) The magnitude of measured UES

anterior/posterior pressure is directly related to the diameter of the measuring device and as such may not reflect the normal physiological tone of the sphincter. (2) An exaggerated anteriorly and posteriorly oriented pressure may be recorded compared with lateral pressures depending on the diameter and nonconforming shape of the recording catheter with respect to the UES producing the appearance of radial asymmetry in the UES HPZ. Use of catheter devices, such as high-resolution manometry which averages the circumferentially recorded pressures, may overestimate the UES pressure depending on their diameter.

Vocal Cord Closure Pressure During Volitional Swallow and Other Voluntary Tasks

Closure of the vocal cords is an integral part of various functions involving the aerodigestive tract including swallowing [16], coughing [17, 18], straining, Valsalva maneuver [19], belching [20], and several airway protective reflexes such as esophagoglottal closure [21], pharyngoglottal closure [22, 23], and intrinsic laryngeal adductor reflexes. Whereas the duration of vocal cord closure during the events can be measured by direct videoendoscopic techniques, the closure pressure that the cords generate during the above functions and whether this closure pressure varies depending on the performed function were not known until videoendoscopic and manometric techniques were combined [16, 19–21].

This study, using concurrent videoendoscopy and manometry, measured the vocal cord closure pressure and its corresponding intra-tracheal pressure during several physiological events such as swallowing, coughing, straining, and phonation [24]. An example of vocal cord closure pressure during a dry swallow is shown in Fig. 18.5. As seen in this swallow the vocal cord closure pressure reached 220 mmHg and was associated with a biphasic pressure wave in the trachea. The original sub-atmospheric pressure of about 4 mmHg was followed by a positive pressure of 6 mmHg in the trachea.

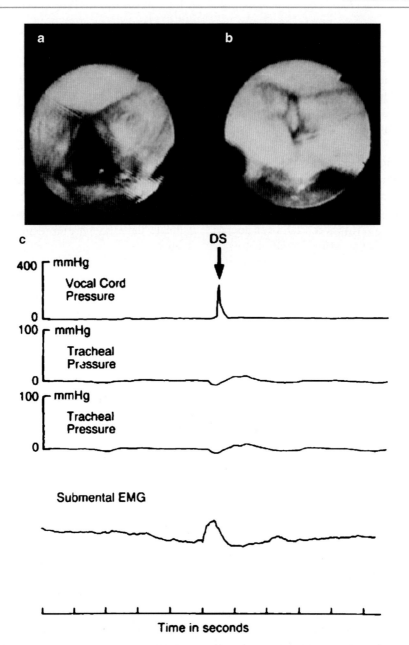

Fig. 18.5 An example of vocal cord closing pressure during a dry swallow. (**a, b**) Still frame from videoendoscopic recording of glottal manometry during dry swallow. (**a**) Vocal cords immediately prior to the onset of their adduction; (**b**) complete closure of the vocal cords just prior to laryngeal elevation. Manometric catheter is seen at the right lower corner of the image. (**c**) Vocal cords and tracheal pressure during maximum deglutitive closure of the cords, just prior to laryngeal elevation. From R. Shaker et al. Dysphagia 2002;17:13–18 with permission

Comparison of inter-cordal and intra-tracheal pressure during straining, swallowing, coughing, and phonation showed that inter-cordal pressure during straining, coughing, and swallowing was significantly higher than that of phonation ($*p < 0.05$). Straining produced pressures significantly higher than coughing ($\#p < 0.05$). Intra-tracheal pressure during coughing induced

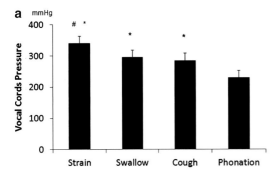

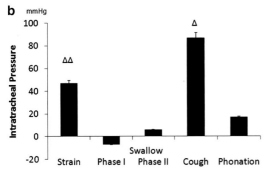

Fig. 18.6 Comparison of inter-cordal and intra-tracheal pressure during straining, swallowing, coughing, and phonation. From R. Shaker et al. Dysphagia 2002;17:13–18 with permission

pressure significantly higher than all other studied events ($\Delta p < 0.05$). Intra-tracheal pressure during straining was significantly higher than those of phonation and swallowing ($\Delta \Delta p < 0.01$). For all studied events, inter-cordal pressures were significantly higher than intra-tracheal pressures (Fig. 18.6).

These studies demonstrate that, the vocal cords generate closure pressures that vary depending on the performed function, i.e., the vocal cord pressure is not stereotyped for all functions. Vocal cord closure pressures are significantly higher than those of the intra-tracheal pressures during various tasks such as coughing, straining, swallowing, and phonation. Considering the fact that the hypo-pharyngeal intra-bolus pressures for crystalloid and semi-solid bolus (mashed potato) in healthy young and elderly, in supine and upright positions, have been reported to range between 5 and 43 mmHg [2, 25], the pressures generated by vocal closures provide a strong barrier against penetration of the swallowed material into trachea.

In summary, the evaluation of pharyngeal pressure phenomena continues to be a powerful research modality. Application of this modality to clinical practice has come of age and can offer useful information in selected conditions. In this regard not only evaluation of peristaltic pressure wave, but also the magnitude of intrabolus pressure in the hypopharynx should be performed. While the information on peristalsis can be helpful in terms of pathophysiology of incomplete pharyngeal bolus clearance, the data on intrabolus pressure provide important insight into pharyngeal outflow resistance induced by abnormalities of UES opening. This technique can provide important information on coordination of pharyngeal peristaltic wave and UES deglutitive relaxation and postrelaxation contraction, which can be helpful in the explanation of some cases of dysphagia and incomplete pharyngeal clearance. In addition, newer recording devices measuring pressure and impedance along with state-of-the-art analysis techniques have recently been introduced with potential to predict aspiration in at-risk individuals [26, 27].

References

1. Pryde A, et al. Radial and axial asymmetry of the pharynx (abstract). Am J Gastrointest Motility. 1991; 3(3):196.
2. Shaker R, et al. Effect of aging and bolus variables on pharyngeal and upper esophageal sphincter motor function. Am J Physiol. 1993;264(3 Pt 1):G427–32.
3. Shaw DW, et al. Influence of normal aging on oral-pharyngeal and upper esophageal sphincter function during swallowing. Am J Physiol. 1995;268(3 Pt 1):G389–96.
4. Shaker R, et al. Pressure-flow dynamics of the oral phase of swallowing. Dysphagia. 1988;3(2):79–84.
5. Bardan E, et al. Effect of aging on bolus kinematics during the pharyngeal phase of swallowing. Am J Physiol Gastrointest Liver Physiol. 2006;290(3): G458–65.
6. Kern MK, et al. Kinematic and dynamic characteristics of solid pellet movement during the pharyngeal phase of swallowing. Ann Otol Rhinol Laryngol. 1996;105(9):716–23.
7. Pal A, et al. Intrabolus pressure gradient identifies pathological constriction in the upper esophageal sphincter during flow. Am J Physiol Gastrointest Liver Physiol. 2003;285(5):G1037–48.

8. Bardan E, et al. Effect of ageing on the upper and lower oesophageal sphincters. Eur J Gastroenterol Hepatol. 2000;12(11):1221–5.

9. Sears Jr VW, Castell JA, Castell DO. Radial and longitudinal asymmetry of human pharyngeal pressures during swallowing. Gastroenterology. 1991;101(6):1559–63.

10. Winans CS. The pharyngoesophageal closure mechanism: a manometric study. Gastroenterology. 1972;63(5):768–77.

11. Sivarao DV, Goyal RK. Functional anatomy and physiology of the upper esophageal sphincter. Am J Med. 2000;108(Suppl 4a):27S–37.

12. Bardan E, et al. Radial asymmetry of the upper oesophageal sphincter pressure profile: fact or artefact. Neurogastroenterol Motil. 2006;18(6):418–24.

13. DiRe C, et al. Manometric characteristics of the upper esophageal sphincter recorded with a microsleeve. Am J Gastroenterol. 2001;96(5):1383–9.

14. Lydon SB, et al. The effect of manometric assembly diameter on intraluminal esophageal pressure recording. Am J Dig Dis. 1975;20(10):968–70.

15. Wallin L, et al. Intraluminal oesophageal manometry. Influence of pressure probe diameter. Scand J Gastroenterol. 1980;15(7):865–8.

16. Shaker R, et al. Coordination of deglutitive glottic closure with oropharyngeal swallowing. Gastroenterology. 1990;98(6):1478–84.

17. Irwin RS, Rosen MJ, Braman SS. Cough. A comprehensive review. Arch Intern Med. 1977;137(9):1186–91.

18. Loudon RD, Shaw GB. Mechanisms of cough in normal subjects and in patients with obstructive respiratory disease. Am Rev Respir Dis. 1967;96:666–77.

19. Martin BJ, et al. Normal laryngeal valving patterns during three breath-hold maneuvers: a pilot investigation. Dysphagia. 1993;8(1):11–20.

20. Shaker R, et al. Mechanisms of airway protection and upper esophageal sphincter opening during belching. Am J Physiol. 1992;262(4 Pt 1):G621–8.

21. Shaker R, et al. Esophagoglottal closure reflex: a mechanism of airway protection. Gastroenterology. 1992;102(3):857–61.

22. Ren J, et al. Glottal adduction response to pharyngeal water stimulation: evidence for a pharyngoglottal closure reflex. Gastroenterology. 1994;106(4–2):A558.

23. Shaker R, et al. Pharyngoglottal closure reflex: identification and characterization in a feline model. Am J Physiol. 1998;275(3 Pt 1):G521–5.

24. Shaker R, et al. Vocal cord closure pressure during volitional swallow and other voluntary tasks. Dysphagia. 2002;17(1):13–8.

25. Cook IJ, et al. Opening mechanisms of the human upper esophageal sphincter. Am J Physiol. 1989;257 (5 Pt 1):G748–59.

26. Omari TI, et al. A method to objectively assess swallow function in adults with suspected aspiration. Gastroenterology. 2011;140(5):1454–63.

27. Omari TI, et al. Reproducibility and agreement of pharyngeal automated impedance manometry with videofluoroscopy. Clin Gastroenterol Hepatol. 2011;9(10):862–7.

Part VI

Esophageal Phase of Deglutition

Development, Anatomy, and Physiology of the Esophagus

19

Kyle Staller and Braden Kuo

Abstract

Esophageal embryonic development and anatomic features play an important role in both normal function and common pathology of the esophagus. The embryonic endoderm provides the scaffolding for the future esophagus, which will ultimately connect the pharynx to the stomach. The developed esophagus has close anatomic relationships with the cervical spine, thoracic aorta, left atrium, and diagphragmatic haitus—relationships associated with esophageal pathology. Esophageal musculature is composed of an external layer of longitudinal fibers and an internal layer of circular fibers which provide peristaltic force; the backflow of food and acidic gastric contents is prevented at the level of two high-pressure regions: the upper and the lower esophageal sphincters. Microscopically, the esophageal wall is composed of four layers: internal mucosa, submucosa, muscularis propria, and adventitia. The esophagus has a segmental arterial supply without dedicated vasculature. Venous drainage is notable for being a portal-caval connection susceptible to portal hypertension. Esophageal innervation occurs via the sympathetic and parasympathetic nervous systems, as well as the intrinsic enteric nervous system.

Keywords

Esophagus • Esophageal Embryology • Muscular Layers • Mucosa • Muscularis Propria • Adventitia • Sympathetic System

K. Staller, MD
Department of Internal Medicine, Resident in Internal Medicine, Massachusetts General Hospital,
55 Fruit Street, GRB 740, Boston, MA 02114, USA

B. Kuo, MD, BSc, MSc (✉)
Department of Gastroenterology, Instructor in Medicine, Harvard Medical School, Massachusetts General Hospital, MGH, Digestive Healthcare Center,
165 Cambridge St 9th floor, Boston, MA 02114, USA
e-mail: bkuo@partners.org

R. Shaker et al. (eds.), *Principles of Deglutition: A Multidisciplinary Text for Swallowing and its Disorders*,
DOI 10.1007/978-1-4614-3794-9_19, © Springer Science+Business Media New York 2013

Esophageal Embryology and Development

The first stages of life are divided into the embryonic and fetal periods. The embryonic period extends from fertilization to week 9. The fetal period lasts from the end of the week 9 to birth. From days 0 to 14, the human embryo develops into a bilaminar disk of ectoderm and endoderm, with the endoderm forming the lining of the yolk sac. The endoderm is the scaffold for the future digestive tract. The ectoderm gives rise to epidermis and neural plates. Through the neurulation process, the neural plates evolve to neural tube and neural crest cells. The neural tube is the precursor for the spinal cord and brain. The neural crest cells, placed between the dorsal neural tube and the overlying epidermis, migrate out to form the peripheral nervous system by week 4. On day 15, the third embryonic layer, the mesoderm, appears and provides the substrate for the connective tissue, angioblasts, smooth muscle, and serosal layers of the gut. By day 21, the mesoderm is thickened and forms longitudinal masses called the paraxial mesoderm. By day 28, the paraxial mesoderm fragments develop progressively from cranial to caudal into cubes of tissue called somites. This process ends with the formation of 33–35 somites by day 31 of embryo development [1].

Mesoderm proliferation and segmentation, which takes place between the endoderm and ectoderm, induces numerous transformations in the endoderm [2]. At the same time, the human embryo elongates craniocaudally and folds laterally. The dorsal part of the yolk sac, composed of endoderm, is compressed by the lateral folding of the embryo and is incorporated as a rim during the fourth week. Thus the human embryo becomes a "body cylinder" dividing the yolk sac into intraembryonic and extraembryonic parts [3]. The intraembryonic part is the origin of digestive tube and its accessory glands. The extraembryonic part regresses and disappears around week 12. At this point, the early digestive system divides into foregut, midgut, and hindgut.

Gut development takes place in four major patterned axes: anterior–posterior, dorsal–ventral, left–right, and craniocaudal. Each axis development is based on the epithelial–mesenchymal interactions mediated by specific molecular pathways [4]. Thus, growth factors such as Wnt5a (expressed by mesoderm), endodermal proteins Six2/Sox2, as well as Hoxa-2, Hoxa-3, and Hoxb-4 control esophageal development in the anterior–posterior axis [5]. These factors affect both the esophageal environment and the neural crest cells by making the environment more permissive for neural crest cells and by preparing the neural crest cells to migrate within the esophagus [4, 5] (Fig. 19.1).

During week 4, the foregut develops a small diverticulum on its ventral surface adjacent to the pharyngeal gut. This tracheobronchial diverticulum subsequently elongates and separates gradually from the dorsal foregut through the formation of the esophagotracheal septum to become the primitive respiratory tract.

The remaining part of the foregut rapidly elongates with the craniocaudal growth of the embryonic body. In the seventh and eighth weeks, the luminal epithelium proliferates and almost completely occludes the foregut with only residual channels persisting. Unlike other species, complete occlusion of the foregut has not been observed in human embryos [6]. By week 10, new vacuoles appear in the luminal cells of the foregut and coalesce to form a single esophageal lumen with a superficial layer of ciliated epithelial cells [1].

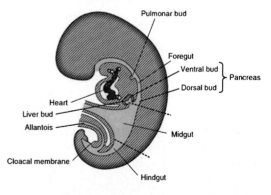

Fig. 19.1 Drawing of median section of the embryo showing the early digestive system. The primordial gut is a long tube extending the length of the embryo

During the fourth month, a stratified squamous epithelium begins to replace the ciliated epithelium, a process that continues until birth. Residual islands of ciliated epithelium at the proximal and distal ends of the esophagus remain and give rise to esophageal glands [1]. Thus the primitive foregut endoderm is the origin for both the future esophageal epithelium and submucosal glands. During week 6 of gestation, the circular muscle coat and ganglion cells of the myenteric plexus form. During week 7, blood vessels enter the submucosa.

The smooth muscle of the lower esophagus and the lower esophageal sphincter (LES) are derived from the mesenchyme of the somites surrounding the foregut. The striated muscle forming the muscularis propria of the upper part of the esophagus and the upper esophageal sphincter (UES) is derived from mesenchyme of the branchial arches 4, 5, and 6. This origin explains the UES innervation by the vagus nerve (the branchial arch 5 nerve) and by the recurrent laryngeal nerve (a branch of the vagus nerve, the branchial arch 6 nerve). The embryologic origin of the gastroesophageal (GE) junction is still controversial, but gastric rotation together with augmentation of the fundus of the stomach is believed to determine its formation [7].

The middle third of esophagus consists of a mixture of smooth and skeletal muscle. The origin of this mixture is controversial, with somites and endoderm influencing each other by molecular mechanisms [4]. It was suggested that esophageal striated muscle arises from the smooth muscle by a process of transdifferentiation; however, it appears that the two muscle types may arise from two distinct differentiation pathways. When definitive endoderm was co-cultured with somitic mesoderm, it stimulated more smooth muscle development than skeletal muscle from the mesenchymal somitic cells [8].

The smooth muscle differentiation begins after the neural crest cells colonize the gut and maturates on the rostrocaudal axis [9]. Whether the circular muscle layer precedes or appears at the same time as the longitudinal muscle layer is still controversial, but both layers have been reported to mature into a rostrocaudal axis by week 9 [9, 10].

At the beginning of week 4, the neural crest cells enter the foregut and migrate rostrocaudally to reach the terminal hindgut by week 7 and give rise to the myenteric plexus [10]. By week 6, the neural crest cells migrate centripetally through the circular muscle layer, giving rise to submucosal plexus.

Interstitial cells of Cajal (ICC) emerge from gut mesenchyme around week 9. By week 14, the ICCs form a network surrounding the myenteric plexus [9, 10]. The ICCs are gut-pacemakers crucial to the generation of slow wave contractions and to neural transmission within the gut. The ICCs form after the differentiation of smooth muscle layers. Whether ICC differentiation requires neural crest cells has not been clearly established yet, and some recent studies identified ICC in the absence of neural crest cells [9, 11, 12].

The development of concentric layers of smooth muscle, ICCs, and neural crest cells (as precursors of the enteric nervous system) is a coordinated process, controlled by numerous genes and signaling molecules including transcription factors (e.g., Phox2b, Sox10, Pax3, Mash1), components of the RET (RET proto-oncogene) and ET(Endothelin)-3/EDNRB (endothelin receptor type B) signaling pathways, secreted proteins [Hedgehog, BMPs(bone morphogenetic proteins)], neurotrophic factors (e.g., neurotrophin-3), and extracellular matrix (ECM) molecules (e.g., laminin) [9, 13–16]. Perturbations in this coordinated process could result in clinical morbidities such as Hirschsprung's disease, where the hindgut (usually colon) is devoid of enteric neurons and glial cells [17].

The myenteric plexus has cholinesterase activity by week 9.5 and ganglion cells are differentiated by week 13. Several investigators have suggested that the esophagus is capable of peristalsis in the first trimester [18]. Three different esophageal motility patterns have been described in the second trimester: simultaneous opening of the esophageal lumen from the oropharynx to the LES, propulsive peristaltic contractions, and reflux from stomach into the esophagus [19]. Although peristaltic movements have been observed in ultrasound images during the second trimester, at birth the propagation of the peristalsis along the esophagus and at the LES is immature, resulting in frequent regurgitation of food during the newborn period. The pressure at the LES approaches that of the adult at 3–6 weeks of age [6].

Anatomic Landmarks

The esophagus is a flattened muscular tube of 18–26 cm in length, from the upper sphincter to the lower sphincter, connecting the pharynx to the stomach (Fig. 19.2). The esophagus starts at approximately 18 cm from the incisors at the pharyngoesophageal junction [20] (C5–6 vertebral interspace at the inferior border of the cricoid cartilage) and descends anteriorly to the vertebral column spanning the superior and then the posterior mediastinum. After traversing the diaphragm at the diaphragmatic hiatus (T10 vertebral level), the esophagus extends through the GE junction to end at the orifice of the cardia of the stomach (T11 vertebral level). Topographically, there are three distinct regions: cervical, thoracic, and abdominal.

The cervical esophagus extends from the pharyngoesophageal junction (C5–C6) to the

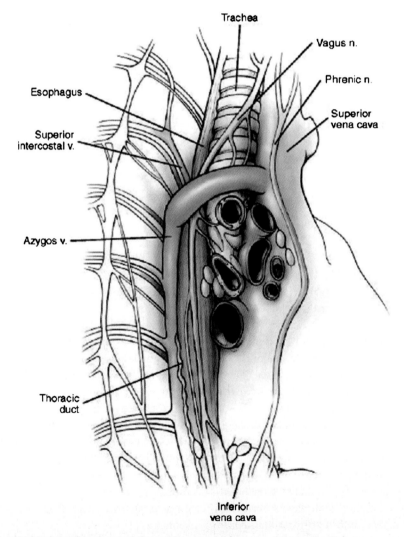

Fig. 19.2 Anatomic relationships between the esophagus and the organs of the mediastinum

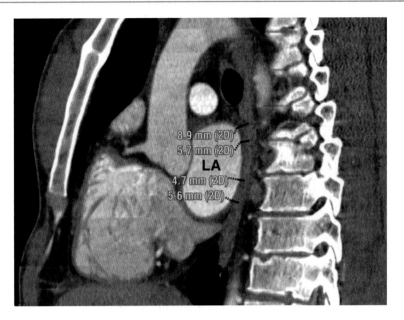

Fig. 19.3 The close relationship between the esophagus and the left atrium (LA)

suprasternal notch (T1) and is about 4–5 cm long. At this level, the esophagus is bordered anteriorly by the trachea, laterally by the carotid sheaths and the thyroid gland, and posteriorly by the vertebral column. The close proximity of the vertebral column to the esophagus can create a unique type of anatomical dysphagia with aspiration events, where cervical osteophytes—either in isolation or as part of a systemic disease (Forestier's disease)—impinge upon the pharynx and cervical esophagus [21].

The thoracic esophagus extends from the suprasternal notch (T1) to the diaphragmatic hiatus (T10), passing posterior to the trachea, the tracheal bifurcation (T4), and the left main stem bronchus. The esophagus lies posterior and to the right of the aortic arch at the T4 vertebral level. From the level of T8 until the diaphragmatic hiatus, the esophagus lies anteriorly and medial to the aorta [22]. The lower part of the thoracic esophagus runs anteriorly to the left atrium, which is the most posterior among all four chambers of the heart (Fig. 19.3). This anatomical location can have important clinical consequences in the setting of mitral stenosis, where the esophagus may be obstructed resulting in dysphagia in advanced stages of mitral stenosis. The dilation of the left atrium in mitral stenosis can be seen on the barium series as an impression on the esophagus. The esophagus also runs between the aorta and the left main bronchus in this region, creating the potential for broncho-aortic constriction known also as thoracic constriction. This is a common area for pill-induced esophagitis and strictures.

The thoracic esophagus lies within a defined fascial compartment, allowing infections from the anterior esophageal wall to spread easily through the peritracheal space down to the pericardium. Noninstrumental or spontaneous perforation of the esophagus (Boerhaave's syndrome) can lead to necrotizing mediastinitis with rapid and disastrous dissemination of the infection and high mortality [23].

The abdominal esophagus is very short and extends from the diaphragmatic hiatus (T10) to the orifice of the cardia of the stomach (T11). The base of the esophagus transitions into the cardia sphincter of the stomach, forming a truncated cone of around 1 cm length. The abdominal esophagus lies in the esophageal groove on the posterior surface of the left lobe of the liver. The anatomic relation of the esophagus with the diaphragmatic

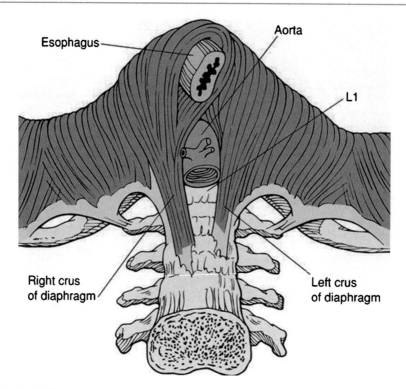

Fig. 19.4 Relationship between the esophagus, the diaphragm, the aorta, and the spine

hiatus is also clinically important (Fig. 19.4). With advancing age, the phreno-esophageal membrane, which has an anchoring role at the distal part of the esophagus, loses its elasticity because the elastic fibers in its structure are replaced by inelastic collagenous fibrous elements [23]. The loss of elasticity in conjunction with a wide diaphragmatic hiatus results in herniation of the GE junction and of the cardia into the thorax—a hiatal hernia.

In the resting state, the esophagus is collapsed in the upper and middle parts and rounded in the lower portion [23]. When the alimentary bolus passes through, the esophagus can distend to approximately 2 cm in the antero-posterior axis and 3 cm in the left–right axis. In the course of the esophagus, three minor curvations are present. The first one, in the upper part, is from the median position toward the medial left. At the level of the T7, the esophagus shifts slightly to the right of the spine. The third angulation and the most important one is at the GE junction, when the esophagus shifts briskly to the left (Fig. 19.5).

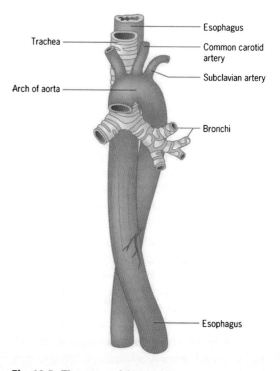

Fig. 19.5 The course of the esophagus

Muscular Layers of the Esophagus

The muscular coat consists of an external layer of longitudinal fibers and an internal layer of circular fibers. The longitudinal fibers are arranged proximally in three fasciculi. The ventral fasciculus is attached to the vertical ridge on the posterior surface of the lamina of the cricoid cartilage by the tendocricoesophageus. The two lateral fasciculi are continuous with the muscular fibers of the pharynx. The longitudinal fibers descend in the esophagus and combine to form a uniform layer that covers the outer surface of the esophagus.

The circular muscle layer provides the sequential peristaltic contraction that propels food toward the stomach. The circular fibers are continuous with the inferior constrictor muscle of the pharynx; they run transverse at the cranial and caudal regions of the esophagus, but oblique in the body of the esophagus. The internal muscular layer is thicker than the external muscular layer. Below the diaphragm, the internal circular muscle layer thickens and the fibers become semicircular and interconnected, constituting the intrinsic component of the LES.

Accessory bands of muscle connect the esophagus and the left pleura to the root of the left bronchus and the posterior pericardium. The muscular fibers in the cranial part of the esophagus consist chiefly of striated muscle; the intermediate part is mixed; and the lower part, with rare exceptions, contains only smooth muscle.

The backflow of food and acidic gastric contents is prevented at the level of two high-pressure regions: the upper and the lower esophageal sphincters. These functional zones are located at the upper and lower ends of the esophagus, but there is not a clear anatomic demarcation of the limits of the sphincters.

The UES is a high-pressure zone situated between the pharynx and the cervical esophagus. The UES is a musculocartilaginous structure composed of the posterior surface of the thyroid and cricoid cartilage, the hyoid bone, and three muscles: cricopharyngeus, thyropharyngeus, and cervical esophagus with contribution from inferior pharyngeal constrictor. Each muscle plays a different role in UES function [24]. These three muscles spread upward, posteriorly, where they insert into the esophageal submucosa after crossing the muscle bundles of the opposite side. The thyropharyngeus muscle is obliquely oriented, whereas the cricopharyngeus muscle is transversely oriented. Between these two muscles, there is a zone of sparse musculature Killian's triangle, of high clinical significance. Because of the low resistance, this region is prone to develop a false diverticulum named Zenker's diverticulum [25], a pulsion diverticulum formed only by the mucosa and submucosa.

The cricopharyngeus (CP) muscle is a striated muscle attached to the cricoid cartilage. It forms a C-shaped muscular band that produces maximum tension in the antero-posterior direction and less tension laterally [26]. Structurally and mechanically, the CP is different from the surrounding pharyngeal and esophageal muscles. It is composed of a mixture of fast- and slow-twitch fibers, with the slow fibers being predominant and having a diameter of 25–35 μm [27]. The CP is suspended between the cricoid processes, surrounds the narrowest part of pharynx, and extends caudally where it blends with the circular muscle of the cervical esophagus.

UES function is controlled by a variety of reflexes that involve afferent inputs to the motor neurons innervating the sphincter. These reflexes elicit either contraction or relaxation of the tonic activity of the UES. Inability of the sphincter to open or discoordination of timing between the opening of the UES with the pharyngeal push of ingested contents leads to difficulty in swallowing known as oropharyngeal dysphagia. The CP muscle component of the UES, in particular, is tonically active, relaxing to allow the opening of the UES and passage of food. Failure of CP relaxation in many cases creates the so-called cricopharyngeal bar, where the contracted CP impedes food bolus passage and creates a sensation of dysphagia [24]. A recent study of elderly cadavers demonstrated that there may be a pure anatomical component of the CP bar as well. One-third of the cadavers examined in the study demonstrated an anatomical cricopharyngeal protrusion on the posterior hypopharyngeal wall, which may have played a role in dysphagia symptoms with normal UES function [28].

The cervical esophagus contains predominantly striated muscle fibers and occasionally smooth fibers [24]. Approximately 4 cm of the proximal end is composed exclusively of striated fibers. Between 4 and 12 cm, a mixture of smooth and striated muscle exists and beginning with the lower border of the cricopharyngeus, only smooth muscle can be seen [20]. Rheumatoid arthritis selectively leads to dysfunction of the predominantly smooth muscle that forms the lower two-thirds of the esophagus, with resultant low peristaltic pressures clinically manifested as dysphagia and/or reflux [29].

The external longitudinal muscle layer of the cervical esophagus originates from the dorsal plane of the cricoid cartilage and because of its lateral and caudal course, delimits a weak space: the Laimer's triangle which is prone to develop a rare type of diverticulum [29]. The external longitudinal layer courses down the length of the entire esophagus. At its distal end the longitudinal fibers become more oblique and end along the anterior and posterior gastric wall [30]. The internal circular layer of muscle originates at the level of cricoid cartilage and while descending, forms incomplete circles [30].

The LES is a high-pressure zone located where the esophagus merges with the stomach. The LES is a functional unit composed of an intrinsic and an extrinsic component. The intrinsic structure of the LES consists of the esophageal muscle fibers and is under neurohormonal influence. The extrinsic component consists of the diaphragm muscle, which functions as an adjunctive external sphincter that raises the pressure in the terminal esophagus related to the movements of respiration. Malfunction in any of these two components can cause GE reflux and its subsequent symptoms and mucosal changes [31].

The intrinsic component of the LES is composed of circular layers of the esophagus, clasp-like semicircular smooth muscle fibers on the right side, and sling-like oblique gastric muscle fibers on the left side [32]. The circular muscles of the LES are thicker than the adjacent esophagus. The clasp-like semicircular fibers have significant myogenic tone but are not very responsive to cholinergic stimulation, whereas the sling-like oblique gastric fibers have little resting tone but contract vigorously to cholinergic stimulation [32].

The extrinsic component of the LES is composed of the crural diaphragm, which forms the esophageal hiatus, and represents a channel through which the esophagus enters into the abdomen. The crural diaphragm encircles the proximal 2–4 cm of the LES and contributes to inspiratory variations in LES pressure noted by esophageal manometry [33] (Fig. 19.6).

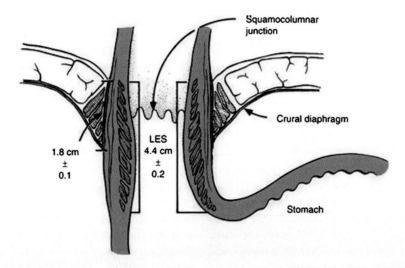

Fig. 19.6 The anatomy of the lower esophageal sphincter (LES), showing the intrinsic and extrinsic components

Histologic Aspects

Macroscopically during endoscopy, the esophageal lumen appears as a smooth, pale pink tube with visible submucosal blood vessels. The transition from esophageal to gastric mucosa is known as the Z-line or squamocolumnar junction and consists of an irregular circumferential line between two areas of different-colored mucosa. The distal gastric mucosa is darker than the more proximal pale pink esophageal mucosa. Microscopically, the esophageal wall is composed of four layers: internal mucosa, submucosa, muscularis propria, and adventitia (Fig. 19.7). Unlike the remainder of the GI tract, the esophagus has no serosa. This allows esophageal tumors to spread more easily and makes them harder to treat surgically [34]. The missing serosal layer also makes luminal disruptions more challenging to repair.

Mucosa

The mucosa is thick and reddish cranially and more pale caudally. It is arranged in longitudinal folds that disappear upon distention. It consists of three sublayers.

The first sublayer is the mucous membrane: a nonkeratinized squamous epithelium. It covers

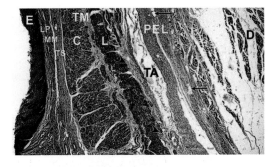

Fig. 19.7 Longitudinal section showing the layers of the esophagus. *C* circular muscle layer, *D* striated muscle cells of the diaphragm, *E* stratified squamous epithelium, *L* longitudinal muscle layer, *LP* lamina propria, *MM* muscularis mucosa, *TA* tunica adventitia, *TM* tunica muscularis, *TS* tunica submucosa, *PEL* phrenicoesophageal ligament, *arrow heads*; the *PEL* attaches to the muscular layer, *arrows*; isolated group of adipose cells

the entire inner surface of the esophagus and at the LES level it may coexist with the columnar, gastric type epithelium. The mucous membrane is composed of stratum basale, stratum intermedium, and stratum superficialis.

Stratum basale (10–15 % of the epithelium) contains cuboidal basophilic cells, low in glycogen attached to the basement membrane by hemidesmosomes. These cells can divide and replenish the superficial layers. In 25 % of the normal population, the stratum basale contains argyrophilic-positive endocrine cells and in 4 % of the normal subjects, it contains melanocytes [35]. The melanocytes from this region account for the occurrence of primary melanoma of the esophagus [36], while the argyrophilic-positive endocrine cells are the potential progenitors of the esophageal small cell carcinoma [35].

Stratum intermedium and stratum superficialis are composed of cells derived from the basal stratum that become more flattened with pyknotic nuclei. These cells may present processes and desmosomal junctions that become fewer and more simplified superficially [37]. Compared with the basal cells, the cells in the stratum intermedium and superficialis are rich in glycogen [38].

The second sublayer forming the mucosa is represented by lamina propria, a thin connective tissue structure containing vascular structures and mucous secreting glands.

The third sublayer of the mucosa is muscularis mucosa. This is a thin layer of longitudinally, irregularly arranged smooth muscle fibers and delicate elastic fibers [39]. The muscularis mucosa extends through the entire esophagus and continues into the rest of the GI tract, being much thinner in the proximal part of the esophagus than in its distal part [40]. At the pharyngeal end of the esophagus, the muscularis mucosa is represented by a few scattered smooth muscle fibers. Caudally, approaching the cardiac orifice, the muscularis mucosa forms a thick layer, so thick that sometimes it may be confused with the muscularis propria on biopsy specimens [38]. The muscularis mucosa separates the lamina propria from the submucosa and retracts when it is sectioned during surgical procedures.

The submucosa contains loose connective tissue as well as lymphocytes, plasma cells, nerve cells (Meissner's plexus), a vascular network (Heller plexus), and submucosal glands. The esophageal submucosal glands are considered to be a continuation of the glands in the oropharynx. They are small racemose glands [38] of the mucous type more concentrated in the upper and lower regions. Their secretion is important in esophageal clearance and tissue resistance to acid [41]. The postobstructive inflammation of the glandular ducts can result in intramucosal pseudo-diverticulosis [42].

Muscularis Propria

The muscularis propria is responsible for motor function. The upper 5–33 % is composed exclusively of striated muscle, and the distal 33 % is composed of smooth muscle. In between there is a mixture of both, called the transition zone. Functionally the transition zone can be observed with manometry as a region where there is no significant pressure noted during a peristaltic contraction that travels down the body of the esophagus [43]. Despite the presence of two different muscle types, they function as a whole unit. Between the longitudinal and circular muscular layers, at this level, the Auerbach's plexus is found. Different pathologic conditions usually affect only one muscular layer, as in sclerodema and achalasia when only the circular layer is involved [38].

Adventitia

The adventitia is an external fibrous layer that covers the esophagus, connecting it with neighboring structures. It is composed of loose connective tissue and contains small vessels, lymphatic channels, and nerve fibers providing a support role. The esophagus does not have a serosal layer except under the diaphragm level where it is formed by the peritoneum [39].

Vascularization

Arteries

The rich arterial supply of the esophagus is segmental (Fig. 19.8). The cervical esophagus is supplied with branches of the left and right superior and inferior thyroid arteries. These branches travel anteriorly toward the lateral aspect of the esophagus and they anastomose on the anterior and posterior esophageal walls. Rarely, the cervical esophagus can be vascularized with branches originating from thyroidea ima artery, common carotid arteries, and subclavian arteries.

The thoracic esophagus is supplied by paired esophageal branches from the tracheo-bronchic arteries. The later ones emerge from the caudal aspect of the aortic arch and are 1–2.5 mm in diameter. They course anteriorly and give off branches to the trachea and esophagus. This region

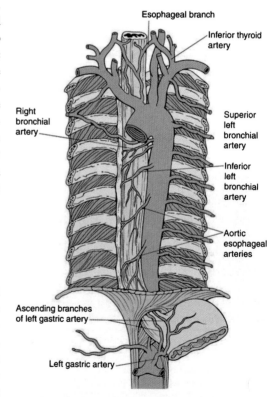

Fig. 19.8 The arterial supply of the esophagus

of the esophagus is also supplied by unpaired esophageal branches of about 1.5–2 mm that arise at variable locations directly from the anterior wall of the aorta and going to the posterior aspect of the esophageal wall [30].

The intra-abdominal esophagus is supplied with branches from the left gastric artery. These vessels travel upward on the anterior aspect of the cardia and they gave off periesophageal tributaries before entering in the muscular wall [23]. The posterior aspect of the abdominal esophagus is supplied by branches of the fundal arteries derived from the splenic artery.

The esophageal vascular system is mainly formed from branches of arteries that supply some other organs, but a dedicated vasculature to the esophagus is less developed. The vessels dip in the esophageal wall creating a network in the submucosa and mucosa, offering an "excellent blood supply" [43].

The vasculature of the esophagus determines a number of surgical particularities. During the pull-through esophagectomy without thoracotomy for excising cancer or tumors, the blood loss is moderate making this procedure relatively safe [44, 45]. Usually if bleeding occurs it is a consequence of the intratumoral or tumoral adhesions hemorrhaging.

Veins

The venous system of the esophagus has two main divisions: the intrinsic division located in the submucosa and the extrinsic division located outside the esophagus and draining blood into larger blood vessels (Fig. 19.9).

The intrinsic venous system is composed of a parallel network located in the esophageal submucosa coursing the whole length of the esophagus [46]. Kitano and colleagues [47] described in detail the intrinsic venous system in the lower part of the esophagus, close to the GE junction (Fig. 19.10). Using resin casting, this group identified four distinct layers forming the intrinsic esophageal venous plexus: (1) Intraepithelial channels, running centrifugally from the epithelium and draining in the superficial venous plexus with a mean diameter of

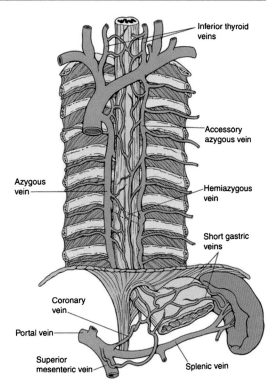

Fig. 19.9 The venous drainage of the esophagus

0.043 mm; (2) Superficial venous plexus located in the mucosa, right below the epithelium, and continuing with a similar plexus at the gastric level (mean diameter=0.188 mm); (3) Deep intrinsic veins, having a higher caliber and draining the blood from the superficial venous plexus (mean diameter=0.442); and (4) Adventitial veins, located more peripherally in the adventitia and also having a higher caliber (mean diameter=0.452 mm). The adventitial veins collect the blood from the deep intrinsic veins through perforating veins that span the muscularis propria layer.

The intrinsic esophageal plexus is of a particular clinical interest because it makes the connection between the portal and the caval venous systems—highly involved in the pathology of esophageal varices. Esophageal varices occur mainly in conditions complicated by portal hypertension such as cirrhosis, schistosomiasis, portal vein thrombosis and rarely occur in the absence of portal hypertension (i.e., superior vena cava syndrome) [48].

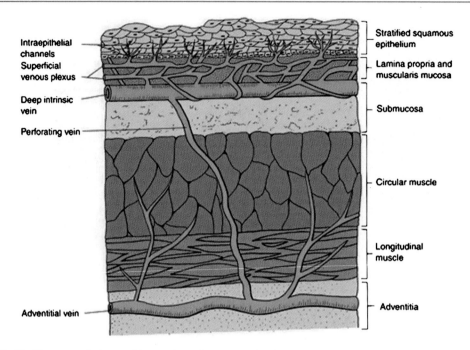

Fig. 19.10 The venous drainage of the esophageal mucosa

The patients with portal hypertension present a specific anatomical pathology. The main changes appear at the level of the deep venous layer that will transform into tortuous variceal structures [47]. Esophageal varices form as backflow pressure increases and may bleed when the intravenous pressure passes over 12 mmHg [49].

The extrinsic venous system of the esophagus drains in large vessels: the upper esophagus blood drains in the azygos and hemiazygos veins, and the mid and low esophagus drain in tributaries of the portal system such as left gastric vein or splenic vein.

Lymphatic System of the Esophagus

Lymphatic drainage in the esophagus consists of two systems: the lymph channels and lymph nodules.

The lymph channels begin in the esophageal tissue space as a network of endothelial channels (20–30 μm) or as blind endothelial sacculations (40–60 μm) [50]. The location of the lymphatic capillary origin is not known precisely. Some authors propose that precapillary spaces exist in the lamina mucosa, but others contend that there is an absence of true lymphatic capillaries in the upper and middle levels of the lamina mucosa [51]. Electron microscopic studies show anastomotic lymph capillaries in the lower mucosal levels and small lymphatic vessels in the submucosa.

From this level fluid, colloid material, cell debris, microorganisms, and sometimes tumor cells are taken and drained into collecting lymph channels (100–200 μm) that continue through the esophageal muscular coat and are distributed parallel to the long axis of the esophagus. Paired semilunar valves within the collecting channels determine the direction of flow. The collecting lymph channels merge into small trunks that open into the regional lymph nodes (Fig. 19.11).

Innervation of the Esophagus

The esophagus, like the rest of the viscera, receives dual motor and sensory innervation supplied by two divisions of the autonomic system: the sympathetic and parasympathetic systems (Fig. 19.12).

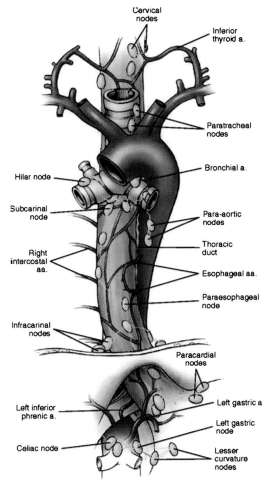

Fig. 19.11 Regional lymph nodes of the esophagus

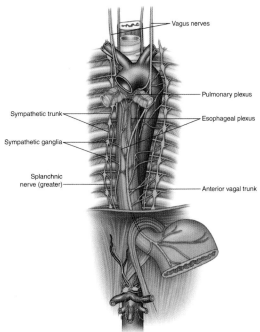

Fig. 19.12 The esophageal plexus of nerves containing the sympathetic and parasympathetic (via the vagus nerve) systems

The Sympathetic System

The afferent system collects the information from the wall of the esophagus using sensorial structures such as osmoreceptors, chemoreceptors, thermoreceptors, and mechanoreceptors [52]. The afferent fibers are dendrites of the unipolar neurons located in the dorsal root ganglion in the thoracic spine (T1–T10). These neurons will synapse with the preganglionic neurons located in the latero-intermedial grey horns from the thoracic spine. The axons of preganglionic neurons leave the spine on the ventral root and they synapse with neurons in the sympathetic paravertebral chain at the same level or they can travel upward or downward to synapse with neurons at different levels.

The axons of these neurons are myelinated and form the white rami communicantes.

The multipolar ganglionic neurons are located in the sympathetic trunk, in the proximity of the spine, against the costal ends and posterior to the costal pleura [53]. The rami emerging from the second to the fifth ganglia form the posterior pulmonary plexus or the deep part of the cardiac plexus. These plexuses can generate small branches that will distribute to the proximal esophagus [23].

The preganglionic fibers deriving from T5 to T9 merge and form the greater splanchnic nerve that descends obliquely in the proximity of the thoracic vertebral bodies and perforates the ipsilateral diaphragmatic crus on its way to the celiac ganglion. Postganglionic fibers from the celiac ganglion distribute as well to the esophagus supplying the sympathetic innervation [53].

The postganglionic fibers influence the activity of the target end-organ glands, muscles, and the enteric nervous system. Throughout these pathways, the sympathetic system generates specific activities such as relaxation of the muscular wall with depression of peristalsis [53, 54] and increase of LES tonus [55].

The sensorial information from the esophageal wall is also transmitted ascending toward supraspinal and cortical centers, where it is interpreted as sensation. The pain, temperature, and visceroceptive information can be transmitted via lamina I Rexed of the spinal cord and spinothalamic pathways in the ventromedial nucleus of the thalamus, projecting to the insular cortex [56, 57]. The information is transmitted through pathways containing numerous small inter-neurons in the laminae VII and X Rexed.

The sympathetic outflow of the neurons from the lateral horn in the spine is also controlled by substantial input from multiple supraspinal structures. Using transneuronal-tracing techniques with pseudorabies virus, it was possible to identify these specific supraspinal structures. After injection of the pseudorabies virus in the celiac and stellate ganglia, five regions were labeled: (1) ventromedial medulla, (2) rostral ventrolateral medulla, (3) caudal raphe nuclei, (4) A5 noradrenergic cell group, and (5) paraventricular nucleus of the hypothalamus [58].

The Parasympathetic System

The parasympathetic system at the esophageal level is mainly represented by the fibers of the vagus nerve. The sensory, afferent fibers of the parasympathetic system are mainly part of the vagus nerve. These fibers are dendritic ends of unipolar neurons located mainly in the nodose (inferior) vagal ganglion and represent approximately 80 % of the vagal trunk [59]. The sensory neurons within the nodose ganglion have a topographic layout suggested by Collman et al. [60]. Using retrograde immunohistochemical techniques, Neuhuber demonstrated that the vagal afferents in the cervical esophagus supplying mucosa and muscularis propria have different origins. The afferent innervation of the muscularis propria originates in nodose ganglion while the fibers supplying the mucosal layer originate mainly from petrosal and jugular ganglion [61]. These

observations are in agreement with some experiments that demonstrate different patterns of stimulation. The *vagal afferents from the muscularis* respond mainly to mechanical distention, while the *afferents in the mucosa* respond to various chemical intraluminal stimulations [52]. The parasympathetic afferents from the esophagus on their way to the sensory ganglion gather and join the superior laryngeal nerve (SLN). The SLN courses along the pharynx, posterior and medial to the internal carotid artery, dividing into internal and external branches. After piercing the inferior constrictor muscle, the internal SLN ascends and gives off branches supplying sensation for the esophagus, especially on the left side [53].

The axons of the primary neurons supplying sensation of the esophagus terminate in different nuclei of the brain stem. The vagal afferents from the proximal striated esophagus project in a specific region on the medial aspect of the solitary tract called the central subnucleus. The afferents from the smooth-muscled part of the esophagus project in the vicinity of the central subnucleus [62, 63].

The efferent fibers supplying the striated and the smooth part of the esophagus also have different origins. The nervous fibers innervating the striated esophagus originate from the rostral part of the nucleus ambiguous [64]. This structure is connected to the ipsilateral central subnucleus of the solitary tract by medullary inter-neurons. The efferent parasympathetic fibers going to the distal smooth-muscled esophagus originate in the medial part of the dorsal nucleus, the largest parasympathetic structure in the brain stem [53]. From the dorsal nucleus, the efferent fibers merge and form the main trunk of the vagus nerve that travels through the jugular foramen. The right vagus nerve courses down on the posterior aspect of the right bronchus and hilum and divides into anterior and posterior subdivision. The posterior subdivision unites with the sympathetic fibers forming the right posterior pulmonary plexus. This plexus will generate in its caudal part rami that innervate the esophagus. These rami join similar rami coming from the left side to form the anterior esophageal plexus.

This plexus continues down along the anterior surface of the esophagus coursing through the diaphragmatic hiatus [53].

At the proximal part of the esophagus at the pharyngeal–esophageal junction, the efferent innervation is supplied with fibers from the recurrent laryngeal nerves. These nerves originate from the vagus nerve curving backward and upward around the subclavian artery on the right side, respectively, around the aortic arch on the left side. In the ascending segments, these nerves travel in the groove formed between trachea and esophagus giving off esophageal branches that participate in the esophageal plexus [53]. The parasympathetic efferent fibers regulate the activity of the esophageal muscle by increasing the peristalsis, decreasing the pressure in the LES, and increasing the secretory activity.

Similar to the sympathetic system, the activity of the parasympathetic system is tonically regulated by supraspinal centers, such as the hypothalamus and cortical areas. Positron emission tomography (PET) and functional magnetic resonance imaging (fMRI) have been used to map the central nervous system projections from the esophagus. Esophageal stimulation at the subliminal and liminal levels is sensed peripherally and transmitted to the brain for further processing and modulation. Esophageal sensory innervation is carried by the vagus nerve to the nodose ganglion and projects through the brainstem, through the thalamus, to terminate in the cortex [60, 65]. Regions that are activated by esophageal stimulation include the secondary sensory and motor cortex, parieto-occipital cortex, anterior and posterior cingulate cortex, prefrontal cortical cortex, and the insula [66].

Enteric Nervous System

Similar to other segments of the gastrointestinal tract, the esophagus has its own neural systems composed of flat networks in the muscular layers that form the myenteric and submucosal enteric plexuses [67, 68]. The thin nerve fibers and numerous

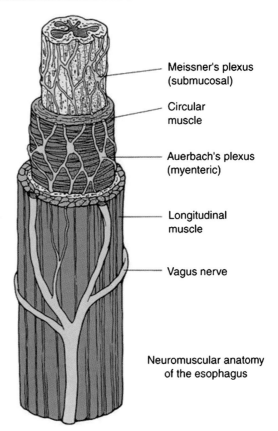

Fig. 19.13 The myenteric (Auerbach's) and submucosal (Meissner's) enteric plexuses, which lie within the muscular layers of the esophagus

ganglia of the intramural myenteric and submucosal plexuses provide the intrinsic innervation of the esophagus (Fig. 19.13). The ganglia that lie between the longitudinal and the circular layers of the tunica muscularis form the myenteric or Auerbach's plexus, whereas those that lie in the submucosa form the submucous or Meissner's plexus. In the smooth-muscled esophagus, the neurons of the myenteric plexus relay between the vagus and the smooth muscle, acting as postganglionic neurons. From here, short motor axons from the ganglia penetrate and innervate the muscle layers [69]. The two intrinsic nervous plexuses have different roles: Auerbach's plexus regulates contraction of the outer muscle layers, whereas Meissner's plexus regulates secretion and the peristaltic contractions of the muscularis mucosae.

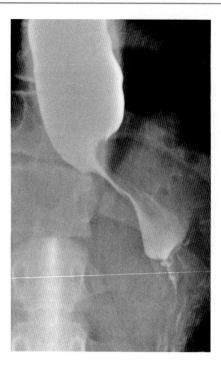

Fig. 19.14 Achalasia on barium swallow. The LES fails to relax, creating a "bird-beak" appearance at the gastroesophageal junction

The neuromuscular activity is regulated by cellular entities within the circular muscular layer of the esophagus: interstitial cells of Cajal (ICC) that form gap junctions with the adjacent smooth muscle cells and play a regulatory role in the neurotransmission. In order to achieve coordinated peristalsis with relaxation of the LES, there are both excitatory and inhibitory inputs from the vagus nerve and the enteric neural plexus. Achalasia, a common worldwide cause of esophageal dysphagia, results from the perturbation of these normal neural inputs that occurs with the selective degeneration of ganglion cells in the myenteric plexus of the esophageal body and the LES [70]. Without this fine balance of neural inputs, esophageal peristalsis is absent and the LES fails to relax (Fig. 19.14).

The recurrent laryngeal nerves and the superior laryngeal nerves have a significant clinical importance. Because of their length and their specific location, they can be easily injured during esophageal resections, thyroid surgery, and left-sided thoracic operations. These injuries

cause a variety of temporary or permanent motor and sensory dysfunctions such as hoarseness and aspiration [23].

References

1. Larsen W. Development of the gastrointestinal tract. In: Sherman LS, Potter SS, Scott WJ, editors. Human embryology. 3rd ed. Philadelphia: Churchill Livingstone; 2001. p. 235–64.
2. Kedinger M, et al. Epithelial-mesenchymal interactions in intestinal epithelial differentiation. Scand J Gastroenterol Suppl. 1988;151:62–9.
3. Larsen W. Embryonic folding. In: Sherman LS, Potter SS, Scott WJ, editors. Human embryology. 3rd ed. Philadelphia: Churchill Livingstone; 2001. p. 133–4.
4. Roberts DJ. Molecular mechanisms of development of the gastrointestinal tract. Dev Dyn. 2000;219(2):109–20.
5. Le Douarin NM, et al. Neural crest cell plasticity and its limits. Development. 2004;131(19):4637–50.
6. Zuidema GD. Shackelford's Surgery of the alimentary tract, vol. 1. Philadelphia: WB Saunders; 1996. p. 1–35.
7. Skandalakis JE, Ellis H. Embryologic and anatomic basis of esophageal surgery. Surg Clin North Am. 2000;80(1):85–155.
8. Kedinger M, et al. Smooth muscle actin expression during rat gut development and induction in fetal skin fibroblastic cells associated with intestinal embryonic epithelium. Differentiation. 1990;43(2):87–97.
9. Wallace AS, Burns AJ. Development of the enteric nervous system, smooth muscle and interstitial cells of Cajal in the human gastrointestinal tract. Cell Tissue Res. 2005;319(3):367–82.
10. Fu M, et al. Embryonic development of the ganglion plexuses and the concentric layer structure of human gut: a topographical study. Anat Embryol (Berl). 2004;208(1):33–41.
11. Newman CJ, et al. Interstitial cells of Cajal are normally distributed in both ganglionated and aganglionic bowel in Hirschsprung's disease. Pediatr Surg Int. 2003;19(9–10):662–8.
12. Ward SM. Interstitial cells of Cajal in enteric neurotransmission. Gut. 2000;47 suppl 4:40–3. discussion iv, 52.
13. Chalazonitis A, et al. Bone morphogenetic protein-2 and -4 limit the number of enteric neurons but promote development of a TrkC-expressing neurotrophin-3-ependent subset. J Neurosci. 2004;24(17): 4266–82.
14. Manie S, et al. The RET receptor: function in development and dysfunction in congenital malformation. Trends Genet. 2001;17(10):580–9.
15. Ramalho-Santos M, Melton DA, McMahon AP. Hedgehog signals regulate multiple aspects of gastrointestinal development. Development. 2000;127(12): 2763–72.
16. Gershon MDV. Genes, lineages, and tissue interactions in the development of the enteric nervous system. Am J Physiol. 1998;275(5 pt 1):G869–73.

17. Amiel J, Lyonnet S. Hirschsprung disease, associated syndromes, and genetics: a review. J Med Genet. 2001;38(11):729–39.
18. Bowie JD, Clair MR. Fetal swallowing and regurgitation: observation of normal and abnormal activity. Radiology. 1982;144(4):877–8.
19. Malinger G, Levine A, Rotmensch S. The fetal esophagus: anatomical and physiological ultrasonographic characterization using a high-resolution linear transducer. Ultrasound Obstet Gynecol. 2004;24(5):500–5.
20. Castell DO, Richter JE. The esophagus. 3rd ed. Philadelphia: Lippincott, Williams & Wilkins; 1999. p. 33.
21. Kos MP, van Royen BJ, David EF, Mahieu HF. Anterior cervical osteophytes resulting in severe dysphagia and aspiration: two case reports and literature review. J Laryngol Otol. 2009;123(10):1169–73.
22. Sobotta J, Putz R, Pabst R. Atlas der anatomie des menschen. 13th ed. Philadelphia: Lippincott, Williams, & Wilkins; 2001. English version.
23. Pearson G, Cooper J, Deslauriers J. Esophageal surgery. 2nd ed. Philadelphia: Churchill. Livingstone; 2002. p. 637–54.
24. Sivarao DV, Goyal RK. Functional anatomy and physiology of the upper esophageal sphincter. Am J Med. 2000;108(Suppl 4a):27S–37.
25. Achkar E. Zenker's Diverticulum. Dig Dis. 1998;16(3):144–51.
26. Gerhardt D, et al. Human upper esophageal sphincter pressure profile. Am J Physiol. 1980;239(1):G49–52.
27. Lang IM, Shaker R. Anatomy and physiology of the upper esophageal sphincter. Am J Med. 1997;103(5A):50S–5.
28. Leaper M, Zhang M, Dawes PJ. An anatomical protrusion exists on the posterior hypopharyngeal wall in some elderly cadavers. Dysphagia. 2005;20(1):8–14. Winter.
29. Ebert EC, Hagspiel KD. Gastrointestinal and hepatic manifestations of rheumatoid arthritis. Dig Dis Sci. 2011;56(2):295–302.
30. Kumoi K, Ohtsuki N, Teramoto Y. Pharyngoesophageal diverticulum arising from Laimer's triangle. Eur Arch Otorhinolaryngol. 2001;258(4):184–7.
31. Liebermann-Meffert D, et al. Muscular equivalent of the lower esophageal sphincter. Gastroenterology. 1979;76(1):31–8.
32. Delattre JF, et al. Functional anatomy of the gastroesophageal junction. Surg Clin North Am. 2000;80(1):241–60.
33. Preiksaitis HG, Diamant NE. Regional differences in cholinergic activity of muscle fibers from the human gastroesophageal junction. Am J Physiol. 1997;272(6 Pt 1):G1321–7.
34. Mittal RK, Balaban DH. The esophagogastric junction. N Engl J Med. 1997;336(13):924–32.
35. Boyce H, Boyce G. Esophagus: anatomy and structureal anomalies. In: Yamada T, Alpers DH, Kaplowitz N, Laine L, Owyang C, Powell DW, editors. Textbook of gastroenterology, vol. 1. 4th ed. Philadelphia: Lippincott William & Wilkins; 2003. p. 1148–65.
36. De La Pava S, et al. Melanosis of the esophagus. Cancer. 1963;16:48–50.
37. DiCostanzo DP, Urmacher C. Primary malignant melanoma of the esophagus. Am J Surg Pathol. 1987;11(1):46–52.
38. Hopwood D, Logan KR, Bouchier IA. The electron microscopy of normal human oesophageal epithelium. Virchows Arch B Cell Pathol. 1978;26(4):345–58.
39. Sternberg S. Histology for pathologists. 2nd ed. New York: Raven Press; 1997.
40. Dellon ES, Aderoju A, Woosley JT, Sandler RS, Shaheen NJ. Variability in diagnostic criteria for eosinophilic esophagitis: a systematic review. Am J Gastroenterol. 2007;102(10):2300–13.
41. Borysenko M, Beringer T. Functional histology. 3rd ed. Boston: Little, Brown & Co.; 1989. p. 20.
42. Christensen J, Wingate DL, Gregory RA. A guide to gastrointestinal motility. Bristol: John Wright & Sons Ltd.; 1983. p. 157–97.
43. Long JD, Orlando RC. Esophageal submucosal glands: structure and function. Am J Gastroenterol. 1999;94(10):2818–24.
44. Ghosh SK, et al. Physiology of the esophageal pressure transition zone: separate contraction waves above and below. Am J Physiol Gastrointest Liver Physiol. 2005;290(3):568–76.
45. Williams DB, Payne WS. Observations on esophageal blood supply. Mayo Clin Proc. 1982;57(7):448–53.
46. Akiyama H. Surgery for carcinoma of the esophagus. Curr Probl Surg. 1980;17(2):53–120.
47. Orringer MB, Orringer JS. Esophagectomy without thoracotomy: a dangerous operation? J Thorac Cardiovasc Surg. 1983;85(1):72–80.
48. Vianna A, et al. Normal venous circulation of the gastroesophageal junction. A route to understanding varices. Gastroenterology. 1987;93(4):876–89.
49. Kitano S, et al. Venous anatomy of the lower oesophagus in portal hypertension: practical implications. Br J Surg. 1986;73(7):525–31.
50. Pashankar D, Jamieson DH, Israel DM. Downhill esophageal varices. J Pediatr Gastroenterol Nutr. 1999;29(3):360–2.
51. Dell'era A, Bosch J. Review article: the relevance of portal pressure and other risk factors in acute gastro-oesophageal variceal bleeding. Aliment Pharmacol Ther. 2004;20 Suppl 3:8–15. discussion 16–7.
52. Zuidema GD. Shackelford's Surgery of the alimentary tract, W.B. Saunders company, Philadelphia, Pennsylvania. 1996. I- esophagus: p. 1–35. World J Surg. 1994;18(2):266–72.
53. Goyal R, Sivarao D. Functional anatomy and physiology of swallowing and esophageal motility. In: Catell OD, Richter JE, editors. The esophagus. 3rd ed. Philadelphia: Lippincott-Raven; 1999. p. 23.
54. Bannister LH, Berry MM, Collins P. Gray's anatomy. 38th ed. New York: Churchill Livingstone; 1995. p. 1637.
55. Robertson D. Primer on the autonomic nervous system. 2nd ed. Boston: Academic; 2004. p. 40.

56. DiMarino AJ, Cohen S. The adrenergic control of lower esophageal sphincter function. An experimental model of denervation supersensitivity. J Clin Invest. 1973;52(9):2264–71.

57. Saper CB. The central autonomic nervous system: conscious visceral perception and autonomic pattern generation. Annu Rev Neurosci. 2002;25: 433–69.

58. Craig AD. An ascending general homeostatic afferent pathway originating in lamina I. Prog Brain Res. 1996;107:225–42.

59. Strack AM, et al. A general pattern of CNS innervation of the sympathetic outflow demonstrated by transneuronal pseudorabies viral infections. Brain Res. 1989;491(1):156–62.

60. Goyal RK, Hirano I. The enteric nervous system. N Engl J Med. 1996;334(17):1106–15.

61. Collman PI, Tremblay L, Diamant NE. The distribution of spinal and vagal sensory neurons that innervate the esophagus of the cat. Gastroenterology. 1992; 103(3):817–22.

62. Wank M, Neuhuber WL. Local differences in vagal afferent innervation of the rat esophagus are reflected by neurochemical differences at the level of the sensory ganglia and by different brainstem projections. J Comp Neurol. 2001;435(1):41–59.

63. Altschuler SM, et al. Viscerotopic representation of the upper alimentary tract in the rat: sensory ganglia and nuclei of the solitary and spinal trigeminal tracts. J Comp Neurol. 1989;283(2):248–68.

64. Cunningham Jr ET, Sawchenko PE. Central neural control of esophageal motility: a review. Dysphagia. 1990;5(1):35–51.

65. Holstege G, et al. Location of motoneurons innervating soft palate, pharynx and upper esophagus. Anatomical evidence for a possible swallowing center in the Pontine reticular formation. An HRP and autoradiographical tracing study. Brain Behav Evol. 1983;23(1–2):47–62.

66. Paintal AS. Vagal afferent fibres. Ergeb Physiol. 1963;52:74–156.

67. Kern MK, et al. Identification and characterization of cerebral cortical response to esophageal mucosal acid exposure and distention. Gastroenterology. 1998; 115(6):1353–62.

68. Christensen J, Robison BA. Anatomy of the myenteric plexus of the opossum esophagus. Gastroenterology. 1982;83(5):1033–42.

69. Christensen J, et al. Arrangement of the myenteric plexus throughout the gastrointestinal tract of the opossum. Gastroenterology. 1983;85(4):890–9.

70. Gabella G. Innervation of the gastrointestinal tract. Int Rev Cytol. 1979;59:129–93.

Normal Aging and the Esophagus

20

Paul Menard-Katcher and Gary W. Falk

Abstract

While changes in normal esophageal function have long been attributed to the aging process, the evidence supporting these changes is mixed. The term presbyesophagus was coined to describe changes in esophageal function with aging. However, studies to date show little evidence for an effect of aging on lower esophageal sphincter (LES) function while changes noted in esophageal motor function with aging are inconsistent. There is, however, good evidence that normal aging does impair esophageal sensory function and results in a stiffer esophageal wall.

Keywords

Esophagus • Motility • Aging • Peristalsis • Lower esophageal sphincter • Esophageal sensation • Presbyesophagus

P. Menard-Katcher, MD
Division of Gastroenterology, Perelman School
of Medicine at the University on Pennsylvania,
9 Penn Tower, One Convention Avenue, Philadelphia,
PA 19104, USA

G.W. Falk, MD, MS (⊠)
Division of Gastroenterology, Department of Medicine,
Perelman School of Medicine at the University
of Pennsylvania, Hospital of the University
of Pennsylvania, 9 Penn Tower, One Convention Avenue,
Philadelphia, PA 19104, USA
e-mail: gary.falk@uphs.upenn.edu

Introduction

Changes in esophageal function associated with aging were first described almost 50 years ago and termed presbyesophagus [1]. However, as techniques for the study of esophageal physiology have advanced, findings once attributed to aging have come into question. Given the aging population and the priority placed on economically sustainable health care costs, along with the impact on quality of life of impaired esophageal function, it is important to examine the current state of knowledge in this field. Considerable uncertainty exists today about what constitutes normal aging of the esophagus. The goal of this chapter is to examine current evidence of changes in esophageal function that occur with aging.

R. Shaker et al. (eds.), *Principles of Deglutition: A Multidisciplinary Text for Swallowing and its Disorders*,
DOI 10.1007/978-1-4614-3794-9_20, © Springer Science+Business Media New York 2013

Presbyesophagus: A Historical Perspective

Presbyesophagus has been defined as a failure of peristalsis in the older esophagus [2]. This term comes from work by Soergel et al. in 1964 from a study of 15 subjects 90 years of age or older who underwent cineradiography and esophageal manometry with systems far more primitive than the high-resolution manometry available today [1]. These subjects included four with dementia as well as others who were bedridden or suffered from diseases such as diabetes mellitus and coronary artery disease. In this small group of elderly patients, cineradiography demonstrated frequent tertiary contractions as well as aperistalsis, delayed esophageal emptying, and dilation of the esophagus. Manometry revealed a disorganized response to swallowing with features such as impaired lower esophageal sphincter (LES) relaxation, nonpropulsive contractions, and an absent motor response to swallows. Normal peristalsis accompanied only 51% of the swallows. As a result, the authors speculated that aging was associated with a progressive decline in esophageal function that they called presbyesophagus, a term that is still in use today. Over the ensuing years, it has become clear that the term presbyesophagus should be discarded, as the changes in esophageal function with normal aging are perhaps more subtle than was conceptualized by Soergel and coworkers.

Structural Changes with Aging

Esophageal smooth muscle and myenteric plexus histology have been examined in an autopsy study of 9 young individuals with a mean age of 29 years compared to 15 older individuals with a mean age of 77 years [3]. Of note, patients with underlying neurologic conditions, diabetes mellitus, and alcoholism were excluded. No difference was found in the smooth muscle thickness between the older and younger individuals. However, there was a decrease in ganglion cells/cm^2 in the older individuals when compared to

the younger group. An inverse correlation of ganglion count with age was also noted. These findings may explain some of the observations described below regarding impairment in sensory function of the esophagus with aging.

Aging may also be associated with a change of biomechanical properties of the esophageal wall. Work by Rao et al. with impedance planimetry found that the cross sectional area in both the striated and smooth muscle part of the esophagus was greater in 11 healthy older subjects, ages 55–82 years, compared to 11 healthy younger subjects, ages 22–45 years (Fig. 20.1) [4]. Furthermore, the tension–strain plot in the smooth muscle portion of the esophagus was shifted to the left in the older individuals suggesting that the esophageal wall also became stiffer with aging (Fig. 20.2). This latter finding has been confirmed by others [5]. Taken together, these two findings suggest that the esophageal wall is associated with a larger but stiffer lumen during the aging process.

Sensory Changes with Aging

In addition to the mechanical changes described above, a number of sensory alterations have been described in the esophagus with aging including changes in chemosensitivity and the response to air and balloon distention.

Sensitivity to acid infusion is clearly impaired with aging in both uncomplicated gastroesophageal reflux disease (GERD) patients and GERD patients complicated with Barrett's esophagus. Fass et al. performed intraesophageal acid infusion with 0.1 N hydrochloric acid in 23 young GERD patients (<age 60 years) and 25 older GERD patients (age≥60 years) [6]. When compared to the younger GERD patients, the older patients had both a longer lag time to initial symptom perception as well as lower symptom intensity rating at the end of the acid perfusion period. Similar findings in response to intraesophageal acid infusion were described by Grade et al. in 10 young Barrett's esophagus patients (≤age 50 years) and 12 older Barrett's esophagus patients (>age 65 years) with comparable segment

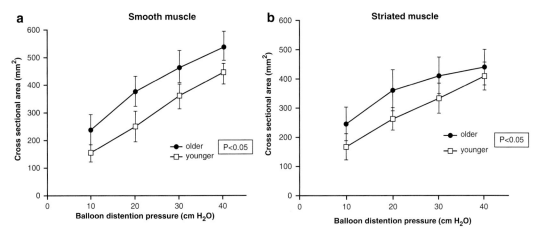

Fig. 20.1 Change in cross sectional area of the smooth muscle part of the esophagus (**a**) and striated muscle part of the esophagus (**b**) in response to balloon distention in younger and older healthy volunteers. From S.S. Rao et al. Am J Gastroenterol 2003;98:1688–95 with permission

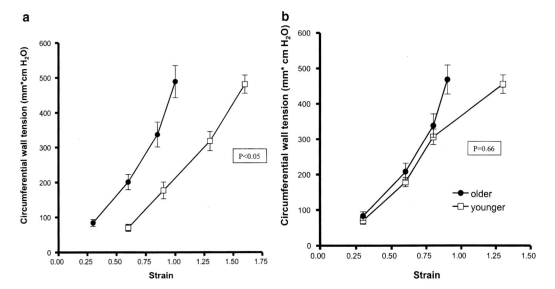

Fig. 20.2 Change in tension–strain association of the smooth muscle part of the esophagus (**a**) and striated muscle part of the esophagus (**b**) in response to balloon distention in younger and older healthy volunteers. From S.S. Rao et al. Am J Gastroenterol 2003;98:1688–95 with permission

lengths [7]. When compared to the younger Barrett's patients, the older patients had both a longer lag time to initial symptom perception as well as lower sensory intensity rating at the end of the acid perfusion period. Five of the older patients did not perceive the acid infusion over a 10-min period whereas all of the younger patients did perceive the acid infusion. These findings are especially interesting given the well-described increase in prevalence of Barrett's esophagus with age [8, 9].

A series of studies have examined the effect of aging on perception of balloon distention in the esophagus. Weusten et al. studied a group of healthy volunteers aged 21–59 years and found that the response to intraesophageal balloon distention was notable for an age-related decrease in sensory perception accompanied by a decrease in amplitude and an increase in latency of cerebral evoked potentials [10]. Additional balloon distention work by Lasch et al. confirmed that older healthy volunteers (mean age 73 years) experienced pain at a higher balloon volume than did young healthy volunteers (mean age 27 years old) (age range 18–37 years) [11]. Furthermore, whereas all of the younger subjects experienced pain at a balloon volume < 28 mL, 10 of 17 older subjects did not have any pain at all with at least one of the two sets of balloon inflation to a maximum volume of 30 mL, and 5 of 17 experienced no pain with both sets of balloon inflation. Similar findings have been noted by others [4, 5]. These findings support an age-related decrease in visceral pain threshold.

Secondary peristalsis, initiated in response to local esophageal stimuli, also may be altered with advancing age. Ren et al. examined secondary esophageal peristalsis in response to intraesophageal air injection and balloon distention in a study of nine healthy young (mean age 35 years) and nine healthy elderly (mean age 74 years) volunteers [12]. They found either absent or less frequent stimulation of secondary peristalsis in the elderly subjects. Elderly patients also experienced less frequent LES relaxation in response to esophageal air distention. While secondary peristalsis was elicited in all of the younger subjects, there was complete failure of secondary peristalsis in four of the elderly subjects. This failure or deterioration of secondary peristalsis in the elderly would suggest impairment in esophageal afferent pathways, a finding that may be supported by the decrease in myenteric neurons described earlier [3].

Taken together, the above data indicate that there is a decrease in esophageal sensation that occurs with increasing age. Whether this impaired sensation is a result of decreased innervation or a failure of appropriate signaling is uncertain.

Esophageal Motility

There is an extensive literature on esophageal manometric findings in elderly individuals. However, the literature needs to be divided into studies of (a) healthy normal volunteers with no esophageal symptoms and (b) individuals referred for esophageal manometric testing for symptoms such as dysphagia, chest pain or GERD. The latter group is by nature much more heterogeneous and any abnormalities seen may be related to an underlying disease process and not simply normal aging. Of note, there are no studies to our knowledge utilizing modern high-resolution manometric techniques to assess esophageal function in the older population.

Lower Esophageal Sphincter

Work by Soergel et al. in 1964 first suggested the possibility of age-dependent changes in LES function, including failure of LES relaxation with swallowing [1]. LES relaxation was encountered in only 44% of swallows and was completely absent in two subjects. As noted earlier, this study was done on 15 individuals older than 90 years of age including some with dementia and diabetes and not in a healthy asymptomatic group of elderly individuals. However, with advances in esophageal physiologic testing in the ensuing years, these findings came into question. Dilation of the esophagus and impaired LES relaxation are seen in achalasia, and the findings seen by Soergel et al. may have been a manifestation of undiagnosed achalasia rather than the aged esophagus. Subsequent esophageal manometry studies in healthy older patients have either failed to reveal similar findings of LES dysfunction, or yielded inconsistent results of uncertain clinical significance.

Multiple studies of healthy volunteers have detected no difference in resting LES pressures or relaxation in older patients compared to younger patients. Hollis et al. examined 21 elderly males between the ages 70 and 87 years and compared them to 11 young healthy males between the ages 19 and 27 years [13]. LES relaxation occurred with 98% of the swallows in both groups. Khan et al. examined 133 healthy asymptomatic volunteers between the ages of 20 and 89 years and found comparable mean resting LES pressures between those below the age of 40 years (24.9±1.2 cm of water) and those over the age of 60 years (25.8±1.6 cm of water) [14]. A landmark study of 95 healthy adult volunteers by Richter et al. that established normal values for esophageal manometry laboratories found no effect of age on LES pressure measurements [15]. In contrast, only one study of healthy volunteers has found an abnormality in LES parameters with aging. Grande et al. studied 79 healthy volunteers with a mean age of 39 years (range 18–73 years) and found an inverse relationship between the lower esophageal resting pressures with age [16].

LES characteristics in symptomatic patients referred for manometry have also been described. In a study of 349 GERD patients who underwent esophageal manometry, Achem et al. found no difference in the resting LES pressures between old (≥65 years old) and young (≤40 years old) patients [17]. Additional work from the same center described similar findings in a study of 470 consecutive patients who underwent esophageal manometry for dysphagia, chest pain, and miscellaneous other indications; no differences were found between groups of older (≥75 years old) vs. younger (≤50 years old) in resting LES pressure (28.6 vs. 27.2 mmHg) or residual LES pressure (2.8 vs. 2.4 mmHg) [18]. Similar findings in a group of dysphagia patients have been described by others as well [19]. On the other hand, one group has described an elevation of basal LES pressure in patients with nonstructural causes of dysphagia referred for manometry [20]. The 23 older patients (≥80 years old) had a mean resting LES pressure of 26.1 mmHg compared to 16.8 mmHg in 23 younger patients (≤46 years old).

Thus, while it has been postulated that LES function deteriorates with age, current evidence suggests that LES dysfunction is not a hallmark of the esophagus in older patients. While abnormal function of the LES may be seen in the elderly, it should be investigated as a manifestation of a disease process such as achalasia or GERD rather than simply as an age-related phenomenon.

Esophageal Body

The studies cited above have also looked at esophageal body motor function in asymptomatic older patients. In Hollis' study of 21 healthy elderly compared to 11 young controls, a number of interesting findings were noted [13]. First, the amplitude of contractions in the distal esophagus was reduced in the elderly compared to the young group, with a marked decline in amplitude after the age of 80 years, both basally and in response to the cholinergic agonist edrophonium. There was no difference between the two groups in peristaltic velocity, duration of contractions, or onset of contractions after a swallow. The work by Khan et al. divided the 135 healthy subjects into two groups: those less than 40 years of age and those greater than 60 years of age [14]. They found that the amplitude of contractions was lower in those over age 60 years (53.9 vs. 74.4 mmHg). Furthermore, more contraction abnormalities were noted in the older subjects, including both an increase in simultaneous contractions and a decrease in peristaltic contractions. Similar findings of a decline in peristaltic amplitude and an increase in simultaneous contractions have been made by others as well [16]. In the Richter study of 95 healthy volunteers, distal contractile amplitude and duration increased with advancing age until peaking in the fifties before declining in the sixties (Fig. 20.3) [15].

Adamek et al. used 24-h esophageal manometry to investigate characteristics of esophageal function during normal diurnal activities of 44 healthy subjects [21]. A comparison of the young group (median age 29 years) with the older group (median age 62 years) found no influence of age on the amplitude and duration of peristaltic waves or the proportion of propulsive or simultaneous contractions.

Also of interest, Nishimura et al. compared findings in four groups in a study of 47 healthy volunteers based on age (<49 years old, 50–59, 60–69, and >70 years old) [22]. Non-propagated peristaltic activity was significantly more frequent in the older groups (60–69 years old and >70 years old) compared to the youngest patients

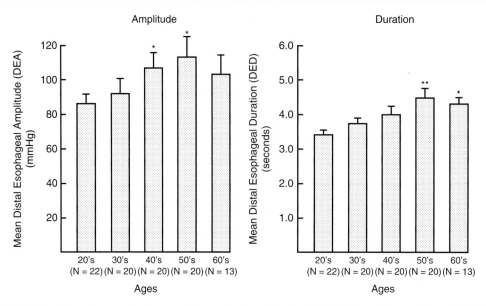

Fig. 20.3 The effect of age on distal contractile amplitude and duration in 95 healthy volunteers. From J.E. Richter et al. Dig Dis Sci 1987;32:583–92 with permission

(<49 years old) and peristaltic amplitude was lower in the group over age 70 years old compared to the group less than 49 years old.

The data are also inconsistent when looking at symptomatic individuals referred for esophageal manometry. The work by Ribeiro et al. examined 470 consecutive esophageal manometry studies in patients referred for a variety of indications [18]. There was a decrease in the frequency of primary peristalsis after wet swallows in older patients (≥75 years) when compared to younger patients (≤50 years) (63 vs. 78% $p < 0.005$). Furthermore, swallows in the older patients were more likely to result in simultaneous contractions than in the younger group (15 vs. 4% $p < 0.02$). However, illustrating the problems in interpreting these data, achalasia was more common in the elderly (15 vs. 4%) as was diffuse esophageal spasm (17 vs. 5%). Given the fact that peristaltic abnormalities such as simultaneous contractions are necessary for the diagnosis of both conditions, the relevance of these findings to normal aging is questionable.

In the study of 349 GERD patients who underwent esophageal manometry, Achem et al. found normal peristalsis after 63% of wet swallows in old (≥65 years old) patients compared to 95% of young (≤40 years old) patients with abnormal acid exposure [17].

Other studies have examined individuals referred for manometry because of nonstructural causes of dysphagia. Robson found no differences in older (>65 years old) vs. younger dysphagia patients (≤45 years old) in the frequency of normal peristalsis as well as contraction amplitude [19]. Andrews et al. in a study of 452 consecutive esophageal manometry studies done on symptomatic patients found that normal motor function was less frequent with aging [23].

Thus while studies are limited and inconsistent, some degree of motility disturbance in the esophageal body of the elderly appears frequent, although physiologic function for the most part remains intact [24]. Most common among these abnormalities seem to be decreased contractile amplitude especially in subjects greater than 80 years of age. The findings of impaired peristaltic activity and increased failure of primary peristalsis are variable. Nevertheless, aperistalsis not explained by achalasia or other connective tissue diseases may be more common in the elderly than in the young [25]. It is important to note that all of these studies were performed with older manometric techniques and not with high-resolution manometry, which provides more information on esophageal physiology than traditional water perfused systems.

Summary

Although motor abnormalities of esophageal function have been attributed in the past to the normal aging process, data supporting these conclusions appear to be lacking. Rather, normal esophageal physiology appears to be the norm in the elderly. Nonetheless, there appear to be consistent changes in esophageal sensation, stiffness, and luminal diameter with aging that may well be related to a decrease in myenteric neurons noted in the esophageal wall with aging. Any changes in LES pressure and relaxation and in the amplitude and duration of contractions as well as contraction abnormalities in the aging esophagus appear to be a manifestation of underlying disease states and not the normal aging process.

References

1. Soergel KH, Zboralske FF, Amberg JR. Presbyesophagus: esophageal motility in nonagenarians. J Clin Invest. 1964;43:1472–9.
2. DeVault KR. Presbyesophagus: a reappraisal. Curr Gastroenterol Rep. 2002;4:193–9.
3. Eckardt VF, LeCompte PM. Esophageal ganglia and smooth muscle in the elderly. Am J Dig Dis. 1978;23:443–8.
4. Rao SS, Mudipalli RS, Mujica VR, et al. Effects of gender and age on esophageal biomechanical properties and sensation. Am J Gastroenterol. 2003;98:1688–95.
5. Gregersen H, Pedersen J, Drewes AM. Deterioration of muscle function in the human esophagus with age. Dig Dis Sci. 2008;53:3065–70.
6. Fass R, Pulliam G, Johnson C, et al. Symptom severity and oesophageal chemosensitivity to acid in older and young patients with gastro-oesophageal reflux. Age Ageing. 2000;29:125–30.
7. Grade A, Pulliam G, Johnson C, et al. Reduced chemoreceptor sensitivity in patients with Barrett's esophagus may be related to age and not to the presence of Barrett's epithelium. Am J Gastroenterol. 1997;92:2040–3.
8. Cameron AJ, Lomboy CT. Barrett's esophagus: age, prevalence, and extent of columnar epithelium. Gastroenterology. 1992;103:1241–5.
9. van Blankenstein M, Looman CW, Johnston BJ, et al. Age and sex distribution of the prevalence of Barrett's esophagus found in a primary referral endoscopy center. Am J Gastroenterol. 2005;100:568–76.
10. Weusten BL, Lam HG, Akkermans LM, et al. Influence of age on cerebral potentials evoked by oesophageal balloon distension in humans. Eur J Clin Invest. 1994;24:627–31.
11. Lasch H, Castell DO, Castell JA. Evidence for diminished visceral pain with aging: studies using graded intraesophageal balloon distension. Am J Physiol. 1997;272:G1–3.
12. Ren J, Shaker R, Kusano M, et al. Effect of aging on the secondary esophageal peristalsis: presbyesophagus revisited. Am J Physiol. 1995;268:G772–9.
13. Hollis JB, Castell DO. Esophageal function in elderly men. A new look at "presbyesophagus.". Ann Intern Med. 1974;80:371–4.
14. Khan TA, Shragge BW, Crispin JS, et al. Esophageal motility in the elderly. Am J Dig Dis. 1977;22:1049–54.
15. Richter JE, Wu WC, Johns DN, et al. Esophageal manometry in 95 healthy adult volunteers. Variability of pressures with age and frequency of "abnormal" contractions. Dig Dis Sci. 1987;32:583–92.
16. Grande L, Lacima G, Ros E, et al. Deterioration of esophageal motility with age: a manometric study of 79 healthy subjects. Am J Gastroenterol. 1999;94:1795–801.
17. Achem AC, Achem SR, Stark ME, et al. Failure of esophageal peristalsis in older patients: association with esophageal acid exposure. Am J Gastroenterol. 2003;98:35–9.
18. Ribeiro AC, Klingler PJ, Hinder RA, et al. Esophageal manometry: a comparison of findings in younger and older patients. Am J Gastroenterol. 1998;93:706–10.
19. Robson KM, Glick ME. Dysphagia and advancing age: are manometric abnormalities more common in older patients? Dig Dis Sci. 2003;48:1709–12.
20. Andrews JM, Fraser RJ, Heddle R, Hebbard G, Checklin H. Is esophageal dysphagia in the extreme elderly (≥ 80 years) different to dysphagia younger adults? A clinical motility service audit. Dis Esophagus. 2008;21:656–9.
21. Adamek RJ, Wegener M, Wienbeck M, et al. Long-term esophageal manometry in healthy subjects. Evaluation of normal values and influence of age. Dig Dis Sci. 1994;39:2069–73.
22. Nishimura N, Hongo M, Yamada M, et al. Effect of aging on the esophageal motor functions. J Smooth Muscle Res. 1996;32:43–50.
23. Andrews JM, Heddle R, Hebbard GS, et al. Age and gender affect likely manometric diagnosis: audit of a tertiary referral hospital clinical esophageal manometry service. J Gastroenterol Hepatol. 2009;24:125–8.
24. Achem SR, DeVault KR. Dysphagia in aging. J Clin Gastroenterol. 2005;39:357–71.
25. Meshkinpour H, Haghighat P, Dutton C. Clinical spectrum of esophageal aperistalsis in the elderly. Am J Gastroenterol. 1994;89:1480–3.

Nascent Esophagus, Sensory-Motor Physiology During Maturation

21

Sudarshan R. Jadcherla

Abstract

The incidence of feeding and airway-related disorders is high, particularly among those neonates that graduate from the intensive care units. Commonly noted neonatal feeding problems that are influenced by esophageal anatomical and pathophysiological considerations include swallowing disorders, gastroesophageal reflux disease, aspiration syndromes, congenital foregut anomalies, and chronic lung disease. The functions of esophagus can be classified into (1) deglutitive peristaltic functions and (2) esophageal protective functions. In contrast to what is known in adult human or animal models, unfortunately, not much is known about these functions relevant to the nascent esophagus. In this chapter, we will explain the developmental physiology of (1) esophageal motility and peristalsis, and (2) sensorymotor aspects of upper esophageal sphincter, lower esophageal sphincter and esophageal body protective reflexes. This chapter follows the pharyngeal functions in relation to deglutition, and therefore the reader should also refer to the former chapter for better understanding of embryology and anatomical considerations.

Keywords

Esophageal and airway protective reflexes • Maturation of upper and lower esophageal sphincter • Nascent esophagus • Premature infants • Sensory-motor physiology

Introduction

This work was supported in part by NIH grants R01 DK 068158 (Jadcherla) and P01 DK 068051 (Jadcherla/Shaker).

S.R. Jadcherla, MD, FRCP (Irel), DCH, AGAF (✉)
Sections of Neonatology, Pediatric Gastroenterology and Nutrition, Nationwide Children's Hospital,
700 Childrens Drive, Columbus, OH 43205, USA
e-mail: Sudarshan.Jadcherla@nationwidechildrens.org

The incidence of feeding and airway-related disorders is high, particularly among those neonates that graduate from the intensive care units. Commonly noted neonatal feeding problems that are influenced by esophageal anatomical and pathophysiological considerations include swallowing disorders, gastroesophageal reflux disease, aspiration syndromes, congenital foregut anomalies, and chronic lung disease. The functions of esophagus can be classified into (1) deglutitive peristaltic functions and (2) esophageal protective functions. In contrast to what is known in adult human or animal models, unfortunately, not much is known about these functions relevant to the nascent esophagus. In this chapter, we will explain the developmental physiology of (1) esophageal motility and peristalsis, and (2) sensory-motor aspects of upper esophageal sphincter, lower esophageal sphincter and esophageal body protective reflexes. This chapter follows the pharyngeal functions in relation to deglutition, and therefore the reader should also refer to the former chapter for better understanding of embryology and anatomical considerations.

This chapter will focus on the physiology of the nascent esophagus in relation to its functions and reflexes. Specifically, we will elucidate how these complex protective and deglutitive esophageal functions are executed by a group of esophageal muscles coordinated by the Vagus.

Neuroanatomical Relationships Within the Aerodigestive Tract

The foregut is a tubular organ comprising inner circular and outer longitudinal muscle layers with myenteric plexus between the muscle layers. The proximal part of foregut is comprised of striated muscle and includes pharynx, upper esophageal sphincter (UES), and proximal third of the esophagus. The UES is characterized by a high pressure zone generated by the cricopharyngeus (the principal muscle), proximal cervical esophagus, and inferior pharyngeal constrictor. The UES is innervated by (1) the Vagus via the pharyngoesophageal, superior laryngeal and recurrent laryngeal branches; (2) the Glossopharyngeal nerve; and (3) the sympathetics via the cranial cervical ganglion. The distal end of the esophagus consists of the specialized smooth muscle, the lower esophageal sphincter, an autonomous contractile apparatus that is tonically active and relaxes periodically to facilitate bolus transit.

The airways and the foregut share common innervations [1–3]. Foregut afferents are derived from both Vagal and dorsal root ganglions with cell bodies in the nodose ganglion. This afferent apparatus conveys signals to the neurons in the nucleus tractus solitarius, located in the dorsomedial medulla oblongata. These signals are integrated in a specific terminal site of the nucleus tractus solitarius, the subnucleus centralis, which is the sole point of termination of esophageal afferents. After sensory integration in the nucleus tractus solitarius, the signals could in turn activate airway motor neurons in the nucleus ambiguous and the dorsal motor nucleus of the Vagus, producing an efferent parasympathetic response and/or nonadrenergic noncholinergic response. In summary, the innervations of the aerodigestive tract are as follows: (a) supraglottal and supra-UES mucosal areas from IX and X nerves, and muscular areas from X nerves; (b) infra-glottal mucosal and muscular areas from X nerve; and (c) pharynx and esophagus from IX and X nerves.

Deglutitive Functions of the Nascent Esophagus

The fetal swallowing ability develops by 11 weeks of embryonic life and fetus swallows amniotic fluid presented into the primitive pharynx. By 18–20 weeks, sucking movements appear, and by full-term gestation fetus can swallow and circulate nearly 500 ml of amniotic fluid. Thus, swallow-induced peristaltic activity begins in fetal life as evidenced by ultrasound studies [4, 5]. Much of the amniotic fluid is produced by the fetal lung, the flow of which is toward the direction of pharynx. However, as sucking, lingual, and oropharyngeal movements evolve, contribution to the amniotic fluid content varies, in that fetal urine and particulate material also are swallowed [6]. The directionality of amniotic fluid movement remains aboral within the fetal foregut and from lung into the pharynx within the airway structure. This balance is maintained until birth or the first breath [7, 8].

Maturation of Upper and Lower Esophageal Sphincter in Premature Infants

Using micromanometry methods, pharyngeal, upper esophageal sphincter (UES), esophageal body, and lower esophageal sphincter (LES) functions have been characterized in neonates [9–11]. Remarkably, the resting UES tone measured as UES pressure in end-expiration increases with maturation and is dependent on the state of alertness and activity. The average resting UES pressure (mean±SD) in preterm-born neonates at 33-week postmenstrual age was 17 ± 7 mmHg, in full-term-born neonates was 26 ± 14 mmHg, whereas in adults it was 53 ± 23 mmHg. With growth and maturation, the muscle mass and therefore the tone and activity of the UES improve. Similarly, changes in LES length and tone have been observed with growth [10, 12, 13]. By determining the lower esophageal sphincter high pressure zone in developing premature infants, others and we have determined changes in esophageal length during postnatal growth in premature and full-term infants. Specifically, the esophageal lengthening occurs in a linear fashion in neonates during growth [10, 12, 13].

Maturation of Esophageal Peristalsis in Premature Infants

During the propagation of the pharyngeal phase of swallow, the UES relaxes, and esophageal body waveforms propulse the bolus from proximal to distal end, which is accompanied by LES relaxation, so as to allow the bolus to enter the stomach. This whole integrated sequence of reflexes constitutes *primary esophageal peristalsis* which is swallow-dependent (Fig. 21.1). Evaluation of consecutive spontaneous solitary swallows during maturation (preterm at 33-week PMA vs. preterm at 36-week PMA) and growth (preterm-born and full-term-born vs. adults) was undertaken. Significant ($P < 0.05$) differences were noted in (1) the basal UES resting pressure, (2) UES relaxation parameters, (3) proximal and distal esophageal body amplitude and duration, (4) magnitude of esophageal waveform propagation, and (5) segmental peristaltic velocity. Specifically, the characteristics of UES and primary esophageal peristalsis exist by 33-week PMA; however, they undergo further maturation and differentiation during the postnatal growth, and are significantly different from that of adults [9].

Airway Protective Functions of the Nascent Esophagus

Esophageal and Airway Protective Reflexes

The esophagus is the frequent target for the anterograde bolus from the oropharynx as in swallowing, and also for the retrograde bolus from the stomach as in gastroesophageal reflux events. During either event, the bolus comes in close proximity to the airway, and evolving postnatal mechanisms facilitate pharyngeal and airway protection. For example, during primary esophageal peristalsis, there is a respiratory pause called deglutition apnea that occurs during the pharyngeal phase of swallow (Fig. 21.1). This brief inhibition in respiration is due to a break in respiratory cycle (inspiratory or expiratory), and is a normal reflex. On the other hand, during esophageal provocation events, esophageal peristalsis occurs independent of pharyngeal swallowing, called *secondary esophageal peristalsis* (Fig. 21.2). During such provocations, proximal esophageal contraction and distal esophageal relaxation will result in the generation of secondary esophageal peristalsis, which occur independent of central swallowing mechanisms. Although the nature and composition of bolus within the pharyngeal or esophageal lumen can vary, peristalsis remains the single-most important function that must occur to favor luminal clearance away from the airway. This reflex peristaltic response and airway protection are the end result of the activation and interaction of receptors–afferents–brain stem mediation–efferents–muscles–effectors. In premature infants, the mechanosensitive, chemosensitive, and osmosensitive stimuli can

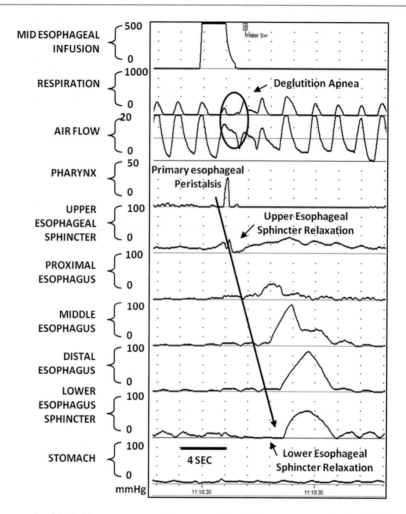

Fig. 21.1 An example of deglutition response or primary peristaltic reflex and deglutition apnea evoked upon mid-esophageal stimulation in a neonate. Note the pharyngeal contraction, UES relaxation, anterograde propagation, and deglutition apnea associated with this event. Note the changes in respiratory phase and air flow during pharyngeal contractile waveform

provoke the esophagus and the resultant reflexes that protect the airway-digestive tract include secondary esophageal peristalsis and UES contractile reflex (Fig. 21.2) [14–16]. These reflexes prevent the ascending spread of the bolus and favor descending propulsion to ensure esophageal clearance.

These reflexes advance during maturation in premature infants. In a study, premature infants were studied twice at 33-week and 36-week mean postmenstrual age. The occurrence of secondary esophageal peristalsis was volume-dependent, and the characteristics were different with advanced maturation. At 36-week postmen-

strual age, (1) completely propagated secondary esophageal peristalsis was greater with liquids than with air, (2) proximal esophageal waveform duration signifying proximal esophageal clearance time was shorter for air and liquids, and (3) the propagating velocity for liquids was faster. Additionally, as the premature infant grew older, the occurrence of secondary esophageal peristalsis increased significantly with increment in dose volumes of air or liquids. These findings are suggestive of the existence of Vago-vagal protective reflex mechanisms that facilitate esophageal clearance in healthy premature neonates, and that these mechanisms improve with growth.

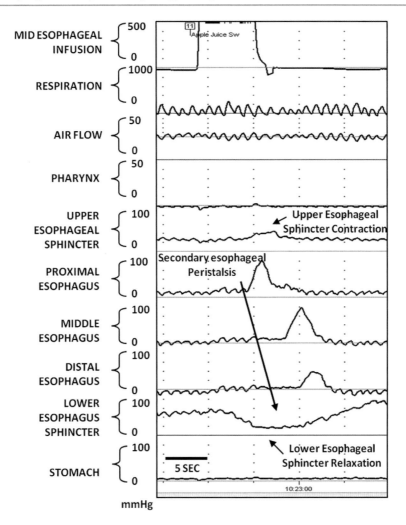

Fig. 21.2 An example of secondary peristaltic reflex along with esophago-upper esophageal sphincter contractile reflex and lower esophageal sphincter relaxation reflex, evoked upon mid-esophageal stimulation. Note the stability of respiration and sustained increase in UES pressure with stimulation

Similar to the occurrence of secondary esophageal peristalsis, esophageal provocation can result in an increase in UES pressure [14, 15]. This reflex is *Esophago-UES-contractile reflex*, and is mediated by the Vagus. We observed that the occurrence of UES contractile reflex was also volume dependent, and the characteristics improved with advanced maturation in healthy premature neonates. This reflex may provide protection to the aerodigestive tract, thus preventing the proximal extent of the refluxate as in spontaneous gastroesophageal reflux events (Fig. 21.2). Concurrently, the LES relaxes to

facilitate bolus clearance. This is called *LES relaxation reflex* response [17].

In summary, we review in this chapter, the developmental neuroanatomy and neurophysiology of esophagus and its aerodigestive relationships that facilitate swallowing, airway protection, and aspiration preventing mechanisms. Maldevelopment and maladaptation of these functions in high-risk infants pose continued threats to swallowing and esophageal functions with the consequence of dysphagia, chronic airway problems, and impaired quality of life. Altered esophageal defenses can occur in conditions such as extreme immaturity, mal-development of the foregut, neurological malfunction, or chronic lung disease. Neonatal maturational delays can result in motility disturbances and may form the basis for infant feeding problems. Important neonatal and infant problems related to the esophagus include dysphagia, gastroesophageal reflux disease, and aggravation of airway injury due to mal-development or malfunctions of the swallowing or airway protection mechanisms.

Acknowledgment This work was supported in part by NIH grant R01 DK 068158 (Jadcherla) and P01 DK 068051 (Jadcherla/Shaker). The author is grateful to Ms. Chin Yee Chan, MS, for assistance with this chapter.

References

1. Goyal R, Sivarao D. Functional anatomy and physiology of swallowing and esophageal motility. Philadelphia: Lippincott Williams and Wilkins; 1999.
2. Goyal RK, Padmanabhan R, Sang Q. Neural circuits in swallowing and abdominal vagal afferent-mediated lower esophageal sphincter relaxation. Am J Med. 2001;111(8A):95S–105.
3. Lang IM, Shaker R. Anatomy and physiology of the upper esophageal sphincter. Am J Med. 1997;103:50S–5.
4. Sase M, Lee JJ, Park JY, et al. Ontogeny of fetal rabbit upper gastrointestinal motility. J Surg Res. 2001;101:68–72.
5. Sase M, Lee JJ, Ross MG, et al. Effect of hypoxia on fetal rabbit gastrointestinal motility. J Surg Res. 2001;99:347–51.
6. Miller JL, Sonies BC, Macedonia C. Emergence of oropharyngeal, laryngeal and swallowing activity in the developing fetal upper aerodigestive tract: an ultrasound evaluation. Early Hum Dev. 2003;71:61–87.
7. Katz C, Bentur L, Elias N. Clinical implication of lung fluid balance in the perinatal period. J Perinatol. 2011;31:230–5.
8. Morrisey EE, Hogan BL. Preparing for the first breath: genetic and cellular mechanisms in lung development. Dev Cell. 2010;18:8–23.
9. Jadcherla SR, Duong HQ, Hofmann C, et al. Characteristics of upper oesophageal sphincter and oesophageal body during maturation in healthy human neonates compared with adults. Neurogastroenterol Motil. 2005;17:663–70.
10. Omari TI, Miki K, Fraser R, et al. Esophageal body and lower esophageal sphincter function in healthy premature infants. Gastroenterology. 1995;109:1757–64.
11. Staiano A, Boccia G, Salvia G, et al. Development of esophageal peristalsis in preterm and term neonates. Gastroenterology. 2007;132:1718–25.
12. Gupta A, Jadcherla SR. The relationship between somatic growth and in vivo esophageal segmental and sphincteric growth in human neonates. J Pediatr Gastroenterol Nutr. 2006;43:35–41.
13. Strobel CT, Byrne WJ, Ament ME, et al. Correlation of esophageal lengths in children with height: application to the Tuttle test without prior esophageal manometry. J Pediatr. 1979;94:81–4.
14. Jadcherla SR, Duong HQ, Hoffmann RG, et al. Esophageal body and upper esophageal sphincter motor responses to esophageal provocation during maturation in preterm newborns. J Pediatr. 2003;143:31–8.
15. Jadcherla SR, Hoffmann RG, Shaker R. Effect of maturation of the magnitude of mechanosensitive and chemosensitive reflexes in the premature human esophagus. J Pediatr. 2006;149:77–82.
16. Gupta A, Gulati P, Kim W, et al. Effect of postnatal maturation on the mechanisms of esophageal propulsion in preterm human neonates: primary and secondary peristalsis. Am J Gastroenterol. 2009;104:411–9.
17. Pena EM, Parks VN, Peng J, et al. Lower esophageal sphincter relaxation reflex kinetics: effects of peristaltic reflexes and maturation in human premature neonates. Am J Physiol Gastrointest Liver Physiol. 2010;299:G1386–95.

Part VII

Esophageal Motility and Its Deglutitive Function

Esophageal Motor Physiology

22

William G. Paterson and Nicholas Evans Diamant

Abstract

The esophagus is a muscular tube that serves to propel the ingested food to the stomach by sequential, aborally progressive contraction of the esophageal circular muscle in concert with shortening of the esophagus effected by longitudinal muscle contraction. Whereas esophageal muscle contraction in the proximal striated muscle segment is activated directly via vagal efferent neurons, control of peristalsis in the distal smooth muscle segment is more complex. Although vagal efferent pathways are necessary for initiating swallow-induced peristalsis, peripheral neuromuscular mechanisms play a key role in generating the sequential contraction of circular muscle in the smooth muscle esophagus, via a complex interplay between cholinergic and nitrergic nerves, as well as the myogenic properties of the muscle.

Keywords

Integration of central and peripheral mechanisms • Longitudinal muscle • Muscularis mucosa • Neurotransmitters • Peripheral innervation • Peripheral neurogenic control • Physiological control of esophageal peristalsis

W.G. Paterson, MD, FRCPC (✉)
Division of Gastroenterology, Department
of Medicine, Hotel Dieu Hospital,
Kingston, ON, Canada
e-mail: patersow@hdh.kari.net

N.E. Diamant, MDCM, FRCP(C)
Department of Medicine/Gastroenterology,
Kingston General Hospital, Kingston, ON, Canada

The main function of the esophagus is to propel swallowed food or fluid into the stomach. This occurs through sequential or "peristaltic" contractions of circular muscle in the esophageal body, in concert with appropriately timed relaxation of the upper and lower esophageal sphincters (UES and LES), and shortening of the esophagus evoked by longitudinal muscle contraction. The esophagus also must clear any refluxed gastric contents back into the stomach and participates in vomiting and belching. This chapter will focus on the peristaltic function of the esophageal body and its control.

R. Shaker et al. (eds.), *Principles of Deglutition: A Multidisciplinary Text for Swallowing and its Disorders*, 303
DOI 10.1007/978-1-4614-3794-9_22, © Springer Science+Business Media New York 2013

Overview of Esophageal Motor Function

The normal swallow-induced contraction of the esophagus is called primary peristalsis. On entry of the bolus into the esophagus the UES closes, and a peristaltic contraction passes distally along the esophageal body to the relaxed LES. The LES then contracts in sequence. Figure 22.1 shows these events as recorded both by conventional and high-resolution manometry. The velocity of the wave varies between 2.5 and 5 cm/s along the esophagus in a bimodal fashion (Fig. 22.2) [1–3]. The normal contraction is usually less than 7 s and contraction amplitudes rarely exceed 200 mmHg [4].

During peristalsis, esophageal shortening of 2–2.5 cm occurs, due to longitudinal muscle contraction that proceeds distally at 2–4 cm/s and onsets slightly in advance of the circular muscle contraction [5–9]. Longitudinal muscle contraction is believed to facilitate bolus transit by two mechanisms: (1) by shortening the esophagus, the esophageal radius must increase, thereby

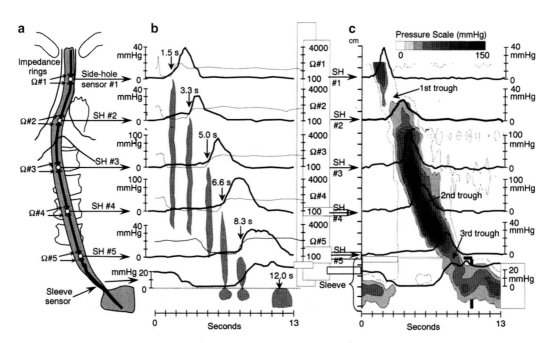

Fig. 22.1 The relationship between videofluoroscopic, manometric, impedance, and topographic representations of esophageal peristalsis. (**a**) Depiction of intraluminal manometry/impedance measurement with five sensors at 4 cm intervals, and a sleeve sensor in the lower esophageal sphincter (LES). (**b**) Representation by overlaying manometry and impedance measurements with videofluoroscopic appearance of a 5-ml swallowed barium bolus. The pressure scale for the *dark thick line* is on the *left* and the impedance scale for the *light thin line* is on the *right*. The *arrows* point to the distribution of the bolus at the times indicated. As the bolus enters the esophagus there is a slight increase in pressure at most sites, the "bolus pressure." As the contraction reaches each site, the pressure increases and the impedance decreases. As the lumen closes and the upstroke of the pressure wave occurs, the tail of the barium bolus is evident. (**c**) Comparison of conventional manometric pressure tracing at five sites and the LES, as positioned in **a**, with the pressure profile obtained with high-resolution manometry and displayed topographically as an isocontour plot. The overlay places the two representations at similar locations. In the isocontour plot deepening shades of *gray* indicate higher pressures. There are three pressure troughs: at the junction of the striated and smooth muscle esophagus; in the mid portion of the smooth muscle portion; and at the end of the peristaltic segment just before the LES. The troughs separate four different pressure segments, the last fronting the contraction that closes the LES. The end of the LES relaxation measured with conventional manometry coincides with arrival of the contraction at the start of the fourth pressure segment and the LES. From J.E. Pandolfino and P.J. Kahrilas. Gastroenterology 2005;128:209–224 with permission from Elsevier Publishing and the American Gastroenterological Association

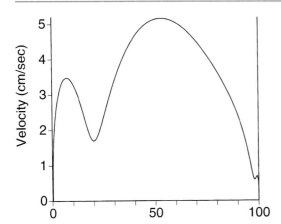

Fig. 22.2 A bimodal velocity pattern of the peristaltic wave front along the esophagus is apparent using axial reconstructions of pressure data. The two modes represent propagation through the proximal striated muscle and distal smooth muscle regions, with deceleration near the lower esophageal sphincter. There is no break in velocity in the smooth muscle region. From R.E. Clouse et al. Dig Dis Sci 1996;41:2369–76 with permission from Plenum publishing

85% and specificity of 66% [15]. Sensory feedback from the esophagus has an effect on the contractions and peristalsis. Larger boluses and greater viscosity increase contraction amplitude and duration, and slow peristaltic velocity [16–18]. Increased intraabdominal pressure and esophageal obstruction also increase amplitude and slow velocity. Gravity facilitates transport, especially of liquids, and distal contraction amplitude can decrease in the more upright position [19].

In addition to the swallow-induced, primary peristaltic wave, local sensory stimulation such as distention from retained food not cleared by the primary wave or from refluxed gastric contents can trigger "secondary peristalsis." This peristaltic wave is similar to that of primary peristalsis but begins in the esophagus slightly above the level of the stimulus. However, distension high in the esophagus can at times initiate the process at the pharyngeal stage [20].

increasing the lumen size ahead of the oncoming bolus [10]; (2) longitudinal contractions tend to slide the esophagus over the bolus and increase the density of the circular muscle fibers orad to the bolus, which in turn increase the efficiency of the circular muscle contraction [11] and reduces stress on the esophageal wall [12].

The amplitude of the circular muscle contraction decreases in a short segment at 4–6 cm below the UES, attributed to the region where striated and smooth muscles intersperse and/or innervation changes from the recurrent laryngeal nerve proximally to the more distal vagal branches. Within the smooth muscle section there is one other region of decreased contraction amplitude about in its middle, and another near the end of the esophageal body and just above the LES [1, 3, 13]. It is not known if these findings are due to separate neuromuscular units governed by output from subunits in the swallowing center, or by peripheral intramural neuromuscular mechanisms.

Contraction amplitude determines the efficiency of bolus propulsion and esophageal emptying, with efficiency decreasing as amplitude decreases [14]. At a threshold of 30 mmHg, incomplete bolus transit can be predicted with a sensitivity of

Physiological Control of Esophageal Peristalsis

Peristalsis in Striated Muscle Esophagus

Like striated muscle in other parts of the body, the striated muscle segment of the esophagus is dependent on excitatory nerve activity from lower motor neurons. The striated muscle of the esophagus is innervated by myelinated vagal lower motor neurons whose cell bodies are located in the nucleus ambiguous and nucleus retrofacialis [21, 22]. A small number of cell bodies may also arise in the dorsal motor nucleus (DMN) of the vagus. These nerve fibers contain choline acetyltransferase and calcitonin gene-related peptide (CGRP) and synapse directly on the motor end plates. Acetylcholine is the primary neurotransmitter involved in activation of esophageal-striated muscle. The role of CGRP is unknown. Bilateral cervical vagotomy above the origin of the pharyngoesophageal branches abolishes peristalsis in the striated muscle esophagus [23, 24]. However, unilateral vagotomy has no effect on peristalsis, presumably because of extensive crossover of vagal innervation within the esophageal wall [25]. Innovative experiments performed by Roman [25] established that vagal efferent neurons destined for the striated muscle esophagus fire sequentially. They used the central portion of the sectioned vagus in sheep to reinnervate the sternocleidomastoid and trapezius muscles from which they were able to record electrical activity. Activation of deglutition-induced sequential contraction of the reinnervated muscles coincided with peristaltic contractions simultaneously measured by intraluminal manometry.

A scant myenteric plexus does exist within the striated muscle esophagus, but its role in esophageal motor function is unclear. Interestingly, it has been demonstrated that motor end plates in the striated muscle esophagus are coinnervated by vagal lower motor neurons and nitrergic myenteric plexus neurons [26–29]. It has been speculated that this myenteric innervation may provide an inhibitory counterbalance to the predominant vagal excitatory innervation [29].

Peristalsis in the Smooth Muscle Esophagus

In this region there are three potential control mechanisms for peristalsis that must interact and integrate effectively: (1) The central swallowing center [30–33] sends sequential efferent signals to the esophagus via the vagus nerves [34–36]; (2) An intramural neural mechanism [37–40]; and (3) A myogenic mechanism [41–43]. All of these mechanisms are influenced by feedback from afferent sensory stimulation.

Central Control Mechanisms

The esophagus receives sequential vagal input to both the striated and smooth muscle segments during both primary and secondary peristalsis. Figure 22.3 demonstrates this vagal activity in the baboon and opossum [34, 35]. The findings in the opossum indicate two different timings of vagal firing patterns, an early rapid-sequence group that would fit with early activation of inhibitory neurons, and a later slower sequence that mirrors the

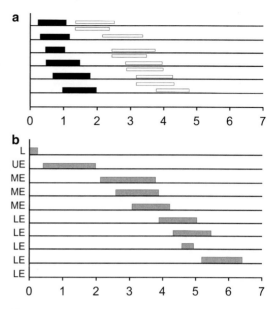

Fig. 22.3 Vagus nerve firing patterns associated with swallow-induced esophageal peristalsis in the opossum (**a**) and the baboon (**b**). In the opossum, there is an early and a late sequential firing pattern. The latter corresponds to the timing and velocity of the esophageal peristaltic wave, whereas the former likely coincides with the initial activation of inhibitory neurons. In the baboon, only a sequential firing pattern timed with the presence of the esophageal contraction along the esophagus was recorded. (**a**) From J.S. Gidda and R.K. Goyal. J Neurophysiol 1984;52:1169–80 with permission from American Physiological Society (**b**) From C. Roman and L. Tieffenbach. J Physiol (Paris)1972;64:479–506 with permission from Elsevier Publishing

timing and velocity of the peristaltic contraction. It is not known if two firing patterns are present in other species. If initial inhibition and subsequent excitation is the function of these two groups, it has been assumed that the early group excites the inhibitory neurons and the later group the excitatory neurons along the smooth muscle esophagus. It is not established if the vagal fibers go directly to these neurons or are routed through interneuronal circuitry.

Peripheral Neurogenic Control

Although sequential firing does occur in vagal efferent nerves, and the vagus is needed for initiation of primary peristalsis, peristalsis can also be induced by local distention and electrical

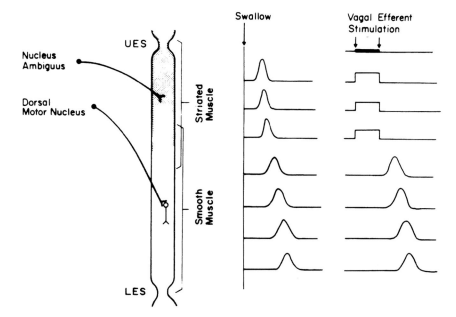

Fig. 22.4 Simultaneous electrical activation of all vagal efferent neurons produces simultaneous contractions in the striated muscle esophagus, which would be expected based on the direct innervation of this muscle by the vagal efferent neurons. However, in the smooth muscle segment a peristaltic wave is induced. This is because intrinsic neurons activated by vagal efferent nerve stimulation are capable of evoking a peristaltic contraction without the need for centrally mediated sequencing. From R.K. Goyal and W.G. Paterson. Handbook of physiology: gastrointestinal system. 1989 with permission from American Physiological Society

stimulation of an esophagus devoid of extrinsic innervation. Furthermore, simultaneous electrical activation of all vagal efferent nerve fibers induces peristalsis after a variable delay, rather than an immediate simultaneous contraction (Fig. 22.4) [39, 44–46]. This indicates the importance of peripheral neuromuscular mechanisms in the generation of peristalsis.

Tension-recording studies of isolated circular smooth muscle strips that have intrinsic but not extrinsic innervation have demonstrated an intrinsic "latency gradient" of contraction along the esophagus that appears to contribute to the generation of the peristaltic wave [47]. Most of these studies have been performed in the opossum model. Short-duration electrical stimulation of the intrinsic nerves of a circular smooth muscle strip results in a contraction that occurs after the stimulus has ended (the so-called off response). The onset of this contraction relative to the stimulus increases in strips taken from more aboral segments of the smooth muscle esophagus (Fig. 22.5). This latency gradient has been shown to relate to

the initial inhibition or hyperpolarization that occurs upon nerve stimulation. In other words, with nerve stimulation there is first release of an inhibitory neurotransmitter (nitric oxide—NO) that causes hyperpolarization of the membrane. The duration of this hyperpolarization is longer aborally [48], so that the ensuing contraction is delayed aborally. This initial hyperpolarization of the circular smooth muscle membrane potential has also been recorded in the opossum in vivo in response to swallows [49]. Furthermore, a wave of initial inhibition can be recorded in humans by creating an artificial high-pressure zone using a partially distended balloon [50]. The reason for the progressive increase in duration of the initial hyperpolarization in the proximal versus distal smooth muscle esophagus is unclear. It could represent a relative increase in the release or local effects of inhibitory neurotransmitter distally, or alternatively, a relative increase in excitatory neurotransmitter release or effects proximally. There is no direct evidence in support of either of these possibilities, but studies in several species

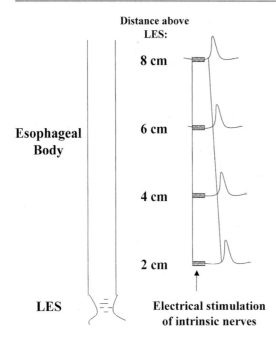

Distance above LES:

Esophageal Body

8 cm

6 cm

4 cm

2 cm

LES   Electrical stimulation
                       of intrinsic nerves

Fig. 22.5 Stimulation electrical stimulation of intrinsic neurons within isolated esophageal circular smooth muscle strips results in phasic contraction after a variable delay. The latency to onset of this contraction increases progressively in strips taken from more aboral segments of the smooth muscle esophagus. This demonstrates the existence of an "intrinsic latency gradient" of contraction along the esophagus, which contributes to the generation of a peristaltic wave. From Paterson. Esophageal peristalsis. GI motility online; 2006 with permission from Nature Publishing Group

[51–62] have shown that atropine delays the onset of peristaltic contractions, with a greater effect in the proximal than distal esophagus, whereas inhibition of NO shortens the latency of contraction, with a more pronounced effect distally than proximally (see below). To date, there has been no morphological evidence of a gradient in the density of cholinergic or nitrergic innervation along the esophagus. This raises the possibility that intrinsic differences in smooth muscle responses along the esophagus may result in a varied response to the same quantum of released neurotransmitter (see below).

Although an aborally increasing gradient in the duration of the initial inhibition is an attractive model to explain peristalsis, the calculated speed of peristalsis based on intrinsic differences in the initial inhibition along the esophagus is on the order of 10 cm/s [48], which is much faster than peristalsis in vivo. Thus, there must be mechanisms other than the intrinsic latency gradient to explain peristalsis. Experiments in which simultaneous electrical and mechanical activity were recorded in both the proximal and distal opossum smooth muscle esophagus have helped clarify the discrepancy between the in vitro and in vivo observations [58]. In this study, it was shown that an initial monophasic inhibitory potential occurs along the esophagus with either swallowing or balloon distention. In keeping with the electrophysiological and muscle strip studies, the duration of the initial hyperpolarization was slightly longer distally than proximally, but this difference was insufficient to explain the marked delay of esophageal contraction in the distal versus the proximal smooth muscle esophagus. Rather, in the distal esophagus the initial monophasic inhibitory potential was followed by a second wave of hyperpolarization before the membrane potential rebounded into depolarization and initiation of spike potentials (Fig. 22.6). It was suggested that this secondary hyperpolarization is likely due to reactivation of descending inhibitory neurons by distention or contraction of the more proximal esophagus in the course of peristalsis (Fig. 22.7). This suggests that intramural descending inhibitory pathways are crucial in generating the peristaltic wave. Subsequent studies in the opossum have demonstrated that localized distention appears to directly activate intrinsic nitrergic inhibitory neurons that send long aboral projections [63, 64]. These long tension-activated descending neurons provide an important intrinsic mechanism to ensure that the distal esophagus remains inhibited as the bolus traverses the esophagus, irrespective of the speed of bolus transit.

Intramural Myogenic (Muscle) Control Mechanisms

With the esophagus isolated in vitro and with nerves blocked, a myogenic peristaltic contraction can be demonstrated in the smooth muscle segment [41–43, 65]. Elsewhere in the gut, a

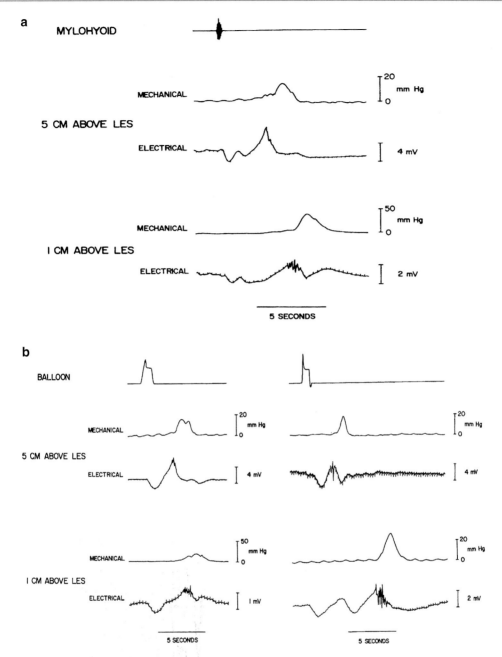

Fig. 22.6 Correlation of electrical and mechanical events during peristalsis evoked by swallowing (**a**) and balloon distention (**b**). The onset of swallowing is marked by the mylohyoid muscle electromyogram. With swallow-induced (primary) peristalsis, note that the delay in onset of depolarization, spike burst, and esophageal contraction in the distal esophagus relates to a marked second wave of hyperpolarization. With mid-esophageal balloon disten-tion in the left tracing, the peristaltic velocity is abnormally fast, and it is apparent that the slight delay in onset of contraction at the distal vs. proximal site is due to an initial hyperpolarization of slightly longer duration. However, when balloon distention induces a secondary peristaltic wave of normal velocity (*right panel*), the marked delay in onset of contraction distally correlates with a second wave of hyperpolarization that is likely due to reactivation of intrinsic descending inhibitory pathways by contractions occurring upstream. From W.G. Paterson. Gastroenterology 1989;97:665–75 with permission from the American Gastroenterological Association; copyright Elsevier

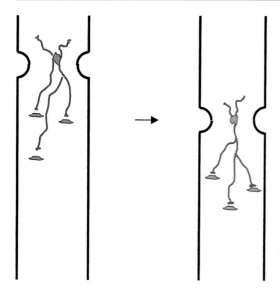

Fig. 22.7 Model to explain the intrinsic neuromuscular mechanisms that mediate normal esophageal peristalsis. With the initial stimulation, be it swallowing or distention, there is a short-lived hyperpolarization that is slightly longer in more aboral region of the esophagus. What then transpires is that intrinsic descending inhibitory neurons are continuously reactivated by contraction and/or bolus distention as it migrates down the esophagus. This mechanism ensures that the esophagus remains inhibited in advance of the oncoming peristaltic contraction and intraluminal bolus. From Paterson. Esophageal peristalsis. GI motility online; 2006 with permission from Nature Publishing Group

myogenic control system has two fundamental characteristics: (1) electrical oscillations of the smooth muscle cells, usually called "slow waves"; and (2) communication among smooth muscle cells allowing the tissue to operate as a functional unit [66, 67]. Both features are present in the esophageal circular smooth muscle, although the former is only manifest with adequate electrical or pharmacological stimulation [42, 43, 65, 68–70]. Spontaneous rhythmic contractions have also been recorded from esophageal longitudinal smooth muscle at rest [42, 71], but their physiological significance is uncertain. In other regions of the gut, interstitial cells of Cajal (ICCs) are believed to play a critical role in myogenic control mechanisms. Appropriately positioned ICCs are also present in the esophagus [72, 73], but their physiological role has yet to be elucidated in this tissue.

It has been assumed that the regional gradients in the cholinergic and nitrergic innervation along the esophagus, discussed above, are sufficient for local control of peristalsis in the smooth muscle section. However, there are also regional differences in the circular smooth muscle along the esophagus that likely contribute significantly to the peristaltic contraction and the delays along the esophagus, including the responses to cholinergic and nitrergic innervation. These differences include a resting membrane potential gradient [74, 75], potassium and calcium ion channel diversity [75–77], and differences in muscle length–tension relationships and responses to cholinergic stimulation [78].

Role of Afferent Sensory Feedback in the Control of Peristalsis

With swallowing the region of the swallowing center that controls the esophageal stage is normally activated [32], but this activation is considerably enhanced when there is greater pharyngeal and esophageal sensory feedback to the swallowing center. Failed esophageal peristalsis in all or part of the esophagus is common in humans, particularly with "dry" swallows. The presence of a bolus increases the frequency and completion of the peristaltic wave [16, 18]. Animal studies have been conflicting in determining the necessity for bolus stimulation of the esophagus for primary peristalsis to occur. In dogs that have a totally striated muscle esophagus, and with diversion of the bolus in the cervical esophagus, primary peristalsis is absent in the distal esophagus [79, 80]. In the decerebrate cat without cortical input, the bolus must be present in the cervical esophagus for peristalsis to proceed in the smooth muscle portion [81]. However, in primates that also have a distal smooth muscle esophagus, the bolus is not always necessary [82]. Transcortical magnetic stimulation in the anesthetized cat [83] or awake dog [84] can itself initiate swallowing, and in the dog produce contraction of the upper esophagus without a bolus. Such cortical stimulation does not appear to initiate swallowing in humans although muscles in the pharynx and upper and lower esophagus can be induced to contract [85–87]. It is clear that the region of the swallowing center controlling the esophageal stage must be adequately activated for primary peristalsis to occur in the esophagus. That is, one or more of the three inputs to the swallowing center, from the cortex, pharynx, or esophagus, must be sufficient for activation, and each can facilitate the other [88]. Normally all three inputs are present. However, involvement of all three may not be necessary depending on species differences and experimental conditions. Regardless, the swallowed bolus is an important component under normal circumstances, and amplitude, duration and velocity of the peristaltic wave are subject to the nature and size of the bolus.

In addition to providing input to the swallowing center, luminal distention by a bolus and/or muscle contraction associated with both primary and secondary peristalsis also provides a sensory stimulus for activation of intrinsic neurons. This sensory input contributes to peristalsis, and in particular the descending inhibitory component [63, 64]. The sensory transduction mechanisms responsible for this are unclear.

Integration of Central and Peripheral Mechanisms

Clearly a central mechanism and peripheral neural and myogenic mechanisms can direct peristalsis in the smooth muscle segment, and must integrate effectively. Which mechanism is dominant under normal circumstances is not established. At rest the esophagus is both mechanically and electrically silent, and some form of stimulus is required for a contraction to occur. With a swallow, the central mechanism initiates and sequences contractions in the striated muscles of the esophagus. For initiation of a contraction in the smooth muscle portion, excitatory cholinergic neurons must be adequately stimulated by central and/or peripheral neural input. The threshold for muscle contraction, its timing in the peristaltic sequence, and contraction amplitude are determined by the balance between excitatory and inhibitory influences at the muscle level.

The swallow or pharyngeal stimulation initiates the swallowing center esophageal stage of control and its vagal output to the smooth muscle. Sensory input from a bolus in the esophagus is not necessary for the occurrence of primary peristalsis in this segment in the human but can alter the intensity and timing of the vagal output that corresponds to the timing and amplitude of the contraction. With secondary peristalsis, the swallowing center behavior is normally similar to that with primary peristalsis. Thus, even though distention-induced peristalsis can occur in the absence of central control, it is likely that under physiological circumstances the central nervous system has significant influence on the secondary peristaltic wave. Indeed, it appears that the proximal excitation component of secondary peristalsis and its occurrence in the striated muscle esophagus are entirely dependent on intact vagal nerves [89]. Vagal inputs also impact directly or indirectly on both excitatory cholinergic and inhibitory nitrergic myenteric neurons and presumably function as the primary control of the peripheral neural network and the network's excitatory and inhibitory outputs to the smooth muscle [90]. Because of its properties, it is likely that the myogenic control mechanism participates in the final contraction pattern, but how this control mechanism might operate or be controlled is not known. When esophageal sensory input is large and has major impact on the local neural mechanism, such as with a large stationary bolus, this neural mechanism itself can have a significant influence on the final contraction pattern. Contraction is enhanced proximally and inhibited distally. Final resolution of how the different control mechanisms operate together is yet to be determined. Thankfully, the presence of more than one control mechanism provides for peristalsis to occur if central control is absent or abnormal.

Neurotransmitters Involved in Esophageal Peristalsis: Evidence of Dual Peripheral Innervation

Vagal efferent neurons involved in esophageal peristalsis synapse on both inhibitory and excitatory myenteric neurons. Ganglionic transmission is predominantly nicotinic, although there may be associated muscarinic and serotonergic transmission [91–93]. A large number of different peptide and nonpeptide neurotransmitters can be detected within the esophageal myenteric plexus using immunohistochemical stains [28, 94–96]. However, it appears that two types of motor nerves predominate. One stains for NO synthase and vasoactive intestinal peptide, and the other for choline acetyl transferase and substance P. NO is the predominant inhibitory neurotransmitter, whereas acetylcholine, acting on either M2 or M3 muscarinic receptors [97–99] is the predominant excitatory neurotransmitter. Evidence for this dual innervation comes from a number of sources. In the opossum model, nerve stimulation of isolated circular smooth muscle strips produces a predominant "off" contraction (i.e., the contraction occurs after the electrical stimulation ends) that is resistant to both adrenergic and cholinergic blockade [47, 100]. Subsequent studies revealed that this off contraction can be blocked by a NO synthase inhibitor [62, 101, 102]. However, depending on the parameters of nerve stimulation, atropine-sensitive contractions may also be induced [37, 103]. Furthermore, in the presence of a NO synthase inhibitor, a predominant cholinergic contraction in response to nerve stimulation becomes unmasked [62]. Similar observations have been made in human esophageal muscle strip studies [104].

These observations are supported by studies using vagal efferent nerve stimulation [39, 51, 62]. With a short train of nerve stimulation, contractions are induced along the smooth muscle esophagus after the stimulus is over. These are often peristaltic in nature, but adjusting the electrical stimulus parameters can influence this. If a long stimulus train is used, however, both an intrastimulus contraction (A wave) and a poststimulus contraction (B wave) are frequently observed [39, 51, 62]. The intrastimulus contraction is usually peristaltic and is blocked by atropine, whereas the poststimulus contraction is blocked by a NO synthase inhibitor and is either simultaneous in onset or has a very rapid -peristaltic velocity. Whether A waves, B waves, or both are induced by long train vagal efferent stimulation depends on the stimulus frequency used. Low-frequency stimulation favors A waves, whereas high-frequency stimulation favors

B waves. Interestingly, administration of atropine not only blocks A waves, but also unmasks or enhances B waves, whereas NO synthase inhibition does the opposite (Fig. 22.8). When both atropine and a NO synthase inhibitor are applied together, both A and B waves are abolished [51]. Similarly, both antagonists are required to completely abolish swallow-induced peristalsis in the opossum model [51]. These studies provide support for the concept that vagal efferent nerve fibers innervate both inhibitory (nitrergic) and excitatory (cholinergic) neurons. It thus appears that the normal peristaltic wave is a result of blended innervation that may vary along the esophagus. Cholinergic neurons activate contraction by directly depolarizing the muscle. On the other hand, nitrergic neurons presumably cause contraction through a "rebound" depolarization following an initial hyperpolarization; that is, NO serves as both an inhibitory and excitatory neurotransmitter. The relative importance of direct cholinergic excitation versus rebound excitation in evoking esophageal contraction varies between species. In the opossum model, rebound excitation following NO-induced inhibition plays a large role, whereas in humans and especially cats, cholinergic excitation is much more dominant [53, 57, 105].

The physiological role of other neurotransmitters found within the smooth muscle esophagus is unclear, as studies often fail to clearly differentiate a pharmacological from a physiological effect. Tachykinins may contribute to part of the noncholinergic excitatory response in human esophageal circular smooth muscle [106]. Enkephalins also may modulate peristalsis by presynaptic inhibition or excitation of neurotransmitters directly responsible for peristalsis [107, 108], whereas catecholamines [109] and CGRP [110] inhibit esophageal contractions.

Role of Longitudinal Muscle and Muscularis Mucosa in Esophageal Peristalsis

To date, studies on the physiology of the longitudinal muscle have focused entirely on the smooth muscle esophagus. As discussed above, the longitudinal muscle also contracts in sequential fashion

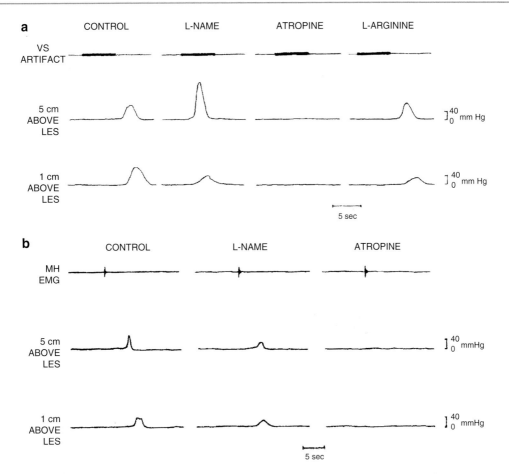

Fig. 22.8 Evidence for dual innervation in the control of esophageal peristalsis in the opossum model. (**a**) Vagal efferent nerve simulation using high stimulus frequency produced only a B-wave (i.e., contraction after the end of stimulation). Following administration of Nω-nitro-L-arginine methyl ester (L-NAME), an inhibitor of NO synthase, the B wave is abolished, and an A wave (i.e., intrastimulus contraction) is unmasked, which in turn is abolished by the administration of atropine. Subsequent administration of L-arginine (a substrate of NO synthase that reverses the effect of L-NAME), results in a return of the B-wave. (**b**) Following the administration of L-NAME, the amplitude of the swallow-induced peristaltic wave is diminished and peristaltic velocity increases owing to a shortening of the onset of contraction in the distal esophageal site (1 cm above the LES). Subsequent administration of atropine abolishes primary peristalsis in the opossum smooth muscle esophagus. From N. Anand and W.G. Paterson. AJP Gastrointest Liver Physiol 1994; modified with permission from American Physiological Society

during peristalsis to facilitate bolus transport [111]. However, it appears that unlike circular smooth muscle, the sequential nature of the esophageal longitudinal smooth muscle contraction is entirely mediated centrally via vagal efferents. Similar to circular muscle, the duration of longitudinal muscle contraction also appears to vary along the esophagus, with contraction lasting longer distally than proximally [111].

In vivo studies in the opossum model have also shown that the primary neurotransmitter involved in longitudinal smooth muscle contrac-tion is acetylcholine. The muscarinic antagonist atropine virtually abolishes longitudinal muscle contraction and esophageal shortening in response to swallowing and vagal stimulation [38, 39, 112]. However, infrequent noncholinergic contractions can be evoked, but the physiological significance of these is unclear [112]. In vitro studies have also shown that longitudinal muscle contraction is predominantly mediated by cholinergic neurons; however, with certain stimulus parameters a slowly developing and sustained longitudinal muscle contraction can be evoked, which is abolished by substance P desensitization [113]. Recent studies suggest that this is mediated by substance P released from capsaicin-sensitive neurons and acting via neurokinin (NK)-2 receptors [114]. It is unlikely that this substance P-mediated contraction is involved in normal peristalsis. However, it may play a role in the reflex longitudinal muscle contraction that occurs with acid reflux into the esophagus [115]. There has been speculation that this substance P-mediated contraction may also be involved in certain esophageal pain syndromes [115, 116].

Although there is evidence that the longitudinal smooth muscle may participate in deglutitive inhibition [117], the phenomenon whereby peristaltic motor activity induced by a swallow is inhibited by a second swallow performed at a closely spaced interval, there is no evidence to date that this is related to direct inhibitory innervation to the longitudinal smooth muscle. Elegant studies in which electrical activity was recorded from a flap of isolated longitudinal smooth muscle in vivo showed no evidence of an inhibitory junction potential occurring during primary peristalsis [118]. Interestingly, NO has been reported to cause paradoxical contraction of esophageal longitudinal smooth muscle [71, 119, 120], but it is unclear whether this neurotransmitter is involved in physiological contraction of this muscle layer [120].

Little is known about the physiological role of the muscularis mucosa during peristalsis. It may contract primarily in response to luminal stimuli, thereby evoking movement of esophageal mucosa. It may also serve to hold the normally loosely attached overlying mucosa in place, thereby preventing excessive movement of the mucosa during bolus movement. Studies on the physiology and pharmacology of this muscle layer have been carried out [121–125]. As with the longitudinal smooth muscle of the muscularis propria, contraction primarily involves cholinergic neurons acting on muscarinic receptors. There also appears to be a more sustained or tonic contraction due to release of substance P [124, 126].

Summary

Although the prime function of esophageal peristalsis is relatively simple (i.e. to propel the ingested food bolus to the stomach), the physiological control mechanisms underlying this function are complex and remain incompletely understood. The inner layer of circular muscle contracts sequentially above the bolus and relaxes distally, thereby pushing the ingested bolus aborally, whereas contraction of the longitudinal muscle layer facilitates bolus transfer by shortening the esophagus and opening up the lumen. Central nervous system control via vagal efferent nerves is essential for initiating the peristaltic wave, and is directly responsible for the sequential activation of circular muscle in the striated muscle segment and longitudinal muscle in both the striated and smooth muscle segments. On the other hand, peripheral neuromuscular mechanisms play a key role in generating the sequential contraction of circular muscle in the smooth muscle esophagus, via a complex interplay between cholinergic and nitrergic nerves, as well as the myogenic properties of the muscle. A better understanding of the physiological control of esophageal peristalsis is essential if we are to optimally manage patients suffering from disorders of esophageal motility.

References

1. Clouse RE, Staiano A. Topography of normal and high-amplitude esophageal peristalsis. Am J Physiol. 1993;265(6 Pt 1):G1098–107.
2. Clouse RE, Staiano A, Bickston SJ, et al. Characteristics of the propagating pressure wave in the esophagus. Dig Dis Sci. 1996;41(12):2369–76.
3. Clouse RE, Alrakawi A, Staiano A. Intersubject and interswallow variability in topography of esophageal motility. Dig Dis Sci. 1998;43(9):1978–85.
4. Richter JE, Wu WC, Johns DN, et al. Esophageal manometry in 95 healthy adult volunteers. Variability of pressures with age and frequency of "abnormal" contractions. Dig Dis Sci. 1987;32(6):583–92.
5. Edmundowicz SA, Clouse RE. Shortening of the esophagus in response to swallowing. Am J Physiol. 1991;260(3 Pt 1):G512–6.

6. Jung HY, Puckett JL, Bhalla V, et al. Asynchrony between the circular and the longitudinal muscle contraction in patients with nutcracker esophagus. Gastroenterology. 2005;128(5):1179–86.

7. Mittal RK, Padda B, Bhalla V, et al. Synchrony between circular and longitudinal muscle contractions during peristalsis in normal subjects. Am J Physiol Gastrointest Liver Physiol. 2006;290(3):G431–8.

8. Nicosia MA, Brasseur JG, Liu JB, et al. Local longitudinal muscle shortening of the human esophagus from high-frequency ultrasonography. Am J Physiol Gastrointest Liver Physiol. 2001;281(4):G1022–33.

9. Roman C, Orengo M, Tieffenbach L. Electromyographic study of esophageal smooth muscle in cats. J Physiol. 1969;61(2):390.

10. Wood JD. Physiology of the enteric nervous system. In: Johnson LR, editor. Physiology of the Gastrointestinal Tract. 2nd ed. New York: Raven; 1987. p. 67–109.

11. Goyal RK, Paterson WG. Esophageal motility. In: Wood JD, editor. Handbook of physiology: the gastrointestinal system. Washington, DC: American Physiology Society; 1989. p. 865–908.

12. Pal A, Brasseur JG. The mechanical advantage of local longitudinal shortening on peristaltic transport. J Biomech Eng. 2002;124(1):94–100.

13. Clouse RE, Staiano A. Topography of the esophageal peristaltic pressure wave. Am J Physiol. 1991;261(4 Pt 1):G677–84.

14. Kahrilas PJ, Dodds WJ, Hogan WJ. Effect of peristaltic dysfunction on esophageal volume clearance. Gastroenterology. 1988;94(1):73–80.

15. Tutuian R, Castell DO. Clarification of the esophageal function defect in patients with manometric ineffective esophageal motility: studies using combined impedance-manometry. Clin Gastroenterol Hepatol. 2004;2(3):230–6.

16. Dodds WJ, Hogan WJ, Reid DP, et al. A comparison between primary esophageal peristalsis following wet and dry swallows. J Appl Physiol. 1973;35(6):851–7.

17. Dooley CP, Schlossmacher B, Valenzuela JE. Effects of alterations in bolus viscosity on esophageal peristalsis in humans. Am J Physiol. 1988;254(1 Pt 1): G8–11.

18. Hollis JB, Castell DO. Effect of dry swallows and wet swallows of different volumes on esophageal peristalsis. J Appl Physiol. 1975;38(6):1161–4.

19. Tutuian R, Elton JP, Castell DO, et al. Effects of position on oesophageal function: studies using combined manometry and multichannel intraluminal impedance. Neurogastroenterol Motil. 2003;15(1):63–7.

20. Seigel Cl, Hendrix TR. Evidence for central mediated secondary peristalsis in the esophagus. Bull Johns Hopkins. 1961;108:297–307.

21. Bieger D, Hopkins DA. Viscerotopic representation of the upper alimentary tract in the medulla oblongata in the rat: the nucleus ambiguus. J Comp Neurol. 1987;262(4):546–62.

22. Collman PI, Tremblay L, Diamant NE. The central vagal efferent supply to the esophagus and lower esophageal sphincter of the cat. Gastroenterology. 1993;104(5):1430–8.

23. Ueda M, Schlegel JF, Code CF. Electric and motor activity of innervated and vagally denervated feline esophagus. Am J Dig Dis. 1972;17(12):1075–88.

24. Vantrappen G, Hellemans J. Diseases of the esophagus. New York: Springer; 1974.

25. Roman C. Nervous control of esophageal peristalsis. J Physiol Paris. 1966;58(1):79–108.

26. Kuramoto H, Kawano H, Sakamoto H, et al. Motor innervation by enteric nerve fibers containing both nitric oxide synthase and galanin immunoreactivities in the striated muscle of the rat esophagus. Cell Tissue Res. 1999;295(2):241–5.

27. Neuhuber WL, Worl J, Berthoud HR, et al. NADPH-diaphorase-positive nerve fibers associated with motor endplates in the rat esophagus: new evidence for co-innervation of striated muscle by enteric neurons. Cell Tissue Res. 1994;276(1):23–30.

28. Singaram C, SenGupta A, Sweet MA, et al. Nitrinergic and peptidergic innervation of the human oesophagus. Gut. 1994;35(12):1690–6.

29. Worl J, Neuhuber WL. Enteric co-innervation of motor endplates in the esophagus: state of the art ten years after. Histochem Cell Biol. 2005;123(2):117–30.

30. Bieger D, Neuhuber W. Neural circuits and mediators regulating swallowing in the brainstem. Part 1 Oral cavity, pharynx and esophagus. GI Motility online 2006; http://www.nature.com/gimo/contents/pt1/full/gimo74.html. Accessed 21 Dec 2010.

31. Jean A. Brain stem control of swallowing: neuronal network and cellular mechanisms. Physiol Rev. 2001;81(2):929–69.

32. Jean A, Dallaporta A. Electrophysiologic characterization of the swallowing pattern generator in the brainstem PART 1 Oral cavity, pharynx and esophagus. GI Motility online 2006; http://www.nature.com/gimo/contents/pt1/full/gimo9.html. Accessed 21 Dec 2010.

33. Lang IM. Brain stem control of the phases of swallowing. Dysphagia. 2009;24(3):333–48.

34. Gidda JS, Goyal RK. Swallow-evoked action potentials in vagal preganglionic efferents. J Neurophysiol. 1984;52(6):1169–80.

35. Roman C, Tieffenbach L. Recording the unit activity of vagal motor fibers innervating the baboon esophagus. J Physiol Paris. 1972;64(5):479–506.

36. Tieffenbach L, Roman C. The role of extrinsic vagal innervation in the motility of the smooth-muscled portion of the esophagus: electromyographic study in the cat and the baboon. J Physiol Paris. 1972;64(3): 193–226.

37. Crist J, Gidda JS, Goyal RK. Intramural mechanism of esophageal peristalsis: roles of cholinergic and

noncholinergic nerves. Proc Natl Acad Sci USA. 1984;81(11):3595–9.

38. Dodds WJ, Stef JJ, Stewart ET, et al. Responses of feline esophagus to cervical vagal stimulation. Am J Physiol. 1978;235(1):E63–73.

39. Dodds WJ, Christensen J, Dent J, et al. Esophageal contractions induced by vagal stimulation in the opossum. Am J Physiol. 1978;235(4):E392–401.

40. Gilbert RJ, Dodds WJ. Effect of selective muscarinic antagonists on peristaltic contractions in opossum smooth muscle. Am J Physiol. 1986;250(1 Pt 1): G50–9.

41. Helm JF, Bro SL, Dodds WJ, et al. Myogenic mechanism for peristalsis in opossum smooth muscle esophagus. Am J Physiol. 1992;263:G953–9.

42. Preiksaitis HG, Diamant NE. Myogenic mechanism for peristalsis in the cat esophagus. Am J Physiol. 1999;277(2 Pt 1):G306–13.

43. Sarna SK, Daniel EE, Waterfall WE. Myogenic and neural control for systems for esophageal motility. Gastroenterology. 1977;73:1345–52.

44. Gidda JS, Goyal RK. Influence of successive vagal stimulations on contractions in esophageal smooth muscle of opossum. J Clin Invest. 1983;71(5):1095–103.

45. Gidda JS, Cobb BW, Goyal RK. Modulation of esophageal peristalsis by vagal efferent stimulation in opossum. J Clin Invest. 1981;68(6):1411–9.

46. Gidda JS, Goyal RK. Regional gradient of initial inhibition and refractoriness in esophageal smooth muscle. Gastroenterology. 1985;89(4):843–51.

47. Weisbrodt NW, Christensen J. Gradients of contractions in the opossum esophagus. Gastroenterology. 1972;62(6):1159–66.

48. Serio R, Daniel EE. Electrophysiological analysis of responses to intrinsic nerves in circular muscle of opossum esophageal muscle. Am J Physiol. 1988;254(1 Pt 1):G107–16.

49. Rattan S, Gidda JS, Goyal RK. Membrane potential and mechanical responses of the opossum esophagus to vagal stimulation and swallowing. Gastroenterology. 1983;85(4):922–8.

50. Sifrim D, Janssens J, Vantrappen G. A wave of inhibition precedes primary peristaltic contractions in the human esophagus. Gastroenterology. 1992;103(3): 876–82.

51. Anand N, Paterson WG. Role of nitric oxide in esophageal peristalsis. Am J Physiol. 1994;266(1 Pt 1):G123–31.

52. Chakder S, Rosenthal GJ, Rattan S. In vivo and in vitro influence of human recombinant hemoglobin on esophageal function. Am J Physiol. 1995;268(3 Pt 1):G443–50.

53. Dodds WJ, Dent J, Hogan WJ, et al. Effect of atropine on esophageal motor function in humans. Am J Physiol. 1981;240(4):G290–6.

54. Dodds WJ, Christensen J, Dent J, et al. Pharmacologic investigation of primary peristalsis in smooth muscle portion of opossum esophagus. Am J Physiol. 1979;237(6):E561–6.

55. Gidda JS, Buyniski JP. Swallow-evoked peristalsis in opossum esophagus: role of cholinergic mechanisms. Am J Physiol. 1986;251(6 Pt 1):G779–85.

56. Murray JA, Ledlow A, Launspach J, et al. The effects of recombinant human hemoglobin on esophageal motor functions in humans. Gastroenterology. 1995; 109(4):1241–8.

57. Paterson WG, Hynna-Liepert TT, Selucky M. Comparison of primary and secondary esophageal peristalsis in humans: effect of atropine. Am J Physiol. 1991;260(1 Pt 1):G52–7.

58. Paterson WG. Electrical correlates of peristaltic and nonperistaltic contractions in the opossum smooth muscle esophagus. Gastroenterology. 1989;97(3):665–75.

59. Paterson WG, Rattan S, Goyal RK. Esophageal responses to transient and sustained esophageal distension. Am J Physiol. 1988;255(5 Pt 1):G587–95.

60. Xue S, Paterson W, Valdez D, et al. Effect of an o-raffinose cross-linked haemoglobin product on oesophageal and lower oesophageal sphincter motor function. Neurogastroenterol Motil. 1999;11(6): 421–30.

61. Xue S, Valdez D, Collman PI, et al. Effects of nitric oxide synthase blockade on esophageal peristalsis and the lower esophageal sphincter in the cat. Can J Physiol Pharmacol. 1996;74(11):1249–57.

62. Yamato S, Spechler SJ, Goyal RK. Role of nitric oxide in esophageal peristalsis in the opossum. Gastroenterology. 1992;103(1):197–204.

63. Muinuddin A, Paterson WG. Initiation of distension-induced descending peristaltic reflex in opossum esophagus: role of muscle contractility. Am J Physiol Gastrointest Liver Physiol. 2001;280(3):G431–8.

64. Paterson WG, Indrakrishnan B. Descending peristaltic reflex in the opossum esophagus. Am J Physiol. 1995;269(2 Pt 1):G219–24.

65. Helm JF, Bro SL, Dodds WJ, et al. Myogenic oscillatory mechanism for opossum esophageal smooth muscle contractions. Am J Physiol. 1991;261(3 Pt 1):G377–83.

66. Bardakjian BL, Diamant NE. Electronic models of oscillator-to-oscillator communication. In: Sperelakis N, Cole W, editors. Cell interactions and gap junctions. Florida: CRC Press; 1989. p. 211–24.

67. Daniel EE, Bardakjian BL, Huizinga JD, et al. Relaxation oscillator and core conductor models are needed for understanding of GI electrical activities. Am J Physiol. 1994;266(3 Pt 1):G339–49.

68. Crist J, Surprenant A, Goyal RK. Intracellular studies of electrical membrane properties of opossum esophageal circular smooth muscle. Gastroenterology. 1987;92(4):987–92.

69. Kannan MS, Jager LP, Daniel EE. Electrical properties of smooth muscle cell membrane of opossum esophagus. Am J Physiol. 1985;248(3 Pt 1):G342–6.

70. Nelson DO, Mangel AW. Acetylcholine induced slow-waves in cat esophageal smooth muscle. Gen Pharmacol. 1979;10(1):19–20.

71. Zhang Y, Paterson WG. Nitric oxide contracts longitudinal smooth muscle of opossum oesophagus via excitation-contraction coupling. J Physiol. 2001; 536(Pt 1):133–40.

72. Faussone-Pellegrini MS, Cortesini C. Ultrastructural features and localization of the interstitial cells of

Cajal in the smooth muscle coat of human esophagus. J Submicrosc Cytol. 1985;17(2):187–97.

73. Huizinga JD, Reed DE, Berezin I, et al. Survival dependency of intramuscular ICC on vagal afferent nerves in the cat esophagus. Am J Physiol Regul Integr Comp Physiol. 2008;294(2):R302–10.

74. Decktor DL, Ryan JP. Transmembrane voltage of opossum esophageal smooth muscle and its response to electrical stimulation of intrinsic nerves. Gastroenterology. 1982;82(2):301–8.

75. Salapatek AM, Ji J, Diamant NE. Ion channel diversity in the feline smooth muscle esophagus. Am J Physiol Gastrointest Liver Physiol. 2002;282(2):G288–99.

76. Muinuddin A, Ji J, Sheu L, et al. L-type Ca(2+) channel expression along feline smooth muscle oesophagus. Neurogastroenterol Motil. 2004;16(3):325–34.

77. Schulze K, Conklin JL, Christensen J. A potassium gradient in smooth muscle segment of the opossum esophagus. Am J Physiol. 1977;232(3):E270–3.

78. Muinuddin A, Xue S, Diamant NE. Regional differences in the response of feline esophageal smooth muscle to stretch and cholinergic stimulation. Am J Physiol Gastrointest Liver Physiol. 2001; 281(6): G1460–7.

79. Janssens J, Valembois P, Hellemans J, et al. Studies on the necessity of a bolus for the progression of secondary peristalsis in the canine esophagus. Gastroenterology. 1974;67(2):245–51.

80. Longhi EH, Jordan Jr PH. Necessity of a bolus for propagation of primary peristalsis in the canine esophagus. Am J Physiol. 1971;220(3):609–12.

81. Lang IM, Medda BK, Shaker R. Mechanisms of reflexes induced by esophageal distension. Am J Physiol Gastrointest Liver Physiol. 2001;281(5): G1246–63.

82. Janssens J, De WI, Vantrappen G. Peristalsis in smooth muscle esophagus after transection and bolus deviation. Gastroenterology. 1976;71(6):1004–9.

83. Hamdy S, Xue S, Valdez D, et al. Induction of cortical swallowing activity by transcranial magnetic stimulation in the anaesthetized cat. Neurogastroenterol Motil. 2001;13(1):65–72.

84. Valdez DT, Salapatek A, Niznik G, et al. Swallowing and upper esophageal sphincter contraction with transcranial magnetic-induced electrical stimulation. Am J Physiol. 1993;264(2 Pt 1):G213–9.

85. Aziz Q, Rothwell JC, Barlow J, et al. Esophageal myoelectric responses to magnetic stimulation of the human cortex and the extracranial vagus nerve. Am J Physiol. 1994;267(5 Pt 1):G827–35.

86. Aziz Q, Rothwell JC, Barlow J, et al. Modulation of esophageal responses to magnetic stimulation of the human brain by swallowing and by vagal stimulation. Gastroenterology. 1995;109(5):1437–45.

87. Aziz Q, Rothwell JC, Hamdy S, et al. The topographic representation of esophageal motor function on the human cerebral cortex. Gastroenterology. 1996;111(4): 855–62.

88. Jordan Jr PH, Longhi EH. Relationship between size of bolus and the act of swallowing on esophageal

peristalsis in dogs. Proc Soc Exp Biol Med. 1971; 137(3):868–71.

89. Paterson WG. Neuromuscular mechanisms of esophageal responses at and proximal to a distending balloon. Am J Physiol. 1991;260(1 Pt 1):G148–55.

90. Hollis JB, Castell DO. Effects of cholinergic stimulation on human esophageal peristalsis. J Appl Physiol. 1976;40(1):40–3.

91. Goyal RK, Rattan S. Nature of the vagal inhibitory innervation to the lower esophageal sphincter. J Clin Invest. 1975;55(5):1119–26.

92. Paterson WG, Anderson MA, Anand N. Pharmacological characterization of lower esophageal sphincter relaxation induced by swallowing, vagal efferent nerve stimulation, and esophageal distention. Can J Physiol Pharmacol. 1992;70(7):1011–5.

93. Rattan S, Goyal RK. Evidence of 5-HT participation in vagal inhibitory pathway to opossum LES. Am J Physiol. 1978;234(3):E273–6.

94. Seelig Jr LL, Doody P, Brainard L, et al. Acetylcholinesterase and choline acetyltransferase staining of neurons in the opossum esophagus. Anat Rec. 1984;209(1):125–30.

95. Singaram C, SenGupta A, Sugarbaker DJ, et al. Peptidergic innervation of the human esophageal smooth muscle. Gastroenterology. 1991;101(5):1256–63.

96. Wattchow DA, Furness JB, Costa M. Distribution and coexistence of peptides in nerve fibers of the external muscle of the human gastrointestinal tract. Gastroenterology. 1988;95(1):32–41.

97. Preiksaitis HG, Laurier LG. Pharmacological and molecular characterization of muscarinic receptors in cat esophageal smooth muscle. J Pharmacol Exp Ther. 1998;285(2):853–61.

98. Preiksaitis HG, Krysiak PS, Chrones T, et al. Pharmacological and molecular characterization of muscarinic receptor subtypes in human esophageal smooth muscle. J Pharmacol Exp Ther. 2000;295(3): 879–88.

99. Sohn UD, Harnett KM, De PG, et al. Distinct muscarinic receptors, G proteins and phospholipases in esophageal and lower esophageal sphincter circular muscle. J Pharmacol Exp Ther. 1993;267(3):1205–14.

100. Christensen J, Arthur C, Conklin JL. Some determinants of latency of off-response to electrical field stimulation in circular layer of smooth muscle of opossum esophagus. Gastroenterology. 1979;77(4 Pt 1):677–81.

101. Conklin JL, Du C, Murray JA, et al. Characterization and mediation of inhibitory junction potentials from opossum lower esophageal sphincter. Gastroenterology. 1993;104(5):1439–44.

102. Murray J, Du C, Ledlow A, et al. Nitric oxide: mediator of nonadrenergic noncholinergic responses of opossum esophageal muscle. Am J Physiol. 1991; 261(3 Pt 1):G401–6.

103. Crist J, Gidda JS, Goyal RK. Characteristics of "on" and "off" contractions in esophageal circular muscle in vitro. Am J Physiol. 1984;246(2 Pt 1):G137–44.

104. Preiksaitis HG, Tremblay L, Diamant NE. Nitric oxide mediates inhibitory nerve effects in human

esophagus and lower esophageal sphincter. Dig Dis Sci. 1994;39(4):770–5.

105. Blank EL, Greenwood B, Dodds WJ. Cholinergic control of smooth muscle peristalsis in the cat esophagus. Am J Physiol. 1989;257(4 Pt 1):G517–23.

106. Krysiak PS, Preiksaitis HG. Tachykinins contribute to nerve-mediated contractions in the human esophagus. Gastroenterology. 2001;120(1):39–48.

107. Stacher G, Bauer P, Steinringer H, et al. Dose-related effects of the synthetic met-enkephalin analogue FK 33-824 on esophageal motor activity in healthy humans. Gastroenterology. 1982;83(5):1057–61.

108. Uddman R, Alumets J, Hakanson R, et al. Peptidergic (enkephalin) innervation of the mammalian esophagus. Gastroenterology. 1980;78(4):732–7.

109. Cohen S, Green F. Force-velocity characteristics of esophageal muscle: effect of acetylcholine and norepinephrine. Am J Physiol. 1974;226(5):1250–6.

110. Rattan S, Gonnella P, Goyal RK. Inhibitory effect of calcitonin gene-related peptide and calcitonin on opossum esophageal smooth muscle. Gastroenterology. 1988;94(2):284–93.

111. Sugarbaker DJ, Rattan S, Goyal RK. Swallowing induces sequential activation of esophageal longitudinal smooth muscle. Am J Physiol. 1984;247(5 Pt 1):G515–9.

112. Paterson WG. Studies on opossum esophageal longitudinal muscle function. Can J Physiol Pharmacol. 1997;75(1):65–73.

113. Crist J, Gidda J, Goyal RK. Role of substance P nerves in longitudinal smooth muscle contractions of the esophagus. Am J Physiol. 1986;250(3 Pt 1):G336–43.

114. Daya F, Miller D, Paterson W. Studies on the neural mechanisms underlying opossum esophageal longitudinal muscle contraction. Neurogastroenterol Motil. 2004;16:674.

115. Paterson WG, Miller DV, Dilworth N, et al. Intraluminal acid induces oesophageal shortening via capsaicin-sensitive neurokinin neurons. Gut. 2007;55:1347–52.

116. Balaban DH, Yamamoto Y, Liu J, et al. Sustained esophageal contraction: a marker of esophageal chest pain identified by intraluminal ultrasonography. Gastroenterology. 1999;116(1):29–37.

117. Shi G, Pandolfino JE, Zhang Q, et al. Deglutitive inhibition affects both esophageal peristaltic amplitude and shortening. Am J Physiol Gastrointest Liver Physiol. 2003;284(4):G575–82.

118. Sugarbaker DJ, Rattan S, Goyal RK. Mechanical and electrical activity of esophageal smooth muscle during peristalsis. Am J Physiol. 1984;246(2 Pt 1):G145–50.

119. Hirano I, Kakkar R, Saha JK, et al. Tyrosine phosphorylation in contraction of opossum esophageal longitudinal muscle in response to SNP. Am J Physiol. 1997;273(1 Pt 1):G247–52.

120. Sifrim D, Lefebvre R. Role of nitric oxide during swallow-induced esophageal shortening in cats. Dig Dis Sci. 2001;46(4):822–30.

121. Bieger D, Triggle C. Pharmacological properties of mechanical responses of the rat oesophageal muscularis mucosae to vagal and field stimulation. Br J Pharmacol. 1985;84(1):93–106.

122. Christensen J, Percy WH. A pharmacological study of oesophageal muscularis mucosae from the cat, dog and American opossum (Didelphis virginiana). Br J Pharmacol. 1984;83(2):329–36.

123. Ohkawa H. Mechanical activity of the smooth muscle of the muscularis mucosa of the guinea pig esophagus and drug actions. Jpn J Physiol. 1980;30(2):161–77.

124. Percy WH, Miller AJ, Brunz JT. Pharmacologic characteristics of rabbit esophageal muscularis mucosae in vitro. Dig Dis Sci. 1997;42(12): 2537–46.

125. Robotham H, Jury J, Daniel EE. Capsaicin effects on muscularis mucosa of opossum esophagus: substance P release from afferent nerves? Am J Physiol. 1985;248(6 Pt 1):G655–62.

126. Domoto T, Jury J, Berezin I, et al. Does substance P comediate with acetylcholine in nerves of opossum esophageal muscularis mucosa? Am J Physiol. 1983;245(1):G19–28.

Sphincter Mechanisms at the Esophago-Gastric Junction

23

Ravinder Mittal

Abstract

Understanding of the sphincter mechanism at the esophago-gastric junction (EGJ) is crucial to the understanding of esophageal motor disorders and gastroesophageal reflux disease. Smooth muscles of the lower end of esophagus (LES) and skeletal muscles of crural diaphragm are the key components of sphincter mechanism at the EGJ. Basal LES tone/contraction is partly myogenic and party neurogenic. LES relaxation is mediated via the vagus nerve, which activates inhibitory motor neurons located in the esophageal wall. Longitudinal muscle contraction of the esophagus appears to play a critical role in the LES relaxation. LES and crural diaphragm relax together during transient LES relaxation (TLESR), which is the major mechanism of gastroesophageal reflux. TLESR is also important during belching, vomiting, and rumination. A large number of pharmacological agents decrease the TLESR frequency and could be potentially useful in the treatment of reflux disease. High-resolution and high-definition manometry has and will continue to improve our understanding of the complex functioning of EGJ.

Keywords

Sphincter mechanisms • Esophago-gastric junction • Lower esophageal sphincter • Extrinsic innervation • Parasympathetic • Sympathetic

R. Mittal, MD (✉)
Department of Medicine, University of California San Diego & San Diego VA Health Care Center,
San Diego, CA, USA
e-mail: rmittal@ucsd.edu

R. Shaker et al. (eds.), *Principles of Deglutition: A Multidisciplinary Text for Swallowing and its Disorders*,
DOI 10.1007/978-1-4614-3794-9_23, © Springer Science+Business Media New York 2013

Introduction and Historical Perspective

A person can stand upside down after eating a large hearty meal, yet no food backs up into the esophagus and mouth. It is intuitively clear that there must be a valve or sphincter mechanism at the lower end of the esophagus. The lower esophageal sphincter or the sphincter mechanism at the esophago-gastric junction (EGJ) has inspired so many and has been an area of intense scrutiny for more than 50 years. One may question if this intense scrutiny of such a small part of the body is really warranted. If one considers that all primary motor disorders of the esophagus are "most likely" secondary to poor relaxation of the EGJ and the majority of gastroesophageal reflux disease is secondary to excessive relaxation of the lower esophageal sphincter (LES), the focus on the sphincter mechanism at the EGJ is quite appropriate and justified. Some call the sphincter mechanism at the lower end of esophagus the LES but it is clear now that it is more appropriate to refer to it as the sphincter mechanism at the EGJ because several anatomical structures contribute to its physiological function. Some of these are intrinsic to the wall of the esophagus and stomach while others are located outside the esophageal wall. In a 1958 review article, Ingelfinger [1] stated that the pinchcock action of the diaphragm was important in the prevention of gastroesophageal reflux. Code et al. [2] were the first to document the intra-luminal high-pressure zone between the esophagus and stomach and suggested that intrinsic muscles of the lower esophagus were entirely responsible for maintaining LES pressure. Definitive evidence of a pinchcock contribution from the diaphragm, however, was not noted until 1985 [2, 3]. Studies conducted during the last 25 years confirm that there are as many as three lower esophageal sphincters. Some have considered clasp and sling fibers of the LES as two separate sphincters because each one has unique anatomical and functional characteristics. The above two constitute the intrinsic or the smooth muscle lower esophageal sphincters. Skeletal muscle fibers of the crural diaphragm that form the esophageal hiatus constitute the extrinsic or the external lower esophageal sphincter. Therefore, current thinking is that the sphincter mechanism at the EGJ consists of three sphincters, "a triple security" mechanism against retrograde movement of gastric content.

Anatomy of the Lower Esophageal Sphincter

Anatomy of the smooth muscle LES has fascinated many because contrary to expected, no consistent thickening of the muscles at the gastroesophageal junction is found on autopsy specimens. Figure 23.1 displays a schematic of the region, based on radiological appearance of human autopsy specimens of the distal esophagus and proximal stomach. Even though in human autopsy specimens no clear evidence of a thick LES muscles exits, in vivo intra-luminal ultrasound imaging in live humans clearly demarcates a region of thick circular and longitudinal muscle layers [4]. The muscle thickness in the middle of the LES is twice that of the adjacent esophagus (Fig. 23.2). Muscle thickness increases and decreases with an increase or decrease in LES pressure, which suggests that the absence of muscle tone in the autopsy specimen accounts for the lack of muscle thickness. Liebermann-Meffert found an oblique gastroesophageal ring (GER) at the junction between the left side of the esophagus and the greater curvature of the stomach, which was the site of greatest muscular thickness. It tapered toward the cephalic and caudal direction, for a length of approximately 31 mm (Fig. 23.3) [5]. These muscle bundles split 10 mm above the GER and extend a length of 25 mm to form short transverse muscle clasps on the right (lesser curvature of the stomach) and oblique fibers on the left (greater curvature of stomach). Oblique fibers form a collar around the left lower end of the esophagus that extends caudally and toward the lesser curvature. The mechanism of how clasp and sling fibers form a circumferential squeeze is currently unclear. As discussed later in the chapter, clasp and sling fibers show marked differences in their functional properties and have

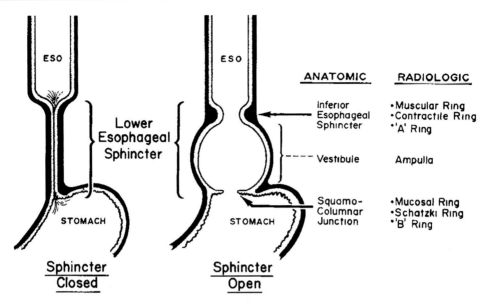

Fig. 23.1 Schematic of the lower esophageal sphincter (by Goyal R.K.)

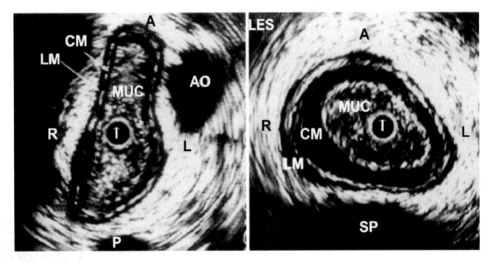

Fig. 23.2 *Asymmetry of the LES shape and LES pressure*. Images were obtained using a 12.5–MHz catheter-based transducer. Circle in the center (T) represents the ultrasound transducer. Note five layers of tissue in the esophagus and LES: *MUC* mucosa, *CM* circular muscle (intermuscular septum is between circular and longitudinal muscle), *LM* longitudinal muscle (outside LM is adventitia), *SP* spine, *A* anterior, *P* posterior, *L* left, *R* right. Images were obtained in resting state. Note the asymmetry of the LES and esophagus. From J. Liu et al. Am J Physiol 1997;272:G1509–17 with permission from American Physiological Society

been referred to as two distinct lower esophageal sphincters [6]. Ultrastructural studies show that the LES muscle, unlike esophageal muscle, shows inward invaginations related to its state of tonic contraction [7]. The nerve varicosities in the LES are no different than that of the esophagus. In addition to circular muscle, the LES also has a longitudinal muscle layer, the fibers of which are inserted in between the fascicles of circular muscles. Unlike circular muscles, which continue into the stomach, longitudinal muscle layers do not extend below the LES.

The crural diaphragm, which forms the hiatus for entry of the esophagus from the chest into

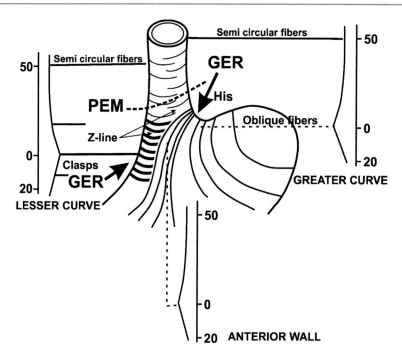

Fig. 23.3 *Anatomy of lower esophageal sphincter.* Note that the muscle fibers of the LES are not circular, rather they are organized as clasp and sling fibers.

From D. Liebermann-Meffert et al. Gastroenterology 1979;76:31–8 with permission

abdomen is formed by the right crus of the diaphragm; its inner or medial fibers are oriented in the circumferential direction and lateral fibers are directed in an oblique cranio-caudal fashion [8]. Embryologically, the crural diaphragm develops in the dorsal mesentery of the esophagus while the costal diaphragm develops from myoblasts originating in the lateral body wall [9]. Also referred to as the pinch cock action of the diaphragm, the crural diaphragm provides a strong sphincter mechanism at the lower end of the esophagus that has been appropriately called the "external lower esophageal sphincter" [10]. The LES and crural diaphragm are anchored to each other by the phrenoesophageal ligament, a condensation of loose areolar tissue. It may form two leaves that extend from the under surface of the diaphragm and attach to the esophagus, approximately at the upper border of the LES (Fig. 23.4). Because of the firm anchoring of the LES and crural diaphragm by the phrenoesophageal ligament, the two structures move together with inspiration and expiration but can separate during longitudinal esophageal muscle contraction related to peristalsis [11] and transient LES relaxation [12].

Extrinsic Innervation: Parasympathetic and Sympathetic

Dorsomotor nucleus of the vagus (DMV) and the nucleus ambiguus (NA) located in the medullary region of brain stem contain cell bodies of neurons whose processes travel in the vagus nerve. The vagus nerve is the major motor nerve of the esophagus and LES. It contains approximately 10,000–50,000 nerves fibers, 90% of which are afferents [13]. The efferent nerve fibers terminate on the myenteric neurons, rather than smooth muscles and therefore are referred to as preganglionic efferents. Vagal branches that innervate the LES actually enter the wall of esophagus several centimeters above the LES. In contrast to the vagus nerve, most fibers present in the splanchnic nerves are motor or efferents (80–90%) [13]. These nerve fibers travel along with the branches of the vagus nerve and blood vessels into the wall of esophagus and LES. The efferent fibers do not terminate on the end organs, i.e., muscle; rather they are involved in the modulation of myenteric neurons. Esophagus and LES are innervated by the vagal and spinal afferents. Vagal afferents

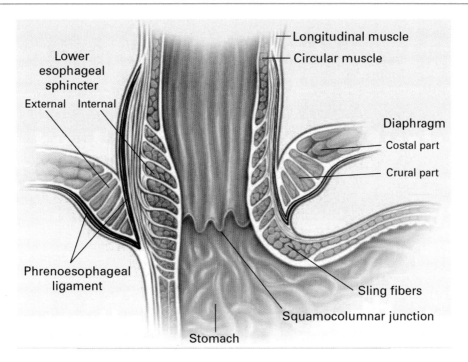

Fig. 23.4 *Anatomy of the esophago-gastric junction.* The lower esophageal sphincter and the crural diaphragm constitute the intrinsic and extrinsic sphincters, respec- tively. The two sphincters are anatomically superimposed and are anchored to each other by the phrenoesophageal ligament

arise from the sensory neurons located in the nodose ganglia in the neck. On the other hand, sympathetic or spinal afferents from the esopha- gus and LES project to the cell bodies in the cer- vical and thoracic dorsal root ganglions (DRG) (from C1 to T9). Spinal afferent fibers innervat- ing the cervical and thoracic esophagus and LES arise from a broad range of DRG but there is some cranio-caudal representation. DRG contain various types of neurons (large, medium, and small) that are mostly pseudo-unipolar [13]. The DRG neurons project to the spinal cord via dorsal nerve roots and travel via spinothalamic tracts and relay visceral afferent input to the CNS.

Intrinsic Innervations of the LES and Esophagus

The truncal portion of neural crest cells contrib- ute to the formation of the enteric nervous system of the esophagus. The Mash-1 gene is essential in the migration of neural crest cells into the foregut (esophagus and cardiac stomach) [14, 15]. Knockout or mutation of Mash-1 genes cause aganglionosis in the esophagus and these mice die soon after birth with no milk in their stomach. The cells proliferate in the neural crest prior to reaching the gut in the presence of appropriate growth factor and transcription factors. Uncommitted progenitors that exit from vagal cells obligatorily express Sox10 and respond to Notch and ET-3/ETB signals (transcription fac- tors). Because Sox10 and Phox2b expression are required by early precursors, the entire gut becomes aganglionic when these transcription factors are deleted. The activation of Ret by GDNF/GFRa, which is essential to the formation of ganglions distal to the cardiac stomach, is not required for the ganglia to form in the esophagus and adjacent stomach. In contrast to Ret, esopha- geal gangliogenesis is Ascl1-dependent [15].

The enteric nervous system of the esophagus is organized into myenteric (located in between the circular and longitudinal muscle) and Meissner's plexus (submucosal), both of which are not as

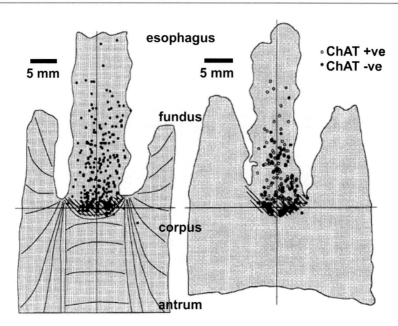

Fig. 23.5 *Location of the inhibitory and excitatory nerves of the lower esophageal sphincter.* (**a**) Computer reconstruction of a preparation opened along the greater curvature after three DiI-coated beads were applied to the right side of the LES (at the origin of the axis, hatched area mark the LES). After 3 days in organotypic culture, 273 labeled motor neuron cell bodies were located in the esophagus and local to the sphincter, but few cells were labeled in the body of the stomach. *Filled dots* represent nerve cell body: –, the orientation of the bundle of smooth muscle fibers in the circular and oblique muscle layers.

(**b**) Distribution of 293 labeled motor neuron cell bodies with and without CHAT immunoreactivity. Each circle represents a single motor neuron to the LES of the guinea pig labeled with DiI after 3 days in organotypic culture. Many of the motor neurons close to the DiI application site on the LES muscle (at the origin of the axes, hatching denotes the region of LES) were immunoreactive for ChAT and, hence likely to be cholinergic excitatory motor neurons, whereas few of the esophageal motor neurons were ChAT immunoreactive. *Filled circles*, motor neurons positive for ChAT; *empty circles*, nonimmunoreactive neurons

developed in the esophagus as in the small and large intestine. Each plexus contain ganglia, collections of neurons (nodes) that are connected with each other by internodal strands or fascicles. Ganglia are more numerous in the smooth muscle portion of the esophagus as compared to the skeletal muscle esophagus [16, 17]. Some of these ganglia lie outside the fascicular tracts (para fascicular). The density of neurons decreases tenfold, from the cranial to the caudal end, reaching a nadir of 100–200 cells/cm [2] at the most distal ends. However, others have argued that this decrease may be related to atypical location of the neurons rather than a true decrease [18]. Details, with regard to various types of cells in the myenteric plexus, are not as well known in the esophagus and LES as is the case in the small and large intestine. In the myeneric plexus of smooth muscle esophagus and LES, there are two major types

of neurons, excitatory and inhibitory. Excitatory ones contain acetylcholine and substance P, and the inhibitory ones contain nitric oxide synthase and vasoactive intestinal peptide. Studies using retrograde axonal dye (DiI) and organ culture technique (Fig. 23.5) show different patterns of innervation of the clasp and sling fibers of the LES, both of which are innervated by cholinergic (excitatory) and nitric oxide (inhibitory) nerves but the dominant ones in the case of clasp fibers are inhibitory neurons with their cell bodies in the esophagus, 2–12 mm above the LES. On the other hand, the cholinergic or excitatory neurons located in the stomach provide dominant innervations to the sling fibers of the LES [19, 20]. This pattern or polarity of neural innervations is similar to the small and large intestine where inhibitory neurons always project in the aboral direction and excitatory neurons in the oral [21]. Inhibitory neurons are generally larger in size than the excitatory ones. Varicosities along the axonal process contain neurotransmitters and these neurotransmitters are released with the passage of action potential in axons. Neurotransmitters diffuse in the spaces around the smooth muscles and act on the receptors present on the surface of smooth muscle cells. In the human esophagus and LES, large numbers of peptide neurotransmitters are present in the neurons and their processes, however, the function and physiological role of these neuropeptides is not clear [22–24].

Interestingly, myenetric neurons are present in the esophagus of animal species that have only skeletal muscle esophagus, as well as in the skeletal muscle portion of the human esophagus. These neurons contain nitric oxide, CGRP, and several other peptides. They are thought to exert inhibitory influences on the skeletal muscle, however definite evidence is lacking. It is possible that they may be left over from the embryonic days, prior to transdifferentiaton of smooth muscle into the skeletal muscle. The other possibility is that they actually innervate the smooth muscles of the LES.

Interstitial Cells of Cajal

Interstitial cells of Cajal (ICCs) are present in the body of the esophagus as well as in the LES. They are dispersed in several different layers and are present in increasing numbers from the cranial to the caudal end of esophagus [25–27]. ICCs make close contact with the smooth muscle cells and neurons. Axonal varicosities (site of storage of neurotransmitters) make closer contact with the ICCs than with the smooth muscle cells. Furthermore, ICCs make gap junctions with the smooth muscles. Based on the above, a large amount of literature during the last 10 years suggest that the ICC serves an intermediary role (between neurons and smooth muscles) in the neuromuscular transmission [28–31]. In addition, ICC contains receptors and signaling pathways for various neurotransmitters. Most direct evidence for the role of ICC in neurotransmission comes from observations that neurotransmission

in the mutant animals lacking ICC (due to the c-Kit receptor deficiency) is impaired. Studies show that both cholinergic and nitrergic neurotransmission in the c-Kit-deficient animals is deficient in the LES [32] and stomach [33]. However, several recent studies suggest that the nitrergic neurotransmission in the LES is actually intact in the ICC-deficient mice [34–36]. It may be that the impaired nitrergic neurotransmission is due to the smooth muscle defect associated with c-Kit receptor deficiency rather than the impaired neuromuscular transmission [37].

Recording Techniques

Any investigator is only as good as his recording technique and fortunately, techniques to study the esophagus and LES have improved tremendously over the years. Original recordings of the esophagus were obtained using balloon and smoke paper kymographs (turn of nineteenth century). These were replaced with water-filled catheters and strip-chart recorders that were in use until early 1970s. Infusion manometry was first introduced and lasted till the beginning of twenty-first century. During the last 5 years, high-resolution manometry with computerized digital recordings has become the gold standard for the esophageal pressure monitoring. In the case of LES, recording techniques have advanced from side-hole sensors (prior to 1980) to Dent sleeve sensor (from 1980s onwards), to electronic sleeve sensor more recently. These improvements have made life simpler for the clinicians and researchers alike [38–42]. Catheters equipped with 36 solid-state transducers that are circumferentially sensitive and span the entire length of the esophagus, EGJ and proximal stomach have replaced infusion manometry recording technique during last 5 years in the most motility laboratories across the country. Topographical visualization of pressure waves recorded by closely spaced sensors has come to age in the first decade of twenty-first century. High-resolution manometry (HRM), seamless color pressure plots using computer algorithms with linear interpolation of pressure between closely spaced transducers, along

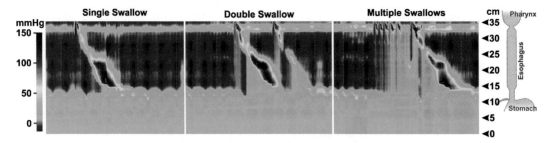

Fig. 23.6 Swallow-induced LES relaxation by the HRM. Also shown is the effect of 2 swallows and multiple swallows spaced at close intervals on the duration of LES relaxation

the entire region of the esophagus, represent significant advance. These plots beautifully show that during peristalsis, a segment rather than a focal point in the esophagus is contracted at any given time during peristalsis (Fig. 23.6). The fidelity of these pressure sensors is significantly better than the infusion manometry and sleeve sensor used earlier. Electronic sleeve sensor of high-resolution manometry is a significant improvement because of its high fidelity. It shows a clear picture of the relationship between swallow and LES relaxation. Closely spaced repeated swallows results in long periods of LES/EGJ relaxation and only one esophageal peristaltic contraction that follows the last swallow. Another advancement in the LES pressure measurement is high-definition manometry technique, which makes it possible to record pressures from 96 transducers at closely spaced intervals (12 rows of 8 circumferential sensors) [43]. The color plots from these recordings show precise axial and circumferential asymmetry of the pressure in the LES/EGJ region (Fig. 23.7).

Recording of longitudinal muscle contraction using catheter-based, intra-luminal ultrasound imaging technique represent another technological advance [44–46]. US imaging can be used with manometry to study anatomy as well as motor function of the LES and esophagus. US imaging can track longitudinal and circular muscle contractions for long periods of time, without radiation hazard inherent to the tracking of implanted radio-opaque markers (another method to measure longitudinal muscle contraction). Under physiological condition, muscles contract either in an isometric or isotonic, or a mixed fashion. Manometry is ideally suited to record isometric contraction of the circular muscle. Longitudinal

muscle contraction occurs under isotonic conditions and US imaging is ideally suited for such recording because it relies on measurement of changes in the muscle cross-sectional area/thickness on tomographic US images. As the esophagus shortens, related to longitudinal muscle contraction, there is a proportional increase in the muscle cross-sectional area/thickness. Consequently, change in the muscle cross-sectional area or thickness on the ultrasound images is a reliable marker of the longitudinal muscle contraction [47]. Tomographic ultrasound images can be displayed as *m-mode* images for the temporal display of changes in the muscle thickness along with the pressure recordings to display circular and longitudinal muscle contraction simultaneously, and provide a complete picture of motor patterns of the esophagus and LES. As discussed later, US imaging has made it possible to understand the role of longitudinal muscles of the esophagus in LES relaxation.

Esophago-Gastric Junction Pressure

Intraluminal pressure at the EGJ, also referred to as the high-pressure zone (HPZ), is a measure of the strength of the sphincter mechanism. It is contributed by the smooth muscles of LES, i.e., clasp and sling fibers along with the skeletal muscles of crural diaphragm. The entire length of HPZ in humans, under normal conditions, is approximately 3.5–4 cm, which is also the length of smooth muscle LES. Crural diaphragm, which forms the esophageal hiatus, is about 2 cm in length and encircles the proximal 2 cm of the HPZ [48]. Therefore, a portion of the LES is intra-abdominal and a portion is located in the hiatus

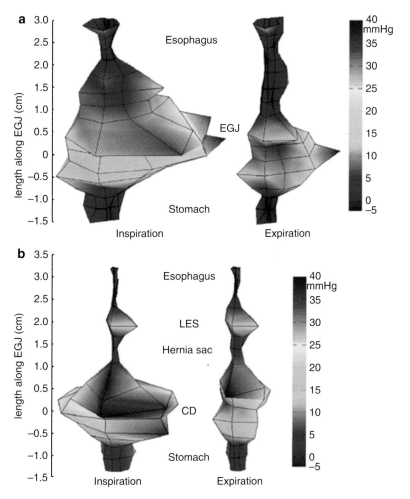

Fig. 23.7 *High-definition manometry of the esophago-gastric junction.* High-definition recordings of the EGJ in a normal individual (**a**) and in a patient with a 2 cm separation between the lower esophageal sphincter (LES) and the crural diaphragm (CD): Pressure is scaled both by color and deflection from the central axis with the deepest blue being −5 mmHg relative to atmospheric pressure. From P.J. Kahrilas et al. Gastroenterology 2008;134:16–18 with permission

itself. The intra-abdominal portion of the LES is frequently termed the submerged segment of the esophagus [49]. Animal studies show that end-expiratory pressure at the EGJ is contributed by the smooth muscles of the LES and the increase with each inspiration is due to the contraction of skeletal muscles of crural diaphragm. Smooth muscles of LES and skeletal muscle of crural diaphragm have also been referred to as the internal and external lower esophageal sphincters [50, 51]. The LES is under the control of autonomic nerves, myenteric plexus and its own myogenic tone. On the other hand, crural diaphragm, like any other skeletal muscles, has no myogenic tone and it

contracts through neural discharges from the somatic nerves (phrenic nerves). Antireflux barrier function and transit (flow) across the esophago-gastric junction requires fine coordination between LES and crural diaphragm, visceral and somatic sphincter respectively, as discussed later.

Asymmetry of Lower Esophageal Sphincter Pressure

The LES pressure profile shows axial and circumferential asymmetry. Axial asymmetry implies that the peak LES pressure is located in the middle of LES and decreases in the orad and aborad direction. On the other hand, circumferential asymmetry means that the side holes of the manometry catheter placed along the circumference of a catheter at the same axial level records different pressures. LES pressures are greater toward the left side than the right side (Fig. 23.7). A number of investigators have provided different explanations for the circumferential asymmetry. Some felt that it is related to the extrinsic compression of the LES by the crus of the diaphragm [5]. In patients with hiatus hernia, LES pressure asymmetry disappears supporting the above hypothesis [52]. Others feel that a greater thickness of the LES muscle on the left compared to the right side is responsible for higher leftwards pressure [5]. Different pharmacological properties of the clasp and sling fibers have also been considered to play an important role in circumferential pressure asymmetry [53]. Ultrasound images of the LES demonstrate that the LES is not circular and it may be that the asymmetry of the LES shape plays a role in the asymmetry of LES pressure [4]. A circular ultrasound probe sits in the LES closer to the left side as compared to the right side of the LES wall. Based on the Laplace law, pressure in a circular tube is inversely proportional to the tube radius. Based on the above, greater LES pressures would be expected on the left side as compared to the right side. The noncircular shape of the LES appears to be related to the basal LES tone. When LES pressure is high, as occurs soon after the swallow, LES shape changes to a perfectly circular shape and circumferential pressure asymmetry disappears. During peristaltic contractions, esophageal shape is perfectly circular and pressures are perfectly symmetrical as well, supporting the hypothesis between shape and pressure asymmetry [4].

Lower Esophageal Sphincter: Genesis of Tone and Neural Control

The LES is a unique muscle; it has its own myogenic tone that is modulated by neural, hormonal, and paracrine factors [54, 55]. Evidence for the myogenic tone comes from following in vitro and in vivo observations, (1) LES muscle strips, devoid of extrinsic innervations and studied in vitro (under no influence of hormonal factors) show steeper length tension characteristics than the muscle strips from the esophagus [56]. Tetrodotoxin (TTX), which abolishes all intrinsic neural activity, does not abolish tone in the LES muscle strips. In the presence of TTX, nitric oxide and other agents that act directly on the muscle reduce LES tone [57]. (2) TTX does not abolish LES pressure in the in vivo studies [58]. Myogenic elements responsible for LES tone maintenance may be due to differences in the structural protein. The LES has proportionally more α-actin and basic essential light chains LC17b, and less of a seven amino acid-inserted myosin isoform and caldesmon than the esophageal body circular muscle [59]. LES muscle utilizes more calcium from the intracellular than extracelluar source as compared to the esophageal muscle [60]. There are also distinct intracellular signaling pathways in the LES as compared to the esophageal body [61].

From an electrophysiological point of view, the LES muscle is in a state of greater depolarization than the esophageal muscle, as evidenced by a higher resting membrane potential than the esophagus [62]. The depolarized state of the sphincter muscle is suggested to be due to the resting chloride conductance [63]. Periodic spike bursts or increase in the depolarization result in an increase in the LES tonic activity. Tonic LES contraction is both spike-dependent and spike-independent [64]. Relative contribution of myogenic tone to the LES pressure differs in different species. In the opossum, myogenic tone dominates under basal resting condition. On the other hand, in cats [65], dogs [66], and humans [67], neural cholinergic drive contributes significantly to the basal LES tone. Atropine (15 μg/kg), which reduces excitatory neural cholinergic drive, reduces LES pressure by 50%–70% in humans [68].

Like stated earlier, LES muscles are made up of clasp and sling fibers [5]. Clasp fibers maintain stronger myogenic tone than the sling fibers [69] and sling fibers respond briskly to cholinergic agonist. Clasp fibers are predominantly innervated by inhibitory neurons located in the body of the esophagus and sling fibers by the excitatory neurons located in the stomach [20, 70]. L-type calcium channels are predominantly seen in the clasp muscle fibers [71] and there are other differences as well in the mechanisms by which sling and clasp muscles contract and relax [72]. Differences in the properties of sling and clasp muscles fibers may be responsible for the greater pressure and greater cholinergic responsiveness of the LES pressure on the left side. Sling fibers are likely to be responsible for the maintenance of angle of HIS and flap valve function both of which are considered to be important in the prevention of reflux.

The myenteric plexus contains both excitatory and inhibitory neurons that have intrinsic activity and are also under the influence of extrinsic vagus and spinal nerves. Excitatory neurons contain acetylcholine and substance P; inhibitory neurons, on the other hand, contain vasoactive intestinal peptide (VIP) and nitric oxide (NO). Electrical stimulation of the LES muscle strip that supposedly stimulates both excitatory and inhibitory neurons elicit relaxation suggesting that inhibitory influence dominates over the excitatory one. Stimulation of the vagus and spinal nerve has opposite effects on the LES pressure. The vagus nerve, which contains fibers that are thought to innervate both excitatory and inhibitory nerves, elicits only relaxation when electrically stimulated [73]. The inhibitory effect is frequency (dose)-dependent and none of the stimulus parameters induces LES contraction. The above does not mean that the vagus does not innervate excitatory neurons to the LES, it may be that when all, i.e., both inhibitory and excitatory vagus nerves fibers, are stimulated, inhibitory influence dominates, just like in vitro muscle strip studies [74]. Motor neurons that supply the LES show topographical localization in the DMV. Stimulation of the rostral neurons elicits LES contraction and caudal neurons cause LES relaxation; both of these effects are blocked by bilateral vagotomy [75]. Above observation suggests that the vagus nerve contains fibers that impinge specifically on either the excitatory or the inhibitory neurons. Electrical stimulation of the sympathetic nerves causes LES contraction that is mediated by α-adrenergic receptors [76, 77]. It is likely that the sympathetic/spinal nerves innervate myenteric neurons rather than the muscles directly. β-Adrenergic stimulation, on the other hand, leads to LES relaxation, an effect that could be mediated through β_1, β_2, or β_3 receptors [78, 79]. β_3-receptor stimulation, unlike β_1 and β_2, does not cause any cardiovascular side effects, which could be relevant for the treatment of esophageal motor disorders and LES hypertension. A large number of neuropeptides, hormones and paracrine substances that modulate LES tone, either increase or decrease LES pressure, as shown in Table 23.1. Whether they play any physiological role, however, is uncertain. Studies in the past investigated the role of various different types of foods including alcohol, smoking and caffeine on the basal LES pressure including their mechanism of action in the hope of understanding how they may elicit gastroesophageal reflux.

Long-term recordings in the animals and humans show fluctuations or phasic pressure changes in the LES. Some of these are related and others unrelated to the gastric component of the migrating myoelectrical complex (MMC) [80–83]. Similar to small intestine, gastric MMC consists of three phases: phase 1 with relatively no contraction in the stomach, phase 2 during which gastric contractions occur at irregular intervals, and phase 3 in which high-amplitude contraction occurs at the regular frequency of 3 cycles/minute. During the first phase of gastric MMC, the LES pressure is relatively stable, but during late phase 2 and throughout phase 3, large-amplitude phasic LES contractions occur without major change in the basal LES pressure. LES pressure increases before the increase in the gastric pressure and thus is important in the prevention of gastroesophageal reflux. These MMC-related contractions are abolished by atropine and anesthesia [82, 84]. Motilin, a neurohumoral agent released into circulation from the specialized cells in the wall of intestine, may be responsible for the MMC-related phasic LES contractions [81]. The LES also contracts in response to increases in intra-abdominal pressure related to abdominal compression or straight leg raise, most likely through a vago-vagal reflex [68, 85].

Table 23.1 Effects of some hormones and putative neurotransmitters on the lower esophageal sphincter and the possible sites of action: From the article Sphincter mechanisms at the lower end of the esophagus. Ravinder K. Mittal and Raj K. Goyal; GI Motility online (2006) doi: 10.1038/gimo14

Site of action					
Agent	Effect	Circular smooth muscle	Inhibitory neurons	Excitatory neurons	Comments
Bombesin	Contraction	√	–	√	Releases norepinephrine from adrenergic neurons
Calcitonin gene-related peptide	Relaxation	√	√	–	
Cholecystokinin	Biphasic	√	√	–	Inhibition overrides excitation, causes paradoxical excitation in achalasia patients
Dopamine	Relaxation (D_2)	√	–	–	
	Contraction (D_1)	√	–	–	
Galanin	Contraction	√	–	–	
Gastric inhibitory polypeptide	Relaxation	?	?	?	
Gastrin	Contraction	√	–	–	
Glucagon	Relaxation	√	–	–	Releases catecholamines from adrenal medulla
Histamine	Contraction	√(H_1)	–	–	
Motilin	Contraction	√	–	√	
Neurotensin	Contraction	√	–	–	
Nitric oxide	Relaxation	√	–	–	
Pancreatic polypeptide	Contraction	√	–		
$PGF_{2\alpha}$	Contraction	√	–	–	
$PGE_{1,2}$	Relaxation	√	–	–	
Progesterone	Relaxation	–	–		
Secretin	Relaxation	√	–	–	
Serotonin	Contraction	√	–	–	
Somatostatin	Contraction	?	?	?	
Substance P	Contraction	√	–	√	
VIP	Relaxation	–	–	–	

PGE prostaglandin E, *PGF* prostaglandin F, *VIP* vasoactive intestinal peptide, √ yes, – no, ? not clear

Swallow-Induced LES Relaxation

LES relaxation dysfunction is an important finding in motor disorders of the esophagus. In fact, it has been suggested that the primary abnormality in all spastic motor disorders of the esophagus is actually impaired LES relaxation [45, 86, 87]. Therefore, understanding of how does a swallow induces LES relaxation is crucial. Swallow-induced LES relaxation is mediated via vagus nerve because bilateral cervical vagotomy and cooling of the cervical vagus nerve abolishes LES relaxation [86, 88, 89]. Electrical stimulation of the vagus nerve causes LES relaxation in a dose-dependent or frequency-dependent fashion [90]. Since extrinsic nerves influence LES muscle through intrinsic or myenteric plexus, it is suggested that the vagus nerve fibers synapse with the inhibitory motor neurons. Acetylcholine is released at the presynaptic nerve endings and acts through the nicotinic (predominantly) and muscrinic (M1) receptors to activate inhibitory motor neurons [91]. What is released by the inhibitory motor neurons that causes LES relaxation was resolved in the 1990s to be nitric oxide. A series of studies in vitro and in vivo including some from humans strongly suggest that NO is

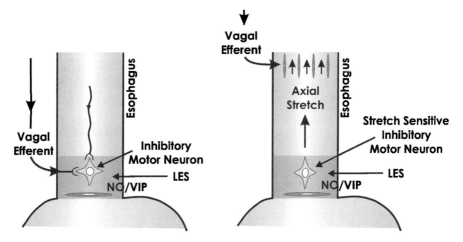

Fig. 23.8 *Vagus nerve-induced relaxation of the lower esophageal sphincter.* Traditional view is that vagal efferent fibers synapses with the inhibitory neuron of the LES, which in turn releases NO that causes LES relaxation (*panel A*). However, based on the recent studies it may be that vagus nerve activates longitudinal muscles of the esophagus, contraction of which in turn activates stretch-sensitive motor inhibitory neuron of the LES. From Y. Jiang et al. Am J Physiol Gastrointest Liver Physiol 2009;297(2):G397–405 with permission

the "noncholinergic, nonadrenergic" inhibitory neurotransmitter [92–96] of the LES. Other neurotransmitters such as VIP, CO, and PCAP likely play a minor role in LES relaxation [97]. Nitric oxide, a gas that diffuses quickly, is not stored in the nerve terminals. It is synthesized quickly by nitric oxide synthase upon neural stimulation. In addition to acting on the smooth muscle, NO may act on the presynaptic nerve terminals to stimulate VIP release [98]. The role of VIP in LES relaxation is not clear because neurally induced LES relaxation is associated with an increase in the intracellular cyclic GMP [99] and VIP-induced stimulation with cyclic AMP [100]. Nitric oxide increases intracellular cyclic GMP and other intracellular messenger system to cause LES muscle relaxation.

All types of LES relaxations in vivo, i.e., swallow-induced, esophageal distension-induced, vagus nerve stimulation-induced, and spontaneous transient LES relaxations are associated with movement of the LES in the cranial direction [12, 101, 102]. Cranial movement with LES relaxation was a major issue in the 1970s because Dodds et al. recognized that it caused relative movement between the side-hole of a manometry catheter (recording pressure sensor) and the LES [11]. In order to prevent the above, animal studies used to pin the catheter and LES together [58]. For the same reasons, Dent devised the sleeve sensor for continuous LES pressure recording in humans [103]. Cranial movement of the LES is caused by longitudinal muscle contraction of the esophagus that is associated with peristalsis and transient LES relaxation, as discussed later. It turns out that a mechanical pull on the LES in the cranial direction, similar to what esophageal longitudinal muscle contraction does to the LES, activates LES relaxation through the activation of inhibitory motor neurons [104]. In mice, with a skeletal muscle esophagus and smooth muscle LES, vagus nerve-stimulated LES relaxation can be blocked by pancuronium (that abolishes esophageal longitudinal muscles contraction) [36]. It is proposed that the vagus nerve fibers, instead of forming synapse with the inhibitory motor neurons are actually destined toward the longitudinal muscles. It may be that the longitudinal muscle contraction activates the stretch-sensitive, inhibitory motor neurons of the LES (Fig. 23.8). In support of the above concept, Nissen fundoplication (used to treat reflux), which restricts cranial stretch on the LES prevents LES relaxation [105]. It is very likely that the above mechanism is crucial in the antireflux action of Nissen fundoplication because it is well known that following Nissen fundoplication the LES does not relax completely.

Crural Diaphragm Contribution to Esophago-Gastric Junction and Neural Control

Crural and costal diaphragms, even though part of the same respiratory diaphragm, are actually two separate muscles [106, 107]. The costal diaphragm is primarily a ventilator muscle. On the other hand, crural diaphragm has two functions, ventilatory and "sphincter-like" action (external lower esophageal sphincter). Both costal and crural diaphragms are supplied by the branches of phrenic nerves, the motor neurons of which are located in the spinal cord, at the level of C5–7 (phrenic nerve nucleus). No topographical localization exists for the neurons of crural and cosal diaphragm in the spinal cord [108, 109]. The respiratory center located in the reticular formation of the medulla innervates the phrenic nerve nucleus in the spinal cord. Recent studies suggest that the vagus nerve also innervates (sensory and motor) the crural but not the costal diaphragm [110]. Retrograde tracer studies have revealed that a tracer injected into the crural diaphragm ends up in the intermediate region of the DMV. Stimulation of the intermediate DMV by glutamate causes relaxation of the LES and crural diaphragm which is mediated by the vagus nerve [111, 112].

Measuring the contribution of the crural diaphragm to the EGJ pressure has been very challenging in humans, especially in the absence of hiatal hernia. LES and diaphragmatic sphincters are anatomically superimposed on each other, thus making differentiation difficult. The crural diaphragm is a skeletal muscle and contracts very quickly. The recording fidelity of manometric pressure sensors needs to be high in order to record the fast contractions of the crural diaphragm. In addition, the crural diaphragm and LES move with respiration and the recording sensor may not necessary move with it. Simultaneous pressure and electromyogram (EMG) recordings using reverse perfuse sleeve

sensors equipped with electrodes greatly improved our understanding of LES biomechanics [68, 113, 114]. Under resting conditions and at end-expiration, the EGJ pressure mostly comes from the smooth muscle contribution to the LES. The increase in EGJ pressure with each inspiration is related to the crural diaphragm contraction (Fig. 23.9). Amplitude of EGJ pressure increase related to inspiration is directly related to the depth of inspiration. With maximal inspiration, the EGJ pressure increases from 20 mmHg to more than 100 mmHg. In addition, crural diaphragm provides tonic and sustained increased in the EGJ pressure during periods of abdominal compression, straight leg raise, and valsalva maneuver [68]. The best evidence for the tonic contraction of the diaphragmatic sphincter comes from a study in patients with a completely absent LES (latter resected due to cancer of the distal esophagus) [115]. In addition to the inspiratory pressure oscillation at the EGJ, a high-pressure zone also exists at end-expiration in these patients, which can only be related to the crural diaphragm contraction. Thus, the significance of the crural diaphragm to the antireflux barrier cannot be overstated. Contractions of the inspiratory muscles of respiration produce negative intra-esophageal pressure and positive intragastric pressure, thus increasing the pressure gradient between stomach and esophagus in favor of gastroesophageal reflux. Contraction of the abdominal wall also increases the pressure gradient between the stomach and esophagus. Therefore, all involuntary/voluntary maneuvers that are associated with inspiratory and abdominal wall muscle contractions (thus an increase in the gastroesophageal pressure gradients) are accompanied by augmentation of EGJ pressure by the crural diaphragm contraction, thus preventing gastroesophageal reflux [50].

The crural diaphragm relaxes along with the LES during swallows [116] and transient LES relaxation (TLESR) [117], less completely with the former than latter. Fine coordination between the visceral (LES) and somatic (crural diaphragm) control mechanism is suggested to occur in the medullary region, like so many other cardiorespiratory reflexes. However, it was found that there

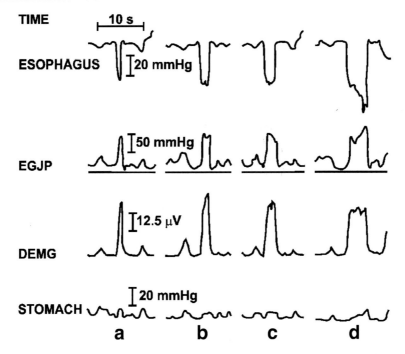

Fig. 23.9 *Diaphragmatic contraction and esophago-gastric junction pressure.* Standardized diaphragmatic contractions of 1, 2, 4, and 6 s duration were performed. Note that each diaphragmatic contract results in a nega- tive esophageal pressure, an increase in the EGJ pressure, and an increase in the integrated crural diaphragm EMG activity (DEMG). From B. Sivri et al. Gastroenterology 1991;101:962–9 with permission

was no inhibition of the spontaneously active inspiratory motor neurons in the medullary region with esophageal distension, when clearly there was inhibition of the crural diaphragm muscle [118] raising doubts if central coordination is the mechanism. A peripheral mechanism located at the level of the crural diaphragm and related to the stretch exerted by the esophageal longitudinal muscle contraction has been proposed, but the precise nature of such a mechanism is not understood [119, 120].

Transient Lower Esophageal Sphincter Relaxation and Pharmacological Inhibition

Motor events associated with the retrograde transport of stomach contents, i.e., belching, gastroesophageal reflux, regurgitation, rumination, and vomiting are distinct from primary and secondary peristalsis. These events begin with spontaneous relaxation of the LES and crural diaphragm (transient LES relaxation), described in exquisite detail in the context of gastroesophageal reflux events. Although transient LES relaxation is the major mechanism of reflux in patients with reflux disease, both TLESR and reflux occur fairly frequently in normal healthy subjects. Transient LES relaxation is also the key motor event during rumination and vomiting (physiological events). Transient LES relaxation is unrelated to swallow and is accompanied by simultaneous relaxation of the LES and crural diaphragm [117] along with the inhibition of contraction in the body of the esophagus [121]. The hallmark of a TLESR is that the relaxation is significantly longer (>10 s) than swallow-induced LES relaxation (<10 s) (Fig. 23.10) [122]. Although there may be minor contraction in the distal esophagus, the esophagus in general remains relatively quiescent during the TLESR [121]. Reverse peristalsis has been described in association with rumination and vomiting, events during which TLESR also occurs [123]. Contractions of the abdominal wall and costal

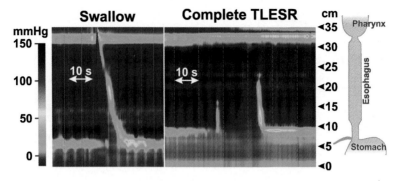

Fig. 23.10 *Swallow-induced and transient relaxation of the LES.* Swallow-induced LES relaxation is brief (6–8 s) and follows swallow-induced pharyngeal contraction. On the other hand, transient LES relaxation is not preceded by a swallow and lasts for longer duration than swallow (>10 s—can last up to 45 s or more)

diaphragm, by reducing the size of the abdominal cavity, increase intra-gastric pressure, which provides propulsion force for the gastric contents to move into the esophagus and pharynx during vomiting and rumination. Generally, there is no increase in gastric pressure in association with gastroesophageal reflux.

Whether refluxed contents into the esophagus travel to the pharynx depends on the state of the upper esophageal sphincter, i.e., contraction or relaxation. It appears that the rapidity of esophageal pressure increase caused by reflux is the major determinant for UES relaxation. Air reflux into the esophagus, especially in the upright position that causes rapid increase in intra-esophageal pressure, is associated with UES relaxation [124]. On the other hand, liquid reflux, especially in the supine position, is associated with slower increase in the esophageal pressure and causes UES contraction [125].

Retrograde transport of gastric contents and transient LES relaxation (TLESR) is associated with a unique and distinct pattern of contraction in the longitudinal muscle layers [12, 126]. The distal esophagus, i.e., just above the LES, shows longitudinal muscle contraction that starts right before the onset of LES relaxation. Longitudinal muscle contraction gets stronger and traverses in an anti-peristaltic fashion toward the proximal esophagus during the entire duration of transient LES relaxation. Circular muscles do not contract during the entire time of TLESR (Fig. 23.11). The LES and crural diaphragm remain relaxed during the entire period of longitudinal muscle contraction and with its cessation there is return of LES basal tone and crural diaphragm activity. During swallow-induced primary peristalsis or esophageal distension-induced secondary peristalsis, circular and longitudinal muscle layers of the esophagus contract synchronously [127]. Therefore, it is clear that the two layers of the esophagus can contract together (during peristalsis) or longitudinal muscle may contract independent of circular muscle (during transient LES relaxation) [126]. Since transient LES relaxation and swallow-mediated peristalsis are mediated via the vagus nerve and brain stem, it is likely that the central program generator (CPG) can initiate two distinct motor patterns in the esophagus: program one—responsible for aboral transport with swallowing, and program 2—responsible for the retrograde transport, of which transient LES relaxation is the key component. As discussed earlier, longitudinal muscle contraction of the distal esophagus is likely a key event that induces LES relaxation through the activation of stretch-sensitive motor neurons of the LES.

Spontaneous TLESRs occur only in the awake state [128, 129]. They are more common in the upright position and general anesthesia appears to suppress them [130–132]. In the experimental setting, gastric distension is the major stimulus to induce transient LES relaxation [133–135]. Distension-activated stretch on the gastric wall [136] activates afferents in the vagus nerve that elicit TLESR through the central pattern

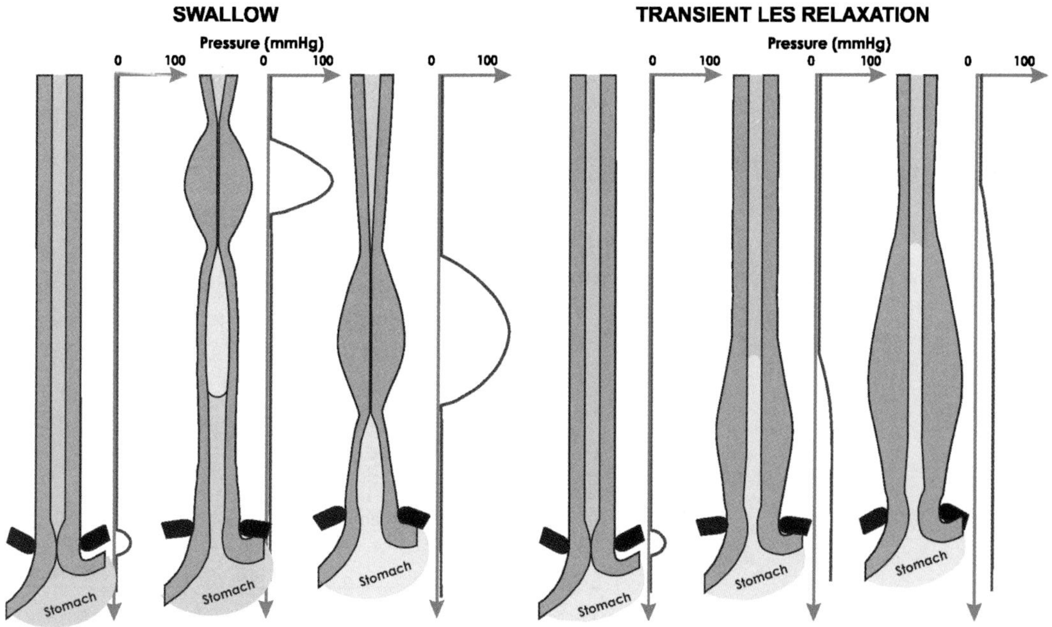

Fig. 23.11 *Patterns of longitudinal muscle contraction during peristalsis and transient LES relaxation.* Peristaltic contraction is associated with an aborally traversing simultaneous contraction of the circular and longitudinal muscle of the esophagus. On the other hand, transient lower esophageal sphincter relaxation (TLESR) is associated with contraction of the longitudinal muscle of the distal esophagus, in the absence of circular muscle contraction. From A. Babaei et al. Gastroenterology 2008;134:1322–31 with permission

generator, DMV, and efferent vagus nerve (vago-vagal reflex) [137]. Therefore, TLESR is blocked by cooling of the cervical vagus nerve [138]. TLESR frequency actually increases in the presence of a catheter in the pharynx, raising the possibility that pharyngeal receptors may be involved [139]. A subthreshold mechanical pharyngeal stimulus and low-frequency electrical stimulation of the superior laryngeal nerve can elicit isolated LES relaxation (without esophageal contractions) even though its phenotypic appearance is different than that of the TLESR [140]. In humans, a subthreshold pharyngeal stimulus provided by injections of small amounts of water induces LES relaxation without crural diaphragm relaxation, a phenotype that also does not resemble TLESR [141, 142]. Furthermore, unlike TLESRs, reflux rarely occurs during pharyngeal stimulated induced LES relaxations. Large numbers of neurotransmitters are involved in the sensory or afferent limb of the vagus nerve, in the motor pattern generator in the brain stem, and in the efferent motor limb of the vagus nerve that mediates TLESR reflex [143]. Therefore, it is possible to interrupt TLESR by many pharmacological agents. GABA(b) agonists have been consistently shown to inhibit TLESR frequency in animal [144, 145] and human studies [146]. Other pharmacological agents that inhibit TLESR are atropine [147, 148], CCK-A receptor antagonists [149], morphine (mu receptor agonist) [150], nitric oxide antagonists, metabotropic glutamate receptor subtype 5 (mGluR5) antagonists [151], and cannabinoid receptor (CBR1) agonists [152]. All of these agents reduce the frequency of TLESR but do not completely abolish them. They also reduce the frequency of spontaneous swallows. None of the above agents completely block swallow reflex and TLESR. Therefore, it is likely that these compounds increase the threshold of activation of the central program generator for swallow and TLESR. The site of action of these agents is shown in Fig. 23.12 [153]. The poor side effect profile of these medications, however, precludes their use in the routine treatment of reflux disease.

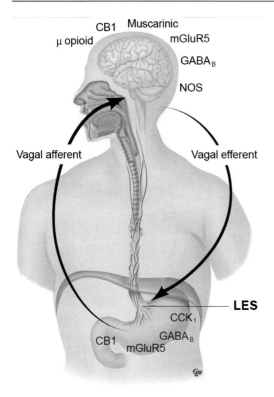

Fig. 23.12 *Site of action of various pharmacological agents known to inhibit TLESR frequency.* From A. Lehmann. Esophageal pain. San Diego, CA: Plural Publishing; 2009 with permission

Compliance of Esophago-Gastric Junction

The EGJ and LES have distinct relaxation and opening functions. X ray studies with fluoroscopy reveal that the bolus arrives at the LES soon after a swallow but it does not flow across it in spite of the fully relaxed LES. A small increase in esophageal pressure (3–10 mmHg) as the peristaltic wave pushes the bolus into the distal esophagus forces open the relaxed LES to the diameter of the distal esophagus. Factors that determine EGJ and LES opening function are likely to be different than relaxation because the latter is an active and nerve-mediated process and the former is a passive or visco-elastic-related property of the tissues. Opening function of the LES/EGJ can be measured by studying its compliance. Later is studied by distending a balloon at the EGJ under fluoroscopy to determine

the pressure–cross-sectional area relationship. Barostat [154], ultrasound imaging of the EGJ [155], and more recently functional luminal imaging probe (FLIP) have also been used [156, 157] to study EGJ compliance. These studies suggest that in normal subjects the hiatus (crural diaphragm) and not the LES is the region of least compliance at the EGJ. Patients with reflux disease have a more compliant EGJ than normal subjects [158, 159]. Some patients with achalasia have normal relaxation [160] but poor compliance of the LES [161]. Dysphagia following surgical fundoplication is also related to the poor EGJ compliance [162, 163].

Acknowledgment   Grant Support: NIH-RO1-DK060733.

References

1. Ingelfinger FJ. Esophageal motility. Physiol Rev. 1958;38:533–84.
2. Code CF, Fyke Jr FE, Schlegel JF. The gastroesophageal sphincter in healthy human beings. Gastroenterologia. 1956;86:135–50.
3. Boyle JT, Altschuler SM, Nixon TE, Tuchman DN, Pack AI, Cohen S. Role of the diaphragm in the genesis of lower esophageal sphincter pressure in the cat. Gastroenterology. 1985;88:723–30.
4. Liu J, Parashar VK, Mittal RK. Asymmetry of lower esophageal sphincter pressure: is it related to the muscle thickness or its shape? Am J Physiol. 1997;272:G1509–17.
5. Liebermann-Meffert D, Allgower M, Schmid P, Blum AL. Muscular equivalent of the lower esophageal sphincter. Gastroenterology. 1979;76:31–8.
6. Brasseur JG, Ulerich R, Dai Q, Patel DK, Soliman AM, Miller LS. Pharmacological dissection of the human gastro-oesophageal segment into three sphincteric components. J Physiol. 2007;580:961–75.
7. Seelig Jr LL, Goyal RK. Morphological evaluation of opossum lower esophageal sphincter. Gastroenterology. 1978;75:51–8.
8. Delattre JF, Palot JP, Ducasse A, Flament JB, Hureau J. The crura of the diaphragm and diaphragmatic passage. Applications to gastroesophageal reflux, its investigation and treatment. Anat Clin. 1985;7:271–83.
9. Langman J. Medical Embryology. Philadelphia: William & Wilkins; 1975.
10. Mittal RK, Goyal RK. Sphincter mechanisms at the lower end of the esophagus. London: Nature Publishing; 2006.
11. Dodds WJ, Walter B. Cannon Lecture: current concepts of esophageal motor function: clinical implications for radiology. AJR Am J Roentgenol. 1977;128:549–61.

12. Pandolfino JE, Zhang QG, Ghosh SK, Han A, Boniquit C, Kahrilas PJ. Transient lower esophageal sphincter relaxations and reflux: mechanistic analysis using concurrent fluoroscopy and high-resolution manometry. Gastroenterology. 2006;131:1725–33.

13. Beyak M, Bulmer D, Jiang W, Keating W, Grundy D. Extrinsic sensory afferent nerves innervating the gastrointestinal tract. New York: Academic; 2006.

14. Gershon MD. Genes and lineages in the formation of the enteric nervous system. Curr Opin Neurobiol. 1997;7:101–9.

15. Gershon MD. Developmental determinants of the independence and complexity of the enteric nervous system. Trends Neurosci. 2010;33:446–56.

16. Christensen J, Robison BA. Anatomy of the myenteric plexus of the opossum esophagus. Gastroenterology. 1982;83:1033–42.

17. Christensen J, Rick GA, Robison BA, Stiles MJ, Wix MA. Arrangement of the myenteric plexus throughout the gastrointestinal tract of the opossum. Gastroenterology. 1983;85:890–9.

18. Sengupta A, Paterson WG, Goyal RK. Atypical localization of myenteric neurons in the opossum lower esophageal sphincter. Am J Anat. 1987;180:342–8.

19. Brookes SJ, Hennig G, Schemann M. Identification of motor neurons to the circular muscle of the guinea pig gastric corpus. J Comp Neurol. 1998;397:268–80.

20. Yuan S, Costa M, Brookes SJ. Neuronal pathways and transmission to the lower esophageal sphincter of the guinea Pig. Gastroenterology. 1998;115:661–71.

21. Porter AJ, Wattchow DA, Brookes SJ, Costa M. The neurochemical coding and projections of circular muscle motor neurons in the human colon. Gastroenterology. 1997;113:1916–23.

22. Singaram C, Sengupta A, Stevens C, Spechler SJ, Goyal RK. Localization of calcitonin gene-related peptide in human esophageal Langerhans cells. Gastroenterology. 1991;100:560–3.

23. Singaram C, Sengupta A, Sugarbaker DJ, Goyal RK. Peptidergic innervation of the human esophageal smooth muscle. Gastroenterology. 1991;101:1256–63.

24. Singaram C, Sengupta A, Sweet MA, Sugarbaker DJ, Goyal RK. Nitrinergic and peptidergic innervation of the human oesophagus. Gut. 1994;35:1690–6.

25. Daniel EE, Posey-Daniel V. Neuromuscular structures in opossum esophagus: role of interstitial cells of Cajal. Am J Physiol. 1984;246:G305–15.

26. Faussone-Pellegrini MS, Cortesini C. Ultrastructural features and localization of the interstitial cells of Cajal in the smooth muscle coat of human esophagus. J Submicrosc Cytol. 1985;17:187–97.

27. Christensen J, Rick GA, Soll DJ. Intramural nerves and interstitial cells revealed by the Champy-Maillet stain in the opossum esophagus. J Auton Nerv Syst. 1987;19:137–51.

28. Sanders KM, Ward SM. Kit mutants and gastrointestinal physiology. J Physiol. 2007;578:33–42.

29. Ward SM, Sanders KM. Involvement of intramuscular interstitial cells of Cajal in neuroeffector transmission in the gastrointestinal tract. J Physiol. 2006;576:675–82.

30. Sanders KM, Ward SM. Interstitial cells of Cajal: a new perspective on smooth muscle function. J Physiol. 2006;576:721–6.

31. Huizinga JD, Zarate N, Farrugia G. Physiology, injury, and recovery of interstitial cells of Cajal: basic and clinical science. Gastroenterology. 2009;137:1548–56.

32. Ward SM, Morris G, Reese L, Wang XY, Sanders KM. Interstitial cells of Cajal mediate enteric inhibitory neurotransmission in the lower esophageal and pyloric sphincters. Gastroenterology. 1998;115:314–29.

33. Burns AJ, Lomax AE, Torihashi S, Sanders KM, Ward SM. Interstitial cells of Cajal mediate inhibitory neurotransmission in the stomach. Proc Natl Acad Sci U S A. 1996;93:12008–13.

34. Sivarao DV, Mashimo HL, Thatte HS, Goyal RK. Lower esophageal sphincter is achalasic in nNOS(-/-) and hypotensive in W/W(v) mutant mice. Gastroenterology. 2001;121:34–42.

35. Farre R, Wang XY, Vidal E, Domenech A, Pumarola M, Clave P, Huizinga JD, Jimenez M. Interstitial cells of Cajal and neuromuscular transmission in the rat lower oesophageal sphincter. Neurogastroenterol Motil. 2007;19:484–96.

36. Jiang Y, Bhargava V, Mittal RK. Mechanism of stretch-activated excitatory and inhibitory responses in the lower esophageal sphincter. Am J Physiol Gastrointest Liver Physiol. 2009;297:G397–405.

37. Zhang Y, Carmichael SA, Wang XY, Huizinga JD, Paterson WG. Neurotransmission in lower esophageal sphincter of W/Wv mutant mice. Am J Physiol Gastrointest Liver Physiol. 2010;298:G14–24.

38. Clouse RE, Staiano A. Topography of the esophageal peristaltic pressure wave. Am J Physiol. 1991;261: G677–84.

39. Clouse RE, Staiano A. Topography of normal and high-amplitude esophageal peristalsis. Am J Physiol. 1993;265:G1098–107.

40. Rohof WO, Boeckxstaens GE, Hirsch DP. High-resolution esophageal pressure topography is superior to conventional sleeve manometry for the detection of transient lower esophageal sphincter relaxations associated with a reflux event. Neurogastroenterol Motil. 2011;23(5):427–32.

41. Jones MP, Sloan SS, Rabine JC, Ebert CC, Huang CF, Kahrilas PJ. Hiatal hernia size is the dominant determinant of esophagitis presence and severity in gastroesophageal reflux disease. Am J Gastroenterol. 2001;96:1711–7.

42. Hong SJ, Bhargava V, Jiang Y, Denboer D, Mittal RK. A unique esophageal motor pattern that involves longitudinal muscles is responsible for emptying in achalasia esophagus. Gastroenterology. 2010; 139:102–11.

43. Kahrilas PJ, Ghosh SK, Pandolfino JE. Challenging the limits of esophageal manometry. Gastroenterology. 2008;134:16–8.

44. Miller LS, Liu JB, Colizzo FP, Ter H, Marzano J, Barbarevech C, Helwig K, Leung L, Goldberg BB, Hedwig K. Correlation of high-frequency esophageal ultrasonography and manometry in the study of

esophageal   motility.   Gastroenterology. 1995;109:832–7.

45. Mittal RK, Liu J, Puckett JL, Bhalla V, Bhargava V, Tipnis N, Kassab G. Sensory and motor function of the esophagus: lessons from ultrasound imaging. Gastroenterology. 2005;128:487–97.

46. Boesmans W, Vanden Berghe P, Farre R, Sifrim D. Oesophageal shortening: in vivo validation of high-frequency ultrasound measurements of oesophageal muscle wall thickness. Gut. 2010;59:433–40.

47. Nicosia MA, Brasseur JG, Liu JB, Miller LS. Local longitudinal muscle shortening of the human esophagus from high-frequency ultrasonography. Am J Physiol Gastrointest Liver Physiol. 2001;281:G1022–33.

48. Heine KJ, Mittal RK. Lower esophageal sphincter: how to quantitate? Gastroenterology. 1992;103:346–7.

49. Ott DJ, Gelfand DW, Wu WC, Castell DO. Esophagogastric region and its rings. AJR Am J Roentgenol. 1984;142:281–7.

50. Mittal RK, Balaban DH. The esophagogastric junction. N Engl J Med. 1997;336:924–32.

51. Mittal RK. The crural diaphragm, an external lower esophageal sphincter: a definitive study. Gastroenterology. 1993;105:1565–7.

52. Kahrilas PJ, Lin S, Chen J, Manka M. The effect of hiatus hernia on gastro-oesophageal junction pressure. Gut. 1999;44:476–82.

53. Preiksaitis HG, Diamant NE. Regional differences in cholinergic activity of muscle fibers from the human gastroesophageal junction. Am J Physiol. 1997;272: G1321–7.

54. Goyal RK, Rattan S. Neurohumoral, hormonal, and drug receptors for the lower esophageal sphincter. Gastroenterology. 1978;74:598–619.

55. Christensen J. Oxygen dependence of contractions in esophageal and gastric pyloric and ileocecal muscle of opossums. Proc Soc Exp Biol Med. 1982;170: 194–202.

56. Biancani P, Goyal RK, Phillips A, Spiro HM. Mechanics of sphincter action. Studies on the lower esophageal sphincter. J Clin Invest. 1973;52:2973–8.

57. Yamato S, Saha JK, Goyal RK. Role of nitric oxide in lower esophageal sphincter relaxation to swallowing. Life Sci. 1992;50:1263–72.

58. Goyal RK, Rattan S. Genesis of basal sphincter pressure: effect of tetrodotoxin on lower esophageal sphincter pressure in opossum in vivo. Gastroenterology. 1976;71:62–7.

59. Szymanski PT, Szymanska G, Goyal RK. Differences in calmodulin and calmodulin-binding proteins in phasic and tonic smooth muscles. Am J Physiol Cell Physiol. 2002;282:C94–104.

60. Biancani P, Hillemeier C, Bitar KN, Makhlouf GM. Contraction mediated by Ca2+ influx in esophageal muscle and by Ca2+ release in the LES. Am J Physiol. 1987;253:G760–6.

61. Biancani P. Signal transduction in lower esophageal sphincter circular muscle. GI Motility online. 2006;doi: 10.1038/gimo24.

62. Papasova M, Milousheva E, Bonev A, Boev K, Kortezova N. On the changes in the membrane potential and the contractile activity of the smooth muscle of the lower esophageal and ileo-caecal sphincters upon increased K in the nutrient solution. Acta Physiol Pharmacol Bulg. 1980;6:41–9.

63. Saha JK, Sengupta JN, Goyal RK. Role of chloride ions in lower esophageal sphincter tone and relaxation. Am J Physiol. 1992;263:G115–26.

64. Asoh R, Goyal RK. Electrical activity of the opossum lower esophageal sphincter in vivo. Its role in the basal   sphincter   pressure.   Gastroenterology. 1978;74:835–40.

65. Behar J, Kerstein M, Biancani P. Neural control of the lower esophageal sphincter in the cat: studies on the excitatory pathways to the lower esophageal sphincter. Gastroenterology. 1982;82:680–8.

66. Martin CJ, Dodds WJ, Liem HH, Dantas RO, Layman RD, Dent J. Diaphragmatic contribution to gastroesophageal competence and reflux in dogs. Am J Physiol. 1992;263:G551–7.

67. Dodds WJ, Dent J, Hogan WJ, Arndorfer RC. Effect of atropine on esophageal motor function in humans. Am J Physiol. 1981;240:G290–6.

68. Mittal RK, Fisher M, McCallum RW, Rochester DF, Dent J, Sluss J. Human lower esophageal sphincter pressure response to increased intra-abdominal pressure. Am J Physiol. 1990;258:G624–30.

69. Preiksaitis HG, Tremblay L, Diamant NE. Cholinergic responses in the cat lower esophageal sphincter show regional variation. Gastroenterology. 1994;106:381–8.

70. Brookes SJ, Chen BN, Hodgson WM, Costa M. Characterization of excitatory and inhibitory motor neurons to the guinea pig lower esophageal sphincter. Gastroenterology. 1996;111:108–17.

71. Muinuddin A, Kang Y, Gaisano HY, Diamant NE. Regional differences in L-type Ca2+ channel expression in feline lower esophageal sphincter. Am J Physiol   Gastrointest   Liver   Physiol. 2004;287:G772–81.

72. L'Heureux MC, Muinuddin A, Gaisano HY, Diamant NE. Feline lower esophageal sphincter sling and circular muscles have different functional inhibitory neuronal responses. Am J Physiol Gastrointest Liver Physiol. 2006;290:G23–9.

73. Goyal RK, Rattan S. Nature of the vagal inhibitory innervation to the lower esophageal sphincter. J Clin Invest. 1975;55:1119–26.

74. Chang HY, Mashimo H, Goyal RK. Musings on the wanderer: what's new in our understanding of vago-vagal reflex? IV. Current concepts of vagal efferent projections to the gut. Am J Physiol Gastrointest Liver Physiol. 2003;284:G357–66.

75. Rossiter CD, Norman WP, Jain M, Hornby PJ, Benjamin S, Gillis RA. Control of lower esophageal sphincter pressure by two sites in dorsal motor nucleus of the vagus. Am J Physiol. 1990;259:G899–906.

76. Fournet J, Snape Jr WJ, Cohen S. Sympathetic control of lower esophageal sphincter function in the cat.

Action of direct cervical and splanchnic nerve stimulation. J Clin Invest. 1979;63:562–70.

77. DiMarino AJ, Cohen S. The adrenergic control of lower esophageal sphincter function. An experimental model of denervation supersensitivity. J Clin Invest. 1973;52:2264–71.

78. Sarma DN, Banwait K, Basak A, DiMarino AJ, Rattan S. Inhibitory effect of beta3-adrenoceptor agonist in lower esophageal sphincter smooth muscle: in vitro studies. J Pharmacol Exp Ther. 2003; 304:48–55.

79. Dimarino M, Banwait K, Rattan S, Cohen S, DiMarino AJ. Beta3 adrenergic stimulation inhibits the opossum lower esophageal sphincter. Gastroenterology. 2002;123:1508–15.

80. Dent J, Dodds WJ, Sekiguchi T, Hogan WJ, Arndorfer RC. Interdigestive phasic contractions of the human lower esophageal sphincter. Gastroenterology. 1983;84:453–60.

81. Holloway RH, Blank E, Takahashi I, Dodds WJ, Layman RD. Motilin: a mechanism incorporating the opossum lower esophageal sphincter into the migrating motor complex. Gastroenterology. 1985;89:507–15.

82. Holloway RH, Blank E, Takahashi I, Dodds WJ, Hogan WJ, Dent J. Variability of lower esophageal sphincter pressure in the fasted unanesthetized opossum. Am J Physiol. 1985;248:G398–406.

83. Itoh Z, Aizawa I, Honda R, Hiwatashi K, Couch EF. Control of lower-esophageal-sphincter contractile activity by motilin in conscious dogs. Am J Dig Dis. 1978;23:341–5.

84. Holloway RH, Blank EL, Takahashi I, Dodds WJ, Dent J, Sarna SK. Electrical control activity of the lower esophageal sphincter in unanesthetized opossums. Am J Physiol. 1987;252:G511–21.

85. Lind JF, Warrian WG, Wankling WJ. Responses of the gastroesophageal junctional zone to increases in abdominal pressure. Can J Surg. 1966;9:32–8.

86. Ryan JP, Snape Jr WJ, Cohen S. Influence of vagal cooling on esophageal function. Am J Physiol. 1977;232:E159–64.

87. Dogan I, Puckett JL, Padda BS, Mittal RK. Prevalence of increased esophageal muscle thickness in patients with esophageal symptoms. Am J Gastroenterol. 2007;102:137–45.

88. Reynolds RP, El-Sharkawy TY, Diamant NE. Lower esophageal sphincter function in the cat: role of central innervation assessed by transient vagal blockade. Am J Physiol. 1984;246:G666–74.

89. Reynolds RP, Effer GW. The effect of differential vagal nerve cooling on feline esophageal function. Clin Invest Med. 1988;11:452–6.

90. Rattan S, Goyal RK. Neural control of the lower esophageal sphincter: influence of the vagus nerves. J Clin Invest. 1974;54:899–906.

91. Gilbert R, Rattan S, Goyal RK. Pharmacologic identification, activation and antagonism of two muscarine receptor subtypes in the lower esophageal sphincter. J Pharmacol Exp Ther. 1984;230: 284–91.

92. Murray JA, Ledlow A, Launspach J, Evans D, Loveday M, Conklin JL. The effects of recombinant human hemoglobin on esophageal motor functions in humans. Gastroenterology. 1995;109:1241–8.

93. Knudsen MA, Svane D, Tottrup A. Action profiles of nitric oxide, S-nitroso-L-cysteine, SNP, and NANC responses in opossum lower esophageal sphincter. Am J Physiol. 1992;262:G840–6.

94. Tottrup A, Svane D, Forman A. Nitric oxide mediating NANC inhibition in opossum lower esophageal sphincter. Am J Physiol. 1991;260:G385–9.

95. Conklin JL, Du C, Murray JA, Bates JN. Characterization and mediation of inhibitory junction potentials from opossum lower esophageal sphincter. Gastroenterology. 1993;104:1439–44.

96. Murray J, Bates JN, Conklin JL. Nerve-mediated nitric oxide production by opossum lower esophageal sphincter. Dig Dis Sci. 1994;39:1872–6.

97. Said SI, Rattan S. The multiple mediators of neurogenic smooth muscle relaxation. Trends Endocrinol Metab. 2004;15:189–91.

98. Murthy KS, Grider JR, Jin JG, Makhlouf GM. Interplay of VIP and nitric oxide in the regulation of neuromuscular function in the gut. Ann N Y Acad Sci. 1996;805:355–62. discussion 362–3.

99. Barnette M, Torphy TJ, Grous M, Fine C, Ormsbee 3rd HS, Cyclic GMP. a potential mediator of neurally- and drug-induced relaxation of opossum lower esophageal sphincter. J Pharmacol Exp Ther. 1989;249:524–8.

100. Torphy TJ, Fine CF, Burman M, Barnette MS, Ormsbee 3rd HS. Lower esophageal sphincter relaxation is associated with increased cyclic nucleotide content. Am J Physiol. 1986;251:G786–93.

101. Dodds WJ, Stewart ET, Hodges D, Zboralske FF. Movement of the feline esophagus associated with respiration and peristalsis. An evaluation using tantalum markers. J Clin Invest. 1973;52:1–13.

102. Paterson WG. Studies on opossum esophageal longitudinal muscle function. Can J Physiol Pharmacol. 1997;75:65–73.

103. Dent J. A new technique for continuous sphincter pressure measurement. Gastroenterology. 1976;71:263–7.

104. Dogan I, Bhargava V, Liu J, Mittal RK. Axial stretch: A novel mechanism of the lower esophageal sphincter relaxation. Am J Physiol Gastrointest Liver Physiol. 2007;292:G329–34.

105. Jiang Y, Sandler B, Bhargava V, Mittal RK. Antireflux action of nissen fundoplication and stretch-sensitive mechanism of lower esophageal sphincter relaxation. Gastroenterology. 2010;140:442–9.

106. De Troyer A, Rosso J. Reflex inhibition of the diaphragm by esophageal afferents. Neurosci Lett. 1982;30:43–6.

107. Pickering M, Jones JF. The diaphragm: two physiological muscles in one. J Anat. 2002;201:305–12.

108. Fournier M, Sieck GC. Somatotopy in the segmental innervation of the cat diaphragm. J Appl Physiol. 1988;64:291–8.

109. Hammond CG, Gordon DC, Fisher JT, Richmond FJ. Motor unit territories supplied by primary branches of the phrenic nerve. J Appl Physiol. 1989;66:61–71.

110. Young RL, Page AJ, Cooper NJ, Frisby CL, Blackshaw LA. Sensory and motor innervation of the crural diaphragm by the vagus nerves. Gastroenterology. 2010;138:1091–101. e1-5.

111. Niedringhaus M, Jackson PG, Evans SR, Verbalis JG, Gillis RA, Sahibzada N. Dorsal motor nucleus of the vagus: a site for evoking simultaneous changes in crural diaphragm activity, lower esophageal sphincter pressure, and fundus tone. Am J Physiol Regul Integr Comp Physiol. 2008;294:R121–31.

112. Niedringhaus M, Jackson PG, Pearson R, Shi M, Dretchen K, Gillis RA, Sahibzada N. Brainstem sites controlling the lower esophageal sphincter and crural diaphragm in the ferret: a neuroanatomical study. Auton Neurosci. 2008;144:50–60.

113. Mittal RK, Rochester DF, McCallum RW. Electrical and mechanical activity in the human lower esophageal sphincter during diaphragmatic contraction. J Clin Invest. 1988;81:1182–9.

114. Sivri B, Mittal RK. Reverse-perfused sleeve: an improved device for measurement of sphincteric function of the crural diaphragm. Gastroenterology. 1991;101:962–9.

115. Klein WA, Parkman HP, Dempsey DT, Fisher RS. Sphincter like thoracoabdominal high pressure zone after esophagogastrectomy. Gastroenterology. 1993;105:1362–9.

116. Altschuler SM, Boyle JT, Nixon TE, Pack AI, Cohen S. Simultaneous reflex inhibition of lower esophageal sphincter and crural diaphragm in cats. Am J Physiol. 1985;249:G586–91.

117. Mittal RK, Fisher MJ. Electrical and mechanical inhibition of the crural diaphragm during transient relaxation of the lower esophageal sphincter. Gastroenterology. 1990;99:1265–8.

118. Altschuler SM, Davies RO, Pack AI. Role of medullary inspiratory neurones in the control of the diaphragm during oesophageal stimulation in cats. J Physiol. 1987;391:289–98.

119. Liu J, Yamamoto Y, Schirmer BD, Ross RA, Mittal RK. Evidence for a peripheral mechanism of esophagocrural diaphragm inhibitory reflex in cats. Am J Physiol Gastrointest Liver Physiol. 2000;278:G281–8.

120. Liu J, Puckett JL, Takeda T, Jung HY, Mittal RK. Crural diaphragm inhibition during esophageal distension correlates with contraction of the esophageal longitudinal muscle in cats. Am J Physiol Gastrointest Liver Physiol. 2005;288:G927–32.

121. Sifrim D, Janssens J, Vantrappen G. Transient lower esophageal sphincter relaxations and esophageal body muscular contractile response in normal humans. Gastroenterology. 1996;110:659–68.

122. Holloway RH, Penagini R, Ireland AC. Criteria for objective definition of transient lower esophageal sphincter relaxation. Am J Physiol. 1995;268: G128–33.

123. Steven C, Seller AF. Rumination. Washington, DC: American Physiological Society; 1968.

124. Kahrilas PJ, Dodds WJ, Dent J, Wyman JB, Hogan WJ, Arndorfer RC. Upper esophageal sphincter function during belching. Gastroenterology. 1986;91:133–40.

125. Babaei A, Bhargava V, Mittal RK. Upper esophageal sphincter during transient lower esophageal sphincter relaxation: effects of reflux content and posture. Am J Physiol Gastrointest Liver Physiol. 2010;298:G601–7.

126. Babaei A, Bhargava V, Korsapati H, Zheng WH, Mittal RK. A unique longitudinal muscle contraction pattern associated with transient lower esophageal sphincter relaxation. Gastroenterology. 2008;134:1322–31.

127. Mittal RK, Padda B, Bhalla V, Bhargava V, Liu J. Synchrony between circular and longitudinal muscle contractions during peristalsis in normal subjects. Am J Physiol Gastrointest Liver Physiol. 2006;290:G431–8.

128. Dent J, Dodds WJ, Friedman RH, Sekiguchi T, Hogan WJ, Arndorfer RC, Petrie DJ. Mechanism of gastroesophageal reflux in recumbent asymptomatic human subjects. J Clin Invest. 1980;65:256–67.

129. Freidin N, Fisher MJ, Taylor W, Boyd D, Surratt P, McCallum RW, Mittal RK. Sleep and nocturnal acid reflux in normal subjects and patients with reflux oesophagitis. Gut. 1991;32:1275–9.

130. Cox MR, Martin CJ, Dent J, Westmore M. Effect of general anaesthesia on transient lower oesophageal sphincter relaxations in the dog. Aust N Z J Surg. 1988;58:825–30.

131. Little AF, Cox MR, Martin CJ, Dent J, Franzi SJ, Lavelle R. Influence of posture on transient lower oesophageal sphincter relaxation and gastro-oesophageal reflux in the dog. J Gastroenterol Hepatol. 1989;4:49–54.

132. Freidin N, Mittal RK, McCallum RW. Does body posture affect the incidence and mechanism of gastro-oesophageal reflux? Gut. 1991;32:133–6.

133. Holloway RH, Hongo M, Berger K, McCallum RW. Gastric distention: a mechanism for postprandial gastroesophageal reflux. Gastroenterology. 1985;89:779–84.

134. Holloway RH, Wyman JB, Dent J. Failure of transient lower oesophageal sphincter relaxation in response to gastric distension in patients with achalasia: evidence for neural mediation of transient lower oesophageal sphincter relaxations. Gut. 1989;30:762–7.

135. Franzi SJ, Martin CJ, Cox MR, Dent J. Response of canine lower esophageal sphincter to gastric distension. Am J Physiol. 1990;259:G380–5.

136. Penagini R, Carmagnola S, Cantu P, Allocca M, Bianchi PA. Mechanoreceptors of the proximal stomach: Role in triggering transient lower esopha-

geal sphincter relaxation. Gastroenterology. 2004;126:49–56.

137. Strombeck DR, Harrold D, Ferrier W. Eructation of gas through the gastroesophageal sphincter before and after truncal vagotomy in dogs. Am J Vet Res. 1987;48:207–10.

138. Martin CJ, Patrikios J, Dent J. Abolition of gas reflux and transient lower esophageal sphincter relaxation by vagal blockade in the dog. Gastroenterology. 1986;91:890–6.

139. Mittal RK, Stewart WR, Schirmer BD. Effect of a catheter in the pharynx on the frequency of transient lower esophageal sphincter relaxations. Gastroenterology. 1992;103:1236–40.

140. Paterson WG, Rattan S, Goyal RK. Experimental induction of isolated lower esophageal sphincter relaxation in anesthetized opossums. J Clin Invest. 1986;77:1187–93.

141. Trifan A, Shaker R, Ren J, Mittal RK, Saeian K, Dua K, Kusano M. Inhibition of resting lower esophageal sphincter pressure by pharyngeal water stimulation in humans. Gastroenterology. 1995;108:441–6.

142. Mittal RK, Chiareli C, Liu J, Shaker R. Characteristics of lower esophageal sphincter relaxation induced by pharyngeal stimulation with minute amounts of water. Gastroenterology. 1996;111:378–84.

143. Mittal RK, Holloway RH, Penagini R, Blackshaw LA, Dent J. Transient lower esophageal sphincter relaxation. Gastroenterology. 1995;109:601–10.

144. Lehmann A, Antonsson M, Bremner-Danielsen M, Flardh M, Hansson-Branden L, Karrberg L. Activation of the GABA(B) receptor inhibits transient lower esophageal sphincter relaxations in dogs. Gastroenterology. 1999;117:1147–54.

145. Blackshaw LA, Staunton E, Lehmann A, Dent J. Inhibition of transient LES relaxations and reflux in ferrets by GABA receptor agonists. Am J Physiol. 1999;277:G867–74.

146. Zhang Q, Lehmann A, Rigda R, Dent J, Holloway RH. Control of transient lower oesophageal sphincter relaxations and reflux by the GABA(B) agonist baclofen in patients with gastro-oesophageal reflux disease. Gut. 2002;50:19–24.

147. Mittal RK, Holloway R, Dent J. Effect of atropine on the frequency of reflux and transient lower esophageal sphincter relaxation in normal subjects. Gastroenterology. 1995;109:1547–54.

148. Fang JC, Sarosiek I, Yamamoto Y, Liu J, Mittal RK. Cholinergic blockade inhibits gastro-oesophageal reflux and transient lower oesophageal sphincter relaxation through a central mechanism. Gut. 1999;44:603–7.

149. Boulant J, Fioramonti J, Dapoigny M, Bommelaer G, Bueno L. Cholecystokinin and nitric oxide in transient lower esophageal sphincter relaxation to gastric distention in dogs. Gastroenterology. 1994;107:1059–66.

150. Penagini R, Bianchi PA. Effect of morphine on gastroesophageal reflux and transient lower esophageal sphincter relaxation. Gastroenterology. 1997;113:409–14.

151. Frisby CL, Mattsson JP, Jensen JM, Lehmann A, Dent J, Blackshaw LA. Inhibition of transient lower esophageal sphincter relaxation and gastroesophageal reflux by metabotropic glutamate receptor ligands. Gastroenterology. 2005;129:995–1004.

152. Lehmann A, Blackshaw LA, Branden L, Carlsson A, Jensen J, Nygren E, Smid SD. Cannabinoid receptor agonism inhibits transient lower esophageal sphincter relaxations and reflux in dogs. Gastroenterology. 2002;123:1129–34.

153. Lehmann A. Es0-hageal Pain. San Diego, CA: Plural Publishing; 2009.

154. Jenkinson AD, Scott SM, Yazaki E, Fusai G, Walker SM, Kadirkamanathan SS, Evans DF. Compliance measurement of lower esophageal sphincter and esophageal body in achalasia and gastroesophageal reflux disease. Dig Dis Sci. 2001;46:1937–42.

155. Liu J, Takeda T, Dogan I, Bhargava V, Mittal RK. Oesophago-gastric junction opening function: assessment using ultrasound imaging and the effects of atropine. Neurogastroenterol Motil. 2006;18: 376–84.

156. McMahon BP, Frokjaer JB, Kunwald P, Liao D, Funch-Jensen P, Drewes AM, Gregersen H. The functional lumen imaging probe (FLIP) for evaluation of the esophagogastric junction. Am J Physiol Gastrointest Liver Physiol. 2007;292:G377–84.

157. Kwiatek MA, Hirano I, Kahrilas PJ, Rothe J, Luger D, Pandolfino JE. Mechanical properties of the esophagus in eosinophilic esophagitis. Gastroenterology. 2010;140:82–90.

158. Pandolfino JE, Shi G, Trueworthy B, Kahrilas PJ. Esophagogastric junction opening during relaxation distinguishes nonhernia reflux patients, hernia patients, and normal subjects. Gastroenterology. 2003;125:1018–24.

159. Pandolfino JE, Shi G, Curry J, Joehl RJ, Brasseur JG, Kahrilas PJ. Esophagogastric junction distensibility: a factor contributing to sphincter incompetence. Am J Physiol Gastrointest Liver Physiol. 2002;282:G1052–8.

160. Katz PO, Richter JE, Cowan R, Castell DO. Apparent complete lower esophageal sphincter relaxation in achalasia. Gastroenterology. 1986;90:978–83.

161. Mearin F, Malagelada JR. Complete lower esophageal sphincter relaxation observed in some achalasia patients is functionally inadequate. Am J Physiol Gastrointest Liver Physiol. 2000;278: G376–83.

162. Blom D, Bajaj S, Liu J, Hofmann C, Rittmann T, Derksen T, Shaker R. Laparoscopic Nissen fundoplication decreases gastroesophageal junction distensibility in patients with gastroesophageal reflux disease. J Gastrointest Surg. 2005;9:1318–25.

163. Kwiatek MA, Kahrilas K, Soper NJ, Bulsiewicz WJ, McMahon BP, Gregersen H, Pandolfino JE. Esophagogastric junction distensibility after fundoplication assessed with a novel functional luminal imaging probe. J Gastrointest Surg. 2010;14: 268–76.

Motility and Pressure Phenomena of the Esophagus

24

Vladimir M. Kushnir and C. Prakash Gyawali

Abstract

The esophagus is a muscular tube consisting of three functional regions: the upper and lower esophageal sphincters, and the esophageal body. On high-resolution manometry, the esophageal body consists of three contracting segments: the proximal striated muscle segment, followed by two smooth muscle segments, separated by pressure troughs. The sphincters and contracting segments function in contiguity to form a chain of relaxing and contracting segments, modulated by cortical, brain stem, and peripheral influences.

Keywords

Motility • Pressure phenomena • Esophagus • Esophageal contraction segments • Striated muscle esophagus • Smooth muscle esophagus

Introduction

The esophagus and its sphincters perform the important function of transport of swallowed food from the pharynx to the stomach. Additionally, these structures are responsible for the prevention of reflux of gastric contents into the esophagus and airways, and for clearing the esophagus of gastroesophageal refluxate. The esophageal phase of deglutition is composed of a series of highly coordinated events that propagates food or fluid bolus from the pharynx into the stomach. Under normal circumstances, this is the result of integration of numerous control mechanisms arising from the central nervous system (CNS), enteric nervous system (ENS), and the musculature of the esophageal body. These control mechanisms also serve as a coordinating mechanism, tying esophageal body motor function to motor phenomena in the oropharynx, lower esophageal sphincter (LES) and the rest of the gut, as well as to the pulmonary and cardiovascular systems [1].

An understanding of normal physiology of the esophageal phase of deglutition is important for the practicing deglutologist, as most disorders of

V.M. Kushnir, MD
Division of Gastroenterology, Barnes Jewish Hospital, Washington University School of Medicine, Campus Box 8124, 660 South Euclid Ave, St. Louis, MO 63112, USA

C.P. Gyawali, MD (✉)
Division of Gastroenterology, Washington University School of Medicine, Campus Box 8124, 660 South Euclid Ave, St. Louis, MO 63124, USA
e-mail: cprakash@wustl.edu

R. Shaker et al. (eds.), *Principles of Deglutition: A Multidisciplinary Text for Swallowing and its Disorders*, DOI 10.1007/978-1-4614-3794-9_24, © Springer Science+Business Media New York 2013

esophageal body motility can be explained by disruption of physiologic mechanisms at various levels. Esophageal motor disorders in turn have helped further our understanding of normal esophageal physiology, especially in the era of high-resolution manometry (HRM) [2, 3]. Clinical assessment of esophageal motor physiology, therefore, gives the clinician insight into the function of these neuromuscular processes, and in some cases allows the diagnosis of specific abnormalities of esophageal motor function.

This chapter will describe normal motility and pressure phenomena in the esophageal body and lay the groundwork for understanding disorders of the esophageal phase of deglutition. Although the oropharynx, upper esophageal sphincter (UES), and LES are structurally and functionally intertwined with esophageal body motility, these are discussed in detail elsewhere in this textbook. Further, cortical, brain stem and local control mechanisms are also discussed elsewhere, but will be mentioned where relevant.

Functional Anatomy and Physiology

The esophagus is a muscular tube composed of three distinct functional regions: the UES, the esophageal body (tubular esophagus), and the LES [4, 5]. The physiologic properties of each region can be evaluated by manometry.

The UES consists of a 2–4 cm zone of elevated pressure located at the junction of the pharynx and esophagus, formed of two striated muscles, the cricopharyngeus and a portion of the inferior pharyngeal constrictor muscle [6]. The cricopharyngeus attaches to the lateral aspects of the cricoid cartilage, resulting in a flat anterior aspect that is resistant to deformation [7, 8]. Therefore, at its resting contracted state, the UES has a crescentic, slit-like appearance [6].

The esophageal body consists of a 20–22 cm muscular tube, originating at the caudal extent of the cricopharyngeus muscle and extending to the proximal margin of the LES. The top 5% of the esophagus—roughly to the level of the aortic arch—consists of striated muscle. The middle 35–40% contains both striated and smooth muscle,

with smooth muscle progressively replacing striated muscle—this part of the esophageal body is sometimes termed the "transition zone." The distal 50–60% of the esophageal body is entirely smooth muscle [9]. The esophageal body is composed of inner circular and outer longitudinal muscle layers, with a neural network called the myenteric plexus sandwiched between the muscular layers [10]. The myenteric plexus receives neural input from the CNS and provides terminal motor innervation to the smooth muscle of the esophagus [11].

The LES consists mainly of a 2–4 cm segment of asymmetrically thickened circular muscle fibers that remain tonically contracted at rest [12]. This resting tone is under neurogenic control through cholinergic innervation mediated by acetylcholine, as well as myogenic tone related to intracellular calcium influx [6, 12]. The LES relaxes with the act of swallowing, and with distension of the esophageal body or the gastric fundus. Relaxation is largely mediated by nonadrenergic noncholinergic (NANC) inhibitory neurons from the vagus nerve and the myenteric plexus, where the main postsynaptic neurotransmitter is nitric oxide [13, 14].

Advances in neuroimaging have shed light into the role of the cerebral cortex in the control of swallowing [15–18]. The internal capsule contains fibers of the corticobulbar tracts responsible for transmitting information from the cortex to the brain stem—emphasizing the importance of cortical input in regulating the brain stem swallowing center [19]. Additional cortical centers participate in the control of swallowing. The efferent motor neurons controlling the oral and pharyngeal phases of deglutition originate in the trigeminal, hypoglossal, and facial nuclei [11]. The "swallowing center," which serves as the central control site for esophageal motor function is located in the brain stem at the junction of the medulla and pons [11, 20]. It is within this center that afferent sensory neurons, efferent motor neurons, and cortical internuclear neurons interact and coordinate all phases of deglutition [11].

The innervation of the striated muscle part of the esophagus is somatic; neurons arising in the nucleus ambiguous travel within the vagus to

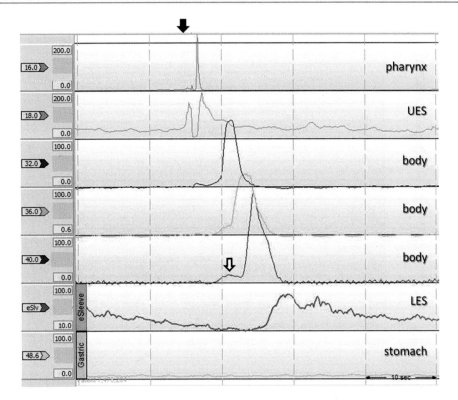

Fig. 24.1 Normal esophageal peristalsis on conventional manometry, displayed as line tracings. Pressure is depicted in mmHg along the *y* axis, and time in seconds along the *x* axis. The *closed arrow* indicates the timing of the swallow, in this instance a 5 mL water bolus. Notations to the *right* indicate the anatomic location of each sensor (*UES* upper esophageal sphincter, *LES* lower esophageal sphincter), and the distances to the *left* indicate distance from the nares. A sleeve was used to obtain LES pressures. Intrabolus pressure preceding peristaltic contraction is depicted by the *open arrow*

synapse directly on striated muscle fibers as motor endplates [21]. Peristalsis in the striated muscle esophagus results from a patterned, sequential activation of these neurons to produce successive activation of striated circular esophageal muscles [21]. The ENS plays an integral role in the control and coordination of esophageal body peristalsis. The extrinsic innervation of the smooth muscle esophagus is derived from the dorsal motor nucleus of the vagus [22]. These parasympathetic preganglionic fibers travel within the vagus to synapse on neurons within the myenteric plexus [23]. Myenteric neurons supply the terminal motor innervation of the smooth muscle esophagus. The programming of peristalsis in the smooth muscle esophagus depends upon a precise interplay among the CNS, myenteric plexus, and smooth muscle of the esophagus. The CNS behaves as a switch that initiates a peripheral program in the myenteric plexus and smooth muscle to produce peristalsis [9]. The neuromuscular mechanisms controlling esophageal motor function are reviewed elsewhere [4, 24].

Esophageal Manometry

Esophageal manometry consists of measurement of pressure phenomena at multiple sites in the esophagus, interpretation of which provides assessment of esophageal sphincters, esophageal muscle function, and esophageal peristalsis. Conventional esophageal manometry consists of esophageal pressure tracings obtained from sensors on a motility catheter placed through the nostril (Fig. 24.1). Typically, conventional catheters have either pressure sensing side holes for

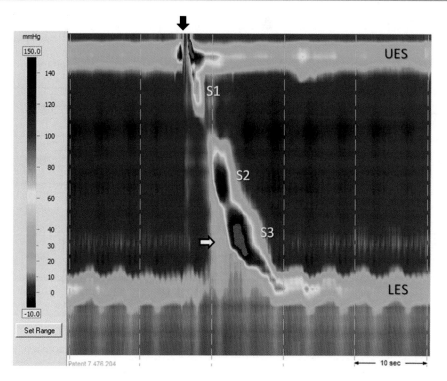

Fig. 24.2 High-resolution manometry (HRM) Clouse plot of normal esophageal peristalsis. Pressure is depicted as colors, *brighter colors* indicating higher amplitudes as described on the scale to the *left*. Distance along the esophagus is depicted along the *y* axis, and time in seconds along the *x* axis. The Clouse plots therefore describe spatio-temporal relationships of pressure events to time and distance along the esophagus. The sphincters (*UES* upper esophageal sphincter, *LES* lower esophageal sphincter) anchor the proximal and distal extents of the esophagus. The peristaltic sequence in the esophageal body consists of three sequentially contracting segments: the striated muscle segment (S1), the proximal smooth muscle segment (S2), and the distal smooth muscle segment (S3). These segments are separated from each other by pressure troughs, and each segment has a peak pressure. Intrabolus pressure exerted by the swallowed bolus is sometimes seen in normal peristalsis as a low-amplitude pressure event preceding smooth muscle contraction; this is accentuated when LES relaxation is incomplete

use with water-perfused systems, or solid-state sensors capable of electronically detecting pressure changes in the esophageal lumen [25]. The sensors are spaced at 3–5 cm intervals depending on the number of sensors incorporated into the catheter, most catheters having eight sensors 3 cm apart [26]. Since single-point sensors have been determined to be inaccurate in assessing sphincter function, a 6 cm sleeve sensor (Dent sleeve) is typically used to interrogate the LES [27].

In the 1990s, a new form of esophageal manometry was introduced by Clouse et al. utilizing pressure tracings from 21 pressure sensors 1 cm apart on a water-perfused motility catheter system [28]. A dedicated prototypic computer program extrapolated "best-fit" pressure data in between the 1 cm data intervals, generating three-dimensional topographic contour plots of esophageal motor function similar to geographic topographic maps [28–30]. This technique, termed HRM, now utilizes as many as 36 high-fidelity circumferential solid-state sensors incorporated into a flexible motility catheter, and provides colorful and easily recognizable topographic contour plots (Clouse plots, Fig. 24.2) of esophageal peristaltic events [31, 32]. Compared to conventional manometry, HRM procedures are considerably shorter in duration, mainly from elimination of the "stationary pull-through" maneuver with the modern solid-state HRM systems [33]. Further, visual recognition of motor patterns on Clouse plots is an important aspect of interpretation [34]. Advances to HRM consist of the addition of electrode pairs to the motility catheter for concurrent impedance measurements to allow assessment of bolus transit termed high resolution impedance manometry (HRIM), and the incorporation of tactile sensor technology to short segments of the HRM catheter for detailed three-dimensional assessment of sphincter anatomy and function (termed high-definition manometry) [35, 36]. These techniques have been used in research studies, and the clinical utility of these advances continues to be assessed.

High-resolution methods offer two basic advances over conventional manometry; first, the increased number of data points obtained with HRM has provided for detailed inspection of pressure phenomena [28, 37, 38]. This advance has allowed detection of subtle pressure changes, and defined peaks and troughs previously unrecognized in esophageal peristaltic function. Esophageal body peristalsis is now understood to be composed of three contracting segments (Fig. 24.2), separated by distinct troughs from adjacent segments and the LES [28]. Further, these contracting segments appear to be under differential control, and may manifest motor disturbances localized to specific segments or troughs [37, 39]. The second advance is the understanding of temporal and spatial relationships between pressure data, made possible by data interpolation and three-dimensional plotting. In particular, detection of abnormal LES relaxation has been enhanced by three-dimensional plotting, which has escalated the accuracy of achalasia diagnosis [3]. Further, HRM has facilitated detailed interrogation of pressure phenomena in the esophageal body and across sphincters, and in conjunction with multichannel esophageal impedance measurements, has improved our understanding of esophageal physiology and pathophysiology.

Esophageal Peristalsis

Esophageal peristalsis is initiated by swallowing, and primary esophageal peristalsis starts when the peristaltic contraction passes from the pharynx into the upper esophagus. Therefore, esophageal peristalsis consists of a wave of circular muscle contraction that proceeds into the proximal esophagus as a continuation of the forceful pharyngeal contraction that initiates relaxation of the UES. Ring-like contraction of the striated muscle in the proximal esophagus propagates seamlessly through the transition zone and down the esophageal body to the level of the LES. While most swallowed food boluses move by gravity, esophageal peristalsis strips the lumen of residual bolus along the esophagus to the stomach [40].

At rest, the musculature of the normal esophageal body generates no rhythmic contractions and little tone. Therefore, most intra-luminal pressure changes recorded in the quiescent esophagus are passive, arising from intra-thoracic pressure changes associated with respiration or with transmitted pressure waves from nearby cardiovascular structures like the heart or aorta. In contrast, both the UES and LES are tonically contracted at rest, generating a baseline pressure profile that is easily recognized on HRM.

Esophageal peristalsis is recorded manometrically as a pressure wave that moves along the length of the esophagus (Fig. 24.1). Motor activity in the esophageal body is described by assessment of pressure waves generated by esophageal contractions. Peristaltic function of the esophagus is a composite of the proportion of wet swallows that produce peristaltic pressure waves, the velocity of propagation of the pressure waves, and the characteristics of the pressure waves themselves [26]. A typical manometric trace is generated by a wet swallow (5 mL water bolus). Under normal circumstances, this generates pharyngeal contraction and UES relaxation which can be identified on the pressure tracing. Esophageal body contraction can be seen as a progressive pressure wave that travels down the esophageal body (Fig. 24.1). The sensor or sleeve sensor at the LES demonstrates relaxation close to the gastric baseline, followed by LES after contraction before pressure settles down to the LES baseline pressure.

The amplitude of the peristaltic wave is defined as the difference between the baseline resting pressure and the pressure at the peak of the pressure wave [26]. To be classified as a pressure wave produced by a contraction, the amplitude of the pressure wave should be at least 20 mmHg. Contractions with amplitudes <30 mmHg are considered by most investigators to be feeble or hypotensive [41–43]. During normal peristalsis, the contractile wave amplitude is typically between 30 and 180 mmHg and rarely exceeds 200 mmHg. Amplitudes >180 mmHg are termed hypertensive [41]. The amplitudes of peristaltic pressure waves vary along the esophagus, with the amplitude being greater in the proximal and distal esophagus than in the mid-esophagus [44]. This diminution in peristaltic pressure appears to occur over the zone of transition from striated to smooth muscle. The amplitudes of peristaltic pressure waves can normally vary from swallow to swallow.

Failure of peristalsis occurs when a wet swallow does not produce an esophageal contraction, when the peristaltic contraction dies out as it progresses down the esophagus, or when an initial peristaltic sequence travels part way down the esophagus and ends as a simultaneous contraction of the remainder of the esophageal body [42]. In each of these instances, bolus transit is abnormal [45]. Repetitive contraction is said to occur when the pressure wave has multiple (≥2) peaks at least 1 s apart, with at least 10 mmHg drop in pressure between peaks [46].

The pressure waves produced by peristaltic contractions traverse the length of the esophageal body in 5–6 s. The velocity of the pressure wave is determined by identifying and following the beginning of the upstroke of the pressure wave through the esophageal body, as the initial upstroke coincides with closure of the esophageal lumen by the peristaltic contraction [45]. Pressure waves progress at about 3 cm/s in the upper esophageal body, 5 cm/s along the middle of the esophageal body, and 2.5 cm/s just above the LES [47]. Most investigators consider propagation rates of greater than 6 cm/s as abnormal, as contractions with faster propagation rates do not propel the bolus effectively [48]. The duration of the peristaltic contraction is defined as the time from the beginning of the upstroke of the pressure wave to the time when the pressure returns

to baseline [26]. Durations of each pressure wave are in the range of 2–4 s, and they tend to be of longer duration in the distal esophagus [44].

The peristaltic pressure wave is sometimes preceded by a transitory fall in intra-esophageal pressure that lasts up to 0.5 s, which may be constantly seen—the mechanism of this pressure drop is unclear. A transient and small increase in intra-luminal pressure may also precede the peristaltic pressure wave, occurring approximately 1.0 s after the swallow initiates. This is thought to represent intrabolus pressure within the swallowed bolus, as the bolus is pushed ahead of the peristaltic wave (Fig. 24.1). The amplitude of this intrabolus pressure is variable, and can be elevated in situations where motor obstruction occurs, such as abnormal LES relaxation [49].

Swallow-induced peristalsis is accompanied by longitudinal muscle contraction that shortens the esophagus by 2–2.5 cm [50–52]. Longitudinal muscle contraction, like peristalsis, begins in the proximal esophagus and progresses in a craniocaudal sequence, but it precedes the peristaltic circular muscle contraction [44]. The process of esophageal shortening is not distinguishable as an intra-luminal pressure change.

Esophageal Contraction Segments

Despite marked regional differences in its neuromuscular makeup and control mechanisms, the esophagus behaves, at least superficially, in a seamless fashion as a single functional unit. However, on detailed evaluation of the peristaltic wave on HRM, esophageal peristalsis consists of a chain of contracting segments (Fig. 24.2), anchored at the top and bottom by relaxing sphincters, the UES and the LES [28]. Peristalsis in the esophagus therefore is segmental in nature, and consequently the amplitude of contractile waves varies along the esophageal body. Identification of contraction segments depends on locating amplitude peaks and troughs within and in-between contraction segments respectively [28, 39, 53]. Much of this variation in contractile amplitudes can be missed when peristalsis is evaluated with conventional esophageal manometry, with a few pressure sensors which are distant from each other. However, this variation in amplitudes can be fully appreciated with HRM (Fig. 24.2). Following initiation of the peristaltic wave at the UES, a high pressure zone can be observed as peristalsis is propagated over the skeletal muscle segment of the esophageal body. This is followed by a conspicuous low pressure zone 4–6 cm below the UES, corresponding to the transition from skeletal to smooth muscle and change in innervations from the recurrent laryngeal nerve to the vagus nerve in the smooth muscle esophagus [54]. When esophageal peristalsis is evaluated using HRM a second, less conspicuous low pressure zone can be seen and divides the smooth muscle esophagus into two roughly equal segments [28].

Upper Esophageal Sphincter

The UES opens during deglutition to allow passage of the swallowed bolus into the esophagus. Closure of the sphincter coincides with arrival of a powerful pharyngeal peristaltic contraction, seen manometrically as a rapid drop in resting UES pressure lasting approximately 0.5 s followed by a rise in pressure that may exceed twice the resting UES pressure. This pressure wave may last for a second or so before returning to resting levels [6].

Striated Muscle Esophagus

Contraction of the striated muscle esophagus is initiated following relaxation of the UES and is directed by sequential activation of vagal fibers via the recurrent laryngeal nerve. The striated muscle corresponds to the first peristaltic segment seen on HRM (S-1) (Fig. 24.2) and is approximately 5–6 cm long, measured from the lower margin of the UES to the first low pressure zone separating the striated and smooth muscle of the esophageal body [53]. The striated muscle segment accounts for approximately a quarter of the length of the esophagus, and is the more consistent peristaltic segment across

multiple swallows with only minor variation between swallows [55]. Peristaltic failure at this level does not usually occur in the absence of a skeletal muscle myopathy (dermatomyositis) or bulbar neurologic dysfunction (amyotrophic lateral sclerosis, myasthenia gravis, cerebrovascular accident, etc.).

Transition Zone

The existence of a pressure trough in the mid-esophagus has long been recognized and corresponds to a transition from skeletal muscle to vagally controlled smooth muscle in the esophageal body. This pressure trough, also termed intersegmental trough (IST, Fig. 24.3), is thought to represent the spatiotemporal handoff of the contraction sequence from the skeletal to the smooth muscle esophagus. The first full description of the transition zone was only possible following the introduction of HRM [56]. The transition zone can be easily identified as the nadir pressure area immediately distal to the first contraction segment on a HRM Clouse plot. The nadir pressure may dip below the 30 mmHg isobaric contour in 60% of swallows in normal subjects [57]. The length of the transition zone is normally 1–2 cm and the peristaltic wave typically traverses this area in less than 1 s. While this pressure trough in the mid-esophagus is physiologic, an abnormally prolonged IST can potentially be associated with abnormal bolus transit or even dysphagia in some individuals, specifically when the pressure trough is temporally prolonged (>1 s) or elongated (>2 cm) on HRM [54, 58].

Smooth Muscle Esophagus

Analysis of peristalsis in the smooth muscle esophagus with HRM has demonstrated that it is separated into two approximately equal segments (S-2 and S-3), first reported by Clouse et al. in 1991 [28]. These smooth muscle contraction segments can be identified as separate, distinct entities in approximately 60% of swallows (Fig. 24.2).

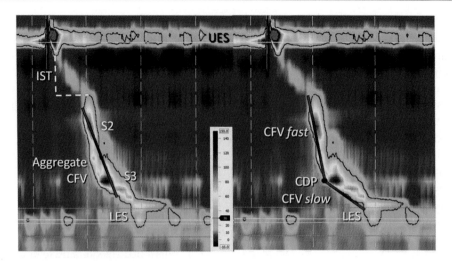

Fig. 24.3 New analysis parameters introduced by high-resolution manometry (HRM). The intersegmental trough (IST, also termed the transition zone) represents a pressure nadir between the skeletal and smooth muscle contraction segments. Normally around 1 cm in length, it can be extensive and can sometime correlate with dysphagia symptoms. Contractile front velocity (CFV) is measured from the proximal extent of smooth muscle contraction (determined by using the 30 mmHg isobaric contour) to the distal most portion adjacent to the lower esophageal sphincter (LES). There are two components to the contractile front, a proximal fast component (CFV *fast*) responsible for bolus propagation, and a distal slow component (CFV *slow*) responsible for esophageal emptying through the LES. The *point* at which CFV slows is termed contractile deceleration point (CDP). Time elapsed from UES relaxation to the CDP (distal contraction latency) may offer an alternate measure of peristaltic progression

Intersubject variability is much more significant that interswallow variability, indicating that the overall peristaltic pattern holds true for any given individual despite variation in the location of peak and trough pressure amplitudes within the smooth muscle esophagus [55]. The two smooth muscle segments (S-2 and S-3) measured 8–9 and 6–7 cm in a small series of 14 normal subjects, accounting for 41% and 31% of esophageal length respectively [53]. The first of the smooth muscle segments is separated from the skeletal muscle segment by the transition zone, which can be detected as a dip in pressure or an actual pressure trough. The two smooth muscle segments are separated by a second pressure trough. When compared to the transition zone, the second trough has higher amplitude, is shorter and has a greater variability in location along the esophageal body. Additionally, this second trough is absent in up to 10% of normal subjects.

There does not appear to be a clear anatomic explanation for the separation of the smooth muscle esophagus into two segments; however the existence of this trough does fit in with the under-standing of esophageal neurophysiology [1, 59]. As described earlier in this chapter, animal studies have demonstrated that both excitatory cholinergic and inhibitory NANC neurons are present in the smooth muscle esophagus [59]. The density of these neurons and their influence on peristalsis is graded throughout the smooth muscle, with cholinergic neurons having a greater influence in the proximal smooth muscle and NANC neurons predominating in the distal smooth muscle and in the LES [39, 59]. Human studies have also demonstrated this gradient; when a cholinergic agonist, cisapride, is administered to normal subjects the contractile amplitude is greatly enhanced in the proximal smooth muscle segment and partially obliterates the pressure trough in the smooth muscle esophagus [39]. Further neurophysiologic studies have suggested that this motor phenomenon may be the result of central separation of esophageal motor control into three neuromuscular units: (1) the UES and upper striated muscle esophagus, (2) proximal smooth muscle of the esophageal body, and (3) distal smooth muscle of the esophageal body and LES [11].

New Insights from HRM

The application of HRM has resulted in new insights into esophageal pressure measurements, and new terms are now being applied to pressure phenomena. At the outset, architecture and integrity of the esophageal body contraction segments can be visually and analytically assessed. A normal pattern of three contracting segments separated by troughs can be quickly identified by simple visual assessment (Fig. 24.2). The onscreen isobaric contour tool can be set at 30 mmHg to assess integrity of the peristaltic sequence. Contracting segments may be fragmented, weak or absent in hypomotility states [29, 60]. In contrast, the segments may be exaggerated, prolonged, and repetitive in hypermotility states [2, 61].

Since the image-based paradigm of HRM displays esophageal smooth muscle peristalsis as a continuous contraction front, the propagation velocity of this contraction front can be calculated (contraction front velocity (CFV), Fig. 24.3) as the slope of the line connecting the start of smooth muscle contraction (proximal smooth muscle contraction segment or S2), and the end of smooth muscle contraction (distal smooth muscle contraction segment or S3) [62]. The 30-mmHg isobaric contour has been used as the pressure threshold for predicting bolus clearance, and consequently, this value is used in determining the proximal and distal extents of the contractile front [45, 62]. Studies in normal volunteers have suggested that the upper limit of mean CFV (95th percentile) is 4.5 cm/s [62]. However, CFV is not uniform throughout the smooth muscle esophagus; wide variations have been documented in normal volunteers, ranging from 0.6 to 12.4 cm/s in one report [63]. Velocity is rapid in the proximal aspect of the contractile front (mean 5.1 cm/s), and slows down as the front approaches the LES (mean 1.7 cm/s) (Fig. 24.3) [64]. Similar variations in propagation velocity were reported using conventional manometry, so this concept is not new [40]. The precise point at which the velocity slows down can be identified in the distal esophagus, and this point is termed the contractile deceleration point (CDP, Fig. 24.3). The CDP occurs at a mean of 6 s after UES relaxation in normal individuals [63, 64]. Using a combination of HRM and fluoroscopy, the roles of both the fast and slow CFV segments have been clarified. The fast proximal smooth muscle segment is instrumental in propagating the bolus through the smooth muscle esophagus, while the slow distal segment allows formation of the phrenic ampulla and assists emptying through the open LES [64]. The CDP therefore demarcates the transition from peristaltic conduction to ampullary emptying of the swallowed bolus [64].

Since CFV is not uniform throughout the esophagus, alternate measures may have better reliability in predicting peristaltic propagation. For instance, distal contraction latency, the time from UES relaxation to the CDP, may allow better characterization of esophageal motor phenomena using physiologic principles [63]. This measure may represent a function of esophageal inhibition, shorter latencies indicating abnormal inhibitory nerve function. If validated, this could serve as a surrogate measure for designation of esophageal motor function as peristaltic and simultaneous.

Vigor of esophageal contraction can be assessed by integrating amplitude and duration of contraction over a length of esophagus, expressed as pressure volume in mmHg/cm/s [55]. This measure assesses cumulative pressure over a defined esophageal length for a specified time duration, using a pressure plane of 10 or 20 mmHg as the bottom of the measurement area [2, 55]. Using onscreen software tools, either or both smooth muscle contraction segments can be analyzed using this tool. When both smooth muscle contraction segments are interrogated simultaneously over a 20 mmHg baseline, this parameter is termed distal contractile integral (DCI). Values higher than 5,000 mmHg/cm/s are considered abnormal, and help in distinguishing hypertensive from normal peristalsis [2]. When each smooth muscle contraction segment is separately interrogated, alterations in individual contraction segments in disease states or with pharmacologic manipulations can be assessed [39, 53]. For instance, cholinomimetic agents such as cisapride have been demonstrated to preferentially augment pressure volume in the proximal smooth muscle contraction segment [39]. Fixed mechanical obstruction in the distal esophagus results in similar augmentation of the proximal smooth muscle segment, which may be a manifestation of a rallying effect in attempting to overcome the obstruction [53]. In contrast, the distal smooth muscle contraction segment shows augmentation of pressure volume in functional LES obstruction from an incompletely relaxing LES [53].

The pressure exerted by the bolus within the lumen of the esophageal body can be visualized on HRM plots as vertical isobaric pressure compartmentalization between the leading edge of the smooth muscle contraction segments and the LES [65]. This pressure is termed "intrabolus pressure," and is best visualized in situations associated with abnormal LES relaxation or other obstructive phenomena at the gastroesophageal junction. With normal LES relaxation, pressure generated by the bolus is rapidly dissipated as the bolus moves past the LES into the stomach. Intrabolus pressure is therefore dependent on the post-deglutitive LES residual pressure, and can be measured when higher than the residual pressure. Consequently, with normal LES relaxation, intrabolus pressures are low, and maximal values are reported in the 11–15 mmHg range [66]. In contrast, when LES relaxation is abnormal or when fixed mechanical obstruction is present at the gastroesophageal junction, the bolus gets compartmentalized between the contracting smooth muscle and the gastroesophageal junction; intrabolus pressures are generally higher than 15 mmHg, and usually greater than 25–30 mmHg [66]. Pan esophageal compartmentalization of intrabolus pressure can be seen in achalasia, where esophageal body peristalsis is absent and the LES does not relax adequately [3].

The combination of high-fidelity pressure sensors and impedance conductors in the same motility catheter has proved invaluable in assessing minimum contraction amplitudes needed for bolus transit. This technique, termed high resolution impedance manometry (HRIM), has demonstrated that an intact 20 mmHg isobaric contour plot in the esophageal body results in complete bolus transit [35, 63]. Breaks in the 20 mmHg isobaric contour plot were associated with incomplete bolus transit, and were seen more frequently when dysphagia symptoms were reported. Both small (2–5 cm) and large (>5 cm) breaks in the 20 mmHg isobaric contour plot are reported in normal volunteers, with frequencies as high as 30% of wet swallows [63]. Such breaks can lead to fragmentation or failure of the peristaltic sequence, which can be seen as part of hypomotile end of the motor disorder spectrum [60]. Further research with the use of HRIM is ongoing in further characterization of hypomotility disorders and weak peristalsis.

Conclusion

Esophageal peristalsis consists of a chain of sphincters and contracting segments, seamlessly coordinated by contractile and inhibitory influences modulated through cortical, brain stem, and peripheral control mechanisms. In recent years, HRM has unveiled more of the intricate mechanisms of peristalsis by providing a novel image-based data acquisition and display system that has simplified assessment of esophageal peristalsis. Newer technologies, including a combination of HRM and impedance measurements, show promise in further definition of peristaltic function, and in better characterization of normal and abnormal esophageal motility.

References

1. Goyal RK, Chaudhury A. Physiology of normal esophageal motility. J Clin Gastroenterol. 2008;42:610–9.
2. Pandolfino JE, Ghosh SK, Rice J, Clarke JO, Kwiatek MA, Kahrilas PJ. Classifying esophageal motility by pressure topography characteristics: a study of 400 patients and 75 controls. Am J Gastroenterol. 2008;103:27–37.
3. Pandolfino JE, Kwiatek MA, Nealis T, Bulsiewicz W, Post J, Kahrilas PJ. Achalasia: a new clinically relevant classification by high-resolution manometry. Gastroenterology. 2008;135:1526–33.
4. Conklin JL, Christensen J. Motor functions of the esophagus. In: Christensen JJ, Alpers D, Jacobsen ED, Walsh J, editors. Physiology of the gastrointestinal tract. Raven Press, New York. 1994. pp. 33–40.
5. Miller A, Bieger MD, Conklin JL. Functional controls of deglutition. In: Perlman A, Schulze-Delrieu K,

editors. Deglutition and its disorders: anatomy, physiology, clinical diagnosis and management. San Diego, CA: Singular Publishing Group, Inc.; 1996. p. 43–97.

6. Kahrilas PJ, Dodds WJ, Dent J, Logemann JA, Shaker R. Upper esophageal sphincter function during deglutition. Gastroenterology. 1988;95:52–62.

7. Sivarao DV, Goyal RK. Functional anatomy and physiology of the upper esophageal sphincter. Am J Med. 2000;108(Suppl 4a):27S–37.

8. Lang IM, Shaker R. Anatomy and physiology of the upper esophageal sphincter. Am J Med. 1997;103:50S–5.

9. Bombeck CT, Dillard DH, Nyhus LM. Muscular anatomy of the gastroesophageal junction and role of phrenoesophageal ligament; autopsy study of sphincter mechanism. Ann Surg. 1966;164:643–54.

10. Christensen J, Robison BA. Anatomy of the myenteric plexus of the opossum esophagus. Gastroenterology. 1982;83:1033–42.

11. Ertekin C, Aydogdu I. Neurophysiology of swallowing. Clin Neurophysiol. 2003;114:2226–44.

12. Mittal RK, Balaban DH. The esophagogastric junction. N Engl J Med. 1997;336:924–32.

13. Goyal RK, Rattan S. Nature of the vagal inhibitory innervation to the lower esophageal sphincter. J Clin Invest. 1975;55:1119–26.

14. Yamato S, Spechler SJ, Goyal RK. Role of nitric oxide in esophageal peristalsis in the opossum. Gastroenterology. 1992;103:197–204.

15. Hamdy S, Mikulis DJ, Crawley A, Xue S, Lau H, Henry S, Diamant NE. Cortical activation during human volitional swallowing: an event-related fMRI study. Am J Physiol. 1999;277:G219–25.

16. Cola MG, Daniels SK, Corey DM, Lemen LC, Romero M, Foundas AL. Relevance of subcortical stroke in dysphagia. Stroke. 2010;41:482–6.

17. Michou E, Hamdy S. Cortical input in control of swallowing. Curr Opin Otolaryngol Head Neck Surg. 2009;17:166–71.

18. Gonzalez-Fernandez M, Kleinman JT, Ky PK, Palmer JB, Hillis AE. Supratentorial regions of acute ischemia associated with clinically important swallowing disorders: a pilot study. Stroke. 2008;39:3022–8.

19. Lowell SY, Poletto CJ, Knorr-Chung BR, Reynolds RC, Simonyan K, Ludlow CL. Sensory stimulation activates both motor and sensory components of the swallowing system. Neuroimage. 2008;42:285–95.

20. Broussard DL, Altschuler SM. Brainstem viscerotopic organization of afferents and efferents involved in the control of swallowing. Am J Med. 2000;108(Suppl 4a):79S–86.

21. Roman C. Nervous control of esophageal peristalsis. J Physiol Paris. 1966;58:79–108.

22. Higgs B, Kerr FW, Ellis Jr FH. The experimental production of esophageal achalasia by electrolytic lesions in the medulla. J Thorac Cardiovasc Surg. 1965;50:613–25.

23. MacGilchrist AJ, Christensen J, Rick GA. The distribution of myelinated nerve fibers in the mature opossum esophagus. J Auton Nerv Syst. 1991;35:227–35.

24. Doty RW. Neural organization of deglutition. In: Code CF, editor. Handbook of physiology, vol. 4. Washington, DC: American Psychological Society; 1968. p. 1861–902.

25. Pandolfino JE, Kahrilas PJ. AGA technical review on the clinical use of esophageal manometry. Gastroenterology. 2005;128:209–24.

26. Murray JA, Clouse RE, Conklin JL. Components of the standard oesophageal manometry. Neurogastroenterol Motil. 2003;15:591–606.

27. Dent J. A new technique for continuous sphincter pressure measurement. Gastroenterology. 1976;71:263–7.

28. Clouse RE, Staiano A. Topography of the esophageal peristaltic pressure wave. Am J Physiol. 1991;261:G677–84.

29. Clouse RE, Prakash C. Topographic esophageal manometry: an emerging clinical and investigative approach. Dig Dis. 2000;18:64–74.

30. Clouse RE, Staiano A, Alrakawi A, Haroian L. Application of topographical methods to clinical esophageal manometry. Am J Gastroenterol. 2000;95:2720–30.

31. Clouse RE, Parks TR, Haroian LR. Novel solid-state technology simplifies high-resolution manometry (HRM) for clinical use. Gastroenterology. 2004;126:A638.

32. Kahrilas PJ. Esophageal motor disorders in terms of high-resolution esophageal pressure topography: what has changed? Am J Gastroenterol. 2010;105:981–7.

33. Salvador R, Dubecz A, Polomsky M, Gellerson O, Jones CE, Raymond DP, Watson TJ, Peters JH. A new era in esophageal diagnostics: the image-based paradigm of high-resolution manometry. J Am Coll Surg. 2009;208:1035–44.

34. Soudagar AS, Sayuk GS, Gyawali CP. Learners Favor High Resolution Esophageal Manometry With Better Diagnostic Accuracy Over Conventional Line Tracings. Gut 2012;61:798–803.

35. Bulsiewicz WJ, Kahrilas PJ, Kwiatek MA, Ghosh SK, Meek A, Pandolfino JE. Esophageal pressure topography criteria indicative of incomplete bolus clearance: a study using high-resolution impedance manometry. Am J Gastroenterol. 2009;104:2721–8.

36. Cheeney G, Remes-Troche JM, Attaluri A, Rao SS. Investigation of anal motor characteristics of the sensorimotor response (SMR) using 3-D anorectal pressure topography. Am J Physiol Gastrointest Liver Physiol. 2011;300:G236–40.

37. Clouse RE, Staiano A. Topography of normal and high-amplitude esophageal peristalsis. Am J Physiol. 1993;265:G1098–107.

38. Li M, Brasseur BJ, Hsieh PY, Nicosia M, Kern MK, Massey BT. A conversion methodology to analyze manometric pressure in space-time. Gastroenterology. 1994;106:A530.

39. Staiano A, Clouse RE. The effects of cisapride on the topography of oesophageal peristalsis. Aliment Pharmacol Ther. 1996;10:875–82.

40. Massey BT, Dodds WJ, Hogan WJ, Brasseur JG, Helm JF. Abnormal esophageal motility. An analysis of concurrent radiographic and manometric findings. Gastroenterology. 1991;101:344–54.

41. Clouse RE, Staiano A. Contraction abnormalities of the esophageal body in patients referred to manometry. A new approach to manometric classification. Dig Dis Sci. 1983;28:784–91.

42. Kahrilas PJ, Dodds WJ, Hogan WJ, Kern M, Arndorfer RC, Reece A. Esophageal peristaltic dysfunction in peptic esophagitis. Gastroenterology. 1986;91:897–904.

43. Richter JE, Wu WC, Johns DN, Blackwell JN, Nelson 3rd JL, Castell JA, Castell DO. Esophageal manometry in 95 healthy adult volunteers. Variability of pressures with age and frequency of "abnormal" contractions. Dig Dis Sci. 1987;32:583–92.

44. Humphries TJ, Castell DO. Pressure profile of esophageal peristalsis in normal humans as measured by direct intraesophageal transducers. Am J Dig Dis. 1977;22:641–5.

45. Kahrilas PJ, Dodds WJ, Hogan WJ. Effect of peristaltic dysfunction on esophageal volume clearance. Gastroenterology. 1988;94:73–80.

46. Clouse RE, Staiano A, Landau DW, Schlachter JL. Manometric findings during spontaneous chest pain in patients with presumed esophageal "spasms". Gastroenterology. 1983;85:395–402.

47. Clouse RE, Hallett JL. Velocity of peristaltic propagation in distal esophageal segments. Dig Dis Sci. 1995;40:1311–6.

48. Hewson EG, Ott DJ, Dalton CB, Chen YM, Wu WC, Richter JE. Manometry and radiology. Complementary studies in the assessment of esophageal motility disorders. Gastroenterology. 1990;98:626–32.

49. Ghosh SK, Kahrilas PJ, Lodhia N, Pandolfino JE. Utilizing intraluminal pressure differences to predict esophageal bolus flow dynamics. Am J Physiol Gastrointest Liver Physiol. 2007;293:G1023–8.

50. Edmundowicz SA, Clouse RE. Shortening of the esophagus in response to swallowing. Am J Physiol. 1991;260:G512–6.

51. Pouderoux P, Lin S, Kahrilas PJ. Timing, propagation, coordination, and effect of esophageal shortening during peristalsis. Gastroenterology. 1997;112:1147–54.

52. Nicosia MA, Brasseur JG, Liu JB, Miller LS. Local longitudinal muscle shortening of the human esophagus from high-frequency ultrasonography. Am J Physiol Gastrointest Liver Physiol. 2001;281:G1022–33.

53. Gyawali CP, Kushnir VM. High-resolution manometric characteristics help differentiate types of distal esophageal obstruction in patients with peristalsis. Neurogastroenterol Motil. 2011;23(6):502-e197.

54. Ghosh SK, Janiak P, Fox M, Schwizer W, Hebbard GS, Brasseur JG. Physiology of the oesophageal transition zone in the presence of chronic bolus retention: studies using concurrent high resolution manometry and digital fluoroscopy. Neurogastroenterol Motil. 2008;20:750–9.

55. Clouse RE, Alrakawi A, Staiano A. Intersubject and interswallow variability in topography of esophageal motility. Dig Dis Sci. 1998;43:1978–85.

56. Ghosh SK, Janiak P, Schwizer W, Hebbard GS, Brasseur JG. Physiology of the esophageal pressure transition zone: separate contraction waves above and below. Am J Physiol Gastrointest Liver Physiol. 2006;290:G568–76.

57. Kumar N, Porter RF, Gyawali CP. Extended intersegmental troughs (ISTs) between skeletal and smooth muscle contraction segments on high resolution manometry (HRM). Neurogastroenterol Motil. 2009;21:A117.

58. Ghosh SK, Pandolfino JE, Kwiatek MA, Kahrilas PJ. Oesophageal peristaltic transition zone defects: real but few and far between. Neurogastroenterol Motil. 2008;20:1283–90.

59. Crist J, Gidda JS, Goyal RK. Intramural mechanism of esophageal peristalsis: roles of cholinergic and noncholinergic nerves. Proc Natl Acad Sci USA. 1984;81:3595–9.

60. Porter RF, Kumar N, Gyawali CP. Fragmented and failed esophageal smooth muscle contraction segments on high resolution manometry. Neurogastroenterol Motil. 2009;21:A185.

61. Clouse RE, Staiano A, Alrakawi A. Topographic analysis of esophageal double-peaked waves. Gastroenterology. 2000;118:469–76.

62. Ghosh SK, Pandolfino JE, Zhang Q, Jarosz A, Shah N, Kahrilas PJ. Quantifying esophageal peristalsis with high-resolution manometry: a study of 75 asymptomatic volunteers. Am J Physiol Gastrointest Liver Physiol. 2006;290:G988–97.

63. Roman S, Lin Z, Pandolfino JE, Kahrilas PJ. Distal contraction latency: a measure of propagation velocity optimized for esophageal pressure topography studies. Am J Gastroenterol. 2011;106(3):443–51.

64. Pandolfino JE, Leslie E, Luger D, Mitchell B, Kwiatek MA, Kahrilas PJ. The contractile deceleration point: an important physiologic landmark on oesophageal pressure topography. Neurogastroenterol Motil. 2010;22:395–400. e90.

65. Pandolfino JE, Fox MR, Bredenoord AJ, Kahrilas PJ. High-resolution manometry in clinical practice: utilizing pressure topography to classify oesophageal motility abnormalities. Neurogastroenterol Motil. 2009;21:796–806.

66. Scherer JR, Kwiatek MA, Soper NJ, Pandolfino JE, Kahrilas PJ. Functional esophagogastric junction obstruction with intact peristalsis: a heterogeneous syndrome sometimes akin to achalasia. J Gastrointest Surg. 2009;13:2219–25.

Part VIII
Oral/Pharyngeal Phase Dysphagia

Symptom Indices for Dysphagia Assessment and Management

25

Jacqueline Allen and Peter C. Belafsky

Abstract

Dysphagia is a symptom and not a disease. The symptom can range from the feeling of a simple lump in the throat with no objective physiologic findings of a swallowing impairment to profound dysfunction necessitating complete reliance on non-oral nutrition via tube feeding. Etiology may offer some indication of the expected level of dysfunction but even in patients suffering the same underlying disease or disorder, symptoms do not always correlate with the level of impairment. Clinicians need to be able to quantify the severity of dysphagia and estimate the effect on quality of life that this symptom causes. Patient reported outcome measures (PROMs) offer a reproducible, safe, and cost-effective method of estimating dysphagia severity, monitoring change over time, and assessing response to treatment. In order to improve the treatment of dysphagia, we must first be able to measure the severity of the symptom. This purpose of this chapter is to review some of the currently available PROMs in the assessment and management of dysphagia and reflux disease.

Keywords

Dysphagia • Reflux • Swallowing • Symptom index • Survey • Questionnaire • Quality of life • Patient reported outcome measure • PROM • Outcome measure • Instrument

J. Allen, MBChB, FRACS
Department of Otolaryngology, North Shore Hospital,
Shakespeare Rd, Takapuna, Auckland 0740,
New Zealand

P.C. Belafsky, MD, MPH, PhD (✉)
Department of Otolaryngology/Head and Neck Surgery
University of California, Davis Medical Center
Sacramento, CA, USA
e-mail: pbelafsky@sbcglobal.net

R. Shaker et al. (eds.), *Principles of Deglutition: A Multidisciplinary Text for Swallowing and its Disorders*,
DOI 10.1007/978-1-4614-3794-9_25, © Springer Science+Business Media New York 2013

Introduction

Oropharyngeal dysphagia is the most common symptom following stroke and has a prevalence of almost 50% in people over the age of 65 years [1, 2]. It is estimated to be present in 16.5 million Americans in 2010 and is correlated with mortality in rest home residents and people in long-term care [3]. The ubiquitous nature of this symptom speaks of the wide variability in expression, i.e., dysphagia may be mild or severe, temporary or permanent, improve or progress over time and may be to solids, liquids, or pills alone or in any combination. Dysphagia may be associated with aspiration, pneumonia, weight loss, malnutrition, pulmonary abscess, and even death [4, 5]. The identification, appreciation, and quantification of dysphagia are crucial in ameliorating this symptom and its potentially catastrophic consequences.

Gastroesophageal reflux disease (GERD) is one of the most prevalent disorders of the twentieth century. Its prevalence has dramatically increased, outstripping even the obesity epidemic, with which it is closely correlated [6, 7]. Population studies report that more than 6% of the population of the Western world suffers daily heartburn or regurgitation, with 14% having weekly symptoms [8, 9]. Prevalence estimates in China range from 3.1 to 5.2% using the symptom-based Montreal definition of GERD [7, 10]. Although 20% of the population in Western societies are said to suffer from GERD, in most cases it is an intermittent phenomenon, which waxes and wanes in a seemingly random fashion [9, 11]. The relationship between GERD and dysphagia is well established. Over 35% of the patients with esophagitis report dysphagia, the presence of swallowing impairment has been associated with the severity of esophageal erosion, and dysphagia resolves in over 80% of the patients with erosive esophagitis who are treated with 4 weeks of proton pump inhibitor [12]. Because of the high prevalence of GERD and its close relationship with dysphagia, an understanding of the utility of Patient reported outcome measures (PROMs) in the treatment of reflux is also necessary.

PROMs are classified as either symptom scores or quality of life (QOL) measures. In addition, they may be part of global self-assessment tools or serve as stand-alone disease-specific instruments. The use of PROMs enhances our diagnostic precision, and provides the ability to document disease severity and monitor treatment efficacy over time. PROMs can assist patients in communicating their experience to clinicians, and may confirm symptoms that a patient may not have volunteered or realized was relevant [13]. This chapter will summarize common instruments currently used in clinical practice, highlighting the advantages and disadvantages inherent in each.

The Ideal Patient Reported Outcome Measure

The ideal outcome measure should be reliable (will consistently reproduce accurate data) and valid (measures what it is intended to measure) [11, 14]. The language used should be clear, concise, and easily understood by patients. Items for inclusion in the instrument are typically proposed by clinician expert input and patient feedback based on item face validity and literature review. The initial comprehensive questionnaire should be piloted in a small number of patients who then provide feedback on the appropriateness of wording and completion time of the survey. Item reduction and revision are achieved after administering the instrument to larger numbers of subjects. After the elimination of redundant and poorly reproducible items, psychometric evaluation is performed on the final iteration of the instrument. The important aspects that will be examined during the psychometric validation include test–retest reliability, responsiveness to change, discriminant validity (the ability to detect the condition in question from other broadly similar diseases), and convergent validity (the instruments' ability in detection or quantification of the disease in question relative to other questionnaires measuring similar constructs) [11, 14–16]. Instruments may be unidimensional, measuring one aspect of disease such as symptoms, or multidimensional measuring multiple aspects, e.g., symptoms and QOL. They may be general or disease specific. Focus on symptoms can generate diagnostic information and severity-scaling information, while QOL measures can assess impact of the disease on one aspect of function or on function as a whole.

Symptom Scores Versus Quality-of-Life Scores

Symptom scores inquire about what the patient is experiencing on a daily, weekly, or monthly basis. The timeframe is called the recall period, and should be tailored to capture enough instances of the symptom in question, while limiting recall bias of very long timeframes. Important information about each symptom that may be used to quantify the symptom impact includes the frequency with which the patient suffers the symptom and at what intensity this occurs. It can be difficult to evenly match and weigh these components, not least due to the fact that the rating is subjective. For instance, does a symptom experienced on a daily basis, at a low intensity create the same impact as a symptom experienced only monthly, but at high intensity? Development of scores should take into account these variables, whilst also bearing in mind that clinicians need a simple tool, with logical overall utility, and are unlikely to remember or use an instrument that needs complex mathematical workings to calculate a score. QOL instruments estimate the overall and/or disease-specific QOL at a single point in time (the survey completion date). Global QOL surveys usually cover several domains that explore the facets of daily living such as physical functioning and emotional well-being, and interaction with others such as communication, eating, and sexual relationships. Disease-specific QOL instruments explore the impact of one pathological process or state, e.g., head and neck cancer, on the biological areas most likely to be affected by it. There is considerable overlap in how the disease can affect life experience, and in what people consider being significant changes. With numerous treatment options available for

the same condition (often with similar cure rates), in many cases the impact of symptoms or QOL is the key factor to consider when choosing between treatment alternatives.

Patient Reported Outcome Measures in Dysphagia

Symptom Instruments for Dysphagia

Numerous symptom scoring instruments have been described for dysphagia (Table 25.1, Appendix A). This section will discuss the benefits and limitations of four validated surveys. Other PROMs not discussed here include the Vanderbilt Head and Neck Symptom Survey, EORTC-C35, EORTC-OES18, and University of Washington Head and Neck questionnaire.

Eating Assessment Tool-10

The Eating Assessment Tool-10 (EAT-10) is a ten-item, validated symptom assessment instrument that asks the patients to estimate how problematic swallowing has been for them [17]. Items are rated on a 5-point Likert scale (0=no problems, 4=severe problem), and the sum total is calculated for an estimation of severity. Validation studies in both dysphagic subjects and normal adults identified a score greater than three as lying more than two standard deviations outside the normal range. The survey takes less than 5 min to complete and is currently being validated in Japanese, Spainish, Portugese, and Chinese [unpublished data]. Development of the survey involved multidisciplinary expert input to item generation and initial item reduction, followed by administration of a 20-item pilot questionnaire to a cohort of 100 normal adults, and 235 adults with either voice or swallowing disorders [17]. The ten most redundant items with poor reliability and weak inter-item correlation were then removed. Internal consistency, by Cronbach's alpha, was 0.96 (highly consistent) and test–retest reliability was excellent (0.72–0.91). The 10-item scale (EAT-10) was then administered to a further normal subject group to establish normative data [mean score ± SD (95% CI), 0.4 ± 1.01]. Finally,

Table 25.1 Summary of selected patient reported outcome measures for dysphagia

Scale name	Number of items	Symptom vs. QOL	Advantages	Disadvantages
EAT-10 (Eating Assessment Tool-10) Belafsky et al. [17]	10	Symptom	Brevity High clinical utility Useful in dysphagia of any etiology Widespread use	Uni-dimensional Does not address symptom frequency
MDADI (MD Anderson Dysphagia Inventory) Chen et al. [18]	20	QOL and Symptom	Multidimensional Brevity High utility validity for head and neck cancer Widespread use	Complex scoring system Limited criterion validation Only validated in head and neck cancer
SSQ (Sydney Swallowing Questionnaire) Wallace et al. [19]	17	Symptom	High face validity Useful in dysphagia of various etiologies Relative brevity	Visual analog scale 10 min completion time
MDQ (Mayo Dysphagia Questionnaire) Grudell et al. [20]	27	Symptom	Evaluates diverse food textures Quantifies symptom duration, frequency, and severity Quantifies heartburn, dysphagia, and regurgitation	Relatively complex scoring 10 min completion time Validity limited to esophageal phase dysphagia
SWAL-QOL McHorney et al. 2000, [21]	44	QOL	Widespread use Thorough research tool Cross cultural application	Lack of symptom quantification Long completion burdeon Limited to oropharyngeal dysphagia

the EAT-10 was administered to patients with swallowing dysfunction prior to treatment, then following treatment, and results compared and assessed for responsiveness. The EAT-10 was elevated in all the patients with dysphagic complaints or with reflux compared to controls. Comparing patients with oropharyngeal dysphagia, head and neck cancer, or esophageal dysphagia to those with reflux disease or voice disorders demonstrated significantly higher EAT-10 scores in the first group. EAT-10 scores improved in all the patients after treatment, but showed greatest improvement in patients undergoing diverticulotomy or balloon disruption of strictures compared to those with reflux disease. This attests to the criterion-based validity of the scale, and to its ability to discriminate patient groups, and document response to treatment. One of the most important aspects of this scale is the ease of completion, with the average time taken to complete the questionnaire being less than 5 min. The lack of subscales in this instrument allows simple summation of each item score to produce the total score, making it easier for the clinician to interpret the results. Advantages of the EAT-10 include its ability to be used in patients with dysphagia from various etiologies, its ease of administration and its simplicity in scoring. The primary limitation of this instrument is the lack of specific QOL domain assessment and the quantification of symptom frequency.

MD Anderson Dysphagia Inventory

The MD Anderson Dysphagia Inventory (MDADI) is a 20-item survey divided into 3 domains and a single global question that was designed to measure the impact of head and neck cancer and its treatment on swallowing [18]. Initial item development was undertaken by physician faculty experts and speech pathologists, followed by several patient focus groups to ensure the face validity and apprehension of the line items. Item reduction was not reported. The instrument was administered to 100 patients diagnosed with head and neck cancer, and test–retest reliability assessed by re-administration of the survey to 29 patients, 2 weeks after initial assessments. The enrolled subjects also completed the Medical Outcomes Study Short Form Healthy Survey (SF-36) as a comparator for discriminant validity. Validity of content was established by the initial focus group input. Criterion validity was reported by comparison of the MDADI score to a clinician-rated Performance Status Scale (PSS) completed by the speech pathologist. The concern with this comparison is that the MDADI is a patient-rated scale, and the PSS in not. Literature suggests that clinician and patient ratings of the same symptoms are not well correlated [11, 16, 22, 23]. Scoring of the MDADI is complex. Eighteen of the 20 items are scored five points for strongly agree and one point for strongly disagree. Two items are scored in reverse. The global score is scored separately. The individual domain's (functional, emotional, physical) questions' are summed, averaged, and then the mean is multiplied by 20. Four separate scores are reported. In the validation paper, a total score is not reported, rather each domain score is reported separately. Internal consistency is confirmed by a Cronbach alpha score of 0.96 for the overall scale. Subscale analysis showed lower but acceptable values (range 0.69–0.88). Criterion validity of the subscales compared to the PSS ranges from 0.47 to 0.61 on the Spearman correlation coefficient. These are reported as acceptable; however, the previous notation regarding comparing a patient-reported scale to a clinician-measured scale calls this into question. Correlation of subscales of MDADI to the SF-36 was modest. Perhaps more clinically relevant was the ability of the MDADI to differentiate patients by the site of tumour and the time elapsed since treatment completion. The MDADI has been validated in Italian [24], used as an outcome measure in assessing patients' symptoms post-glossectomy [25], used to compare the effects of chemoradiation to surgery plus radiation for upper aerodiges-

tive tract cancer [26], and used to assess elderly rest home residents for dysphagic complaints [27]. The advantage of the MDADI is its utility and evaluation in a specific dysphagic population (head and neck cancer), its multidimensional QOL assessment, and its relative ease of administration. The primary disadvantages of the instrument include the lack of utility outside of head and neck cancer and the complexity of the scoring system.

Sydney Swallowing Questionnaire

Developed and reported by Wallace et al. in 2000, the Sydney Swallowing Questionnaire contains 17 questions regarding physiologic swallowing functions [19]. It was designed to report mechanical swallow ability and severity of dysfunction in oropharyngeal dysphagia, and to assist clinicians in assessing response to treatment. The items were generated then assessed for face validity by 25 experts in dysphagia. Initially it was tested in 45 patients with neuromyogenic dysphagia. This confirmed internal consistency and test–retest reliability. Factor analysis supported construct validity and association of the individual items to dysphagia as a whole. Scoring is by visual analog scale, with each item scored out of 100 and a cumulative total calculated by summation. A higher score indicates worse swallow function. Discriminant validity was established by pre- and post-operative administration in 11 patients undergoing surgery for Zenker diverticulum [19]. The SSQ has recently been further validated by Dwivedi and colleagues in a cohort of 54 patients treated for oral and oropharyngeal cancer [28]. In Dwivedi's validation study, test–retest reliability was high (Spearman's rank correlation: 0.83), internal consistency was excellent (Cronbach's alpha: 0.95), and convergent validity compared to the MDADI was moderately high for both total score and general subscale scores, confirming its utility in head and neck cancer patients as well as neuromyogenic dysphagic subjects [28]. Average completion time is approximately 10 min. Responsiveness of the survey to treatment in the head and neck population is yet to be reported. The primary advantages of this survey are its ability to provide accurate disease specific information regarding oropharyngeal dysphagia, ease of completion for patients, and simple scoring for the clinician. The limitations of the survey are the use of visual analog scales to score each component except one, and the lack of further validation in other dysphagic patient populations.

The Mayo Dysphagia Questionnaire

Developed and reported by Grudell et al. in 2007, the Mayo Dysphagia Questionnaire (MDQ) is a 27-item disease-specific symptom survey for esophageal dysphagia [20]. Many of the items were taken from other previously validated questionnaires [21, 29, 30]. The initial instrument used a 1 year to lifetime recall period. Subsequent iterations have used a 2 weeks and 30 days recall period (MDQ-2; MQD-30). The instrument uses a combination of dichotomous, Likert, and non-hierarchical questions divided into three symptom domains of heartburn, dysphagia, and regurgitation. Symptom duration, frequency, and severity are quantified. Concurrent validity, time of survey completion, and test–retest reproducibility were evaluated. Kappa values evaluating concurrent validity between physician patient interview and survey results ranged from 0.42 to 0.97 with a mean of 0.63. Test–retest analysis revealed a median kappa value of 0.76 indicating substantial agreement. The reliability and validity of the MDQ-30 were recently evaluated by McElhiney et al. [31]. The authors reported good agreement between physician interview and patient survey results and good test–retest reproducibility. The instrument took 10 min to complete on average. The advantages of the MDQ include the inclusion of specific domains, its relative ease of administration, the evaluation of various food consistencies, and the incorporation of previously validated items. The inclusion of non-hierarchal and multiple hierarchal items makes scoring slightly complex. The other disadvantages include its 10-min time of completion, the lack of normative data, its limitation to esophageal phase dysphagia, and the lack of a thorough construct, content, and criterion-based validity analysis.

Quality of Life Instruments for Dysphagia

General QOL Instruments utilized most commonly in dysphagia studies have been the Medical Outcomes Study Short Form-36, and the Work Productivity and Activity Impairment-GERD [32]. Although general QOL instruments have been widely validated in a variety of disease states, in most cases they contain only one or two questions that might capture information about the impact of dysphagia or reflux on an individual's QOL. Disease-specific surveys have been preferred due to a better ability to examine multiple facets of dysphagia impact [16] (Table 25.2, Appendix A).

Swallowing Quality of Life

The SWAL-QOL (Swallowing Quality of Life) is a 44-item self-assessment, outcomes tool specifically designed to measure the impact of oropharyngeal dysphagia on daily QOL [21, 40–42]. It was developed via a three-phase process utilizing psychometric tests and patient input. A multicenter study recruited outpatients with oropharyngeal dysphagia (of any cause) that were considered stable by speech pathologist evaluation. Initial patient focus groups were conducted, some of which also involved caregivers, to help the study developers' produce items with patient-friendly wording and ensure coverage of those areas the patients felt were most affected. Nineteen domains were identified and 185 items generated for initial testing. This preliminary questionnaire was administered to 106 subjects who were predominantly elderly white males (average age 68 years; 75% male; 90% Caucasian). Average test completion time was 56 min. Examination of items for convergent validity and floor and ceiling effects led to exclusion of 92 questions, leaving a total of 93 items in the Phase 3 survey. During Phase 3 of survey development, the original 93 items were separated into two distinct surveys—the SWAL-QOL (44-items; 10 domains) and the SWAL-CARE (15 items; 3 domains). Although the SWAL-QOL is widely inclusive and informative, there is a need to balance the burden of completing the survey with its information. Investigators felt that reducing the

Table 25.2 Summary of selected patient reported outcome measures for reflux

Scale name	Number of items	Symptom vs. QOL	Advantages	Disadvantages
RDQ (Reflux Disease Questionnaire), Shaw et al. [33]	12	Symptom	Potential diagnostic utility Widespread use, cross-cultural application Heartburn, regurgitation, dyspepsia subscales	Variable scoring system Questionable diagnostic utility over physician assessment
GIS (GERD Impact Scale) Jones et al. [13]	9	Symptom	Brevity Multidimensional High clinical utility	Questionable diagnostic precision
GERD-Q (Gastroesophageal Reflux Disease Questionnaire), Jones et al. [34]	6	Symptom	Brevity Use of questions from other validated scales High clinical utility Easy scoring system	Limited sensitivity and specificity in diagnosis of GERD Uni-dimensional assessment
Chinese GerdQ, Wong et al. [35]	7	Symptom	Brevity Multidimensional frequency and severity evaluation Easy scoring system High diagnostic sensitivity/ specificity	Variable recall period Lack of widespread use and cross-cultural validation
GSRS (Gastrointestinal Symptom Rating Scale), Revicki et al. 1998	15 Five sub-scales	Symptom	Multiple GI disorders—reflux, abdominal pain, constipation, diarrhea, indigestion Widespread use, cross-cultural application	Inclusion of domains unrelated to reflux Long completion time Limited diagnostic utility
Carlsson/Dent questionnaire, QUEST, Carlsson et al. [36]	7	Symptom	Brevity Widespread use	Relatively complex scoring system Limited diagnostic utility Lack of improvement with reflux treatment
QOL-RAD (Quality Of Life in Reflux And Ayspepsia) Wiklund et al. 1998	25 Five sub-scales	QOL	Multidimensional Extensive validation Widespread use Cross-cultural application	Relatively long instrument Includes dyspepsia
GERD-QOL, Chan et al. [37]	16	QOL	Brevity Multidimensional	Complex scoring system
GIQLI (Gastrointestinal Quality of Life Index), Eypasch et al. [38]	36 Five sub-scales	QOL	Multidimensional Broad GI disturbance assessment Cross-cultural application	Relatively long instrument Non-specific for GERD
GERD-HRQL, Velanovich et al. [39]	11	Symptom	Brevity Simple scoring system Cross-cultural application	Limited QOL assessment

size of the instrument would improve the utility of the survey overall. The shortened version was administered to 386 dysphagic subjects and 40 normal swallowing subjects. Extensive psycho-metric testing supported test–retest reliability, discriminant and convergent validity, and internal consistency of the final instruments. Additionally all items were weighted with equal significance to allow simple summation of each subscale and total scores. The scales displayed significantly different scores in subjects that were dysphagic compared to those without this symptom, and also differentiated between oral eaters and those reliant on tube feeds. Despite this extensive and thorough development process, the SWAL-QOL was not able to support tests of responsiveness as it was not administered pre- and post-treatments. In a subsequent study, McHorney and colleagues compared SWAL-QOL scores to videofluoroscopic swallowing study measures [22]. Only modest correlation was seen relating to oral and total transit times. This divergence of results reinforces that significant physiologic changes are not always associated with self-reported QOL. How one functions on a day-to-day basis may be more clinically relevant than actual physiologic variance from normal values. The SWAL-QOL has now been validated and translated into French, Dutch, and Chinese [43–45], and has been utilized in patients with both neurogenic dysphagia, and head and neck cancer [42, 46–49]. The primary advantage of this survey is the very thorough symptom-specific documentation of an individual's dysphagia that is gathered by the questionnaire due to the inclusive and complete coverage of symptoms. Additionally, the survey has had extensive psychometric testing and is valid across cultures. It remains the only survey expressly developed to assess QOL in oropharyngeal dysphagia. The primary limitations of this survey are the long completion time which limits application in daily practice, the initial validation in a selective patient group (although cross-cultural studies support generalizability of the survey), and the lack of reported responsiveness to treatment.

Assessment, Outcome, and Quality of Life Tools for Reflux

The need for self-reported assessment tools in Gastroesophageal and Extra-esophageal reflux is illustrated by the very number of instruments reported and by several large multicenter, multinational trials that attest to the impact that these chronic conditions have on patients' well-being [8, 16, 50–54]. There are a multitude of different survey instruments relating to GERD and extra-esophageal reflux. We have selected several of the most frequently utilized scales (Table 25.2), but recognize that there are many that are not discussed here (GSAS, GERDyzer, ReQuest, ReQuest in Practice, Quality of Life after Anti-reflux surgery (QOLARS), Heartburn QOL, Reflux-Qual (RQS), Reflux Questionnaire, EORTC-QLQ-C30, EORTC-OES18, PAGI-QOL).

Symptom Assessment Tools for Reflux

Symptom inquiry tools have been developed to gauge the frequency and severity of symptoms experienced by patients. In addition to these PROMs, various "diagnostic" instruments have been developed to predict esophageal findings at endoscopy and pH testing. Reflux symptom scoring systems were published as early as 1983 [55]. A clinical assessment questionnaire for esophageal symptoms was reported by Greatorex and Thorpe in *British Journal of Clinical Practice* as a guide for general practitioners regarding which patients may have significant esophageal pathology. The instrument inquired about six symptoms (heartburn, regurgitation, dysphagia, bleeding, dyspepsia/indigestion, and vomiting) each rated on a 0–3 scale of no symptoms to worst symptoms. Scores greater than 4 correlated with the findings at ambulatory pH testing and manometry [55]. The scale was not diagnostic or prognostic, but was utilized as a guide to direct further investigation. The recognition of extra-esophageal manifestations of reflux, often termed laryngopharyngeal reflux (LPR), has complicated the picture further and leads to additional diagnostic dilemmas [7, 52]. Classic GERD symptoms are often lacking in the extra-esophageal symptom complex, with chest pain, cough, throat clearing, laryngeal disorders, and asthma being listed as the most common reflux complaints [7, 52, 53]. The remainder of this chapter will focus on PROMs and diagnostic surveys for GERD (Table 25.2).

Reflux Disease Questionnaire

Designed to act as a diagnostic tool for GERD, the 12-item reflux disease questionnaire (RDQ) has now been used as both an outcome measure and as a diagnostic tool [33, 56–58]. Developed by Shaw et al., items were generated after a literature search and refined by expert opinion and cognitive interviews with patients. The initial survey contained 22 items and was administered to 200 consecutive patients in primary care settings on two occasions. All questions were scored by Likert scale (either 0–5 or 0–7), and the recall period was 4 weeks. At the second interview, an overall treatment effect (OTE) question was also included. Patients also completed the digestive health status instrument (DHSI) as a comparator. Factor analysis, intraclass correlations for internal consistency, and convergent and discriminant item validities were calculated and resulted in the removal of 10 items from the survey. The remaining 12 items were grouped into three subscales—heartburn, regurgitation, and dyspepsia. Convergent validity was assessed compared to the DHSI with moderate correlation (0.52). Responsiveness was established using the OTE as a guide. Those patients reporting no change in symptoms (as per the OTE rating) at second visit ($n=58$) were used to estimate test–retest reliability, and those reporting at least moderate change ($n=59$) acted as subjects for calculation of responsiveness. All three subscales demonstrated significant alterations in keeping with the reported OTE change ($p<0.0029$). The RDQ has subsequently been translated and validated in Swedish and Norwegian [56]. It has been used as a symptom survey to monitor symptom severity over time in patients enrolled in the ProGERD study in Europe, showing useful stability and reproducibility [57] and in the Diamond study comparing diagnostic tools in reflux disease [58]. One interesting aspect of this survey instrument is the lack of use of the word "heartburn." Initial development suggested that this term was poorly understood by most patients, and that a "word picture" was better in conveying the symptom, i.e., burning feeling rising up from the stomach behind the breastbone [33]. The primary advantages of this survey are its conciseness, short completion time, adapted patient wording describing symptoms clearly, and cross-cultural validation. The primary limitations are inclusion of more than one disease profile (i.e., GERD and dyspepsia), long recall period, uncontrolled treatment in the patient validation population, diagnostic accuracy equal to that of physician assessment, and variable scoring system.

GERD Impact Scale

Jones and colleagues proposed the Gastroesophageal Reflux Disease Impact Scale (GIS) as a management tool for primary care physicians [13]. The survey aims to assist patients in conveying GERD severity and impact, and to prompt clinicians to inquire about reflux-related symptoms [13]. Patient and clinician (primary care physicians and gastroenterologists) inputs were used to review three draft questionnaires. GIS comprises nine questions with a 1-week recall period that may be completed in a matter of minutes, primarily focused on measuring frequency of symptom occurrence on a 4-point Likert scale (1 = daily, 2 = often, 3 = sometimes, 4 = never) for several items thought to be related to GERD (acid-related symptoms, chest pain, extra-esophageal symptoms, use of additional medication, the impact of symptoms on sleep, work, meals, and social occasions). Primary content validity was tested in 13 volunteers with GERD. The survey was then administered to 205 GERD patients (new diagnoses and chronic stable disease). Convergent and discriminant validity were assessed by comparison to the RDQ and QOLRAD (quality of life in reflux and dyspepsia) questionnaires, and responsiveness assessed by repetition of the survey after 2 weeks of medical treatment. Internal consistency was satisfactory (Cronbach's alpha = 0.68–0.82), and responsiveness was confirmed by inter-visit changes (effect size −0.32 to −1.49). Primary care physicians using the scale found it helped direct treatment decisions and assess treatment effectiveness. It has been utilized and reported by Gisbert et al. as part of the multi-national European RANGE (Retrospective Analysis of GERD) study [50]. In the 2,678 patients completing the survey, the average GIS score ranged from

3.30 to 3.15 (lower score equals greater impact of symptoms). Louis et al. reported the GIS correlated well with physician-assessed GERD severity, and was sensitive to treatment changes over time [59]. The primary advantages of this survey are the multidimensionality of the survey (symptoms and impact of GERD) and the brevity of the survey. The primary limitations of this survey are the tendency for results to cluster around the middle of the scale that does not allow separation of severity and lack of diagnostic precision (GER vs. dyspepsia vs. functional heartburn).

Gastroesophageal Reflux Disease Questionnaire

Planned as a diagnostic and management tool for primary care physicians, the gastroesophageal reflux disease questionnaire (GERD-Q) is a distillation of three previously validated scales—the RDQ, Gastrointestinal Symptom Rating Scale (GSRS), and GIS (see below), wherein six items were selected from these scales as being the most specific and sensitive for the diagnosis of GERD in the primary practice population [34]. Receiver operator analysis indicated a sensitivity of 65% and specificity of 71% for the diagnosis of GERD compared to pH-metry and symptom association probability (SAP), endoscopy, and trial of proton pump inhibitor. Development of the instrument occurred during the DIAMOND study—a multinational study of patients in primary care settings presenting with upper abdominal symptoms [34, 58]. The scale assesses the frequency of symptoms alone, graded by patients on a 4-point scale (no symptoms, 1 day, 2–3 days, and 4–7 days) over a 1-week recall period. Four items document reflux symptoms (heartburn, regurgitation, sleep disturbance due to the symptoms, and use of over-the-counter medications) scored positively from 0 to 3 (higher score demonstrates worse symptoms) and two items thought to be negative predictors of GERD (nausea and epigastric pain) scored negatively from 3 to 0 (with 3 = none, 0 = worst symptoms). The total score is obtained by summation (range 0–18). When administered to 308 patients with upper abdominal symptoms, a cut-off score of 8 predicted high likelihood of GERD with 71% specificity and 65% sensitivity. There was also good correlation between heart-burn severity at baseline and the GerdQ score. Responsiveness was estimated from distribution-based analysis not a trial of treatment [34]. The primary advantages of this survey are the brevity of the instrument and the use of previously validated items. The primary limitations of this survey include moderate sensitivity and specificity in diagnosis (equal to clinical judgment in controlled trials), uni-dimensional assessment, and lack of published reports of responsiveness in clinical treatment trials.

Chinese GERDQ

Reported in 1993, this 7-item questionnaire was written and developed in Chinese, then back-translated to English [35]. It has no relationship to the GERD-Q (above) reported by Jones et al. The aim of the survey was to establish the diagnosis of GERD. Items were selected by a literature review, expert opinion, and patient focus group interviews. Scoring was on a 5-point Likert scale of symptom severity where 1 = none (no symptoms) and 5 = incapacitating (incapacitating symptoms with inability to perform daily activities or requiring a day off work $\geq$ once daily). Each symptom severity rating used a different time period: 1 = no symptoms in the past year, 2 = symptoms less than once a month, 3 = symptoms greater than once a month, 4 = symptoms greater than weekly, and 5 = incapacitation (daily symptoms). This may introduce recall bias. Validation was undertaken in 201 subjects (100 patients with pH-positive or endoscopically proven GER) and 101 controls. The initial 20 items were reduced to 7 items through factor and principal component analysis (frequency and severity of heartburn, frequency and severity of feeling of acidity in the stomach, frequency and severity of acid regurgitation, and frequency of use of "antacids"). Receiver operator characteristics identified a score of 12 (sum of 7 items) as having 82% sensitivity and 84% specificity for identification of GERD subjects. Internal consistency (Cronbach's alpha = 0.90), test–retest reliability, responsiveness, and discriminant validity were reported as acceptable. The survey was quick to complete and was suggested as a method to monitor frequency and severity of GERD symptoms, or for estimating treatment efficacy.

The primary advantages of this survey are dual frequency and severity information obtained in a simple, easily administered scale, the higher sensitivity and specificity of the tool for diagnostic use, use of pH or endoscopically proven GERD as the gold standard, and the easy scoring system for clinicians. The primary limitations are the variable recall period, lack of widespread use in the literature, and lack of cross validation of the survey among other groups.

Gastrointestinal Symptom Rating Scale

This disease-specific symptom scale contains 15 items that are grouped into five subscales—reflux, abdominal pain, constipation, diarrhea, and indigestion. The recall period is 1 week and patients are asked to rate how bothersome each symptom has been over that time period. Scoring is by 7-point Likert scale (0=no discomfort, 7=very severe discomfort) with higher scores indicating worse symptom severity [60]. The GSRS has been validated in German and Italian, Afrikaans, Hungarian, Polish, and Spanish [61–64]. Attwood and colleagues utilized the GSRS (and QOL-RAD) survey to assess treatment effects of medical therapy for GERD vs. laparoscopic fundoplication [51]. Interestingly, pH studies showed a marked difference between these two treatments although the patient-reported symptom scales did not differ significantly between treatment groups [51]. The GSRS has also been used as a comparator for the development of other surveys such as the QOL-RAD [61], and as a measure of impact of GERD in many studies [54, 61, 65]. The primary advantage of this survey is the widespread use allowing comparison of scores. The primary limitations are the inclusion of domains unrelated to reflux, the broad scoring scale (0–7) where a differentiation between severe and very severe and mild and very mild may not be clinically relevant or detectable, and possibly low sensitivity to change in reflux severity suggested by lack of correlation to pH studies.

Carlsson–Dent Questionnaire

Reported in 1998, prior to many other scales, the Carlsson–Dent questionnaire (QUEST) was devised to assist diagnosis of GERD in primary practice [36]. Expert consensus was used in item generation. The 7-item scale begins with an orientating question (really the diagnostic item) then enquires about exacerbating factors, relieving factors, effect of medications, and timing of the symptom. Scoring is different from question to question (see Appendix A), but summation is used to achieve a total score (range −7 to +18). Validation and accuracy studies were conducted in two studies recruiting subjects (439 and 538 patients) in Sweden and the United Kingdom. Although scores were higher in patients with endoscopically proven esophagitis, the difference was not statistically significant. Sensitivity in identifying esophagitis by a cutoff score of 4 or greater was 70% but specificity was only 46%. A description of heartburn as a burning feeling rising from the stomach or lower chest up towards the neck' was more readily identified by patients rather than "heartburn" and this symptom alone had a sensitivity of 73% and specificity of 43% for reflux disease diagnosis. Response to omeprazole in a double-blind study failed to correlate with questionnaire scores [36]. Test–retest reliability, internal consistency, and discriminant validity were not reported [36]. Numans and De Wit performed another study that demonstrated poor diagnostic performance of the QUEST [66]. Danjo and colleagues in Japan compared the QUEST to a Japanese questionnaire [frequency scale for symptoms of gastroesophageal reflux disease (FSSG)] and found equal sensitivity, specificity, and accuracy between the scales [67]. The primary advantage of this survey is its widespread usage allowing comparison of scores. The primary limitations of this survey are the poor diagnostic performance, the weak psychometric properties, lack of correlation with proton pump inhibitor treatment, and complex scoring system.

Quality of Life Tools: Reflux

GERD and LPR have been demonstrated to substantially reduce health-related quality of life (HRQL) [16, 23, 68, 69]. As there is no gold standard for diagnosis of GER or LPR, and as endoscopic damage is relatively rare in patients with reflux in general, amelioration of symptoms and improvement in QOL may be the best measure of treatment success. To date, QOL ratings by patients do not seem to be associated with endoscopic mucosal injury [8, 11, 16, 23, 52]. Ronkainen and colleagues report that in more than one-third of patients with endoscopic esophagitis, there was no reported heartburn or regurgitation in the 3 months prior to endoscopy [8]. Impaired QOL now forms part of a definition of gastroesophageal disease [10] and it seems that clinicians and patients' estimation of the effect of GERD are not equivalent, with most clinicians underestimating the QOL detriment [8, 10, 11, 16, 23, 70]. Studies suggest that a clinically meaningful impairment in QOL can be detected in patients suffering reflux symptoms on a weekly basis [8, 65].

General Quality of Life Instruments for GERD

General QOL Instruments utilized most commonly in GERD studies have been the Medical Outcomes Study Short Form-36, Work Productivity and Activity Impairment-GERD, and the Psychological General Well-Being Index (PGWBI) [8, 23, 32, 54, 71–73]. Although general QOL instruments have been widely validated in a variety of disease states, in most cases they contain only one or two questions that might capture information about the impact of reflux on a subject's QOL. Disease-specific surveys have been developed for reflux and are preferred due to a better ability to discriminate the effect of GERD on QOL [11, 16, 23], (Table 25.2, Appendix A).

Disease-Specific Quality of Life Instruments for GERD

Quality of Life in Reflux and dyspepsia

The QOLRAD or Quality of Life in Reflux and Dyspepsia survey is a multidimensional disease-specific 25-item, validated questionnaire developed by Wiklund et al. [61]. It has a 1-week recall period and divides the 25 items into five dimensions—emotional distress, sleep disturbance,

vitality, food/drink problems, and physical/social functioning. Scoring is on a 7-point Likert scale with lower values demonstrating more severe impact of disease on daily life. In validation studies, high internal consistency (Cronbach's alpha = 0.88–0.97), good test–retest reliability ($r = 0.93$), and convergent and discriminant validity have been demonstrated [11, 61, 74]. A change of 0.5 points has previously been reported to be clinically meaningful and of 1.0 point to be clinically important [11, 62–64, 74]. The QOLRAD has been validated in German and Italian, Afrikaans, Hungarian, Polish, and Spanish patients [61–64]. The survey shows significant correlation with SF-36 domains in multiple languages supporting its construct validity. QOLRAD has been used as an outcome tool to assess the efficacy of medical vs. surgical treatment for GERD and Barrett's esophagus [51], as a symptom severity index for dyspepsia, and to assess proton pump inhibitor effect on QOL in GERD patients [75]. The primary advantages of this survey are the robust psychometric validation in multiple languages, the consistent clinical meaningful change value, easy scoring system, multidimensionality, and low completion burden. The primary limitations of this survey include encompassing dyspepsia in the survey although this does not seem to diminish the responsiveness or accuracy of the instrument in GERD patients.

GERD-QOL

This 16-item, 4-domain instrument with a 7-day recall period was developed initially in the Chinese language then translated to English, and is designed to specifically measure HRQOL in patients with non-erosive and erosive GERD [37]. Item generation was through expert consensus combined with patient feedback, and then factor analysis was used to remove redundant or poor items. The GERD-QOL was then administered to 316 patients with reflux, of whom 11 repeated the questionnaire 2 weeks later (test–retest reliability) and 17 repeated the questionnaire after esomeprazole treatment (responsiveness). Items were presented as statements and patients were asked to choose a response from 0 to 4 that indicated their level of agreement with the statement (0 = strongly agree, 1 = somewhat agree, 2 = neutral, 3 = somewhat disagree, 4 = strongly disagree). Low total scores represent worse GERD impact. Subjects in the validation study also completed the SF-36, and a VAS scale for each item statement in the GERD-QOL. Finally, subjects were asked to rate how bad their acid regurgitation and heartburn had been in the last 7 days on a 4-point scale (0 = asymptomatic, 1 = mild, 2 = moderate, 3 = severe). Internal consistency (Cronbach's alpha = 0.64–0.88; intraclass correlation coefficient = 0.73–0.94), construct validity (Pearson's correlation $r = 0.23$–0.49), and responsiveness (t-test $p < 0.001$) were reported and adequate. Although endoscopy was performed in all cases, no correlation was reported between endoscopy results and scale scores. Scoring requires addition of items in each domain (daily activity, treatment effect, diet, psychological well-being) multiplied by 100 and divided by $4 \times n$ (items) (for example, there are eight items in the daily activity scale; so the subscale score is determined by DA = (Q2 + Q4 + Q5 + Q8 + Q10 + Q11 + Q12 + Q13) × 100/32. The total GERD-QOL score is then achieved by summing the domain scores. The primary advantage of this survey is the multidimensional QOL assessment with one total survey score. The primary limitation is the complex scoring system.

Gastrointestinal Quality of Life Index

The Gastrointestinal Quality of Life Index (GIQLI) assesses five dimensions (core symptoms, social integration, physical function, emotions, and gastrointestinal symptoms) through 36 questions, asking subjects to rate how frequently (on a 5-point Likert scale) a symptom has interfered with their life in the past 2 weeks. Subscale and total scores are calculated by summation. Due to its breadth, it may discriminate between healthy subjects and those affected by GI diseases, but not between GI diseases. Internal consistency, test–rest reliability, and content validity were demonstrated, and the GIQLI has been validated in French, German, Chinese, and Spanish [11, 38, 76–78]. Utilization of the GIQLI in patients undergoing Nissen fundoplication dem-

onstrated low pre-operative GIQLI scores when compared to normal subjects, with significant improvements in all dimensions following surgery for up to 72 months [79]. Despite marked improvements, GIQLI scores for post-operative subjects remained below normal values, even more than 5 years after surgery [79]. The primary advantage of this survey is the multidimensional nature of symptom assessment. The primary limitations include inclusion of non-GERD symptoms, inability to discriminate between different GI disorders, and the length of the survey (completion burden).

GERD-Health Related Quality of Life

Initially proposed in 1996 by Velanovich, the GERD-HRQL was designed to quantify typical GERD symptoms, and to allow assessment of change over time (with treatment or without) [39]. It has undergone minor adjustment to become an 11-item scale, where 10 items are scored by the patients from 0 to 5 (0 = no symptoms, to 5 = incapacitating) and a single global satisfaction item regarding overall disease status is rated as satisfied, neutral, or dissatisfied (and not included in the total score) [39, 80]. Total score can range from 0 to 50. Convergent and discriminant validities were evaluated against the QOLARS and SF-36 surveys. Test–retest reliability was confirmed and responsiveness tested with both medical and surgical therapies for GERD with good response. The survey has been translated into several languages, and is short, resulting in low patient completion burden. The primary advantages of this survey are the ease of completion and scoring system. The primary limitations are the limited multidimensional data regarding QOL and lack of questions about atypical GERD symptoms.

Summary

Dysphagia is a symptom. In order to adequately care for persons with disorders of deglutition, the clinician must be able to quantify the symptom of dysphagia and its effect on the patient's daily life. PROMs can not only assist with the diagnosis but also can help determine disease severity, document the effect on QOL, and evaluate treatment efficacy. Well-constructed, validated PROMs are inexpensive, efficacious, and reproducible and offer insights on which to base management decisions. The diversity and capacious number of dysphagia and reflux-specific PROMs attest to their utility in the diagnosis and management of these disorders. We have outlined some of the PROMs commonly used in assessment, diagnosis, quantification, and management of dysphagia and reflux. There is no single flawless tool, rather several complementary instruments that may, in combination, give a complete picture of burden of disease, progression or resolution of symptoms, and treatment effect.

Appendix: Dysphagia and GER Indices

Eating Assessment Tool-10 (Belafsky et al. [17])

Patient scores each statement "To what extent are these scenarios problematic for you?"

  0 = no problem, 4 = severe problem
1. My swallowing problem has caused me to lose weight.
2. My swallowing problem interferes with my ability to go out for meals.
3. Swallowing liquids takes extra effort.
4. Swallowing solids takes extra effort.
5. Swallowing pills takes extra effort.
6. Swallowing is painful.
7. The pleasure of eating is affected by my swallowing.
8. When I swallow food sticks in my throat.
9. I cough when I eat.
10. Swallowing is stressful.

MD Anderson Dysphagia Inventory (Chen et al. [18])

The following statements have been made by people who have problems with their swallowing. Some of the statement may apply to you. Please read each statement and circle the response which best reflects your experience in the past week.

(Response options are strongly agree, agree, no opinion, disagree, or strongly disagree).

My swallowing ability limits my day-to-day activities.
E2. I am embarrassed by my eating habits.
F1. People have difficulty cooking for me.
P2. Swallowing is more difficult at the end of the day.
E7. I do not feel self-conscious when I eat.
E4. I am upset by my swallowing problem.
P6. Swallowing takes great effort.
E5. I do not go out because of my swallowing problem.
F5. My swallowing difficulty has caused me to lose income.
P7. It takes me longer to eat because of my swallowing problem.
P3. People ask me "Why can't you eat that?"
E3. Other people are irritated by my eating problem.
P8. I cough when I try to drink liquids.
F3. My swallowing problems limit my social and personal life.
F2. I feel free to go out to eat with my friends, neighbours, and relatives.
P5. I limit my food intake because of my swallowing difficulty.
P1. I cannot maintain my weight because of my swallowing problem.
E6. I have low self-esteem because of my swallowing problem.
P4. I feel that I am swallowing a huge amount of food.
F4. I feel excluded because of my eating habits.

  First question scored alone. E = emotional, F = functional, P = physical. Items added together for each domain and then mean score of each scale multiplied by 20 to give range 0–100 for each scale (higher scores show better QOL).

Sydney Swallowing Questionnaire (Wallace et al. [19])

Patient scores each statement on a 100 mm VAS scale with left end = no difficulty at all and right end = unable to swallow at all.

1. How much difficulty do you have swallowing at present?
2. How much difficulty do you have swallowing thin liquids? (e.g., tea, soft drink, beer, coffee)
3. How much difficulty do you have swallowing thick liquids? (e.g., milkshakes, soups, custard)
4. How much difficulty do you have swallowing soft foods? (e.g., mornays, scrambled egg, mashed potato)
5. How much difficulty do you have swallowing hard foods? (e.g., steak, raw fruit, raw vegetables)
6. How much difficulty do you have swallowing dry foods? (e.g., bread, biscuits, nuts)
7. Do you have any difficulty swallowing your saliva?
8. Do you have any difficulty starting a swallow? (never—occurs every time I swallow)
9. Do you ever have a feeling of food getting stuck in your throat when you swallow? (never—occurs every time I swallow)
10. Do you ever cough or choke when swallowing solid foods? (never—occurs every time I swallow)
11. Do you ever cough or choke when swallowing liquids? (never—occurs every time I drink)
12. How long does it take you to eat an average meal? Less than 15 min/15–30 min/30–45 min/45–60 min/>60 min/unable to swallow
13. When you swallow does food or liquid go up behind your nose or come out of your nose? (never—occurs every time I swallow)
14. Do you ever need to swallow more than once for your food to go down? (never—occurs every time)
15. Do you ever cough up or spit out food or liquids during a meal? (never—occurs every time)
16. How do you rate the severity of your swallowing problem today? (no problem—extremely severe problem)
17. How much does your swallowing problem interfere with your enjoyment or quality of life? (no interference—extreme interference)

Mayo Dysphagia Questionnaire-30 Days/2 Weeks (MDQ-30; MDQ-2) (McElhiney et al. [31]; Grudell et al. [20])

Multiple different scoring systems for groups of items (Likert scale, dichotomous scales, hierarchical scales). Some questions are stem-leaf arrangements where patient only answers further questions if the stem question is positive. Subject may answer anywhere from 14 to 55 queries.

Onset of dysphagia
Dysphagia
Change in dysphagia
Change—to what degree
Severity of dysphagia (categorical)
Severity of dysphagia (linear analog scale)
Degree of dysphagia today
Frequency of dysphagia
Dysphagia for liquids
Cold liquids, warm liquids
Solid food dysphagia
Liquid dysphagia following solid bolus impaction
Avoids oatmeal
Avoids banana
Avoids apple
Avoids ground meat
Avoids bread
Avoids steak/chicken
Dysphagia w/oatmeal
Dysphagia w/banana
Dysphagia w/apple
Dysphagia w/ground meat
Dysphagia w/bread
Dysphagia w/dry fibrous solid
Food modifications
Modifies oatmeal
Modifies banana
Modifies apple
Modifies ground meat
Modifies bread
Modifies steak/chicken
Pace compared to others
Minutes to complete a meal
Dysphagia for pills
Impaction
Impaction >5 min
Odynophagia

Odynophagia following solid bolus impaction
Lack of odynophagia
Heartburn composite
Acid regurgitation composite
GERD composite
Seasonal allergies
Food allergies
Childhood asthma
Adult asthma
Antacids
H2 blockers
PPIs
Fundoplication
Fundoplication in the last 30 days
Esophagectomy
Esophagectomy in the last 30 days
Dilation
Dilation in the last 30 days

Swallowing Quality of Life (McHorney et al. [21])

Ten domains and symptom frequency (SP = swallowing problem)
Burden
  Dealing with my SP is very difficult.
  SP is a major distraction in my life.
Eating duration
  It takes me longer to eat than other people.
  It takes me forever to eat a meal.
Eating desire
  Most days, I don't care if I eat or not.
  I don't enjoy eating anymore.
  I'm rarely hungry anymore.
Food selection
  Figuring out what I can eat is a problem for me.
  It is difficult to find food I both like and can eat.
Communication
  People have a hard time understanding me.
  It's been difficult for me to speak clearly.
Fear
  I fear I may start choking when I eat food.
  I worry about getting pneumonia.
  I am afraid of choking when I drink liquids.
  I never know when I am going to choke.

Mental health
  My SP depresses me.
  I get impatient dealing with my SP.
  Being so careful when I eat or drink annoys me.
  My SP frustrates me.
  I've been discouraged by my SP.
Social
  I do not go out to eat because of my SP.
  My SP makes it hard to have a social life.
  My usual activities have changed because of my SP.
  Social gatherings are not enjoyable because of my SP.
  My role with family/friends has changed because of my SP.
Fatigue
  Feel exhausted
  Feel weak
  Feel tired
Sleep
  Have trouble falling asleep.
  Have trouble staying asleep.
Symptom frequency
  Coughing
  Choking when you eat food
  Choking when you take liquids
  Having thick saliva or phlegm
  Gagging
  Having excess salvia or phlegm
  Drooling
  Problems chewing
  Food sticking in your throat
  Food sticking in your mouth
  Food/liquid dribbling out your mouth
  Food/liquid coming out your nose
  Coughing food/liquid out your mouth

Reflux Disease Questionnaire (Shaw et al. [33])

Three domains (heartburn, regurgitation, dyspepsia)
  Acid taste frequency
  Acid taste severity
  Movement of materials severity
  Movement of materials frequency

Frequency of pain behind the breastbone
Frequency of burning behind the breastbone
Severity of burning behind the breastbone
Severity of pain behind the breastbone
Upper stomach burning severity
Upper stomach burning frequency
Upper stomach pain frequency
Upper stomach pain severity

GERD Impact Scale (Jones et al. [13])

Subjects make one of four responses—daily, often, sometimes or never
1. How often have you had the following symptoms:
   Pain in your chest or behind the breastbone?
   Burning sensation in your chest or behind the breastbone?
   Regurgitation or acid taste in your mouth?
   Pain or burning in your upper stomach?
   Sore throat or hoarseness that is related to your heartburn or acid reflux?
2. How often have you had difficulty getting a good night's sleep because of your symptoms?
3. How often have your symptoms prevented you from eating or drinking any of the foods you like?
4. How frequently have your symptoms kept you from being fully productive in your job or daily activities?
5. How often do you take additional medication other than what the physician told you to take (such as Tums, Rolaids, Maalox)?

GerdQ (Jones et al. [34])

1. How often did you have a burning feeling behind your breastbone (heartburn)?
2. How often did you have stomach contents (liquid or food) moving upwards to your throat or mouth (regurgitation)?
3. How often did you have a pain in the centre of the upper stomach?
4. How often did you have nausea?

5. How often did you have difficulty getting a good night's sleep because of your heartburn and/or regurgitation?
6. How often did you take additional medication for your heartburn and/or regurgitation, other than what the physician told you to take? (such as Tums, Rolaids, Maalox?)
Scored—0=0 day, 1=1 day, 2=2–3 days, 3=4–7 days

Chinese GERDQ (Wong et al. [35])

Subjects grade each item on 5-point Likert scale (1=none/no symptoms past year, 2=mild: symptoms can be easily ignored/less than once per month, 3=moderate: awareness of symptoms but easily tolerated/≥ once per month, 4=severe: symptoms sufficient to cause an interference with normal activities/≥ once daily)
1. Frequency of heartburn
2. Severity of heartburn
3. Frequency of feeling of acidity in stomach
4. Severity of feeling of acidity in stomach
5. Frequency of acid regurgitation
6. Severity of acid regurgitation
7. Frequency of "use of antacids"

GSRS (Gastrointestinal Symptom Rating Scale) Revicki et al. [60]

Response scale for patients
1. No discomfort at all
2. Slight discomfort
3. Mild discomfort
4. Moderate discomfort
5. Moderately severe discomfort
6. Severe discomfort
7. Very severe discomfort.
GSRS items
1. Have you been bothered by stomach ache or pain during the past week? (Stomach ache refers to all kinds of aches or pains in your stomach or belly.)
2. Have you been bothered by heartburn during the past week? (By heartburn we mean a burning pain or discomfort behind the breastbone in your chest.)

3. Have you been bothered by acid reflux during the past week? (By acid reflux we mean regurgitation or flow of sour or bitter fluid into your mouth.)
4. Have you been bothered by hunger pains in the stomach or belly during the past week? (This hollow feeling in the stomach is associated with the need to eat between meals.)
5. Have you been bothered by nausea during the past week? (By nausea we mean a feeling of wanting to be sick.)
6. Have you been bothered by rumbling in your stomach or belly during the past week? (Rumbling refers to vibrations or noise in the stomach.)
7. Has your stomach felt bloated during the past week? (Feeling bloated refers to swelling in the stomach or belly.)
8. Have you been bothered by burping during the past week? (Burping refers to bringing up air or gas through the mouth.)
9. Have you been bothered by passing gas or flatus during the past week? (Passing gas or flatus refers to the release of air or gas from the bowel.)
10. Have you been bothered by constipation during the past week? (Constipation refers to a reduced ability to empty the bowels.)
11. Have you been bothered by diarrhoea during the past week? (Diarrhoea refers to frequent loose or watery stools.)
12. Have you ever been bothered by loose stools during the past week? (If your stools have been alternately hard and loose, this question only refers to the extent you have been bothered by the stools being loose.)
13. Have you been bothered by hard stools during the past week? (If your stools have been alternately hard and loose, this question only refers to the extent you have been bothered by the stools being hard.)
14. Have you been bothered by an urgent need to have a bowel movement during the past week? (This urgent need to open your bowels makes you rush to the toilet.)
15. When going to the toilet during the past week, have you had the feeling of not completely emptying your bowels? (The feeling

that after finishing a bowel movement, there is still more stool that needs to be passed.)

Carlsson–Dent Questionnaire/QUEST (Carlsson et al. [36]) [Item Scoring in Parentheses]

1. Which one of these four statements best describes the main discomfort you get in your stomach or chest? (A burning feeling rising from your stomach or lower chest up towards your neck [5], feelings of sickness or nausea [0], pain in the middle of your chest when you swallow [2], none of the above [0])
2. Having chosen one of the above, please now choose which one of the next three statements best describes the timing of your main discomfort? (any time [−2], most often within 2 h of taking food [3], always at a particular time of day or night without any relationship to food [0])
3. How do the following affect your main discomfort?
   Larger than usual meals (worsens [1], improves [−1], no effect [0])
   Food rich in fat (worsens [1], improves [−1], no effect [0])
   Strongly flavoured or spicy food (worsens [1], improves [−1], no effect [0])
4. Which one of the following best describes the effect of indigestion medicines on your main discomfort? (no benefit [0], definite relief within 15 min [3], definite relief after 15 min [0], not applicable [I don't take indigestion medicines] [0])
5. Which of the following best describes the effect of lying flat, stooping, or bending on your main discomfort? (no effect [0], brings it on or makes it worse [1], gives relief [−1], don't know [0])
6. Which of the following best describes the effect of lifting or straining (or any other activity that makes you breathe heavily) on your main discomfort? (no effect [0], brings it on or makes it worse [1], gives relief [−1], don't know [0])
7. If food or acid-tasting liquid returns to your throat or mouth what effect does it have on

your main discomfort? (no effect [0], brings it on or makes it worse [1], gives relief [−1], don't know [0])

Quality of Life in Reflux and Dyspepsia (Wiklund et al. [61])

Subscales (5)
  Emotional distress
  Sleep disturbance
  Food/drink problems
  Physical/social functioning
  Vitality
Total score

GERD-QOL (Chan et al. [37])

Patients indicate rating from 0 to 4 for each item. (0 = strongly agree, 1 = somewhat agree, 2 = neutral, 3 = somewhat disagree, 4 = strongly disagree).
  1. Afraid to eat
  2. Unable to sleep
  3. Inconvenient to take medication regularly
  4. Discomfort when exercise
  5. Reduced social activity
  6. Afraid to eat or drink too much
  7. Disturbed by side effect of medication
  8. Avoided bending over
  9. Afraid to have favourite food and drinks
  10. Needed to be careful of sleeping posture
  11. Could not concentrate on work
  12. Affected sexual life
  13. Disturbed postprandial activities
  14. Frustrated to take medications regularly
  15. Worry that the disease will turn into a serious disease
  16. Feel anxious and distressed

Gastrointestinal Quality of Life Index (Eypasch et al. [38])

Five domains and total score, 36 items
  Symptoms
  Emotion
  Physical function

Social function
Medical treatment
Total Score

GERD-HRQL (Velanovich et al. [39])

Subjects rate the first 10 items (0 = no symptoms, 1 = symptoms noticeable but not bothersome, 2 = symptoms noticeable and bothersome, but not every day, 3 = symptoms bothersome every day, 4 = symptoms affect daily activities, 5 = symptoms incapacitating, unable to do daily activities) and final item as satisfied/neutral/dissatisfied.
  1. How bad is your heartburn?
  2. Heartburn when lying down?
  3. Heartburn when standing up?
  4. Heartburn after meals?
  5. Does heartburn change your diet?
  6. Does heartburn wake you from sleep?
  7. Do you have difficulty swallowing?
  8. Do you have pain with swallowing?
  9. Do you have bloating or gassy feelings?
  10. If you take medication, does this affect your daily life?
  11. How satisfied are you with your present condition?

References

1. Meng NH, Wang TG, Lien IN. Dysphagia in patients with brainstem stroke: incidence and outcome. Am J Phys Med Rehabil. 2000;79:170–5.
2. Robbins J, Langmore S, Hinds JA, Erlichman M. Dysphagia research in the 21st century and beyond: proceedings from Dysphagia Experts Meeting, August 21, 2001. J Rehabil Res Dev. 2002;39:543–8.
3. Shariatzadeh MR, Huang JQ, Marrie TJ. Differences in the features of aspiration pneumonia according to site of acquisition: community or continuing care facility. J Am Geriatr Soc. 2006;54(2):362–4.
4. Altman KW, Yu GP, Schaefer SD. Consequence of dysphagia in the hospitalized patient. Impact on prognosis and hospital resources. Arch Otolaryngol Head Neck Surg. 2010;136:784–9.
5. Ramsey DJC, Smithard DG, Kalra L. Early assessments of dysphagia and aspiration risk in acute stroke patients. Stroke. 2003;34:1252–7.
6. Lien HC, Wang CC, Hsu JY, Sung FC, Cheng KF, Liang WM, Kuo HW, Lin PH, Chang CS. Classical

reflux symptoms, hiatal hernia and overweight independently predict pharyngeal acid exposure in patients with suspected reflux laryngitis. Aliment Pharmacol Ther. 2011;33(1):89–98. doi:10.1111/j.1365-2036.2010.04502.x.

7. He J, Ma X, Zhao Y, Wang R, Yan X, Yan H, Yin P, Kang X, Fang J, Hao Y, Dent J, Sung JJY, Wallander MA, Johansson S, Liu W, Li Z. A population-based survey of the epidemiology of symptom-defined gastroesophageal reflux disease: the Systematic Investigation of Gastrointestinal disease in China. BMC Gastroenterol. 2010;10:94.

8. Ronkainen J, Aro P, Storskrubb T, Lind T, Bolling-Sternevald E, Junghard O, Talley NJ, Agreus L. Gastro-oesophageal reflux symptoms and health-related quality of life in the adult general population—the Kalixanda study. Aliment Pharmacol Ther. 2006;23:1725–33.

9. Lacy B, Weiser K, Chertoff J, Fass R, Pandolfino JE, Richter JE, Rothstein RI, Spangler C, Vaezi MF. The diagnosis of gastroesophageal reflux disease. Am J Med. 2010;123:583–92.

10. Vakil N, van Zanten SV, Kahrilas P, Dent J, Jones R. Global consensus group. The Montreal definition and classification of gastroesophageal reflux disease: a global evidence-based consensus. Am J Gastroenterol. 2006;101:1900–20.

11. Chassany O, Holtmann G, Malagelada J, Gebauer U, Doerfler H, Devault K. Systematic review: health-related quality of life (HRQOL) questionnaires in gastro-oesophageal reflux disease. Aliment Pharmacol Ther. 2008;27:1053–70.

12. Vakil NB, Traxler B, Levine D. Dysphagia in patients with erosive esophagitis: prevalence, severity, and response to proton pump inhibitor treatment. Clin Gastroenterol Hepatol. 2004;2(8):665–8.

13. Jones R, Coyne K, Wiklund I. The gastro-oesophageal reflux disease impact scale: a patient management tool for primary care. Aliment Pharmacol Ther. 2007;25:1451–9.

14. Branski RC, Cukier-Blaj S, Pusic A, Cano SJ, Klassen A, Mener D, Patel S, Kraus DH. Measuring quality of life in dysphonic patients: a systematic review of content development in patient-reported outcomes measures. J Voice. 2008;24:193–8.

15. Cano SJ, Browne JP, Lamping DL. The patient outcomes of surgery—head/neck (POS-head/neck): a new patient-based outcome measure. J Plast Reconstr Aesthet Surg. 2006;59:65–73.

16. Quigley EMM, Hungin APS. Review article: quality of life issues in gastro-oesophageal reflux disease. Aliment Pharmacol Ther. 2005;22 Suppl 1:41–7.

17. Belafsky PC, Mouadeb DA, Rees CJ, Allen JE, Leonard RJ. Validity and reliability of the Eating Assessment Tool (EAT-10). Ann Otol Rhinol Laryngol. 2008;117:919–24.

18. Chen AY, Frankowski R, Bishop-Leone J, Hebert T, Leyk S, Lewin J, Geopfert H. The development and validation of a dysphagia-specific quality-of-life questionnaire for patients with head and neck cancer. Arch Otolaryngol Head Neck Surg. 2001;127:870–6.

19. Wallace KL, Middleton S, Cook IJ. Development and validation of a self-report symptom inventory to assess the severity of oral-pharyngeal dysphagia. Gastroenterology. 2000;118:678–87.

20. Grudell AB, Alexander JA, Enders FB, Pacifico R, Fredericksen M, Wise JL, Locke 3rd GR, Arora A, Zais T, Talley NJ, Romero Y. Validation of the Mayo Dysphagia Questionnaire. Dis Esophagus. 2007;20(3):202–5.

21. McHorney CA, Robbins J, Lomax K, Rosenbek JC, Chignell KA, Kramer AE, Bricker DE. The SWAL-QOL and SWAL-CARE outcomes tool for oropharyngeal dysphagia in adults: III. Documentation of reliability and validity. Dysphagia. 2002;17:97–114.

22. McHorney CA, Martin-Harris B, Robbins J, Rosenbek JC. Clinical validity of the SWAL-QOL and SWAL-CARE outcomes tool with respect to bolus flow measure. Dysphagia. 2006;21:141–8.

23. Ofman JJ. The economic and quality of life impact of symptomatic gastroesophageal reflux disease. Am J Gastroenterol. 2003;98(Suppl):S8–14.

24. Schindler A, Borghi E, Tiddia C, Ginocchio D, Felisati G, Ottaviani F. Adaptation and validation of the Italian MD Anderson Dysphagia Inventory (MDADI). Rev Laryngol Otol Rhinol (Bord). 2008;129:97–100.

25. Kazi R, Prasad V, Venkitaraman R, Nutting CM, Clarke P, Rhys-Evans P, Harrington KJ. Questionnaire analysis of swallowing-related outcomes following glossectomy. ORL J Otorhinolaryngol Relat Spec. 2008;70:151–5.

26. Gillespie MB, Brodsky MB, Day TA, Lee FS, Martin-Harris B. Swallowing-related quality of life after head and neck cancer treatment. Laryngoscope. 2004;114:1362–7.

27. Chen PH, Golub JS, Hapner ER, Johns 3rd MM. Prevalence of perceived dysphagia and quality-of-life impairment in a geriatric population. Dysphagia. 2009;24:1–6.

28. Dwivedi RC, St Rose S, Toe JWG, Khan AS, Pepper C, Nutting CM, Clarke PM, Kerawala CJ, Rhys-Evans PH, Harrington KJ, Kazi R. Validation of the Sydney Swallow Questionnaire (SSQ) in a cohort of head and neck cancer patients. Oral Oncol. 2010;46:e10–4.

29. Locke GR, Talley NJ, Weaver AL, Zinsmeister AR. A new questionnaire for gastroesophageal reflux disease. Mayo Clin Proc. 1994;69:539–47.

30. Dauer E, Thompson D, Zinsmeister AR, Dierkhising R, Harris A, Zais T, Alexander J, Murray JA, Wise JL, Lim K, Locke 3rd GR, Romero Y. Supraesophageal reflux: validation of a symptom questionnaire. Otolaryngol Head Neck Surg. 2006;134(1):73–80.

31. McElhiney J, Lohse MR, Arora AS, Peloquin JM, Geno DM, Kuntz MM, Enders FB, Fredericksen M, Abdalla AA, Khan Y, Talley NJ, Diehl NN, Beebe TJ, Harris AM, Farrugia G, Graner DE, Murray JA, Locke 3rd GR, Grothe RM, Crowell MD, Francis DL, Grudell AM, Dabade T, Ramirez A, Alkhatib M,

Alexander JA, Kimber J, Prasad G, Zinsmeister AR, Romero Y. The Mayo Dysphagia Questionnaire-30: documentation of reliability and validity of a tool for interventional trials in adults with esophageal disease. Dysphagia. 2010;25(3):221–30. Epub 2009 Oct 24.

32. Brozek JL, Guyatt GH, Heels-Ansdell D, Degl'Innocenti A, Armstrong D, Fallone CA, Wiklund I, van Zanten SV, Chiba N, Barjun AN, Akl EA, Schunemann HJ. Specific HRQL instruments and symptom scores were more responsive than preference-based generic instruments in patients with GERD. J Clin Epidemiol. 2009;62:102–10.

33. Shaw MJ, Talley NJ, Beebe TJ, Rockwood T, Carlsson R, Adlis S, Fendrick M, Jones R, Dent J, Bytzer P. Initial validation of a diagnostic questionnaire for gastroesophageal reflux disease. Am J Gastroenterol. 2001;96:52–7.

34. Jones R, Junghard O, Dent J, Vakil N, Halling K, Wernersson B, Lind T. Development of the GerdQ, a tool for the diagnosis and management of gastro-oesophageal reflux disease in primary care. Aliment Pharmacol Ther. 2009;30:1030–8.

35. Wong WM, Lam KF, Lai KC, Hui WM, Hu WCH, Lam CLK, Wong NYH, Xia HHX, Huang JQ, Chan AOO, Lam SK, Wong BCY. A validated symptoms questionnaire (Chinese GERDQ) for the diagnosis of gastro-oesophageal reflux disease in the Chinese population. Aliment Pharmacol Ther. 2003;17:1407–13.

36. Carlsson R, Dent J, Bolling-Sternevald E, Johnsson F, Junghard O, Lauritsen K, Riley S, Lundell L. The usefulness of a structured questionnaire in the assessment of symptomatic gastroesophageal reflux disease. Scand J Gastroenterol. 1998;33:1023–9.

37. Chan Y, Ching JYL, Cheung CMY, Tso KKF, Polder-Verkeil S, Pang SHY, Quan WL, Kee KM, Chang FKL, Sung JJY, Wu JCY. Development and validation of a disease-specific quality of life questionnaire for gastro-oesophageal reflux disease: the GERD-QOL questionnaire. Aliment Pharmacol Ther. 2009;31:452–60.

38. Eypasch E, Williams JI, Wood-Dauphinee S, Ure BM, Schmülling C, Neugebauer E, Troidl H. Gastrointestinal quality of life index: development validation and application of a new instrument. Br J Surg. 1995;82:216–22.

39. Velanovich V, Vallance SR, Gusz JR, Tapice FV, Hurkabus MA. Quality of life scale for gastroesophageal reflux disease. J Am Coll Surg. 1996;183:217–24.

40. McHorney CA, Bricker DE, Kramer AE, Rosenbek JC, Robbins J, Chignell KA, Logemann JA, Clarke C. The SWAL-QOL outcomes tool for oropharyngeal dysphagia in adults: I. Conceptual foundation and item development. Dysphagia. 2000;15:115–21.

41. McHorney CA, Bricker DE, Robbins J, Kramer AE, Rosenbek JC, Chignell KA. The SWAL-QOL outcomes tool for oropharyngeal dysphagia in adults: II. Item reduction and preliminary scaling. Dysphagia. 2000;15:122–33.

42. Rinkel RN, Verdonck-de-Leeuw IM, Langendijk JA, Van Reij EJ, Aaronson NK, Leemans CR. The psychometric and clinical validity of the SWAL-QOL questionnaire in evaluating swallowing problems experienced by patients with oral and oropharyngeal cancer. Oral Oncol. 2009;45:e67–71.

43. Khaldoun E, Woisard V, Verin E. Validation in French of the SWAL-QOL scale in patients with oropharyngeal dysphagia. Gastroenterol Clin Biol. 2009;33:167–71.

44. Bogaardt HC, Speyer R, Baijens LW, Fokkens WJ. Cross-cultural adaptation and validation of the Dutch version of SWAL-QOL. Dysphagia. 2009;24:66–70.

45. Lam PM, Lai CK. The validation of the Chinese version of the swallow quality-of-life questionnaire (SWAL-QOL) using exploratory and confirmatory factor analysis. Dysphagia. 2011;26(2):117–24.

46. Leow LP, Huckabee ML, Anderson T, Beckert L. The impact of dysphagia on quality of life in ageing and Parkinson's disease as measure by the swallowing quality of life (SWALQOL) questionnaire. Dysphagia. 2010;25:216–20.

47. Costa Bandeira AK, Azevedo EH, Vartanian JG, Nishimoto IN, Kowalski LP, Carrara-de Angelis E. Quality of life related to swallowing after tongue cancer treatment. Dysphagia. 2008;23:183–92.

48. Roe JW, Leslie P, Drinnan MJ. Oropharyngeal dysphagia: the experience of patients with head and neck cancers receiving specialist palliative care. Palliat Med. 2007;21:567–74.

49. Lovell SJ, Wong HB, Loh KS, Ngo RY, Wilson JA. Impact of dysphagia on quality of life in nasopharyngeal carcinoma. Head Neck. 2005;27:864–72.

50. Gisbert JP, Cooper A, Karagiannis D, Hatlebakk J, Agréus L, Jablonowski H, Zapardiel J. Impact of gastro-oesophageal reflux disease on patients' daily lives: a European observational study in the primary care setting. Health Qual Life Outcomes. 2009;7:60.

51. Attwood SE, Lundell L, Hatlebakk JG, Eklund S, Junghard O, Galmiche J-P, Ell C, Fiocca R, Lind T. Medical or surgical management of GERD patients with Barrett's esophagus: the LOTUS trial 3-year experience. J Gastrointest Surg. 2008;12:1646–55.

52. Richter JE. Review article: extraesophageal manifestations of gastro-oesophageal reflux disease. Aliment Pharmacol Ther. 2005;22 Suppl 1:70–80.

53. Jaspersen D, Kulig M, Labenz J, Leodolter A, Lind T, Meyer-Sabellek W, Vieth M, Willich SN, Lindner D, Stolte M, Malfertheiner P. Prevalence of extraesophageal manifestations in gastroesophageal reflux disease: an analysis based on the ProGERD Study. Aliment Pharmacol Ther. 2003;17:1515–20.

54. Wiklund I, Carlsson J, Vakil N. Gastroesophageal reflux symptoms and well-being in a random sample of the general population of a Swedish community. Am J Gastroenterol. 2006;101:18–28.

55. Greatorex R, Thorpe JAC. Clinical assessment of gastro-oesophageal reflux by questionnaire. Br J Clin Pract. 1983;37:133–5.

56. Shaw M, Dent J, Beebe T, Junghard O, Wiklund I, Lind T, Johnsson F. The Reflux Disease Questionnaire:

a measure for assessment of treatment response in clinical trials. Health Qual Life Outcomes. 2008;6:31.

57. Nocon M, Labenz J, Jaspersen D, Leodolter A, Richter K, Vieth M, Lind T, Malfertheiner P, Willich SN. Health-related quality of life in patients with gastro-oesophageal reflux disease under routine care: 5-year follow-up results of the ProGERD study. Aliment Pharmacol Ther. 2008;29:662–8.

58. Dent J, Vakil N, Jones R, Bytzer P, Schoning U, Halling K, Junghard O, Lind T. Accuracy of the diagnosis of GORD by questionnaire, physicians and a trial of proton pump inhibitor treatment: the Diamond Study. Gut. 2010;59:7114–721.

59. Louis E, Tack J, Vandenhoven G, Taeter C. Evaluation of the GERD Impact Scale, an international, validated patient questionnaire, in daily practice. Results of the ALEGRIA study. Acta Gastroenterol Belg. 2009;72:3–8.

60. Revicki DA, Wood M, Wiklund I, Crawley J. Reliability and validity of the gastrointestinal symptom rating scale in patients with gastroesophageal reflux disease. Qual Life Res. 1998;7:75–83.

61. Wiklund IK, Junghard O, Grace E, Talley NJ, Kamm M, Veldhuyzen van Zanten S, Chiba N, Leddin DS, Bigard MA, Colin R, Schoenfeld P. Quality of life in reflux and dyspepsia patients. Psychometric documentation of a new disease-specific questionnaire (QOLRAD). Eur J Surg Suppl. 1998;583:41–9.

62. Kulich KR, Malfertheiner P, Madisch A, Labenz J, Bayerdörffer E, Miehlke S, Carlsson J, Wiklund IK. Psychometric validation of the German translation of the gastrointestinal symptom rating scale (GSRS) and quality of life in reflux and dyspepsia (QOLRAD) questionnaire in patients with reflux disease. Health Qual Life Outcomes. 2003;1:62.

63. Kulich KR, Calabrese C, Pacini F, Vigneri S, Carlsson J, Wiklund IK. Psychometric validation of the Italian translation of the gastrointestinal symptom rating scale (GSRS) and quality of life in reflux and dyspepsia (QOLRAD) questionnaire in patients with gastro-oesophageal reflux disease. Clin Drug Investig. 2004;24:205–15.

64. Kulich KR, Madisch A, Pacini F, Piqué JM, Regula J, Van Rensburg CJ, Újszászy L, Carlsson J, Halling K, Wiklund IK. Reliability and validity of the Gastrointestinal Symptom Rating Scale (GSRS) and Quality of Life in Reflux and dyspepsia (QOLRAD) questionnaire in dyspepsia: a six-country study. Health Qual Life Outcomes. 2008;6:12.

65. Hansen JM, Wildner-Christensen M, Schaffalitzky de Muckadell OB. Gastroesophageal reflux symptoms in a Danish population: a prospective follow-up analysis of symptoms, quality of life, and health-care use. Am J Gastroenterol. 2009;104:2394–403.

66. Numans ME, De Wit NJ. Reflux symptoms in general practice: diagnostic evaluation of the Carlsson-Dent gastro-oesophageal reflux disease questionnaire. Aliment Pharmacol Ther. 2003;17:1049–55.

67. Danjo A, Yamaguchi K, Fujimoto K, Saitoh T, Inamori M, Ando T, Shimatani T, Adachi K, Fukunori K, Kuribayashi S, Mitsufuji S, Fujiwara Y, Koyama S, Akiyama J, Takagi A, Manabe N, Miwa H, Shimoyama Y, Kusano M. Comparison of endoscopic findings with symptom assessment systems (FSSG and QUEST) for gastroesophageal reflux disease in Japanese centres. J Gastroenterol Hepatol. 2009;24:633–8.

68. Kulig M, Leodolter A, Vieth M, Schulte E, Jaspersen D, Labenz J, Lind T, Meyer-Sabellek W, Malfertheiner P, Stolte M, Willich SN. Quality of life in relation to symptoms in patients with gastro-oesophageal reflux disease—an analysis based on the Pro-GERD initiative. Aliment Pharmacol Ther. 2003;18:767–76.

69. Revicki DA, Wood BAM, Maton MDPN, Sorensen MPHS. The impact of gastro-esophageal reflux disease on health-related quality of life. Am J Med. 1998;104:252–8.

70. McColl E, Junghard O, Wiklund I, Revicki DA. Assessing symptoms in gastroesophageal reflux disease: how well do clinicians' assessments agree with those of their patients? Am J Gastroenterol. 2005;100:11–8.

71. Havelund T, Lind T, Wiklund I, Glise H, Hernqvist H, Lauritsen K, Lundell L, Pedersen SA, Carlsson R, Junghard O, Stubberöd A, Anker-Hansen O. Quality of life in patients with heartburn but without esophagitis: effects of treatment with omeprazole. Am J Gastroenterol. 1999;94:1782–9.

72. Wiklund I, Bardhan KD, Muller-Lissner S, Bigard MA, Bianchi Porro G, Ponce J, Hosie J, Scott M, Weir D, Fulton C, Gillon K, Peacock R. Quality of life during acute and intermittent treatment of gastro-oesophageal reflux disease with omeprazole compared with ranitidine. Results from a multicentre clinical trial. Ther European Study Group. Ital J Gastroenterol Hepatol. 1998;30:19–27.

73. Mathias SD, Colwell HH, Miller DP, Pasta DJ, Henning JM, Ofman JJ. Health-related quality-of-life and quality-days incrementally gained in symptomatic nonerosive GERD patients treated with lansoprazole or ranitidine. Dig Dis Sci. 2001;46:2416–23.

74. Talley NJ, Fullerton S, Junghard O, Wiklund I. Quality of life in patients with endoscopy-negative heartburn: reliability and sensitivity of disease-specific instruments. Am J Gastroenterol. 2001;96:1998–2004.

75. Aanen MC, Weusten BL, Numans ME, de Wit NJ, Samsom M, Smout AJ. Effect of proton-pump inhibitor treatment on symptoms and quality of life in GERD patients depends on the symptom-reflux association. J Clin Gastroenterol. 2008;42:441–7.

76. Slim K, Bousquet J, Kwiatkowski F, Lescure G, Pezet D, Chipponi J. First validation of the French version of the gastrointestinal quality of life index (GIQLI). Gastroenterol Clin Biol. 1999;23:25–31.

77. Quintana JM, Cabriada J, Lopez de Tejada I, Varona M, Oribe V, Barrios B, Perdigo L, Bilbao A. Translation and validation of the gastrointestinal qual-

ity of life index (GIQLI). Rev Esp Enferm Dig. 2001;93:693–706.

78. Lien HH, Huang CC, Wang PC, Chen YH, Huang CS, Lin TL, Tsai MC. Validation assessment of the Chinese (Taiwan) version of the gastrointestinal quality of life index for patients with symptomatic gallstone disease. J Laparoendosc Adv Surg Tech A. 2007;17(4):429–34.

79. Borie F, Glaise A, Pianta E, Veyrac M, Millat B. Long-term quality-of-life assessment of gastrointestinal symptoms before and after laparoscopic Nissen fundoplication. Gastroenterol Clin Biol. 2010;34:397–402.

80. Velanovich V. The development of the GERD-HRQL symptom severity instrument. Dis Esophagus. 2007;20:130–4.

Cerebro-Vascular Accidents and Dysphagia

Allison R. Gallaugher, Carol-Leigh Wilson, and Stephanie K. Daniels

Abstract

Dysphagia is common following stroke. Appropriate management begins with the evaluation and should be based on the specific swallowing impairment. Cognitive and communication functioning must be considered when determining compensatory and rehabilitative approaches.

Keywords

Stroke • Dysphagia • Lesion location • Dysphagia screening • Clinical swallowing evaluation • Videofluoroscopic swallow study • Cognitive and communication influences • Compensatory strategies • Rehabilitation exercises

Definition

Defining dysphagia is controversial, and there is limited agreement as to what measure(s) one should use to identify it. Swallowing is generally measured in terms of speed of bolus movement through the oropharynx and structural movement (onset, extent, duration) [1–3]. These measures, in turn, impact safety and efficiency. Whatever measure is used, it is important to balance over-identification with under-identification. Understanding performance related to healthy aging is critical to prevent overidentification. This is supported by recent research demonstrating that the onset of the pharyngeal swallow can occur caudal to the anterior faucial arch and, indeed, can occur inferior to the angle of the mandible in healthy adults, particularly as age increases, with increased incidence of airway invasion [4–6]. These studies suggest that a specific swallowing impairment (e.g., delayed pharyngeal swallow, decreased hyolaryngeal elevation), which does not impact safety (airway invasion) or efficiency (postswallow residual), may not represent a clinically significant impairment. Recent research has suggested that determining dysphagia based on a single swallow does not distinguish between healthy adults and individuals following stroke with and without dysphagia [7, 8]. Abnormality across multiple swallows appears to be a more robust method of defining dysphagia. An exception to this rule would be an individual whose swallowing on a single trial is deemed so severe

A.R. Gallaugher, MA • C.-L. Wilson, MA
• S.K. Daniels, PhD (✉)
Communication Sciences and Disorders,
University of Houston, Houston, TX 77204, USA
e-mail: skdaniels@uh.edu

R. Shaker et al. (eds.), *Principles of Deglutition: A Multidisciplinary Text for Swallowing and its Disorders*,
DOI 10.1007/978-1-4614-3794-9_26, © Springer Science+Business Media New York 2013

that the patient's safety is compromised with continued administration of that volume or consistency.

Prevalence/Incidence

Stroke is a major medical problem in the United States affecting approximately 700,000 individuals annually and is the third leading cause of death [9]. The incidence of stroke is increased with advancing age and in particular racial groups such as African Americans. African Americans are also are more likely to have stroke at a younger age than Caucasians [10]. The reported incidence of dysphagia in stroke is variable due, in part, to patient selection methods (i.e., consecutive patients, case series) and evaluation methods (i.e., questionnaire, clinical swallowing evaluation (CSE), instrumental methods), and as noted previously, how one defines dysphagia. Determination of dysphagia based on patient complaint or the CSE generally underestimates the incidence. Dysphagia, as identified on a videofluoroscopic swallow study (VFSS), occurs in approximately 50% of acute stroke patients [11–13] with the incidence of aspiration occurring in about half of those with dysphagia [12, 14]. Of acute stroke patients who aspirate, 40–70% do so silently [11, 15]. That is, there is no overt sign of aspiration such as cough or voice change when material contacts the true vocal folds or enters the trachea.

Pathophysiology

The central pattern generator for swallowing is located in the medulla, and damage to this region can result in profound dysphagia. Acute and chronic dysphagia, however, can occur following a single unilateral stroke to either hemisphere. Similar regions important in swallowing have been identified with functional imaging studies in

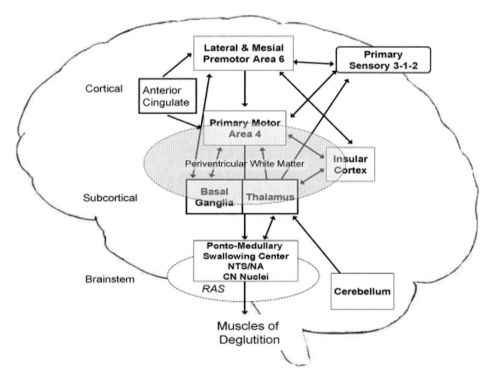

Fig. 26.1 Proposed neuroanatomical model of swallowing. From S.K. Daniels and M.L. Huckabee. Dysphagia following stroke. San Diego, CA: Plural Publishing; 2008 with permission. *CN* cranial nerve, *NTS* nucleus tractus solitarius, *NA* nucleus ambiguus, *RAS* reticular activating system

healthy adults and lesion studies in stroke patients. These regions include the primary motor, supplementary motor, and primary somatosensory cortices, insula, anterior cingulated, basal ganglia, internal capsule, as well as white matter pathways that connect these regions (for review [16]). See Fig. 26.1 for a proposed neuroanatomical model of swallowing.

It was previously thought that dysphagia characteristics were dependent on the hemisphere lesioned. That is, individuals with right hemispheric stroke would demonstrate pharyngeal stage dysfunction and a greater occurrence of aspiration, whereas individuals with left hemispheric stroke would demonstrate oral stage dysfunction and infrequent aspiration [18]. Recent research, however, contradicts this notion as similar patterns of swallowing are evident following left and right hemispheric stroke [19, 20]. Differences in functional swallowing, however, may appear worse in individuals with right hemispheric damage due to cognitive deficits and reduced awareness of swallowing problems.

Diagnosis

Dysphagia Screening

Early detection of dysphagia in acute stroke is critical as it allows for immediate intervention, thereby reducing mortality, morbidity, length of hospitalization, and healthcare costs [21–23]. These findings have led to the recommendation to screen swallowing ability in all acute stroke patients, regardless of stroke severity [21]. Rapid administration of aspirin following stroke onset is associated with reduced mortality and has resulted in the American Heart Association/American Stroke Association (AHA/ASA) to recommend the administration of aspirin within 24–48 h of stroke onset [24]. Timing of aspirin administration, however, is dependent upon screening of swallowing as AHA/ASA recommends that dysphagia screening must be completed prior to the administration of food, liquid, or any medication, including aspirin. Completion of dysphagia screening prior to administration of

oral intake was a Joint Commission guideline until 2010. It was removed due, in part, to a lack of systematically defined standards as to what constitutes a valid dysphagia screening tool [25].

While many screening dysphagia tools are available, few have been validated. Five recent dysphagia screening tools have been developed, validated at some level, and undergone peer review; four of which focus on stroke [26–30]. Each screening tool has strengths and weaknesses. When evaluating a screening test for implementation, important factors to consider are (1) comparison of the screening against a gold standard (VFSS, videoendoscopic evaluation of swallowing), (2) a balance between sensitivity and specificity in order not to underidentify patients with dysphagia but also not to overidentify patients, (3) blinding, that is, the person who administers the screening should not be the same person who interprets the gold-standard instrumental examination, (4) risk of dysphagia, not aspiration, is the outcome measured, and (5) feasibility in implementation and administration. Refer to volume II, chapter 2 for a review of specific swallowing screening tools.

Clinical Swallowing Examination

Once a screening has been completed and a patient is identified to be at risk of dysphagia, speech pathologists are consulted and typically conduct a CSE. The purposes of the CSE are to (1) determine which patient warrants an instrumental evaluation, (2) determine if a diet should be initiated, maintained, or discontinued depending on the patient's oral intake status and need for an instrumental swallowing evaluation, and (3) develop a hypotheses concerning the underlying swallowing impairment and potential management strategies.

Chart Review

Prior to completing the CSE, it is essential to conduct a thorough chart review. This will provide a clear picture of the patient and aid in formulating an evaluation plan. Key pieces of information to glean from the chart review include:

- Admitting primary and co-occurring diagnosis
- Medical history
  - Particularly previous strokes
- Previous and/or current history of dysphagia or aspiration pneumonia
- Prior swallowing evaluations and/or treatment
- Current stroke lesion site
- Nutritional status
- Status of ambulation and activities of daily living
- Respiratory status/recent chest X-rays
- Medications, paying particular attention to medications that can affect swallowing and or arousal/mental status

Communication/Cognitive Screening

Evaluation of cognitive, speech, voice, language, and praxis status is important in stroke patients as function in these areas may have significant impact on the evaluation and treatment of swal-

lowing disorders. The depth of the evaluation is dependent upon the cognitive-communication functioning of the patient. At minimum, a screening of cognition and communication should be completed during the initial evaluation of all acute stroke inpatients. Important areas to screen/test are:

- Level of consciousness
- Attention
  - Focus/concentration
  - Neglect
- Memory
- Auditory comprehension
- Verbal expression
- Motor speech
- Voice
- Buccofacial apraxia
- Limb apraxia

Specific cognitive/communication patterns are evident dependent on lesion location (Table 26.1). It should be noted that this is by no means a comprehensive list, and a patient's cognitive/communication pattern resemblance to these patterns will vary depending on lesion location (i.e., Brodmann's area) and lesion size.

Table 26.1 Lesion location and associated cognitive/communication deficits and effects on swallowing

Lesion location	Cognitive	Expressive language	Receptive language	Nonlanguage impairments	Effects on swallowing
Left hemisphere	Not typical	Impaired verbal output Jargon/Logorrhea Phonemic or semantic paraphasias	Impaired auditory comprehension	Apraxia of speech Dysarthria Limb apraxia	Unable to follow directions in evaluation or during treatment Difficulty with using utensils to eat
Right hemisphere	Reduced attention Impaired executive function Impulsivity Anosognosia/ Prosopagnosia Memory impairment Left neglect		Impaired recognition/ interpretation of paralinguistic features	Dysarthria	Unaware of coughing/ choking during meals Limited monitoring of volume or pace of oral intake Unable to implement compensatory strategies due to poor memory Not eating food on the left side of the tray
Brainstem	Reduced arousal Impaired initiation			Dysarthria	No oral intake if unable to maintain alertness
				Dysarthria	Weak cough

Cranial Nerve Examination

Prior to completing a cranial nerve examination, an assessment of the integrity of oral structures should be made. One should note any missing structures or surgical repairs. The mucosa of the oral cavity should be inspected in terms of color and salivation. Dentition should be inspected for the number and appearance of teeth as well as for evidence of dental prostheses.

Next the clinician should evaluate the patient as he/she performs various motor and sensory tasks to determine cranial nerve function. Performance provides inferred insights into unobservable pharyngeal functioning [17]. Table 26.2 provides details in completing the cranial nerve examination and potential associated oropharyngeal abnormalities.

Oral Intake

A thorough CSE will assess the patient's ability to swallow liquids, semisolids, and solids. For safety, particularly for acute stroke patients, starting the clinical evaluation of oral intake with small liquid volumes is advisable to prevent complications. The safety of stroke patients initially self-regulating large volumes should be monitored as many individuals, particularly those with a right hemispheric stroke, may be unaware of their dysphagia and continue to swallow even though coughing/choking may be present [31]. For consistency across and within patients, using calibrated volumes is advised; however, the patient's self-regulation of large volumes should be evaluated if swallowing of smaller volumes appears safe. Depending on results and the patient's medical status, multiple trials of each consistency should be administered. Ideally, the examination of oral intake should begin with 5 ml of water/liquid, followed by 10 ml, and self-regulated single cup sips. If signs/symptoms of aspiration are present with these discrete swallows, the clinician may then also wish to evaluate sequential swallowing of thin liquids. The clinician should also evaluate ingestion of semisolid, solids, and any particular food in which a patient/family reports to be problematic. The clinician should palpate submental musculature and the thyroid cartilage with each swallow. Although submental and thyroid palpation may assist in identifying onset of the pharyngeal swallow, even the most skilled clinician is unable to determine the location of the bolus within the oropharynx in relation to onset of the pharyngeal swallow. Palpation of the thyroid cartilage can also provide information on the number of swallows required to clear the bolus. In addition, the clinician should monitor vocal quality for any changes after each swallow and should identify throat clear, coughing, or choking which may be signs of aspiration. Last, with each swallow, the clinician should monitor labial seal, postswallow oral residual, and any complaints the patient may have.

Individual or a cluster of features from the CSE have been identified to be associated with dysphagia and/or aspiration. Dysphonia, dysarthria, weak volitional cough, abnormal gag reflex, cough, or throat clear after trial water swallows, and voice change after trial water swallows were each identified to be predictive of risk of aspiration (penetration with laryngeal residual) in acute stroke patients [11]. However, specificity for each item was reduced, indicating that each of these clinical features had the potential to overidentify risk of aspiration. Continued research revealed that identification of any two of these six clinical features identified earlier provided the best yield of sensitivity (e.g., not under-identifying patients with actual risk of aspiration) and specificity [14]. Further research in this area has revealed other features such as response to a 3-oz water swallow test (i.e., cough, wet voice), dysphonia, and jaw weakness to be the best predictors of aspiration in stroke patients [32].

Instrumental Evaluation

If dysphagia is suspected, an instrumental evaluation is warranted and should be completed before any management recommendations are made, including implementation of compensatory strategies. Swallowing treatment should always be based on the results of the instrumental examination. The purpose of the instrumental evaluation is to evaluate biomechanic and physiologic

Table 26.2 Cranial nerve assessment

Cranial nerve	Tested by	Motor innervation	Potential implications

V Trigeminal	Motor
	Jaw open to resistance
	Jaw lateralization, bite
	Sensory
	Sensory to face, hard palate anterior tongue
		Temporalis
		Masseters
		Medial and lateral pterygoids
		Anterior belly of digastric
		Mylohyoid
		Tensor veli palatini
			Bolus breakdown and preparation of solids
			Reduced anterior hyoid movement with consequent
			  Decreased epiglottic deflection with intra-swallow aspiration 2° impaired supraglottic closure
			  Decreased opening of the upper esophageal sphincter with pyriform sinus residual and postswallow aspiration
			  Decreased bolus recognition/awareness

VII Facial	Motor
	Close eyes, wrinkle brow
	Smile, kiss, whistle
	Flatten cheeks, Lateralize lips
	Sensory
	Taste to anterior 2/3 tongue
	Sensory to soft palate and Adjacent pharyngeal wall
		Posterior belly of digastric
		Stylohyoid
		Submandibular and sublingual glands
		Muscles of face and lips (orbicularis oris)
			Reduced elevation of hyoid
			  Decreased pharyngeal shortening and supraglottic compression with risk of intra-swallow aspiration
			Reduced superior, posterior displacement of tongue, hyoid, larynx
			  May have 2° implications for oral containment of the bolus with premature spillage and preswallow pooling
			  Base of tongue to posterior pharyngeal wall approximation with postswallow vallecular residual
			Decreased salivation

IX Glosso-pharyngeal	Motor
	Gag reflex[a]
	Sensory
	Gag reflex[a]
	Estimation of onset of swallow[b]
		Stylopharyngeus
		Taste and sensation to posterior
		1/3 tongue and oral cavity, faucial arches
			Reduced pharyngeal motility and reduced pharyngeal shortening
			  Postswallow diffuse residual
			2° Reduced supraglottic compression
			  Risk of intra-swallow aspiration
			Decreased base of tongue to posterior pharyngeal wall approximation
			  Postswallow vallecular residual
			Decreased bolus recognition/awareness

X Vagus	Motor
	Vocal quality
	Volitional cough, glottal coup
	Sensory
	Reflexive cough
	Inhalation cough challenge
		Cricothyroid
		Intrinsic/extrinsic laryngeal muscles (interarytenoid, lateral cricoarytenoid)
		Sensory input to lower pharynx, larynx
		Cricopharyngeus
			Diminished capacity for laryngeal adduction
			  Intra-swallow aspiration
			Decreased effectiveness of cough on aspiration (motor)
			Silent aspiration (sensory)
			Impairment opening of the upper esophageal sphincter
			  Postswallow pyriform residual
			  Postswallow aspiration

IX & X Pharyngeal plexus	See IX, X	Superior, middle and inferior pharyngeal constrictor
		Palatoglossus
		Palatopharyngeus
		Salpingopharyngeus
		Levator veli palatini
			Poor preswallow bolus containment
			  Premature spillage and preswallow pooling
			  Preswallow aspiration
			Decreased pharyngeal shortening and supraglottic compression
			  Risk of intra-swallow aspiration

(continued)

Table 26.2 (continued)

Cranial nerve	Tested by	Motor innervation	Potential implications

XII Hypo-glossal	Motor only
	Lingual movement-superior, lateral
	Protrusion, retraction
		Intrinsic/extrinsic muscles of tongue
		Genioglossus, styloglossus
		Hyoglossus
		Strap muscles, thyrohyoid, and geniohyoid when paired with C1–2 (ansa cervicalis)
			Poor bolus manipulation, preparation, and transfer
			  Lack of cohesive bolus
			  Postswallow oral residual (buccal and sublingual)
			Decreased base of tongue to posterior pharyngeal wall approximation
			  Postswallow vallecular residual

From [17], used with permission
[a]High risk of false positive
[b]Very difficult to assess clinically

function and dysfunction, determine swallowing safety and efficiency, identify effects of compensatory strategies on swallowing, and determine the appropriate diet consistency. VFSS and videoendoscopic evaluation of swallowing are the two typical instrumental evaluations performed by speech pathologists to evaluate oropharyngeal dysphagia. Pharyngeal manometry may be employed to evaluate pharyngeal pressure. See Table 26.3 for advantages and disadvantages of each evaluation, particularly as they pertain to individuals with stroke.

Videofluoroscopic Swallowing Study

During the VFSS, clinicians should observe timing, direction, and clearance of the bolus as well as the integrity of structural movement. Any anatomical abnormalities should also be noted. To minimize the patient's radiation exposure, swallowing tasks should be limited to three consistencies (liquid, solid, semisolid) unless additional consistencies are needed for testing specific swallowing complaints or for use as compensatory strategies. The evaluation should begin with the patient in the lateral view. An anterior–posterior view can be obtained to distinguish between unilateral and bilateral pyriform sinus residual. Whenever possible, the patient should self-administer the trials as this is the most natural condition and will provide the best representation of typical feeding behaviors.

If the patient is capable of self-administration, then the clinician should premeasure bolus volumes and present them to the patient to ensure safe and consistent trials. This is of particular concern when evaluating individuals with frontal lobe or right hemisphere lesions as they can exhibit reduced inhibition, judgment, and impulse control. Two to three trials of each volume and consistency should be presented [33]. Bolus administration should begin with 5 ml of thin liquid barium. As a verbal cue to swallow can affect timing of oral and pharyngeal transfer [34], this should be omitted if at all possible. If significant aspiration or postswallow residual is not identified with the 5 ml volume, continue with 10 ml of thin liquid, followed by self-regulated cup sip (or straw sip if this is how the patient normally ingests liquid). Next, proceed to 5 ml of a puree/semisolid texture. Finally, present the solid texture consisting of half of a cookie or cracker topped with barium. Depending on the result of the liquid trials and if significant aspiration is not evident, the patient should sequentially swallow a large volume (e.g., 100 ml) of thin liquid barium as the biomechanics of sequential swallowing has been proven to be different than discrete swallows [4, 35]. If the patient demonstrates consistent airway invasion or postswallow residual, then evaluate the effects of applied compensatory strategies. Figure 26.2 provides an example of a VFSS protocol. Progression through the flowchart is, of course, dependent upon each patient's specific characteristics.

Table 26.3 Advantages and disadvantages of various instrumental assessments

Instrumentation	Strengths	Weaknesses	When to use
Videofluoroscopic swallowing study	Direct assessment of oral, pharyngeal, and esophageal stages Evaluate bolus flow, temporal and spatial structural movement Determine the effects of compensatory strategies	Radiation exposure that limits the length of the examination Patient positioning, especially those with cognitive problems, hemiplegia or contractures Nonnatural environment may exacerbate cognitive problems Use of barium as opposed to real food	Need assessment of all three stages of swallowing Wish to distinguish between a delayed pharyngeal swallow and reduced oral control Evaluate what happens during the swallow
Videoendoscopic evaluation of swallowing	Completed at bedside Use of real food No time constraints No radiation exposure Direct visualization of the larynx	No ability to assess oral or esophageal functioning No visualization of the actual swallow due to "white out" Unable to analyze the timing or extent of structural movement	Physical or cognitive limitations would significantly restrict VFSS findings Evaluation of secretion management Patient is ventilator dependent or in the intensive care unit Follow-up assessments to restrict radiation exposure
Pharyngeal manometry	Quantification of observed pharyngeal biomechanics No time constraints No radiation exposure Not subjective	Does not visualize the timing or extent of structural movement or evaluate swallowing safety Scope of evaluation limited to pharyngeal pressure	Differential diagnosis of pharyngeal motility disorders following completion of primary instrumental tests

Modified from [17], used with permission

Videoendoscopic Evaluation of Swallowing

As noted in Table 26.3, VFSS allows the clinician to evaluate the oral, pharyngeal, and esophageal stages of swallowing. The oral stage of swallowing, in particularly can be affected by stroke and negatively impact pharyngeal functioning. Hence, an instrumental evaluation that allows for examination of all swallowing stages may be preferred by some clinicians. Videoendoscopy, however, has very specific advantages and may be the preferred evaluation method. Patients that are too medically fragile to transport to radiology or who are ventilator dependent may be eligible for videoendoscopy, as it is portable and can be administered at bedside. Moreover, there is no time limitation, real food can be administered, and secretion management can be evaluated.

Patients should be positioned sitting as upright as possible, but unlike VFSS, exact positioning is much more flexible. Once inserted, the scope itself may need to be repositioned to obtain the ideal view of laryngeal and pharyngeal structures. Prior to administering actual food and/or liquid, it is important to observe the appearance and symmetry of all structures and the location, quantity, and consistency of secretions. Integrity of structures should be assessed as well, including velopharyngeal competence/sufficiency, true vocal fold adduction, ability and duration of breath holding, and sensation (response to aspiration, pooling, or residual material in the pharynx). The same bolus presentation guidelines for VFSS should be followed for the videoendoscopic evaluation of swallowing.

Management

Treatment can be thought of in terms of compensation and rehabilitation. There is, however, not always a clear distinction between the two types of treatments (Table 26.4). Depending on how

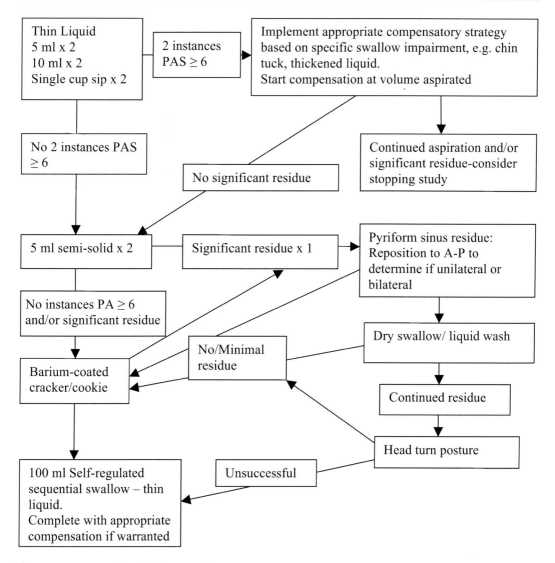

Fig. 26.2 Flowchart of an idealized videofluoroscopic swallow study protocol. *PAS* penetration–aspiration scale [36]

specific management techniques are implemented, some treatments may be considered as both compensatory and rehabilitative. For example, the Mendelsohn maneuver may be considered compensatory if a patient implements this strategy during mealtime to facilitate bolus clearance through the UES and prevent post-swallow aspiration. Repeated practice of this technique as part of dysphagia therapy outside of mealtime may result in long-term improvement in hyolaryngeal elevation thereby facilitating UES opening and bolus clearance [37, 38]. This,

in turn, would result in no need for the compensatory strategy to be used during mealtime.

Compensatory management is meant to immediately and temporarily eliminate a patient's symptoms in order to facilitate swallowing efficiency and safety and maintain the patient on some form of oral intake. Compensatory strategies do not alter swallowing physiology or provide any long-term benefit. Only when a patient exhibits significant cognitive impairments would treatment consist solely of compensatory management.

The effects of compensatory strategies should be based on the specific swallowing impairment and evaluated in the instrumental examination prior to implementation during the meal. Table 26.5 provides a list of compensatory strategies and the specific swallowing impairment for which they were intended.

Rehabilitative exercises, unlike compensatory strategies, aim to positively alter swallowing physiology over time resulting in permanent improvement in swallowing function. Most rehabilitation techniques require good comprehension and cognition. Frail patients may require increased time to build endurance in order to obtain the targeted repetitions. As with compensatory strategies, rehabilitation exercises should address the specific swallowing impairment identified during the instrumental examination. Table 26.6 provides a list of rehabilitation exercises and the associated specific swallowing impairment for which they were designed.

Studies of the effects of rehabilitative swallowing treatment are primarily limited to case studies or small case series; however, larger studies and clinical trials have recently being conducted. A recent randomized controlled trial investigated the effects of high intensity treatment (rehabilitation exercises), low intensity exercises (compensatory strategies), and usual care (physician recommendation) in stroke patients [39]. Results revealed that that the number of stroke patients who returned to a normal diet at 6 months was greater for individuals who underwent high-intensity treatment as compared to those who underwent low-intensity treatment which, in turn, was greater than in patients who underwent usual care. Return to functional swallowing was significantly greater in the active treatment groups, and chest infection and complications related to dysphagia were significantly less in these two treatment groups compared to the control group.

The neural plastic effect of rehabilitative swallowing therapy is an important concept to consider when designing and recommending treatment approaches. Plasticity is the capacity of a system to be altered. It is known that some treatments can improve airway protection, improve timing, and movement of structures; however, it is unclear if our swallowing therapy can change neural pathways and synapses of the central nervous system. Neuroplastic changes, at least in terms of the motor map reorganization, are different for the limb as compared to midline structures. That is, for the limb, reorganization is to the ipsilesional hemisphere, whereas for midline structures, like those involved in swallowing, reorganization is to the contralesional hemisphere.

Peripheral electrical stimulation (PES) and repetitive transcranial magnetic stimulation (rTMS), both treatments for dysphagia, have been shown to produce neuroplastic changes. PES consists of electrodes housed in an intraluminal catheter that is inserted into the pharynx. The device is set at 5 Hz at 75% maximum tolerated stimulation and the length of stimulation is 10 min. Results in stroke patients revealed increased excitability of response in the contralesional hemisphere and significant changes for temporal and airway invasion measures [40]. rTMS has been studied

Table 26.4 Management approaches for dysphagia

Compensation	Both	Rehabilitation
Posture	Thermal tactile stimulation	Lingual strengthening
Sensory enhancement	Effortful swallow	Tongue-hold maneuver
Breath holding techniques	Mendelsohn maneuver	Shaker exercise
Bolus modification		NMES
		EMST
		LSVT

NMES neuromuscular electrical stimulation, *EMST* expiratory muscle strength training, *LSVT* Lee Silverman voice treatment

Table 26.5 Compensation approach to management

The symptoms of	Secondary to physiologic abnormality of	Compensation
Anterior leakage	Poor orolingual control	Thickened liquid
Inadequate bolus preparation	Poor orolingual control	Chopped or pureed diet
Discoordinated oral transfer	Poor orolingual control	3-s prep
Oral residual	Poor orolingual control	Cyclic ingestion
Pharyngeal pooling to the level of____	Poor orolingual control	Thickened liquid Volume regulation Chin tuck
Pharyngeal pooling to the level of____	Delayed pharyngeal swallow	Thickened liquid Volume regulation 3-s prep Increased taste-sour bolus Thermal-tactile stimulation Chin tuck[a]
Nasal regurgitation	Poor pharyngeal motility	Thick consistencies
Inadequate epiglottic deflection	Decreased anterior hyoid movement Intrinsic structural changes in supportive tissue	No identified compensatory strategy
Vallecular residual	Decreased base of tongue to posterior pharyngeal wall approximation	Cyclic ingestion Chin tuck Carbonation-physiology of residual not specified
Vallecular residual	Inadequate epiglottic deflection	Cyclic ingestion Carbonation-physiology of residual not specified
Inadequate opening of the UES	Decreased anterior hyoid movement Intrinsic structural functional changes in cricopharyngeus	Head turn
Unilateral pharyngeal residue	Pharyngeal hemiparesis	Head turn to weaker side
Pyriform sinus residual	Inadequate opening of the UES	Cyclic ingestion Carbonation-physiology of residual not specified Head turn
Penetration	Preswallow pharyngeal pooling	Thickened liquids Volume regulation 3-s prep Chin tuck[a] Increased taste-sour bolus Thermal-tactile stimulation
Penetration	Inadequate epiglottic deflection	No identified compensatory strategy
Penetration	Oral residual	Cyclic ingestion
Penetration	Pharyngeal residual	Cyclic ingestion Chin tuck Carbonation
Penetration	Reduced laryngeal valving	Super-supraglottic swallow
Penetration	Preswallow pharyngeal pooling	Same as for penetration Supraglottic or super-supraglottic swallow
Aspiration	Physiology not specified	Carbonation
Aspiration	Reduced laryngeal valving	Super-supraglottic swallow
Aspiration	Inadequate true vocal fold closure	Supraglottic swallow
Aspiration	Oral residual	Same as for penetration
Aspiration	Pharyngeal residual	Same as for penetration

From [17], used with permission

UES upper esophageal sphincter

[a]Precaution-use chin tuck only with pooling to valleculae. Use with pooling more inferior may increase airway invasion

Table 26.6 Rehabilitation approach to management

The symptoms of	Secondary to physiologic abnormality of	Rehabilitation approach	Other considerations
Anterior leakage Inadequate bolus preparation Inadequate bolus formation Oral residual	Poor orolingual control	Oral motor exercises Tongue to palate pressure Tongue to tongue depressor pressure	Biofeedback device: IOPI or other oral pressure measurement device
Pharyngeal pooling to the level of ___	Delayed pharyngeal swallow	No known rehabilitation techniques at this time	
Nasal regurgitation	Poor pharyngeal motility	Effortful swallow Masako maneuver	Biofeedback device: sEMG of submental muscle group Precautions: attend to hyoid movement, may wish to add head lift maneuver as prophylactic
Inadequate epiglotic deflection	Decreased anterior hyoid movement	Head lift maneuver	
Inadequate epiglotic deflection	Intrinsic structural changes in supportive tissue	No rehabilitation techniques at this time	
Vallecular residual	Decreased base of tongue to posterior pharyngeal wall approximation[a]	Masako maneuver Effortful swallow Oral motor exercises	Biofeedback device: sEMG of submental muscle group Precautions: attend to hyoid movement, may wish to add head lift maneuver as prophylactic
Vallecular residual	Inadequate epiglottic deflection[a]	See rehabilitation approaches for physiologic abnormalities resulting in inadequate epiglottic deflection above.	
Inadequate opening of the UES[a]	Decreased anterior hyoid movement[a]	Head lift maneuver	
Inadequate opening of the UES[a]	Intrinsic structural functional changes in cricopharyngeus	Mendelsohn maneuver	Biofeedback device: sEMG of submental muscle group Precautions: attend to hyoid movement, may wish to add head lift maneuver as prophylactic
Pyriform sinus residual	Inadequate opening of the UES[a]	See rehabilitation approaches for physiologic abnormalities resulting in inadequate opening of the UES above	
Penetration	Preswallow pharyngeal pooling[a] Inadequate epiglottic deflection[a] Inadequate supraglottic shortening/laryngeal elevation[a] Oral residual[a] Pharyngeal residual[a]	Refer to rehabilitation approaches associated with physiologic abnormalities underlying penetration	
Aspiration	Preswallow pharyngeal pooling[a]	Refer to rehabilitation approaches associated with physiologic abnormalities underlying aspiration	
Aspiration	Inadequate true vocal fold closure	Vocal adduction exercises	
Aspiration	Oral residual[a] Pharyngeal residual[a]	Refer to rehabilitation approaches associated with physiologic abnormalities underlying aspiration	

From [17] used with permission

sEMG,surface electromyography, *UES* upper esophageal sphincter

[a]Occasionally a symptom will be caused by another symptom, which requires the clinician to problem solve through to the initial presenting physiologic abnormality

primarily in healthy individuals and involves delivering trains of magnetic pulses to the motor cortex. Results suggest increased excitability of corticobulbar projections to the pharynx [41].

Behavior treatment (i.e., compensatory and rehabilitative therapy) has not been studied in terms of neuroplastic effects. This type of treatment can be thought of in terms of sensory treatment (bolus effects, thermal tactile application), motor training with swallowing, which involves skill plus strength training (e.g., effortful swallow), and motor training without swallowing, which is pure strength training (e.g., Shaker exercise) [42]. Currently, it is unclear if neuroplastic effects would be different in skill training versus strength training, when one should target one type of training over the other, and when strength or skilled training is not indicated.

Key Points

- Dysphagia is common following stroke.
- Single, unilateral supratentorial lesions can produce acute and protracted dysphagia.
- Swallowing should be screened in all acute stroke patients prior to any oral intake.
- Cognitive and communication status must be considered when evaluating and treating patients.
- Treatment begins with the instrumental study, and any recommended compensatory strategy must be tested in the instrumental examination.
- Neuroplastic effects of treatment are important to consider when designing and implementing treatment studies.

Acknowledgment The authors would like to acknowledge Dr. Joe Murray's assistance with conceptualization and design of Fig. 26.2.

References

1. Logemann JA. Swallowing disorders. 2nd ed. Austin, TX: Pro-ED; 1999.
2. Martin-Harris B, Brodsky MB, Michel Y, et al. MBS measurement tool for swallow impairment—MBSImp: establishing a standard. Dysphagia. 2008;23:392–405.
3. Robbins J, Hamilton JW, Lof GL, et al. Oropharyngeal swallowing in normal adults of different ages. Gastroenterology. 1992;103:823–9.
4. Daniels SK, Corey DM, Hadskey LD, et al. Mechanism of sequential swallowing during straw drinking in healthy young and older adults. J Speech Lang Hear Res. 2004;47:33–45.
5. Martin-Harris B, Brodsky MB, Michel Y, et al. Delayed initiation of the pharyngeal swallow: normal variability in adult swallows. J Speech Lang Hear Res. 2007;50:585–94.
6. Stephen JR, Taves DH, Smith RC, et al. Bolus location at the initiation of the pharyngeal stage of swallowing in healthy older adults. Dysphagia. 2005;20:266–72.
7. Daniels SK, Schroeder MF, DeGeorge PC, et al. Defining and measuring dysphagia following stroke. Am J Speech Lang Pathol. 2009;18:74–81.
8. Daniels SK, Schroeder MF, McClain M, et al. Dysphagia in stroke: development of a standard method to examine swallowing recovery. J Rehabil Res Dev. 2006;43:347–56.
9. Broderick J, Brott T, Kothari R, et al. The Greater Cincinnati/Northern Kentucky Stroke Study: preliminary first-ever and total incidence rates of stroke among blacks. Stroke. 1998;29:415–21.
10. Kleindorfer DO, Lindsell C, Broderick J, et al. Impact of socioeconomic status on stroke incidence: a population-based study. Ann Neurol. 2006;60:480–4.
11. Daniels SK, Brailey K, Priestly DH, et al. Aspiration in patients with acute stroke. Arch Phys Med Rehabil. 1998;79:14–9.
12. Mann G, Hankey GJ, Cameron D. Swallowing function after stroke: prognosis and prognostic factors at 6 months. Stroke. 1999;30:744–8.
13. Smithard DG, O'Neill PA, Parks C, et al. Complications and outcome after acute stroke. Does dysphagia matter? Stroke. 1996;27:1200–4.
14. Daniels SK, McAdam CP, Brailey K, et al. Clinical assessment of swallowing and prediction of dysphagia severity. Am J Speech Lang Pathol. 1997;6:17–24.
15. Splaingard ML, Hutchins B, Sulton LD, et al. Aspiration in rehabilitation patients: videofluoroscopy vs bedside clinical assessment. Arch Phys Med Rehabil. 1988;69:637–40.
16. Leopold NA, Daniels SK. Supranuclear control of swallowing. Dysphagia. 2010;25:250–7.
17. Daniels SK, Huckabee ML. Dysphagia following stroke. San Diego, CA: Plural; 2008.
18. Robbins J, Levine R. Swallowing after lateral medullary syndrome plus. Clin Commun Disord. 1993;3:45–55.
19. Daniels SK, Foundas AL. Lesion localization in acute stroke patients with risk of aspiration. J Neuroimaging. 1999;9:91–8.
20. Theurer JA, Johnston JL, Taves DH, et al. Swallowing after right hemisphere stroke: oral versus pharyngeal deficits. Can J Speech Lang Pathol Audiol. 2008;32:114–22.
21. Hinchey JA, Shephard T, Furie K, et al. Formal dysphagia screening protocols prevent pneumonia. Stroke. 2005;36:1972–6.
22. Martino R, Pron G, Diamant N. Screening for oropharyngeal dysphagia in stroke: insufficient evidence for guidelines. Dysphagia. 2000;15:19–30.

23. Odderson IR, McKenna BS. A model for management of patients with stroke during the acute phase. Outcome and economic implications. Stroke. 1993;24:1823–7.

24. Adams Jr HP, del Zoppo G, Alberts MJ, et al. Guidelines for the early management of adults with ischemic stroke: a guideline from the American Heart Association/American Stroke Association Stroke Council, Clinical Cardiology Council, Cardiovascular Radiology and Intervention Council, and the Atherosclerotic Peripheral Vascular Disease and Quality of Care Outcomes in Research Interdisciplinary Working Groups: the American Academy of Neurology affirms the value of this guideline as an educational tool for neurologists. Stroke. 2007;38:1655–711.

25. Lakshminarayan K, Tsai AW, Tong X, et al. Utility of dysphagia screening results in predicting poststroke pneumonia. Stroke. 2010;41:2849–54.

26. Antonios N, Carnaby-Mann G, Crary M, et al. Analysis of a physician tool for evaluating dysphagia on an inpatient stroke unit: the modified mann assessment of swallowing ability. J Stroke Cerebrovasc Dis. 2010;19:49–57.

27. Martino R, Silver F, Teasell R, et al. The Toronto Bedside Swallowing Screening Test (TOR-BSST): development and validation of a dysphagia screening tool for patients with stroke. Stroke. 2009;40:555–61.

28. Suiter DM, Leder SB, Karas DE. The 3-ounce (90-cc) water swallow challenge: a screening test for children with suspected oropharyngeal dysphagia. Otolaryngol Head Neck Surg. 2009;140:187–90.

29. Trapl M, Enderle P, Nowotny M, et al. Dysphagia bedside screening for acute-stroke patients: the gugging swallowing screen. Stroke. 2007;38:2948–52.

30. Turner-Lawrence DE, Peebles M, Price MF, et al. A feasibility study of the sensitivity of emergency physician dysphagia screening in acute stroke patients. Ann Emerg Med. 2009;54:344-8–48 e1.

31. Parker C, Power M, Hamdy S, et al. Awareness of dysphagia by patients following stroke predicts swallowing performance. Dysphagia. 2004;19:28–35.

32. McCullough GH, Rosenbek JC, Wertz RT, et al. Utility of clinical swallowing examination measures for detecting aspiration post-stroke. J Speech Lang Hear Res. 2005;48:1280–93.

33. Lazarus CL, Logemann JA, Rademaker AW, et al. Effects of bolus volume, viscosity, and repeated swallows in nonstroke subjects and stroke patients. Arch Phys Med Rehabil. 1993;74:1066–70.

34. Daniels SK, Schroeder MF, DeGeorge PC, et al. Effects of verbal cue on bolus flow during swallowing. Am J Speech Lang Pathol. 2007;16:140–7.

35. Daniels SK, Foundas AL. Swallowing physiology of sequential straw drinking. Dysphagia. 2001;16:176–82.

36. Rosenbek JC, Robbins JA, Roecker EB, et al. A penetration-aspiration scale. Dysphagia. 1996;11:93–8.

37. Logemann JA, Kihrilas PJ. Relearning to swallow after stroke-application of maneuvers and indirect feedback: a case study. Neurology. 1990;40:1136–38.

38. Kahrilas PJ, Logemann JA, Krugler C, et al. Volitional augmentation of upper esophageal sphincter opening during swallowing. Am J Physiol. 1991;260:G450–56.

39. Carnaby G, Hankey GJ, Pizzi J. Behavioural intervention for dysphagia in acute stroke: a randomised controlled trial. Lancet Neurol. 2006;5:31–7.

40. Fraser C, Power M, Hamdy S, et al. Driving plasticity in human adult motor cortex is associated with improved motor function after brain injury. Neuron. 2002;34:831–40.

41. Gow D, Rothwell J, Hobson A, et al. Induction of long-term plasticity in human swallowing motor cortex following repetitive cortical stimulation. Clin Neurophysiol. 2004;115:1044–51.

42. Robbins J, Butler SG, Daniels SK, et al. Swallowing and dysphagia rehabilitation: translating principles of neural plasticity into clinically oriented evidence. J Speech Lang Hear Res. 2008;51:S276–300.

Progressive Neurologic Disease and Dysphagia (Including Parkinson's Disease, Multiple Sclerosis, Amyotrophic Lateral Sclerosis, Myasthenia Gravis, Post-Polio Syndrome)

27

John C. Rosenbek and Michelle S. Troche

Abstract

This chapter's purposes are to provide a compact review of eleven progressive neurologic conditions' effects on swallowing dysfunction and to briefly discuss management options specific to each. They were selected because dysphagia, with subsequent influences on health and quality of life, is nearly inevitable during the course of each. The conditions include eight syndromes, among them Parkinson's disease, amyotrophic lateral sclerosis, and multiple sclerosis and three movement abnormalities-ataxia, dystonia, and chorea. Each syndrome or movement abnormality is defined, then prevalence/incidence, pathophysiology, evaluation, complications such as aspiration pneumonia, and team management are described. The emphasis is on focused evaluation and rehabilitation of the dysphagia.

Keywords

Progressive neurologic disease • Dysphagia • Parkinson's disease • Multiple sclerosis • Amyotrophic lateral sclerosis • Myasthenia gravis • Post-polio syndrome • Introduction

Approximately 600 neurologic syndromes have been identified. Oropharyngeal dysphagia may result from any neurologic disease affecting neural networks. It is difficult in a chapter-length discussion to select the disorders to incorporate and with what detail they should be addressed. A second, and overlapping, challenge is to avoid a simple encyclopedic listing of disease. Categorizing neurologic disease is challenging. Grouping by neuroanatomical site of lesion is difficult because the majority of neurologic diseases involve multiple system impairment (e.g., Parkinson's disease, multiple sclerosis, multisystem atrophy). Ordering by underlying pathophysiology such as rigidity, spasticity, weakness, or dyscoordination is also unsatisfactory because as diseases develop, multiple symptoms may become affected. Limited data make organization

J.C. Rosenbek, PhD
University of Florida, Speech, Language
Hearing Sciences, 101 S. Newell, Rm 2128,
Gainesville, FL 32610-0174, USA

M.S. Troche, PhD (✉)
Department of Speech, Language,
and Hearing Sciences, University of Florida,
PO Box 117420, Gainesville, FL 32611, USA
e-mail: michi81@phhp.ufl.edu

based on neuropathology such as abnormalities of the tau protein untenable, and the neuropathology data available in some instances are incompatible with traditional clinical diagnosis as when progressive supranuclear palsy (PSP) defined pathophysiologically is diagnosed clinically as PD. Consensus conferences [1] have improved the correlation of clinical and pathophysiological diagnosis but have left some clinicians (and neuropathologists) unsure about traditional clinical syndromes. What remains is a traditional hybrid approach to the ordering of the disease content mixing clinical diagnoses such as PD and Parkinson plus syndromes with sections based on the primary pathophysiology such as dystonia and ataxia. This approach affords the most common progressive neurologic diseases supplemented by brief, presentation of rarer conditions such as Wilson's disease, Guillan–Barre, and post-polio syndrome. The purpose of this chapter is to provide a comprehensive review of the effect of progressive neurologic disease on swallowing dysfunction and briefly discuss management options.

Parkinson's Disease

Definition

Parkinson's disease (PD) has long been considered an illness caused by dopamine depletion in the substantia nigra that affects only motor function, but the current conceptualization of PD acknowledges that it affects distributed neuroanatomical regions, disrupting multiple motor and nonmotor systems [2]. The cardinal symptoms include bradykinesia, rigidity, resting tremor, and postural instability. In addition to basal ganglia-specific changes, it is now recognized that the PD process begins in the dorsal motor nucleus of the vagal nerve and, from there, proceeds upward until it arrives at the cerebral cortex [2].

Prevalence/Incidence of Swallowing Dysfunction

The incidence of dysphagia in persons with PD established by careful clinical and instrumental examination has been reported to be between

18.5% and 100% [3–6] with silent aspiration occurring in at least one-third of patients [7]. Not surprisingly, many PD patients report no swallowing impairment presumably due to their frequent lack of insight about their neurologic changes [8].

Pathophysiology

The etiology of swallowing dysfunction in persons with PD has not been well defined. Changes have been attributed to the cardinal symptoms of PD from dopaminergic pathway abnormality: rigidity, hypokinesia, and tremor [9]. Rigidity and bradykinesia have been implicated specifically as responsible for difficulty chewing and drooling. Eadie and Tyrer [10] and Ertekin et al. [11] hypothesized that the hypokinetic, reduced rate of spontaneous swallowing movements, and the "slowness of segmented but coordinated sequential movements" (p 948), may be the most significant cause of swallowing dysfunction in PD. Lastly, swallowing dysfunction in PD has also been attributed to the involvement of the dorsal motor nucleus of the vagus nerve and of "Lewy bodies in the myenteric plexus of the esophagus" [12] (p 730).

Diagnosis

Widespread impairment in PD results in swallowing deficits of every stage of swallowing, and therefore, in addition to a complete history, videofluoroscopy seems to be the best method for assessing both motor and sensory involvement of the entirety of the swallowing mechanism. Dysfunction is commonly seen in oral manipulation of the bolus including lingual pumping, labial bolus leakage, lingual tremor, slowed or limited mandibular function, piecemeal deglutition, pre-swallow spill, delayed swallow triggering, and post-swallow residue [4, 11, 13–20]. Changes to the pharyngeal phase of swallow include slow pharyngeal transit, abnormal/delayed contraction of the pharyngeal wall, coating of the pharyngeal walls with bolus material, deficient epiglottic positioning, decreased epiglottic range of motion, stasis in the vallecula and pyriform sinuses, slow laryngeal elevation and excursion, penetration, aspiration, and upper esophageal sphincter (UES) discoordination [4, 8, 13–21]. Other associated impairments include vocal fold bowing, drooling, and difficulty swallowing saliva in up to 78% of persons with PD, and deficits in swallow–respiratory relationships as evidenced by more swallowing during inhalation and swallowing at low tidal volume [22–24]. Further complicating the management of persons with PD and dysphagia are the associated gastrointestinal symptoms which often accompany PD [25]. These in conjunction with oropharyngeal dysphagia can result in reduced oral intake.

Complications

The risk of death secondary to pneumonia in PD is six times greater than in those without PD [26], with aspiration pneumonia being the leading cause of death [27–31]. This risk is probably a consequence of chronic immobilization and swallowing impairment, particularly in later stages of the disease [32].

Management

Levodopa (L-Dopa), the gold standard for the treatment of PD related symptoms, has not been found to be efficacious for the treatment of dysphagia in PD [5, 15, 16, 33], nor does L-Dopa improve/influence respiratory–swallow relationships [23]. A study testing the effects of various compensatory strategies (i.e., chin tuck, nectar and honey-thickened liquids) on occurrence of pneumonia in persons with dementia and PD found significantly higher incidence of pneumonia in persons given honey-thickened liquids versus nectar-thickened liquids [34]. Additionally, a recent randomized clinical trial found 4 weeks of treatment with an expiratory muscle training device resulted in significantly improved swallowing safety (i.e., reductions in penetration/aspiration) and improved cough effectiveness [35]. Other smaller scale non-randomized studies have identified LSVT [36], verbal cueing [24], traditional swallowing exercises (e.g., Mendelsohn, range of motion) [37], and bolus modification [38] as possible treatment modalities for dysphagia in PD. Surgical management with cricopharyngeal sphincterotomy and myotomy for

cricopharyngeal dysfunction have been discussed in the literature with good results on selected patients [15, 39].

Parkinsonian Syndromes

Definition

Depending on the source, 12 or more conditions are included among the parkinsonian syndromes [40]. Multiple system atrophy (MSA) and progressive supranuclear palsy (PSP) are discussed in this section. Gilman and colleagues [41] define MSA as a "progressive neurodegenerative disease of unknown etiology. The disease occurs sporadically and causes parkinsonism with cerebellar, autonomic, urinary and pyramidal dysfunction in many combinations" [41]. Three syndromes are traditionally identified: (1) MSA-P (also called striatonigral degeneration or SND) in which parkinsonian features predominate, (2) MSA-C (also called OPCA) in which cerebellar features predominate, and (3) MSA-A (called Shy–Drager syndrome, an increasingly infrequent label) in which autonomic features predominate. Signs of all three types appear in more than 25% of patients with disease progression. See Higo [42] for more details. PSP, also called Richardson's disease, is a progressive neurologic disorder of middle age often beginning with gait abnormality and frequent falls. Litvan and colleagues [43] outline criteria for diagnosis.

Prevalence and Incidence

The estimated prevalence for MSA, without regard for subtypes, is 4.0 per 100,000 people [44]. Ben-Shlomo et al. [45] report onset at an average age of 54 years and a median survival of 6.2 years. Dysphagia occurs earlier and with greater severity in MSA than in Parkinson's disease. Shulman et al. [46] call dysphagia a "pervasive" sign. Using videofluoroscopy, Higo and colleagues [47] identified at least one sign of dysphagia in approximately 75% of patients with MSA referred for swallowing evaluation. Prevalence of PSP is estimated at 3.9 per 100,000 persons in the United States [48]. Onset usually occurs between ages of 55 and 70 and death for most occurs 5–7 years after diagnosis. Litvan et al. [49] reported a variety of oral and pharyngeal stage symptoms in 26 of 27 patients with PSP, including coughing and choking and signs on videofluoroscopic swallowing examination including delayed swallow initiation.

Pathophysiology

Pathophysiology is complex in MSA. Delayed initiation of movement, slowed movement, and rigidity are the most frequent parkinsonian signs. Hypotonicity and dyscoordination are likely with cerebellar involvement. Hypertonicity and affective disorders and additional cognitive changes impacting swallowing can also occur. Rigidity, bradykinesia, spasticity, and dystonia are common features of PSP and are often accompanied by general cognitive slowness and behavioral abnormalities [43].

Diagnosis

The definitive diagnosis of MSA requires autopsy. The clinical diagnosis of PSP requires the presence of gait instability, early falls, rigidity, bradykinesia, vertical gaze abnormality, spastic dysarthria, profound dysphagia, and frontal lobe abnormalities [49]. The swallowing clinician is often working with a tentative diagnosis. The swallowing evaluation can accomplish the following: (1) establish the signs of dysphagia and its severity, (2) support hypotheses about the usually complex underlying pathophysiology as a focus of treatment, (3) determine the probable quality of life and health impact of the dysphagia, (4) identify potential affective and cognitive influences on the swallowing and on treatment, (5) attend carefully to laryngeal stridor secondary to vocal fold immobility which may be more common in MSA than in other neurodegenerative diseases, and (6) contribute to differential diagnosis by identifying the onset and features of the dysphagia. Both oral and pharyngeal deficits are often observed. According to Higo and colleagues [47] the most common signs are delayed initiation of the swallow, reduced posterior tongue movement, and "disturbance of bolus holding" (p 632). Residuals in the pyriform sinuses and valleculae

and reduced opening of the UES are among the most frequent pharyngeal signs [50, 51].

Complications

Higo's group [52] says dysphagia "is the most critical complication of MSA" (p 647). Muller et al. [53] report an average duration of 15 months from a patient's recognizing swallowing changes to death. Twenty-four percent of Higo et al.'s [47] patients had a history of aspiration pneumonia. Muller and colleagues [53] identify dysphagia as a bad prognostic sign in PSP. Aspiration, dehydration, malnutrition, and prolonged eating with attendant caregiver stress are among the complications.

Management

Because medical and surgical management of parkinsonian syndromes is often of limited usefulness for all but general symptom reduction, dysphagia management is especially critical. If the underlying pathophysiology is assumed to be rigidity, hypotonia, and/or weakness then a variety of the strengthening techniques may be appropriate. If dyscoordination, delayed initiation, or slow movement predominates, the skill building techniques may be appropriate. Combinations will likely be necessary as will be a concerted behavioral effort to improve cognitive deficits that include attention and general responsiveness. While these efforts are ongoing, compensations will also be useful.

Multiple Sclerosis

Definition

Multiple sclerosis (MS) is an inflammatory process in which the myelin surrounding the axons of the brain and spinal cord is damaged leading to demyelinating and lesions throughout the neuroaxis [54]. There are four main types of MS: (1) relapsing/remitting, (2) secondary progressive, (3) primary progressive, and (4) progressive relapsing. Relapsing/remitting, the most prevalent of the subtypes, is characterized by acute attacks of MS followed by periods of remission. This is in contrast to secondary progressive MS that also involves acute attacks, but in these cases there is a progression of disease between attacks as well. Those with primary progressive MS have a steady decline of symptoms from onset of disease and those with progressive relapsing experience a steady decline of disease, but with superimposed attacks throughout the disease process [55].

Prevalence/Incidence of Dysphagia

The prevalence of dysphagia in MS is estimated between 30% and 43% [56, 57], although some have suggested that this figure is likely underestimated [57]. The incidence of dysphagia in MS increases to 65% in those most severely disabled (as measured by the Expanded Disability Status Scale (EDSS)). It is important to note, though, that 17% of patients with low disability will also have dysphagia [56].

Pathophysiology

The inflammatory processes involved in MS affect a variety of areas of the central nervous system, thus making the pathophysiology of dysphagia in MS variable from patient to patient [58]. Longer disease duration in addition to involvement of cerebellar, brainstem, and cognitive regions has been found to better predict the presence of dysphagia in MS [56]. Therefore, it can be postulated that dyscoordination of the swallowing mechanism secondary to cerebellar lesions, weakness of the swallowing mechanism from brainstem involvement, and/or disruption of the swallowing mechanism secondary to diminished cognitive resources during swallowing most often characterize the pathophysiology underlying dysphagia in MS.

Diagnosis

As described above, dysphagia in persons with MS varies greatly in its presentation depending on the areas of the neuroaxis which have been most affected by the disease. Therefore, a complete history identifying specific swallowing changes in conjunction with instrumental assessment of swallowing with videofluoroscopy is recommended. This will help identify loci of dysfunction and any sensory changes as well. In general, all phases of swallowing are affected with the greatest percentage of patients with dysphagia and MS, demonstrating pharyngeal phase disorders (28.7%), oral stage disorders in 5% of patients, and aspiration in 6.9% [57]. There also appears to be particular cricopharyngeal dysfunction in persons with MS and dysphagia. A study by Abraham and Yun [59] found impairment of the UES in 100% of a small group of persons with MS with moderate impairment as measured by the EDSS.

Complications

In addition to reductions in quality of life, dysphagia in MS has been linked with enhanced risk for dehydration and aspiration pneumonia [60, 61]. These complications result in enhanced morbidity and ultimately death in late stages of MS [60–63].

Management

There are no pharmacologic treatments found to be efficacious for the treatment of dysphagia in persons with MS. Surgical myotomy has been used to treat UES hyperactivity [64–66] and a recent study found that botulinum neurotoxin type A injection of the CP is also effective for the treatment of oropharyngeal symptoms in select persons with MS [58]. It has been demonstrated that given the very low referral rates, only 2% of patients with MS and dysphagia receive behavioral treatment [67]. This is further complicated by a complete paucity of literature on the efficacy and effectiveness of swallowing rehabilitation in MS. It is considered that in milder cases of dysphagia, the treatment should focus on improvement of oral bolus control with later therapy focused on improved function of the pharyngeal mechanism [68]. A study investigating the effects of neuromuscular electrostimulation (NMES) on swallowing dysfunction in patients with MS demonstrated improvements in swallowing function. Following NMES these participants were found to have significantly less pooling of saliva in the pyriform sinuses and less incidence of aspiration [69].

Amyotrophic Lateral Sclerosis and Motor Neuron Disease

Definition

ALS, the most common of the motor neuron diseases, is a rapidly progressing neurodegenerative condition affecting both upper and lower motor neurons [70]. ALS is fatal and characterized by progressive muscular paralysis reflecting degeneration of motor neurons in the motor cortex, corticospinal tract, brainstem, and spinal cord. The clinical picture most often includes progressive limb weakness, respiratory insufficiency, spasticity, hyperreflexia, and bulbar symptoms [71]. Survival is about 2–5 years after confirmatory diagnosis, with death usually resulting from respiratory failure [70]. Motor neuron disease is sometimes used as a general classification comprising (1) ALS; (2) primary lateral sclerosis, with deterioration confined at least initially to the upper motor neurons of the spinal, bulbar, or both systems; and (3) lower motor neuron variants called spinal muscular atrophy when the spinal system is exclusively involved and progressive bulbar palsy when the bulbar system is the focus of disease. Life expectancy is longest for primary lateral sclerosis with severe dysphagia primarily involving delayed initiation of the pharyngeal swallow. Progressive bulbar palsy can have devastating and early effects on all stages of swallowing. Even when the disease is confined to the spinal system respiration can be affected especially in the lower motor neuron variant of the disease resulting in impaired ability to coordinate respiration, swallowing, and cough [72]. This section will focus on ALS, as most literature on dysphagia and motor neuron disease pertains to ALS versus other variations of motor neuron disease.

Prevalence/Incidence of Dysphagia

The incidence of ALS is about 2 in 100,000 [70]. Bulbar dysfunction is the presenting symptom in one-third of cases with ALS, but the incidence is markedly increased in later stages of the disease [73, 74]. It has been reported that 86% of those with ALS and bulbar involvement have dysphagia [75, 76].

Pathophysiology

Both upper and lower motor neuron involvement in ALS can result in dysphagic symptoms. Pseudobulbar palsy, or upper motor neuron involvement in ALS, often results in spasticity of the bulbar musculature. Degeneration of cranial nuclei in the brainstem results in flaccid pareses, muscular atrophy, and fasiculations and/or tongue fibrillations. Degeneration of motor neurons in the spinal cord can also result in dysphagic symptoms secondary to changes in the respiratory–swallow coordination and inefficiency of cough function [71, 77, 78].

Diagnosis

Motor neuron degeneration will result in changes to the spectrum of oropharyngeal swallowing which may begin with difficulty in lip control and end with cricopharyngeal dysfunction. A complete history identifying nutritional needs, current feeding strategies, and long-term plans for feeding and respiratory support is important to identify during the clinical evaluation. Instrumental assessment with videofluoropscopy seems to be most appropriate for identification of possible silent aspiration and involvement of all swallowing phases. With the possibility of reductions in motility, strength, and coordination of orofacial structures come likely impairments of bolus preparation, mastication, and oral transport. The patient with ALS will likely demonstrate dysfunction of the pharyngeal phase of swallowing, specifically poor pharyngeal stripping, poor laryngeal elevation, incomplete laryngeal closure, reduced extent and duration of cricopharyngeal opening, and reduced sensation in the laryngopharynx [79–84], especially if lower motor neuron deficits predominate. Reduced cough effectiveness is also likely [72].

Complications

Malnutrition has been identified as an independent risk factor for death in ALS. This, combined with the increased risk for airway obstruction and aspiration, results in markedly reduced life expectancy in patients with ALS [85, 86]. During the course of the disease, these marked changes of swallowing and feeding function adversely affect quality of life [87, 88].

Management

At all levels of management, care is often proactive and palliative in nature, and a multidisciplinary approach is considered a necessity. Most swallowing management is going to be compensatory in nature, with changes to position during feeding along with dietary modifications. The speech pathologist will often identify when it is no longer safe for the patient to eat orally, in cases where the patient has decided not to consider non-oral feeding, decisions regarding the safest possible diet should be made. In addition to education regarding proper diet, it is essential that the clinician educate the patient and family regarding the benefits of early PEG placement. This is especially salient given the data suggesting that PEG placement once the patient becomes nutrionally compromised may be inappropriate and even unsafe [89]. The safety and efficacy of behavioral swallowing therapy in ALS has been challenged; however, sensorimotor exercises in ALS have been considered to improve sensory response to the bolus in the oral and pharyngeal cavities [71]. The utility and safety of other rehabilitative swallowing exercises for ALS have not been well studied, but evidence from the training of the limbs in ALS would suggest that modest stretching, gentle strengthening, and even skill training as with a hard swallow may be beneficial [90].

Ataxia

Definition

Ataxia is characterized by dyscoordination manifest as irregular, erratic, jerky, and incomplete movements. Rate, range, and force of movement across structures such as the tongue, larynx, and velopharynx may be abnormal. These abnormal patterns, leading to over and undershooting of targets, have also been called asynergia or dyssynergia.

Any process damaging the cerebellum or pathways connecting cerebellum to other portions of the nervous system can cause ataxia. Common in clinical practice are the autosomal-dominant and autosomal-recessive ataxias. The spinocerebellar atrophies are autosomal-dominant. Dysphagia is especially likely in SCA-1 and SCA-3, also known as Machado–Joseph disease. Friedreich's ataxia (FRDA) and ataxia telangiectasia (AT) are among the most frequent autosomal-recessive ataxias, and dysphagia is a risk in both.

Prevalence/Incidence of Dysphagia

The prevalence of hereditary ataxias is estimated to be 6 per 100,000 [44]. FRDA is the most common inherited ataxia with an estimated prevalence of 1 per 30,000–50,000 Europeans [91]. Jardin and colleagues [92] report that 30 of 47 patients (64%) with Machado–Joseph disease (SCA-3) had dysphagia. Nagaya and colleagues [93] report aspiration in 30% of a heterogeneous group of ataxic patients. Twenty-one of 23 patients described in the study by Ramio-Torrenta et al. [94] complained of swallowing difficulty. All 23 had abnormal instrumental examinations.

Pathophysiology

Dyscoordination and hypotonia are the major influences on swallowing function in pure ataxia. Because other portions of the nervous system such as the brain stem, cortical, and subcortical structures may also be involved resulting in weakness, spasticity, hypokinesia, and cognitive deficits. Cognitive deficits including impaired learning ability may further complicate swallowing rehabilitation and its management. Dyscoordination alone may produce no or only a mild and functionally insignificant swallowing impairment.

Diagnosis

The medical diagnosis primarily depends on the neurologic examination and special imaging and genetic testing. The swallowing evaluation's purposes are to (1) establish the presence, signs, and severity of dysphagia, (2) assess the quality of life and health consequences, (3) hypothesize the specific underlying pathophysiology, and (4) determine patient's motivation, insight, and ability to learn

Complications

In a study of SCA-1, pulmonary complications, presumably at least in part resulting from dysphagia, were the major cause of death [95]. This and other health and quality of life consequences can be expected whenever severe dysphagia is present especially if mobility and independence are also compromised.

Management

Paulson and Ammache [96] identify speech therapy for dysphagia in ataxic disorders as being "especially helpful" (p 779) in part because medical and surgical treatment options are limited. Skill building treatments will be important because, depending on severity, patients may be able to compensate for their dysfunction by consciously trying to modify their behavior. Accompanying weakness or hypotonia will require simultaneous strengthening approaches. In our experience, intense and lengthy treatment duration is required.

Dystonia

Definition

Dystonia is a heterogenous pattern of involuntary, sustained, and repetitive muscle contractions resulting in abnormal postures and twisting movements of involved body parts. Dystonia is classified by age of onset—early versus late; by etiology—primary (idiopathic) or secondary (symptomatic); and by distribution—generalized, multifocal, segmental, or focal [97]. Regardless of onset, etiology, or distribution, swallowing will be altered if respiratory or bulbar musculature is affected. Among the dystonias of greatest significance to the swallowing specialist or deglutologist are spasmodic torticollis [98] and the oromandibular dystonias (OMDs) [99], including Meige syndrome sometimes called Brueghel's syndrome [100]. These distinctions are important because different sites of dystonic involvement may lead to different signs of dysphagia.

Prevalence/Incidence of Dysphagia

The prevalence for early onset dystonia ranges from 3 to 50 cases per 1,000,000 [97]. The range for late onset is 30–7,320 cases per 1,000,000. Focal dystonia is more common than generalized

dystonia and cervical dystonia is the most common of the focal dystonias. The incidence of oromandibular dystonia derived from a population study in Iceland was 2.8 per 1,000,000 [101]. Dystonia occurs more often in women than in men and varies by ethnicity. In a typical study, Ertekin and colleagues [98] report dysphagia in 76% of a mixed group of 25 dystonic patients. Oral abnormalities are more frequent than pharyngeal ones.

Pathophysiology

The simultaneous co-contraction of agonist and antagonistic muscle groups that defines dystonia disrupts the skilled movements necessary to normal swallowing. The cause may be genetic, sporadic, or secondary to acquired nervous system damage from trauma, disease, toxins, or medications. For a recent summary of the genetics of dystonia see Bruggemann and Klein [102]. Dystonia can also occur as an accompaniment to a variety of basal ganglia diseases including Parkinson's disease, Wilson's disease, corticobasal degeneration, and progressive supranuclear palsy.

Diagnosis

The medical diagnosis rests primarily on a history and neurologic examination supplemented by genetic testing and imaging. The swallowing diagnosis will include history; physical examination of the respiratory and bulbar musculature including non-speech and speech tasks; a clinical swallowing examination; and an instrumented evaluation, in most instances the videofluoroscopic swallowing examination. Evaluation's goals are to (1) establish the likelihood that a patient has dystonia alone or in combination with other neurologic abnormalities, (2) define the dystonia's distribution across the respiratory and swallowing structures, and (3) identify the resulting swallowing abnormalities. During the instrumented examination special attention should be paid to the influence of sensory tricks and posture and to teasing out the influence of dystonia on the interaction of oral and pharyngeal stages. In cervical dystonia, oral stage abnormalities include abnormal bolus preparation [103]. In Meige syndrome pre-swallow spill is a common finding [104]. Pharyngeal abnormalities in both cervical and oromandibualr dystonia include post-swallow pharyngeal residue particularly in the vallecula. Asymmetric bolus transport is more likely to occur in cervical dystonia [105, 106].

Complications

Embarrassment, social isolation, weight loss, and aspiration are possible functional consequences with the psychosocial implications often outweighing the physical.

Management

The primary treatments of dystonia are botulinum toxin injection and deep brain stimulation (DBS) [100]. DBS's positive effects for Meige syndrome are reported by Ghang and colleagues [107] and Lyons et al. [108]. Transcranial magnetic stimulation (TMS) to somatosensory cortex is promising [109].

Behavioral therapy for dysphagia secondary to dystonia has been compensatory. Postural stabilization may reduce swallowing symptoms secondary to abnormal posture. In addition, because enhanced sensory input (geste antagoniste) such as touching the cheek, neck, jaw, or other bulbar structures can sometimes reduce dystonia, it behooves the clinician to inquire if a patient has discovered such methods and furthermore to evaluate the effects of touching the neck, face, and head. The array of rehabilitation techniques can be employed, but recent data on neurorehabilitation and treatments for focal dystonia of the hand should motivate new treatments. For example, Candia and colleagues [110] base a treatment on principles of neural reorganization and functional imaging data of cortical maps in cases of focal hand dystonia. Their method, SMR, involves splinting different combinations of non-dystonic fingers and then having the participant use the dystonic finger(s) in various skilled movements with various combinations of normal fingers. The goal is reestablishment of the normal patterns of cortical finger representation and an accompanying improvement in dystonic finger movement. The hypothesis that dystonia results in part from alterations in what Vitek [111] calls somatosensory responsiveness should motivate research into sensory stimulation as part of dysphagia treatment.

Chorea

Definition

Chorea is defined as a series of quick, unpredictable, irregular, jerking movements. Impaired voluntary movements, delayed initiation, and slowness of movement are also features of chorea and may involve one or multiple body parts. Chorea can occur in a number of syndromes such as Wilson's disease (discussed later in this chapter), but occurs primarily in two conditions—Huntington's disease (HD) and Sydenham's chorea (SC). SC is a rare condition that is the result of infection in children and usually resolves spontaneously. HD is an inherited disorder of adults with chorea beginning often in the hands and face and generalizing to other body parts. Behavior change and dementia are also hallmarks of this relentlessly progressive disease that ends in severe dementia, anarthria, and aphagia.

Prevalence/Incidence

HD occurs with a prevalence of 2–12 persons per 100,000 [44]. Klasner [112], referencing National Institutes of Health data, says approximately 30,000 new cases of HD are diagnosed in the United States each year. Age of onset is typically between 30 and 45, although earlier or later onset is possible. Disease duration is usually 15–20 years [113]. Eating and swallowing abnormalities occur in nearly 100% of patients at some time during the disease's course. More specifically, Yorkston et al. [114] describe choreatic involvement of the respiratory mechanism in 40%, aspiration and aerophagia in 10%, and excessive belching or eructation in 40%.

Pathophysiology

Pathophysiology of dysphagia in HD is complex. Patients may be primarily hyperkinetic, hypokinetic, or both. Dyscoordination may be a major or secondary influence on skilled eating and swallowing movements. Affective disorders, including apathy, and other cognitive abnormalities, including impulsivity, may complicate swallowing signs, evaluation, and treatment.

Diagnosis

Aims of diagnosis are the same as for previously discussed conditions. Of special importance in chorea are clinical and eating evaluations. Tachyphagia or fast eating and belching are among the signs that may be missed with an instrumented examination although such an examination may inform the clinician about underlying swallowing physiology. Chorea makes patience and special positioning during instrumental examination a necessity. Allowing self-administered boluses may inform the clinician about the difference between caregiver and self-administered bolus consumption. A substantial challenge is identifying the focus of abnormality, whether it is respiratory, oral, or pharyngeal involvement alone or in combination.

Complications

Common health consequences include aspiration pneumonia, dehydration, malnutrition, and weight loss. The medications utilized to treat chorea may further degrade swallowing [115]. Tachyphagia, belching, and abnormal movements may lead to social isolation and a host of other psychosocial consequences. The incidence of fatal airway obstruction may be elevated.

Management

Bilney, Morris, and Perry [116] found only "a small amount of evidence to support the use of speech pathology services or that of a swallowing specialist for the management of eating and swallowing disorders" in HD (p 12). Nonetheless, treatment can be offered. Kagel and Leopold [117] support the use of a variety of compensations including the use of a weighted cup and wrist and leg weights. If the patient has a more rigid form of HD, maximum performance and even muscle strengthening exercises may be appropriate. The affective and behavioral abnormalities make treatment difficult, and the clinician must consider the cost–benefit ratio of introducing treatment.

Myasthenia Gravis

Definition

Myasthenia graves (MG) is a rare auto-immune disease affecting the neuromuscular junction. MG can be classified as either ocular or generalized. Ocular MG affects extraocular muscles specifically, but can often develop into generalized MG at which time the oropharygeal musculature may be involved [118]. Presentation of MG usually occurs with ocular symptoms (60%), but there have been cases of oropharyngeal muscle weakness as the presenting symptom [119].

Prevalence/Incidence

One in every 5,000 people will develop MG [120, 121]. Forty percent of persons with MG will develop dysphagia during the course of the disease [122]. Only 6–15% will present with dysphagia [123].

Pathophysiology

Weakness and fatiguability of facial, jaw, buccal, lingual, and pharyngeal muscles are thought to contribute to the etiology of swallowing dysfunction in MG. Electrophysiological studies of laryngeal function have demonstrated abnormalities suggesting that the neuromuscular junctions of the corticobulbar tract can be affected by MG [124]. It is considered that antibodies working against the acetylcholine receptors result in deficits to neuromuscular transmission [125, 126]. The relapsing and remitting of swallowing disturbance in this population is often observed, and relapse usually signals worsening of overall condition.

Diagnosis

When gathering the patient history it is important to identify changes in swallowing function that may occur as the day and time spent in eating progress. VFES is the gold standard as changes are evident throughout the swallowing mechanism. In some cases dysfunction will be specific to orofacial structures, but the pharyngeal phase of swallowing seems to be the most significantly impaired in MG with pharyngeal phase delay and particular impairment in laryngeal elevation and epiglottic inversion [127]. Abbreviated videofluoroscopic swallowing examinations before and after tensilon testing may contribute both diagnostic and prognostic information.

Complications

Dysphagia with aspiration is often a source of morbidity and mortality in MG [119]. Additionally, the strain of intermittent and often embarrassing swallow disturbance can be detrimental to quality of life.

Management

MG is a treatable disease, and pharmacological management is the first line of treatment. Treatments, however, are often more effective for corticospinal than corticobulbar symptoms. Both compensatory and restorative swallow-specific treatments can be utilized. Given the worsening of symptoms with continued muscle fatigue, smaller more frequent meals are essential for maintaining swallowing safety and good nutritional state. Exercises aimed at increasing muscle strength of the oropharyngeal mechanism are limited by fatiguing of muscles and in some cases may be inappropriate [127]. Skill-based treatments may be an alternative to strengthening but have not been well studied in this population. Compensatory treatments are frequently offered and include diet modification, postural adjustment, and in severely affected individuals, non-oral feeding. Exacerbations or relapsing of dysphagia in MG will often result in changes to pharmacological management with increased doses of cholinergic agents, immunomodulatory therapies, and even initiation of plasma exchange.

Rare Disorders

There is a subset of rarer neurodegenerative disorders that may lead to dysphagia and for which we provide a more cursory review below.

Wilson's Disease

Wilson disease is an autosomal-recessive genetic disorder that can result in neurodegeneration

[128]. The disease is characterized primarily by a disorder of copper metabolism which can result in a build up of copper in the liver, eyes, and central nervous system at times manifesting as a movement disorder. Unless WD is diagnosed and treated early in the disease's course, muscular discoordination, tremor, muscle stiffness, behavioral changes, and resultant dysarthria and dysphagia can occur [129]. Imaging studies have identified lesions throughout the neuroaxis including cerebral cortex, white matter, cerebellum, thalamus, and basal ganglia all of which might result in dysphagia [130, 131]. Swallow-specific symptoms include prolonged oral transit times and greater percentage of oral residue when compared to age-matched healthy individuals [132]. Additional parkinsonian swallowing deficits are also common. Lifelong treatment is required to control the disease, but if identified promptly and treated appropriately patients can maintain function long term. Therefore, treatment of swallowing dysfunction should have marked impact for health and quality of life.

Post-polio Syndrome

Post-polio syndrome is a neurologic disorder occurring in about 5% of individuals at least 15 years after infection with the polio virus. PPS has been reported to result in weakness, fatigue, and reduced endurance of limbs, trunk, respiratory, and oropharyngeal musculature [133, 134] with subsequent muscle atrophy, respiratory insufficiency, dysphonia, and dysphagia [135, 136]. As in other neurodegenerative diseases, dysphagia in PPS is the result of a slow progressive deterioration to bulbar functioning [135–138]. The proper management of dysphagia in PPS requires further investigation.

Guillain–Barre Syndrome

Guillain–Barre syndrome (GBS) is an acute, immune-based disorder of the peripheral nervous system usually following an infectious process. GBS results in a paralysis beginning in the lower extremities which quickly ascends to the upper extremities and bulbar musculature [139]. Management in the acute phases of the syndrome is centered on sustaining life through control of autonomic dysfunction. Management of insidious swallowing dysfunction is secondary. Following the acute phase of the disease, patients may have mild to severe changes to the swallowing mechanism and respiration. The manifestation of swallowing dysfunction will depend on the affected cranial and/or spinal nerves involved with impairments including difficulty with bolus formation and aspiration/penetration. If respiration is also involved, coordination of swallowing and respiration may be disrupted. For example the person may have difficulty prolonging the apneic period of swallow sufficiently to allow safe, adequate oral feeding. Swallowing management may include compensatory or behavioral techniques. Treatment effects must be carefully monitored, as efficacy data is limited.

References

1. Gelb DJ, Oliver E, Gilman S. Diagnostic criteria for Parkinson disease. Arch Neurol. 1999;56(1): 33–9.
2. Braak H, et al. Stages in the development of Parkinson's disease-related pathology. Cell Tissue Res. 2004;318(1):121–34.
3. Bassotti G, et al. Esophageal manometric abnormalities in Parkinson's disease. Dysphagia. 1998;13(1):28–31.
4. Coates C, Bakheit AM. Dysphagia in Parkinson's disease. Eur Neurol. 1997;38(1):49–52.
5. Hunter PC, et al. Response of parkinsonian swallowing dysfunction to dopaminergic stimulation. J Neurol Neurosurg Psychiatry. 1997;63(5):579–83.
6. Logemann JA, Blonsky ER, Boshes B. Editorial: dysphagia in parkinsonism. J Am Med Assoc. 1975;231(1):69–70.
7. Mari F, et al. Predictive value of clinical indices in detecting aspiration in patients with neurological disorders. J Neurol Neurosurg Psychiatry. 1997; 63(4):456–60.
8. Bushmann M, et al. Swallowing abnormalities and their response to treatment in Parkinson's disease. Neurology. 1989;39(10):1309–14.
9. Lieberman AN, et al. Dysphagia in Parkinson's disease. Am J Gastroenterol. 1980;74(2):157–60.
10. Eadie MJ, Tyrer JH. Radiological abnormalities of the upper part of the alimentary tract in parkinsonism. Australas Ann Med. 1965;14:23–7.
11. Ertekin C, et al. Electrophysiological evaluation of pharyngeal phase of swallowing in patients with Parkinson's disease. Mov Disord. 2002;17(5): 942–9.
12. Edwards LL, Quigley EM, Pfeiffer RF. Gastrointestinal dysfunction in Parkinson's disease: frequency and pathophysiology. Neurology. 1992;42(4):726–32.
13. Ali GN, et al. Mechanisms of oral-pharyngeal dysphagia in patients with Parkinson's disease. Gastroenterology. 1996;110(2):383–92.
14. Blonsky ER, et al. Comparison of speech and swallowing function in patients with tremor disorders and in normal geriatric patients: a cinefluorographic study. J Gerontol. 1975;30(3):299–303.
15. Born LJ, et al. Cricopharyngeal dysfunction in Parkinson's disease: role in dysphagia and response to myotomy. Mov Disord. 1996;11(1):53–8.
16. Leopold NA, Kagel MC. Laryngeal deglutition movement in Parkinson's disease. Neurology. 1997;48(2):373–6.
17. Leopold NA, Kagel MC. Pharyngo-esophageal dysphagia in Parkinson's disease. Dysphagia. 1997;12(1):11–8. discussion 19–20.
18. Leopold NA, Kagel MC. Prepharyngeal dysphagia in Parkinson's disease. Dysphagia. 1996;11(1):14–22.
19. Nagaya M, et al. Videofluorographic study of swallowing in Parkinson's disease. Dysphagia. 1998;13(2): 95–100.
20. Stroudley J, Walsh M. Radiological assessment of dysphagia in Parkinson's disease. Br J Radiol. 1991;64(766):890–3.
21. Eadie MJ, Tyrer JH. Alimentary disorder in parkinsonism. Australas Ann Med. 1965;14:13–22.
22. Gross RD, et al. The coordination of breathing and swallowing in Parkinson's disease. Dysphagia. 2008;23(2):136–45.
23. Lim A, et al. A pilot study of respiration and swallowing integration in Parkinson's disease: "on" and "off" levodopa. Dysphagia. 2008;23(1):76–81.
24. Pinnington LL, et al. Non-invasive assessment of swallowing and respiration in Parkinson's disease. J Neurol. 2000;247(10):773–7.
25. Salat-Foix D, et al. Gastrointestinal symptoms in Parkinson disease: clinical aspects and management. Can J Neurol Sci. 2011;38(4):557–64.
26. Morgante L, et al. Parkinson disease survival: a population-based study. Arch Neurol. 2000;57(4): 507–12.
27. Fernandez HH, Lapane KL. Predictors of mortality among nursing home residents with a diagnosis of Parkinson's disease. Med Sci Monit. 2002;8(4): CR241–6.
28. Gorell JM, Johnson CC, Rybibki BA. Parkinson's disease and its comorbid disorders: an analysis of Michigan mortality data, 1970 to 1990. Neurology. 1994;44:1865–8.
29. Hoehn MM, Yahr MD. Parkinsonism: onset, progression, and mortality. Neurology. 1967;17(5): 427–42.

30. Shill H, Stacy M. Respiratory complications of Parkinson's disease. Semin Respir Crit Care Med. 2002;23(3):261–5.

31. Singer RB. Mortality in patients with Parkinson's disease treated with dopa. J Insur Med. 1992;24(2):126–7.

32. Fall PA, et al. Survival time, mortality, and cause of death in elderly patients with Parkinson's disease: a 9-year follow-up. Mov Disord. 2003;18(11):1312–6.

33. Menezes C, Melo A. Does levodopa improve swallowing dysfunction in Parkinson's disease patients? J Clin Pharm Ther. 2009;34(6):673–6.

34. Robbins J, et al. Comparison of 2 interventions for liquid aspiration on pneumonia incidence: a randomized trial. Ann Intern Med. 2008;148(7):509–18.

35. Troche MS, et al. Aspiration and swallowing in Parkinson disease and rehabilitation with EMST: a randomized trial. Neurology. 2010;75(21):1912–9.

36. El Sharkawi A, et al. Swallowing and voice effects of Lee Silverman voice treatment (LSVT): a pilot study. J Neurol Neurosurg Psychiatry. 2002;72(1):31–6.

37. Nagaya M, Kachi T, Yamada T. Effect of swallowing training on swallowing disorders in Parkinson's disease. Scand J Rehabil Med. 2000;32(1):11–5.

38. Troche MS, Sapienza CM, Rosenbek JC. Effects of bolus consistency on timing and safety of swallow in patients with Parkinson's disease. Dysphagia. 2008;23(1):26–32.

39. Byrne KG, Pfeiffer R, Quigley EM. Gastrointestinal dysfunction in Parkinson's disease. A report of clinical experience at a single center. J Clin Gastroenterol. 1994;19(1):11–6.

40. Watts CC, Whurr R, Nye C. Botulinum toxin injections for the treatment of spasmodic dysphonia. Cochrane Database Syst Rev. 2004;3:CD004327.

41. Gilman S, et al. Consensus statement on the diagnosis of multiple system atrophy. J Neurol Sci. 1999;163(1):94–8.

42. Higo H. Multiple system atrophy (MSA). In: Jones HN, Rosenbek JC, editors. Dysphagia in rare conditions: an encyclopedia. San Diego: Plural Publishing; 2010. p. 385–91.

43. Litvan I, et al. Clinical research criteria for the diagnosis of progressive supranuclear palsy (Steele-Richardson-olszewski syndrome): report of the NINDS-SPSP international workshop. Neurology. 1996;47(1):1–9.

44. Fernandez HH, et al. Movement disorders: diagnosis and surgical and medical management. New York: Demos Medical Publishing; 2007.

45. Ben-Shlomo Y, et al. Survival of patients with pathologically proven multiple system atrophy: a meta-analysis. Neurology. 1997;48(2):384–93.

46. Shulman LM, Minagar A, Weiner WJ. Multiple-system atrophy. In: Watts RL, Koller WC, editors. Movement disorders: neurologic principles and practice. New York: McGraw-Hill; 2004. p. 359–69.

47. Higo R, et al. Videofluoroscopic and manometric evaluation of swallowing function in patients with multiple system atrophy. Ann Otol Rhinol Laryngol. 2003;112(7):630–6.

48. Golbe LI. The epidemiology of PSP. J Neural Transm Suppl. 1994;42:263–73.

49. Litvan I, Sastry N, Sonies BC. Characterizing swallowing abnormalities in progressive supranuclear palsy. Neurology. 1997;48(6):1654–62.

50. Merlo IM, et al. Not paralysis, but dystonia causes stridor in multiple system atrophy. Neurology. 2002;58(4):649–52.

51. Alfonsi E, et al. Electrophysiologic patterns of oral-pharyngeal swallowing in parkinsonian syndromes. Neurology. 2007;68(8):583–9.

52. Higo R, Nito T, Tayama N. Swallowing function in patients with multiple-system atrophy with a clinical predominance of cerebellar symptoms (MSA-C). Eur Arch Otorhinolaryngol. 2005;262(8):646–50.

53. Muller J, et al. Progression of dysarthria and dysphagia in postmortem-confirmed parkinsonian disorders. Arch Neurol. 2001;58(2):259–64.

54. Compston A, Coles A. Multiple sclerosis. Lancet. 2008;372(9648):1502–17.

55. Lublin FD, Reingold SC. Defining the clinical course of multiple sclerosis: results of an international survey. National multiple sclerosis society (USA) advisory committee on clinical trials of New agents in multiple sclerosis. Neurology. 1996;46(4):907–11.

56. Abraham S, et al. Neurologic impairment and disability status in outpatients with multiple sclerosis reporting dysphagia symptomatology. J Neurol Rehabil. 1997;11:7–13.

57. Poorjavad M, et al. Oropharyngeal dysphagia in multiple sclerosis. Mult Scler. 2010;16(3):362–5.

58. Restivo DA, et al. Botulinum toxin improves dysphagia associated with multiple sclerosis. Eur J Neurol. 2010;18:486–90.

59. Abraham SS, Yun PT. Laryngopharyngeal dysmotility in multiple sclerosis. Dysphagia. 2002;17(1):69–74.

60. Marchese-Ragona R, et al. Evaluation of swallowing disorders in multiple sclerosis. Neurol Sci. 2006;27:335–7.

61. Calcagno P, et al. Dysphagia in multiple sclerosis—prevalence and prognostic factors. Acta Neurol Scand. 2002;105(1):40–3.

62. Restivo DA, Marchese-Ragona R. Botulinum toxin treatment for oropharyngeal dysphagia due to tetanus. J Neurol. 2006;253(3):388–9.

63. Thomas FJ, Wiles CM. Dysphagia and nutritional status in multiple sclerosis. J Neurol. 1999;246(8):677–82.

64. McKenna JA, Dedo HH. Cricopharyngeal myotomy: indications and technique. Ann Otol Rhinol Laryngol. 1996;101:216–21.

65. Duranceau A. Cricopharyngeal myotomy in the management of neurogenic and muscular dysphagia. Neuromusc Disord. 1997;7:S85–95.

66. Fradet G, et al. Upper esophageal sphincter myotomy in oculopharyngeal muscular dystrophy: long-term clinical results. Neuromusc Disord. 1997;7:S90–5.

67. Hartelius L, Svensson P. Speech and swallowing symptoms associated with Parkinson's disease and multiple sclerosis: a survey. Folia Phoniatr Logop. 1994;46(1):9–17.

68. Giusti A, Giambuzzi M. Management of dysphagia in patients affected by multiple sclerosis: state of the art. Neurol Sci. 2008;29 Suppl 4:S364–6.

69. Bogaardt H, et al. Use of neuromuscular electrostimulation in the treatment of dysphagia in patients with multiple sclerosis. Ann Otol Rhinol Laryngol. 2009;118(4):241–6.

70. Mitsumoto H, Przedborski S, Gordon PH. Amyotrophic lateral sclerosis. New York: Taylor and Francis; 2006.

71. Kuhnlein P, et al. Diagnosis and treatment of bulbar symptoms in amyotrophic lateral sclerosis. Nat Clin Pract Neurol. 2008;4(7):366–74.

72. Miller RM, Britton D. Dysphagia in neuromuscular diseases. San Diego: Plural Publishing; 2011.

73. Haverkamp LJ, Appel V, Appel SH. Natural history of amyotrophic lateral sclerosis in a database population. Validation of a scoring system and a model for survival prediction. Brain. 1995;118(Pt 3):707–19.

74. Oliver D. The quality of care and symptom control–the effects on the terminal phase of ALS/MND. J Neurol Sci. 1996;139(Suppl):134–6.

75. Carpenter 3rd RJ, McDonald TJ, Howard Jr FM. The otolaryngologic presentation of amyotrophic lateral sclerosis. Otolaryngology. 1978;86(3 Pt 1): ORL479–84.

76. Chen A, Garrett CG. Otolaryngologic presentations of amyotrophic lateralsclerosis. Otolaryngol Head Neck Surg. 2005;132(3):500–4.

77. Lowe JS, Leigh N. Disorders of movement and system degenerations. In: Graham DI, Lantos PL, editors. Greenfield's neuropathology. London: Arnold; 2010. p. 325–430.

78. Strand EA, et al. Management of oral-pharyngeal dysphagia symptoms in amyotrophic lateral sclerosis. Dysphagia. 1996;11(2):129–39.

79. Hillel AD, et al. Amyotrophic lateral sclerosis severity scale. Neuroepidemiology. 1989;8(3):142–50.

80. Higo R, Tayama N, Nito T. Longitudinal analysis of progression of dysphagia in amyotrophic lateral sclerosis. Auris Nasus Larynx. 2004;31(3):247–54.

81. Kawai S, et al. A study of the early stage of dysphagia in amyotrophic lateral sclerosis. Dysphagia. 2003;18(1):1–8.

82. Robbins J. Swallowing in ALS and motor neuron disorders. Neurol Clin. 1987;5(2):213–29.

83. Newall AR, Orser R, Hunt M. The control of oral secretions in bulbar ALS/MND. J Neurol Sci. 1996;139(Suppl):43–4.

84. Amin MR, et al. Sensory testing in the assessment of laryngeal sensation in patients with amyotrophic lateral sclerosis. Ann Otol Rhinol Laryngol. 2006;115(7):528–34.

85. Desport JC, et al. Nutritional status is a prognostic factor for survival in ALS patients. Neurology. 1999;53(5):1059–63.

86. Kasarskis EJ, et al. Nutritional status of patients with amyotrophic lateral sclerosis: relation to the proximity of death. Am J Clin Nutr. 1996;63(1): 130–7.

87. Bourke SC, et al. Effects of non-invasive ventilation on survival and quality of life in patients with amyotrophic lateral sclerosis: a randomised controlled trial. Lancet Neurol. 2006;5(2):140–7.

88. Worwood AM, Leigh PN. Indicators and prevalence of malnutrition in motor neurone disease. Eur Neurol. 1998;40(3):159–63.

89. Beggs K, Choi M, Travlos A. Assessing and predicting successful tube placement outcomes in ALS patients. Amyotroph Lateral Scler. 2010;11(1–2): 203–6.

90. Cup EH, et al. Exercise therapy and other types of physical therapy for patients with neuromuscular diseases: a systematic review. Arch Phys Med Rehabil. 2007;88(11):1452–64.

91. Victor M, Ropper AH. Principles of neurology. New York: McGraw-Hill; 2001.

92. Jardim LB, et al. Neurologic findings in Machado-Joseph disease: relation with disease duration, subtypes, and (CAG)n. Arch Neurol. 2001;58(6): 899–904.

93. Nagaya M, et al. Videofluorographic observations on swallowing in patients with dysphagia due to neurodegenerative diseases. Nagoya J Med Sci. 2004;67(1–2):17–23.

94. Ramio-Torrenta L, Gomez E, Genis D. Swallowing in degenerative ataxias. J Neurol. 2006;253(7): 875–81.

95. Genis D, et al. Clinical, neuropathologic, and genetic studies of a large spinocerebellar ataxia type 1 (SCA1) kindred: (CAG)n expansion and early premonitory signs and symptoms. Neurology. 1995;45(1):24–30.

96. Paulson H, Ammache Z. Ataxia and hereditary disorders. Neurol Clin. 2001;19(3):759–82. viii.

97. Tagliati M, et al. Deep brain stimulation for dystonia. Expert Rev Med Devices. 2004;1(1):33–41.

98. Ertekin C, et al. Oropharyngeal swallowing in craniocervical dystonia. J Neurol Neurosurg Psychiatry. 2002;73(4):406–11.

99. Papapetropoulos S, Papapetropoulos N, Salcedo AG. Oromandibular dystonia (OMD). In: Jones HN, Rosenbek JC, editors. Dysphagia in rare conditions: an encyclopedia. San Diego: Plural Publishing; 2010. p. 443–8.

100. Jones HN. Meige syndrome. In: Rosenbek IHJJ, editor. Dysphagia in rare conditions: an encyclopedia. San Diego: Plural Publishing; 2010. p. 361–8.

101. Asgeirsson H, et al. Prevalence study of primary dystonia in Iceland. Mov Disord. 2006;21(3): 293–8.

102. Bruggemann N, Klein C. Genetics of primary torsion dystonia. Curr Neurol Neurosci Rep. 2010;10(3):199–206.

103. Horner J, et al. Swallowing in torticollis before and after rhizotomy. Dysphagia. 1992;7(3):117–25.

104. Cersosimo MG, et al. Swallowing disorders in patients with blepharospasm. Medicina (B Aires). 2005;65(2):117–20.
105. Horner J, et al. Swallowing, speech, and brainstem auditory-evoked potentials in spasmodic torticollis. Dysphagia. 1993;8(1):29–34.
106. Riski JE, Horner J, Nashold Jr BS. Swallowing function in patients with spasmodic torticollis. Neurology. 1990;40(9):1443–5.
107. Ghang JY, et al. Outcome of pallidal deep brain stimulation in Meige syndrome. J Kor Neurosurg Soc. 2010;48(2):134–8.
108. Lyons MK, et al. Long-term follow-up of deep brain stimulation for Meige syndrome. Neurosurg Focus. 2010;29(2):E5.
109. Havrankova P, et al. Repetitive TMS of the somatosensory cortex improves writer's cramp and enhances cortical activity. Neuro Endocrinol Lett. 2010;31(1):73–86.
110. Candia V, et al. Sensory motor retuning: a behavioral treatment for focal hand dystonia of pianists and guitarists. Arch Phys Med Rehabil. 2002;83(10):1342–8.
111. Vitek JL. Pathophysiology of dystonia: a neuronal model. Mov Disord. 2002;17 Suppl 3:S49–62.
112. Klasner ER. Huntington disease. In: Jones HN, Rosenbek JC, editors. Dysphagia in rare conditions: an encyclopedia. San Diego: Plural Publishing; 2010. p. 267–72.
113. Rosenbek J, Jones H. Dysphagia in movement disorders. San Diego: Plural Publishing; 2008.
114. Yorkston KM, Miller RM, Strand EA. Management of speech and swallowing in degenerative diseases. 2nd ed. San Antonio: Communication Skill Builders; 2004.
115. Walker FO. Huntington's disease. Semin Neurol. 2007;27(2):143–50.
116. Bilney B, Morris ME, Perry A. Effectiveness of physiotherapy, occupational therapy, and speech pathology for people with Huntington's disease: a systematic review. Neurorehabil Neural Repair. 2003;17(1):12–24.
117. Kagel MC, Leopold NA. Dysphagia in Huntington's disease: a 16-year retrospective. Dysphagia. 1992;7(2):106–14.
118. Juel VC, Massey JM. Myasthenia gravis. Orphanet J Rare Dis. 2007;2(44):1–13.
119. Thomas CE, et al. Myasthenic crisis: clinical features, mortality, complications, and risk factors for prolonged intubation. Neurology. 1997;48(5):1253–60.
120. Vincent A. Unravelling the pathogenesis of myasthenia gravis. Nat Rev Immunol. 2002;2(10):797–804.
121. Conti-Fine BM, Milani M, Kaminski HJ. Myasthenia gravis: past, present, and future. J Clin Invest. 2006;116(11):2843–54.
122. Huang MH, King KL, Chien KY. Esophageal manometric studies in patients with myasthenia gravis. J Thorac Cardiovasc Surg. 1988;95(2):281–5.
123. Grob D, et al. The course of myasthenia gravis and therapies affecting outcome. Ann N Y Acad Sci. 1987;505:472–99.
124. Xu W, et al. Clinical and electrophysiological characteristics of larynx in myasthenia gravis. Ann Otol Rhinol Laryngol. 2009;118(9):656–61.
125. Hughes BW, Moro De Casillas ML, Kaminski HJ. Pathophysiology of myasthenia gravis. Semin Neurol. 2004;24(1):21–30.
126. Vincent A, Newsom DJ. Anti-acetylcholine receptor antibodies. J Neurol Neurosurg Psychiatry. 1980;43(7):590–600.
127. Colton-Hudson A, et al. A prospective assessment of the characteristics of dysphagia in myasthenia gravis. Dysphagia. 2002;17(2):147–51.
128. Ferenci P. Wilson's disease. Clin Liver Dis. 1998;2(1):31–49. v-vi.
129. Ferenci P. Review article: diagnosis and current therapy of Wilson's disease. Aliment Pharmacol Ther. 2004;19(2):157–65.
130. Oder W, et al. Wilson's disease: evidence of subgroups derived from clinical findings and brain lesions. Neurology. 1993;43(1):120–4.
131. van Wassenaer-van Hall HN, et al. Wilson disease: findings at MR imaging and CT of the brain with clinical correlation. Radiology. 1996;198(2):531–6.
132. da Silva-Junior FP, et al. Swallowing dysfunction in Wilson's disease: a scintigraphic study. Neurogastroenterol Motil. 2008;20(4):285–90.
133. Sonies B. Postpolio syndrome. In: Jones HN, Rosenbek JC, editors. Dysphagia in rare conditions: an encyclopedia. San Diego: Plural Publishing; 2010. p. 465–6.
134. Halstead LS. Diagnosing postpolio syndrome: inclusion and exclusion criteria. In: Silver JK, Gawne AC, editors. Postpolio syndrome. Philadelphia: Hanley and Belfus; 2004. p. 1–20.
135. Sonies BC, Dalakas MC. Dysphagia in patients with the post-polio syndrome. N Engl J Med. 1991;324(17):1162–7.
136. Sonies BC, Dalakas MC. Progression of oral-motor and swallowing symptoms in the post-polio syndrome. Ann N Y Acad Sci. 1995;753:87–95.
137. Sonies BC. Speech and swallowing in post-polio syndrome. In: Halstead LS, Grimby G, editors. Postpolio syndrome. Philadelphia: Hanley and Belfus; 2004. p. 105–16.
138. Sonies BC. Oropharyngeal dysphagia in the elderly. Clin Geriatr Med. 1992;8(3):569–77.
139. Dikeman K, Kazandjian M. Guillain-Barre syndrome (GBS). In: Jones HN, Rosenbek JC, editors. Dysphagia in rare conditions: an encyclopedia. San Diego: Plural Publishing; 2010. p. 243–8.

Disorders of Appetite, Eating, and Swallowing in the Dementias

28

Manabu Ikeda and John Hodges

Abstract

It is well known that eating problems occur in association with cognitive dysfunction, psychiatric problems, and decline of daily activity in individuals with dementia. Feeding and eating difficulties leading to weight loss are common in the advanced stages of dementia. In contrast to the wealth of information on advanced dementia, relatively few studies have addressed the eating problems in mild dementia and disease-specific behaviors. As the disease progresses, patients with Alzheimer's disease (AD) have difficulty swallowing due to sensory impairment secondary to dysfunctions in the temporoparietal areas. Vascular dementia patients showed more deficits in bolus formation and mastication of semisolid food, hyolaryngeal excursion, epiglottic inversion, and silent aspiration caused by motor impairments due to disruptions in the corticobulbar tract. The frequencies of appetite change, alterations in food preference toward sweet foods and changed eating habits, are greater in Frontotemporal lobar degeneration (FTLD) than in AD. Appetite increase in FTLD seem to be exacerbated by cultural factors in Western countries. Dementia with Lewy bodies patients showed a higher incidence of swallowing problems and anorexia than AD patients.

Keywords

Eating behavior • Swallowing problem • Dementia • Alzheimer's disease • Vascular dementia • Frontotemporal lobar degeneration • Dementia with Lewy bodies • Introduction

M. Ikeda, MD, PhD (✉)
Department of Neuropsychiatry, Kumamoto University,
1-1-1 Honjo, Kumamoto 860-8556, Japan
e-mail: mikeda@kumamoto-u.ac.jp

J. Hodges, MBBS, MD, FRCP
Neuroscience Research, Frontier Barker Street,
Randwick, Sydney, NSW 2031, Australia

R. Shaker et al. (eds.), *Principles of Deglutition: A Multidisciplinary Text for Swallowing and its Disorders*, 411
DOI 10.1007/978-1-4614-3794-9_28, © Springer Science+Business Media New York 2013

It is well known that eating problems occur in association with cognitive dysfunction, psychiatric problems, and decline of daily activity in individuals with dementia [1, 2]. Among the daily activities in older people, eating is fundamental to independence and a good quality of life. A survey by the Alzheimer's Society (2000) revealed a high level of concern among caregivers about problems such as poor appetite and weight loss [3]. Several studies have reported the pattern and prevalence of eating disturbance in severe dementia. Patients with dementia have difficulty understanding the concept of meal times, frequently become confused and forgetful, and as a consequence, stop eating. Dysphagia may lead to aspiration pneumonia, a common cause of death in the later stage of dementia. A study of nursing home residents with advanced dementia showed that more than half had episodes of chest infection, and 86% had eating problems over the course of 18 months [4]. A study of nurses and other caregivers revealed that feeding was a daily problem in severe dementia [5]. In contrast to the wealth of information on advanced dementia, relatively few studies have addressed the eating problems in mild dementia and disease-specific behaviors.

Eating behaviors are modulated by many factors including personal habits, ethnic culture, and climate. Food culture, meal styles, and customs differ substantially between Western Countries and Japan. For example, bread is a staple in the West while rice is a staple in Japan and Japanese use chopsticks instead of forks and knives. People in the UK eat more sweets/candies and a higher total daily calorific intake than Japanese people. Calorie intakes are 3,227 kcal/day on average in the UK population while only 2,622 kcal/day in Japan. Sugar and sweetener consumption are 43.7 kg/person/year on average in the UK population compared to 29.4 kg/person/year in Japan [6]. Eating behaviors in demented patients may, therefore, differ from other behavioral and psychiatric features such as loss of insight, apathy, mood change, and hallucinations. A cross-cultural perspective is of particular importance when investigating eating behaviors in dementia patients.

The purpose of this chapter is to review the unique characteristics of swallowing dysfunction and eating behavior for various dementia syndromes and discuss issues from a socio-cultural perspective.

Alzheimer's Disease

Alzheimer's disease (AD) is the most prevalent form of dementia, accounting for approximately 50% of all dementias in the elderly. In addition to cognitive decline, particularly memory loss, behavioral disturbances such as apathy, irritability, and delusions are common symptoms.

Eating comprises two independent processes: self-feeding and swallowing. AD patients rely on partner-initiated cues or direct assistance in self-feeding. Eating problems have been shown to be mild and infrequent in early-stage AD patients [7–9], although eating and swallowing impairments are well documented in late-stage AD. When dysphagia occurs in early-stage AD, it is characterized by delayed onset of the pharyngeal swallow and reduced lingual movement. Moderate AD presents as difficulty with oral preparation of the bolus, pharyngeal clearance, upper esophageal sphincter opening, and visible aspiration on video fluoroscopy (Fig. 28.1) [10, 11]. Compared to patients with mild/moderate AD, the mean latency of the swallowing reflex is significantly longer in severe AD patients. The prolongation of swallowing latency is exacerbated by use of neuroleptics [12]. Swallowing therapy in AD should focus on enhancing the sensory aspects of deglutition. For example, dysphagia management techniques such as oral stage sensory stimulation, which can be achieved by changes of texture, taste, or temperature of food to enhance the awareness of food substance in their mouths, may be beneficial [10].

As the disease progresses, patients with AD start to have difficulty swallowing and may lose interest in eating [13]. Aspiration pneumonia in ambulatory AD patients is significantly and independently associated with severity of dementia, silent brain infarction in the basal ganglia, neuroleptic medication, and male gender [14].

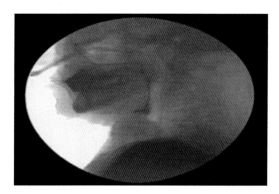

Fig. 28.1 Lateral image of an Alzheimer's disease patient taken during a videofluoroscopic swallowing study. It shows the patient holding thick liquid in the anterior portion of the oral cavity, resulting in delayed oral transit. Owing to the delay in oral transit, the patient is asked to tilt his head backward, resulting in spillage of some of the liquid substance into the vallecular space. From M.K. Suh et al. Alzheimer Dis Assoc Disord 2009;23:178–84 with permission

Some patients with moderate AD cannot remember that they have eaten and continuously demand food from caregivers. Despite this, weight loss and low body weight are commonly reported. Overall, approximately 40% of AD patients have significant weight loss. This may result from a variety of factors including changes in eating habits and access to inadequate nutrition due to memory impairment. Weight loss was found to be a predictor of mortality, while weight gain appeared to have a protective effect in AD [1]. In terms of the neural basis, hypoperfusion to the left orbitofrontal cortex and left anterior cingulate cortex and relative sparing of right orbitofrontal, right anterior cingulate, and left middle mesial temporal cortex emerged as predictors of appetite loss in one study of AD patients [15].

Another related topic is the relationship between body mass index (BMI) and dementia risk. A recent longitudinal study showed that declining BMI was associated with increased risk of incident AD [16], although the opposite has also been reported [17]. A recent longitudinal study, involving community-dwelling elderly African–Americans, found that participants with incident dementia or MCI had accelerated weight loss from as early as 6 years before diagnosis of AD [18]. Similarly, dementia-associated weight

loss was found 2–4 years prior to the onset of the clinical syndrome in Japanese American men which then accelerated around the time of diagnosis [19]. Loss of BMI may reflect the locus of pathological changes in AD, but this has not been investigated systematically. Level of AD pathology has been shown to be associated with changes in BMI, while Lewy body pathology and cerebral infarctions were not [20].

Stroke and Vascular Dementia

Stroke produces a range of deficits that could interfere with normal eating, including impaired arm movement, posture, lip closure, chewing, swallowing, sensation, perception, attention, and cognition. Moreover, depression and apathy are frequent problems. The assessment of the contribution of these factors in stroke patients is, therefore, highly complex. Not surprisingly more than 80% of the stroke patients in nursing homes have some sort of eating disturbance [21]. Physical and cognitive impairments known to influence eating were most severe in patients who were severely dependent for eating. Dysphagia was reported in almost a quarter and poor food intake or poor appetite in 30% of the patients.

A comparison of swallowing in AD and vascular dementia (VaD) using video fluoroscopy to assess separate oral, pharyngeal, and laryngeal phases of deglutition revealed that the AD patients were significantly more impaired in "oral transit delay over 5 s" with liquids, whereas the VaD patients showed more deficits in bolus formation and mastication of semisolid food, hyolaryngeal excursion, epiglottic inversion, and silent aspiration (Fig. 28.2) [10]. These results suggest that the swallowing disorder in AD results from sensory impairment secondary to damage of temporoparietal areas, whereas dysphagia in the VaD group is more likely to be the result of corticobulbar tract damage. These results have clinical implications for feeding modification and dysphagia therapy in patients with dementia. In VaD patients, treatment methods focusing on oral and pharyngeal motor aspects of swallow, for example, oromotor-strengthening exercise for

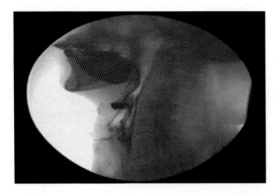

Fig. 28.2 Lateral image of a vascular dementia patient taken during a videofluoroscopic swallowing study. The image shows residue in the lateral sulcus, indicating weakness of the buccal muscles. It also reveals residue in the valleculae and pyriform sinus, resulting from reduced pharyngeal peristalsis, hyolaryngeal excursion, epiglottic inversion, and relaxation of the upper esophageal sphincter. The image also shows penetration to the level of the vocal folds. From M.K. Suh et al. Alzheimer Dis Assoc Disord 2009;23:178–84 with permission

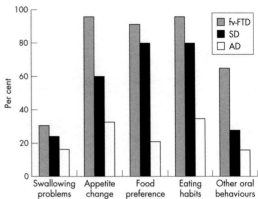

Fig. 28.3 Frequency of each symptom domain in frontal variant frontotemporal dementia (fv-FTD), semantic dementia (SD), and Alzheimer's disease (AD) groups. From M. Ikeda et al. J Neurol Neurosurg Psychiatry 2002;73:371–6 with permission

enhancing bolus control or mastication abilities, may be appropriate. To help with the laryngeal elevation (i.e., hyolaryngeal elevation and epiglottic inversion), the Mendelsohn maneuver or swallowing therapy methods using the electrical stimulation could be used [22].

Frontotemporal Lobar Degeneration

Frontotemporal lobar degeneration (FTLD) is the currently preferred term for primary cerebral degeneration involving the frontal and/or anterior temporal lobes associated with non-Alzheimer type pathology, characterized by behavioral changes, including loss of insight, disinhibition, apathy, mood changes, stereotypic behavior, and abnormal eating behavior [7]. Although many studies have highlighted the high prevalence of alterations in food preference and eating habits in FTLD [23], there have been few systematic studies comparing FTLD subgroups, or contrasting AD and FTLD [8, 24].

To investigate the frequency of changes in eating behaviors and the sequence of development of eating behaviors in FTLD and AD, we utilized a newly created caregiver questionnaire [8]. Three groups of patients were studied: FTD (frontal

variant frontotemporal dementia; fv-FTD), semantic dementia (SD), and AD. The questionnaire consisted of 36 questions investigating five domains: swallowing problems, appetite change, food preference, eating habits, and other oral behaviors. The frequencies of symptoms in all five domains, except swallowing problems, were higher in FTD than in AD, and changes in food preference and eating habits were greater in SD than in AD (Fig. 28.3). In SD, the developmental pattern initially revealed a change in food preference, followed by appetite increase and altered eating habits, other oral behaviors, and finally swallowing problems. In FTD, the first symptom altered was eating habits or appetite increase. In AD, the pattern was not clear although swallowing difficulties developed in relatively early stages (Fig. 28.4). Change in eating behavior was significantly more common in both of the FTLD groups than in AD.

Dietary or eating behavioral disturbances have been found to correlate with the degree of atrophy on MRI of the right lateral orbitofrontal cortex and the adjacent insula [25]. A voxel-based morphometry study in FTLD patients showed that hyperphagia was associated with gray matter loss in anterior lateral orbitofrontal cortices and a sweet tooth with gray matter loss in posterior lateral orbitofrontal cortices and the right anterior insula [26].

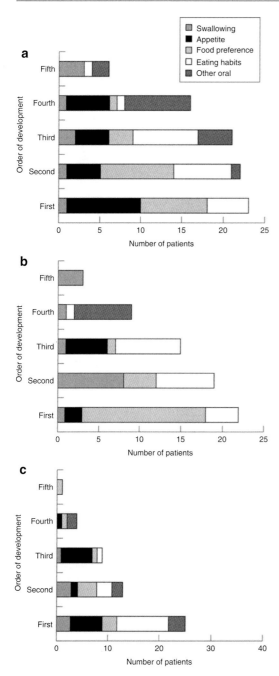

Fig. 28.4 The development order of abnormal eating symptom in (**a**) frontal variant frontotemporal dementia, (**b**) semantic dementia, and (**c**) Alzheimer's disease. From M. Ikeda et al. J Neurol Neurosurg Psychiatry 2002;73:371–6 with permission

A fiberoptic endoscopic examination of swallowing revealed moderate swallowing abnormality in 57% of FTLD patients without known

amyotrophic lateral sclerosis (ALS), PSP, or CBD [27]. There were significant differences between the FTLD and control subjects on five variables, all relating to swallowing: leakage time during mastication, swallow onset time, typical and lowest bolus location at swallow onset, and reduced bolus clearance. These abnormalities were not explained by compulsive eating behaviors, but seemed to reflect deficits in cortical and subcortical pathways connecting with the brainstem swallowing centers. Aspiration pneumonia is a common cause of death in FTLD [28] and the early detection of swallowing problems in patients with FTLD had prognostic implications.

It is important to note that there is considerable overlap both clinically and pathologically between FTLD and ALS. Between 10% and 20% of patients with FTLD develop frank ALS, which is typically of the bulbar type with significant dysphagia and dysarthria [29]. It is possible, therefore, that a much higher proportion of patients have more subtle but significant involvement of bulbar motor neurons.

Taking a cross-cultural and ethnological viewpoint, we used an identical methodology of the UK study [8] to examine changes in eating behaviors in patients with FTLD and AD in Japan and to compare directly with those in the UK [30]. On the whole, the findings in a Japanese cohort were similar to those previously reported in the UK. Changes in eating behaviors in Japanese patients with both SD and FTD were significantly more common than in AD patients, as was the case in the UK. Changes in eating behaviors in FTLD appear to be universal, although ethniccultural factors might modulate these results to some extent. Changes in eating behaviors seem to be a direct consequence of the pathology of FTLD rather than being an expression of other neuropsychiatric features in a specific socio-cultural context. There is a possibility that abnormal eating behaviors such as appetite increase are exacerbated by cultural factors in Western countries. This hypothesis was supported by the fact that weight gain of more than 7.5 kg was found in approximately 30% of FTD and SD cases in the UK, while less than 10% of FTD and SD cases in Japan gained weight. As described

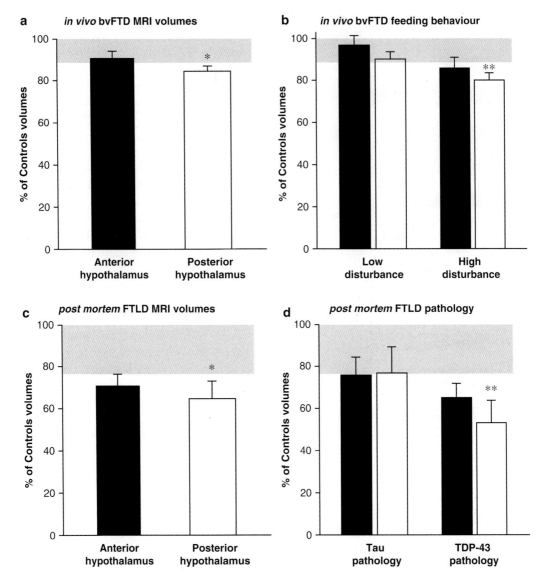

Fig. 28.5 Volumetric changes in the hypothalamus of patients with behavioral-variant frontotemporal dementia (bvFTD) compared to healthy controls. Volumes are standardized to a percentage of the mean hypothalamic volume of the healthy control group (*the gray band* reflecting the standard deviation). (**a**) In vivo anterior and posterior hypothalamic volumes in bvFTD corrected for head size. Significant atrophy in the posterior hypothalamus atrophy is observed in bvFTD at presentation. (**b**) In vivo hypothalamic volumes in bvFTD patients exhibiting high or low feeding disturbance corrected for head size. Greater atrophy of the posterior hypothalamus (*white bar, right*) is present in bvFTD patients with high feeding disturbances at presentation compared to bvFTD patients with low feeding disturbance and compared with healthy controls.

(**c**) Postmortem absolute anterior and posterior hypothalamic volumes in frontotemporal lobar degeneration (FTLD). Significant posterior hypothalamic atrophy in FTLD is observed. (**d**) Postmortem absolute hypothalamic volumes in FTLD patients exhibiting different inclusion pathologies. More severe posterior hypothalamic atrophy is observed in the FTLD-TDP group (*white bar, right*) compared with the FTLD-tau group, and compared with healthy controls. *MRI* magnetic resonance imaging, *TDP-43* TAR-DNA-binding protein 43. *Posterior hypothalamus in this group is significantly smaller than that of healthy controls; **posterior hypothalamus in this group is significantly smaller than those of the other two groups. From O. Piguet et al. Ann Neurol 2011;69:312–9 with permission

above, sugar intake and total calorie consumption differ significantly in the general population between Japan and the UK. It may be, therefore, that Japanese FTLD patients did not manifest severe weight gain because their eating behaviors were not amplified by cultural factors.

Relatively little was known about the pathological mechanisms that underlie the appetite change and weight gain in FTLD until recently. The neuroendocrinology of satiety is complex. In brief, nuclei in the hypothalamus play a key role and are modulated by levels of leptin and ghrelin produced by body fat and the stomach wall, respectively. These hypothalamic nuclei regulate energy levels and feeding behavior through the autonomic nervous system. Using high-resolution MRI, Piguet et al. [31] showed that selective early atrophy of the posterior hypothalamus in FTD was correlated with the degree of eating dysregulation (Fig. 28.5). A parallel neuropathological study demonstrated significant neuronal loss in posterior hypothalamic nuclei at postmortem.

Dementia with Lewy Bodies

Dementia with Lewy bodies (DLB) is the third most common form of dementia accounting for 15–20% of cases in pathological studies. DLB is clinically characterized by marked fluctuations in cognition, visual hallucinations, extrapyramidal signs (EPS), and sensitivity to neuroleptics [32]. It is well established that approximately one-half of patients with Parkinson's disease (PD) have swallowing problems. Since DLB is clinically and pathologically related to PD, it is reasonable to assume that eating/swallowing problems are also common in DLB patients. Indeed, in a recent report from the DLB consortium, "eating and swallowing difficulties" were described as part of the supportive diagnostic features [33]. There have, however, been few systematic studies of eating problems in DLB patients.

To address this deficiency, the author's group in Japan assessed a series of consecutive DLB and AD patients using a revised version of the compre-

hensive questionnaire originally designed for patients with FTD/AD [8, 30]. Four new questions were added and seven FTD-specific questions were deleted. DLB patients showed significantly higher scores than AD patients for "difficulty in swallowing foods," "difficulty in swallowing liquids," "coughing or choking when swallowing," "taking a long time to swallow," "suffering from sputum," "loss of appetite," "need watching or help," and "constipation" (Table 28.1). The Unified Parkinson disease Rating Scale (UPDRS) score correlated significantly with "difficulty in swallowing foods," "taking a long time to swallow" and "needs watching or help," whereas the neuropsychiatric inventory (NPI) score correlated with "loss of appetite." The UPDRS, NPI, and CDR were associated with scores for "difficulty in swallowing liquids." No significant independent variables affected the scores for "coughing or choking when swallowing," "suffering from sputum," and "constipation." EPS, psychiatric symptoms and severity of dementia did not affect these scores, and they may reflect some other mechanism such as autonomic dysfunction. No significant independent variables affected the "constipation" score, because constipation may be the direct result of autonomic dysfunction [34]. A previous study noted that 83% of patients with pathologically confirmed DLB showed constipation [35], and our results also support this high frequency of constipation in DLB patients. There was an interesting difference between difficulty swallowing liquids and solids. The former was modulated by UPDRS, NPI and CDR scores, whereas the later was affected by the UPDRS only. Swallowing liquids may require more accurate control of muscles than swallowing solids. Clinicians should be aware of this difference, and ask caregivers which problems predominate in DLB patients.

Yamamoto et al. [36] investigated the time from scanning until pneumonia onset or discontinuation of oral intake using video fluorography in patients with idiopathic Parkinson's disease (IPD) and DLB. Aspiration during video fluorography was a risk factor for pneumonia onset in these patients. Aspiration and Hoehn-Yahr stage (scale for defining the severity stages

Table 28.1 The scores (frequency×severity) for each symptom domain in the DLB and AD groups (Shinagawa et al. [9])

		DLB	AD	*p* value
Swallowing problems	Difficulty in swallowing food	1.71	0.03	0.002
	Difficulty in swallowing liquids	0.61	0.03	0.043
	Coughing or choking when swallowing	0.96	0.24	0.013
	Taking a long time to swallow	1.57	0.00	0.000
	Placing food in mouth but not chewing it	0.29	0.00	NS
	Chewing food but not swallowing it	0.04	0.03	NS
	Suffering from sputum	0.86	0.12	0.011
	Fluctuation in swallowing ability	0.18	0.00	NS
Appetite change	Loss of appetite	1.79	0.15	0.000
	Increase in appetite	0.04	0.33	NS
	Seeking out food between meals	0.00	0.64	NS
	Overeating at meal time	0.07	0.03	NS
	Reporting hunger or requesting more food	0.04	0.03	NS
	Reporting being overfull	0.00	0.00	NS
	Needs to limit food	0.00	0.12	NS
	Fluctuation in appetite	0.64	0.03	NS
Food preference	Preferring sweet foods more than before	0.07	0.18	NS
	Drinking more soft or sweet drinks	0.07	0.06	NS
	Drinking more tea/coffee or water	0.18	0.24	NS
	"Taste" in food changed in some way	0.00	0.00	NS
	Adding more seasoning to their food	0.04	0.00	NS
	Developing other food fads	0.00	0.00	NS
	Hoarding foods	0.00	0.00	NS
	Drinking more alcohol	0.11	0.00	NS
Eating habits	Wants to cook or eat the same food every day	0.04	0.21	NS
	Tends to eat foods in the same order	0.00	0.03	NS
	Wants to eat at the same time every day	0.00	0.00	NS
	Decline in table manners	0.36	1.12	NS
	Eating with hands	0.18	0.52	NS
	Takes a long time to eat	1.32	0.42	NS
	Getting drowsy at meal time	0.39	0.03	NS
	Needs watching or help	2.32	0.00	0.000
Other eating behaviors	Tends to overfill mouth	0.00	0.24	NS
	Chewing or sucking without trying to eat them	0.00	0.00	NS
	Eats nonedible foodstuffs	0.25	0.18	NS
	Tends to snatch or grasp any food items	0.00	0.27	NS
	Becomes a heavier smoker or takes up smoking	0.00	0.00	NS
	Episodes of vomiting	0.04	0.00	NS
	Fever with a meal	0.21	0.00	NS
	Constipation	3.39	0.21	0.000

of Parkinson's disease) were risk factors for discontinuing oral intake.

Visual hallucinations, which are the most common psychiatric symptom in DLB, may lessen the patients' appetite. It has been pointed out that visual hallucinations disturb the patients' concentration while eating food [37].

Conclusions

Recent studies highlight the importance of careful observation and assessment of eating behaviors of dementia taking a disease and stage-specific viewpoint. Although patients with each of the dementia syndromes discussed here show many eating problems, the cause of these varies across diseases and depends on a number of complex factors.

The potentially life threatening complications of dysphagia can be postponed if physicians are aware of the symptom(s) in their patients early in the course of their disease, and if the problem is managed by a speech pathologist specializing in dysphagia. Aspiration pneumonia is significantly and independently associated with severe dementia and intake of neuroleptics. As soon as the behavioral and psychiatric problems ameliorate, drug tapering or discontinuation should be considered in order to prevent aspiration pneumonia. To prevent the pervasive symptom of weight loss, caregivers of patients with AD and DLB should focus on support during and between meals with a special attention on the amount of food and fluid take. Weight gain in patients with moderate and severe dementia can be achieved by adjusting the meal environment to the individual's needs [38]. Regular inspection of the patient's oral cavity and lubrication of the mucosa of the mouth are also important [1]. In FTD there is often weight gain that can be controlled by limiting the range of available food in the environment. Appetite-suppressing drugs such as antidepressant serotonin reuptake blockers may be helpful [39, 40]. A proportion of patients with FTD develop severe dysphagia and clinicians should evaluate for features of bulbar ALS such as tongue wasting or fasciculation.

For caregivers, it may be difficult to understand and recognize eating/swallowing problems in neurodegenerative disorders such as AD, FTD, and DLB. Education of family caregivers and care staff about eating/swallowing problems is important.

Key Points

- Feeding and eating difficulties leading to weight loss are common in the advanced stages of dementia.
- As the disease progresses, patients with AD have difficulty swallowing due to sensory impairment secondary to dysfunctions in the temporoparietal areas.
- VaD patients showed more deficits in bolus formation and mastication of semisolid food, hyolaryngeal excursion, epiglottic inversion, and silent aspiration caused by motor impairments due to disruptions in the corticobulbar tract.
- The frequencies of appetite change, alterations in food preference toward sweet foods and changed eating habits, are greater in FTD and in SD than in AD. A proportion of patients with FTD develop bulbar palsy in the context of ALS.
- DLB patients showed a higher incidence of swallowing problems and anorexia than AD patients.
- A cross-cultural perspective is of particular importance when investigating eating behaviors in dementias.

Acknowledgments The present study was undertaken with the support of grants provided by the Ministry of Health, Labor and Welfare (Research on dementia) and by the Ministry of Education, Culture, Sports, Science and Technology (Grant no. 23591718) for MI.

References

1. Holm B, Söderhamn O. Factors associated with nutritional status in a group of people in an early stage of dementia. Clin Nutr. 2003;22:385–9.
2. Correia Sde M, Morillo LS, Jacob Filho W, Mansur LL. Swallowing in moderate and severe phases of Alzheimer's disease. Arq Neuropsiquiatr. 2010;68:855–61.
3. Alzheimer's Society. Food for thought. London: Alzheimer's Society; 2000.
4. Mitchell SL, Teno JM, Kiely DK, et al. The clinical course of advanced dementia. N Engl J Med. 2009;361:1529–38.
5. Pasman HR, The BA, Onwuteaka-Philipsen BD, et al. Feeding nursing home patients with severe dementia: a qualitative study. J Adv Nurs. 2003;42:304–11.
6. Food and Agriculture Organization of the United Nations 2002. http://faostat.fao.org/.
7. Bozeat S, Gregory CA, Lambon Ralph MA, et al. Which neuropsychiatric and behavioural features distinguish frontal and temporal variants of Frontotemporal dementia from Alzheimer's disease? J Neurol Neurosurg Psychiatry. 2000;69:178–86.
8. Ikeda M, Brown J, Holland AJ, et al. Changes in appetite, food preference, and eating habits in frontotem-

poral dementia and Alzheimer's disease. J Neurol Neurosurg Psychiatry. 2002;73:371–6.

9. Shinagawa S, Adachi H, Toyota Y, et al. Characteristics of eating and swallowing problems in patients who have dementia with Lewy bodies. Int Psychogeriatr. 2009;21:520–5.

10. Suh MK, Kim H, Na DL. Dysphagia in patients with dementia: Alzheimer versus vascular. Alzheimer Dis Assoc Disord. 2009;23:178–84.

11. Humbert IA, McLaren DG, Kosmatka K, et al. Early deficits in cortical control of swallowing in Alzheimer's disease. J Alzheimers Dis. 2010;19: 1185–97.

12. Wada H, Nakajoh K, Satoh-Nakagawa T, et al. Risk factors of aspiration pneumonia in Alzheimer's disease patients. Gerontology. 2001;47:271–6.

13. Kalia M. Dysphagia and aspiration pneumonia in patients with Alzheimer's disease. Metabolism. 2003; 52 Suppl 2:36–8.

14. Chouinard J. Dysphagia in Alzheimer disease: a review. J Nutr Health Aging. 2000;4:214–7.

15. Ismail Z, Herrmann N, Rothenburg LS, et al. A functional neuroimaging study of appetite loss in Alzheimer's disease. J Neurol Sci. 2008;271: 97–103.

16. Buchman AS, Wilson RS, Bienias JL, et al. Change in body mass index and risk of incident Alzheimer disease. Neurology. 2005;65:892–7.

17. Gorospe EC, Dave J. The risk of dementia with increased body mass index. Age Ageing. 2007;36: 23–9.

18. Gao S, Nguyen JT, Hendrie HC, et al. Accelerated weight loss and incident dementia in an elderly African–American cohort. J Am Geriatr Soc. 2011;59:18–25.

19. Stewart R, Masaki K, Xue QL, et al. A 32-year prospective study of change in body weight and incident dementia: the Honolulu-Asia aging study. Arch Neurol. 2005;62:55–60.

20. Buchman AS, Schneider JA, Wilson RS, et al. Body mass index in older persons is associated with Alzheimer disease pathology. Neurology. 2006;12(67):1949–54.

21. Kumlien S, Axelsson K. Stroke patients in nursing homes: eating, feeding, nutrition and related care. J Clin Nurs. 2002;11:498–509.

22. Burnett TA, Mann EA, Cornell SA, et al. Laryngeal elevation achieved by neuromuscular stimulation at rest. J Appl Physiol. 2003;94:128–34.

23. Snowden JS, Bathgate D, Varma A, et al. Distinct behavioural profiles in frontotemporal dementia and semantic dementia. J Neurol Neurosurg Psychiatry. 2001;70:323–32.

24. Mendez MF, Licht EA, Shapira JS. Changes in dietary or eating behavior in frontotemporal dementia versus Alzheimer's disease. Am J Alzheimers Dis Other Demen. 2008;23:280–5.

25. Woolley JD, Gorno-Tempini ML, Seeley WW, et al. Binge eating is associated with right orbitofrontal-insular-striatal atrophy in frontotemporal dementia. Neurology. 2007;69:1424–33.

26. Whitwell JL, Sampson EL, Loy CT, et al. VBM signatures of abnormal eating behaviours in frontotemporal lobar degeneration. Neuroimage. 2007;35: 207–13.

27. Langmore SE, Olney RK, Lomen-Hoerth C, Miller BL. Dysphagia in patients with frontotemporal lobar dementia. Arch Neurol. 2007;64:58–62.

28. Grasbeck A, Englund E, Horstmann V, et al. Predictors of mortality in frontotemporal dementia: a retrospective study of the prognostic influence of pre-diagnostic features. Int J Geriatr Psychiatry. 2003;18:594–601.

29. Lillo P, Garcin B, Hornberger M, et al. Neurobehavioral features in frontotemporal dementia with amyotrophic lateral sclerosis. Arch Neurol. 2010;67:826–30.

30. Shinagawa S, Ikeda M, Nestor PJ, et al. Characteristics of abnormal eating behaviours in frontotemporal lobar degeneration: a cross-cultural survey. J Neurol Neurosurg Psychiatry. 2009;80:1413–4.

31. Piguet O, Petersén A, Yin Ka Lam B, et al. Eating and hypothalamus changes in behavioral-variant frontotemporal dementia. Ann Neurol. 2011;69:312–9.

32. McKeith IG. Consensus guidelines for the clinical and pathologic diagnosis of dementia with Lewy bodies (DLB): report of the consortium on DLB international workshop. J Alzheimers Dis. 2006;9 Suppl 3:417–23.

33. McKeith IG, Dickson J, Lowe M, et al. Diagnosis and management of dementia with Lewy bodies third report of the DLB consortium. Neurology. 2005;65: 1863–72.

34. Thaisetthawatkul P, Boeve BF, Benarroch EE, et al. Autonomic dysfunction in dementia with Lewy bodies. Neurology. 2004;62:1804–9.

35. Horimoto Y, Matsumoto M, Akatsu H, et al. Autonomic dysfunctions in dementia with Lewy bodies. J Neurol. 2003;250:530–3.

36. Yamamoto T, Kobayashi Y, Murata M. Risk of pneumonia onset and discontinuation of oral intake following videofluorography in patients with Lewy body disease. Parkinsonism Relat Disord. 2010;16:503–6.

37. Kindell J. Feeding and swallowing disorders in dementia. UK: Speechmark Publishing Ltd; 2002.

38. Mamhidir AG, Karlsson I, Norberg A, Mona K. Weight increase in patients with dementia, and alteration in meal routines and meal environment after integrity promoting care. J Clin Nurs. 2007;16:987–96.

39. Ikeda M, Shigenobu K, Fukuhara R, et al. Efficacy of fluvoxamine as a treatment for behavioral symptoms in FTLD patients. Dement Geriatr Cogn Disord. 2004;17:117–21.

40. Lebert F, Stekke W, Hasenbroekx C, et al. Frontotemporal dementia: a randomized controlled trial with trazodone. Dement Geriatr Cogn Disord. 2004;17:355–9.

Dystrophies and Myopathies (Including Oculopharyngeal)

29

Safwan Jaradeh

Abstract

As previous chapters have illustrated, the oropharyngeal swallow is the end result of several coordinated neuromuscular elements: velopharyngeal closure, tongue loading, tongue pulsion, closure of the laryngeal vestibule, upper esophageal sphincter opening, and pharyngeal clearance. It is estimated that more than 30 muscles are involved in the various stages of the swallow. Muscular disorders leading to impairment in any of these steps can cause dysphagia. A better understanding of the swallowing problems associated with these conditions may help in guiding treatment, choosing technical aids, modifying the consistency of foods, swallowing rehabilitation, and nutritional support by the non-oral route.

Keywords

Duchenne muscular dystrophy (DMD) • Dystrophies • Hereditary muscle diseases • Myopathies • Myotonic dystrophy (MD) • Oculopharyngeal muscular dystrophy (OPMD) • Steinert's disease

Definition

Prevalence/Incidence, Pathophysiology, Diagnosis, Complications, Management

The potential muscular causes of oropharyngeal dysphagia may not be readily apparent at first. When faced with dysphagia, clinicians often consider at first neurogenic dysphagia secondary to upper or lower motor neuron dysfunction, since it is statistically more frequent. Myopathies and neuromuscular junction disorders are often considered after that.

Disordered swallowing can develop over the course of many myopathies. Deglutition may be impaired because of weakness or inflammation of the oropharyngeal and esophageal musculature. Dysphagia may appear variably among patients in parallel to the pattern of weakness of the various muscles.

S. Jaradeh, MD (✉)
Professor of Neurology and Neurological Sciences,
Stanford University Medical Center,
300 Pasteur Drive, Room A347,
Stanford, CA 94305-5235, USA
e-mail: jaradeh@mcw.edu

R. Shaker et al. (eds.), *Principles of Deglutition: A Multidisciplinary Text for Swallowing and its Disorders*,
DOI 10.1007/978-1-4614-3794-9_29, © Springer Science+Business Media New York 2013

Prevalence/Incidence

Feeding problems in patients with neuromuscular diseases are often underestimated. In a survey of 451 patients by the French Muscular Dystrophy Association, 409 patients responded, and swallowing difficulties were reported by at least 35% of patients [1]. Among these responders, 38 had spinal muscular atrophy, 139 had myasthenia, but the remaining 232 patients had various myopathies. In further analysis, impaired swallowing was reported in 37–41% of hereditary muscular dystrophies, and in 30% of acquired inflammatory myopathies. Difficulties in the oral phase were encountered primarily in Duchenne muscular dystrophy (DMD), limb-girdle muscular dystrophy (LGMD), and facio-scapulo-humeral muscular dystrophy (FSHMD). The pharyngeal phase was particularly affected in dermatomyositis, polymyositis, and LGMD. The survey was limited to the above-mentioned diagnoses and did not include other inflammatory myopathies, such as inclusion body myositis, or other hereditary myopathies, such as oculopharyngeal muscular dystrophy (OPMD).

Pathophysiology

When diagnosticians approach muscular disorders leading to dysphagia, it is useful to consider two major categories: genetic and acquired. While it is intuitive that any muscular disorder may present with dysphagia, abnormalities of deglutition tend to predominate in some types of myopathies. These include oculopharyngeal muscular dystrophy (OPMD), myotonic dystrophy (MD), patients in the advanced stages of Duchenne muscular dystrophy (DMD), inflammatory myopathies, such as polymyositis (PM), dermatomyositis (DM), and inclusion body myositis (IBM), and certain metabolic myopathies, particularly mitochondrial myopathies. Thyroid disorders and certain iatrogenic myopathies can also lead to prominent dysphagia.

When myopathic patients present with dysphagia, their complaints range widely. Some describe mild choking on solids, while others have complete inability to swallow their food. Some patients have to chew carefully and swallow slowly, while others cough frequently particularly when drinking liquids. With progression, there is pooling of secretions and weight loss. In a subset of patients, the dysphagia is associated with impaired cricopharyngeal muscle function and its ability to relax, which prevents the food from leaving the hypopharynx into the esophagus (cricopharyngeal achalasia). Patients with myopathy may describe tightness in the throat, while others may point to the upper cervical region or to the mid-sternal region depending on whether the esophagus is involved.

Hereditary Muscle Diseases

Oculopharyngeal muscular dystrophy was first described by Taylor in 1915. In OPMD, patients usually develop symptoms after the fourth decade. Dysphagia is frequent and may be the presenting symptom; it is usually progressive. Ptosis may occur early, but weakness of other extraocular muscles occurs much later in the course of the disease; diplopia and total ophthalmoplegia are rare. The dysphagia is due mainly to the pharyngeal weakness, but the lingual and oral phases are also affected. With disease progression, patients develop dysphonia and aspiration, as well as proximal muscle weakness particularly in the lower limbs. Life span is usually normal, unless repeated aspiration occurs, or in rare patients who develop cardiac conduction block. In rare cases of OPMD, a distal neuropathy has been reported (references); the neuropathy is axonal. CK level almost never exceeds 1,000 U/L and may be normal in mild cases. On routine histochemical studies, a muscle biopsy obtained from a weak muscle reveals rimmed vacuoles. Electron microscopy shows intranuclear inclusions made of tubular filaments measuring 8.5 nm in diameter. In older patients, concomitant mitochondrial changes may appear, including occasional ragged red fibers and paracrystalline mitochondrial inclusions [2, 3].

Though OPMD has a worldwide incidence, it is more common in certain ethnic communities, particularly the French Canadian population and the Jewish populations of Bukhara and Uzbekistan. Genetically, the disease is autosomal dominant and is caused by expansion of a GCG repeat sequence located within the polyadenylate binding protein nuclear 2 gene (PABP2) on chromosome 14q11.2-13. In normal subjects, only six GCG repeats are expressed and code for alanine. Expansion beyond eight repeats results in OPMD. The severity of the phenotype usually parallels the size of expansion, so in patients who are homozygous for this expansion, the onset of dysphagia occurs 10–20 years earlier than in heterozygotes [3]. On the other hand, patients with a smaller expansion manifest a more benign phenotype, where limb weakness is very mild and dysphagia may be the only clinical manifestation. The PABP2 protein is expressed in the nuclei of skeletal muscle. The expansion of the GCG repeat sequence causes abnormal lengthening and misfolding of the PABP polyalanine tail, leading to its intranuclear accumulation as inclusions [4]. This aberrant protein interferes with normal mRNA function, and because of its resistance to degradation, this accumulation causes toxicity to muscle cells.

Certain patients with *Mitochondrial myopathies*, such as Kearns–Sayre, chronic progressive external ophthalmoplegia and MNGIE syndrome (mitochondrial myopathy, peripheral neuropathy, gastrointestinal disease, and encephalopathy) present with dysphagia [5, 6]. The swallowing impairment is mainly due to weak pharyngeal constrictor muscles, but there is also weakness of the oropharyngeal musculature. In one study of 12 patients, cricopharyngeal achalasia was present in 9, and deglutitive incoordination was found in one patient. In MNGIE syndrome, there is additional smooth muscle involvement, which may result in intestinal pseudo-obstruction due to the visceral neuropathy [6]. Clinically, extraocular muscle involvement is earlier and much greater than in OPMD, and some patients have sensorineural hearing loss as well as mild peripheral neuropathy involving the large or small nerve fibers. On routine histochemical studies, a muscle biopsy often shows ragged red fibers (Fig. 29.1) and cytochrome oxidase negative fibers. Electron microscopy shows paracrystalline mitochondrial inclusions. Given the potential clinical overlap with OPMD [7, 8] it is important to search for the intranuclear tubulo-filamentous inclusions that are specific to the latter diagnosis. Otherwise, genetic testing may be necessary.

Myotonic dystrophy (MD, Steinert's disease) is the most common muscular dystrophy in adults. In the United States it has an incidence of 13.5 per 100,000 live births. Patients often complain of distal weakness. In the arms, the hand intrinsic muscles and the extensors of the fingers and wrist are preferentially affected; in the legs, patients may develop foot drop. Proximal limb muscles may become affected later. There is weakness of the facial muscles and atrophy of the temporalis, masseter, and sternocleidomastoid muscles leading to a characteristic "hatchet face". Ptosis and frontal balding are common. There is frequent weakness of the palatal and pharyngeal muscles leading to dysarthria and dysphagia. The dysphagia is worsened by involvement of the smooth musculature of the esophagus. Radiologic evaluation of swallowing shows impairment of all phases: oral, pharyngeal, and esophageal. Impairment of other smooth muscles (gallbladder, intestines) causes additional GI issues (gallstones and intestinal pseudo-obstruction). Cardiac involvement is common and is a major source of

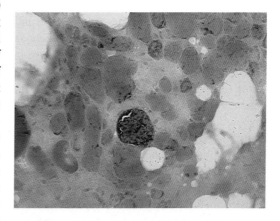

Fig. 29.1 Biopsy of the vastus muscle in a patient with dysphagia and mitochondrial myopathy showing a ragged red fiber. Trichrome stain × 200

mortality: EKG is abnormal in 65%, and Holter monitoring is abnormal in 29% of patients [9]. First-degree atrioventricular block is the most common abnormality. Clinically, myotonia is an important diagnostic clue. In myotonia, there is impaired relaxation of muscle after forceful voluntary contraction. This causes difficulty releasing their handgrip after a handshake, unscrewing a bottle top, or opening their eyelids after forceful eyeclosure. Myotonia classically improves with repeated exercise, and worsens with exposure to cold. It can be demonstrated at the bedside by percussion of the thenar eminence, wrist extensors, or tongue. While patients may subjectively complain of muscle stiffness or tightness, muscle weakness is usually a greater concern of theirs. Electromyography (EMG) reveals myotonic discharges with the character- istic "dive-bomber" sound. CK level is normal or minimally elevated. Other common problems are bilateral posterior subcapsular cataracts, insulin resistance, testicular atrophy, and uterine hypotonia. Lower IQ occurs particularly with earlier age of symptom onset. MRI of the brain can reveal hyperintense white matter lesions or cortical atrophy [10].

On muscle biopsy, there is type I fiber atrophy, relative type II hypertrophy, several ring fibers, and a significant increase in the number of myofibers containing internal nuclei. Cardiac histopathology shows fibrosis, primarily in the conducting system and sino-atrial node, myocyte hypertrophy, and fatty infiltration. MD is an auto- somal-dominant disease due to an abnormal expansion of a CTG trinucleotide repeat sequence located on chromosome 19q13.2 [11]. There is genetic anticipation, with an increase of the repeat size and worse phenotype in subsequent generations. The repeat sequence lies in the myotonin protein kinase (DMPK) gene. Normal controls have less than 35 repeats. Like OPMD, there is some correlation between the number of repeats and the phenotype. The most severe form of congenital MD appears in infants born to an affected mother; they generally have over 1,000 repeats. They present with neonatal hypotonia and may require mechanical ventilation because of respiratory distress. All infants have bifacial

weakness and feeding difficulties. Examination of the mother is helpful for the diagnosis, which is confirmed by genetic testing. Once children survive the infantile period, progressive muscle weakness appears later, and up to one half are mentally retarded. Genetic testing has lessened the need for muscle biopsy in MD.

Duchenne muscular dystrophy (DMD) is the most common muscular dystrophy in children. The inheritance is X-linked, with female carriers and affected males. The incidence of DMD is approximately 1:3,500 live births. DMD is caused by mutations in the dystrophin gene, located on the short arm of the X chromosome (Xp21.2). This gene codes for dystrophin, a large intracel- lular protein that provide stability to the muscle membrane by linking the intracellular cytoskel- eton and extracellular matrix. Boys are normal at birth, but childhood motor milestones become somewhat delayed. By the age of 5 years, they experience difficulty running, climbing stairs, or arising from the floor (Gowers' sign). Calf hyper- trophy is an early sign. CK levels are markedly elevated. With advanced disease, there is involve- ment of the oropharyngeal muscles. The later occurrence of macroglossia further complicates the oral phase of swallowing. Some may have impaired gastric motility due to the involvement of smooth muscles. This may lead in advanced stages to esophageal dysmotility, gastric dilata- tion, and intestinal pseudo-obstruction [12]. The average IQ is one standard deviation below the mean. Boys often become wheelchair-bound before 12 years of age. Scoliosis complicates the respiratory dysfunction in these patients. Cardiomyopathy occurs in the late teenage years, and is a frequent source of morbidity and mortality. Most often, it is of the dilated type, but hypertro- phic cardiomyopathy may also occur. Patients die before their third decade.

Dysphagia may also occur in *Limb girdle muscular dystrophy* (LGMD), but it is not as common as it is in the above-mentioned dystro- phies. In one systematic study of 20 LGMD patients [13], two (10%) reported some swallow- ing difficulties. But when swallowing was evaluated by conventional cineradiography and manometry, an abnormal radiologic study was found in 6 patients (30%), and an abnormal manometric study in 4 patients (20%) even without complaints of dysphagia. Mean manometric pressures were not significantly different when patients were compared with a healthy, age- and sex-matched volunteer group. In the two symptomatic patients, the dysphagia was mainly due to dysfunction of the pharyngeal muscle.

Oculopharyngodistal myopathy is a rare type of hereditary myopathy that present with external ophthalmoplegia, dysphagia, and distal weakness in all limbs [14]. Serum CK level is mildly elevated. EMG shows a myopathic pattern but with myotonic discharges. A muscle biopsy reveals dystrophic changes with rimmed vacuoles. Ultrastructural examination reveals tubulofilamentous inclusions in both sarcoplasm and nucleus. While the phenotype may resemble OPMD, the distal weakness and myotonic discharges differ. Genetic testing for OPMD is negative. No mutations have been identified.

Congenital muscular dystrophy is a childhood disease characterized by severe muscle weakness and inability to achieve independent ambulation. The condition is due to deficiency in merosin, another muscle membrane protein. In a study of 14 children (age range: 2–14 years), parents of 12 children reported feeding difficulties, and their children were below the third centile for weight [15]. On videofluoroscopy, 13/14 children had abnormal oral phase, and 9/14 had abnormal pharyngeal phase with a delayed swallow reflex; 6 of these 9 patients had recurrent chest infections, and the imaging showed laryngeal pooling in 3 and frank aspiration in 3. Eight children had pH monitoring study, and 6/8 had gastro-oesophageal reflux. In 5 children, the placement of a gastrostomy tube stopped the chest infections and improved weight gain.

Among *Congenital myopathies*, nemaline rod myopathy is probably the one most associated with dysphagia. Most cases present during early childhood with neonatal hypotonia; muscle stretch reflexes are absent. Respiratory distress may be present and leads to death in the first year of life. Otherwise, the child grows but there is delay of motor milestones during childhood. Children have significant facial weakness, a high arched palate, micrognathia, and weak masseter and pterygoid muscles. The pharyngeal and laryngeal muscles may also be affected, but extraocular muscles are spared. Skeletal anomalies such as scoliosis, pectus excavatum, clubfoot, and pes cavus are common. Dysphagia does not occur in the adult form, which presents with a limb-girdle phenotype. CK levels are normal, but the EMG shows myopathic changes. The condition derives its name from the histological finding of rods (red clusters) in the subsarcolemmal zone of muscle fibers. Ultrastructurally, the nemaline rods arise from the Z disk. Inheritance is usually autosomal dominant and rarely autosomal recessive. To date, mutations have affected genes encoding for various skeletal proteins, such as tropomyosin-3, actin, and nebulin [16].

Acquired Muscle Diseases

Primary inflammatory muscle diseases represent the largest group of acquired and potentially treatable myopathies. There are three main subsets: polymyositis (PM), dermatomyositis (DM), and inclusion body myositis (IBM). Cutaneous involvement is specific to DM, which may have infantile or adult onset. PM and IBM are disorders of adults.

In PM and DM, proximal weakness develops in weeks to months, and CK levels are often elevated. In some patients, specific autoantibodies may be detected in the serum; the most common antibodies are antisynthetase or anti-Jo1 in PM\DM with interstitial lung disease, and anti-Mi-1 and 2 in DM [17]. EMG and muscle biopsy are important for the diagnosis. Adult PM and DM may be associated with connective-tissue disease (overlap syndrome) or cancers. Some cases of PM are secondary to infections (HIV, HTLV1, and toxoplasmosis). Idiopathic PM is probably less common than other types of inflammatory myopathy, such as IBM, DM, or overlap PM [18]. In a longitudinal study of 100 consecutive adult patients with inflammatory myopathies, PM was the most common diagnosis at presentation, accounting for 45% of the cohort. Patients were then reclassified based on their clinical, antibody, and biopsy data. After complete workup, the frequency of idiopathic PM fell to 14%, while the frequency of myositis associated with connective tissue disease increased from 24 to 60% [19]. In that particular series, systemic sclerosis was the most common connective tissue disease associated with PM, accounting for 29% of the cohort.

Swallowing impairment may be severe in these patients [20]. Dysphagia is due primarily to the involvement of striated muscles, but the upper third of the esophagus may be affected in some patients, particularly in overlap PM seen with systemic sclerosis or mixed connective tissue disorders. In a study of 62 patients with overlap PM (systemic sclerosis or related disorders) referred for a gastrointestinal (GI) evaluation, dysphagia was present in 61% of patients. In addition to the dysphagia, patients may have deglutitive pharyngeal and laryngeal pain, and may develop aspiration of their food. Manometric studies in 36 patients showed antral hypomotility and reduced amplitude and frequency of intestinal contractions [21].

IBM is the most frequently acquired myopathy after 50 years of age. It is characterized by distal greater than proximal muscle weakness, slow course, and suboptimal response to corticosteroid and immunosuppressive agents. Histologically, the muscle biopsy shows rimmed vacuoles and filamentous inclusions in addition to the cytotoxic inflammatory process. On immunofluorescence, beta secretases that cleave amyloid-beta-precursor protein co-localize with amyloid beta in IBM vacuolated muscle fibers [22]. There is accumulation of tau protein in the inclusions [23]. Dysphagia may be a prominent and an early feature in older patients with IBM [24]. In some cases, dysphagia may be the presenting symptom. Laryngoscopy reveals pooling of saliva in the pharyngeal recesses. Videofluoroscopy shows a prominent cricopharyngeus muscle, and biopsies of the cricopharyngeus muscle may show the inflammatory changes [20].

Immunological stains reveal that DM is a microangiopathy affecting skin and muscle; there are perivascular B and CD4 lymphocytic infiltrates, and activation and deposition of complement that causes lysis of endomysial capillaries and muscle ischemia. In PM and IBM, CD8-positive cytotoxic T cells invade muscle fibers and lead to fiber necrosis mainly via the perforin pathway. In IBM, there is formation of vacuoles with amyloid deposits as well. The responsible antigen has not yet been identified. The upregulation of various cell adhesion molecules and cytokines contribute to the immunopathological process in all three conditions. Early diagnosis and initiation of therapy is essential, since both PM and DM respond to immunosuppressive agents. As stated above, IBM tends to be less responsive to treatment [17].

In *Thyrotoxic myopathy*, dysphagia is uncommon, but may occur. In the majority, dysphagia is preceded by proximal limb muscle weakness. Dysphagia is slow, but may appear abruptly. The dysphagia is usually due to oropharyngeal dysfunction, but some have esophageal dysmotility. Secondary hypokalemia may compound the weakness. Aspiration pneumonia may occur. Impaired swallowing may resolve 3–4 weeks after treatment for thyrotoxicosis with antithyroid agents and beta-blockers [25].

Dysphagia is not common in *Iatrogenic myopathies*, but there are rare reports involving patients with chronic renal insufficiency who were given procainamide hydrochloride for arrhythmia [26]. The dysphagia is mainly due to esophageal dysmotility, but there is also some bulbar and proximal muscle weakness. The myopathy resolves gradually after drug discontinuation. The disorder is likely due to impaired clearance leading to accumulation of the drug.

Diagnosis and Differential Diagnosis

The diagnosis depends on detailed medical history, family history, and physical and neurological examination. Elevated muscle enzymes and the presence of certain inflammatory markers aid in the diagnosis. Electrodiagnostic testing with routine nerve conduction studies, repetitive motor nerve stimulation, and needle electromyography are helpful in establishing the presence and extent of the myopathy. Muscle biopsy and genetic testing may be needed for diagnostic confirmation.

Disorders of neuromuscular transmission can present with bulbar weakness and dysphagia, and may be difficult to differentiate clinically from bulbar myopathies. In myasthenia gravis, swallowing difficulties are usually intermittent and typically worsen throughout the meal or throughout the day, but may become constant. There are often oculomotor abnormalities (diplopia, ptosis) and facial muscle weakness, and there may be dysphonia. When present, fatigable muscle weakness is often a clue to the diagnosis. The risk of aspiration is significant. Measurement of acetylcholine receptor antibodies, anti-MuSK (muscle-specific receptor tyrosine kinase) antibodies, and single fiber EMG establish the diagnosis [27]. Treatment includes cholinesterase inhibitors, corticosteroids, and plasmapheresis with occasional use of intravenous gammaglobulins [28].

The bulbar muscles can be affected in polyradiculoneuropathies, both acute (Guillain–Barré syndrome, GBS) and chronic (chronic inflammatory demyelinating polyradiculoneuropathy, CIDP). There is frequent involvement of other cranial nerves, particularly facial [29, 30]. CSF protein is elevated. Nerve conduction testing and needle EMG differentiate them from myopathy. The treatment is by preventing other medical complications, such as aspiration, and using various immune-modulating and immunosuppressive therapies.

Motor neuron disorders such as amyotrophic lateral sclerosis involve the bulbar muscles and lead to progressive dysphagia. There is weakness of the oro-lingual as well as the pharyngeal muscles. Muscle fasciculations (tongue, face) are common. These patients develop swallowing difficulties mainly to solids, but given the frequent presence of an upper motor neuron dysfunction, they may choke on liquids. Dysphagia occurs in up to 20% of the patients after 1 year of diagnosis and increases steadily with disease progression. The risk for aspiration pneumonia is high, and these patients should be counseled regarding the insertion of a gastric feeding tube.

Among hereditary motor neuron disorders, dysphagia tends to occur early in bulbospinal muscular atrophy (Kennedy's disease). This is an X-linked disorder in which a triple CAG repeat on the long arm of the X chromosome leads to degeneration of bulbar motor neurons and reduced tissue responsiveness to androgen. The syndrome should be suspected in a middle-aged man who presents with dysphagia and gynecomastia. Genetic testing is confirmatory [31].

Management

The discussion of management will focus on the appropriate intervention in patients with chronic, untreatable, non-inflammatory muscle disease.

The primary objective should be the reduction in laryngeal penetration of bolus, reduction in aspiration and chest infections, stabilization or reversal of progressive weight loss, and improvement in the quality of life.

The initial evaluation should ascertain safe swallowing. While bedside assessment is frequently done as first step, it may underestimate the degree of swallowing impairment. Therefore, a videofluoroscopic swallowing study should be performed. The videofluoroscopic imaging also assists in selecting optimal food texture and consistency. The patient should be instructed in the importance of positioning for safe swallowing; the patient should be seated upright with the head tilted slightly forward and the neck flexed. If there is unilateral pharyngeal paresis, head turning may allow the bolus to traverse the intact side [32].

Nasogastric tube feeding or peripheral intravenous feeding are temporary measures, and if the patient's condition does not improve, long-term nutritional approaches become necessary. In these cases, the wishes of the patient and family must be considered. The most common procedure performed is that of percutaneous endoscopic gastrostomy (PEG). The procedure can be performed quickly with minimal sedation. There is the potential for gastropharyngeal reflux and aspiration particularly if pharyngeal weakness coexists; this risk can be reduced by feeding the patient upright and by using a slow-rate of infusion.

In patients with slowly progressive myopathies who aspirate, the procedures to protect the airway should be discussed. Tracheostomy is probably the most common procedure performed in these patients. Other procedures, such as laryngeal closure or diversion procedures, are more aggressive but may be necessary in the few refractory cases.

In a large percentage of myopathic patients, cricopharyngeal dysfunction contributes significantly to the dysphagia. Upper esophageal sphincter dilatation and botulinum toxin injections may provide temporary relief [32–34]. Cricopharyngeal myotomy is the operation performed most frequently to correct dysphagia in these patients. This procedure seems to be particularly successful in oculopharyngeal dystrophy [35, 36]. The presence of a significant gastroesophageal reflux is a relative contraindication to this procedure. The Cochrane Data Base reviewed various trials of adults and children with chronic untreatable non-inflammatory muscle disease [37]. The interventions included dietary modification, swallowing maneuvers, enteral feeding, and other surgical interventions including cricopharyngeal myotomy. The unfortunate conclusion was the lack of adequate trials to evaluate the efficacy of treatments in the management of chronic myopathic dysphagia.

Dysphagia rehabilitation methods include muscle strengthening, compensatory methods (such as head turning and double swallowing), sensory stimulation, and dietary modification. However, these methods tend to more successful in neurogenic than in myopathic dysphagia. Therefore, the rehabilitation plan is individualized.

References

1. Willig TN, Paulus J, Lacau Saint Guily J, et al. Swallowing problems in neuromuscular disorders. Arch Phys Med Rehabil. 1994;75:1175–81.
2. Tome FM, Chateau D, Helbling-Leclerc A, Fardeau M. Morphological changes in muscle fibers in oculopharyngeal muscular dystrophy. Neuromuscul Disord. 1997;7 Suppl 1:S63–69.
3. Blumen SC, Brais B, Korczyn AD, et al. Homozygotes for oculopharyngeal muscular dystrophy have a severe form of the disease. Ann Neurol. 1999;46:115–8.
4. Calado A, Tome FM, Brais B, et al. Nuclear inclusions in oculopharyngeal muscular dystrophy consist of poly(A) binding protein 2 aggregates which sequester poly(A) RNA. Hum Mol Genet. 2000;9:2321–8.
5. Clay AS, Behnia M, Brown KK. Mitochondrial disease: a pulmonary and critical-care medicine perspective. Chest. 2001;120:634–48.
6. Kornblum C, Broicher R, Walther E, et al. Cricopharyngeal achalasia is a common cause of dysphagia in patients with mtDNA deletions. Neurology. 2001;56:1409–12.
7. Alusi GH, Grant WE, Quiney RE. Oculopharyngeal myopathy with sensorineural hearing loss. J Laryngol Otol. 1996;110:567–9.
8. Wong KT, Dick D, Anderson JR. Mitochondrial abnormalities in oculopharyngeal muscular dystrophy. Neuromuscul Disord. 1996;6:163–6.
9. Groh WJ, Lowe MR, Zipes DP. Severity of cardiac conduction involvement and arrhythmias in myotonic dystrophy type 1 correlates with age and CTG repeat length. J Cardiovasc Electrophysiol. 2002;13(5): 444–8.
10. Censori B, Provinciali L, Danni M, et al. Brain involvement in myotonic dystrophy: MRI features and their relationship to clinical and cognitive conditions. Acta Neurol Scand. 1994;90:211–7.
11. Harley HG, Rundle SA, MacMillan JC, et al. Size of the unstable CTG repeat sequence in relation to phenotype and parental transmission in myotonic dystrophy. Am J Hum Genet. 1993;52:1164–74.
12. Barohn RJ, Levine EJ, Olson JO, et al. Gastric hypomotility in Duchenne's muscular dystrophy. N Engl J Med. 1988;319:15–8.
13. Stübgen JP. Limb girdle muscular dystrophy: a radiologic and manometric study of the pharynx and esophagus. Dysphagia. 1996;11:25–9.
14. Lu H, Luan X, Yuan Y, et al. The clinical and myopathological features of oculopharyngodistal myopathy in a Chinese family. Neuropathology. 2008;28: 599–603.
15. Philpot J, Bagnall A, King C, et al. Feeding problems in merosin deficient congenital muscular dystrophy. Arch Dis Child. 1999;80:542–7.
16. Ryan MM, Schnell C, Strickland CD, et al. Nemaline myopathy: a clinical study of 143 cases. Ann Neurol. 2001;50(3):312–20.
17. Dalakas MC, Hohlfeld R. Polymyositis and dermatomyositis. Lancet. 2003;362(9388):971–82.
18. Van der Meulen MF, Bronner IM, Hoogendijk JE, et al. Polymyositis: a diagnostic entity reconsidered. Neurology. 2003;61:316–21.
19. Trotanov Y, Tremblay JL, Goulet JR, et al. Novel classification of idiopathic inflammatory myopathies based on overlap syndrome features and autoantibodies: analysis of 100 French Canadian patients. Medicine. 2005;84:231–49.
20. Shapiro J, Martin S, DeGirolami U, Goyal R. Inflammatory myopathy causing pharyngeal dysphagia: a new entity. Ann Otol Rhinol Laryngol. 1996;105:331–5.
21. Weston S, Thumshirn M, Wiste J, Camilleri M. Clinical and upper gastrointestinal motility features in systemic sclerosis and related disorders. Am J Gastroenterol. 1998;93:1085–9.

22. Vattemi G, Engel WK, McFerrin J, et al. Presence of BACE1 and BACE2 in muscle fibres of patients with sporadic inclusion-body myositis. Lancet. 2001;358(9297):1962–4.

23. Salajegheh M, Pinkus JL, Taylor PJ, et al. Sarcoplasmic redistribution of nuclear TDP-43 in inclusion body myositis. Muscle Nerve. 2009;40:19–31.

24. Verma A, Bradley WG, Adesina AM, Sofferman R, Pendlebury WW. Inclusion body myositis with cricopharyngeus muscle involvement and severe dysphagia. Muscle Nerve. 1991;14(5):470–3.

25. Chiu WY, Yang CC, Huang IC, Huang TS. Dysphagia as a manifestation of thyrotoxicosis: report of three cases and literature review. Dysphagia. 2004;19:120–4.

26. Miller CD, Oleshansky MA, Gibson KF, Cantilena LR. Procainamide-induced myasthenia-like weakness and dysphagia. Ther Drug Monit. 1993;15:251–4.

27. Vincent A, Bowen J, Newsom-Davis J, McConville J. Seronegative generalized myasthenia gravis: clinical features, antibodies, and their targets. Lancet Neurol. 2003;2:99–106.

28. Richman DP, Agius MA. Treatment of autoimmune myasthenia gravis. Neurology. 2003;61:1652–61.

29. Ropper AH. Unusual clinical variants and signs in Guillain–Barré syndrome. Arch Neurol. 1986;43:1150–2.

30. Dyck PJ, Prineas J, Pollard J. Chronic inflammatory demyelinating polyradiculoneuropathy. In: Dyck PJ, Thomas PK, Griffin JW, Low PA, Poduslo JF, editors.

Peripheral Neuropathy. 3rd ed. Philadelphia, PA: WB Saunders; 1993. p. 1498–517.

31. Parboosingh JS, Figlewicz DA, Krizus A, Meininger V, Azad NA, Newman DS, Rouleau GA. Spinobulbar muscular atrophy can mimic ALS: the importance of genetic testing in male patients with atypical ALS. Neurology. 1997;49(2):568–72.

32. Sonies BC. Evaluation and treatment of speech and swallowing disorders associated with myopathies. Curr Opin Rheumatol. 1997;9:486–95.

33. Mathieu J, Lapointe G, Brassard A, et al. A pilot study on upper esophageal sphincter dilatation for the treatment of dysphagia in patients with oculopharyngeal muscular dystrophy. Neuromuscul Disord. 1997;7 Suppl 1:S100–104.

34. Restivo DA, Marchese Ragona R, Staffieri A, de Grandis D. Successful botulinum toxin treatment of dysphagia in oculopharyngeal muscular dystrophy. Gastroenterology. 2000;119:1416–6.

35. Duranceau A. Cricopharyngeal myotomy in the management of neurogenic and muscular Dysphagia. Neuromusc Disord. 1997;7(1):S85–9.

36. Fradet G, Pouliot D, Robichaud R, et al. Upper esophageal sphincter myotomy in oculopharyngeal muscular dystrophy: long-term clinical results. Neuromuscul Disord. 1997;7 Suppl 1:S90–95.

37. Hill M, Hughes T, Milford C. Treatment for swallowing difficulties (dysphagia) in chronic muscle disease. Cochrane Database Syst Rev. 2004;2(CD004303):1–17.

Cathy Lazarus

Abstract

This chapter reviews the effects of chemotherapy and radiotherapy on swallowing in treated head and neck cancer patients. Early and late effects of radiotherapy on tissues are described. Specific effects of chemotherapy and radiotherapy on oropharyngeal swallowing are reviewed. Behavioral, medical, and surgical management of dysphagia in this population are discussed.

Keywords

Chemoradiotherapy • Dysphagia • Head and neck cancer • Radiotherapy • Rehabilitation • Swallowing

Dysphagia is a common consequence after treatment for head and neck cancer and has been found in up to 40 % of head and neck cancer survivors [1]. Further, the incidence of aspiration pneumonia due to dysphagia in the patient treated with chemoradiotherapy has been found to range from 22 to 89 % [2–6], with silent aspiration occurring in up to 100 % [2]. Organ preservation treatment by radiotherapy and chemoradiotherapy has been found to result in cure rates comparable to those after surgery and radiation therapy for head and neck cancer [7–12]. Further, chemoradiotherapy has resulted in significantly improved locoregional control as compared to induction chemotherapy followed by radiotherapy or radiotherapy alone [13–15]. However, when comparing chemoradiotherapy, induction chemotherapy followed by concomitant chemoradiotherapy, and surgery and radiotherapy treatments, the mucosal toxicity of concomitant chemoradiotherapy has been found to be nearly twice as great as that seen after the other two treatments [13]. Altered fractionation (i.e., hyperfractionation and/or acceleration) schedules can improve locoregional control and overall survival [16, 17]. However, side effects, both acute and chronic have been found to be more severe [16].

C. Lazarus, PhD., CCC-SLP, BRS-S, ASHA Fellow (✉)
Department of Otolaryngology Head & Neck Surgery,
Beth Israel Medical Center, 10 Union Square East,
New York, NY, USA

Department of Otorhinolaryngology Head & Neck
Surgery, Albert Einstein College of Medicine,
New York, NY, USA
e-mail: clazarus@chpnet.org

Radiotherapy Physiologic Effects

The effects of external beam irradiation on tissues have been well documented. The acute and late effects of high-dose irradiation on nerves, muscles, and the vascular system have been studied extensively in animals. High-dose radiation to the mouse tongue has resulted in injury to the neuromuscular junctures and produced wider synaptic cleft width [18]. Radiation-induced neuropathy has resulted in widened motor end-plate zones and atrophied muscle fibers, with an increase in connective tissue [19]. Fewer motor end-plate potentials due to chronic impairment in nerve conduction have also been observed [19]. Muscle fiber atrophy, necrosis, degeneration of the T tubes and alteration of sarcoplasmic reticulum, the latter resulting in impairment of sarcomere contraction have been found [19, 20]. Vascular changes following irradiation have been found which result in replacement of muscle and tissue fibrosis [21] as well as loss of muscle fibers, decreased fiber size, and necrosis [21]. Inflammation has been seen as an early effect and atrophic fibrosis has been observed as a late radiation effect.

Early and late effects of radiation have also been examined in humans. Early effects, which typically occur during treatment or within the first 1–2 months of radiation exposure, include erythema, resulting from dilatation of capillaries, tissue ulceration and mucositis. Mucositis can result in pain, soreness, and ulceration [22]. Changes to the mucosa can also include erythema and desquamation following radiotherapy to the oral cavity and oropharynx [23]. In addition to tissue effects, other physiologic effects of radiotherapy, particularly to the oral and oropharyngeal regions, can include burning sensation, altered tactile sensation, altered or reduced taste sensation, reduced dental sensation, xerostomia, and changes in the oral flora.

Late effects of radiotherapy can include bone changes, such as osteoradionecrosis, trismus (restriction in mouth opening), and worsening of xerostomia [23–28]. In addition, impaired pharyngeal and laryngeal sensation has been found

postradiotherapy [29]. Older age, advanced T stage, larynx/hypopharynx primary sites, and neck dissection after chemoradiotherapy have been associated with increased risk of late toxicities [30]. Radiotherapy can also result in peripheral neuropathy [31–33]. An additional late effect of radiotherapy, which typically occurs after 6 months, is tissue fibrosis. Radiation fibrosis is characterized by damage to arteries, arterioles, and capillaries, with capillary occlusion and collagen replacement, which reduces the blood supply to the muscles, further interfering with muscle functioning. Fibrosis is characterized by changes in vascular connective tissue tissues that involve excessive extracellular matrix deposition, fibroblast proliferation, and an inflammatory process [34, 35] causing persistent induration and fibrosis [36–38]. Fibrosis has been associated with stiffness of tissues in the neck soft tissue, with a more severe degree of fibrosis resulting in increased stiffness that can result in reduced range of motion [39]. Lingual necrosis has been observed following high-dose radiotherapy to the tongue base with interstitial implantation of the tumor [40].

Both acute and late effects of radiotherapy to the oral cavity, oropharynx, and pharynx appear to be dose dependent, including total dose, dose per fraction, and total treatment time [41–44]. Shorter latency to onset of side effects with increasing intensity of radiotherapy has been found, with tissue changes occurring up to 15 years after irradiation [43]. Less severe acute effects and reduced risk for late effects have been found with extension of overall treatment time [42].

Radiotherapy can also affect muscle strength, though much of the research has focused on the limbs. Studies have shown a reduction in muscle strength with radiotherapy which persists over time [45, 46], with reductions in muscle strength of up to 25 % following radiotherapy [45]. Muscle wasting and loss of movement have also been observed as early and late complications following radiotherapy to skeletal muscle [38]. Lingual muscle strength has been found to be reduced following chemoradiotherapy in oral and oropharyngeal cancer patients as compared to healthy individuals [5].

Radiotherapy Effects on Salivary Function

Reduced salivary flow in the irradiated head and neck cancer patient can have a major impact on swallow functioning. Saliva plays a critical role in maintaining and protecting the oral tissues. This is accomplished by lubricating the mucosal tissues, which provides a barrier to injury and providing salivary proteins, which protect against candida and which modulate the bacterial and fungal colonization within the oral cavity [47]. In addition, saliva provides lubrication to assist in bolus formation, manipulation, and propulsion [48, 49]. Reduced salivary flow can result in increased oral transit times in individuals with salivary dysfunction [49]. In addition, saliva is necessary for triggering of the pharyngeal swallow [50]. Xerostomia results in elimination of salivary bicarbonate and contributes to GERD and extraesophageal reflux in some patients [51]. Irradiated head and neck cancer patients have been found to exhibit markedly reduced unstimulated salivary flow rates when compared to normal controls [27, 52]. Further, there is often no recovery of salivary function over time in these patients [52]. Interestingly although perception of reduced salivary flow correlates well with measured salivary production, reduced salivary flow does not affect oral phase physiology in terms of bolus transport through the oral cavity (i.e., oral transit times and percent oral residue) [53].

Chemo and Radiotherapy Effects on Quality of Life

Inability to eat, either due to physiologic swallow impairment, or due to nausea, lack of appetite, lack of or altered taste, xerostomia, and mucositis can have a devastating impact on quality of life [54–57]. Alterations in taste after radiotherapy can play a major role in appetite and the pleasure of eating [54–56]. Patients often complain of difficulty chewing, increased meal time, reduced pleasure eating, as well as sticky saliva, and food sticking in the mouth and throat, all of which can also result in a major negative impact on quality of life [54–58]. Malnutrition and weight loss are an additional problem in this population and can result in prolonged dependence on nonoral means of nutrition, such as gastrostomy or PEG feedings [57, 59, 60]. Patients have been found to lose 10 % of their pretreatment weight and demonstrate a decline in eating ability [59]. However, eating ability has been found to improve over the course of the first year after chemoradiation in a group of oral and oropharyngeal cancer patients, with all patients able to take at least 50 % of nutrition by mouth [61].

Weight loss has been found to influence outcomes with chemoradiotherapy, including treatment interruption [62]. It has been shown that weight loss greater than 20 % of prediagnosis weight significantly correlates with treatment interruptions [62]. Further, PEG insertion at the onset of treatment has been found to result in smaller reduction in body mass index at 12 months posttreatment than in a similar group of patients who did not undergo PEG placement [63]. Not all patients, however, require PEG tube placement at the onset of treatment and nutritional outcomes have been found comparable in patients undergoing prophylactic PEG vs. no PEG prior to radiotherapy [64]. In a group of 90 consecutive patients who underwent chemoradiotherapy, 60 % of the patients did not require PEG tube placement [65]. Adding oral nutritional supplementation can have a positive impact on outcomes regarding weight loss and can result in lower rate of PEG tube placement [66]. Lee and colleagues [66] found a 37 % reduction in weight loss in patients treated with chemoradiotherapy who received nutritional supplementation. Others have found placement of NG tubes only when needed during treatment to be an effective method for managing malnutrition in those treated with concomitant chemoradiotherapy to the head and neck [67]. These authors found a median duration of NG tube placement to be 40 days [67].

Chemo and Radiotherapy Effects on Swallowing Pathophysiology

Radiotherapy and chemoradiotherapy can have a profound impact on swallowing. Swallowing impairment following primary radiotherapy or chemoradiotherapy has been observed in head and neck cancer patients treated with chemoradiotherapy to tumor sites including oral cavity, oropharynx, nasopharynx, hypopharynx, and larynx [2, 3, 5, 6, 13, 61, 68–72]. Both oral and pharyngeal phase function can become impaired. Oral phase swallow impairment can include reduced ability to manipulate and propel a bolus, reduced lingual strength, increased oral transit times, and increased oral residue in patients treated with primary chemoradiotherapy [2, 3, 5, 61, 73]. Reduced lingual strength has been found to correlate with increased oral residue, prolonged oral transit times, and reduced oropharyngeal swallow efficiency (OPSE, a global measure of swallowing safety and efficiency) [74] in patients treated with chemoradiotherapy to the oral cavity or oropharynx [5]. Tongue strength has been found to significantly correlate with percent oral intake in oral and oropharyngeal cancer patients treated with chemoradiotherapy [61]. The pharyngeal swallow has been found to trigger late in these patients [2, 4, 73], likely due to peripheral sensory changes due to the radiotherapy [23, 25].

Pharyngeal phase swallow impairment has been observed across head and neck tumor sites and can include one or more of the muscular components of the pharyngeal motor response, including reduced tongue base posterior movement, velopharyngeal closure, delayed triggering of the pharyngeal swallow, reduced pharyngeal contraction, reduced hypo-laryngeal motion, reduced laryngeal vestibule and glottic closure, and reduced opening of the upper esophageal sphincter, all of which can contribute to reduced bolus clearance through the pharynx and subsequent aspiration [2–4, 6, 69, 70, 73]. Both speed of motion, timing and extent of pharyngeal structural movement have been found to be reduced as compared to healthy control subjects [4]. Aspiration typically occurs after the swallow,

due to pharyngeal residue, and is often silent, due to reduced cough reflex as well as reduced laryngopharyngeal sensation in these irradiated patients [23, 29]. Pharyngeal manometry has revealed reduced tongue base and pharyngeal wall pressures that correlate with impaired bolus clearance and pharyngeal residue in irradiated head and neck cancer patients [75]. Stenosis or stricture within the oropharynx and pharyngoesophageal (PE) region has also been observed in patients treated with high-dose chemoradiation [1, 68, 76].

Although swallow impairment can be seen during and soon after radiotherapy, patients often demonstrate swallowing impairment as a late effect of radiotherapy, due to the later effects of tissue fibrosis [5, 37, 46, 77, 78], with impairment in pharyngeal constrictor motion, reduced laryngeal motion for airway protection and upper esophageal sphincter opening, and reduced bolus clearance through the pharynx [5, 77–79]. These late effects of radiation fibrosis can occur up to 40 years posttreatment. In a group of patients having undergone radiotherapy at least 10 years previously, all patients demonstrated pharyngeal phase motility disorders including reduced laryngeal elevation, reduced cricopharyngeal opening, reduced laryngeal vestibule closure, and impaired tongue base to pharyngeal wall contact during the swallow [80].

There is disagreement in the literature as to the course of swallow functioning after concomitant chemoradiotherapy treatment. Swallowing has been found to improve over the course of 12 months in a group of oral and oropharyngeal cancer patients treated with primary chemoradiotherapy, with a significant drop in ability to eat 1 month posttreatment and 100 % of patients able to take at least half of their nutrition by mouth by 12 months posttreatment [61]. However, Logemann and colleagues [73] found that patients treated with primary chemoradiotherapy demonstrated an increase in frequency of oral and pharyngeal phase swallow motility disorders over time and a significant decrease in frequency of functional swallow from baseline to 3 months postchemoradiotherapy, with some improvement was seen by 12 months.

High-dose rate (HDR) intraoperative radio-therapy (IORT) and interstitial radiotherapy (i.e., brachytherapy) have been utilized with surgery and chemoradiotherapy with good out-comes in terms of disease control and long-term survival in new and recurrent head and neck tumors [81–84]. Both IORT and brachytherapy were developed to deliver high-dose radiotherapy into the tumor bed in order to minimize dosage to surrounding healthy tissue and also preserve salivary function [85].

A new subset of patients with oropharynx tumors have been identified that are nonsmokers and nondrinkers but have human papillomavirus (HPV) tumor markers [86–88]. Response to chemoradiotherapy regimens in these patients has been better than that seen in comparable patients who have HPV-negative tumors [86]. A 58 % reduction in risk of death posttreatment has been found in HPV-positive cancers as compared to HPV-negative tobacco-related cancers [86, 89]. Thus, newer radiotherapy treat-ment regimens are currently being developed to deintensify radiotherapy treatment for this subset of patients.

Evaluation and Treatment of Swallowing Problems After Chemoradiotherapy

Instrumental assessment of swallowing is critical to define the physiologic swallowing abnormali-ties and determine whether therapeutic strategies might improve swallow efficiency and safety. Instrumental techniques include the Modified Barium Swallow (videofluoroscopic swallow study) [90, 91] and Flexible Endoscopic Evalu-ation of swallowing (FEES) [92–94]. Assessment should utilize calibrated bolus volumes as well as varied bolus viscosities, including liquids, pudding, and a masticated consistency to assess the impact of bolus variables on oropharyngeal swallow functioning. Therapeutic strategies should be a component of the instrumental assess-ment, and can include postures, swallow maneu-vers, and sensory enhancements to improve swallow functioning [95, 96]. Manometry can be

employed to assess oral and pharyngeal pressure generation and upper esophageal sphincter func-tion during swallowing [75, 97–99]. When paired with fluoroscopy, pressure information can be correlated with physiologic events that occur (i.e., reduced UES opening, reduced tongue base and pharyngeal constrictor motion, both of which can result in reduced bolus clearance and residue) in the oral and pharyngeal phases of swallowing.

Swallow maneuvers can modify various aspects of the pharyngeal motor response, specifically, modifying extent, timing, and/or coordination of pharyngeal structural movement. The Mendelsohn maneuver and Shaker exercise both focus on increasing the extent and duration of hyo-laryngeal movement, thereby increasing the width and duration of upper esophageal sphincter opening [100–103]. The super supra-glottic swallow maneuver assists in early airway entrance and glottic closure for added airway protection for those with reduced or slowed air-way closure, as is often seen in patients after chemoradiotherapy [104, 105]. The Effortful swallow is designed to improve tongue base posterior motion to improve contact with the posterior pharyngeal wall and thereby improve bolus clearance through the upper pharynx [80, 106–110]. This maneuver has been found to generate higher velocity bolus driving forces to propel the bolus into and through the pharynx for improved bolus clearance through the oral cavity and pharynx [80, 106, 107]. The tongue-hold maneuver is designed to improve pharyngeal constrictor motion (i.e., anteriorward), which is frequently impaired in these patients [90, 111, 112]. The pharyngeal squeeze maneuver is an addi-tional maneuver that may improve pharyngeal constrictor motion for swallowing [113]. These maneuvers cannot only improve the extent of pharyngeal structural movement, but also improve timing and coordination of the pharynx l during swallowing [80, 106].

Postures do not alter swallow physiology; rather, they can change bolus flow through the oral cavity and pharynx [95]. These include chin tuck, head back, head tilt, head rotation, and lying down to improve bolus flow and clearance through the oral cavity and pharynx. They also afford improved airway protection (i.e., chin tuck, head rotation) as well as improved bolus clearance in unilateral oral and pharyngeal impairment [95]. The Modified Barium Swallow study and the FEES examination both are useful for determining the effects of postures and maneuvers, once the specific physiologic disorders are identified.

Prevention of Swallowing Problems for Patients Undergoing Chemoradiotherapy

Since approximately 44 % of patients experience difficulty swallowing following chemoradiotherapy [114], clinicians have begun to provide prophylactic, pretreatment swallow exercise programs to patients. These exercises are designed to preserve range of motion, rate, coordination, and flexibility of the vocal tract musculature involved in swallowing [95]. These exercises focus on maintaining tongue, jaw, and pharyngeal constrictor strength, hyo-laryngeal elevation and anterior motion, airway closure, and upper esophageal sphincter opening. This treatment regimen typically includes tongue range of motion, tongue strengthening, tongue base range of motion (i.e., effortful swallow, tongue-hold maneuver, and tongue base retraction exercise (gargle) [115]), jaw range of motion (as indicated), pharyngeal constrictor exercise (tongue-hold maneuver), hyo-laryngeal elevation/upper esophageal sphincter opening exercises (Mendelsohn maneuver, Shaker exercise), and airway closure exercises (i.e., super supraglottic swallow). A range of motion and strengthening exercises have been found to improve lingual function and swallowing [116–119]. Patients are instructed to perform these exercises on a daily basis during chemoradiotherapy.

There are recent studies that support the use of swallow exercise programs during radio/chemoradiotherapy. Two studies have shown potential benefit to patients undergoing primary radio/chemoradiotherapy, with improvement in both quality of life and pharyngeal phase swallow functioning as compared to control (no-exercise) groups [120, 121]. A randomized study examined the effects of tongue strengthening exercise on swallowing during chemoradiotherapy in oral/oropharyngeal cancer patients. Although these authors found no change in tongue strength when comparing the two groups (exercise vs. no exercise), they found significantly improved quality of life in the treatment group as compared to the controls, perhaps because the treatment group was doing an exercise protocol [122]. A recent randomized clinical trial examined the effects of two exercise regimens: (1) "standard" rehabilitation exercise (i.e., range of motion and strengthening (effortful, tongue-hold, and super supraglottic swallow); and (2) experimental rehabilitation exercise: "standard" exercise plus passive mouth opening using a mobilization device [123] combined with a suprahyoid muscle strengthening task [124]. These authors found significantly less residue based on MBS evaluation in the experimental exercise arm [124]. These authors also observed good ability to perform the exercises and fairly good compliance with the exercise programs during chemoradiotherapy [124], providing support for the use of exercise programs during treatment. Further, research has shown that delayed swallow therapy is not as useful as therapy within the first year of treatment [125].

Since swallowing impairment can last up to a year, patients should be followed with the eventual goal of maximizing diet type and removal of PEG tubes. Clinicians should work with nutritionists to determine best caloric and nutritional needs when PEG feedings are weaned and oral intake is increased. Nutritional counseling with added oral nutritional supplementation can improve outcomes related to weight loss and PEG tube placement [62]. Further, nutritional supplementation has been associated with a 37 % relative reduction in weight loss in patients treated with chemoradiotherapy [62].

As patients may experience dysphagia long after chemoradiotherapy treatment, patients should be monitored yearly for changes in swallowing for at least 5 years posttreatment.

In addition, patients should be encouraged to continue performing swallowing exercises given during treatment with the goal of preventing additional fibrotic changes to the oral and pharyngeal tissues that may have a negative impact on swallowing [126]. However, research is needed to examine treatment efficacy for prevention of late onset dysphagia with use of these exercises. A newer strategy to improve oropharyngeal swallow functioning includes neuromuscular surface electrode electrical stimulation (NMES); however, the majority of data currently do not support its use [127]. However, randomized clinical trials are currently under way examining the effects of NMES on swallowing in treated head and neck cancer patients. Electrical stimulation has been utilized with good results to improve neck range of motion in patients treated with radiotherapy to the head and neck [128].

A newer technique, expiratory muscle strength training, designed to improve respiratory strength has been found to improve swallowing and cough [129–132]. This technique has only been investigated in neurologically impaired patients, but warrants investigation in the treated head and neck cancer population.

In addition to swallowing management, newer treatments have shown some promise in the management of oral mucosal fibrosis. Trental (Pentoxifylline) has been found to reduce some of the symptoms of fibrosis [133]. Specifically, in a randomized clinical trial, this medication has been found to result in improved mouth opening, improved tongue range of motion, reduced intolerance to spicy foods, and reduce the symptoms of dysphagia and difficulty speaking [133]. Treatment of lymphedema with manual lymphatic drainage and complex decongestive therapy has been utilized to reduce lymphatic pooling for other tumor sites, such as the limbs following radiotherapy in breast cancer patients [134]. These techniques have been advocated to improve swallow functioning in treated head and neck cancer patients. However, no data to date have examined the efficacy of these techniques in the irradiated head and neck cancer population.

Prevention of Dysphagia

Intensity-modulated radiotherapy (IMRT) has been developed to spare structures related to swallowing as well as spare salivary function. Pharyngeal phase abnormalities, as identified by videoflouroscopy, have been found to correlate with anatomic changes in pharyngeal structures in patients after chemoradiotherapy to the head and neck [135]. Specifically, structural damage to the pharyngeal constrictors and larynx correlated with impairment in pharyngeal contraction, laryngeal elevation, and closure and contributed to aspiration in these patients [135]. In these same patients having undergone IMRT, they demonstrated sparing of the pharyngeal constrictors and larynx as compared to standard three-dimensional radiotherapy. Further, dosage of radiotherapy was found to correlate with swallow functioning and aspiration [135]. A similar study examining dose sparing to the superior constrictors and protection of glottic larynx with IMRT found only one instance of aspiration and feeding tube dependence 24 months after treatment in a cohort of 31 patients treated for oropharyngeal cancer [136]. A similar study in a group of nasopharynx and oropharynx cancer patients found that higher doses to the pharyngeal constrictors and laryngeal region significantly correlated with impairment in bolus clearance through the pharynx due to reduced tongue base, pharyngeal constrictor, and laryngeal elevation for swallowing [137]. Reduced rates of dermatitis as well as lower rates of gastrostomy tube placement have been found in patients treated with IMRT vs. conventional radiotherapy [44].

Medical and Other Management of Chemoradiotherapy Side Effects

Patients can develop late onset debilitating problems related to high-dose radiotherapy. These can include pharyngeal and/or esophageal stricture, due to tissue fibrosis, osteoradionecrosis of the mandible, chronic xerostomia, and trismus. For those patients who develop pharyngo-esophageal stricture, esophageal dilation has been employed, including antegrade, retrograde, and combined antegrade and retrograde endoscopic dilation, with good results [138–141]. However, patients often require multiple dilations [141]. Therefore, pharyngeal and pharyngo-esophageal reconstruction with microvascular free flaps has been utilized to improve swallow functioning with good reported results [142–145]. Jaw range of motion exercises are typically prescribed for those patients with trismus [95]. These are designed to improve maximal opening, lateral motion, and rotary motion for chewing. Mobilization regimens that mechanically assist jaw opening have been found to significantly improve jaw range of motion in the radiated patient as compared to both unassisted exercise and mechanically assisted exercise with stacked tongue depressors [123]. Artificial saliva products are often used to compensate for xerostomia. In addition, reflux medications to suppress acid production and hopefully decrease stricture formation are often prescribed for the irradiated patient. Acupuncture has been used to treat xerostomia, with improved salivary flow reported [146–148]. However a recent systematic review of the acupuncture literature to treat radiation-induced xerostomia has shown limited evidence of its benefit [149]. Osteoradio-necrosis can occur as a sequela of high-dose radiotherapy to the mandible, where bone can become devitalized and exposed, with infection and pathologic fracture development [150, 151]. Hyperbaric oxygen (HBO) treatment has been utilized to increase the diffusion of oxygen into hypoxic tissues, which can stimulate fibroblast proliferation and collagen formation [152, 153]. However, HBO does not necessarily result in favorable outcomes, particularly in those patients with severe ORN [154, 155]. Mandibular reconstruction with microvascular surgery utilizing free tissue transfer with bone can replace devascularized bone and improve outcome, including elimination of infection, restoring mandibular continuity, dental occlusion, and allowing for dental rehabilitation [156]. Osteocutaneous-free flaps can include scapula, fibula, and iliac crest [156].

The effects of radiotherapy and chemoradiotherapy can have a major impact on swallowing and quality of life. Future studies are needed to determine optimal swallow therapy regimens during and after completion of radiotherapy or chemoradiotherapy to maximize and maintain swallow functioning. Timing, duration, frequency, dosage, and overall treatment time need to be examined. Further, future studies should examine the utility of swallow exercise programs on a long-term basis, such as 5–10 years to determine whether swallow function and oral intake can be maintained over time. In addition, the effects of these exercise regimens on prevention of tissue fibrosis need to be examined. Radiation treatment regimens and adjuvant chemotherapy agents need to be refined to minimize damage to oral, pharyngeal and laryngeal structures, as well as to minimize side effects of xerostomia, mucositis, altered taste and sensation.

References

1. Francis DO, et al. Dysphagia, stricture, and pneumonia in head and neck cancer patients: does treatment modality matter? Ann Otol Rhinol Laryngol. 2010;119(6):391–7.
2. Hughes PJ, et al. Dysphagia in treated nasopharyngeal cancer. Head Neck. 2000;22(4):393–7.
3. Carrara-de Angelis E. Voice and swallowing in patients enrolled in a larynx preservation trial. Arch Otolaryngol Head Neck Surg. 2003;129(7):733–8.
4. Lazarus CL, et al. Swallowing disorders in head and neck cancer patients treated with radiotherapy and adjuvant chemotherapy. Laryngoscope. 1996;106(9 Pt 1):1157–66.
5. Lazarus CL, et al. Swallowing and tongue function following treatment for oral and oropharyngeal cancer. J Speech Lang Hear Res. 2000;43(4):1011–23.
6. Kotz T, et al. Pharyngeal transport dysfunction consequent to an organ-sparing protocol. Arch Otolaryngol Head Neck Surg. 1999;125(4):410–3.
7. Mendenhall WM, et al. Is radiation therapy a preferred alternative to surgery for squamous cell carcinoma of the base of tongue? J Clin Oncol. 2000;18(1):35–42.
8. Sessions DG, et al. Analysis of treatment results for base of tongue cancer. Laryngoscope. 2003;113(7): 1252–61.
9. Vokes EE, et al. Induction chemotherapy followed by concomitant chemoradiotherapy for advanced

head and neck cancer: impact on the natural history of the disease. J Clin Oncol. 1995;13(4):876–83.

10. Lefebvre JL, et al. Larynx preservation in pyriform sinus cancer: preliminary results of a European Organization for Research and Treatment of Cancer phase III trial EORTC Head and Neck Cancer Cooperative Group. J Natl Cancer Inst. 1996;88(13):890–9.

11. The Department of Veterans Affairs Laryngeal Cancer Study Group. Induction chemotherapy plus radiation compared with surgery plus radiation in patients with advanced laryngeal cancer. N Engl J Med. 1991;324(24):1685–90.

12. Harrison LB, et al. Performance status after treatment for squamous cell cancer of the base of tongue–a comparison of primary radiation therapy versus primary surgery. Int J Radiat Oncol Biol Phys. 1994;30(4):953–7.

13. Forastiere AA, et al. Concurrent chemotherapy and radiotherapy for organ preservation in advanced laryngeal cancer. N Engl J Med. 2003;349(22): 2091–8.

14. Calais G, et al. Randomized trial of radiation therapy versus concomitant chemotherapy and radiation therapy for advanced-stage oropharynx carcinoma. J Natl Cancer Inst. 1999;91(24):2081–6.

15. Adelstein DJ, et al. An intergroup phase III comparison of standard radiation therapy and two schedules of concurrent chemoradiotherapy in patients with unresectable squamous cell head and neck cancer. J Clin Oncol. 2003;21(1):92–8.

16. Budach W, et al. A meta-analysis of hyperfractionated and accelerated radiotherapy and combined chemotherapy and radiotherapy regimens in unresected locally advanced squamous cell carcinoma of the head and neck. BMC Cancer. 2006;6:28.

17. Mendenhall WM, et al. Altered fractionation and/or adjuvant chemotherapy in definitive irradiation of squamous cell carcinoma of the head and neck. Laryngoscope. 2003;113(3):546–51.

18. Gorodetsky R, Amir G, Yarom R. Effect of ionizing radiation on neuromuscular junctions in mouse tongues. Int J Radiat Biol. 1992;61(4):539–44.

19. Love S, Gomez S. Effects of experimental radiation-induced hypomyelinating neuropathy on motor endplates and neuromuscular transmission. J Neurol Sci. 1984;65(1):93–109.

20. Khan MY. Radiation-induced changes in skeletal muscle. An electron microscopic study. J Neuropathol Exp Neurol. 1974;33(1):42–57.

21. Remy J, et al. Long-term overproduction of collagen in radiation-induced fibrosis. Radiat Res. 1991;125(1):14–9.

22. Treister N, Sonis S. Mucositis: biology and management. Curr Opin Otolaryngol Head Neck Surg. 2007;15(2):123–9.

23. Arcuri MR, Schneider RL. The physiological effects of radiotherapy on oral tissue. J Prosthodont. 1992;1(1):37–41.

24. Knowles JC, Chalian VA, Shidnia H. Pulp innervation after radiation therapy. J Prosthet Dent. 1986;56(6): 708–11.

25. Aviv JE, et al. Surface sensibility of the floor of the mouth and tongue in healthy controls and in radiated patients. Otolaryngol Head Neck Surg. 1992;107(3): 418–23.

26. Ichimura K, Tanaka T. Trismus in patients with malignant tumours in the head and neck. J Laryngol Otol. 1993;107(11):1017–20.

27. Schwartz LK, et al. Taste intensity performance in patients irradiated to the head and neck. Physiol Behav. 1993;53(4):671–7.

28. Abu Shara KA, et al. Radiotherapeutic effect on oropharyngeal flora in patients with head and neck cancer. J Laryngol Otol. 1993;107(3):222–7.

29. Nguyen NP, et al. Effectiveness of the cough reflex in patients with aspiration following radiation for head and neck cancer. Lung. 2007;185(5):243–8.

30. Machtay M, et al. Factors associated with severe late toxicity after concurrent chemoradiation for locally advanced head and neck cancer: an RTOG analysis. J Clin Oncol. 2008;26(21):3582–9.

31. Gillette EL, et al. Late radiation injury to muscle and peripheral nerves. Int J Radiat Oncol Biol Phys. 1995;31(5):1309–18.

32. Johansson S, Svensson H, Denekamp J. Dose response and latency for radiation-induced fibrosis, edema, and neuropathy in breast cancer patients. Int J Radiat Oncol Biol Phys. 2002;52(5):1207–19.

33. Lin YS, Jen YM, Lin JC. Radiation-related cranial nerve palsy in patients with nasopharyngeal carcinoma. Cancer. 2002;95(2):404–9.

34. Denham JW, Hauer-Jensen M. The radiotherapeutic injury–a complex "wound". Radiother Oncol. 2002;63(2):129–45.

35. Burger A, et al. Molecular and cellular basis of radiation fibrosis. Int J Radiat Biol. 1998;73(4):401–8.

36. Ben-Yosef R, Kapp DS. Persistent and/or late complications of combined radiation therapy and hyperthermia. Int J Hyperthermia. 1992;8(6):733–45.

37. Bentzen SM, Thames HD, Overgaard M. Latent-time estimation for late cutaneous and subcutaneous radiation reactions in a single-follow-up clinical study. Radiother Oncol. 1989;15(3):267–74.

38. Brown AP, Fixsen JA, Plowman PN. Local control of Ewing's sarcoma: an analysis of 67 patients. Br J Radiol. 1987;60(711):261–8.

39. Huang YP, Zheng YP, Leung SF. Quasi-linear viscoelastic properties of fibrotic neck tissues obtained from ultrasound indentation tests in vivo. Clin Biomech. 2005;20(2):145–54.

40. Lazarus CL, et al. Swallow recovery in an oral cancer patient following surgery, radiotherapy, and hyperthermia. Head Neck. 1994;16(3):259–65.

41. Karasek K, Constine LS, Rosier R. Sarcoma therapy: functional outcome and relationship to treatment parameters. Int J Radiat Oncol Biol Phys. 1992;24(4): 651–6.

42. Maciejewski B, et al. Dose fractionation and regeneration in radiotherapy for cancer of the oral cavity and oropharynx. Part 2. Normal tissue responses: acute and late effects. Int J Radiat Oncol Biol Phys. 1990;18(1):101–11.

43. Bentzen SM, Turesson I, Thames HD. Fractionation sensitivity and latency of telangiectasia after postmastectomy radiotherapy: a graded-response analysis. Radiother Oncol. 1990;18(2):95–106.

44. Salama JK, et al. Induction chemotherapy and concurrent chemoradiotherapy for locoregionally advanced head and neck cancer: a multi-institutional phase II trial investigating three radiotherapy dose levels. Ann Oncol. 2008;19(10):1787–94.

45. Jentzsch K, et al. Leg function after radiotherapy for Ewing's sarcoma. Cancer. 1981;47(6):1267–78.

46. Stinson SF, et al. Acute and long-term effects on limb function of combined modality limb sparing therapy for extremity soft tissue sarcoma. Int J Radiat Oncol Biol Phys. 1991;21(6):1493–9.

47. Fox PC, et al. Xerostomia: evaluation of a symptom with increasing significance. J Am Dent Assoc. 1985;110(4):519–25.

48. Abd-El-Malek S. Observations on the morphology of the human tongue. J Anat. 1939;73(Pt 2):201–10. 3.

49. Sonies BC, Ship JA, Baum BJ. Relationship between saliva production and oropharyngeal swallow in healthy, different-aged adults. Dysphagia. 1989;4(2):85–9.

50. Mansson I, Sandberg N. Oro-pharyngeal sensitivity and elicitation of swallowing in man. Acta Otolaryngol. 1975;79(1–2):140–5.

51. De Fede O, et al. Oral manifestations in patients with gastro-oesophageal reflux disease: a single center case-control study. J Oral Pathol Med. 2008;37:336–40.

52. Kuo WR, et al. The effects of radiation therapy on salivary function in patients with head and neck cancer. Gaoxiong Yi Xue Ke Xue Za Zhi. 1993;9(7):401–9.

53. Logemann JA, et al. Effects of xerostomia on perception and performance of swallow function. Head Neck. 2001;23(4):317–21.

54. Hammerlid E, et al. A prospective quality of life study of patients with laryngeal carcinoma by tumor stage and different radiation therapy schedules. Laryngoscope. 1998;108(5):747–59.

55. de Graeff A, et al. A prospective study on quality of life of laryngeal cancer patients treated with radiotherapy. Head Neck. 1999;21(4):291–6.

56. List MA, et al. Quality of life and performance in advanced head and neck cancer patients on concomitant chemoradiotherapy: a prospective examination. J Clin Oncol. 1999;17(3):1020–8.

57. Oates JE, et al. Prospective evaluation of quality of life and nutrition before and after treatment for nasopharyngeal carcinoma. Arch Otolaryngol Head Neck Surg. 2007;133(6):533–40.

58. Boscolo-Rizzo P, et al. Long-term quality of life after total laryngectomy and postoperative radiotherapy versus concurrent chemoradiotherapy for laryngeal preservation. Laryngoscope. 2008;118(2):300–6.

59. Newman LA, et al. Eating and weight changes following chemoradiation therapy for advanced head and neck cancer. Arch Otolaryngol Head Neck Surg. 1998;124(5):589–92.

60. Garcia-Peris P, et al. Long-term prevalence of oropharyngeal dysphagia in head and neck cancer patients: impact on quality of life. Clin Nutr. 2007;26(6):710–7.

61. Lazarus C, et al. Effects of radiotherapy with or without chemotherapy on tongue strength and swallowing in patients with oral cancer. Head Neck. 2007;29(7):632–7.

62. Capuano G, et al. Influence of weight loss on outcomes in patients with head and neck cancer undergoing concomitant chemoradiotherapy. Head Neck. 2008;30(4):503–8.

63. Morton RP, et al. Elective gastrostomy, nutritional status and quality of life in advanced head and neck cancer patients receiving chemoradiotherapy. ANZ J Surg. 2009;79(10):713–8.

64. Chang JH, et al. Prophylactic gastrostomy tubes for patients receiving radical radiotherapy for head and neck cancers: a retrospective review. J Med Imaging Radiat Oncol. 2009;53(5):494–9.

65. McLaughlin BT, et al. Management of patients treated with chemoradiotherapy for head and neck cancer without prophylactic feeding tubes: the University of Pittsburgh experience. Laryngoscope. 2010;120(1):71–5.

66. Lee H, et al. Effect of oral nutritional supplementation on weight loss and percutaneous endoscopic gastrostomy tube rates in patients treated with radiotherapy for oropharyngeal carcinoma. Support Care Cancer. 2008;16(3):285–9.

67. Clavel S, et al. Enteral feeding during chemoradiotherapy for advanced head-and-neck cancer: a single-institution experience using a reactive approach. Int J Radiat Oncol Biol Phys. 2011;79(3):763–9.

68. Dworkin JP, et al. Swallowing function outcomes following nonsurgical therapy for advanced-stage laryngeal carcinoma. Dysphagia. 2006;21(1):66–74.

69. Smith RV, et al. Long-term swallowing problems after organ preservation therapy with concomitant radiation therapy and intravenous hydroxyurea: initial results. Arch Otolaryngol Head Neck Surg. 2000;126(3):384–9.

70. Kendall KA, et al. Structural mobility in deglutition after single modality treatment of head and neck carcinomas with radiotherapy. Head Neck. 1998;20(8):720–5.

71. Murry T, et al. Acute and chronic changes in swallowing and quality of life following intraarterial chemoradiation for organ preservation in patients with advanced head and neck cancer. Head Neck. 1998;20(1):31–7.

72. Hutcheson KA, et al. Swallowing outcomes after radiotherapy for laryngeal carcinoma. Arch Otolaryngol Head Neck Surg. 2008;134(2):178–83.

73. Logemann JA, et al. Swallowing disorders in the first year after radiation and chemoradiation. Head Neck. 2008;30(2):148–58.

74. Rademaker AW, et al. Oropharyngeal swallow efficiency as a representative measure of swallowing function. J Speech Hear Res. 1994;37(2):314–25.

75. Pauloski BR, et al. Relationship between manometric and videofluoroscopic measures of swallow function in healthy adults and patients treated for head and neck cancer with various modalities. Dysphagia. 2009;24(2):196–203.

76. Vu KN, et al. Proximal esophageal stenosis in head and neck cancer patients after total laryngectomy and radiation. ORL J Otorhinolaryngol Relat Spec. 2008;70(4):229–35.

77. Watkin KL, et al. Ultrasonic quantification of geniohyoid cross-sectional area and tissue composition: a preliminary study of age and radiation effects. Head Neck. 2001;23(6):467–74.

78. Eisele DW, et al. Case report: aspiration from delayed radiation fibrosis of the neck, Dysphagia. 1991;6(2):120–2.

79. Pauloski BR, Logemann JA. Impact of tongue base and posterior pharyngeal wall biomechanics on pharyngeal clearance in irradiated postsurgical oral and oropharyngeal cancer patients. Head Neck. 2000;22(2):120–31.

80. Lazarus CL. Effects of radiation therapy and voluntary maneuvers on swallow functioning in head and neck cancer patients. Clin Commun Disord. 1993;3(4):11–20.

81. Schuller DE, et al. Multimodal intensification regimens for advanced, resectable, previously untreated squamous cell cancer of the oral cavity, oropharynx, or hypopharynx: a 12-year experience. Arch Otolaryngol Head Neck Surg. 2007;133(4):320–6.

82. Malone JP, et al. Disease control, survival, and functional outcome after multimodal treatment for advanced-stage tongue base cancer. Head Neck. 2004;26(7):561–72.

83. Grecula JC, et al. Long-term follow-up on an intensified treatment regimen for advanced resectable head and neck squamous cell carcinomas. Cancer Invest. 2001;19(2):127–36.

84. Garrett P, et al. Intraoperative radiation therapy for advanced or recurrent head and neck cancer. Int J Radiat Oncol Biol Phys. 1987;13(5):785–8.

85. Ship JA, Hu K. Radiotherapy-induced salivary dysfunction. Semin Oncol. 2004;31(6 Suppl 18):29–36.

86. Kumar B, et al. EGFR, p16, HPV Titer, Bcl-xL and p53, sex, and smoking as indicators of response to therapy and survival in oropharyngeal cancer. J Clin Oncol. 2008;26(19):3128–37.

87. Gillison ML, et al. Evidence for a causal association between human papillomavirus and a subset of head and neck cancers. J Natl Cancer Inst. 2000;92(9):709–20.

88. D'Souza G, et al. Case-control study of human papillomavirus and oropharyngeal cancer. N Engl J Med. 2007;356(19):1944–56.

89. Ang KK, et al. Human papillomavirus and survival of patients with oropharyngeal cancer. N Engl J Med. 2010;363(1):24–35.

90. Logemann JA. Approaches to management of disordered swallowing. Baillieres Clin Gastroenterol. 1991;5(2):269–80.

91. Martin-Harris B, et al. MBS measurement tool for swallow impairment–MBSImp: establishing a standard. Dysphagia. 2008;23(4):392–405.

92. Aviv JE, et al. Fiberoptic endoscopic evaluation of swallowing with sensory testing (FEESST) in healthy controls. Dysphagia. 1998;13(2):87–92.

93. Langmore SE, Schatz K, Olsen N. Fiberoptic endoscopic examination of swallowing safety: a new procedure. Dysphagia. 1988;2(4):216–9.

94. Leder SB. Serial fiberoptic endoscopic swallowing evaluations in the management of patients with dysphagia. Arch Phys Med Rehabil. 1998;79(10):1264–9.

95. Lazarus CL. Management of swallowing disorders in head and neck cancer patients: optimal patterns of care. Semin Speech Lang. 2000;21(4):293–309.

96. Logemann JA. Rehabilitation of oropharyngeal swallowing disorders. Acta Otorhinolaryngol Belg. 1994;48(2):207–15.

97. McConnel FM, Mendelsohn MS, Logemann JA. Manofluorography of deglutition after supraglottic laryngectomy. Head Neck Surg. 1987;9(3):142–50.

98. McConnel FM, et al. Manofluorography of deglutition after total laryngopharyngectomy. Plast Reconstr Surg. 1988;81(3):346–51.

99. Lazarus C, et al. Effects of voluntary maneuvers on tongue base function for swallowing. Folia Phoniatr Logop. 2002;54(4):171–6.

100. Kahrilas PJ, et al. Volitional augmentation of upper esophageal sphincter opening during swallowing. Am J Physiol. 1991;260(3 Pt 1):G450–6.

101. Shaker R, et al. Augmentation of deglutitive upper esophageal sphincter opening in the elderly by exercise. Am J Physiol. 1997;272(6 Pt 1):G1518–22.

102. Logemann JA, et al. A randomized study comparing the Shaker exercise with traditional therapy: a preliminary study. Dysphagia. 2009;24(4):403–11.

103. Easterling C. Does an exercise aimed at improving swallow function have an effect on vocal function in the healthy elderly? Dysphagia. 2008;23(3):317–26.

104. Martin BJ, et al. Normal laryngeal valving patterns during three breath-hold maneuvers: a pilot investigation. Dysphagia. 1993;8(1):11–20.

105. Logemann JA, et al. Closure mechanisms of laryngeal vestibule during swallow. Am J Physiol. 1992;262(2 Pt 1):G338–44.

106. Steele CM, Huckabee ML. The influence of orolingual pressure on the timing of pharyngeal pressure events. Dysphagia. 2007;22(1):30–6.

107. Hind JA, et al. Comparison of effortful and noneffortful swallows in healthy middle-aged and older adults. Arch Phys Med Rehabil. 2001;82(12):1661–5.

108. Takasaki K, et al. Influence of effortful swallow on pharyngeal pressure: evaluation using a high-resolution manometry. Otolaryngol Head Neck Surg. 2011;144(1):16–20.

109. Huckabee ML, et al. Submental surface electromyographic measurement and pharyngeal pressures during normal and effortful swallowing. Arch Phys Med Rehabil. 2005;86(11):2144–9.

110. Huckabee ML, Steele CM. An analysis of lingual contribution to submental surface electromyographic measures and pharyngeal pressure during effortful swallow. Arch Phys Med Rehabil. 2006;87(8): 1067–72.

111. Fujiu M, Logemann J, Pauloski B. Increased postoperative posterior pharyngeal wall movement in patients with anterior oral cancer: preliminary findings and possible implications for treatment. Am J Speech Lang Pathol. 1995;4:24–30.

112. Fujiu M, Logemann J. Effect of a tongue-holding maneuver on posterior pharyngeal wall movement during deglutition. Am J Speech Lang Pathol. 1996;5:23–30.

113. Fuller SC, et al. Validation of the pharyngeal squeeze maneuver. Otolaryngol Head Neck Surg. 2009;140(3):391–4.

114. Eisbruch A, et al. Can IMRT or brachytherapy reduce dysphagia associated with chemoradiotherapy of head and neck cancer? The Michigan and Rotterdam experiences. Int J Radiat Oncol Biol Phys. 2007;69(2 Suppl):S40–2.

115. Veis S, Logemann JA, Colangelo L. Effects of three techniques on maximum posterior movement of the tongue base. Dysphagia. 2000;15(3):142–5.

116. Logemann JA. Rehabilitation of head and neck cancer patients. Cancer Treat Res. 1999;100:91–105.

117. Lazarus C, et al. Effects of two types of tongue strengthening exercises in young normals. Folia Phoniatr Logop. 2003;55(4):199–205.

118. Robbins J, et al. The effects of lingual exercise on swallowing in older adults. J Am Geriatr Soc. 2005;53(9):1483–9.

119. Robbin J, et al. The effects of lingual exercise in stroke patients with dysphagia. Arch Phys Med Rehabil. 2007;88(2):150–8.

120. Carroll WR, et al. Pretreatment swallowing exercises improve swallow function after chemoradiation. Laryngoscope. 2008;118(1):39–43.

121. Kulbersh BD, et al. Pretreatment, preoperative swallowing exercises may improve dysphagia quality of life. Laryngoscope. 2006;116(6):883–6.

122. Chang CW, et al. Early radiation effects on tongue function for patients with nasopharyngeal carcinoma: a preliminary study. Dysphagia. 2008;23(2): 193–8.

123. Buchbinder D, et al. Mobilization regimens for the prevention of jaw hypomobility in the radiated patient: a comparison of three techniques. J Oral Maxillofac Surg. 1993;51(8):863–7.

124. van der Molen L, et al. A randomized preventive rehabilitation trial in advanced head and neck cancer patients treated with chemoradiotherapy: feasibility, compliance, and short-term effects. Dysphagia. 2011;26(2):155–70.

125. Waters TM, et al. Beyond efficacy and effectiveness: conducting economic analyses during clinical trials. Dysphagia. 2004;19(2):109–19.

126. Lazarus CL. Effects of chemoradiotherapy on voice and swallowing. Curr Opin Otolaryngol Head Neck Surg. 2009;17(3):172–8.

127. Ludlow CL. Electrical neuromuscular stimulation in dysphagia: current status. Curr Opin Otolaryngol Head Neck Surg. 2010;18(3):159–64.

128. Lennox AJ, et al. Pilot study of impedance-controlled microcurrent therapy for managing radiation-induced fibrosis in head-and-neck cancer patients. Int J Radiat Oncol Biol Phys. 2002;54(1):23–34.

129. Pitts T, et al. Impact of expiratory muscle strength training on voluntary cough and swallow function in Parkinson disease. Chest. 2009;135(5): 1301–8.

130. Sapienza CM, Wheeler K. Respiratory muscle strength training: functional outcomes versus plasticity. Semin Speech Lang. 2006;27(4):236–44.

131. Sapienza CM. Respiratory muscle strength training applications. Curr Opin Otolaryngol Head Neck Surg. 2008;16(3):216–20.

132. Saleem AF, Sapienza CM, Okun MS. Respiratory muscle strength training: treatment and response duration in a patient with early idiopathic Parkinson's disease. NeuroRehabilitation. 2005;20(4):323–33.

133. Rajendran R, Rani V, Shaikh S. Pentoxifylline therapy: a new adjunct in the treatment of oral submucous fibrosis. Indian J Dent Res. 2006;17(4): 190–8.

134. Korpan M, Crevenna R, Fialka Moser V. Lymphedema: a therapeutic approach in the treatment and rehabilitation of cancer patients. Am J Phys Med Rehabil. 2011;90(5 Suppl 1):S69–75.

135. Eisbruch A, et al. Dysphagia and aspiration after chemoradiotherapy for head-and-neck cancer: which anatomic structures are affected and can they be spared by IMRT? Int J Radiat Oncol Biol Phys. 2004;60(5):1425–39.

136. Schwartz DL, et al. Candidate dosimetric predictors of long-term swallowing dysfunction after oropharyngeal intensity-modulated radiotherapy. Int J Radiat Oncol Biol Phys. 2010;78(5):1356–65.

137. Feng FY, et al. Intensity-modulated radiotherapy of head and neck cancer aiming to reduce dysphagia: early dose-effect relationships for the swallowing structures. Int J Radiat Oncol Biol Phys. 2007;68(5):1289–98.

138. Bueno R, et al. Combined antegrade and retrograde dilation: a new endoscopic technique in the management of complex esophageal obstruction. Gastrointest Endosc. 2001;54(3):368–72.

139. Goguen LA, et al. Combined antegrade and retrograde esophageal dilation for head and neck cancer-related complete esophageal stenosis. Laryngoscope. 2010;120(2):261–6.

140. Lew RJ, et al. Technique of endoscopic retrograde puncture and dilatation of total esophageal stenosis in patients with radiation-induced strictures. Head Neck. 2004;26(2):179–83.

141. Sullivan CA, et al. Endoscopic management of hypopharyngeal stenosis after organ sparing therapy for head and neck cancer. Laryngoscope. 2004;114(11):1924–31.

142. Amin AA, et al. Fasciocutaneous free flaps for hypopharyngeal reconstruction. J Reconstr Microsurg. 2002;18(1):1–5.

143. Lorenz RR, Alam DS. The increasing use of enteral flaps in reconstruction for the upper aerodigestive tract. Curr Opin Otolaryngol Head Neck Surg. 2003;11(4):230–5.

144. Delaere P, et al. Reconstruction for postcricoid pharyngeal stenosis after organ preservation protocols. Laryngoscope. 2006;116(3):502–4.

145. Urken ML, Jacobson AS, Lazarus CL. Comprehensive approach to restoration of function in patients with radiation-induced pharyngoesophageal stenosis: report of 31 patients and proposal of new classification scheme. Head and neck. 2011.

146. Johnstone PA, Niemtzow RC, Riffenburgh RH. Acupuncture for xerostomia: clinical update. Cancer. 2002;94(4):1151–6.

147. Garcia MK, et al. Acupuncture for radiation-induced xerostomia in patients with cancer: a pilot study. Head Neck. 2009;31(10):1360–8.

148. Blom M, Lundeberg T. Long-term follow-up of patients treated with acupuncture for xerostomia and the influence of additional treatment. Oral Dis. 2000;6(1):15–24.

149. O'Sullivan EM, Higginson IJ. Clinical effectiveness and safety of acupuncture in the treatment of irradiation-induced xerostomia in patients with head and neck cancer: a systematic review. Acupunct Med. 2010;28(4):191–9.

150. Teng MS, Futran ND. Osteoradionecrosis of the mandible. Curr Opin Otolaryngol Head Neck Surg. 2005;13(4):217–21.

151. Bras J, de Jonge HK, van Merkesteyn JP. Osteoradionecrosis of the mandible: pathogenesis. Am J Otolaryngol. 1990;11(4):244–50.

152. Marx RE. Osteoradionecrosis: a new concept of its pathophysiology. J Oral Maxillofac Surg. 1983;41(5):283–8.

153. Marx RE, Johnson RP. Studies in the radiobiology of osteoradionecrosis and their clinical significance. Oral Surg Oral Med Oral Pathol. 1987;64(4):379–90.

154. Annane D, et al. Hyperbaric oxygen therapy for radionecrosis of the jaw: a randomized, placebo-controlled, double-blind trial from the ORN96 study group. J Clin Oncol. 2004;22(24):4893–900.

155. Mounsey RA, et al. Role of hyperbaric oxygen therapy in the management of mandibular osteoradionecrosis. Laryngoscope. 1993;103(6):605–8.

156. Bak M, et al. Contemporary reconstruction of the mandible. Oral Oncol. 2010;46(2):71–6.

Swallow Syncope

Samer Gawrieh

Abstract

Swallow or deglutition syncope is a rare condition characterized by loss of consciousness that is preceded by or associated with swallowing. Dysphagia or underlying esophageal disease may not be present in all patients. The majority of patients experience brady-arrhythmias with the event. The diagnosis is suspected from the temporal relation between swallowing and the syncopal event, and confirmed by documenting concomitant swallow-induced symptoms with cardiac arrhythmias. Effort should be made to correct any underlying esophageal disease. Recurrent syncopal symptoms can be effectively prevented by placement of a cardiac pacemaker. The prognosis of deglutition syncope is generally benign although occurrence of symptoms during certain activities may subject patients to significant physical injuries.

Keywords

Swallow • Deglutition • Syncope • Dysphagia • Schatzki's ring

Swallow or deglutition syncope is characterized by temporary loss of consciousness that occurs during or immediately following swallowing.

Despite increasing awareness of this rare condition, there are less than 100 reported cases in the English literature since the condition was first described by Spens in 1793 [1].

S. Gawrieh, MD (✉)
Division of Gastroenterology and Hepatololgy,
Froedtret Hospital, Medical College of Wisconsin,
9200 W. Wisconsin Ave, Milwaukee, WI 53226, USA
e-mail: sgawrieh@mcw.edu

Clinical Presentation

Affected patients report a variety of symptoms that include lightheadedness, dizziness, weakness, near-fainting, or complete temporary loss of consciousness that accompany or shortly follow swallowing. These intermittent symptoms may be present for decades before patients seek medical attention or diagnosis is made [2–4]. The syncopal symptoms may be associated with odynophagia or dysphagia in some patients. Other symptoms such as throat or chest pain may be part of the presentation [5–12].

Swallow syncope occurs with various food consistencies (solid, liquid, carbonated or

R. Shaker et al. (eds.), *Principles of Deglutition: A Multidisciplinary Text for Swallowing and its Disorders*,
DOI 10.1007/978-1-4614-3794-9_31, © Springer Science+Business Media New York 2013

noncarbonated beverages, water, soup) and temperatures (hot or cold) [8, 9, 12–20].

Conditions Associated with Swallow Syncope

Only about 40% of the reported cases had under-lying gastroesophageal disorder. Therefore, gas-troesophageal pathology is not a prerequisite for development of swallow syncope. Structural and functional gastroesophageal conditions reported in association with swallow syncope are listed in Table 31.1. These include esophageal web, gas-troesophageal reflux disease, esophagitis, peptic stricture, Schatzki's ring, esophageal diverticu-lum, esophageal carcinoma, achalasia, diffuse or focal esophageal spasm, Nutcracker's esophagus, hiatal hernia, and gastric banding [5–15, 17–19, 21–31].

Extra-digestive conditions have also been reported in association with swallow syncope (Table 31.1): periodontitis, carotid endarterec-tomy, lung cancer, thoracic aortic aneurysm, and thoracic surgery [3, 9, 32–35].

Underlying cardiac disease is not present in most patients. However, coronary artery disease,

Table 31.1 Conditions associated with swallow syncope

Gastroesophageal
Esophageal web
Gastroesophageal reflux disease
Esophagitis
Esophageal peptic stricture
Schatzki's ring
Esophageal diverticulum
Esophageal carcinoma
Achalasia
Esophageal spasm (diffuse or focal)
Nutcracker's esophagus
Hiatal hernia
Gastric banding
Non-gastroesophageal
Periodontitis
Carotid endarterectomy
Lung cancer
Thoracic aortic aneurysm
Thoracic surgery

congestive heart failure, atrial fibrillation, and sick-sinus syndrome have been described in some patients [3, 4, 8, 12, 17, 34, 36, 37].

Mechanism

Swallow syncope is a neurally mediated situational syncope [38]. The afferent limb of the reflex likely originates from the esophageal branches of the vagus, whereas the efferent limb of the reflex likely involves the cardiac branches of the vagus, as atropine had been reported to effectively abolish the cardiac arrhythmia and subsequent symptoms [2, 3, 7, 9, 11, 15, 37, 39].

Diagnosis

The diagnosis is suspected from the history, and confirmed by documenting cardiac arrhythmias in association with swallow-induced symptoms. Underlying esophageal structural pathology should be investigated by barium esophogram and endoscopy. If these investigations are unre-vealing and the symptoms include dysphagia, heartburn, or regurgitation, esophageal manome-try, pH, and impedance studies should be consid-ered to determine the presence of esophageal dysmotility or reflux.

The majority of arrhythmias associated with swallow syncope are brady-arrhythmias: sinus bradycardia, junctional bradycardia, atrial and ventricular asystole, and varying degrees of atrio-ventricular block [4, 7, 8, 10–12, 15, 17, 19, 34]. Rarely, swallow syncope may be associ-ated with atrial fibrillation and rapid ventricular rate [5, 18, 25].

Management

Therapy involves identification and correction of any underlying esophageal pathology. Drugs that result in cardiac conduction delay should be dis-continued. Despite reported efficacy, the side effects of atropine or propantheline limit their use in this condition [2, 11, 37]. Selective vagotomy had been described but is rarely necessary [39]. Placement of a cardiac pacemaker is the most efficacious intervention at preventing recurrence of presyncopal and syncopal attacks, even if the underlying esophageal condition cannot be treated or corrected [4, 18, 36, 40, 41].

Prognosis

Swallow syncope may result in significant physical injuries if it occurs without warning or at critical times, such as operating heavy machinery, driving, or exercise. Although affected patient's survival has not been reported to be decreased, the quality of life may be negatively impacted especially if the clinical course is marked by recurrent syncopal attacks.

References

1. Spens T. Medical commentary 7:463,1793. In: Major RH, editor. Classic descriptions of disease. 2nd ed. Springfield, IL: Charles C. Thomas; 1939. P. 355.
2. Bortolotti M, Cirignotta F, Labo G. Atrioventricular block induced by swallowing in a patient with diffuse esophageal spasm. J Am Med Assoc. 1982;248(18): 2297–9.
3. Haumer M, Geppert A, Karth GD, et al. Transient swallow syncope during periods of hypoxia in a 67-year-old patient after self-extubation. Crit Care Med. 2000;28(5):1635–7.
4. Gawrieh S, Carroll T, Hogan WJ, Soergel KH, Shaker R. Swallow syncope in association with Schatzki ring and hypertensive esophageal peristalsis: report of three cases and review of the literature. Dysphagia. 2005;20(4):273–7.
5. Schima W, Sterz F, Pokieser P. Syncope after eating. N Engl J Med. 1993;328(21):1572.
6. Tolman KG, Ashworth WD. Syncope induced by dysphagia. Correction by esophageal dilatation. Am J Dig Dis. 1971;16(11):1026–31.
7. Tomlinson IW, Fox KM. Carcinoma of the oesophagus with "swallow syncope". Br Med J. 1975;2 (5966):315–6.
8. Waddington JK, Matthews HR, Evans CC, Ward DW. Letter: carcinoma of the oesophagus with "swallow syncope". Br Med J. 1975;3(5977):232.
9. Nakano T, Okano H, Konishi T, Ma W, Takezawa H. Swallow syncope after aneurysmectomy of the thoracic aorta. Heart Vessels. 1987;3(1):42–6.
10. Golf S, Forfang K. Congenital swallowing-induced symptomatic heart block: a case report of a probably

hereditary disorder. Pacing Clin Electrophysiol. 1986;9(4):602–5.
11. Guberman A, Catching J. Swallow syncope. Can J Neurol Sci. 1986;13(3):267–9.
12. Armstrong PW, McMillan DG, Simon JB. Swallow syncope. Can Med Assoc J. 1985;132(11):1281–4.
13. Kunis RL, Garfein OB, Pepe AJ, Dwyer Jr EM. Deglutition syncope and atrioventricular block selectively induced by hot food and liquid. Am J Cardiol. 1985;55(5):613.
14. Kakuchi H, Sato N, Kawamura Y. Swallow syncope associated with complete atrioventricular block and vasovagal syncope. Heart. 2000;83(6):702–4.
15. Antonelli D, Rosenfeld T. Deglutition syncope associated with carotid sinus hypersensitivity. Pacing Clin Electrophysiol. 1997;20(9 Pt 1):2282–3.
16. Olshansky B. A Pepsi challenge. N Engl J Med. 1999;340(25):2006.
17. Shapira Y, Strasberg B, Ben-Gal T. Deglutition syncope with coexistent carotid sinus hypersensitivity. Chest. 1991;99(6):1541–3.
18. Omi W, Murata Y, Yaegashi T, Inomata J, Fujioka M, Muramoto S. Swallow syncope, a case report and review of the literature. Cardiology. 2006;105(2): 75–9.
19. Marshall TM, Mizgala HF, Yeung-Lai-Wah JA, Steinbrecher UP. Successful treatment of deglutition syncope with oral beta-adrenergic blockade. Can J Cardiol. 1993;9(10):865–8.
20. Wik B, Hillestad L. Deglutition syncope. Br Med J. 1975;3(5986):747.
21. Ausubel K, Gitler B. Swallow syncope in an otherwise healthy young man. Am Heart J. 1987;113(3): 831–2.
22. Alstrup P, Pedersen SA. A case of syncope on swallowing secondary to diffuse oesophageal spasm. Acta Med Scand. 1973;193(4):365–8.
23. Drake CE, Rollings HE, Ham Jr OE, Heidary DH, Yeh TJ. Visually provoked complete atrioventricular block: an unusual form of deglutition syncope. Am J Cardiol. 1984;53(9):1408–9.
24. Farb A, Valenti SA. Swallow syncope. Md Med J. 1999;48(4):151–4.
25. Gordon J, Saleem SM, Ngaage DL, Thorpe JA. Swallow syncope associated with paroxysmal atrial fibrillation. Eur J Cardiothorac Surg. 2002;21(3):587–90.
26. Deguchi K, Mathias CJ. Continuous haemodynamic monitoring in an unusual case of swallow induced syncope. J Neurol Neurosurg Psychiatry. 1999;67(2):220–2.
27. Kunimoto S, Sibata S, Abiru M, et al. A case of swallow syncope induced by vagovagal reflex. Jpn J Med. 1990;29(2):199–202.
28. Maekawa T, Suematsu M, Shimada T, Go M, Shimada T. Unusual swallow syncope caused by huge hiatal hernia. Intern Med. 2002;41(3):199–201.
29. Lichstein E, Chadda KD. Atrioventricular block produced by swallowing, with documentation by His bundle recordings. Am J Cardiol. 1972;29(4):561–3.

30. Bortolotti M, Sarti P, Brunelli F, Mazza M, Barbara L. Abnormal esophagocardiac inhibitory reflex in patients with diffuse esophageal spasm. Digestion. 1995;56(6):488–92.

31. Leitman M, Zyssman I, Abuhatzera S, Vasserman M, Ben Baruh C, Vered Z. A 37-year-old man with recurrent fainting: a short communication. Eur J Echocardiogr. 2010;11(7):E30.

32. Endean ED, Cavatassi W, Hansler J, Sorial E. Deglutition syncope: a manifestation of vagal hyperactivity following carotid endarterectomy. J Vasc Surg. 2010;52(3):720–2.

33. Favaretto E, Schenal N, Russo N, Buja G, Iliceto S, Bilato C. An uncommon case of right-sided throat pain and swallow syncope. J Cardiovasc Med (Hagerstown). 2008;9(11):1152–5.

34. Levin B, Posner JB. Swallow syncope. Report of a case and review of the literature. Neurology. 1972;22(10):1086–93.

35. Patsilinakos SP, Antonatos DG, Spanodimos S, et al. Swallow syncope in a patient with esophageal stenosis caused by an ascending aorta aneurysm: differential diagnosis from postprandial hypotension: a case report. Angiology. 2007;58(1):126–9.

36. Casella F, Diana A, Bulgheroni M, et al. When water hurts. Pacing Clin Electrophysiol. 2009;32(11):e25–7.

37. Sy AO, Plantholt S. Swallowing-induced atrioventricular block. South Med J. 1991;84(10):1274–5.

38. Benditt DG. Neurally mediated syncopal syndromes: pathophysiological concepts and clinical evaluation. Pacing Clin Electrophysiol. 1997;20(2 Pt 2):572–84.

39. Sapru RP, Griffiths PH, Guz A, Eisele J. Syncope on swallowing. Br Heart J. 1971;33(4):617–22.

40. Tuzcu V, Halakatti R. Swallow syncope associated with complete atrioventricular block in an adolescent. Pediatr Cardiol. 2007;28(5):409–11.

41. Srivathsan K, Lee RW. Swallow syncope. Pacing Clin Electrophysiol. 2003;26(3):781–2.

Globus Pharyngeus

32

Ian J. Cook

Abstract

Globus is an extremely common, benign condition in the community. Surprisingly little is known about its aetiology. While reflux disease can be a contributory factor in a proportion of patients, there is no high level evidence that reflux causes globus. Controlled, carefully conducted radiological and manometric studies have failed to demonstrate consistent underlying motor dysfunction of the pharynx, cricopharyngeus or oesophagus. Oscillatory, inspiration-related augmentation in upper oesophageal sphincter pressure has been demonstrated but the pathogenetic relevance of this finding is unclear. Oesophageal hypersensitivity and aberrant viscerosomatic referral of oesophageal sensation to the neck has been demonstrated suggesting upregulation of oesophageal visceral afferents might be implicated. Clinical assessment in cases where globus is the sole symptom and in which there are no "alarm" symptoms (dysphagia, weight loss, pain, hoarseness), could be confined to nasolaryngoscopic examination of the larynx and pharynx. While current guidelines recommend a trial of PPI therapy in globus, there is no high level evidence to support this recommendation. A randomised controlled study has shown APC ablation of cervical oesophageal inlet patch mucosa, when present, can alleviate globus. Adoption of such therapy, however, must balance the risk of potential complications with a very common benign sensory symptom.

Keywords

Globus pharyngeus • Antireflux therapy • Argon plasma coagulation (APC) ablation • Visceral hypersensitivity • Dysphagia • Odynophagia

I.J. Cook, MBBS, MD(Syd), FRACP (✉)
Department of Gastroenterology and Hepatology,
St George Hospital,
Kogarah, NSW 2217, Australia
e-mail: i.cook@unsw.edu.au

Symptom-Based Definition

The term "globus" is derived from the Latin meaning "ball". It was originally termed globus hystericus implying a female preponderance and psychogenic aetiology. Appropriately, the

R. Shaker et al. (eds.), *Principles of Deglutition: A Multidisciplinary Text for Swallowing and its Disorders*, 449
DOI 10.1007/978-1-4614-3794-9_32, © Springer Science+Business Media New York 2013

qualifier "hystericus" has been dropped. Currently, the most widely accepted, consensus-based diagnostic definition is provided by the Rome III diagnostic criteria (Table 32.1) [1].

Typically the symptom is perceived as a sense of a lump or retained food bolus or tightness in the throat. A range of additional foreign body-like descriptors is reported by patients including a sense of retained particulate matter, mucus accumulation or a restrictive or choking sensation. The sensation is usually localised to the midline between the thyroid cartilage and the manubriosternal notch but in 20 % of cases it is perceived in the paramedian position [2]. There is reasonably good broad agreement among investigators on the types of sensations that constitute globus. Furthermore, factor analysis confirms that this patient population is clearly distinguishable from dysphagia and throat pain [3]. As the pathophysiology of globus remains unknown, and as there is no current biological marker for the condition, the diagnosis remains a clinical one. There are additional qualifiers on which there seems to be broad agreement. The symptom is non-painful, frequently improves with eating, and is frequently episodic [2–5]. Conversely, there are a number of features which most would agree incompatible with the diagnosis such as constant or intermittent pain or weight loss [4, 6]; dysphagia or odynophagia [3, 7]. Reflux disease can cause varying symptoms in the neck and throat and some cases of globus are associated with reflux disease (see below).

Table 32.1 Rome III: diagnostic criteria for globus [1]

At least 12 weeks, which need not be consecutive, in the preceding 6 months of
 Persistent or intermittent, non-painful, sensation of a lump or foreign body in the throat
 Occurrence of the sensation between meals
 Absence of dysphagia, odynophagia
 Absence evidence that gastroesophageal reflux is the cause of the symptom
 Absence of histopathology-based oesophageal motility disorders

Epidemiology

Globus is extremely common being reported in 7–46 % of apparently healthy individuals with the peak incidence in middle age and very uncommon in individuals under 20 [2, 4, 8–10]. Overall, the symptom accounts for around 4 % of ENT referrals [11]. The symptom in healthy individuals who are not seeking health care for it shares an equal prevalence between males and females [4, 6, 12]. There is a higher prevalence of females among those seeking health care for globus [2] and female gender appears to be a risk factor for globus in patients undergoing upper gastrointestinal endoscopy [13].

Diagnosis and Evaluation

The diagnosis is made on clinical history. It is important to distinguish globus from dysphagia at the outset as the diagnostic algorithms will differ markedly [14]. The impression that this distinction can be made reliably on clinical grounds has been backed up by systematic analysis of symptoms. Factor analysis, utilising a self-report (ten-item) symptom scale, the Glasgow–Edinburgh throat scale, derived from 105 consecutive patients found that globus sensation could be segregated from dysphagia and pain in those seeking health care [3] and in those not seeking health care [15].

Physical examination of the neck followed by nasolaryngoscopic examination of the pharynx and larynx are advised. The risk of cancer is very low in globus and it remains unproven whether nasolaryngoscopy should be done routinely [5, 16–18]. It is very rare for globus to be the sole presenting symptom of pharyngolaryngeal malignancy and cancer is usually accompanied by pain, dysphagia or hoarseness. A series of 120 globus patients undergoing rigid oesophagoscopy under general anaesthesia showed hypopharyngeal cancer in two, but both of these had additional symptoms including dysphagia and hoarseness [16]. Timon et al. reported a tongue base tumour in 1 of 83 prospective cases referred to an ENT clinic [17]. Furthermore, long-term follow-up studies out to 7 years do not report the later appearance of upper aerodigestive tract malignancy in patients with simple globus sensation [5].

Beyond nasolaryngoscopy currently there is no uniformly agreed policy on investigation or treatment [19]. That study found, at least in a survey of ENT surgeons in the UK, that 14 % do not perform any investigations (apart from nasolaryngoscopy) on these patients. Of the remainder, the most common investigation is rigid oesophagoscopy (61 %) followed by barium swallow (56 %). The argument for reflux notwithstanding, and the potential for finding heterotopic gastric mucosa in the cervical oesophagus in a minority of patients (see below), there is little evidence to support the need for routine oesophagoscopy in the evaluation of simple globus sensation in the absence of additional symptoms that might suggest oesophageal neoplasia (e.g. pain, dysphagia or weight loss). Barium swallow, while detecting incidental findings in some, adds little of diagnostic value in globus [20]. At present, in lieu of clear guidelines, it would seem reasonable to perform outpatient nasolaryngoscopy for the isolated symptom of globus and reserve oesophagoscopy for cases in whom there are additional alarm symptoms such as dysphagia, pain, hoarseness or weight loss [21].

uncontrolled studies of globus patients (30–50 %) [6, 23] is comparable to that estimated in the general population [25, 26]. The cricopharyngeal bar, found in up to 17 % of individuals undergoing contrast radiography [27, 28], is no more prevalent in globus [6].

There are a number of recent case reports of a suspected association between globus and cervical oesophageal inlet patch (heterotopic gastric mucosa) [18, 29–31]. These small case reports do not tell us much as the majority of globus sufferers do not have an inlet patch. Furthermore, the prevalence of an inlet patch ranges from 1 to 5 % in unselected endoscopies. The true prevalence may be greater as its detection depends on the level of endoscopist vigilance [32–35]. Nonetheless, a prospective cross-sectional survey of 2,053 consecutive endoscopies, aided by narrow band imaging, reported the prevalence of globus symptom to be 5.8 % and a prevalence of inlet patch of 13.8 % [13]. After excluding those who had been using PPIs, and by applying multivariate analysis that group found that both nonerosive reflux disease (NERD) and inlet patch were independent risk factors for globus [13]. Interestingly they also found that asymptomatic erosive GERD was inversely related to globus postulating that oesophageal hypersensitivity rather than acid reflux *per se*, might be more important than acid reflux itself.

Associated Conditions

A number of radiographic findings have been reported in association with globus, largely in retrospective studies. Hiatus hernia, cervical osteophytes, cricopharyngeal bar, cervical web, peptic ulcer and gallstones have been reported, but the prevalence of such findings varies dramatically among such studies; probably because a subset had additional dysphagia [6, 22, 23]. A well designed prospective analysis of 77 consecutive cases found normal radiological examinations in 53 % and hiatus hernias in only 13 % [24]. Hiatus hernia is unlikely to have aetiological significance as the reported prevalence of hiatus hernia in

Pathogenesis of Globus

A wide range of pathogenic mechanisms have been proposed to account for globus. These include gastroesophageal reflux, cricopharyngeal spasm, pharyngeal or oesophageal dysmotility, pharyngeal or oesophageal visceral hypersensitivity. While many of these are plausible, high level evidence for a direct causative link between any of them and globus remains to be demonstrated.

Cricopharyngeal hypertonicity was initially suspected to be a cause of globus when an early study, using a posteriorly oriented perfused catheter and pull-through technique, found higher resting upper oesophageal sphincter (UES)

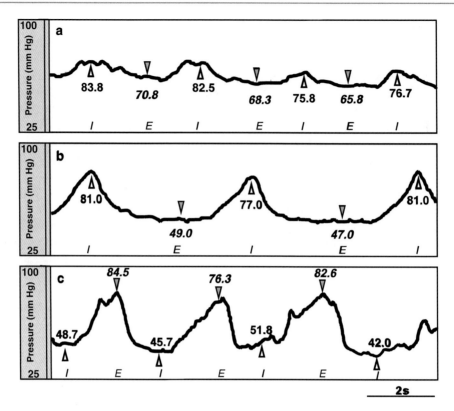

Fig. 32.1 Exaggerated respiratory oscillatory augmentation of UES pressure in globus. Shown are pressure–time plots of resting upper oesophageal sphincter (UES) pressure during respiration in (**a**) an asymptomatic control, (**b**) a globus patient with hyperdynamic respiratory UES augmentation and (**c**) a globus patient with a phase-shifted respiratory augmentation such that maximal augmentation occurred during expiration. Note that despite the significantly larger oscillations of pressure in tracings panels (**b**) and (**c**) compared with the control (**a**), the maximal pressure recorded is similar between the three subject types. (*White* and *black arrows mark* the midpoints of inspiration (I) and expiration (E), respectively). From M. Kwiatek et al. Am J Gastroenterol 2009;104:289–98 with permission (Fig. 2)

pressures when compared with controls [36]. However, UES pressure is labile and both responsive to emotional stress and to local physical stimulation. Hence this finding may better reflect an abnormal response to the mechanical stimulation induced by the pull-through itself or the attendant discomfort in the process [37]. Accordingly, subsequent studies, either using stationary sleeve sensors [12, 38] or non-perfused manometric catheters and a station pull-through technique to measure UES tone [12, 39], or solid-state high-resolution manometry [40] found no difference in resting UES pressure in globus when compared with healthy controls. The notion that UES hyper-reactivity might be implicated in globus has been formally evaluated in response to physiological phenomena and experimental stimuli known to augment upper sphincter tone including emotional stress, mechanical oesophageal distension and respiratory oscillation of resting UES pressure. Although the symptom of globus is anecdotally precipitated by deep emotion, and while the UES normally contracts in response to emotional stress [37], such stress-induced augmentation in UES tone in these patients is normal [38]. The physiological augmentation of UES pressure in response to oesophageal balloon distension in globus patients has been shown to be comparable to that seen in healthy controls [41]. More recently, Kwiatek et al. found exaggerated respiratory oscillatory augmentation of UES pressure in globus when compared with controls (Fig. 32.1) [40]. The significance of this finding is unclear. While transient changes in

UES tone do not underpin the symptom of globus, the findings of Kwiatek et al. may represent an upregulation of vagal neural pathways that are likely to share a common mechanism with perception of globus sensation.

Based on videoradiographic and most manometric assessments, the pharyngeal swallow mechanism is normal in globus [22, 40–42]. This is not surprising as these patients do not have dysphagia and symptoms generally improve during the meal. Reports from manometric studies are discrepant. Wilson et al. [12] reported these patients to have higher hypopharyngeal and UES after-contraction pressures when compared with controls. However, in that study, mean hypopharyngeal amplitudes in controls was only 40 mmHg which is substantially lower than normal pharyngeal pressures reported by others [43]. One study reported that the urge to swallow, and hence the swallow frequency increases between meals in these patients. It is uncertain whether this habitual dry swallowing, presumably to "dislodge" the apparent bolus, is a result of the foreign body sensation or whether it contributes to the sensation by periodically causing air entrapment in the proximal oesophagus [44].

Given the observed oesophageal hypersensitivity to distension in this group (see below), it might be argued that oesophageal motor or sensory dysfunction may better account for globus than pharyngo-cricopharyngeal dysfunction. A tertiary referral centre, which carefully examined physiological and psychometric variables in globus patients, reported approximately 25 % of those presenting with globus to have manometrically proven achalasia [42, 45]. However, 21 of 24 of such patients had one or more of the typical symptoms of achalasia. This is not a consistent finding among other studies. Other motor disorders, including diffuse oesophageal spasm and non-specific motor disorders have been reported in a small proportion of patients [46–48] although the prevalence among such studies varies widely [12]. One controlled study found no difference in the prevalence of these motility abnormalities (25 %) between globus patients and controls [48]. On the basis of current evidence, it is possible that oesophageal dysmotility might have globus as one of its manifestations, but there is certainly no oesophageal motor pattern which characterises globus and the majority of globus sufferers do not have significant oesophageal dysmotility.

Although some evidence exists to suggest the cervical oesophageal inlet patch might be a risk factor in globus [13], it is difficult to contemplate a mechanism by which the inlet patch could mediate the symptom as none of the columnar mucosa biopsied in these studies demonstrated acid-secreting parietal cells [13, 49]. Argon plasma coagulation (APC) ablation of the heterotopic gastric mucosa in one controlled study demonstrated symptom improvement in the majority [49]. From these observations, it is currently impossible to know whether the inlet patch somehow causes globus in a subset of patients or whether APC damage to the cervical oesophagus modulates the sensory pathways mediating the symptom.

Gastroesophageal reflux is the most favoured aetiology for globus, although the evidence for a causative link between these conditions is far from convincing. A range of plausible mechanisms have been proposed which might link gastroesophageal reflux with globus including: referred sensation from the oesophagus to the neck (perhaps mediated by hypersensitisation of oesophageal afferents); reflexive contraction of the UES in response to oesophageal acidification or distension; oesophago-pharyngeal regurgitation causing direct laryngo-pharyngeal damage and/or sensitisation; reflexive cough or habitual throat clearing in response to oesophageal acidification.

Globus is very common (see above) and the prevalence of reflux symptoms in those not seeking health care is also high ranging from 15 to 39 % [4, 9, 26, 50–52]. In one Scandinavian population survey, 20 % had heartburn and 20 % had globus, while half of those with heartburn reported globus [52]. Report of a high association between the two is very weak evidence for causation because the two entities will frequently coexist by chance. However, two studies using multivariate analysis confirm that reflux symptoms are a risk factor for globus. A population survey in Olmstead county found a prevalence for heartburn or regurgitation of 42 % and for globus of 7 %. More relevant, heartburn or regurgitation was reported in 86 % of those with globus. The odds ratio of someone with reflux symptoms experiencing globus was 1.9 (95 % CI, 1.0–3.6) times that of someone without reflux symptoms [9]. A prospective endoscopic survey found the odds ratio for reflux symptoms in those with globus to be 11.6 (95 % CI 7.1–19.1) [13].

Pooling data from studies utilising ambulatory 24 h pH monitoring, an increased oesophageal acid exposure is present in around one-third of patients with globus [22, 47, 48, 53–57]. The two key issues, however, are whether excessive oesophageal acid exposure is over-represented in globus when compared with appropriate controls and whether oesophageal acidification causes the symptom (either directly or indirectly). There are only two adequately controlled studies that addressed these issues and they had conflicting results [22, 48]. Wilson et al. found that 24 h oesophageal acid profile did not differ between those with globus and appropriate controls nor was there any temporal relationship identified between globus sensation and actual reflux events [22]. Hill et al., in a Chinese population, found an abnormal pH profile in a significantly higher proportion (31 %) of globus patients compared with controls (5 %) [48]. Curran et al. found 61 % of 21 patients with globus had a positive symptom index on ambulatory pH testing [55]. However, there are substantial inherent difficulties in attributing temporal association between globus sensation, which is frequently present continuously for hours, and discrete transient reflux events.

Is there a dose–response relationship and a close temporal relationship between reflux and the symptom of globus to strengthen the case for causation? One prospective study found a strong statistical correlation between frequency of reflux symptoms and the likelihood of reporting globus sensation. That study found globus reported by 8.7 % of those with infrequent GERD and 14.2 % of those with frequent GERD symptoms [9]. While this could be evidence supporting a causative link between acid reflux and globus, it could equally well reflect oesophageal hypersensitivity as an aetiological factor in presence and severity of each symptom.

In examining any potential temporal relationship, the disappearance of symptoms on treatment might provide the best indirect evidence of a causative link. Unfortunately, the available efficacy data for antisecretory medication in globus are limited, conflicting and largely uncontrolled (see below). Despite the clinical belief that globus is frequently reflux-related and the current recommendation that a trial of high-dose PPI is appropriate, there is no high level evidence to support this recommendation.

In conclusion, there appears to be a reasonably strong, although quite variable, association between globus and reflux. However, a large proportion of the globus population do not have reflux and there is currently no high level evidence supporting a causative relationship between reflux and globus. Therefore, at best we can say currently is that a subset of globus is likely to be attributable to GERD, but proof of this assertion is still required.

Visceral Hypersensitivity

Visceral hypersensitivity has been demonstrated in a wide range of functional gastrointestinal disorders including functional heartburn and functional dyspepsia. Chen et al. examined this hypothesis in globus patients using balloon distension and electrical stimulation to the oesophagus as stimuli and compared sensory thresholds and viscerosomatic referral patterns with healthy controls [58]. They found that globus patients demonstrated lowered thresholds (heightened perception) to non-painful and painful oesophageal sensation induced by mid-oesophageal balloon distension (Fig. 32.2). They also demonstrated that the pattern and site of viscerosomatic referral of oesophageal sensations in patients differed markedly from controls. Virtually all patients experienced symptom referral to or above the suprasternal notch (Fig. 32.3). These data suggest that globus sensation could arise from oesophageal rather than pharyngeal afferent receptors and that oesophageal hypersensitivity might be important in the genesis of the symptom and its localisation to the neck.

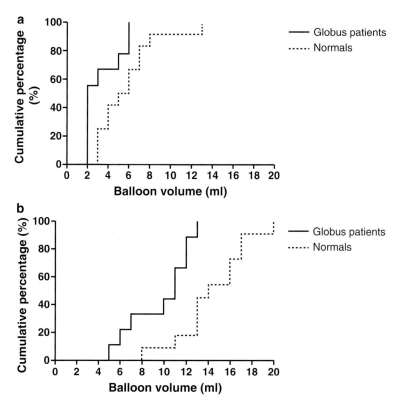

Fig. 32.2 Oesophageal sensory thresholds to balloon distension showing cumulative response rates for: (**a**) first perception and (**b**) pain threshold, to balloon distension. When compared with controls, note the left shift in perception ($P=0.03$) and pain thresholds ($P=0.001$) of globus patients. From C.L. Chen et al. Neurogastroenterol Motil 2009;21(11):1142–e96 with permission (Fig. 2)

Psychological Features

A number of studies have demonstrated higher levels of anxiety and depression, greater introversion and neuroticism in affected patients when compared with healthy controls [38, 59–62]. However, psychoneurosis has not been causally linked to the symptom and may simply reflect health care seeking behaviour or self-referral bias as less than 10 % of sufferers seek medical advice for it. For example, using the DSM III-R criteria a psychiatric diagnosis can be attached to 25–60 % of these patients [42, 47], but these studies revealed no more anxiety and depression than was found in patients in a general medical outpatient clinic [17, 42]. Up to 96 % of sufferers report symptoms exacerbated by strong emotion [4]. Acute experimental stress has also been shown to augment UES tone but, at least in the laboratory, does not induce globus in these patients nor does the UES pressure response to acute stress differ from that seen in healthy controls [37, 38].

Life stress events might precipitate globus. Deary et al. found, when compared with controls, that significantly more globus patients had life stress events (e.g. death of close relative, loss of job) within 2 months of symptom onset [61]. This phenomenon was confirmed by a subsequent controlled study of life events, which found that globus patients reported significantly more severe life events than controls over the preceding year and fewer close confiding relationships than controls [63]. Personality traits that might influence ones responses to life events have been assessed in 121 globus patients and found low extraversion levels in females but largely normal personality traits in

a

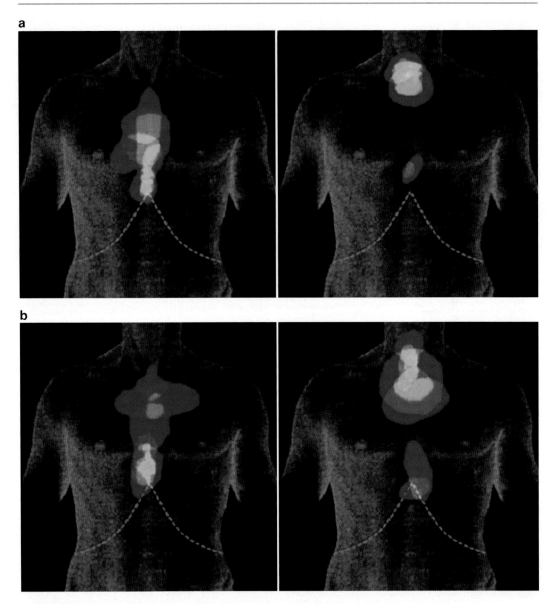

b

Fig. 32.3 Patterns of viscerosomatic referral of pain in response to mid-oesophageal stimulation by: (**a**) balloon distension and (**b**) electrical stimulation in healthy controls (*left*) and in patients with globus (*right*). (**a**) In response to balloon distension none of the controls and seven of nine globus patients ($P=0.001$) reported pain referred to a site at or above the suprasternal notch. (**b**) In response to electrical stimulation, there was a similar tendency for pain referral to the neck in globus patients, but there was much greater overlap when compared with healthy controls

males [64]. Systematic studies have failed to demonstrate hysterical features in globus patients. Appropriately, the qualifier "hystericus" has been dropped from the term since the early 1970s.

In summary, there is no psychometric or personality profile that is specific for globus, nor is it necessary for such abnormalities to be present in all sufferers. Life stress might be a cofactor in genesis of or exacerbation of the symptom. A proportion of the psychiatric diagnoses evident in clinic presenters may reflect health care seeking behaviour.

Treatment

Given the benign nature of the condition, the likelihood of persistent symptoms long term, and the absence of high level efficacy data for pharmacotherapy, the mainstay of treatment rests with explanation and reassurance. The high proportion in whom symptoms persist for years should urge the patient to adopt realistic expectations for the future. There are grounds for a trial of a PPI, particularly where typical reflux symptoms coexist. However, prior warning of the likelihood of persistence of globus sensation would seem prudent.

Antireflux Therapy

Examining the literature back to 1990, there are only two randomised controlled therapeutic trials of acid suppressive therapy for globus which found benefit neither for cimetidine [65] nor for lansoprazole [66] when compared with placebo. Dumper et al. studied 40 globus patients in a randomised controlled study with follow-up over 3 months. Using the Glasgow–Edinburgh throat scale [15], they found no significant differences in symptom scores on treatment with lansoprazole 30 mg daily when compared with placebo [66]. In a small, controlled but non-randomised study, the response to omeprazole 20 mg daily (in those with coexistent heartburn) was equivalent to that of reassurance alone (25 % in both patients and controls) [48]. Considering the remaining prospective uncontrolled, open-label studies of antisecretory therapy (five evaluating PPIs, two H_2 receptor antagonists), the response rate ranged widely from 25 to 77 % [17, 55, 57, 67–70]. Larger randomised controlled trials of twice daily PPI need to be done as the long-term remission rate, irrespective of antireflux treatment is only 20–50 % in globus [5]. An uncontrolled trial of cisapride showed marginal symptomatic benefit over 14 weeks [71]. Hence, notwithstanding the widely held but anecdotal belief that acid suppressive therapy is effective in treating globus, there is no high level efficacy data to support this contention.

Argon Plasma Coagulation Ablation of Cervical Oesophageal Inlet Patch

A small pilot study [72] and a prospective randomised controlled study [49] evaluating APC ablation of cervical oesophageal heterotopic gastric mucosa (inlet patch) have shown symptomatic improvement in globus symptoms. In 21 patients with globus who were unresponsive to PPI therapy and who had an inlet patch identified were randomised to sham or APC ablation. There was no a priori definition of a primary outcome measure of improvement. However, globus score and total symptom score reduction were significantly greater in APC when compared to sham arm [49]. I believe it is premature to consider APC as a valid treatment in cases of globus with inlet patch based on one small randomised controlled trial because APC is not without complication (e.g. oesophageal stricture); globus is an extremely common and benign condition and the majority of sufferers do not have an inlet patch.

Behavioural and Psychotropic Therapies

There are no controlled trials of antidepressants, but there is some anecdotal evidence for the efficacy of tricyclic antidepressants [73]. A recent, small ($n=29$) open-label study from China reported the SSRI paroxetine superior to esomeprazole over a limited 3 weeks follow-up [74].

A recent small ($n=10$) uncontrolled pilot study found that hypnotherapy-assisted relaxation therapy was well accepted and significantly reduced globus mean symptom severity score in those who had failed to respond to trial of PPI therapy [75]. The data at present are too sparse to make firm recommendations about psychotherapeutic approaches.

Natural History and Prognosis

There are some data evaluating prognosis. An early longitudinal study found symptoms persist in 23 % of patients at 3 years [76]. Later studies reported persistence of globus in around 75 % at

2–3 years although one-third reported improvement over this time [17]. Interestingly, that study found that neither the presence or absence of reflux, nor antireflux therapy, had any correlation with symptom resolution. The longest duration of follow-up found that while symptoms tended to improve with time, symptoms did persist in 45 % of sufferers at 8 years [5].

Summary of Key Points

- Globus is an extremely common, benign condition in the community.
- Globus is a clinical diagnosis which is distinct from dysphagia.
- While a wide spectrum of conditions have been reported in association with globus, high level evidence supporting a causative link between any of these and globus is lacking.
- Reflux disease can be a contributory factor in a proportion of patients. There is no high level evidence that reflux causes globus.
- Pharyngeal and upper oesophageal tone and UES relaxation are normal.
- Oscillatory upper oesophageal sphincter, inspiration-related augmentation in pressure has been demonstrated but the pathogenic relevance of this finding is unclear.
- Oesophageal hypersensitivity and aberrant viscerosomatic referral of oesophageal sensation to the neck have been demonstrated suggesting upregulation of oesophageal visceral afferents may be implicated.
- Clinical assessment in cases where globus is the sole symptom and in which there are no "alarm" symptoms (dysphagia, weight loss, pain, hoarseness) could be confined to nasolaryngoscopic examination of the larynx and pharynx.
- There are no firm guidelines on the need for, nor value of radiological examination or oesophagoscopy. It would seem reasonable to perform outpatient nasolaryngoscopy for the isolated symptom of globus and reserve oesophagoscopy for cases in whom there are additional alarm symptoms such as dysphagia, pain, hoarseness or weight loss.

- There is no psychometric or personality profile that is specific to patients with globus.
- A randomised controlled study has shown APC ablation of cervical oesophageal inlet patch mucosa, when present, can alleviate globus.
- While current guidelines recommend a trial of PPI therapy in globus, there is no high level evidence to support this recommendation.

References

1. Galmiche JP, Clouse RE, Balint A, Cook IJ, Kahrilas PJ, Paterson WG, et al. Functional esophageal disorders. Gastroenterology. 2006;130(5):1459–65.
2. Batch AJG. Globus pharyngeus (part I). J Laryngol Otol. 1988;102:152–8.
3. Deary IJ, Wilson JA, Harris MB, MacDougall G. Globus pharyngis: development of a symptom assessment scale. J Psychosom Res. 1995;39(2):203–13.
4. Thompson W, Heaton K. Heartburn and globus on apparently healthy people. CMAJ. 1982;126:46–8.
5. Rowley H, O'Dwyer TP, Jones AS, Timon CI. The natural history of globus pharyngeus. Laryngoscope. 1995;105(10):1118–21.
6. Malcomson K. Radiological findings in globus hystericus. Br J Radiol. 1966;39:583–6.
7. Ravich WJ, Wilson RS, Jones B, Donner MW. Psychogenic dysphagia and globus: reevaluation of 23 patients. Dysphagia. 1989;4:35–8.
8. Drossman DA, Li Z, Andruzzi E, Temple RD, Talley NJ, Thompson JG, et al. US householders survey of functional gastrointestinal disorders: prevalence, sociodemography and health impact. Dig Dis Sci. 1993;38:1569–80.
9. Locke GR, Talley NJ, Fett SL, Zinsmeister AR, Melton LJ. Prevalence and clinical spectrum of gastroesophageal reflux: a population-based study in Olmsted County, Minnesota. Gastroenterology. 1997;112:1448–56.
10. Ruth M, Mansson I, Sandberg N. The prevalence of symptoms suggestive of esophageal disorders. Scand J Gastroenterol. 1991;26(1):73–81.
11. Moloy P, Charter R. The globus symptom. Arch Otolaryngol. 1982;108:740–4.
12. Wilson J, Pryde A, Piris J, Allan P, Macintyre C, Maran A, et al. Pharyngoesophageal dysmotility in globus sensation. Arch Otolaryngol Head Neck Surg. 1989;115:1086–90.
13. Hori K, Kim Y, Sakurai J, Watari J, Tomita T, Oshima T, et al. Non-erosive reflux disease rather than cervical inlet patch involves globus. J Gastroenterol Hepatol. 2010;45:1138–45.
14. Cook IJ. Diagnostic evaluation of dysphagia. Nat Clin Pract Gastroenterol Hepatol. 2008;5(7):393–403.

15. Ali KHM, Wilson JA. What is the severity of globus sensation in individuals who have never sought health care for it? J Laryngol Otol. 2007;121:865–8.
16. Wilson JA, Murray JM, Haacke NPV. Rigid endoscopy in ENT practice: appraisal of the diagnostic yield in a district general hospital. J Laryngol Otol. 1987;101:286–92.
17. Timon C, O'Dwyer T, Cagney D, Walsh M. Globus pharyngeus: long-term follow-up and prognostic factors. Ann Otol Rhinol Laryngol. 1991;100:351–4.
18. Alaani A, Jassar P, Warfield AT, Gouldesbrough DR, Smith I. Heterotopic gastric mucosa in the cervical oesophagus (inlet patch) and globus pharyngeus—an under-recognised association. J Laryngol Otol. 2007;121:885–8.
19. Webb CJ, Makura ZG, Fenton JE, Jackson SR, McCormick MS, Jones AS. Globus pharyngeus: a postal questionnaire survey of UK ENT consultants. Clin Otolaryngol Allied Sci. 2000;25(6):566–9.
20. Back GW, Leong P, Kumar R, Corbridge R. Value of barium swallow in investigation of globus pharyngeus. J Laryngol Otol. 2000;114(12):951–4.
21. Harar RP, Kumar S, Saeed MA, et al. Management of globus pharyngeus: review of 699 cases. J Laryngol Otol. 2004;118:522–7.
22. Wilson J, Heading R, Maran A, Pryde A, Piris J, Allan P. Globus sensation is not due to gastro-oesophageal reflux. Clin Otolaryngol. 1987;12:271–5.
23. Delahunty J, Ardran G. Globus hystericus—a manifestation of reflux oesophagitis? J Laryngol Otol. 1970;84:1049–55.
24. Mair IWSS, Schroder KE, Modalsli B, Maurer HJ. Aetiological aspects of the globus symptom. J Laryngol Otol. 1974;88:1033–40.
25. Dyer WH, Pridie RB. Incidence of hiatus hernia in asymptomatic subjects. Gut. 1968;9:696–9.
26. Wienbeck M, Barnert J. Epidemiology of reflux disease and reflux esophagitis. Scand J Gastroenterol. 1989;156 Suppl 24:7–13.
27. Clements JL, Cox GW, Torres WE, Weens HS. Cervical esophageal webs: a roentgen anatomic correlation. Am J Roentgenol. 1974;121(2):221–31.
28. Curtis DJ, Cruess DF, Berg T. The cricopharyngeal muscle: a videorecording review. Am J Roentgenol. 1984;142:497–500.
29. Lancaster JL, Gosh S, Sethi R, Tripathi S. Can heterotopic gastric mucosa present as globus pharyngeus? J Laryngol Otol. 2006;120:575–8.
30. Akbayir N, Sokmen HM, Calis AB, Bolukbas C, Erdem L, Alkim C, et al. Heterotopic gastric mucosa in the cervical esophagus: could this play a role in the pathogenesis of laryngopharyngeal reflux in a subgroup of patients with posterior laryngitis? Scand J Gastroenterol. 2005;40:1149–56.
31. Chong VH, Jalihal A. Cervical inlet patch: case series and literature review. South Med J. 2006;99:865–9.
32. Akbayir N, Alkim C, Erdem L, Sökmen HM, Sungun A, Basak T, Turgut S, Mungan Z. Heterotopic gastric mucosa in the cervical esophagus (inlet patch): endoscopic prevalence, histological and clinical characteristics. J Gastroenterol Hepatol. 2004;19:891–6.
33. Azar C, Jamali F, Tamim H, Abdul-Bak iH, Soweid A. Prevalence of endoscopically identified heterotopic gastric mucosa in the proximal esophagus: endoscopist dependent? J Clin Gastroenterol. 2007;41:468–71.
34. Tang P, McKinley MJ, Sporrer M, Kahn E. Inlet patch: prevalence, histologic type, and association with esophagitis, Barrett esophagus, and antritis. Arch Pathol Lab Med. 2004;128:444–7.
35. Alagozlu H, Simsek Z, Unal S, Cindoruk M, Dumulu S, Dursun A. Is there an association between Helicobacter pylori in the inlet patch and globus sensation? World J Gastroenterol. 2010;7:42–7.
36. Watson W, Sullivan S. Hypertonicity of the cricopharyngeal sphincter: a cause of globus sensation. Lancet. 1974;2:1417–9.
37. Cook IJ, Dent J, Shannon S, Collins SM. Measurement of upper esophageal sphincter pressure: effect of acute emotional stress. Gastroenterology. 1987;93:526–32.
38. Cook IJ, Dent J, Collins SM. Upper esophageal sphincter tone and reactivity to stress in patients with a history of globus sensation. Dig Dis Sci. 1989;34:672–6.
39. Linsell J, Anggiansah A, Owen W. Manometric findings in patients with the globus sensation. Gut. 1987;28:A1378.
40. Kwiatek M, Mirza F, Kahrilas PJ, Pandolfino JE. Hyperdynamic upper esophageal sphincter pressure: a manometric observation in patients reporting globus sensation. Am J Gastroenterol. 2009;104:289–98.
41. Cook I, Shaker R, Dodds W, Hogan W, Arndorfer R. Role of mechanical and chemical stimulation of the esophagus in globus sensation. Gastroenterology. 1989;96:A99.
42. Moser G, Wenzel-Abatzi TA, Stelzeneder M, Wenzel T, Weber U, Wiesnagrotzki S, et al. Globus sensation: pharyngoesophageal function, psychometric and psychiatric findings, and follow-up in 88 patients. Arch Intern Med. 1998;158(12):1365–73.
43. Kahrilas P, Dodds W, Dent J, Haeberle B, Hogan W, Arndorfer R. Effect of sleep, spontaneous gastroesophageal reflux, and a meal on upper esophageal sphincter pressure in normal human volunteers. Gastroenterology. 1987;92:466–71.
44. Gray L. The relationship of the "inferior constrictor swallow" and globus hystericus or the hypopharyngeal syndrome. J Laryngol Otol. 1993;97:607–18.
45. Moser G, Vacariu-Granser G, Schneider C, Abatzi T, Pokieser P, Stacher-Janotta G, et al. High incidence of esophageal motor disorder in consecutive patients with globus sensation. Gastroenterology. 1991;101:1512–21.
46. Leelamanit V, Geater A, Sinkitjaroenchai W. A study of 111 cases of globus hystericus. J Med Assoc Thai. 1996;79(7):460–7.
47. Farkkila MA, Ertama L, Katila H, Kuusi K, Paavolainen M, Varis K. Globus pharyngis, commonly associated with esophageal motility disorders. Am J Gastroenterol. 1994;89(4):503–8.

48. Hill J, Stuart RC, Fung HK, Ng EK, Cheung FM, Chung CS, et al. Gastroesophageal reflux, motility disorders, and psychological profiles in the etiology of globus pharyngis. Laryngoscope. 1997;107(10):1373–7.

49. Bajbouji M, Becker V, Eckel F, Miehlke S, Pech O, Prinz C, et al. Argon plasma coagulation of cervical heterotopic gastric mucosa as an alternative treatment for globus sensations. Gastroenterology. 2009;137(2): 440–4.

50. Andersen LIB, Madsen PV, Dalgaard P, Jensen G. Validity of clinical symptoms in benign esophageal disease, assessed by questionnaire. Acta Med Scand. 1987;221:171–7.

51. Ollyo JB, Monnier P, Fontolliet C, Savary M. The natural history, prevalence and incidence of reflux oesophagitis. Gullet. 1993;3(Suppl):1–10.

52. Lindgren MD, Janzon L. Prevalence of swallowing complaints and clinical findings among 50–79 year old men and women in an urban population. Dysphagia. 1991;6:187–92.

53. Ott DJ, Ledbetter MS, Koufman JA, Chen MY. Globus pharyngeus: radiographic evaluation and 24-hour pH monitoring of the pharynx and esophagus in 22 patients. Radiology. 1994;191(1):95–7.

54. Corso MJ, Pursnani KG, Mohiuddin MA, Gideon RM, Castell JA, Katzka DA, et al. Globus sensation is associated with hypertensive upper esophageal sphincter but not with gastroesophageal reflux. Dig Dis Sci. 1998;43(7):1513–7.

55. Curran AJ, Barry MK, Callanan V, Gormley PK. A prospective study of acid reflux and globus pharyngeus using a modified symptom index. Clin Otolaryngol Allied Sci. 1995;20(6):552–4.

56. Woo P, Noordzij P, Ross JA. Association of esophageal reflux and globus symptom: comparison of laryngoscopy and 24-hour pH manometry. Otolaryngol Head Neck Surg. 1996;115(6):502–7.

57. Chevalier JM, Brossard E, Monnier P. Globus sensation and gastroesophageal reflux. Eur Arch Otorhinolaryngol. 2003;260(5):273–6.

58. Chen CL, Szczesniak MM, Cook IJ. Evidence for oesophageal visceral hypersensitivity and aberrant symptom referral in patients with globus. Neurogastroenterol Motil. 2009;21(11):1142–e96.

59. Puhakka H, Lehtinen V, Aalto T. Globus hystericus—a psychosomatic disease? J Laryngol Otol. 1976;90: 1021–6.

60. Pratt LW, Tobin WH, Gallagher RA. Globus hystericus—office evaluation by psychological testing with the MMPI. Laryngoscope. 1976;86:1540–51.

61. Deary IJ, Smart A, Wilson JA. Depression and "hassles" in globus pharyngis. Br J Psychiatry. 1992; 161:115–7.

62. Deary IJ, Wilson JA, Kelly SW. Globus pharyngis, personality, and psychological distress in the general population. Psychosomatics. 1995;36(6):570–7.

63. Harris MB, Deary IJ, Wilson JA. Life events and difficulties in relation to the onset of globus pharyngis. J Psychosom Res. 1996;40(6):603–15.

64. Deary IJ, Wilson JA, Mitchell L, et al. Covert psychiatric disturbance in patients with globus pharyngis. Br J Med Psychol. 1989;62:381–9.

65. Kibblewhite DJ, Morrison MD. A double-blind controlled study of the efficacy of cimetidine in the treatment of the cervical symptoms of gastroesophageal reflux. J Otolaryngol. 1990;19(2):103–9.

66. Dumper J, Mechor B, Chau J, Allegretto M. Lansoprazole in globus pharyngeus: double blind, randomized, placebo-controlled trial. J Otolaryngol Head Neck Surg. 2008;37:657–63.

67. Koufman JA. The otolaryngologic manifestations of gastroesophageal reflux disease (GERD): a clinical investigation of 225 patients using ambulatory 24-hour pH monitoring and an experimental investigation of the role acid and pepsin in the development of laryngeal injury. Laryngoscope. 1991;101(4 pt 2 Suppl 53):1–78.

68. Tokashiki R, Yamaguchi H, Nakamura K, Suzuki M. Globus sensation caused by gastroesophageal reflux disease. Auris Nasus Larynx. 2002;29(4): 347–51.

69. Dore MP, Pedroni A, Pes GM, Maragkoudakis E, Tadeu V, Pirina P, et al. Effect of antisecretory therapy on atypical symptoms in gastroesophageal reflux disease. Dig Dis Sci. 2007;52:463–8.

70. Sinn DH, Kim JH, Son HJ, Kim JJ, Rhee JC, Rhee PL. Response rate and predictors of response in a short-term empirical trial of high-dose rabeprazole in patients with globus. Aliment Pharmacol Ther. 2008;27(12):1275–81.

71. Leelamanit V, Geater A, Ovartlarnporn T. Cisapride in the treatment of globus hystericus. Adv Otorhinolaryngol. 1997;51:112–24.

72. Meining A, Bajbouji M, Preeg M, et al. Argon plasma ablation of gastric inlet patches in the cervical esophagus may alleviate globus sensation: a pilot trial. Endoscopy. 2006;38:566–70.

73. Brown SR, Schwartz JM, Summergrad P, et al. Globus hystericus syndrome responsive to antidepressants. Am J Psychiatry. 1986;143:917–8.

74. Wang T, Hou P. A clinical prospective study: based on between esomeprazole and paroxetine in the oral treatment for globus pharyngis. Chin J Clinicians. 2010;4(6):772–5.

75. Kiebles JL, Kwiatek M, Pandolfino JE, Kahrilas PJ, Keefer L. Do patients with globus sensation respond to hypnotically assisted relaxation therapy? A case series report. Dis Esophagus. 2010;23(7):545–53.

76. Freeland AP, Ardran GM, Emrys-Roberts E. Globus hystericus and reflux esophagitis. J Laryngol Otol. 1974;88:1025–31.

Deglutition in Patients with Tracheostomy, Nasogastric Tubes, and Orogastric Tubes

33

Steven B. Leder and Debra M. Suiter

Abstract

Swallowing, in both normal and disordered populations, with regard to the presence of a tracheotomy tube, one-way tracheotomy tube speaking valve, nasogastric tube, and orogastric tube is described. Specific subject areas include swallowing and tracheotomy tube use across the age span from pediatric to adult populations and swallowing success when mechanical ventilation via tracheotomy is required. Additional topics include swallowing success dependent on tracheotomy tube cuff status, i.e., inflated versus deflated, tracheotomy tube occlusion status, i.e., occluded versus open, and the presence versus absence of a tracheotomy tube itself. Also, current data and a discussion on swallowing and one-way tracheotomy tube speaking valve use are addressed. Lastly, nasogastric and orogastric tubes, by traversing the same path as a food bolus, can potentially impact on swallowing and information regarding their effect on swallowing is presented.

Keywords

Deglutition • Deglutition disorders • Aspiration • Tracheotomy • Tracheotomy tube • Nasogastric tube • Orogastric tube

S.B. Leder, PhD (✉)
Department of Surgery, Section of Otolaryngology,
Yale University School of Medicine,
New Haven, CT 06520-8041, USA
e-mail: Steven.Leder@yale.edu

D.M. Suiter, PhD
Department of Speech Pathology,
VA Medical Center-Memphis,
Surgical Service (112), AE127, 1,030 Jefferson Ave,
Memphis, TN 38104, USA

Introduction

Tracheotomy, the creation of a surgical airway, is beneficial in a wide variety of conditions, including acute upper airway obstruction secondary to infection or edema, chronic upper airway obstruction secondary to a neoplasm, tracheostenosis, and tracheomalacia, obstructive sleep apnea, acute trauma, chronic respiratory failure requiring prolonged ventilator support, and intractable chronic aspiration. Despite its widespread use and the fact that the overwhelming majority of patients who require a tracheotomy tube swallow successfully, the purported impact of a tracheotomy tube on related anatomic structures and their physiological and biomechanical relationships has often been incorrect. The purpose of this chapter is to present the latest evidence in an attempt to resolve misconceptions and highlight areas that may require further research.

Advances in critical care medicine have led to increased survival rates among individuals who experience respiratory insufficiency severe enough to require a surgical airway. The decision of when to transition from an endotracheal tube to a tracheotomy and placement of a tracheotomy tube occurs at three distinct time intervals. Immediate tracheotomy placement or early transition to a tracheotomy, i.e., 0–3 days post-intubation, is performed as a result of major trauma or other severe respiratory conditions when patients are deemed as having no chance for early ventilator weaning. Mid-transition to a tracheotomy occurs at approximately 2 weeks post-intubation for patients who were thought to have the potential to be weaned from mechanical ventilation but have not made adequate respiratory progress towards this goal. Late transition for conversion to a tracheotomy occurs after approximately 4–6 weeks of mechanical ventilation due to severe respiratory compromise not allowing for weaning trials, that is when progress towards weaning is progressing too slowly, or the duration off ventilator support cannot be advanced beyond short time periods.

Swallowing After Tracheotomy and Placement of a Tracheotomy Tube

Respiration and Swallowing

In humans, the mutually exclusive but overlapping functions of respiration and swallowing share the same anatomic structures in the upper aerodigestive tract. Breathing and swallowing are well coordinated in healthy adults, and this coordination is most evident at the level of the larynx. Swallowing is composed of a highly complex

neuromuscular system requiring exquisite coordination between neural commands and anatomic structures in order to precisely sequence physiological and respiratory events with the goal of minimizing aspiration risk.

Any interruption in the ability to coordinate airway closure and swallowing has the potential to lead to airway compromise and place individuals at risk for aspiration. Physiological conditions such as pulmonary disease, aging, neurological disease, and head and neck cancer have the potential to disrupt coupling of respiration with swallowing. In young, healthy individuals, swallowing most often interrupts expiration followed by resumption of expiration after the swallow, whereas in the healthy elderly, swallowing most often interrupts inspiration followed by expiration after the swallow [1]. Individuals with physiological conditions such as pulmonary disease, advanced age, neurological disease, and head and neck cancer often demonstrate a different pattern of breathing–swallowing coordination in which swallows are initiated in and followed by an inspiration [2, 3]. Swallows initiated in this manner may potentially compromise airway protection and place individuals at risk for aspiration.

Swallowing Physiology and Tracheotomy

Glottal Reflexes and Tracheotomy

Three seminal papers, using the canine model, investigated the effect of tracheotomy on abductor and adductor glottic reflexes. Aspiration was not investigated but the information specific to control of laryngeal opening and closing is invaluable [4]. Sasaki et al. found that reduction in airflow through the larynx resulted in diminished abductor, i.e., posterior cricoarytenoid muscle, activity and that total absence of ventilatory resistance results in complete inactivity of the laryngeal abductor during phasic respiration. Sasaki et al. [5] reported that chronic upper airway bypass via tracheotomy results in a weakened and ill-coordinated adductor response, i.e., predominately by the thyroarytenoid muscle, with concomitant coordination of respiratory protection temporarily lost. Importantly, when airflow is restored through the larynx, by decannulation or tracheotomy tube capping, both the laryngeal opening and closure reflexes return to normal. Ikari and Sasaki [6] found that deflation of the lungs enhances adductor excitability of respiratory neurons while inflation reduces excitability. Therefore, negative intra-thoracic pressure facilitates glottic closure while positive intra-thoracic pressure inhibits glottic closure. The findings of Ikari and Sasaki [6] are critical in our discussion of the role of subglottic air pressure and use of one-way tracheotomy tube speaking valves.

- Glottic closure is facilitated by
  - Expiratory phase of respiration
  - Decreased arterial partial pressure of carbon dioxide
  - Increased arterial pressure of oxygen
  - Negative intra-thoracic pressure
- Glottic closure is inhibited by
  - Inspiratory phase of respiration
  - Increased arterial partial pressure of carbon dioxide
  - Decreased arterial pressure of oxygen
  - Positive intra-thoracic pressure

Presence or Absence of a Tracheotomy Tube and Aspiration Status

Although evidence in the literature is equivocal, it has been suggested that the presence of a tracheotomy tube is associated with a high incidence of pharyngeal dysphagia and aspiration [7–9]. The number of individuals with tracheotomy and concomitant oropharyngeal dysphagia has been reported to be as high as 87% [10]. Normal swallowing occurs within a closed aerodigestive system. Tracheotomy inherently violates the closed aerodigestive system and has the potential to alter the precise inter-related coordination involved in respiration and swallowing [11, 12]. However, swallowing is also controlled by highly redundant [13] and adaptable neural mechanisms that allow for successful swallowing despite disordered neurological conditions or anatomical changes.

Purported effects of tracheotomy on swallow biomechanics and physiology include decreased elevation and anterior rotation of the larynx [9, 14]; esophageal compression due to the tracheotomy tube cuff [7]; disordered abductor and adductor laryngeal reflexes due to chronic upper airway bypass [4–6]; desensitization of the oropharynx and larynx as a result of airflow diversion through the tracheotomy tube [9]; reduced effectiveness of the cough reflex to clear accumulated supra-glottic secretions [15, 16]; reduced subglottal air pressure [17, 18]; and disuse atrophy of the laryngeal muscles [14]. Additional disturbances of swallowing that have been reported include difficulty with bolus formation, delayed initiation of the pharyngeal phase of swallowing, increased residual in the pharynx, and silent aspiration [19]. However, as will be shown, these abnormalities may or may not be associated with the presence of a tracheotomy tube.

Many assumptions regarding a tracheotomy tube's impact on swallowing have not been supported. Two long-held traditional opinions regarding effects of tracheotomy tubes on swallowing are that the tracheotomy tube cuff impedes hyolaryngeal excursion and that the tracheotomy tube cuff impinges on the esophageal wall. Betts [7] attributed the presence of dysphagia in some patients with tracheotomy to tracheotomy cuff impingement on the esophagus. However, this was based on anecdotal, rather than empirical, evidence, as this evidence was reported in a Letter to the Editor rather than in a scientifically-based manuscript. Bonanno [9] suggested that the presence of an inflated tracheotomy tube cuff inhibited elevation and anterior rotation of the larynx. However, of the 43 participants in the study, only 3 (7%) actually demonstrated this effect.

In a prescient paper, Conley [20] stated, "Tracheostomy is often the key to survival in situations where the act of swallowing has compromised the airway system. Decannulation … should be delayed until the swallowing act is effectively rehabilitated." The literature has too often erroneously attributed aspiration to the most obvious variable, i.e., the tracheotomy tube, and not to important co-morbidities that may cause dysphagia [15, 21–25], e.g., respiratory failure [23–25], trauma [26], head and neck cancer [11], stroke [27, 28], altered mental status [29], advanced age [30], reduced functional reserve [14, 30], and medications used to treat the critically ill [31].

These people may well exhibit undocumented aspiration pre-tracheotomy due to their medical, neurological or surgical conditions that necessitated consideration for a tracheotomy in the first place [15, 21, 22, 24, 25].

Leder et al. [11] investigated the effects that presence of a tracheotomy tube had on aspiration status in early, postsurgical, head and neck cancer patients. Twenty-two adult, postoperative, head and neck cancer patients were evaluated with fiberoptic endoscopic evaluation of swallowing (FEES) under three conditions: (1) tracheotomy tube present; (2) tracheotomy tube removed and tracheostoma covered with gauze sponge; and (3) tracheotomy tube removed and tracheostoma left open and uncovered. For each condition, the endoscope was first inserted transnasally to determine aspiration status during FEES and then inserted through the tracheostoma to corroborate aspiration status by examining the distal trachea inferiorly to the carina. Two experienced examiners determined aspiration status under each condition and endoscope placement. There was 100% agreement on aspiration status between FEES results and endoscopic examination through the tracheostoma. Specifically, 13 of 22 (59%) patients swallowed successfully and 9 of 22 (41%) patients aspirated. There was also 100% agreement on aspiration status among the three conditions, i.e., tracheotomy tube present, tracheotomy tube removed and tracheostoma covered by gauze sponge, and tracheotomy tube removed and tracheostoma left open and uncovered. Neither presence of a tracheotomy nor decannulation affected aspiration status in early, postsurgical, head and neck cancer patients.

There are a number of possible reasons for the disagreement over aspiration results between the early and late postsurgical patients with regard to tracheotomy tube presence. First, Leder et al. [32] included a larger number of consecutive patients than reported previously [33]. Second, unlike previous studies, any bias to identifying aspiration was eliminated [15]. Third, early postsurgical patients may exhibit different dysphagia patterns compared to late postsurgical patients [15, 33] due to the length of time a tracheotomy tube is present, early postoperative edema, more impaired lingual and mandibular range of motion, and greater oropharyngeal sensitivity and pain. Fourth, it is also understood that physiological impairment of adductor laryngeal reflexes may not occur for 6–8 months after tracheotomy [5, 34]. Fifth, differences in bolus volumes used, i.e., 5 mL in the Leder et al. [32] and 10 mL in the scintigraphy studies [15, 33]. Similarly, Donzelli et al. [12] investigated what effects, if any, the presence of a tracheotomy tube had on incidence of laryngeal penetration and aspiration in patients with known or suspected dysphagia. FEES was used to determine aspiration status in 37 participants (23 M/14 F; mean age 64.4 years; range 34–85 years) using four different tracheotomy tubes, i.e., Bivona, Shiley, Portex, and Jackson. Swallowing was evaluated first with the tracheotomy tube open and then with the tube occluded with a cap, one-way speaking valve, and finger. The tracheotomy tube was then removed, the tracheostoma covered gently with a gauze pad, and swallowing evaluated again. Lastly, swallowing was re-evaluated with the tracheotomy removed and the tracheostoma uncovered. Direct confirmation of aspiration was made by inserting the endoscope into the tracheostoma after swallowing trials. Tracheotomy tube occlusion status and tracheotomy tube removal status had no immediate effect on incidence of laryngeal penetration or aspiration.

The fundamental flaw in all research methodologies was that no *pre-tracheotomy* aspiration data were collected [7–10, 14, 35, 36]. Although difficult, since it cannot be predicted who will undergo a tracheotomy in the future and once the decision to perform a tracheotomy has been made the patient is either too medically compromised to have a dysphagia evaluation or an endotracheal tube is present, collecting pre-tracheotomy data is crucial in order to determine causality. Therefore, aspiration status must be investigated both pre- and post-tracheotomy in the same person [21, 22].

In the initial study investigating whether there is a direct causal relationship between presence of a tracheotomy tube and aspiration [21], FEES [37, 38] was performed in the same 20 patients, aged 47–84 years, first pre- and then post-tracheotomy. Findings indicated that 100% (12 of 12) of participants who aspirated pre-tracheotomy also aspirated post-tracheotomy and 87.55% (7 of 8) of participants who did not aspirate pre-tracheotomy also did not aspirate post-tracheotomy.

Although no causal relationship was found between tracheotomy tube use and aspiration status [21], debate continues regarding an association between tracheotomy and placement of a tracheotomy tube and aspiration risk [39, 40]. Therefore, a direct replication study with a larger sample size was completed [22]. Replication provides two basic functions essential for the foundation of any scholarly field: verification or disconfirmation, i.e., a fact is not a fact until it is replicable [41]. Specific to the current issue, a causal relationship exists when presence of a tracheotomy tube is a sufficient condition for the occurrence of aspiration. That is, a causal relationship does not exist if the effect (aspiration) occurs before its cause (tracheotomy tube) [42].

Results of the direct replication study [22] found that 88% (22 of 25) of participants exhibited the same aspiration status or resolved aspiration pre- versus post-tracheotomy tube use. Three participants exhibited new aspiration post-tracheotomy tube placement due to worsening medical conditions. Conversely, four participants exhibited resolved aspiration post-tracheotomy tube placement due to improved medical conditions. Excluding these seven participants, all nine participants who aspirated pre- also aspirated post-tracheotomy tube placement and all nine participants who did not aspirate pre- also did not aspirate post-tracheotomy tube placement ($p>0.05$). No statistically significant differences were found between aspiration status and days since tracheotomy ($X^2=0.08$, $p>0.05$) or age and aspiration status ($p>0.05$). The absence of a causal relationship between tracheotomy tube use and aspiration status was confirmed. In addition, there was no statistically significant difference for the number of days between pre-tracheotomy FEES and post-tracheotomy FEES based on aspiration status ($N=13$ non-aspirators, $\bar{X}=21.5$ days, sd 20.72, range 6–69 days versus $N=12$ aspirators, $\bar{X}=25.7$, sd 22.13, range 3–86 days, $p>0.05$).

Combined Data from Direct Replication Study with Leder and Ross [21] Study

Results from the direct replication study [22] ($N=25$) were combined with results from the initial study ($N=20$) [21], thereby strengthening the analysis due to use of a much larger sample size, i.e., total $N=45$; 26 males and 19 females; $X=65.8$ years, and range$=43$–84 years. This allowed for achievement of an important goal of the current direct replication study, i.e., verification of facts [41] from the original study [21]. Results of aspiration status pre- versus post-tracheotomy tube placement indicated that 91% of (41 of 45) participants exhibited either the same aspiration status or resolved aspiration pre- versus post-tracheotomy tube use. Similar to both the initial and direct replication studies, number of days post-tracheotomy was not significantly different ($p>0.05$) for participants who aspirated ($\bar{X}=13.3$ days) versus participants who did not aspirate ($\bar{X}=11.3$ days). Participants who aspirated pre-tracheotomy were not significantly older than participants who aspirated post-tracheotomy ($\bar{X}=66.4$ years, sd 10.85 versus 67.4 years, sd 10.66, $p>0.05$). Similarly, participants who did not aspirate pre-tracheotomy were not significantly older than participants who did not aspirate post-tracheotomy ($\bar{X}=65.1$ years, sd 12.26 versus $\bar{X}=63.8$ years, sd 12.21, $p>0.05$).

The consensus of results from the initial study [21], the direct replication study [22], and the combined data all agree that there is no causal relationship between presence of tracheotomy tube and aspiration status. Over 90% of participants exhibited the same or resolved aspiration status pre- and post-tracheotomy tube placement, confirming the lack of a causal relationship.

What is of importance is that resolution of aspiration in this population is due primarily to improvement in medical condition, mental status, and physical strength [26] and discontinuance of medications used to treat the critically ill, i.e., high-dose corticosteroids, neuromuscular blocking agents, and sedatives [31, 43]. The finding of the absence of a causal relationship between presence of a tracheotomy tube and aspiration leads directly to the conclusion that presence or absence of a tracheotomy tube is irrelevant to swallowing success or failure [11, 12, 44]. This is supported further by research which reported that swallowing dysfunction can continue following decannulation [45] and, conversely, swallowing improvement can occur when the tracheotomy tube remains in place [31]. The latter is corroborated by the direct replication study [22] as four participants exhibited resolution of aspiration with the tracheotomy tube in place due to improvement in their general medical condition. In summary, the presence of tracheotomy tube is not causative for aspiration. Neither aspiration status nor successful swallowing is influenced by presence or absence of a tracheotomy tube.

Since neither short- [11] nor long-term [12] differences regarding swallowing success and tracheotomy tube removal were observed it would be of interest to determine if removal of a tracheotomy tube after even longer use, i.e., years, would result in similar findings regarding dysphagia and aspiration status. To summarize:

- Many individuals with tracheotomy have co-existing medical conditions that could predispose them to dysphagia.
- Aspiration in individuals with tracheotomy tubes is often erroneously attributed to the tracheotomy tube rather than co-existing medical conditions.
- Studies in which pre- and post-tracheotomy conditions have been compared have found no causal effect of tracheotomy tubes on aspiration status.
- Dysphagia in patients with tracheotomy is a multi-faceted issue resulting from medical comorbidities necessitating tracheotomy tube placement rather than presence of the tracheotomy tube itself.
- Recent research findings do not support the notion that presence of a tracheotomy tube results in disordered swallowing or increased aspiration risk.

Age, Tracheotomy Tubes, and Swallowing

Older individuals appear to be at increased risk for oropharyngeal dysphagia associated with tracheotomy because of increased incidence of age-related reductions in cardiopulmonary function, neuromuscular disease, and metabolic changes and disease as well as changes in swallowing associated with normal aging (e.g., slowed pharyngeal transit and delayed initiation of the pharyngeal swallow) [14, 30]. Completed videofluoroscopic swallow studies (VFSS) with 83 mechanically ventilated individuals with tracheotomy. Half of the participants aspirated during VFSS. Those who aspirated were significantly older (mean age = 72.5 years) than those who did not aspirate (mean age = 64.8 years). Leder [23] reported similar findings. FEES were performed with 52 mechanically ventilated adults with tracheotomy. Seventeen (33%) participants aspirated. Those who aspirated were significantly older (mean age = 73) than those who did not aspirate (mean age = 59). It was hypothesized that decreased functional reserve, i.e., the ability to adapt to stress [46], led to the higher incidence of aspiration in older subjects. Although there are normal age-related changes in biomechanical coordination of swallowing, in the absence of illness or other stressors, these do not typically lead to an increased incidence of aspiration. However, when stress, e.g., illness requiring mechanical ventilation via tracheotomy, is introduced, the time course of these deteriorating capacities can accelerate, which leads to rapid declines in functional reserve and impaired ability to complete activities of daily living.

The benefit of tracheotomy in older individuals with respiratory insufficiency has been questioned because short-term mortality rates are high and long-term outcomes are poor. Possible complications associated with tracheotomy include pneumothorax, infection, sinusitis, and tracheal damage. Older individuals appear to be particularly at risk for complications from tracheotomy [24]. Baskin et al. [24] completed a retrospective study of 78 older individuals (mean age = 77.6) who underwent tracheotomy. Results indicated that tracheotomy was associated with a high incidence of death (56%), increased need for gastrostomy tube placement (71%), and impaired laryngeal function (87%). The authors concluded that older, severely ill individuals experience poor outcomes following tracheotomy, and stricter criteria need to be imposed for performing tracheotomy in this population.

Hyoid Bone and Laryngeal Excursion and Presence of a Tracheotomy Tube

Current knowledge of the synergy between hyoid bone and laryngeal movement when a tracheotomy tube is present has been based on inadequate data. To wit, it has been conjectured that placement of a tracheotomy tube increases aspiration risk by limiting the rostrocaudal movement of the hyolaryngeal complex and, therefore, the opening of the upper esophageal sphincter (UES) [8, 9, 36]. To illustrate this point, the literature begins with conjectures from two often cited case reports, i.e., "…presence of a tracheotomy tube *may* alter the mechanics of deglutition to prevent proper elevation of the larynx on swallowing…" [47] and "Fixation of the larynx by the tracheostomy…*might* prevent normal elevation of the larynx…" leading to "…a disorder of swallowing *produced by* the tracheostomy" [8]. This implied and unsubstantiated causal relationship between presence of a tracheotomy tube and swallowing success has been erroneously perpetuated until shown to be erroneous only recently [21, 22].

There have been attempts to investigate pharyngeal swallow biomechanics using objective techniques. Two radiographic studies reported reduced laryngeal elevation during swallowing and attributed the resultant dysphagia to an anchoring effect caused by the presence of a tracheotomy tube [9, 14]. In both studies, however, no objective procedure for actually measuring laryngeal movement was reported. Rather, laryngeal movement was subjectively "eye-balled" and since no measurements were made statistical analysis was not performed. In addition, no other potential etiologies for dysphagia were investigated.

Despite its methodological flaws and the overlooked fact that 93% (40 of 43) of participants with a tracheotomy tube swallowed successfully, the previously mentioned study by Bonanno [9] has been cited in all subsequent investigations of swallowing, laryngeal movement, and tracheotomy [10, 15, 17, 31, 33, 35, 45, 48–50]. Further, the unsubstantiated finding that a tracheotomy tube has an anchoring effect and impairs normal elevation and anterior excursion of the hyoid bone and larynx during swallowing has been perpetuated by inclusion in review articles [34, 36], a dysphagia diagnostic manual [51], and contemporary dysphagia books [52–54].

The investigation of pharyngeal biomechanics during swallowing when a tracheotomy tube is present has been investigated with videofluoroscopy [50]. Videofluoroscopic analysis indicated that light digital occlusion placed on the external hub of the tracheotomy tube resulted in mixed results for improvement in swallowing. Potential benefits for swallowing success were increased hyoid bone and laryngeal excursion. Potential detriments were reduced base of tongue contact to posterior pharyngeal wall and late onset of anterior movement of posterior pharyngeal wall relative to onset of UES opening. Tracheotomy tube occlusion eliminated aspiration in 50% (two of four) of subjects, resulted in no change in the third subject, and actually worsened swallowing in the fourth subject [50]. The small sample size and the equivocal results regarding swallowing success with light digital occlusion of the tracheotomy tube prevent generalizable interventions. Individualized evaluation remains necessary to determine whether tracheotomy tube occlusion status has the potential to reduce aspiration risk.

Terk et al. [55] were the first group to objectively measure hyoid bone and laryngeal excursion dependent on the presence or absence of a tracheotomy tube in the same individual. Specifically, they examined the biomechanical effects on movement of the hyoid bone and larynx during swallowing under different conditions, i.e., presence/absence of a tracheotomy tube, inflated/deflated cuff status, and capped/

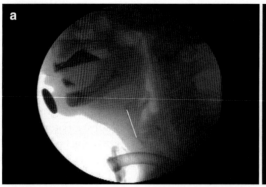
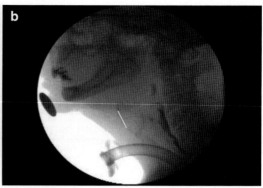

Fig. 33.1 Larynx to hyoid approximation (HLhold-HLmax): (**a**) The distance between the anterior margin of the hyoid bone and the anterior thyroid cartilage is measured at "hold" position with the bolus in the oral cavity. (**b**) From this measurement, the distance between the hyoid and the thyroid at "max" position is subtracted. From A.R. Terk. Dysphagia 2007;22:89–93 with permission from Springer

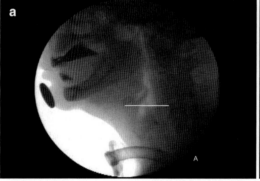
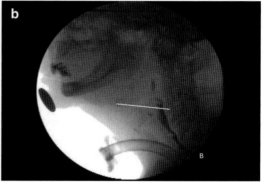

Fig. 33.2 Maximum hyoid discursion (Hmax): defined as the difference between the hyoid at bolus hold to its position when maximally displaced superiorly and anteriorly ("max.") (**a**) In the frame corresponding to bolus hold position, the distance between the hyoid and anterior C4 verte- bra is measured. (**b**) In the frame corresponding to hyoid "max" position, the distance is measured again between the same two points. The difference between these two measures is the maximum hyoid discursion. From A.R. Terk. Dysphagia 2007;22:89–93 with permission from Springer

uncapped tracheotomy tube. Seven adults (5 M/2 F; age range from 46 to 82 years; mean 63 years) with tracheotomy tubes participated. All participants completed VFSS under three randomized conditions: tracheotomy tube in and open with 5 cc air in cuff, tracheotomy tube in and capped with deflated cuff, and tracheotomy tube out. Larynx to hyoid approximation (HLhold-HLmax) was defined as the difference between the distance between the anterior margin of the hyoid bone and a clear and consistent landmark on the anterior thyroid cartilage at bolus hold position (HLhold) and the distance between the above two points at the maximum hyoid excursion both anteriorly and superiorly (HLmax) (Fig. 33.1). Maximum hyoid displacement (Hmax) was defined as the difference between the distance between the anterior margin of the hyoid bone and the anterior aspect of the C4 vertebral body at bolus hold position and at maximum position (Fig. 33.2) [56]. No significant differences ($p > 0.05$) were found for both maximum hyoid bone displacement and larynx-to-hyoid bone approximation during swallowing based on tracheotomy tube presence, tube cuff status, or tube capping status. For the first time with objective data, it was shown that the presence of a tracheotomy tube did not significantly alter pharyngeal swallow biomechanics. This agrees with both objective fluoroscopic data [57] and clinical observations, i.e., persistent dysphagia following decannulation cannot be attributed to either laryngeal tethering or obstruction by an inflated tracheotomy tube cuff [45]. The hypothesis that a tracheotomy tube limits the rostrocaudal movement of the hyolaryngeal complex and, consequently, the opening of the UES during swallowing was not supported.

Tracheotomy Tube Cuff Deflation and Swallowing

Some have conjectured that the presence of an inflated tracheotomy tube cuff disrupts swallow function by either tethering the larynx and thereby reducing hyolaryngeal excursion during the swallow or by inhibiting the flow of food or liquid through the esophagus, such as would occur in the presence of an overinflated tracheotomy tube cuff. Several studies have sought to determine effects of the tracheotomy cuff on swallow safety and physiology.

Tippett and Siebens [58] investigated the effects of tracheotomy tube cuff status during swallowing in five adults, aged 21–70 years, who were ventilator-dependent. The results of the study were mixed from this very small sample, i.e., three participants were able to swallow safely following cuff deflation and adjustment of their ventilator settings. However, because adjustments in ventilator settings and cuff status were not individually controlled, it is unclear if cuff deflation alone had any significant effect on swallowing success or failure. Due to inadequate sample size, the influence of age could not be assessed.

Suiter et al. [57] employed VFSS to examine the biomechanical effects of cuff deflation on swallow function in 14 adults, aged 19–80 years, with tracheotomy tubes. Cuff deflation resulted in increased pharyngeal transit duration, increased duration of hyoid maximum anterior excursion, and increased mean maximum anterior hyoid movement. Cuff deflation also resulted in a

significantly shorter duration of cricopharyngeal opening. However, oropharyngeal residue and penetration–aspiration scores were not significantly affected by cuff deflation. Thus, cuff deflation did not result in functional improvements in swallowing success or improved swallowing safety. There were not enough subjects in any one age group to determine age-related effects.

In a retrospective study, Ding and Logemann [59] reviewed 623 adult participants (mean age $= 52 \pm 19$ years) who underwent one VFSS with their tracheotomy tube cuff either inflated or deflated. Participants who had their tracheotomy cuffs inflated exhibited reduced laryngeal elevation which resulted in a higher incidence of aspiration and greater incidence of silent aspiration. Due to the retrospective nature of the study design and methodology that allowed for only one VFSS to be evaluated, it was, therefore, not possible to assess swallow physiology in the same subject under both cuff-inflated and cuff-deflated conditions. However, only by doing so can the effect, if any, of cuff inflation status on swallow physiology be determined.

Research does not support the notion that an inflated cuff prevents aspiration [35, 57, 59]. It is important to note that, by definition, when food or liquid falls below the level of the true vocal folds, aspiration has occurred [54]. An inflated cuff may prevent material from immediately spilling farther into the trachea or lungs, but because tracheotomy cuffs are compliant and do not form a water-tight seal between the cuff and tracheal wall, material will inevitably seep around the cuff and fall into the lower airway. In addition, an inflated cuff does not permit coughing to clear material from the upper airway. In summary:

- Presence of a tracheotomy tube may lead to declines in functional reserve in older individuals and increase the likelihood of aspiration.
- An inflated tracheotomy tube cuff does not appear to result in functional improvement in swallowing.
- Deflating the tracheotomy tube cuff does not result in increased hyolaryngeal excursion during the swallow.

Tracheotomy Tube Occlusion Status and Swallowing

It has been suggested that tracheotomy tube occlusion, either digitally with a finger or mechanically with a cap, may improve pharyngeal swallow biomechanics and improve swallowing success by reducing incidence of aspiration. Tracheotomy tube occlusion necessitates tracheotomy cuff deflation, thereby reestablishing airflow through the larynx and upper airway. In addition, tracheotomy tube occlusion has been suggested as an intervention to improve swallowing success by increasing subglottal air pressure [60, 61].

Muz et al. [33] completed scintigraphic assessment of swallowing in seven individuals, aged 44–66 years, with head and neck cancer who required a tracheotomy tube. In this study individuals were given one 10-mL bolus to swallow under two conditions, i.e., first with and then without the tracheotomy tube occluded by an obturator. Results indicated that tracheotomy tube occlusion resulted in significant reductions in the incidence and severity of aspiration. However, because participants were given only one presentation of a thin liquid, it is impossible to determine whether tracheotomy tube occlusion would have similar effects for thickened liquid, puree, or solid bolus consistencies or for boluses with different volumes.

Muz et al. [15] used scintigraphy to examine swallow function in 18 patients with head and neck cancer first with and then without occlusion of their tracheotomy tubes. As with the previous study, participants were given only one presentation of a 10 mL liquid bolus. Results indicated a statistically significant reduction in the percentage of aspirated material during the tracheotomy occluded condition when compared to the open tracheotomy condition. Interestingly, although reduced, aspiration occurred under both conditions.

Logemann et al. [50] examined the biomechanical effects of light digital occlusion of the tracheotomy tube in eight patients with head and neck cancer. A total of 20 specific temporal and distance measures were assessed from videofluorographic images. Light digital occlusion of the tracheotomy tube resulted in significant changes for five measures, but not all changes appeared to be beneficial for safe swallowing. Specific changes in swallowing biomechanics that were potentially beneficial for swallowing success were increased hyoid bone and laryngeal movement. However, detrimental biomechanical changes included reductions in both base of tongue contact to posterior pharyngeal wall and onset of anterior movement of posterior pharyngeal wall relative to onset of UES opening occurred later. Tracheotomy tube occlusion eliminated aspiration in two of four aspirating subjects, resulted in no change in the third subject, and worsened the swallow in the fourth subject. It was concluded that although light digital occlusion changed some biomechanical aspects of the swallow, the results were not generalizable and, therefore, individualized assessment was necessary to determine whether tracheotomy tube occlusion could potentially reduce aspiration.

A number of studies have reported that tracheotomy tube occlusion status does not affect aspiration status when swallowing real food of different consistencies. Leder et al. [62] investigated the effect of occlusion of a tracheotomy tube on aspiration in medical, i.e., nonsurgical, patients ($N=20$; age range 17–85 years). The tracheotomy tubes were occluded for 3–5 min prior to VFSS and three swallows each of liquid and puree consistencies were given, first with an occluded tracheotomy tube (six swallows) and then with an unoccluded tracheotomy tube (six swallows). In no case did a subject aspirate first with an occluded tracheotomy tube and then not aspirate with an unoccluded tube or, conversely, the patients did not aspirate with an occluded tube and then aspirate when the tube was unoccluded. Therefore, it was concluded that the occlusion status of the tracheotomy tube did not influence swallowing success or aspiration status. It is of interest to note that 90% (nine of ten) of the participants who exhibited aspiration were over 65 years of age. Conversely, only 25% (3 of 12) of the 65+-year-old participants did not exhibit aspiration following placement of a tracheotomy tube.

Leder et al. [32] utilized VFSS to investigate tracheotomy tube occlusion status on the incidence of aspiration in adult patients with head and neck cancer after surgery, i.e., 6–44 days postoperatively. Ten of 16 patients (62.5%) aspirated both with thin liquid and puree consistency foods under both occluded and unoccluded conditions; two subjects (12.5%) aspirated thin liquids but did not aspirate with puree consistency under both conditions; while four subjects (25%) did not aspirate any consistency under either condition. It was concluded that tracheotomy tube occlusion status did not affect incidence of aspiration.

Leder et al. [63] investigated the effect of light digital occlusion of the tracheotomy tube during swallowing on UES and pharyngeal pressures in both aspirating and nonaspirating patients. Aspiration was determined objectively with FEES; pharyngeal and UES pressures were measured by manometry. A total of 11 adult individuals with tracheotomy participated; 7 swallowed successfully and 4 exhibited aspiration. Light digital occlusion of the tracheotomy tube, for either aspirating or nonaspirating individuals, did not significantly change UES and pharyngeal pressure recordings. It was concluded that the swallow biomechanics, UES and pharyngeal pressure measures were not changed significantly by occlusion of the tracheotomy tube for both those who aspirated and those who did not aspirate. These results are consistent with previous findings that tracheotomy tube occlusion status did not influence the incidence of aspiration in medical patients [62], and early postsurgical head and neck cancer patients [32]. In summary:

- Tracheotomy tube occlusion necessitates cuff deflation thereby restoring airflow through the larynx and upper airway.
- Occluding the tracheotomy tube may result in improved swallow function for some individuals.
- Both positive and negative effects of tracheotomy tube occlusion on swallow biomechanics have been found.
- Individualized assessment is important to determine whether patients benefit from tracheotomy tube occlusion.

One-Way Tracheotomy Tube Speaking Valves and Swallowing

The purpose of a one-way tracheotomy tube speaking valve is to allow individuals who require a tracheotomy tube. Airflow through the larynx for voice and speech production in there are a number of manufacturers of one-way tracheotomy tube speaking valves, i.e., the Passy–Muir Tracheostomy Speaking Valve (Passy–Muir, Inc., Irvine, CA); Shiley Phonate speaking valve (Mallinckrodt, Inc., St. Louis, MO); and Blom speaking valve (Pulmodyne, India Napolis IN). The most widely used one-way speaking valve is a bias-closed valve that opens only upon inspiration and is closed during exhalation (Passy–Muir, Inc.). Escape of exhaled air through the tracheotomy tube is prevented as the closed valve mandates diversion of airflow between the tube and tracheal walls and then caudally through the upper respiratory system. However, a number of additional benefits of the one-way valve have been reported. These include decreased oral and nasal secretions, increased food intake, and increased energy levels [64–66].

Placement of a one-way speaking valve has also been used to facilitate weaning from mechanical ventilation as half of the respiratory cycle is normalized, i.e., inhalation is accomplished through the tracheotomy with exhalation through the upper airway [67]. Specific to the goal of decannulation, the use of a one-way speaking valve offers several advantages over digital (finger) occlusion of a tracheotomy tube. The advantages include decreased risk of infection by elimination of possible contamination with digital occlusion, improved patient compliance and speaking effort.

An ancillary function of a one-way speaking valve has been proposed, i.e., to improve swallow function in select individuals who require a tracheotomy tube and exhibit dysphagia. It has been suggested that a one-way speaking valve may potentially assist in eliminating or reducing aspiration. Research investigating the use of a one-way speaking valve and its effect on improvement of swallow function is needed.

Prior to placement of the valve on a cuffed trach, the tracheotomy tube cuff must be deflated. Cuff deflation allows air to flow through the upper airway, specifically the larynx and true vocal folds, which may restore laryngeal sensation and facilitate airway clearance. In addition, cuff deflation and speaking valve placement reportedly restores subglottal air pressure [18, 61]. Although the role of subglottic air pressure in swallowing is not fully understood, it has been suggested that a reduction in subglottic air pressure is the primary mechanism affecting swallow function in patients with open tracheotomy tubes [18].

The following is a review of the literature regarding the variable effects of one-way tracheotomy tube speaking valve placement has on swallow function. Dettelbach et al. [17] performed a VFSS to evaluate 11 patients, aged 43–85 years, with tracheotomy. Swallowing was analyzed both with and without a one-way valve in place. Aspiration was experienced by four (36%) patients, although all patients had a reduction in the observed volume of aspiration following valve placement. It is difficult to determine the volume of aspirated material using videofluoroscopy [68]. It is unclear how the authors determined the reduction in volume of aspiration with a one-way valve in place.

Stachler et al. [16] completed simultaneous scintigraphy and VFSS with and without a one-way speaking valve in place. Eleven patients who were either pre- or posttreatment for head and neck cancer participated. Presence of a one-way speaking valve did not eliminate aspiration for any of the patients, but the amount of aspirate was significantly reduced with the one-way speaking valve.

Elpern et al. [69] studied 15 patients, aged 32–84 years, with tracheotomy tubes using VFSS swallowing thin liquid to determine the incidence of aspiration with and without a one-way speaking valve. During the valve off condition, seven participants aspirated during at least one presentation. Of the seven who aspirated, five aspirated with the one-way valve off and two aspirated during both the valve off and valve on conditions. Aspiration was less frequent with the valve on, i.e., 3 of 43 swallows, versus the valve off condition, i.e., 13 of 44 swallows.

Gross et al. [61] evaluated four patients with tracheotomy tubes under two conditions with VFSS. With the speaking valve on, all participants exhibited a reduction in bolus transit times and duration of pharyngeal biomechanics. In addition, scores on an eight-point penetration–aspiration scale [70] improved for three of four participants during the speaking valve on condition. Two of the participants who demonstrated changes in penetration–aspiration scale scores exhibited only very minimal improvements in swallow function, i.e., scores improved by 0.5 points.

Suiter et al. [57] used VFSS to examine the biomechanical effects of speaking valve placement on swallow function in 18 patients requiring a tracheotomy tube. Fourteen patients had cuffed tracheotomy tubes and completed the VFSS under three conditions: (1) cuff inflated, (2) cuff deflated, and (3) cuff deflated with speaking valve in place. Four participants had cuffless tracheotomy tubes and completed the VFSS under two conditions: (1) no speaking valve and (2) speaking valve in place. Results for the cuff inflated versus speaking valve indicated that penetration–aspiration scale [70] scores were significantly reduced, i.e., improved, for the liquid bolus during speaking valve placement. Results for the cuff deflated versus cuffless-speaking valve showed significantly improved penetration–aspiration scale scores for liquid boluses with valve placement. There were no significant changes in duration of swallow biomechanical measures or hyolaryngeal excursion with either condition. However, there was an increase in the amount of residue observed on the tongue base, on the posterior pharyngeal wall, and at the UES with the speaking valve placement. The reason for reduction in aspiration remains unclear.

The specific effects of one-way speaking valve placement on swallow physiology remain unknown. Speaking valve placement may restore subglottal air pressure, which is reduced as a consequence of an open tracheotomy tube. It has been conjectured that this reduction in subglottal pressure without the one-way valve in place leads to an increased incidence of aspiration [18].

Gross et al. [60] measured subglottal air pressure with the tracheotomy tube open versus with placement of speaking valve and found a tenfold increase in subglottal pressure during swallowing with the speaking valve in place. Increased subglottal air pressure due to placement of the one-way speaking valve does not appear to necessarily result in significant improvements in swallowing safety, as only minor improvements in penetration–aspiration scale scores have been reported [61]. It therefore continues to be unclear whether increases in subglottal air pressure associated with one-way speaking valve use result in functional improvements in swallowing safety.

Speaking valve placement may also be beneficial in restoring laryngeal sensation by diverting airflow back through the upper airway rather than through the tracheotomy tube. When airflow is restored through the larynx, by decannulation, tracheotomy tube capping, or placement of a one-way speaking valve, both the laryngeal opening and closure reflexes return to normal. Restoration of both abductor [4] and adductor glottal reflexes [5] has the potential to improve sensation and restore the protective cough reflex, both of which contribute to a safe swallow. Further research is needed to determine the specific effects of speaking valve placement on laryngeal and pharyngeal sensation.

Although there is emerging evidence indicating improved swallow safety following one-way speaking valve placement, the research remains contradictory. Leder [71] used FEES to evaluate swallowing in 20 patients, 14 men (mean age 66 years) and 6 women (mean age 72 years) who had tracheotomies. Swallowing was evaluated first with and then without a one-way speaking valve in place. Puree consistency food was used. It was found that all subjects who aspirated without the valve in place also aspirated with the valve in place. Conversely, subjects who presented with no aspiration with the valve removed also did not aspirate with the valve in place. Thus, one-way speaking valve placement had no effect on aspiration status. An explanation for this finding may be the bolus consistency used. That is, with the

patients studied and timing of their aspiration with puree consistency they would have invariably aspirated the liquid consistency as well [72]. However, if puree consistency is swallowed successfully and only thin liquid consistency is aspirated, then placement of a one-way speaking valve may be of some benefit in selected individuals [57]. Additional research with a much larger sample size is needed to determine the interaction of bolus consistency, bolus volume, and use of a one-way speaking valve in regards to improving swallowing success.

Ohmae et al. [73] hypothesized that airflow directed through the larynx due to placement of a one-way speaking valve would allow for clearance of any residual bolus remaining in the subglottis, laryngeal vestibule, and pharynx, thereby preventing laryngeal penetration and aspiration. Sixteen patients with tracheotomies underwent a FEES and a VFSS. Swallowing parameters were compared first with and then without a one-way valve in place. Valve placement improved laryngeal residue clearance and the incidence of laryngeal penetration during swallowing. However, it did not affect pharyngeal bolus residue, laryngeal elevation, pharyngeal delay, or, most importantly, incidence of aspiration. These results add to the growing consensus that a one-way valve, with redirection of exhaled air through the larynx and upper airway, improves the patient's ability to clear bolus residue from the laryngeal vestibule. Findings, however, do not support use of a one-way valve as a primary means of improving actual pharyngeal swallow functioning or elimination of aspiration altogether.

Overall, evidence in the research literature supports the notion that one-way speaking valve placement may improve swallow safety for selected patients and/or selected food consistencies. Further research is needed to determine the specific effects of speaking valve placement on swallow function.

The current body of research pertaining to swallow-related responses with speaking valve placement has included small sample sizes and homogeneous age groups. To determine age and gender effects, large group studies should be undertaken.

The clinician who treats patients with tracheotomy tubes and speaking valves should be aware that age influences swallowing success, i.e., older individuals aspirate with greater frequency, and aspiration status has more to do with the severity and chronic nature of an individual's illness rather than presence of a tracheotomy tube [21, 22].

In summary, the results of the current research indicate that placement of a speaking valve improves swallow function for some, but not all individuals, and for some (specifically thin liquids) bolus consistencies but not others (puree). Some research indicates that speaking valve placement may increase oral and pharyngeal residue [57] or negatively affect the biomechanical aspects of swallowing [50]. Therefore, caution should be taken when making decisions regarding whether to feed a patient with a speaking valve in place. It is imperative that a complete instrumental swallow evaluation be performed for those patients who have a tracheotomy. The evaluation should include several food and/or liquid consistency presentations with both the one-way speaking valve in place and removed prior to making decisions regarding the use of the valve as a means for reducing aspiration and improving swallow function.

Some patients may not be able to tolerate valve placement for a period of time sufficient to complete a meal. Clinicians working with these patients should perform the swallow evaluation under the same conditions as the patient would normally eat. In other words, if the tracheotomy cuff is inflated during mealtimes, the patient should complete the swallow evaluation with the cuff inflated.

Clinical Tips

- An instrumental assessment by the SLP is required prior to determining valve on or valve off oral intake condition and recommendations.
- Determine for each individual patient which aspect(s) of swallowing improve during each of the following conditions: tube occlusion,

wearing a speaking valve, cuff status inflated or deflated. After this determination, be consistent in the use of this strategy during eating.
- Consider the age of the patient as it may affect swallowing safety and impact of the tracheotomy.
- Consider the patient's underlying disease on swallow function as it may make more difference than the presence of a tracheotomy or may compound the effects of the tracheotomy.

Mechanical Ventilation via Tracheotomy Tube and Swallowing

Patients who require mechanical ventilation via a tracheotomy tube may be successful with oral alimentation. Since the tracheotomy tube cuff cannot be deflated, these patients cannot produce a cough to clear aspirated material from the airway above the inflated cuff. To evaluate and treat patients who require mechanical ventilation, a clinical bedside swallowing assessment is inadequate and must be done in conjunction with an objective instrumental FEES or VFSS in order to make a diagnosis and recommendation regarding oral feeding.

Incidence and type (timing) of aspiration in patients requiring mechanical ventilation via tracheotomy is of great interest. Determination of the renewed ability to swallow safely is often the first step towards recovery and is a huge boon to quality-of-life enhancement for patients, families, and caregivers. The literature on this topic is sparse and includes primarily case studies [8, 48] and studies that did not perform a swallow evaluation to assess aspiration [35] and those with results using data that grouped patients who were both mechanically ventilated and breathing without mechanical ventilation [10, 31]. Only one study investigated aspiration status in patients requiring long-term mechanical ventilation via tracheotomy (range 25–547 days; mean 112 days) [14]. Based on VFSS evaluation, it was reported that 50% of the subjects aspirated and 77% of those had silent aspiration. Subjects who aspirated were significantly older (mean age: 72.5 versus 64.8 years) than those who did not aspirate.

Incidence and type of aspiration following tracheotomy and long-term mechanical ventilation [14] may be different from that found in acutely ill patients requiring tracheotomy for short-term mechanical ventilation. Therefore, the incidence of aspiration and type of aspiration found in acutely ill patients requiring 2 months or less mechanical ventilation via a tracheotomy was studied [23]. Fifty adult inpatients referred for a FEES participated. Results indicated that 34 of 50 (68%) patients did not aspirate while 16 of 50 (32%) aspirated. Thirteen of 16 (81%) patients who aspirated were silent aspirators. Patients who aspirated were significantly older (mean 72 years, range 48–87 years) than those who did not aspirate (mean 59 years, range 20–83 years) ($p < 0.05$), and since females in this sample were older than males more females aspirated than males. Patients who aspirated were post-tracheotomy for significantly less time (mean 14.4 days, range 3–48 days) than those who did not aspirate (mean 23.5 days, range 2–62 days) ($p < 0.05$). No significant difference was found when comparing duration of translaryngeal intubation for aspirators (mean 14.2 days, range 0–31 days) versus non-aspirators (mean 14.2 days, range 0–29 days) ($p > 0.05$).

Normal aging with resulting changes manifest from sarcopenia may decrease cardiopulmonary, neuromuscular, and metabolic capacities resulting in a progressive loss of functional reserve, and the reduced ability to adapt to stress [46]. Aging also alters the intricate biomechanical coordination of swallowing. Although in healthy elderly the incidence of aspiration does not increase, the oral–pharyngeal stage transition has been shown to increase significantly at ~70 years of age [30, 74]. When a stressor such as respiratory failure requiring mechanical ventilation via tracheotomy is introduced in an otherwise healthy older adult, for example, it may accelerate deterioration of systems resulting in functional reserve below the level required for activities of daily living [46].

When patients with tracheotomy and long-term mechanical ventilation needs were investigated, it was found that older patients, i.e., mean age 72.5 years, aspirated significantly more often than younger patients [14]. These results were corroborated for patients requiring mechanical ventilation via a new tracheotomy tube. Specifically, a mean age of 72 years differentiated patients who aspirated versus patients who swallowed successfully [23]. Therefore, decreased functional reserve due to advanced age is an important variable for increased risk of aspiration in patients who require mechanical ventilation.

Swallowing in Infants Requiring Mechanical Ventilation via Tracheotomy Tube

On the opposite end of the age spectrum, medically and respiratory fragile infants with long-term need for tracheotomy and taking nothing by mouth, are at risk for developing feeding difficulties independent of their mechanical ventilation status [75]. Dysphagia diagnostic testing and feeding intervention are integral components of the plan of care for these infants [76]. Early feeding habilitation can potentially decrease development of resistance to oral feeding and behavioral feeding issues, i.e., oral aversion [77].

The incidence of dysphagia and aspiration following tracheotomy and mechanical ventilation in infants is of great interest as there may be differences from those found in adults who required either short- or long-term mechanical ventilation via tracheotomy. Leder et al. [78] performed FEES and VFSS to diagnose dysphagia and establish goals to initiate safe oral alimentation in medically stable infants who required mechanical ventilation via tracheotomy. Ten males (mean chronological age 8.0 months, range 3–14 months; mean gestational age 28.9 weeks, range 24–39 weeks) and four females (mean chronological age 8.3 months, range 3–13 months; mean gestational age 27.3 weeks, range 25–30 weeks) participated. Thirteen of 14 (93%) infants swallowed successfully, and although some exhibited an oral dysphagia, none experienced aspiration. No infant exhibited aspiration when a feeding tube was present. Only one infant exhibited pharyngeal dysphagia with aspiration and a recommendation of nil-by-mouth status was made from FEES and VFSS evaluation. Ninety-three percent of the medically stable infants who required mechanical ventilation via tracheotomy swallowed successfully without aspirating indicating that it may be advantageous to evaluate swallowing function in this patient population. Although dependent on different criteria than adults, timing of the swallow evaluation for infants is also critical for success. Noting the improved physical condition and medical progress, the stable ventilator settings over a period of 7–14 days, and absence of tachypnea proved to be good prognostic indicators for recommendation to evaluate swallowing function with the goal to initiate oral alimentation.

The low incidence of aspiration (7%) in infants requiring mechanical ventilation via tracheotomy [78] differed from the 50% incidence of aspiration reported in adult patients with long-term [14] and 33% incidence of aspiration reported in adult patients with short-term [23] mechanical ventilation requirements.

The principal findings when studying swallow function with mechanical ventilation via a tracheotomy tube were:

- Sixty-eight percent of adult patients requiring short-term mechanical ventilation via a new tracheotomy swallowed successfully.
- Type of aspiration noted in patients with tracheotomy and mechanical ventilation was predominately silent.
- Age appears to be a determining factor in differentiation of aspiration status.
- Incidence of aspiration differed in patients with short-term versus long-term ventilation use.

Effect of Nasogastric Tubes on Aspiration Status

Nasogastric (NG) tube feeding is the most widely used nonoral feeding method for patients unable to eat by mouth and those patients unable to take adequate oral nutrition [79–81]. NG tube placement is relatively atraumatic, minimally invasive, and usually well tolerated [82]. Enteral nutrition delivered via NG tube can be given to patients of all ages and spanning all medical specialties [83].

A common but major complication often coinciding with NG tube use is aspiration [80, 81, 83, 84]. However, due to the multifactorial nature of aspiration pneumonia, no specific causative effect has been documented among presence of an NG tube, aspiration, and development of aspiration pneumonia [80, 83, 84]. Specifically, neither the contribution of anterograde aspiration (defined as aspiration during oral alimentation due to oropharyngeal dysphagia) nor retrograde aspiration (defined as aspiration of refluxed gastric contents) concurrent with NG tube use are known [83, 84].

Since an NG tube is a foreign object that traverses the same path as a food bolus in the pharynx and esophagus it could be assumed to potentially impact negatively on safe and efficient swallowing ability. A number of studies have investigated this assumption. Manometry tube placement in 80 normal volunteers resulted in longer durations for hyoid bone excursion and UES opening dependent on bolus consistency, age, and gender, but no aspiration was observed on any swallows [30]. NG tube placement was investigated in before–after feeding trials with 10 normal adults [85] and 22 [86] and 25 [87] stroke patients, respectively. No significant differences in aspiration rates were reported in either normal or stroke patients. Lastly, when a 3.6 mm diameter flexible fiberoptic endoscopic was present versus absent in the nasopharynx of 14 healthy normal adult volunteers, there was no significant alteration of duration of swallowing stage transitions, pharyngeal transit timing, or extent of maximum hyoid bone elevation, and, consistent with all other reports, there was no effect on incidence of aspiration [88].

Therefore, although aspiration may occur coincident with NG tube use [80, 81, 83, 84], no causal relationship was demonstrated in both normal and disordered populations [85–88], and even tubes of differing diameters were all associated with a safe swallow without aspiration. However, due to small sample sizes, non-comparable population samples, and differing methodologies there is need for a large-scale study to provide a definitive answer as to whether or not an NG tube affects swallowing success.

Leder and Suiter [89] investigated the effect an NG tube had on occurrence of anterograde aspiration of both liquid and puree bolus consistencies during objective evaluation of swallowing with FEES. A referred sample of 1,260 consecutively enrolled inpatients participated. Group 1 ($N=630$; 346 M; 284 F) had an NG tube present at the time of referral for a dysphagia evaluation while Group 2 ($N=630$; 360 M; 270 F) did not have an NG tube at the time of referral. Approximately 61% had small-bore tubes (8 Fr., 2.65 mm diameter) and 39% had large-bore tubes (18 Fr., 6.0 mm diameter). There were no significant differences ($p>0.05$) in incidence aspiration of either liquid (24 versus 23%) or puree (14 versus 15%) food consistencies dependent on the presence or absence of an NG tube. In addition, no significant interactions ($p>0.05$) were found between NG tube status and gender, age, or diagnostic category. Interestingly, older subjects, between 60 and 90 years of age, and regardless of NG tube status were noted to aspirate more frequently than younger subjects.

For the first time with both an adequately large and heterogeneous population sample and objective dysphagia testing, incidence of aspiration with either liquid or puree consistencies was not affected by the presence of an NG tube. Specifically, the occurrence of aspiration for both liquid and puree food consistencies was the same between two separate but comparable groups, i.e., one with and one without an NG tube in place. Although prior studies reported minor differences in temporal measurements during swallowing, there was no reported increase in the most important nontemporal swallowing indicator, i.e., aspiration, when an NG tube was present in the pharynx and esophagus [30, 85, 86, 88, 89] and confirmed that a safe and successful swallow, defined as no aspiration during FEES, was not affected by the presence of an NG tube.

Fattal et al. [90] investigated waht effect, if any, the presence or absence of an NG tube in the same person had on the incidence of aspiration. Sixty-two consecutively enrolled adult inpatients with both small-bore (8 Fr., external diameter 2.65 mm) and large-bore (18 Fr., external diameter 6.0 mm) NG tubes participated. Group 1 had

FEES first with the NG tube in place and a second FEES after NG tube removal while Group 2 did not have an NG tube and had FEES first without an NG tube and a second FEES after placement of a small-bore NG tube. There were no significant differences (p > 0.05) in aspiration status for both liquid and puree consistencies in the same person dependent on presence or absence of either a small-bore or large-bore NG tube.

It is important to note that although an NG tube did not increase the occurrence of aspiration, this does not mean that all aspiration events are equally important. Patients who received NG tube feeding were usually older and, regardless of NG tube status, it was found that patients between 60 and 90 years of age aspirated more frequently than younger subjects. Also, patients who required NG tube feeding prior to FEES presented with risk factors that predisposed them to the development of an aspiration pneumonia, e.g., dementia, nonambulatory/bed-bound, severely ill, malnourishment, postsurgery, and poor functional reserve [80–82]. Therefore, whenever an NG tube is used an appropriate assessment followed by implementation of measures to reduce aspiration risk is necessary [80, 83].

Nasogastric Tubes and Swallowing Success

In summary:

- No statistically significant differences were found regarding aspiration status for liquid or puree food consistencies between two separate but comparable groups, i.e., one with and one without an NG tube, regardless of gender, age or diagnostic category.
- Given that an objective swallowing evaluation, i.e., either fiberoptic or fluoroscopic, can be performed with an NG tube in place, it is not necessary to remove an NG tube to evaluate dysphagia.
- Similarly, there is no contraindication to leaving an NG tube in place to supplement oral alimentation until prandial nutrition is adequate.
- Future research should explore NG tube placement and aspiration status in very young

478   S.B. Leder and D.M. Suiter

(0–10 years) and very old (90–100+ years) individuals and the impact of duration of NG tube use on swallowing success.

Effect of Orogastric Tubes on Aspiration Status

An orogastric (OG) tube is used frequently in both the adult and pediatric intensive care units. The reasons being that a large-bore OG tube is often more easily placed than a small-bore NG tube, and facial trauma or surgery often precludes placement via the nasal route. Since an OG tube is a foreign object that traverses the *entire* pathway a food bolus travels during all three stages of swallowing (from the oral cavity through the pharynx and into the esophagus), there is a corresponding a priori assumption that its presence can have a negative impact on safe and efficient swallowing. In the only study published to date, Leder et al. [91] investigated what effect, if any, the presence of an OG tube had on incidence of anterograde aspiration of both liquid and puree bolus consistencies as determined by objective evaluation, i.e., FEES and VFSS, and if diet recommendations can be made successfully for patients who require an OG tube.

Ten patients (two pediatric, age 17 days and 3 months, and eight adults, mean 63 years) were enrolled prospectively. Two swallow studies were performed within a 5-min time interval. An OG tube was present for the first FEES or VFSS and then removed for the second swallow study. Adult participants had large-bore OG tubes (18 Fr., 6.0 mm diameter) and when an NG tube was also present it was always a small-bore tube (8 Fr., 2.7 mm diameter). Pediatric participants had pediatric OG feeding tubes (5 Fr., 1.7 mm diameter). There were no significant differences ($p > 0.05$) for either overall incidence of aspiration or aspiration by food consistency (liquid or puree) dependent on OG tube presence. Also, all nine participants recommended for an oral diet ate successfully. Interestingly, four of five (80%) participants swallowed successfully without aspiration despite the presence of two tubes, i.e., OG and NG, plus the fiberoptic endoscope required

for FEES. It was concluded that objective dysphagia testing with either FEES or VFSS can be performed with an OG tube in place and there is no contraindication to keeping an OG tube to supplement oral alimentation until prandial nutrition is adequate.

Orogastric Tubes and Swallowing Success

- No statistically significant differences were found regarding aspiration status for liquid or puree food consistencies based on the presence or absence of either an NG or OG tube regardless of gender, age, or diagnostic category.
- Given that an objective swallowing evaluation, i.e., either fiberoptic or fluoroscopic, can be performed with both an NG and OG tube in place, it is not necessary to remove either tube to evaluate dysphagia.
- Similarly, there is no contraindication to leaving an NG or OG tube in place to supplement oral alimentation until prandial nutrition is adequate.
- Future research should explore NG and OG tube placement and aspiration status in very young (0–10 years) and very old (90–100+ years) individuals and the impact of duration of NG or OG tube use on swallowing success.

Assessment of Swallowing in Patients Requiring Tracheotomy Tubes

Clinical Swallow Examination

Modified Evans Blue Dye Test
The modified Evans blue dye test (MEBDT) has been proposed as an adjunct to the clinical swallow assessment of individuals with tracheotomy. As originally described [35], the blue dye test involved placing four drops of a 1% solution of Evans blue dye on the patient's tongue every 4 h followed by tracheal suctioning at set intervals. Although concerns regarding the safety of blue dye have been raised recently [92–94], the blue dye test continues to be used by many clinicians.

In clinical practice, the blue dye test has been modified to include the presentation of blue dye-tinged foods or liquids during the bedside swallow assessment. Aspiration is assumed if blue dye is present in the tracheal secretions.

Subsequent research has questioned the accuracy of the blue dye test for determining tracheal aspiration. Cameron [35] stated that an inflated tracheotomy tube cuff had no effect on the incidence of aspiration. However, the subjects were not comparable, i.e., 69% of patients with a tracheotomy tube aspirated while 0% of patients with an endotracheal tube aspirated; aspiration status was assessed from 1 to 28 days in patients with a tracheotomy tube but only up to 48 h in patients with an endotracheal tube; and ~50% of patients with a tracheotomy had neurological or trauma as an etiology versus 0% of patients with an endotracheal tube. Therefore, subject, time, and inclusion criteria confounded the findings.

The accuracy of the blue dye test for determining tracheal aspiration is questionable. Thompson-Henry and Braddock [95] examined five patients with tracheotomy and found that the MEBDT failed to identify five of five individuals who subsequently aspirated during a follow-up instrumental swallow evaluation. However, it is important to note that average time from MEBDT to instrumental assessment was 11.6 days. To accurately determine test accuracy, concurrent MEBDT and instrumental assessments should have been performed. It cannot be assumed that patients behave similarly during two separate swallow examinations.

Subsequent investigations have improved upon the methodology in the Thompson Braddock and Henry study. Brady et al. [96] completed simultaneous blue dye test with VFSS. Eight of 20 (40%) subjects aspirated during VFSS. Findings were equivocal. Although the MEBDT detected aspiration in 100% of cases in which aspiration was greater than trace, it failed to identify 100% of those with trace aspiration.

Similar results were found in a follow-up investigation [97] in which 15 patients underwent simultaneous endoscopy (through the stoma) and blue dye test. Aspiration occurred in eight (53%) of studies. Blue tracheal secretions were present

in only 50%. Of the examinations in which more than trace aspiration was observed, 67% showed blue tracheal secretions on endoscopy and suctioning. None of the studies with trace aspiration showed blue secretions.

Belafsky et al. [98] completed MEBDT followed by a subsequent endoscopic examination of swallowing in 30 individuals. Twenty-two (73%) aspirated on FEES; 23 (77%) aspirated on MEBDT. Sensitivity of MEBDT for predicting puree aspiration on FEES was 93%; specificity was 33%. Sensitivity of MEBDT for predicting liquid aspiration on FEES was 86%; specificity was 43%. Overall sensitivity of the MEBDT was 82%; specificity was 38%. For those on mechanical ventilation, sensitivity was 100%; for those not on mechanical ventilation, sensitivity was 76%. Specificity was low overall. The authors concluded that their results validated the use of the MEBDT as a screening tool for detection of aspiration in individuals with tracheotomy. However, as with the Thompson-Braddock and Henry study [95], examinations were not completed simultaneously, and individuals cannot be assumed to behave similarly across examination times.

Instrumental Assessment

Since over two-thirds of the patients with tracheotomy and mechanical ventilation included in the study by Leder were found to swallow successfully and without significant dysphagia, it is advantageous to assess swallowing function in the acute care setting [23]. Timing of the swallow evaluation is critical for success. Patients who require transition from endotracheal intubation to tracheotomy exhibit respiratory failure that does not permit weaning from mechanical ventilation. Post-tracheotomy these patients continue with the same degree of respiratory compromise and it is not surprising that aspiration occurs during the immediate post-tracheotomy period, i.e., 14 days or less. As respiratory function improves, while still requiring mechanical ventilation, the majority of patients swallow successfully. Specifically, ~3 weeks post-tracheotomy is the optimal time to perform a swallow evaluation. Some patients, however, swallowed successfully earlier post-tracheotomy, i.e., 7 days or less. Clinical judgment based on age, medical progress, and respiratory recovery rate should be used to determine when best to perform a swallowing evaluation.

It is important to note that the majority of patients with tracheotomy who aspirate do so silently. This is why a clinical assessment must be done in conjunction with, not independent of, an objective instrumental swallowing evaluation [99]. Patients who require a tracheotomy tube, with or without mechanical ventilation, have diminished laryngeal protective reflexes [4, 5, 34] due to bypassing of the laryngeal airway and desensitization due to chronic aspiration of oral–pharyngeal secretions. An objective assessment of swallowing function, either FEES or videofluoroscopy, is needed to accurately determine aspiration status and make appropriate diet recommendations [23].

In summary:

- Clinical predictors of aspiration clinicians look for during traditional bedside swallow assessment may not be reliable predictors of aspiration risk in individuals with tracheotomy.
- The blue dye test has been found to have relatively high sensitivity but low specificity for detection of aspiration. Therefore, there is the potential for a high rate of false-negative findings when administering the blue dye test.
- Ideally, instrumental assessment (videofluoroscopy or FEES) should be used in the evaluation of patients with tracheotomy who are considered to be at risk for oropharyngeal dysphagia.
- It is contraindicated to use the 3 oz water swallow challenge for patients who require a tracheotomy tube and/or mechanical ventilation.

References

1. Shaker R, Li Q, Ren J, Townsend WF, Dodds WJ, Martin BJ, et al. Coordination of deglutition and phases of respiration: effect of aging, tachypnea, bolus volume, and chronic obstructive pulmonary disease. Am J Physiol. 1992;263:G750–5.
2. Martin-Harris B. Clinical implications of respiratory-swallowing interactions. Curr Opin Otolaryngol Head Neck Surg. 2008;16:194–9.
3. Brodky MB, McFarland DH, Dozier TS, Blair J, Ayers C, Michel Y, Gillespie MB, Day TA, Martin-Harris B. Respiratory-swallow phase patterns and their relationship to swallowing impairment in patients treated for oropharyngeal cancer. Head Neck. 2010; 32:481–9.
4. Sasaki CT, Fukuda H, Kirchner JA. Laryngeal abductor activity in response to varying ventilator resistance. Trans Am Acad Ophthalmol Otolaryngol. 1973;77:403–10.
5. Sasaki CT, Suzuki M, Horiuchi M, Kirchner JA. The effect of tracheostomy on the laryngeal closure reflex. Laryngoscope. 1977;87:1428–33.
6. Ikari T, Sasaki CT. Glottic closure reflex: control mechanisms. Ann Otol Rhinol Laryngol. 1980;89:220–4.
7. Betts RH. Post-tracheostomy aspiration. N Engl J Med. 1965;273:155.
8. Feldman SA, Deal CW, Urquhart W. Disturbance of swallowing after tracheostomy. Lancet. 1966;1:954–5.
9. Bonanno PC. Swallowing dysfunction after tracheostomy. Ann Surg. 1971;174:29–33.
10. Elpern EH, Jacobs ER, Bone RC. Incidence of aspiration in tracheally intubated adults. Heart Lung. 1987;16:527–31.
11. Leder SB, Joe JK, Ross DA, Coelho DH, Mendes J. Presence of a tracheotomy tube and aspiration status in early, postsurgical head and neck cancer patients. Head Neck. 2005;27:757–61.
12. Donzelli J, Brady S, Wesling M, Theisen M. Effects of the removal of the tracheotomy tube on swallowing during the fiberoptic endoscopic exam of the swallow (FEES). Dysphagia. 2005;20:283–9.
13. Peck KK, Branski RC, Lazarus C, Cody V, Kraus D, Haugage S, Ganz C, Holodny AI, Kraus DH. Cortical activation during swallowing rehabilitation maneuvers: a functional MRI study of healthy controls. Laryngoscope. 2010;120:2153–9.
14. Elpern EH, Scott MG, Petro L, Ries MH. Pulmonary aspiration in mechanically ventilated patients with tracheostomies. Chest. 1994;105:563–6.
15. Muz J, Hamlet S, Mathog R, Farris R. Scintigraphic assessment of aspiration in head and neck cancer patients with tracheostomy. Head Neck. 1994;16:17–20.
16. Stachler RJ, Hamlet SL, Choi J, Fleming S. Scintigraphic quantification of aspiration reduction with the Passy-Muir valve. Laryngoscope. 1996;106:231–4.
17. Dettelbach MA, Gross RD, Mahlmann J, Eibling DE. Effect of the Passy-Muir valve on aspiration in patients with tracheostomy. Head Neck. 1995;17:297–302.
18. Eibling DE, Gross RD. Subglottic air pressure: a key component of swallowing efficiency. Ann Otol Rhinol Laryngol. 1996;105:253–8.
19. Davis LA, Thompson Stanton S. Characteristics of dysphagia in elderly patients requiring mechanical ventilation. Dysphagia. 2004;19:7–14.

20. Conley JJ. Swallowing dysfunctions associated with radical surgery of the head and neck. Arch Surg. 1960;80:602–12.

21. Leder SB, Ross DA. Investigation of the causal relationship between tracheotomy and aspiration in the acute care setting. Laryngoscope. 2000;110:641–4.

22. Leder SB, Ross DA. Confirmation of no causal relationship between tracheotomy and aspiration status: a direct replication study. Dysphagia. 2010;25:35–9.

23. Leder SB. Incidence and type of aspiration in acute care patients requiring mechanical ventilation via a new tracheotomy. Chest. 2002;122:1721–6.

24. Baskin JZ, Panagopoulos G, Parks C, Komisar A. Predicting outcome in aged and severely ill patients with prolonged respiratory failure. Ann Otol Rhinol Laryngol. 2005;114:902–6.

25. Norton SA, Quill TE. Complex questions embedded in tracheotomy decisions. Head Neck. 2004;26: 75–6.

26. Leder SB, Cohn SM, Moller BA. Fiberoptic endoscopic documentation of the high incidence of aspiration following extubation in critically ill trauma patients. Dysphagia. 1998;13:208–12.

27. Daniels SK, Ballo LA, Mahoney MC, Foundas AL. Clinical predictors of dysphagia and aspiration risk: outcome measures in acute stroke patients. Arch Phys Med Rehabil. 2000;81:1030–3.

28. Leder SB, Espinosa JF. Aspiration risk after acute stroke: comparison of clinical examination and fiberoptic endoscopic evaluation of swallowing. Dysphagia. 2002;17:214–8.

29. Leder SB. Fiberoptic endoscopic evaluation of swallowing in patients with acute traumatic brain injury. J Head Trauma Rehabil. 1999;14:448–53.

30. Robbins J, Hamilton JW, Lof GL, Kempster GB. Oropharyngeal swallowing in normal adults of different ages. Gastroenterology. 1992;103:823–9.

31. Tolep K, Getch CL, Criner GJ. Swallowing dysfunction in patients receiving prolonged mechanical ventilation. Chest. 1996;109:167–72.

32. Leder SB, Ross DA, Burrell MI, Sasaki CT. Tracheotomy tube occlusion status and aspiration in early post-surgical head and neck cancer patients. Dysphagia. 1998;13:167–71.

33. Muz J, Mathog RH, Nelson R, Jones Jr LA. Aspiration in patients with head and neck cancer and tracheostomy. Am J Otolaryngol. 1989;10:282–6.

34. Buckwalter JA, Sasaki CT. Effect of tracheotomy on laryngeal function. Otolaryngol Clin North Am. 1984;17:41–8.

35. Cameron JL, Reynolds J, Zuidema GD. Aspiration in patients with tracheostomies. Surg Gynecol Obstet. 1973;136:68–70.

36. Nash M. Swallowing problems in the tracheotomized patient. Otolaryngol Clin North Am. 1988;21:701–9.

37. Langmore SE, Schatz K, Olsen N. Fiberoptic endoscopic examination of swallowing safety: a new procedure. Dysphagia. 1988;2:216–9.

38. Langmore SE, Schatz K, Olson N. Endoscopic and videofluoroscopic evaluations of swallowing and aspiration. Ann Otol Rhinol Laryngol. 1991;100: 678–81.

39. Hammond CAS, Goldstein LB. Cough and aspiration of food and liquids due to oral-pharyngeal dysphagia. Chest. 2006;129:154S–68.

40. Shama L, Connor NP, Ciucci MR, McCulloch TM. Surgical treatment of dysphagia. Phys Med Rehabil Clin N Am. 2008;19:817–35.

41. Muma JR. The need for replication. J Speech Hear Res. 1993;36:927–30.

42. Heise DR. Causal analysis. New York, NY: Wiley; 1975.

43. Ashley J, Duggan M, Suitcliffe N. Speech, language, and swallowing disorders in the older adult. Clin Geriatr Med. 2006;22:291–310.

44. Sharma OP, Oswanski MF, Singer D, Buckley B, Courtright B, Raj SS, Waite PJ, Tatchell T, Gandaio A. Swallowing disorders in trauma patients: impact of tracheostomy. Am Surg. 2007;73:1117–21.

45. DeVita MA, Spierer-Rundback L. Swallowing disorders in patients with prolonged orotracheal intubation or tracheostomy tubes. Crit Care Med. 1990;18:1328–30.

46. Pendergast DR, Fisher NM, Calkins E. Cardiovascular, neuromuscular, and metabolic alterations with age leading to frailty. J Gerontol. 1993;48(Spec No):61–7.

47. Kremen AJ. Cancer of the tongue—a surgical technique for a primary combined en bloc resection of tongue, floor of mouth, and cervical lymphatics. Surgery. 1951;30:227–40.

48. Pinkus NB. The dangers of oral feeding in the presence of cuffed tracheostomy tubes. Med J Aust. 1973;1:1238–40.

49. Leverment JN, Pearson FG, Rae S. A manometric study of the upper oesphagus in the dog following cuffed-tube tracheostomy. Br J Anaesth. 1976;48:83–9.

50. Logemann JA, Pauloski BR, Colangelo L. Light digital occlusion of the tracheostomy tube: a pilot study of effects on aspiration and biomechanics of the swallow. Head Neck. 1998;20:52–7.

51. Logemann JA. Manual for the videofluorographic study of swallowing. 2nd ed. Austin, TX: Pro-Ed; 1993.

52. Dikeman KJ, Kazandjian MS. Communication and swallowing management of tracheostomized and ventilator-dependent adults. 2nd ed. Clifton Park, NY: Thomson Delmar Learning; 2003.

53. Perlman AL, Schulze-Delrieu K. Deglutition and its disorders: anatomy, physiology, clinical diagnosis, and management. San Diego, CA: Singular Publishing Group; 1997.

54. Logemann JA. Evaluation and treatment of swallowing disorders. 2nd ed. Austin, TX: Pro-Ed; 1998.

55. Terk AR, Leder SB, Burrell MI. Hyoid bone and laryngeal movement dependent upon presence of a tracheotomy tube. Dysphagia. 2007;22:89–93.

56. Leonard RJ, Kendall KA, McKenzie S, Goncalves MI, Walker A. Structural displacements in normal swallowing: a videofluoroscopic study. Dysphagia. 2000;15:146–52.

57. Suiter DM, McCullough GH, Powell PW. Effects of cuff deflation and one-way tracheostomy speaking valve placement on swallow physiology. Dysphagia. 2003;18:284–92.

58. Tippett DC, Siebens AA. Using ventilators for speaking and swallowing. Dysphagia. 1991;6:94–9.

59. Ding R, Logemann JA. Swallow physiology in patients with trach cuff inflated or deflated: a retrospective study. Head Neck. 2005;27:809–13.

60. Gross RD, Dettelbach M, Zajac D, Eibling D. Measure of subglottic air pressure during swallowing in a patient with tracheotomy. San Diego, CA: Ame Acad Otolaryngol Head Neck Surg; 1994.

61. Gross RD, Mahlmann J, Grayhack JP. Physiologic effects of open and closed tracheostomy tubes on the pharyngeal swallow. Ann Otol Rhinol Laryngol. 2003;112:143–52.

62. Leder SB, Tarro JM, Burrell MI. Effect of occlusion of a tracheotomy tube on aspiration. Dysphagia. 1996;11:254–8.

63. Leder SB, Joe JK, Hill SE, Traube M. Effect of tracheotomy tube occlusion on upper esophageal sphincter and pharyngeal pressures in aspirating and nonaspirating patients. Dysphagia. 2001;16:79–82.

64. Manzano JL, Lubillo S, Henriquez D, Martin JC, Perez MC, Wilson DJ. Verbal communication of ventilator-dependent patients. Crit Care Med. 1993;21:512–7.

65. Passy V, Baydur A, Prentice W, Darnell-Neal R. Passymuir tracheostomy speaking valve on ventilator-dependent patients. Laryngoscope. 1993;103:653–8.

66. Lichtman SW, Birnbaum IL, Sanfilippo MR, Pellicone JT, Damon WJ, King ML. Effect of a tracheostomy speaking valve on secretions, arterial oxygenation, and olfaction: a quantitative evaluation. J Speech Hear Res. 1995;38:549–55.

67. Frey JA. Weaning from mechanical ventilation augmented by the Passy-Muir speaking valve. New York, NY: American Lung Association American Thoracic Society; 1991.

68. Muz J, Mathog RH, Miller PR, Rosen R, Borrero G. Detection and quantification of laryngotracheopulmonary aspiration with scintigraphy. Laryngoscope. 1987;97:1180–5.

69. Elpern EH, Borkgren Okonek M, Bacon M, Gerstung C, Skrzynski M. Effect of the Passy-Muir tracheostomy speaking valve on pulmonary aspiration in adults. Heart Lung. 2000;29:287–93.

70. Rosenbek JC, Robbins JA, Roecker EB, Coyle JL, Wood JL. A penetration-aspiration scale. Dysphagia. 1996;11:93–8.

71. Leder SB. Effect of a one-way tracheotomy speaking valve on the incidence of aspiration in previously aspiration patients with tracheotomy. Dysphagia. 1999;14:73–7.

72. Suiter DM, Leder SB. Clinical utility of the 3-ounce water swallow test. Dysphagia. 2008;23:244–50.

73. Ohmae Y, Adachi Z, Isoda Y, et al. Effects of one-way speaking valve placement on swallowing physiology for tracheostomized patients: impact on laryngeal clearance. Nippon Jibiinkoka Gakkai Kaiho. 2006;109:594–9.

74. Rademaker AW, Pauloski BR, Coleangelo LA, Logemann JA. Age and volume effects on liquid swallowing function in normal women. J Speech Lang Hear Res. 1998;41:275–84.

75. Wetmore R, Handler S, Potsic W. Pediatric tracheostomy experience during the past decade. Ann Otol Rhinol Laryngol. 1982;91:628–32.

76. Abraham SS, Wolf EL. Swallowing physiology of toddlers with long-term tracheostomies: a preliminary study. Dysphagia. 2000;15:206–12.

77. Simon BM, McGowan JS. Tracheostomy in young children: implications for assessment and feeding disorders. Inf Young Children. 1989;1:1–9.

78. Leder SB, Baker KE, Goodman TR. Dysphagia testing and aspiration status in medically stable infants requiring mechanical ventilation via tracheotomy. Pediatr Crit Care Med. 2010;11:484–7.

79. Finucane P, Aslan SM, Duncan D. Percutaneous endoscopic gastrostomy in elderly patients. Postgrad Med J. 1991;67:371–3.

80. DiSario JA. Future considerations in aspiration pneumonia in the critically ill patient: what is not known, areas for future research, and experimental methods. JPEN J Parenter Enteral Nutr. 2002;26 Suppl 6:S75–8. discussion S79.

81. Dennis MS, Lewis SC, Warlow C, FOOD Trial Collaboration. Effect of timing and method of enteral tube feeding for dysphagic stroke patients (FOOD): a multicentre randomized controlled trial. Lancet. 2005;365:764–72.

82. Dhamarajan TS, Unnikrishnan D. Tube feeding in the elderly; the technique, complications, and outcome. Postgrad Med. 2004;115:58–61.

83. McClave SA, DeMeo MT, DeLegge MH, et al. North American summit on aspiration in the critically ill patient: consensus statement. JPEN J Parenter Enteral Nutr. 2002;26 Suppl 6:S80–5.

84. Gomes GF, Pisani JC, Macedo ED, et al. The nasogastric feeding tube as a risk factor for aspiration and aspiration pneumonia. Curr Opin Clin Nutr Metab Care. 2003;6:327–33.

85. Huggins PS, Tuomi SK, Young C. Effects of nasogastric tubes on the young, normal swallowing mechanism. Dysphagia. 1999;14:157–61.

86. Wang TG, Wu M-C, Chang Y-C, et al. The effect of nasogastric tubes on swallowing function in persons with dysphagia following stroke. Arch Phys Med Rehabil. 2006;87:1270–3.

87. Dziewas R, Warnecke T, Hamacher C, et al. Do nasogastric tubes worsen dysphagia in patients with acute stroke? BMC Neurol. 2008;8:28.

88. Suiter DM, Moorhead MK. Effects of flexible fiberoptic endoscopy on pharyngeal swallow physiology. Otolaryngol Head Neck Surg. 2007;137:956–8.

89. Leder SB, Suiter DM. Effect of nasogastric tubes on incidence of aspiration. Arch Phys Med Rehabil. 2008;89:648–51.

90. Fattal M, Suiter DM, Warner HL, Leder SB. Effect of presence/absence of a nasogastric tube in the same person on incidence of aspiration. Otolaryngol Head Neck Surg. 2011;145:796–800.

91. Leder SB, Lazarus CL, Suiter DM, Acton LM. Effect of orogastric tubes on aspiration status and recommendations for oral feeding. Otolaryngol Head Neck Surg. 2011;144:372–5.

92. File Jr TM, Tan JS, Thomson Jr RB, Stephens C, Thompson P. An outbreak of Pseudomonas aeruginosa ventilator-associated respiratory infections due to contaminated food coloring dye–further evidence of the significance of gastric colonization preceding nosocomial pneumonia. Infect Control Hosp Epidemiol. 1995;16:417–8.

93. Gaur S, Sorg T, Shukla V. Systemic absorption of FD&C blue dye associated with patient mortality. Postgrad Med J. 2003;79:602–3.

94. Maloney JP, Halbower AC, Fouty BF, Fagan KA, Balasubramaniam V, Pike AW, et al. Systemic absorption of food dye in patients with sepsis. N Engl J Med. 2000;343:1047–8.

95. Thompson-Henry S, Braddock B. The modified Evan's blue dye procedure fails to detect aspiration in the tracheostomized patient: five case reports. Dysphagia. 1995;10:172–4.

96. Brady SL, Hildner CD, Hutchins BF. Simultaneous videofluoroscopic swallow study and modified Evans blue dye procedure: an evaluation of blue dye visualization in cases of known aspiration. Dysphagia. 1999;14:146–9.

97. Donzelli J, Brady S, Wesling M, Craney M. Simultaneous modified Evans blue dye procedure and video nasal endoscopic evaluation of the swallow. Laryngoscope. 2001;111:1746–50.

98. Belafsky PC, Blumenfeld L, LePage A, Nahrstedt K. The accuracy of the modified Evan's blue dye test in predicting aspiration. Laryngoscope. 2003;113:1969–72.

99. Leder SB, Suiter DM, Warner HL, Kaplan LJ. Initiating safe oral feeding in critically ill intensive care and step-down unit patients based on passing the 3-ounce (90 cc) water swallow challenge. J Trauma. 2011;70(5):1203–7.

Dysphagia Secondary to Systemic Diseases

34

Olle Ekberg and Thomas Mandl

Abstract

Systemic disease may cause dysphagia by several mechanisms, such as salivary gland impairment causing xerostomia, and painful mucosal blisters and ulcers impairing oral, pharyngeal, and esophageal function. In addition acute and chronic mucosal and submucosal inflammation may result in strictures in the esophagus and pharynx. Altered biomechanics of oral and pharyngeal musculature may be due to cervical spine abnormalities in patients with rheumatoid arthritis. Finally, vasculitides might involve vessels in the central nervous system and thereby lead to cortical and brainstem ischemia and thus neurological impairment which may cause dysphagia.

Keywords

Primary Sjögren's syndrome • Scleroderma • Systemic lupus erythematosus • Pemphigus • Pemphigoid • Epidermolysis bullosa dystrophica • Lichen planus • Behçet disease • Sarcoidosis • Rheumatoid arthritis • Xerostomia • Stricture • Vasculitis

O. Ekberg, MD, PhD
Department of Diagnostic Radiology, Diagnostic Centre of Imaging and Functional Medicine,
Skåne University Hospital,
S Förstadsgatan 101, Malmö 205 02, Sweden

T. Mandl, MD, PhD (✉)
Department of Rheumatology,
Skåne University Hospital,
Entrance 25, Malmö 205 02, Sweden
e-mail: Thomas.Mandl@med.lu.se

Primary Sjögren's Syndrome

Primary Sjögren's syndrome (pSS) is an autoimmune disease primarily affecting the salivary and lacrimal glands, thereby impairing salivary and lacrimal secretion resulting in mucosal dryness. Various non-exocrine organs may also be involved including the gastrointestinal tract and the nervous system.

Genetic factors increase the risk of developing pSS as reflected by an increased prevalence in patients with certain HLA-DR2 and DR3 genes. In addition, several non-HLA genes may be involved including genes coding for cytokines

R. Shaker et al. (eds.), *Principles of Deglutition: A Multidisciplinary Text for Swallowing and its Disorders*,   485
DOI 10.1007/978-1-4614-3794-9_34, © Springer Science+Business Media New York 2013

and second messengers. Furthermore, a disturbance of the androgen/estrogen balance may also be of importance in the pathogenesis of pSS.

pSS is a rheumatic disease characterized by lymphocytic infiltration and hypofunction of the exocrine glands, particularly the salivary and lacrimal glands, resulting in dryness of the mouth and eyes without other coexisting connective tissue diseases (CTD), whilst secondary Sjögren's syndrome is when the syndrome is associated with a CTD such as rheumatoid arthritis (RA), systemic lupus erythematosus (SLE), or scleroderma.

Due to the decreased production of saliva, xerostomia is the most common gastrointestinal symptom in pSS patients [1–6]. However, esophageal dysmotility and esophageal webs have also been reported [3, 5, 7–9]. The lack of saliva makes swallowing difficult by interfering with bolus manipulation and bolus movement in the mouth, pharynx, and esophagus. The sialometric measurements of the parotid gland may be close to 0mL/5min after masticatory stimulation (normal value >3.5 ml/5min).

One-third of pSS patients show varying degrees of esophageal dysmotility including weak contractions, aperistalsis, and tertiary contractions as well as differences in peristaltic velocity and duration, and some patients may have a decrease in the lower esophageal sphincter pressures [10].

In a recent study, Mandl et al. found that 65 % of pSS patients reported dysphagia in an interview/questionnaire [11] including a variety of symptoms, such as solid and/or liquid food dysphagia, globus sensation, regurgitation, and pyrosis. However, some pSS patients also had misdirected swallowing, coughing after swallowing, hawking when eating, and even food and fluid coming out of their nose during or after eating. Some had experienced painful swallowing, a feeling of obstruction when swallowing and episodes of acute obstruction. The majority of patients had an increased liquid intake when eating. This can be regarded as a compensation maneuver.

In any pSS patient who complains of dry mouth, a sialometric evaluation is of value [12]. Pharyngeal and esophageal function is best evaluated with a barium swallow or fiberoptic examination of swallowing. For the esophagus, manometry can be of value. In patients with abnormal motor function of the pharynx, a CT or MRI of the brain is recommended.

Systemic treatment in pSS includes secretagogues such as pilocarpine and cevimeline, which exert their effect by stimulating the muscarinic-3 receptor (M3R), thereby increasing salivary flow. Due to the presence of M3R in other parts of the body, subjects using these drugs may experience adverse effects, e.g., abdominal distress, irritable bladder, and sweating [13]. Biological agents such as TNF-alpha blockers have not been convincing in the treatment of pSS [14], whilst B-cell targeting therapies, e.g., rituximab, have shown more promising results [15].

Local treatment of dry mouth includes an increased water intake lubricating the dry mucosal surfaces of the oral cavity thus improving chewing and swallowing. Lozenges and chewing gums may also stimulate salivary secretion even in hypofunctional salivary glands. Finally, meticulous dental hygiene and fluoride substitution are mandatory since the lack of saliva leads to and accelerates tooth decay including caries development. Fluoridation of water is known to prevent tooth decay.

Scleroderma (Systemic Sclerosis)

Systemic sclerosis (SSc), also known as scleroderma, is a systemic disorder characterized by functional and structural abnormalities of small blood vessels and by fibrosis of the skin and internal organs. The etiology is largely unknown.

The affected tissues undergo varying degrees of inflammation, fibrosis, and atrophy. SSc may appear as a diffuse cutaneous affliction and is characterized by symmetric distal and truncal skin sclerosis with early involvement of internal organs. A subset of patients with SSc may have only visceral organ involvement without any skin lesions. Raynaud's phenomenon is common and the presence of anti-nuclear antibodies, sometimes with a centromere pattern, as well as anti-Scl-70 antibodies, support the diagnosis.

In the oral and pharyngoesophageal area, sclerosis of mucosa, mastication muscles, and

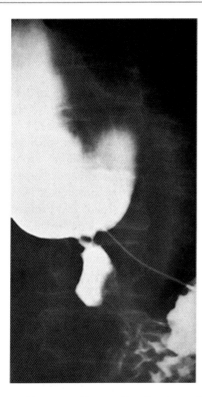

Fig. 34.1 Sixty-year-old man with scleroderma. Barium esophagram shows a dilated esophagus without peristalsis. There is a tight stricture in the distal esophagus

salivary glands may result in changes of voice and mouth function [16, 17]. A classical finding in SSc is microstomia, i.e., fibrosis of the perioral tissues leading to a small mouth [18, 19]. In the esophagus, there is progressive destruction of smooth muscle leading from abnormal peristalsis to aperistalsis. There is also an extreme lack of tonicity in the lower esophageal sphincter leading to massive gastroesophageal reflux disease. This causes major changes due to gastroesophageal reflux disease including tight strictures (Fig. 34.1).

Patients present with a multitude of symptoms. Microstomia (small mouth opening) makes for mechanical reason intake of food difficult. Fibrosis in the perioral muscles results in a stiffness of the cheeks and tongue. Masticatory muscles have a reduced elasticity. Due to decreased salivary production, i.e., secondary Sjögren's syndrome, patients may experience xerostomia. The patients also have esophageal dysphagia.

When strictures have developed, this may present with characteristic obstruction for solid foods. The disease may also affect the stomach and small bowel resulting in dysmotility and thereby impaired transportation at various gastrointestinal levels that may add considerably to the patient's complex symptomatology.

In those patients who present without skin lesions, the diagnosis may be spurious. The best method is to perform a biopsy and look for smooth muscle degeneration. In patients who have the typical microstomia, the diagnosis can be obvious. Due to the high prevalence of reflux and its consequences, the patients should undergo evaluation for GERD.

Whilst treatment of several other rheumatological diseases have developed considerably over the last years, current therapies for SSc are still disappointing. Today, treatment of SSc mainly consists of symptomatic treatment of the consequences of the disease with, e.g., various vasodilatory drugs, gastrointestinal prokinetic drugs, and proton pump inhibitors. Immunomodulatory treatment has limited use in SSc.

There are several means to try to slow the progression of microstomia [20]. No specific treatment is available for muscle fibrosis and muscle degeneration. However, treatment of the patient's GERD is paramount in order to avoid the development of strictures. In addition, the use of prokinetic drugs, antibiotics and vitamin and mineral supplementation may play a role in the treatment of bowel dysmotility, bacterial overgrowth, and malabsorption.

Systemic Lupus Erythematosus

SLE is an autoimmune, inflammatory progressive systemic disease of connective tissues including the skin and internal organs. Various antibodies directed against nuclear antigens may be encountered in the disease.

SLE is a connective tissue disease with several clinical manifestations in the skin. There are widespread endothelial changes in small blood vessels and changes in the collagen fibers of the connective tissue. Fibrinoid degeneration and collagen sclerosis are present [21, 22]. Anti-double-stranded deoxyribonucleic acid (dsDNA) antibodies are more specific for SLE than the anti-nuclear antibodies (ANA), used when screening for the disease. Fairly pathognomonic for SLE is the butterfly shaped malar rash on skin exposed to the sun usually appearing on the cheeks and nose bilaterally.

The patient may present with oral and pharyngeal ulcers, including ulcers on the palate. When the salivary glands are involved, i.e., when the patient has secondary Sjögren's syndrome, xerostomia may appear.

Up to 10 % of patients with SLE experience dysphagia [23]. Erythematous oral ulcers may be due to xerostomia and salivary gland involvement. Symptoms of xerostomia are dealt with under Sjögren's syndrome. Ulcerations in the pharynx may extend into the nasopharynx and larynx. Gastrointestinal dysmotility may include the esophagus as well as more distal parts of the gastrointestinal system. The underlying cause is not clear but might be due to submucosal fibrosis and ulceration. In addition, patients with SLE might have central nervous involvement that may cause motor or sensory impairment, particularly in the face, i.e., trigeminal and facial nerve involvement. There is also a high percentage of cerebrovascular complications in patients with SLE. Assessment of swallowing function may include a combination of fluoroscopic imaging and endoscopy for the assessment of mucosal lesions.

Medical treatment includes corticosteroids and disease-modifying anti-rheumatic drugs, e.g., antimalarials, azathioprine, cyclosporine, mycophenolat mofetil, and cyclophosphamide as well as more modern B-cell targeting therapies such as rituximab. There is no specific treatment for swallowing impairment in SLE other than those described under the specific dysfunction.

Pemphigus and Pemphigoid

Bullous pemphigoid is a chronic subepidermal blistering skin disease that may involve mucous membranes. Acantholysis is present in pemphigus but not in pemphigoid. Pemphigus and pemphigoid are both autoimmune diseases characterized by presence of antibodies directed against hemidesmosomal bullous pemphigoid antigens BP230 (BPAg1) and BP180 (BPAg2). IgG-autoantibodies bind to the skin basement membrane and cause blistering by separation of the dermis and epidermis. This may also affect the mucosa in the mouth and pharynx [24, 25].

The patient's mucosal abnormalities may cause odynophagia, i.e., painful swallowing. Secondary infection of the ruptured blisters may aggravate the pain. The infection of the blisters may then cause fibrosis and eventually stricture formation. Radiologic swallowing studies and/or endoscopy are often necessary in order to detect or rule out pharyngeal and esophageal involvement such as webs and strictures.

Patients with advanced disease can be treated with corticosteroids and immunosuppressive agents. Careful oral hygiene is important including prevention of secondary infections. In patients with oral mucous involvement, eating hard and crunchy foods such as chips, raw fruits, or vegetables may cause symptoms like odynophagia to flair. Localized disease in the oral cavity can be treated by topical steroids.

Epidermolysis Bullosa Dystrophica

Epidermolysis bullosa dystrophica (EBD) is an inherent disease affecting the skin and other organs including the mucosa of the oropharynx. EBD is an autoimmune disease caused by genetic defects within the human COL-7A-1 that encodes the production of collagen. The collagen VII forms a structural link between the epidermal basement membrane and the collagen fibrils in the upper dermis.

Mucosal abnormalities are due to sloughing of the mucosa resulting in ulcers that are painful and easily infected. The oral mucosa is mostly affected but laryngeal, esophageal, and conjunctival mucosa can also be involved. These blisters, erosions, and ulcers in the pharynx and esophagus may lead to scars, webs, and strictures. It has even been reported that such scarring can lead to esophageal shortening. This may promote development of hiatal hernia and gastroesophageal reflux disease [26]. Odynophagia is common. Topical corticosteroids are often used and endoscopic dilatation may be necessary if esophageal strictures develop.

Lichen Planus

Lichen planus is a chronic mucocutaneous disease in the form of papules, lesions or rashes involving the skin, mucous membranes, nails, and genitals. It has been suggested the lichen planus is an autoimmune disease that involves CD4+ and CD8+ T lymphocytes. In the esophageal epithelium, parakeratosis and atrophy are present. Strictures may form and in the proximal esophagus, and besides for their location, can be difficult to distinguish from those secondary to gastroesophageal reflux disease [27–30]. Other endoscopic findings include elevated lacy white papules, esophageal webs, erosions, and pseudomembranes. Although the entire esophagus may be involved, the disease is most frequent in the proximal and mid-esophagus. The lichenoid lesions may be painful, and can cause dysphagia and odynophagia from lesions in the oral cavity and esophagus. Spicy food may exacerbate pain.

Therapeutic options include systemic corticosteroids, cyclosporine, and azatioprin. Topical steroids can also be used. When strictures occur, endoscopic dilatation is beneficial.

Behçet Disease

Behçet disease is a vasculitis localized to the mucous membrane in the mouth and on the genitals. It may also include a systemic involvement of visceral organs, musculoskeletal apparatus, and central nervous system. There is a genetic predisposition in individuals who have the gene HLA-B51. The vasculitis causes recurrent oral and genital ulcers. Moreover, uveitis and erythema nodosum, folliculitis, thrombophlebitis and venous thrombosis, meningitis and central nervous system vasculitis, and arthritis may also be present [31–34].

The oral mucocutaneous ulcerations in the form of aphthoid ulcers may be very painful. The aphthoid ulcers can be found on the lips, tongue, and inside of the cheeks. They may occur as single lesions or in clusters. Ulcerations may also be found in the esophagus. Both the ulcers in the oral cavity and esophagus are painful and may evolve after slight trauma.

Treatment of the mucosal ulcers includes colchicine whilst more systemic disease is treated with steroids and immunomodulatory drugs. Oral hygiene is important to prevent secondary infection of the ulcers that per se are sterile. Acidic food should be avoided as it may cause pain.

Sarcoidosis

Sarcoidosis is a granulomatous disease characterized by non-caseating epithelioid granulomas. The lungs and mediastinum are the predominant locations, but may affect any organ. The etiology is unknown but an autoimmune predisposition has been suggested. There is an increased B-cell activity with hypergammaglobulinemia but also a reduced delayed-type hypersensitivity response in many patients with sarcoidosis. The non-caseating epithelial granulomas may also occur in the gastrointestinal tract.

The epitheloid granulomas may occur in the mucosa where they may cause superficial nodules and ulcerations that may be painful. When larger granulomas occur, these may result in irregular strictures and obstruction. An achalasia-like dysmotility secondary to esophageal sarcoidosis has also been reported [35]. Gingival sarcoidosis may be painful and cause odynophagia. Superficial nodules in the esophagus may also cause odynophagia. Irregular strictures in the esophagus may cause an obstruction for bolus transit.

The patient should undergo endoscopy or barium/iodine contrast radiologic evaluation. In patients with a feeling of obstructed swallowing, a solid bolus test should be included [36–38].

Oral corticosteroids are the treatment of choice. More advanced disease can be treated with immunomodulatory drugs and with the TNF-alpha blocker infliximab in severe refractory cases. Oral mucosal involvement can be treated with topical steroids. Esophageal strictures can either be treated with balloon dilatation or if not successful, with surgical resection.

Rheumatoid Arthritis

RA is an autoimmune disorder, characterized by a small joint synovitis resulting in swelling, pain, stiffness, and loss of function in joints. The synovitis may, if not sufficiently treated, eventually lead to permanent damage to cartilage, bones, and surrounding tissue. RA is an autoimmune disease. The predisposition is genetically inherited but is also triggered by environmental factors such as smoking and infections. The synovia is invaded by lymphocytes activated by cytokines such as TNF.

Dysphagia may be due to swelling of the synovial membrane in the cricothyroid and cricoarytenoid joints [39]. Subluxation of the atlantoaxial joint may lead to medullary compression of the odontoid process and cause brainstem symptoms. Moreover, subluxation of the atlantoaxial joint may cause altered biomechanics of the swallowing musculature. Abnormal temporomandibular joints may cause mastication problem. Anterior cervical spine pannus may cause compression of the cervical esophagus. Many patients with RA also have xerostomia. In patients with juvenile rheumatoid arthritis, dysphagia may be due to micrognathia [40, 41]. Dysphagia in RA has a multitude of presentations from dry mouth to delayed initiation of the pharyngeal stage of swallow. Painful swallowing may also be present [41–44]. Therefore the clinical evaluation including imaging should be done with a broad approach.

Modern treatment of RA includes early initiation of treatment with disease-modifying antirheumatic drugs (DMARD), where methotrexate is the most commonly used. It has been shown that early initiation of DMARDs improves the prognosis and stops or delays the joint destruction that otherwise is the consequence of the disease. In case of an inadequate response to the first-line DMARD, a combination of older DMARDs may be used or biological DMARDS where the TNF-alpha blockers are the most widely used. Corticosteroids and NSAIDs are mainly used to alleviate symptoms while waiting for DMARDs to start exerting their effects, which may take a couple of weeks after initiating treatment. In patients with xerostomia, increased water intake and artificial saliva can be utilized.

Systemic disease may cause dysphagia by several mechanisms, namely
- Xerostomia due to salivary gland impairment.
- Odynophagia due to mucosal blisters, ulcers, and other abnormalities of the tongue, gingiva, and cheeks.
- Mucosal and submucosal strictures in the esophagus and/or pharynx due to acute or chronic inflammation, particularly in patients with strictures of the esophagus, the major differential diagnosis is strictures caused by gastroesophageal reflux disease.
- Altered biomechanics of oral and pharyngeal musculature due to cervical spine abnormalities.
- Cortical and brain stem ischemia due to central nervous system vasculitis leading to neurological impairment.

References

1. Türk T, Pirildar T, Tunc E, Bor S, Doganavsargil E. Manometric assessment of esophageal motility in patients with primary Sjögren's syndrome. Rheumatol Int. 2005;25:246–9.
2. Kjellen G, Fransson SG, Lindström F, Sokjer H, Tibblin L. Esophageal function, radiography and dysphagia in Sjögren's syndrome. Dig Dis Sci. 1986;31:225–9.
3. Anselmino M, Zaninotto G, Constantini M, Ostuni P, Ianiello A, Boccu C, et al. Esophageal motor function in primary Sjögren's syndrome. Dig Dis Sci. 1997;42:113–8.
4. Rosztóczy A, Kovács L, Wittmann T, Lonovics J, Pokorny G. Manometric assessment of impaired esophageal motor function in primary Sjögren's syndrome. Clin Exp Rheumatol. 2001;19:147–52.
5. Tsianos EB, Vasakos S, Drosos AA, Malamou-Mitsi VD, Moutsopoulos HM. The gastrointestinal involvement in primary Sjögren's syndrome. Scand J Rheumatol. 1986;Suppl 61:151–5.
6. Hradsky M, Hybasek J, Cernoch V, Sazmova V, Juran J. Oesophageal abnormalities in Sjögren's syndrome. Scand J Gastroenterol. 1967;2:200–3.

7. Volter F, Fain O, Mathieu E, Thomas M. Esophageal function and Sjögren's syndrome. Dig Dis Sci. 2004;49:248–53.

8. Palma R, Freire J, Freitas J, Morbey A, Costa T, Saraiva F, et al. Esophageal motility disorders in patients with Sjögren's syndrome. Dig Dis Sci. 1994;38:758–61.

9. Tsianos EB, Chiras CD, Drosos AA, Moutsopoulos HM. Oesophageal dysfunction in patients with primary Sjögren's syndrome. Ann Rheum Dis. 1985;44:610–3.

10. Anselmino M, Zaninotto G, Costantini M, et al. Esophageal motor function in primary Sjögren's syndrome. Correlation with dysphagia and xerostomia. Dig Dis Sci. 1997;42:113–8.

11. Mandl T, Ekberg O, Wollmer P, Manthorpe R, Jacobsson LTH. Dysphagia and dysmotility of the pharynx and oesophagus in patients with primary Sjögren's syndrome. Scand J Rheumatol. 2007;36:394–401.

12. Liquidato BM, Bussoloti Filho I. Evaluation of sialometry and minor salivary gland biopsy in classification of Sjögren's syndrome patients. Rev Bras Otorrinolaringol. 2005;71(3):346–54. doi:10.1590/S0034-72992005000300014.

13. Thanou-Stavraki A, James JA. Primary Sjögren's syndrome: current and prospective therapies. Semin Arthritis Rheum. 2008;37:273–92.

14. Ramos-Casals M, Brito-Zerón P. Emerging biological therapies in primary Sjögren's syndrome. Rheumatology. 2007;46:1389–96.

15. Meijer JM, Meiners PM, Vissink A, Spijkervet FK, Abdulahad W, Kamminga N, Brouwer E, Kallenberg CG, Bootsma H. Effectiveness of rituximab treatment in primary Sjögren's syndrome: a randomized, double-blind, placebo-controlled trial. Arthritis Rheum. 2010;62:960–8.

16. Ntoumazios SK, Voulgari PV, Potsis K, Koutis E, Tsifetaki N, Assimakopoulos DA. Esophageal involvement in scleroderma: gastroesophageal reflux, the common problem. Semin Arthritis Rheum. 2006;36:173–81.

17. Rout PG, Hamburger J, Potts AJ. Orofacial radiological manifestations of systemic sclerosis. Dentomaxillofac Radiol. 1996;25:193–6.

18. Pizzo G, Scardina GA, Messina P. Effects of a nonsurgical exercise program on the decreased mouth opening in patients with systemic scleroderma. Clin Oral Investig. 2003;7:175–8.

19. Menditti D, Palomba F, Rullo R, Minervini G. Progressive systemic sclerosis (sclerodermal): oral manifestations. Arch Stomatol. 1990;31:537–48.

20. Prithviraj DR, Ramaswamy S, Romesh S. Prosthetic rehabilitation of patients with microstomia. Indian J Dent Res. 2009;20:483–6.

21. Virella G. Introduction. In: Virella G, editor. Introduction to medical immunology. 3rd ed. New York, NY: Dekker; 1993. p. 1–8.

22. Goust J, Tsokos G. Systemic lupus erythematosus. In: Virella G, editor. Introduction to medical immunology. 3rd ed. New York, NY: Dekker; 1993. p. 437–50.

23. Pope J. Other manifestations of mixed connective tissue disease. Rheum Dis Clin North Am. 2005;31:519–33.

24. Yeh SW, Ahmed B, Sami N, Ahmed AR. Blistering disorders: diagnosis and treatment. Dermatol Ther. 2003;16:214–23.

25. International Pemphigus & Pemphigoid Foundation. What is pemphigus? http://www.pemphigus.org/index.php?option=com_content&view=article&id=364&Itemid=100073/.

26. Agah FP, Francis IR, Ellis CN. Esophageal involvement in epidermolysis bullosa dystrophica: clinical and roentgenographic manifestation. Gastrointest Radiol. 1983;8:111–7.

27. Chandan VS, Murray JA, Abraham SC. Esophageal lichen planus. Arch Pathol Lab Med. 2008;132:1026–9.

28. Madhusudhan KS, Sharma R. Esophageal lichen planus: a case report and review of literature. Ind J Dermatol. 2008;53:26–7.

29. Sugerman PB, Porter SR. Oral lichen planus. http://www.emedicine.medscape.com/article/1078327-overview.

30. Katzka DA, Smyrk TC, Bruce AJ, Romero Y, Alexander JA, Murray JA. Variations in presentations of esophageal involvement in lichen planus. Clin Gastroenterol Hepatol. 2010;8:777–82.

31. Brookes GB. Pharyngeal stenosis in Behcet's syndrome. The first reported case. Arch Otolaryngol. 1983;109:338–40.

32. Levack B, Hanson D. Behcet's disease of the esophagus. J Laryngol Otol. 1979;93:99–101.

33. Demetriades N, Hanford H, Laskarides C. General manifestations of Behcet's syndrome and the success of CO_2-laser as treatment for oral lesions: a review of the literature and case presentation. J Mass Dent Soc. 2009;58:24–7.

34. Messadi DV, Younai F. Aphthous ulcers. Dermatol Ther. 2010;23:281–90.

35. Bredenoord AJ, Jafari J, Kadri S, et al. Achalasia-like dysmotility secondary to oesophageal involvement of sarcoidosis. Gut. 2011;60(2):153–5. doi:10.1136/gut.2010.227868.

36. Levine MS, Ekberg O, Rubesin SE, Gatenby RA. Gastrointestinal sarcoidosis: radiographic findings. AJR Am J Roentgenol. 1989;153:293–5.

37. Hardy WE, Tulgan H, Haidak G, Budnitz J. Sarcoidosis: a case presenting with dysphagia and dysphonia. Ann Intern Med. 1967;66:353–7.

38. Cook DM, Dines DE, Dycus DS. Sarcoidosis: report of a case presenting as dysphagia. Chest. 1970;57:84–6.

39. Chen JJ, Branstetter IV BF, Myers EN. Cricoarytenoid rheumatoid arthritis: an important consideration in aggressive lesions of the larynx. AJNR Am J Neuroradiol. 2005;26:970–2.

40. Lindqvist C, Santavirta S, Sandelin J, Konttinen Y. Dysphagia and micrognathia in a patient with juvenile rheumatoid arthritis. Clin Rheumatol. 1986;5:410–5.

41. Ekberg O, Redlund-Johnell I, Sjöblom KG. Pharyngeal function in patients with rheumatoid arthritis of the cervical spine and temporomandibular joint. Acta Radiol. 1987;28:35–9.

42. Geterud A, Bake B, Bjelle A, Jonsson R, Sandberg N, Ejnell H. Swallowing problems in the rheumatoid arthritis. Acta Otolaryngol. 1991;111:1153–61.

43. Erb N, Pace V, Delamere JP, Kitas GD. Dysphagia and stridor caused by laryngeal rheumatoid arthritis. Rheumatology. 2001;40:952–3.

44. Sun DCH, Roth SH, Mitchell CS, Englund DW. Upper gasatrointestinal disease in rheumatoid arthritis. Dig Dis. 1974;19:405–10.

Part IX

Upper Esophageal Sphincter Opening Dysfunction

Zenker's Diverticulum

Ian J. Cook

Abstract

There is now strong evidence that acquired Zenker's diverticulum arises in most cases secondary to a poorly compliant, but normally relaxing, UES which cannot fully distend during the process of sphincter opening. This gives rise to increased hypopharyngeal intrabolus pressure during the phase of *trans*-sphincteric bolus flow; pressure which is imparted to the area of relative muscular weakness (Killian's dehiscence) just proximal to the cricopharyngeus. This combination of factors gives rise to posterior herniation of the pouch over many years. The restricted opening of the cricopharyngeus is a result of muscle fibre degeneration and fibroadipose tissue replacement. For this reason, cricopharyngeal myotomy is the essential component for successful surgical treatment of the condition. The precise aetiology of this myopathic process affecting the cricopharyngeus is unknown and may be multifactorial. However, an underlying myositis with a predilection for the cricopharyngeus muscle is likely to be one such factor in some cases.

Keywords

Zenker's diverticulum • Bilobed pharyngeal pouches • Bilobed with one opening • Pouches with separate necks • Bilobed pouch • Laryngocoele • Upper oesophageal sphincter (UES) • Dysphagia • Swallowing • Pathophysiology

I.J. Cook, MBBS, MD(Syd), FRACP(✉)
Director Neurogastroenterology and Motility Service and Swallow Centre, Department of Gastroenterology and Hepatology, St George Hospital, Sydney, Australia

Professor of Medicince, Faculty of Medicine, University of New South Wales, Sydney, Australia
e-mail: i.cook@unsw.edu.au

Introduction and Historical Perspective

The first reported case of a posterior pharyngeal diverticulum was published by Ludlow [1]. He reported the case of a 65-year-old man with emaciation and progressive dysphagia resulting in his demise 13 days after presentation; arguably hastened by attempted therapies which included blind dilatations with a whale bone and swallowing a "great quantity of quicksilver". It was not until a century later that a systematic anatomical description of the entity was published by Zenker and von Zeimsen in 1878 [2]. They reviewed 22 cases from the literature, all confirmed by autopsy and an additional five of their own cases (Fig. 35.1). They elegantly showed that the sac constitutes a herniation of mucosa and submucosa posteriorly between the inferior constrictor and cricopharyngeus muscles at a point of the pharynx that "...*has lost the support of the muscular fibres which usually sustain it, in consequence of some local influence upon the same*" and that there are no muscle fibres on the diverticulum itself. The focal region of relative lack of muscular support was subsequently termed Killian's dehiscence; the roughly triangular region bounded by the inferior fibres of the inferior constrictor and the superior fibres of the cricopharyngeus [3].

Definition and Anatomical Considerations

Pharyngeal diverticula are most conveniently classified according to their anatomical site. Broadly speaking, these anatomical structures can be lateral or posterior and they can lie above (pharyngeal) or below the cricopharyngeus (cervical oesophageal). The lateral pharyngeal diverticula are quite distinct entities from the posterior (Zenker's) diverticulum.

The typical Zenker's diverticulum herniates posteriorly just proximal to the cricopharyngeus (Fig. 35.2). Although it protrudes posteriorly, as it grows in size it may track to one side or the

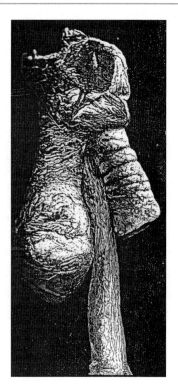

Fig. 35.1 Preserved autopsy specimen of a large diverticulum from the first case series described by Zenker and von Zeimsen [2]. This specimen currently resides in the Museum of Pathological Anatomy, Erlangen. (The autopsy specimen of the very first case described by Ludlow still exists in the pathological collection of the Royal Infirmary, Glasgow)

other but tends to be left sided in the majority. The reason for this is unclear but an anatomical consideration that may explain it in part is the greater potential space between the concavity of the cervical oesophagus and the left carotid artery compared with the right [4]. While the pouch generally has a single opening into the hypopharynx, a number of anatomical variations have been reported including three different types of bilobed pharyngeal pouches: bilobed with one opening [5]; two separate pouches with separate necks [6] and a bilobed pouch separated by a septum with two necks [7] (Fig. 35.3).

Histopathological studies confirm the original descriptions of Zenker and von Ziemsen that the pouch itself is lined by stratified squamous epithelial mucosa and submucosa which is often surrounded by fibrous tissue [8]. Muscle fibres

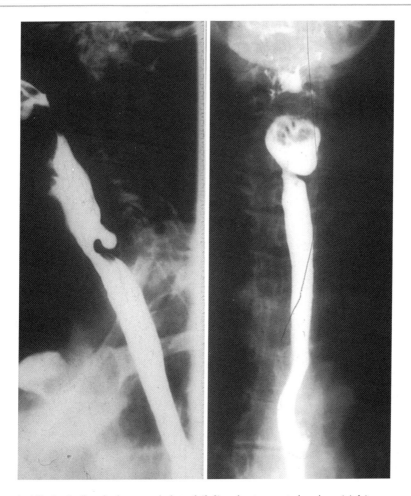

Fig. 35.2 A typical Zenker's diverticulum seen in lateral (*left*) and anteroposterior views (*right*)

are notably absent except in some cases in the region of the neck of the diverticulum. Rarely, a squamous carcinoma or carcinoma *in situ* is found (see below).

Proximal, lateral pharyngeal diverticula are frequently bilateral, are more common in the elderly and occur at the level of the vallecula in an area of relative weakness through the thyrohyoid membrane at a site that is relatively poorly supported by cartilage or muscle (Fig. 35.4). Lateral diverticula may be a congenital pharyngocele or, more commonly, acquired pulsion diverticula. Congenital lateral pouches are true branchial cleft cysts representing an embryological remnant of the third pharyngeal pouch corresponding to the thyrohyoid membrane [9]. The area of relative weakness is bounded by the hyoid bone superiorly, at a site where there is incomplete overlap of the thyrohyoid muscle anteriorly and the inferior constrictor muscle inferiorly [10]. At this site the thyrohyoid membrane is also perforated by the superior laryngeal artery, and the internal laryngeal branch of the superior laryngeal nerve. Lateral pharyngeal diverticula rarely cause symptoms and they are a common incidental finding [10, 11]. However, there are sporadic case reports of successful alleviation of dysphagia following surgical ligation or removal of a lateral pharyngeal diverticulum [12, 13].

Occasionally lateral diverticula can originate just below the cricopharyngeus and herniate through an area of relative weakness lateral to the point of insertion of the longitudinal muscle of the oesophagus

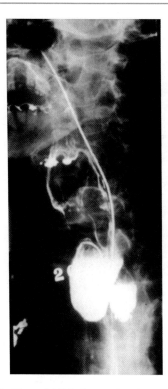

Fig. 35.3 Unusual bilobed posterior pharyngeal pouch seen in an oblique view with single neck arising proximal to the cricopharyngeus

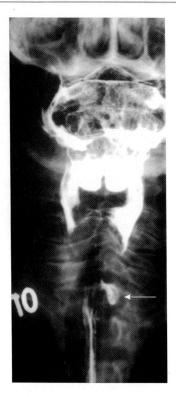

Fig. 35.5 Lateral cervical (Killian–Jamieson) diverticulum. This pouch protrudes laterally and below the cricopharyngeus (see text)—not to be confused with a posterior (Zenker's) diverticulum

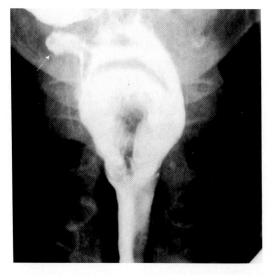

Fig. 35.4 Lateral pharyngeal pouch seen in the proximal pharynx—a distinct entity not to be confused with a posterior (Zenker's) diverticulum

onto the cricoid cartilage [14]. These proximal lateral cervical pouches are sometimes termed Killian–Jamieson diverticula and may be confused with a true Zenker's because of their close proximity to the cricopharyngeus (Fig. 35.5). However, they generally extend anterior to the cervical oesophagus as it enlarges while a Zenker's will not. Killian–Jamieson diverticula are much less common than Zenker's and are also less likely to cause symptoms with one study attributing symptoms to this diverticulum in 19 % of patients studied [15].

Epidemiology

A community study in the UK reported an annual incidence of 2 per 100,000 people per year [16]. However, the true prevalence is unknown and may be higher than this as many have minimal or no symptoms. For example,

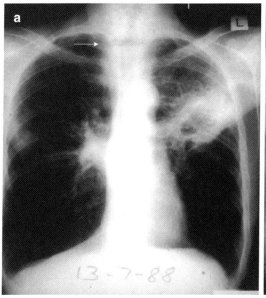 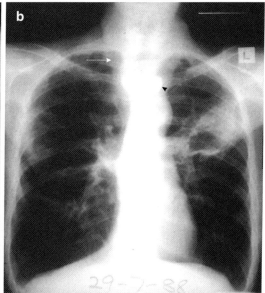

Fig. 35.6 CXR of patient presenting with "vomiting", unexplained recurrent bouts of pneumonia and weight loss. (**a**) A plain CXR demonstrates pneumonic changes and a fluid level can be seen within the upper mediastinum (*white arrow*). (**b**) After swallowing barium, the inferior margin of the diverticulum is more clearly outlined (*black arrow head*)

several radiological studies report 0.1–2 % incidence in otherwise asymptomatic individuals [17, 18]. Zenker's diverticulum is more common in males than females by a factor of 3:1 [19]. The condition is very uncommon under the age of 40; extremely rare under the age of 30 and is generally confined to the geriatric population with a median age of presentation in the seventh to eighth decades in various studies [20, 21]. However, congenital pharyngeal pouches have been reported, some with a family history, suggesting that a congenitally enlarged or weakened Killian's triangle may be a factor in some [22–24]. There are few reports of racial differences but it appears to be more common in Europeans than Asians, possibly related to differences in neck length and it is more common in Northern than Southern Europe [25].

Clinical Features

Presenting symptoms include dysphagia combined with varying degrees of regurgitation depending on the size of the pouch. Regurgitation of undigested food is very common (80 %) [19]. While this is more frequent immediately after the meal, patients will often describe regurgitation of food ingested many hours earlier or at night. Aspiration symptoms, such as deglutitive cough, as well as chronic cough, recurrent chest infections and weight loss are common features. Occasionally recurrent pneumonia and weight loss may be the predominant presenting feature particularly if the pouch is large (Fig. 35.6). Audible gurgling during the swallow may be present. Halitosis, due to stasis in the pouch, can be a feature. The duration of symptoms prior to presentation varies from weeks to many years. There is little published data on the natural history of this entity but the available evidence suggest that the diverticulum develops over many years with little or minor demonstrable change in pouch size over 8 years in one small, longitudinal radiological study [26]. However, even in the context of a known long-standing pouch, rapid escalation of symptoms can be a feature even without appreciable change in pouch size (Cook unpublished). The reason for the apparent increase in symptoms is not known. However, based on our current understanding of the biomechanics of the pharynx and sphincter in this condition, a likely explanation for this observation might be that a critical level of cricopharyngeal fibrosis and stenosis is reached.

Physical examination is usually non-contributory although rarely, a palpable lump in the neck which gurgles on palpation may be evident. Features that might suggest possible malignant change include rapid symptom progression, or bleeding. Pain is rarely reported but its presence is highly suggestive of malignant change [27].

Complications

Squamous carcinoma complicating a pouch is rare but is well described with an incidence possibly between 0.4 and 1.5 % [27, 28]. Analogous with achalasia of the cardia, chronic stasis is believed to underpin the malignant change.

Haemorrhage from the pouch is rare. Benign ulceration of the mucosa within the pouch can occur and this can result in significant bleeding. Ulceration is potentially related to acid reflux [29], aspirin-induced mucosal ulceration [30], or carcinoma [27].

Bezoar formation in the diverticulum has been reported in large pouches [31]. Fistula formation, either spontaneous between pouch and trachea or unintentional, secondary to instrumentation has been reported [31].

Diagnosis

The most useful diagnostic test is a barium swallow, which usually readily demonstrates the diverticulum. The radiographic study should also carefully examine the oesophagus to identify coexistent pathology that might account for or contribute to the patient's dysphagia and regurgitation. For example, a large hiatal hernia or oesophageal achalasia is an alternative cause of regurgitation and dysphagia. If a diverticulum is known or suspected, a dynamic videoradiographic swallow study is preferable to standard static films for a number of reasons. Very small diverticula (as well as subtle cervical webs) are sometimes only seen transiently during deglutition and are best detected on dynamic studies replayed in slow motion. The timing and extent of aspiration, usually immediately post-swallow in a pure Zenker's, is better appreciated in a dynamic study. Finally, if there is concomitant neuromyogenic pharyngeal dysfunction (e.g. myopathy) the only way to detect this with certainty is with a videofluoroscopic study (Fig. 35.7) [32]. Concurrent neuromuscular dysfunction, if present, is important to detect as it has diagnostic and prognostic implications (see below). If there is any doubt about the possible coexistence of a neuromuscular disorder (e.g. myositis), in addition to a careful neurological examination, preliminary testing should include a plasma CPK level [32–34].

Endoscopic techniques have limited diagnostic capability as the opening of the pouch is not always apparent endoscopically. If a constant filling defect is seen radiographically, then pharyngoscopy may be useful in ruling out a complicating carcinoma. However, examination by nasolaryngoscopy [flexible endoscopic evaluation of swallowing (FEES)] frequently does not detect a diverticulum. FEES will often demonstrate regurgitation from the pouch but if a pouch is suspected, barium radiography is still indicated. In deciding upon the mode of therapy, it is important to estimate the size (predominantly depth) of the pouch which can be "sized" in cms or relative to vertebral width [35]. For example, transoral diverticulostomy may not be feasible if the pouch is not sufficiently deep to accommodate the tip of the instrument (refer Chap. 59).

Pathogenesis and Pathophysiology

Zenker and von Ziemssen in 1878 hypothesised that the pouch arises primarily due to relative lack of muscular support in the region immediately proximal to the cricopharyngeus [2]. This roughly triangular section of the posterior pharyngeal wall was well described by Killian (and subsequently termed "Killian's dehiscence") to

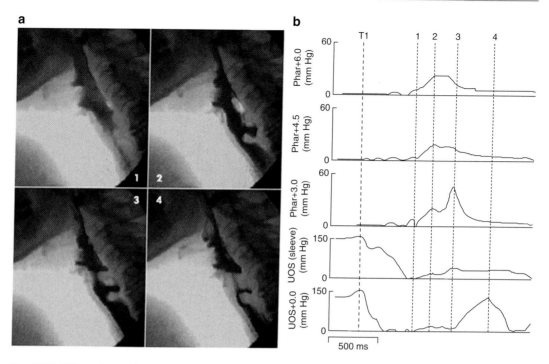

Fig. 35.7 Videoradiographic sequence (**a**) and corresponding pharyngeal manometry (**b**) in a patient presenting with dysphagia, aspiration and who was found to have polymyositis and an early Zenker's diverticulum. Each *vertical dashed line* in (**b**) represents the time corresponding to the numbered radiographic frames in (**a**). While the sphincter relaxes completely (**b**) it has markedly restricted opening as evident by the prominent cricopharyngeal bar (**a**). Note the weak pharyngeal stripping wave, incomplete contact of tongue base with pharyngeal wall and resulting poor pharyngeal clearance. Hypopharyngeal intrabolus pressure (frame 2, channel 3) is increased due to the restricted opening of the upper oesophageal sphincter (UES). From R.B. Williams et al. Gut 2003;52:471–8 with permission (Fig. 3, page 474)

be bounded by the oblique fibres of the inferior constrictor muscle above and the transverse fibres of the cricopharyngeus below [36]. Zenker believed that if the region were to sustain an insult that might render it even weaker, the likelihood of herniation would be greater. Zenker went on to say, somewhat perspicaciously, that *"if there is already a stenosis of the upper end of the esophagus before the occurrence of any of these causes, it may be readily understood that this would favour the formation of a diverticulum, for not only would a foreign body in this case be more easily detained in the canal, but also, in consequence of the stasis of food caused by the stenosis, the pressure on the weak spot must be increased"* [2]. Over the next century following that statement, there has been much debate about the pathogenesis of the diverticulum. Furthermore, while Zenker and those following postulated that

elevated hypopharyngeal pressures might have pathogenic significance, this phenomenon was not demonstrated until 114 years later [20].

Numerous hypotheses have been put forward that might account for the proposed increased hypopharyngeal pressure. Initially it was believed that upper oesophageal sphincter (UES) incoordination, specifically premature sphincter closure, in some cases combined with early UES relaxation, would cause elevated hypopharyngeal pressure [37–39]. The validity of those early observations is questionable. The radiographic studies were semi-quantitative. In the manometric studies, the UES relaxation profiles were recorded by a discrete perfused side-hole positioned within the sphincter without appreciation of the deglutitive axial mobility of the UES, which is known to profoundly influence temporal swallowing measures [40–42]. Other theories proposed included resting

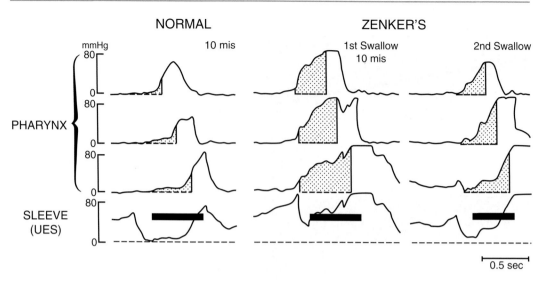

Fig. 35.8 Intraluminal manometric traces in a patient with Zenker's diverticulum (two *right* panels) showing much higher intrabolus pressure waves (*stippled*) than those seen in the healthy aged control subject (*left* panel). Note that when the patient swallowed the second time to clear residual bolus from the pharynx, this lower volume bolus was associated with a lower (but still abnormal) intrabolus pressure and a shorter interval of trans-sphincteric bolus flow (*black bar*). From I.J. Cook et al. Gastroenterology 1992;103:1229–35 with permission (Fig. 3, page 1,232)

UES hypertonia [43], failure of UES relaxation [44], and a second swallow against a closed sphincter [38, 45]. There has been no consistent demonstration of any of these phenomena and a number of early manometric studies reported normal UES tone, deglutitive relaxation and coordination [46, 47]. Indeed a number of subsequent manometric studies, accounting for sphincter radial asymmetry and axial mobility, reported normal or low basal UES tone, normal UES relaxation, and normal pharyngo-sphincteric coordination during the swallow [20, 48].

A combined videoradiographic and manometric study in which 14 patients were compared with nine age-matched healthy controls demonstrated that the maximal opening of the UES, in both sagittal and transverse planes, is significantly restricted in patients with Zenker's diverticulum [20]. That study also demonstrated conclusively a markedly increased hypopharyngeal intrabolus pressure during the phase of trans-sphincteric bolus flow and that this elevated pressure domain is in continuity with the neck of the diverticulum (Figs. 35.8 and 35.9). That study also demonstrated normal resting UES tone and complete sphincter relaxation during the swallow.

Additionally, they found no sphincter incoordination between pharyngeal contraction and sphincter relaxation and opening. These findings confirm that the underlying disorder is one of loss of muscle compliance of the UES but that the innervation and central control of the constrictors and cricopharyngeus muscle is normal as evidenced by complete and normally coordinated deglutitive sphincter relaxation.

Further confirmatory evidence for the primary defect being a loss of UES compliance came from histopathological and *in vitro* muscle studies. In a prospective histopathological study, cricopharyngeus and inferior constrictor muscle specimens obtained at the time of cricopharyngeal myotomy from patients with Zenker's were compared with control tissue obtained at autopsy from non-dysphagic individuals [49]. When compared with controls, the cricopharyngeus muscle from Zenker's patients demonstrated marked fibroadipose tissue replacement, muscle fibre degeneration, and segmental necrosis with macrophage myophagia (Fig. 35.10). Two of 14 specimens demonstrated additional inflammatory changes. Although healthy cricopharyngeus muscle has markedly different morphological

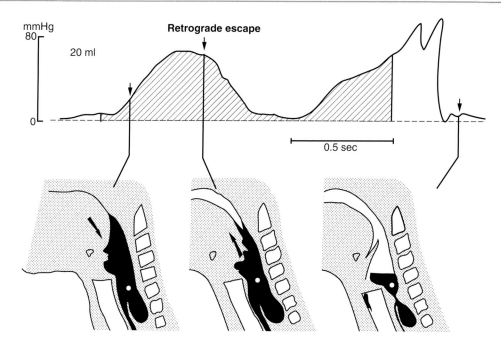

Fig. 35.9 Correlation of manometry (*top*) and radiographic tracings (*bottom*) from the same patient as previous figure during a larger (20 mL) barium bolus swallow. Note the extremely high intrabolus pressure (*left*) in continuity with the open sphincter and the neck of the pouch (*white dot* represents pressure recording site). Indeed, the intrabolus pressure in this case exceeds the peak pha- ryngeal contractile pressure which results in peristaltic "failure" and retrograde escape of the bolus (*centre* panel). The patient swallowed a second time shortly thereafter (*right* panel) and cleared most of the residual bolus but not before a small amount of aspiration occurred. From I.J. Cook et al. Gastroenterology 1992;103:1229–35 with permission (Fig. 4, page 1,233)

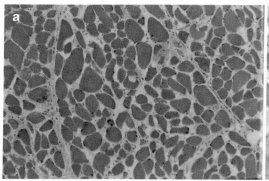
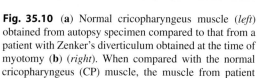
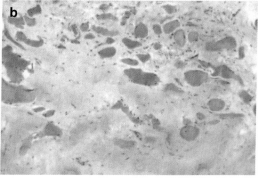

Fig. 35.10 (**a**) Normal cricopharyngeus muscle (*left*) obtained from autopsy specimen compared to that from a patient with Zenker's diverticulum obtained at the time of myotomy (**b**) (*right*). When compared with the normal cricopharyngeus (CP) muscle, the muscle from patient with Zenker's demonstrates muscle fibre dropout (due to necrosis, as evidenced by scattered degenerative fibres); greater fibre size variability and a markedly increased fibroadipose tissue replacement. (H & E×200)

and histological appearances to limb skeletal muscle [49, 50], the degenerative and fibrotic changes identified in the muscle from Zenker's patients, if present in a limb muscle, would be consistent with a primary myopathic process and accounts for the previously demonstrated loss of compliance of the UES in these patients. Lerut et al. also showed abnormal contractile properties

BEFORE SURGERY   AFTER SURGERY

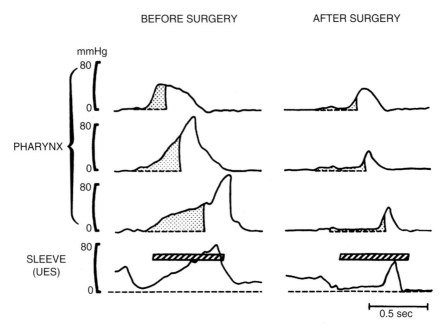

Fig. 35.11 Pharyngeal manometric tracings from a patient with Zenker's diverticulum before and after cricopharyngeal myotomy. The stippled segment of the pres- sure trace represents the hypopharyngeal intrabolus pressure domain which is very prominent preoperatively and which normalises after myotomy

in isolated cricopharyngeal muscle from patients with Zenker's in that stimulated isolated cricopharyngeus muscle strips *in vitro* demonstrated diminished time to peak twitch, reduced contractile velocity and lower amplitude contractions when compared with control tissue [51]. These alterations in biomechanical properties would also be consistent with the observed muscle fibre drop out and fibrosis.

Further evidence that poor cricopharyngeal compliance underpins Zenker's diverticulum and accounts for the observed increase in deglutitive intrabolus pressure comes from systematic examination of the biomechanical properties of the pharyngo-oesophageal junction before and after cricopharyngeal myotomy. Cricopharyngeal myotomy, effectively a curative surgical procedure, normalises both the extent of UES opening and hypopharyngeal intrabolus pressure in these patients (Fig. 35.11) [52]. In that study, the relationship between maximal UES calibre and hypopharyngeal intrabolus pressure only approximated that of healthy aged controls following the surgery consistent with normalisation of UES compliance

by myotomy (Fig. 35.12). That study also demonstrated that an adequate myotomy is the essential component of treatment, irrespective of what is done with the pouch itself. Unless the intrabolus pressure is normalised by myotomy, the clinical result may be suboptimal (Fig. 35.13).

Aetiology

A wide range of conditions have been reported in association with Zenker's [31]. Some of these may be chance associations and for most, supportive evidence for a causative link is lacking or minimal. Laryngocoele, benign tumours of pharynx or oesophagus have been reported rarely. Myositis has been reported and systematically studied (see below). There are several case reports of a pouch developing after anterior cervical spine fusion [53, 54]. Presumably this relates in part to a degree of adhesive fixation of the posterior pharyngeal wall to the cervical prevertebral fascia inducing a traction component to the region. The long-standing associations among

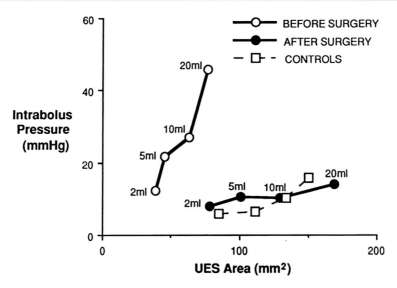

Fig. 35.12 Plot of relationship between upper oesophageal sphincter (UES) opening and hypopharyngeal intrabolus pressure before and after surgery. Note that the preoperative compliance curve is shifted to the left and is steeper—indicative of poor sphincter compliance. Following surgery, the location and gradient of the curve is indicative of normalisation of sphincter compliance following myotomy

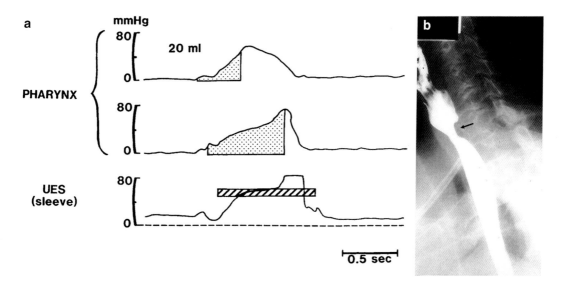

Fig. 35.13 Postoperative manometric tracing (**a**) and barium radiograph (**b**) in a patient who underwent diverticulectomy but in whom dysphagia was only partially relieved. Note the persistent post-cricopharyngeal restriction (*arrow*) indicating that the myotomy was incomplete. Note the manometric tracing showing persistently elevated intrabolus pressure (*stippled*) indicating persistently poor sphincter compliance

hiatal hernia, reflux and pharyngeal pouch, as well as the significance of it, remain unresolved.

Although inflammatory changes were found in only 14 % of myotomy specimens in those undergoing surgery [49], these samples are likely to represent a late stage in the condition in which fibrosis predominates. The cricopharyngeus would appear to be quite sensitive to inflammation as evidenced by the loss of UES compliance in patients presenting with dysphagia in whom myositis was subsequently found to be the cause [32]. The mean time from symptom onset to diagnosis of inflammatory myopathy in that study was 55 months. Of even greater potential relevance in that retrospective case–control study was that 69 % of myositis cases had a restrictive disorder of the cricopharyngeus (bar or circumferential stenosis) and 24 % of all patients had Zenker's diverticulum; a significantly greater proportion than was seen in controls (6 %) with a neurogenic pharyngeal dysphagia [32]. There is an additional case report of a Zenker's associated with polymyositis [55]. However, a number of case reports in patients coming to myotomy for dysphagia suggest that myositis can be very focal, apparently confined to the cricopharyngeus and can cause stenosis of the sphincter [56–58].

There are a number of reports of an apparent increased association with hiatal hernia, including one case–control study [59, 60]. A number of studies report an association with reflux disease [43, 60–63]. Reflux and hiatal hernias are very common conditions; the latter particularly in the geriatric population in which pharyngeal pouches are most prevalent. Hence, a chance association among these conditions will be common. The mechanisms potentially responsible for such a putative link are speculative and, as yet, lack proof. One notion is that the hiatal hernia alone or reflux *per se* increases resting tone within the UES. While abrupt pressurisation of the oesophagus during spontaneous reflux events generally triggers reflexive UES relaxation, some reflux events can induce increased basal UES tone [64, 65]. However, these events do not impair deglutitive UES relaxation—the critical time domain during which the swallow-related increased intraluminal pressure is acting on the posterior pharyngeal wall [65]. Others have postulated that oesophageal shortening, as a consequence of reflux events and/or in association with hiatus hernia formation, put differential axial traction on the relatively untethered cricopharyngeus compared with the inferior constrictors [63]. They postulate that this differential axial mobility, due to the better anchoring of the inferior constrictors through its median raphe, would tend to open up the region of Killian's triangle. In the absence of more plausible pathogenetic mechanisms and until objective demonstration of such mechanisms is found, the potential causative link with GERD must remain highly speculative [66].

Summary

There is now strong evidence that acquired Zenker's diverticulum arises in most cases secondary to a poorly compliant, but normally relaxing, UES which cannot fully distend during the process of sphincter opening. This gives rise to increased hypopharyngeal intrabolus pressure during the phase of *trans*-sphincteric bolus flow; pressure which is imparted to the area of relative muscular weakness (Killian's dehiscence) just proximal to the cricopharyngeus. This combination of factors gives rise to posterior herniation of the pouch over many years. The restricted opening of the cricopharyngeus is a result of muscle fibre degeneration and fibroadipose tissue replacement. For this reason, cricopharyngeal myotomy is the essential component for successful surgical treatment of the condition. The precise aetiology of this myopathic process affecting the cricopharyngeus is unknown and may be multifactorial. However, an underlying myositis with a predilection for the cricopharyngeus muscle is likely to be one such factor in some cases.

References

1. Ludlow A. A case of obstructed deglutition from a preternatural dilatation of and bag formed in the pharynx. Med Observ Inq. 1764;3:85–101.
2. Zenker FA, von Ziemssen H. Dilatations of the esophagus. In: Cyclopaedia of the practice of medicine. London: Low, Marston, Searle and Rivington; 1878. p. 46–68.
3. Killian G. The mouth of the oesophagus. Laryngoscope. 1907;17:421–8.
4. Westrin KM, Ergun S, Carlsoo B. Zenker's diverticulum—a historical review and trends in therapy. Acta Otolaryngol. 1996;116:351–60.
5. Izzat AB, Dezso A, Hardingham M. Bilobed pharyngeal pouch: a very rare finding. J Laryngol Otol. 2000;114:802–4.

6. Stafford N, Frootko N. Doubel pharyngeal pouch. Ann Otol Rhinol Laryngol. 1987;96:127.

7. Meehan T, Henein R. An unusual pharyngeal pouch. J Laryngol Otol. 1992;106:1002–3.

8. Fenoglio-Preiser CM, Noffsinger AE, Stemmermann GN, Lantz PE, Listrom MB, Rilke FO. Gastrointestinal pathology. An atlas and text. 2nd ed. Philadelphia, PA: Lippincott Williams and Wilkins; 1999.

9. Bachman AL, Seaman WB, Macken KL. Lateral pharyngeal diverticula. Radiology. 1968;91:774–82.

10. Liston SL. Lateral pharyngeal diverticula. Otolaryngol Head Neck Surg. 1985;93:582–5.

11. Curtis DJ, Cruess DF, Crain M, Sivit C, Winters C, Dachman AH. Lateral pharyngeal outpouchings: a comparison of dysphagic and asymptomatic patients. Dysphagia. 1988;2:156–61.

12. Mantoni M, Ostri B. Acquired lateral pharyngeal diverticulum. J Laryngol Otol. 1987;101:1092–4.

13. Pace-Balzan A, Habashi SMZ, Nassar WY. View from within: radiology in focus lateral pharyngeal diverticulum. J Laryngol Otol. 1991;105:793–5.

14. Ekberg O, Nylander G. Lateral diverticula from the pharyngoesophageal junction area. Radiology. 1983;146:117.

15. Rubesin SE, Levine MS. Killian–Jamieson diverticula: radiographic findings in 16 patients. AJR Am J Roentgenol. 2001;177:85–9.

16. Laing MR, Murthy P, Ah-See KW, et al. Surgery for pharyngeal pouch: audit of management with short and long term follow up. J R Coll Surg Edinb. 1995;40:315–8.

17. Holmgren BS. Inkonstante hypopharynx-divertikel. Eine roentgenologische Untersuchung. Acta Radiol. 1946;61:129–36.

18. Wheeler D. Diverticula of the fore-gut. Radiology. 1947;49:476–81.

19. Jamieson GG, Duranceau AC, Payne WS. Pharyngo-oesophageal diverticulum. In: Jamieson GG, editor. Surgery of the oesophagus. Edinburgh: Churchill Livingstone Press; 1988. p. 435–43.

20. Cook IJ, Gabb M, Panagopoulos V, Jamieson GG, Dodds WJ, Dent J, et al. Pharyngeal (Zenker's) diverticulum is a disorder of upper esophageal sphincter opening. Gastroenterology. 1992;103:1229–35.

21. Maran AG, Wilson JA, Muhanna AH. Pharyngeal diverticula. Clin Otolaryngol. 1986;11:219–25.

22. Britnall ES, Kridelbaugh WW. Congenital diverticulum of the posterior phyopharynx simulating atresia of the oesophagus. Ann Surg. 1950;131:564–74.

23. Groves LK. Pharyngoesophageal diverticulum in each of three sisters. Report of cases. Cleve Clin Q. 1978;35:207–14.

24. Nelson AR. Congenital true osophageal diverticulum of the posterior hypopharynx: report of a case unassociated with other oesophagotrachal abnormality. Ann Surg. 1957;145:258–64.

25. van Overbeek JJ. Pathogenesis and methods of treatment of Zenker's diverticulum. Ann Otol Rhinol Laryngol. 2003;112:583–93.

26. Einharssen S. On the treatment of esophageal diverticula. Acta Otolaryngol (Stockholm). 1967;64:30–6.

27. Bowdler DA, Stell PM. Carcinoma arising in posterior pharyngeal pulsion diverticulum (Zenker's diverticulum). Br J Surg. 1987;74:561–3.

28. Bradley PJ, Kochaar A, Quraishi MS. Pharyngeal pouch carcinoma: real of imaginary risks? Ann Otol Rhinol Laryngol. 1999;108:1027–32.

29. Shirazi KK, Daffner RH, Gaede JT. Ulcer occurring in Zenker's diverticulum. Gastrointest Radiol.77;25:117–8.

30. Vaghei R, Harrison I, Ortiz RA. Massive bleeding from the pharyngoesophageal diverticulum. Am Surg. 1976;42:917–9.

31. Sen P, Kumar G, Bhattacharyya AK. Pharyngeal pouch: associations and complications. Eur Arch Otorhinolaryngol. 2006;263:463–8.

32. Williams RB, Grehan MJ, Hersch M, Andre J, Cook IJ. Biomechanics, diagnosis, and treatment outcome in inflammatory myopathy presenting as oropharyngeal dysphagia. Gut. 2003;52:471–8.

33. Cook IJ, Kahrilas PJ. Medical position statement on management of oropharyngeal dysphagia. Gastroenterology. 1999;116:452–4.

34. Cook IJ, Kahrilas PJ. AGA technical review on management of oropharyngeal dysphagia. Gastroenterology. 1999;116(2):455–78.

35. van Overbeek JJ, Groote AD. Zenker's diverticulum. Curr Opin Otolaryngol Head Neck Surg. 1994;2: 55–8.

36. Killian G. Uber den mund der speiserohre. Zschr Ohrenheilk. 1908;55:1.

37. Ardran GM, Kemp FH, Lund WS. The aetiology of the posterior pharyngeal diverticulum: a cineradiographic study. J Laryngol Otol. 1964;78:333–49.

38. Lichter I. Motor disorder in pharyngoesophageal pouch. J Thorac Cardiovasc Surg. 1978;76:272–5.

39. Ellis FH, Schlegal JF, Lynch VP, Payne WS. Cricopharyngeal myotomy for pharyngoesophageal diverticulum. Ann Surg. 1969;170:340–9.

40. Isberg A, Nilsson ME, Schiratzki H. Movement of the upper esophgeal sphincter and a manometric device during deglutition, a cineradiographic investigation. Acta Radiol Diagn. 1985;26:381–8.

41. Cook IJ, Dodds WJ, Dantas RO, Kern MK, Massey BT, Shaker R, et al. Timing of videofluoroscopic, manometric events, and bolus transit during the oral and pharyngeal phases of swallowing. Dysphagia. 1989;4:8–15.

42. Cook IJ, Dodds WJ, Dantas RO, Massey B, Kern MK, Lang IM, et al. Opening mechanisms of the human upper esophageal sphincter. Am J Physiol. 1989;257: G748–59.

43. Hunt PS, Connell AM, Smiley TB. The cricopharyngeal sphincter in gastric reflux. Gut. 1970;11:303–6.

44. Hurwitz AL, Nelson JA, Haddad JK. Oropharyngeal dysphagia: manometric and cine-esophagographic findings. Am J Dig Dis. 1975;20:313–24.

45. Wilson CP. Pharyngeal diverticula, their cause and treatment. J Laryngol Otol. 1962;76:151–80.

46. Kodicek JM, Creamer B. A study of pharyngeal pouches. J Laryngol Otol. 1961;75:406–11.

47. Pedersen AS, Hansen JB, Alstrup P. Pharyngo-esophageal diverticula: a manometric follow up study of ten cases treated by diverticulectomy. Scand J Thorc Cardiovasc Surg. 1973;7:87–92.
48. Knuff TE, Benjamin SB, Castell DO. Pharyngoesophageal (Zenker's) diverticulum: a reappraisal. Gastroenterology. 1982;82:734–6.
49. Cook IJ, Blumbergs P, Cash K, Jamieson GG, Shearman DJ. Structural abnormalities of the cricopharyngeus muscle in patients with pharyngeal (Zenker's) diverticulum. J Gastroenterol Hepatol. 1992;7:556–62.
50. Bonington A, Mahon M, Whitmore I. A histological and histochemical study of the cricopharyngeus muscle in man. J Anat. 1988;156:27–37.
51. Lerut T, Guelinckx P, Dom P, Geboes K, Gruwez J. Does the musculus cricopharyngeus play a role in the genesis of Zenker's diverticulum? Enzyme histochemical and contractility properties. In: Siewart JR, Holscher AH, editors. Diseases of the esophagus. Berlin: Springer; 1988. p. 1018–23.
52. Shaw DW, Cook IJ, Jamieson GG, Gabb M, Simula ME, Dent J. Influence of surgery on deglutitive upper esophageal sphincter mechanics in Zenker's diverticulum. Gut. 1996;38:806–11.
53. Salam MA, Cable HR. Acquired pharyngeal diverticulum following anterior cervical fusion operation. Br J Clin Pract. 1994;48:109–10.
54. Sood S, Henein RR, Girgis B. Pharyngeal pouch following anterior cervical fusion. J Laryngol Otol. 1998;112:1085–6.
55. Georgalas C, Baer ST. Pharyngeal pouch and polymyositis: association and implications for aetiology of Zenker's diverticulum. J Laryngol Otol. 2000;114(10):805–7.
56. Shapiro J, Martin S, DeGirolami U, Goyal R. Inflammatory myopathy causing pharyngeal dysphagia: a new entity. Ann Otol Rhinol Laryngol. 1996; 105(5):331–5.
57. Horvath OP, Zombari J, Halmos L, Bozoky B, Olah T. Pharyngeal dysphagia caused by isolated myogen dystrophy of musculus cricopharyngeus. Acta Chir Hung. 1998;37(1–2):51–8.
58. Bachmann G, Streppel M, Krug B, Neuen-Jacob E. Cricopharyngeal muscle hypertrophy associated with florid myositis. Dysphagia. 2001;16(4):244–8.
59. Gage-White L. Incidence of Zenker's diverticulum with hiatus hernia. Laryngoscope. 1988;98:527–30.
60. Smiley TB, Caves PK, Porter DC. Relationship between posterior pharyngeal pouch and histus hernia. Thorax. 1970;25:725–31.
61. Resouly A, Braat J, Jackson A, Evans H. Pharyngeal pouch: link with reflux and oesophageal dysmotility. Clin Otolaryngol. 1994;19:241–2.
62. Delahunty JE, Margulies SI, Alonso WA, Knudson DH. The relationship of reflux esophagitis to pharyngeal pouch (Zenker's diverticulum) formation. Laryngoscope. 1971;81:570–7.
63. Sasaki CT, Ross DA, Hundal J. Association between Zenker's diverticulum and gastroesophageal reflux disease: development of a working hypothesis. Am J Med. 2003;115(Suppl 3A):169S–71.
64. Lang IM, Medda BK, Shaker R. Mechanisms of reflexes induced by esophageal distension. Am J Physiol Gastrointest Liver Physiol. 2001;281(5): G1246–63.
65. Szczesniak MM, Fuentealba SE, Burnett A, Cook IJ. Differential relaxation and contractile responses of the human upper esophageal sphincter mediated by interplay of mucosal and deep mechanoreceptor activation. Am J Gastroenterol. 2008;294:G982–8.
66. Feussner H, Siewert JR. Zenker's diverticulum and reflux [see comments]. Hepatogastroenterology. 1992; 39(2):100–4.

Cricopharyngeal Bar

36

Roberto Oliveira Dantas

Abstract

A cricopharyngeal bar on lateral radiographs of barium swallows is noted in some of patients who undergo pharyngeal and esophageal radiographic examination. Reduced compliance by fibrosis has been the explanation for the bar. The bolus flow through the upper esophageal sphincter is the same as that observed in healthy subjects. The increased resistance to flow markedly raises the forces required to drive bolus passage. The intrabolus pressure in the hypopharynx of these patients is higher than in healthy subjects. The increase in intrabolus pressure depends on the distended pharyngoesophageal segment during swallows, with a more significant increase associated with a smaller upper esophageal sphincter diameter and an increase of bolus volume. Most of the time, cricopharyngeal bar is an unexpected and incidental observation on an esophageal radiologic examination. The bar may not cause symptoms, but when it is present dysphagia is the most frequent complaint. However, the cause of dysphagia may be pharyngeal and esophageal motor abnormalities and not the cricopharyngeal bar, a possibility that should be investigated. If the patient has dysphagia, he should be investigated by radiologic, endoscopic and manometric examinations. The treatment involves some options, as surgery, dilatation or botulin toxin.

Keywords

Zenker's diverticulum • Cricopharyngeal bar • Upper esophageal sphincter (UES) • Pharyngoesophageal segment (PES) • Cricopharyngeal (CP) muscle

R.O. Dantas, MD (✉)
Department of Medicine, Medical School
of Ribeirão Preto, University of São Paulo,
14049-900 Ribeirão Preto, SP, Brazil
e-mail: rodantas@fmrp.usp.br

R. Shaker et al. (eds.), *Principles of Deglutition: A Multidisciplinary Text for Swallowing and its Disorders*, 509
DOI 10.1007/978-1-4614-3794-9_36, © Springer Science+Business Media New York 2013

The major component of the upper esophageal sphincter (UES), often termed the pharyngoesophageal segment or PES, is the cricopharyngeal (CP) muscle, a 1–2 cm wide muscle that does not account for the entire UES high-pressure zone, but which also includes the participation of the inferior pharyngeal constrictor and the cranial cervical esophageal muscles. The CP muscle is located in the transition between pharynx and esophagus and is distinct from the surrounding pharyngeal and esophageal muscles. It is composed of striated muscle of small average diameter fibers which are not oriented in a parallel fashion [1] and contains a large proportion of connective tissue. The CP muscle is tonically active, has a high degree of elasticity, does not develop maximal tension at basal length, and is composed of a mixture of slow- and fast-twitch fibers, with the former predominating [1, 2]. This permits the CP muscle to be able to be stretched open by distracting forces, such as a swallowed bolus and hyoid and laryngeal excursion [2]. The passive elasticity of the tissues is responsible for part of the UES pressure.

The UES must open adequately to permit transfer of the bolus from pharynx to esophagus. The opening mechanism of this sphincter involves sphincter relaxation, anterior hyo-laryngeal traction, and intrabolus pressure [3]. Sphincter relaxation occurs during laryngeal elevation and precedes opening by a mean period of 0.1 s. UES opening is an active mechanical event rather than simply a consequence of CP relaxation [4], with the sphincter diameter during opening also being a function of bolus volume and consistency [3, 5]. Sufficient opening of the sphincter is necessary for the complete transit of the bolus, otherwise the bolus flow will not be complete and the subject may complain of dysphagia and have residues in the pharynx.

A CP bar on lateral radiographs of barium swallows is noted in some patients who undergo pharyngeal and esophageal radiographic examination, almost always in elderly subjects (Fig. 36.1) [6], seen as a posterior indentation of the esophageal lumen between cervical vertebrae 3 and 6. This may be manifested as an anatomical protrusion in elderly cadavers [7]. Most of the

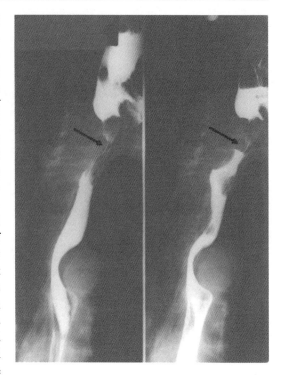

Fig. 36.1 A 72-year-old woman with a marked cricopharyngeal bar (*arrow*) narrowing the UES opening

time the CP bar does not cause symptoms, but dysphagia may be reported by some subjects. The terms achalasia, spasm, and hypertrophy are inappropriate to describe this radiologic finding. The CP bar is seen as a prominence in the UES lumen, different from the circumferential reduction in sphincter lumen which indicates CP stenosis.

Reduced compliance by fibrosis has been the explanation for CP bar. It has not been demonstrated that these patients have impaired relaxation of the UES. Investigations showed that the UES relaxes normally and the magnitude of hyoid and laryngeal movement is normal, suggesting that the major abnormality in the CP bar is reduced passive compliance of the relaxed UES [5] similar to that seen in patients with a Zenker's diverticulum.

There are descriptions of a transverse ridge on the posterior hypopharyngeal wall of elderly cadavers [7]. On the median sagittal plane, the muscular layer of the ridge was thicker than that of adjacent parts of the wall. Histologic sections through the ridge revealed four tissue layers: mucosa, fibrous, muscular, and adventitial. The fibrous layer contained collagen and elastin fibers which mainly ran longitudinally underneath the mucosa and were continuous with the horizontal fibrous septa in the muscular layer. The muscular layer appeared as a partial fold on the sections. The superior part did not continue with the muscular layer in the pharyngeal wall, and the inferior part of the ridge gradually became thinner. Other described alterations are degeneration and regeneration in the muscle fibers with interstitial fibrosis [8]. Alterations of the UES opening have been described in elderly subjects, even those without a CP bar. Elderly subjects have a lower UES pressure than young individuals and delayed UES relaxation [9]. The anteroposterior UES diameter and hyoid and anterior laryngeal excursion are shorter in the elderly compared to the young [10]. The intrabolus pressure in the pharynx of elderly subjects is higher than that of young subjects, suggesting a higher pharyngeal outflow resistance in the elderly [10]. The intrabolus pressure is the positive hypopharyngeal pressure that precedes the peristaltic pressure wave, with its onset coincident with the arrival of the bolus head at the hypopharynx [3].

The CP bar in some individuals represents a pharyngeal outflow resistance to flow. However, the flow through the UES is the same as that observed in healthy subjects [11]. The increased resistance to flow observed in the presence of abnormal structure or function of the pharyngeal–esophageal transition markedly raises the forces required to drive bolus passage [12]. The intrabolus pressure in the hypopharynx of patients with a CP bar is higher than in healthy subjects, and is almost four times higher than in healthy subjects when the volume of liquid bolus swallowed is 20 mL compared with two times higher when the volume is 2 mL [11]. Intrabolus pressure reflects locally the existence of UES constriction with resistance to flow [12]. The increase in intrabolus pressure depends on the distended pharyngoesophageal segment during swallows, with a more significant increase associated with a smaller UES diameter [13].

As the CP bar is more frequently seen in older subjects, the alterations of pharyngeal transit and contraction that may be observed in CP bar patients are the same as those of older subjects without a CP bar. Compared with younger subjects, elderly individuals have longer hypopharyngeal transit time, longer UES opening [6], increased amplitude and duration of the peristaltic pressure wave in the hypopharynx, a decrease in UES resting pressure [14], an increase in pharyngeal residues, and longer oral and pharyngeal transit time and pharyngeal clearance time [15]. The differences between the patients with symptomatic CP bar and older healthy subjects is the smaller sagittal and transverse diameter seen during radiologic examination [6, 11, 13], and an increase in intrabolus pressure proximal to the UES [11, 12]. The increase in intrabolus pressure should preserve the normal flow rates even though the UES does not open normally. This situation may be a contributor to the development of Zenker's diverticulum in some patients [12, 16].

Diagnosis

Most of the time, CP bar is an unexpected and incidental observation on an esophageal radiologic examination. The bar may not cause symptoms, but when it is present, and symptomatic, dysphagia is the most frequent complaint. The dysphagia may only be manifested by dietary modifications and prolonged meal time, but some patients may have severely decompensated abnormal swallowing and weight loss. However, the cause of dysphagia may be pharyngeal and esophageal motor abnormalities and not the CP bar, a possibility that should be investigated. The CP bar is more frequently associated with dysphagia when there is a marked obstructive bar with a small UES diameter narrowing the lumen [13], when a Zenker's diverticulum is present, or when the patient also has pharyngeal weakness or neuromuscular dysfunction.

If the patient has dysphagia, it should be investigated by radiologic, endoscopic, and manometric examinations. The CP bar is seen as a posterior indentation of the esophageal lumen between cervical vertebrae 3 and 6, as visualized in the lateral view X-ray, not related to a cervical osteophyte [6], and may be mild, moderate, or marked, as exemplified in several papers [6, 11–13, 17]. A marked CP bar is shown in Fig. 36.1, with a restricted UES opening in the radiologic examination of a 72-year-old woman with severe dysphagia.

The introduction of high-resolution manometry (HRM) has improved our understanding of motility alterations of the pharynx, UES, and esophagus [17]. Manometry is not essential for the diagnosis, but will show an increase in intrabolus pressure that represents the resistance to flow across the UES [12, 17]. The UES relaxation is normal. Generally there are no further abnormalities in pharyngeal, UES, or proximal esophagus motility, but weak pharyngeal constrictors have been described [13]. Other motility abnormalities may be found in the pharynx and esophagus because dysphagia is a common problem in older subjects. Changes in physiology with aging are seen in the pharynx, UES, and esophagus of both symptomatic and asymptomatic older individuals [18].

A CP bar is difficult to evaluate on endoscopic examination, but rigid or flexible endoscopy may be of benefit in some patients by excluding malignancies as the cause of dysphagia.

Treatment

The objective of the treatment of a CP bar is to create conditions that increase the sphincter diameter during swallowing. If the subjects do not have symptoms or if the symptoms are not a consequence of the CP bar, there is no need to treat the bar. Surgical intervention is only appropriate for selected patients after careful evaluation. The patients should not have other clinical conditions, which might be responsible for the symptoms. In this situation, the treatment of these other clinical conditions should come first.

There are no sufficient controlled investigations about therapy of the CP bar with botulin toxin and CP dilatation, but some investigations have reported good results.

Botolinum toxin injection, either endoscopically or transcutaneously, has been reported to be of benefit. With the injection of 30 units into the CP muscle of 10 selected patients with dysphagia and pure UES dysfunction, the relative opening of the sphincter improved from 47 ± 14 % before treatment to 71 ± 24 % after treatment. Hypopharyngeal retention or laryngeal penetration was significantly reduced in four of seven patients. Clinical symptom scores improved in all of them [19]. A single injection of botulinum toxin into the CP muscle has long-lasting effectiveness in patients with neurologic dysphagia caused by alteration in the UES opening and with pharyngeal contraction, but it is not possible to rule out the effect of potential spontaneous improvement of neurologic injury [20]. This option best serves cases of failed relaxation of the CP muscle, which is usually not the case in patients with CP bar. Diffusion of the toxin to adjacent muscles may worsen dysphagia or cause vocal cord dysfunction as well. Controlled trials are needed to determine the safety and efficacy of the use of the toxin.

CP dilatation is a possibility but there are few studies showing results of this treatment in patients with a CP bar. In a study of six patients with CP bar and dysphagia, all subjects experienced immediate relief, five showed continued improvement at 1–4 weeks, and three still showed complete resolution of dysphagia at long-term follow-up ranging from 8 to 27 months [21]. This therapy should be an option only for elderly patients who are in no condition to undergo surgical treatment. Repeated dilatation over many years may be required for about half the patients, and some of them eventually require surgery [22]. Balloon dilatation of the UES is a low-risk option that works best in patients with fibrosis of the CP [23], which is the case for the CP bar.

The most important option to treat patients with structural disorders that limit the opening of the UES, such as a symptomatic CP bar, is cricopharyngeal myotomy [22]. CP myotomy is indicated when there is a limitation in UES opening, but the laryngo-hyoid complex elevated in an anterosuperior direction to open the sphincter and the pharyngeal pressure is sufficient to propel a bolus through the open sphincter [23]. CP myotomy helps to normalize the UES opening [24, 25] and may improve pharyngeal contraction [24]. In 20 patients with cricopharyngeal dysfunction, 12 with Zenker's diveticulum, the UES opening for a 3 mL bolus was 3.0 ± 1.7 mm before myotomy and 5.1 ± 1.5 mm after myotomy, corresponding to normal values (5.2 ± 0.2 mm) [25]. Pharyngeal size was unchanged, but UES opening showed better improvement with CP myotomy than with dilatation or botulinum toxin, suggesting that CP myotomy is more effective than the latter procedures in relieving obstruction [24]. Endoscopic cricopharyngeal myotomy is a safe and effective treatment option for patients with cricopharyngeal dysphagia [26], with most surgeons using a laser to perform the myotomy [27]. The evaluation of symptoms in 14 patients with a CP bar, with normal or low pharyngeal pressure contraction, using the Functional Outcome Swallowing Scale (FOSS) found a significant decrease of symptoms in all of them after endoscopic laser CP myotomy, with normal physiologic function without symptoms in five [27]. The improvement after this treatment was significant in patients with normal pharyngeal contraction and in patients with a weak pharyngeal contraction. There was an increase from 32.8 to 123.5 mm^2 in the mean cross-sectional CP (or UES) area after endoscopic laser myotomy. The intrabolus-pressure gradient (the difference between the intrabolus pressure recordings from above and below the 3 cm UES region) decreased from 25.4 to 13.2 mmHg 6 months postoperatively. Both the groups with normal and with weak pharyngeal driving force had the same results, suggesting that a weak pharyngeal pressure is not a problem for myotomy [27]. The laser technique is at least as effective as the transcervical approach for CP myotomy to improve dysphagia in properly selected patients, with a lower risk of major complications.

Key Points

1. CP bar may be found in radiologic examination of elderly subjects with no complaints.
2. CP bar is seen as a posterior indentation of the esophageal lumen between cervical vertebrae 3 and 6, causing a reduction of the upper esophageal sphincter diameter during opening.
3. CP bar is more frequently seen in older subjects.
4. Reduced compliance by fibrosis has been the explanation for CP bar.
5. During pharyngeal and upper esophageal sphincter bolus flow, there is an increase in hypopharyngeal intrabolus pressure that represents the resistance to flow across the upper esophageal sphincter.
6. The best option to treat patients with structural disorders that limit the opening of the upper esophageal sphincter, such as a symptomatic or obstructive CP bar, is cricopharyngeal myotomy.

References

1. Singh S, Hamdy S. The upper oesophageal sphincter. Neurogastroenterol Motil. 2005;17 Suppl 1:3–12.
2. Sivarao DV, Goyal RK. Functional anatomy and physiology of the upper esophageal sphincter. Am J Med. 2000;104:27S–37.
3. Cook IJ, Dodds WJ, Dantas RO, Massey B, Kern MK, Lang IM, Brasseur JG, Hogan WJ. Opening mechanisms of the human upper esophageal sphincter. Am J Physiol. 1989;257:G748–59.
4. Jacob P, Kahrilas PJ, Logemann JA, Shah V, Ha T. Upper eophageal sphincter opening and modulation during swallowing. Gastroenterology. 1989;97:1469–78.
5. Dantas RO, Kern MK, Massey BT, Dodds WJ, Kahrilas PJ, Brasseur JG, Cook IJ, Lang IM. Effect of swallowed bolus variables on oral and pharyngeal phases of swallowing. Am J Physiol. 1990;258:G675–81.
6. Leonard R, Kendall K, McKenzie S. UES opening and cricopharyngeal bar in nondysphagic elderly and nonelderly adults. Dysphagia. 2004;19:182–91.
7. Leaper M, Zhang M, Daves PJD. An anatomical protrusion exists on the posterior hypopharyngeal wall in some elderly cadavers. Dysphagia. 2005;20:8–14.
8. Cruse JP, Edwards DA, Smith JF, Wyllie JH. The pathology of a cricopharyngeal dysphagia. Hystopathology. 1979;3:223–32.
9. Fulp SR, Dalton CB, Castell JA, Castell DO. Aging-related alterations in human upper esophageal sphincter function. Am J Gastroenterol. 1990;85:1569–72.
10. Kern M, Bardan E, Arndorfer R, Hofmann C, Ren J, Shaker R. Comparison of upper esophageal sphincter opening in healthy asymptomatic young and elderly volunteers. Ann Otol Rhinol Laryngol. 1999;108:982–9.
11. Dantas RO, Cook IJ, Dodds WJ, Kern MK, Lang IM, Brasseur JG. Biomechanics of cricopharyngeal bars. Gastroenterology. 1990;99:1269–74.
12. Pal A, Williams RB, Cook IJ, Brasseur JG. Intrabolus pressure gradient identifies pathological constriction

in the upper esophageal sphincter during flow. Am J Physiol. 2003;285:G1037–48.

13. Olsson R, Ekberg O. Videomanometry of the pharynx in dysphagic patients with a posterior cricopharyngeal indentation. Acta Radiol. 1995;2:597–601.

14. Shaker R, Ren J, Podvrsan B, Dodds WJ, Hogan WJ, Kern M, Hoffmann R, Hintz J. Effect of aging and bolus variables on pharyngeal and upper esophageal sphincter motor function. Am J Physiol. 1993;264:G427–32.

15. Cook IJ, Weltman MD, Wallace K, Shaw DW, McKay E, Smart RC, Butler SP. Influence of aging on oral-pharyngeal bolus transit and clearance during swallowing: scintigraphic study. Am J Physiol. 1994;266:G972–7.

16. Cook IJ, Gabb M, Panagopoulos V, Jamieson GG, Dodds WJ, Dent J, Shearman DJ. Pharyngeal (Zenker's) diverticulum is a disorder of upper esophageal sphincter opening. Gastroenterology. 1992;103:1229–35.

17. Fox MR, Bredenoord AJ. Oesophageal high-resolution manometry: moving from research into clinical practice. Gut. 2008;57:405–23.

18. Achem SR, DeVault KR. Dysphagia in aging. J Clin Gastroenterol. 2005;39:357–71.

19. Alberty J, Oelerich M, Ludwig K, Hartmann S, Stow W. Efficacy of botulinum toxin A for treatment of upper esophageal sphincter dysfunction. Laryngoscope. 2000;110:1151–6.

20. Terre R, Valles M, Panades A, Mearin F. Long-lasting effect of a single botulinum toxin injection in the treatment of oropharyngeal dysphagia secondary to upper esophageal sphincter dysfunction: a pilot study. Scand J Gastroenterol. 2008;43:1286–303.

21. Wang AY, Kadkade R, Kahrilas PJ, Hirano I. Effectiveness of esophageal dilation for symptomatic cricopharyngeal bar. Gastrointest Endosc. 2006;61:148–52.

22. Cook IJ. Oropharyngeal Dysphagia. Gastroenterol Clin North Am. 2009;38:411–31.

23. Kelly JH. Management of upper esophageal sphincter disorders: indications and complications of myotomy. Am J Med. 2000;108(Suppl):43S–6.

24. Allen J, White CJ, Leonard R, Belafsky PC. Effect of cricopharyngeal muscle surgery on the pharynx. Laryngoscope. 2010;120:1498–503.

25. Yip HT, Leonard R, Kendall KA. Cricopharyngeal myotomy normalizes the opening size of the upper esophageal sphincter in cricopharyngeal dysfunction. Laryngoscope. 2006;116:93–6.

26. Lawson G, Remacle M. Endoscopic cricopharyngeal myotomy: indications and technique. Curr Opin Otolaryngol Head Neck Surg. 2006;14:437–41.

27. Ozgursoy OB, Salassa JR. Manofluorographic and functional outcomes after endoscopic laser cricopharyngeal myotomy for cricopharyngeal bar. Otolaryngol Head Neck Surg. 2010;142:735–40.

Cricopharyngeal Achalasia

Benson T. Massey

Abstract

Cricopharyngeal achalasia is a disorder characterized by an abnormal pattern of deglutitive inhibition of tone in the cricopharyngeus muscle. The condition is distinct from abnormalities of the normal relaxation response to esophageal air distension (termed here cricopharyngismus) and elevated resting tone. Diverse etiologies may cause the disorder, and a sequence of tests is usually necessary to confirm the diagnosis and exclude other conditions that might cause similar symptoms. Guidance on treatment options is limited due to the lack of controlled trials for the disorder as well as concern about accuracy of the diagnosis in prior publications.

Keywords

Cricopharyngeus muscle • Cricopharyngeal achalasia • Upper esophageal sphincter • Manometry • Electromyography • Videofluoroscopy • Eructation • Belch • Globus • Dysphagia

Introduction

Cricopharyngeal achalasia is a somewhat confusing entity that suffers from an inconsistent definition throughout the relatively sparse medical literature (at the time of this publication only 120 articles are detected in PUBMED using this as a search term). The term "achalasia" derives from the ancient Greek *a*-(not)+*khalasis* (relaxation) and was coined early in the twentieth century to indicate the failure of the normal relaxation response of the lower esophageal sphincter in response to deglutition. However, the lower esophageal sphincter and the upper esophageal sphincter have fundamentally different compositions, innervations, and mechanisms of action.

The lower esophageal sphincter (LES) is a smooth muscle structure that generates spontaneous tone, independent of neural excitation. Activation of vagal neural input (from the dorsal motor nucleus) is transmitted via synapses to neurons having an intramural location in the esophagus. The subsequent activation of these postsynaptic neurons releases nitric oxide, resulting in hyperpolarization and relaxation of the

B.T. Massey, MD, FACP (✉)
Division of Gastroenterology and Hepatology,
Medical College of Wisconsin,
9200 W. Wisconsin Avenue, Milwaukee,
WI 53226, USA
e-mail: bmassey@mcw.edu

R. Shaker et al. (eds.), *Principles of Deglutition: A Multidisciplinary Text for Swallowing and its Disorders*,
DOI 10.1007/978-1-4614-3794-9_37, © Springer Science+Business Media New York 2013

LES. Distension of the esophagus can activate local intramural or vago-vagal reflex arcs to inhibit the lower esophageal sphincter also. There is also a chronic excitatory innervation to the LES, involving the neurotransmitter acetylcholine acting at muscarinic receptors in the smooth muscle cells. Blockade of this excitatory input by use of muscarinic antagonists, such as atropine, results in a fall in resting tone. However, the inhibitory innervation is normally dominant, so that when the vagus nerve is electrically stimulated, the net result of activation of both excitatory and inhibitory postganglionic neurons is LES relaxation. Achalasia of the LES occurs when there is loss of its inhibitory innervation. An achalasia-like condition can also be induced pharmacologically by agents that block the synthesis of nitric oxide.

In contrast, the upper esophageal sphincter (UES) is a skeletal muscle structure. Its innervation is from excitatory motor neurons residing in the nucleus ambiguus. The excitatory neurotransmitter is again acetylcholine, but this acts on nicotinic receptors at the neuromuscular junction. There is no spontaneous tone in these skeletal muscle cells. Resting tone in the UES is dependent on tonic input from the excitatory motor neurons. Temporal variations in the UES tone, as occur with phasic contractions, reflect variations in the recruitment and activation of the motor neurons supplying the UES. Destruction of these motor neurons or pharmacologic blockade of nicotinic transmission results in a flaccid UES. Relaxation of the UES with deglutition results from inhibition of the tonic firing of the excitatory motor neurons. The first order of control for these motor neurons resides in the interneurons comprising the swallowing central pattern generator in the brainstem. Distension of the esophageal body can alter the tone of the UES via reflex arcs involving the afferent vagal pathways. Whether the UES contracts or relaxes depends upon the physical parameters of the stimulus. For example, focal distension of the esophagus (as occurs with a distending balloon) causes UES contraction. However, abrupt gaseous distension of most of the esophagus (as occurs during gastroesophageal reflux of gas) results in UES relaxation.

During the act of deglutition, normal relaxation of the UES is not just a matter of the completeness and duration of the inhibition of muscle tone. This relaxation has to occur at the correct time in the swallow cycle. This occurs after elevation and anterior movement of the larynx (and with it movement of the UES). The relaxation occurs during the apogee of UES movement, which facilitates entry of the bolus into the UES. The bolus is being propelled into the pharyngoesophageal segment by the organized contractions of the tongue and pharyngeal constrictors. Premature or delayed relaxation of the UES relative to the action of the other muscles of deglutition can have effects similar to no deglutitive relaxation in terms of impairing bolus transit into the esophagus.

Unfortunately, the literature on cricopharyngeal achalasia has been made confusing by the lack of a uniform definition of the condition. In addition, the presence of cricopharyngeal achalasia has been inferred from diagnostic testing modalities without an appreciation of alternative disorders that could produce findings that have been attributed to achalasia. Ideally, detection of abnormalities in the deglutitive inhibition would be accomplished by direct recordings from the motor neurons supplying the CP muscle or from the muscle itself. Such techniques either are not available clinically or the availability is confined to a few tertiary centers.

In an attempt to develop some consistency within the field, the following definitions are proposed:

Cricopharyngeal achalasia: A condition in which, during deglutition, the CP muscle or the motor neurons supplying it exhibit one or more of the following abnormal patterns of activity: (1) incomplete inhibition of activation; (2) abnormally short duration of complete activation inhibition; (3) abnormal timing of inhibited activation, relative to the activation of other motor neurons controlled by the swallowing central pattern generator; (4) increased activation during the normal interval of inhibition.

Cricopharyngismus: A condition in which the CP muscle or the motor neurons supplying it exhibit either an increased activation or a reduced deactivation in response to an esophageal stimulus that normally results in an inhibition of activity.

Cricopharyngeal hypertonicity: A condition in which the CP muscle or the motor neurons supplying it exhibit abnormally elevated activity during interdeglutitive intervals.

Cricopharyngeal Achalasia

Etiopathogenesis

The pathogenesis of cricopharyngeal achalasia is largely unknown, due to the rarity of the condition, lack of precision in the diagnosis, difficulties in instrumental investigation, and unavailability of a reliable animal model (sporadic cases have been reported in dogs naturally, but these have not been characterized systematically). Based upon the clinical conditions associated with the disorder, the most likely causes are destruction of portions of the neuronal circuitry that comprises the central pattern generator for swallowing, which resides within the medullary brainstem. Destruction could involve any of the following: medullary interneurons, efferent pathways having input from cortical swallowing centers, and afferent pathways conveying sensory information to the central pattern generator and cortex. Complete destruction of the primary motor neurons or their axons that supply the CP muscle is unlikely to be a major mechanism for cricopharyngeal achalasia, as this would render the UES flaccid, rather than spastic.

It is important to recognize that the abnormal deglutitive response of the UES may be a somewhat isolated phenomenon, and the function of the UES during other processes, such as respiration may remain intact. For example, this author has observed that most patients with abnormal deglutitive UES responses maintain a UES relaxation response to esophageal air distension or gastroesophageal reflux of air (Fig. 37.1a, b). Likewise, many patients with deglutitive UES

dysfunction continue to have this function modified by sensory input. Thus, patients with impaired relaxation or paradoxical contraction with dry swallows show improved relaxation parameters with wet swallows (Fig. 37.2) [1].

A list of conditions presumptively associated with cricopharyngeal achalasia is shown in Table 37.1. The term presumptive is used, because in the majority of cases the findings upon which the diagnosis of cricopharyngeal achalasia was based (reduced opening of the pharyngoesophageal segment on videofluoroscopy) may have instead resulted from another pathophysiology (e.g., pharyngeal myopathy or paralysis). This is almost certainly the case for the reports of cricopharyngeal achalasia with mitochondrial myopathies, such as Kearns–Sayre syndrome, so that these conditions are not included in the list of etiologies at this time. In many cases, the etiology remains unknown.

Clinical Presentation

Cricopharyngeal achalasia has been reported in all age groups. Symptoms may have an abrupt or gradually progressive onset, depending on whether the etiology is a vascular/traumatic catastrophe or results from an ongoing neurodegenerative process. The symptoms associated with cricopharyngeal achalasia are nonspecific and listed in Table 37.2. In many cases, the symptoms reflect the effects of additional disorders that are present conjointly with cricopharyngeal achalasia, such as pharyngeal paralysis or laryngeal sensory neuropathy. Solid dysphagia is usually more common than liquid dysphagia. "Stringy" foods, such as noodles and vegetable leaves, seem to be particularly challenging. In addition to foods, pills often hang up. Solids provoking dysphagia can take several swallows to get down; failing this, they may be coughed back into the oral cavity and expectorated. Prolonged retention of caustic pills, such as potassium chloride or aspirin, may cause a pill-induced mucosal injury in the hypopharynx, resulting in symptoms of odynophagia. Dysphagia with liquids in isolation is more likely to occur when there are concomitant disturbances in the function of other

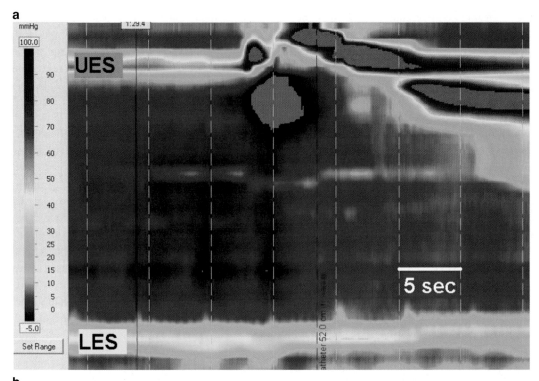

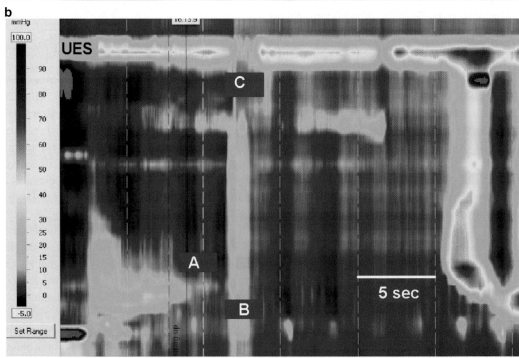

Fig. 37.1 (a) Contour plot from a high-resolution solid-state manometry study in a patient with cricopharyngeal achalasia. At the start of a dry swallow the upper esophageal sphincter (UES) contracts briefly, then as it moves orad, the pressure remains considerably elevated above the intra-esophageal pressure. *LES* lower esophageal sphincter. (b) Same patient as in a. However, after the patient sits up there is a transient lower esophageal sphincter relaxation (A). This is followed by an abdominal strain event (B), which is associated with a non-deglutitive relaxation of the UES (C) that is accompanied by a belch

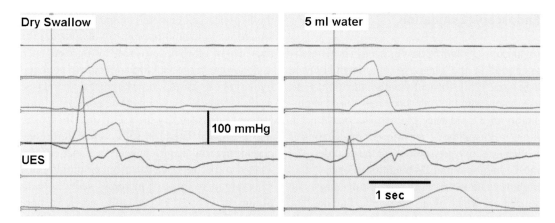

Fig. 37.2 Manometric tracings from a study using a perfused sleeve to record from the *upper* esophageal sphincter UES. The *left panel* shows a dry swallow. The UES fails to relax. The early dramatic pressure spike results from the non-relaxing UES pushing fluid back on the sleeve during its orad ascent. The second panel shows a complete UES relaxation with a 5 ml water swallow, although the duration of relaxation remains abnormally short

Table 37.1 Conditions associated with cricopharyngeal achalasia

Cortical stroke
Lateral medullary stroke (Wallenberg's syndrome)
Parkinson's disease
Cerebral palsy
Multiple sclerosis
Amyotrophic lateral sclerosis
Alzheimer's disease
Myasthenia gravis
Primary central nervous system or metastatic cancer
Arnold–Chiari malformation
Myotonic dystrophy
Multiple system atrophy
Ataxia telangiectasia
Trauma/surgical injury
Inclusion body myositis
Post-polio syndrome

Table 37.2 Symptoms associated with cricopharyngeal achalasia

Solid dysphagia
Liquid dysphagia
Odynophagia
Globus sensation
Cough/choking/stridor/hoarseness
Nasopharyngeal regurgitation
Starvation/dehydration

swallowing structures, such as tongue or inferior constrictor weakness.

Respiratory symptoms typically result from the aspiration of ingesta retained within the hypopharynx above the non-relaxing UES. This is more likely to occur during oropharyngeal multitasking, such as when the patient is both conversing and eating. Respiratory symptoms provoked by undistracted deglutition suggest that additional sensorimotor deficits may be present, including those affecting supraglottic and glottic structures.

Physical Examination

There are no findings on physical examination that support the diagnosis of cricopharyngeal achalasia. The purpose of the physical examination is to assess for the presence of findings that might offer a clue to the underlying etiology. Given the most common etiologies, a meticulous neurologic examination, particularly of structures innervated by the cranial nerves, is paramount. Detection of oral and cervical masses or lymphadenopathy may be the first clue of an underlying malignancy. Scars from previous trauma or surgery may point to the etiology. The cardiovascular system is assessed for sources of stroke. The pulmonary examination is important to detect complications, such as aspiration pneumonia.

Endoscopic Evaluation

Endoscopy (including laryngoscopy) is generally unhelpful in the diagnosis of cricopharyngeal achalasia. While difficulty with intubation of the esophagus with the endoscope may raise the possibility of the presence of cricopharyngeal achalasia, in this author's experience, this finding is neither sensitive nor specific for the disorder. The most common finding is retention of excess fluid or particulate debris in the pyriform sinuses and valleculae, which is a nonspecific finding. The main role of endoscopy is to exclude other conditions which might cause similar symptoms (such as tumors of the larynx, pharynx, and cervical esophagus) and to survey for other conditions whose presence may complicate the treatment plans for cricopharyngeal achalasia (such as severe gastroesophageal reflux disease). Endoscopy can identify additional disorders that may be present, either incidentally or as part of the process that caused the cricopharyngeal achalasia. These can include esophageal webs or inlet patches, laryngeal paresis, and vocal cord lesions. Depending upon the instrument used, mucosal lesions can be biopsied and stenoses dilated during the endoscopic examination.

Particularly with smaller caliber endoscopes, intubation of the esophagus can be difficult in patients with cricopharyngeal achalasia. Because the UES fails to relax, or even contracts, during its orad excursion with deglutition, it tends to knock the endoscope away from the lumen of the pharyngoesophageal segment. Endoscopic intubation is often more successful by using slow but steady pressure to advance the endoscope tip into the esophageal inlet between swallows, particularly in older subjects who have lower resting tone in the UES.

Videofluoroscopic Evaluation

Videofluoroscopy remains the mainstay for evaluating the patient with symptoms suggestive of cricopharyngeal achalasia. It can demonstrate reduced opening of the pharyngoesophageal segment and post-deglutitive bolus retention within the hypopharynx that are commonly seen in this condition. Videofluoroscopy can also detect the presence of other disturbances in function, such as abnormal tongue strength or control, impaired hyolaryngeal elevation, pharyngeal paralysis, nasopharyngeal regurgitation, aspiration, and esophageal spasm. By the use of anterior–posterior as well as lateral images, videofluoroscopy can detect unilateral defects in function [2]. Videofluoroscopy can detect other intraluminal disorders that cause symptoms, such as neoplasms or cervical osteophytes, and it is more sensitive than endoscopy for detecting subtle webs in the proximal esophagus. Because relatively flat mucosal lesions can also be missed on videofluoroscopy, it is never satisfactory as the sole modality for evaluating patients with possible cricopharyngeal achalasia.

Videofluoroscopy suffers from two fundamentally diametric limitations in the diagnosis of cricopharyngeal achalasia. The first is that pharyngoesophageal segment opening does not depend solely upon UES relaxation. The degree of opening is also determined by (1) traction on the larynx by the contraction of the thyrohyoid muscle (serving to pull open the UES), (2) strength of the pulsion forces transmitted through the bolus by pharyngeal muscle contraction (serving to push open the UES), (3) size of the bolus being swallowed, and (4) distensibility properties of the CP muscle tissue. Thus, reduced pharyngoesophageal segment opening and post-deglutitive bolus retention in the hypopharynx can be seen with other conditions besides cricopharyngeal achalasia. These include pharyngeal paresis, reduced distensibility of the CP (as occurs with muscular inflammation, fibrosis, or neoplastic infiltration), and impairment of the hyolaryngeal muscle complex that serves to pull open the UES during deglutition. Completely normal deglutitive relaxation of the UES may still be associated with abnormal pharyngoesophageal segment opening and bolus transit if one or more of these other factors is abnormal. Of course, cricopharyngeal achalasia may co-occur with these other abnormalities.

Conversely, intact function of the other muscles of deglutition may be sufficient to overcome the non-relaxing UES, resulting in seemingly normal bolus clearance, particularly with the relatively low viscosity liquid boluses that are routinely used [3]. In this author's experience, nearly half of patients with manometrically documented deglutitive UES dysfunction have no abnormalities detected on videofluoroscopy [4]. Thus, videofluoroscopy is neither sensitive nor specific for the diagnosis of cricopharyngeal achalasia.

Cricopharyngeal *achalasia* should be distinguished from cricopharyngeal *bar*, which is the appearance of a focal indentation of the barium column at the level of the cricopharyngeus muscle during a fluoroscopic examination (see separate section on Cricopharyngeal Bar). While a cricopharyngeal bar can be observed in patients with cricopharyngeal achalasia, this finding is neither sensitive nor specific, as the above discussion indicates.

CT/MRI Imaging

Imaging by CT or MRI is not helpful in diagnosing cricopharyngeal achalasia. Within the neck, the main purpose of such imaging is to identify extra-luminal processes such as neoplasms, abscesses, osteophytes, vascular aneurysms/anomalies, and surgical or traumatic changes that could cause or mimic cricopharyngeal achalasia. Imaging within the central nervous system is directed toward identifying pathologic processes and lesions that could result in cricopharyngeal achalasia.

Intraluminal Manometry

Intraluminal manometry is covered in more detail in other sections. With the use of adequate methodology, manometry can detect the impairment of the degree and duration of deglutitive relaxation of the UES, as well as inappropriate contraction during the normal period of motor quiescence. It can assess the coordination of this relaxation with proximal pharyngeal muscle contraction. Finally, with some manometric equipment, concurrent assessment of esophageal motor

function is also possible, and esophageal body/LES dysfunction is observed frequently in patients with UES dysfunction, in this author's experience [5].

The caveat is that the above are possible only when the manometric equipment is adequate and appropriately utilized. Unfortunately, the literature is replete with studies using techniques that cannot track the axial movement of the UES with deglutition. When a point sensor is placed in the UES high-pressure zone at rest, during deglutition, this sensor will be displaced into the proximal esophagus. Thus, the manometric recording will display a spurious interval of relaxation, when what is actually being recorded is the time of UES axial excursion. This can result in a false-negative study in terms of detecting cricopharyngeal achalasia. Because of this limitation, many studies having taken elevated "resting" UES pressure as evidence of cricopharyngeal achalasia. The discomfort from this test itself in a patient with cricopharyngeal achalasia may be enough to elevate this resting pressure, which is not a reliable predictor of impaired deglutitive UES relaxation.

A more fundamental difficulty for intraluminal manometry is that the pressure recorded does not always reflect the state of contraction of the adjacent musculature. Intraluminal manometric evaluation of UES function may also infer the presence of abnormal UES relaxation erroneously. There are two situations where this may occur. First, even when the CP muscle are paralyzed, a manometric sensor (depending upon its size and configuration) may detect an intraluminal pressure of up to 25 mmHg, resulting from passive stretch of the muscle by the manometric probe [6]. Further fall from this pressure during deglutition depends upon the anterior traction forces acting upon the CP. Loss of these traction forces could result in elevated deglutitive residual pressures in the UES that are misinterpreted as demonstrating abnormal UES relaxation.

Second, the period of deglutitive UES relaxation overlaps the interval of pharyngoesophageal segment opening and bolus flow into the esophagus. Hence, during this period, an intraluminal manometer is usually recording an intrabolus pressure. This intrabolus pressure does not directly reflect the contractile state of musculature in the adjacent wall. Normally, this intrabolus pressure is relatively low and the manometric signal indicates complete UES relaxation. However, if there is impediment to normal bolus flow, there will be an elevation of intrabolus pressure, which will give the manometric appearance of impaired UES relaxation. While abnormal UES relaxation can be a mechanism for abnormally elevated intrabolus pressure, several other processes can cause this also. These include constriction of the lumen through which the bolus must pass (such as reduced distensibility of the CP or a proximal cervical esophageal web) and elevation of downstream intraluminal pressures in the esophagus (as occurs frequently with esophageal achalasia).

Finally, commercially available manometric probes at this time are laterally indiscriminate. Thus, they are unable to demonstrate that in some patients UES dysfunction is unilateral.

As is the case with smaller caliber endoscopes, advancement of the manometric catheter across the UES may be difficult with ongoing deglutition. Availability of, and experience with, manometric recording equipment that meets requirements for reliable assessment of UES sphincter function is largely limited to tertiary referral centers. Because manometry cannot assess for the presence of many other conditions that can cause symptoms similar to those of cricopharyngeal achalasia, it is never by itself sufficient for clinical evaluation. Manometry is better employed to confirm that suggestive findings on videofluoroscopy do indeed result from cricopharyngeal achalasia and not from another disorder.

Electromyography

Electromyography (EMG) of the CP muscle can detect loss of the normal inhibition of electrical activity with deglutition. When combined with concurrent EMG of the inferior constrictor muscles, it is possible to assess the appropriate coordination of CP inhibition with pharyngeal activation. Use of concentric needle EMG recordings also allows the ability to detect neuropathic and myopathic changes in the muscle, including evidence for ongoing denervation [7]. EMG recordings also allow detection of unilateral cricopharyngeal abnormalities. Of course, this means that EMG recordings need to be performed bilaterally to avoid missing a unilateral abnormality, unless other clinical information supports a unilateral disorder beforehand.

A potential limitation of EMG recordings from the cricopharyngeus muscle is the orad movement of the muscle during deglutition by as much as 2 cm. Unless the electrode is inserted in such a way that it can travel within the muscle during this excursion, the period of electric silence that is observed will simply reflect temporary displacement of the electrode from the muscle, analogous to displacement of point sensors on manometric probes. This difficulty is not well addressed in the EMG literature in terms of recognition of the problem or methods to detect this problem.

EMG recordings are most helpful when videofluoroscopy suggests the possibility of cricopharyngeal achalasia, and subsequent manometric assessment is either unavailable or non-diagnostic. When prior studies have made the diagnosis of cricopharyngeal achalasia fairly certain, EMG may have additional value in detecting associated myopathy, myotonia, or neuropathy. Most neurologists do not have expertise in cricopharyngeal EMG recordings, and availability of this technique currently is confined to a few tertiary referral centers.

Therapy

Optimal treatment of cricopharyngeal achalasia remains uncertain. First, it is often unclear whether the treatments described in the literature were applied to true cases of cricopharyngeal achalasia. Second, published studies of treatment are mostly anecdotal and of limited case series at best. There are no randomized, placebo-controlled trials or even trials comparing one treatment modality to another. Follow-up data are extremely limited.

Dietary modifications are a reasonable first-line approach, especially if bothersome symptoms are provoked by a limited range of foods. These should simply be avoided or their consistency modified. Similarly, many troublesome pills may be crushed or switched to a liquid formulation. For patients with predominant solid food and pill dysphagia, liberal use of liquid washes may provide an afferent sensory stimulation that drives the swallow central pattern generator toward more normal function.

Swallow therapy exercises are appealing because of their safety and low cost. None of these have been evaluated specifically in cricopharyngeal achalasia. Head-raising exercises, such as the Shaker exercise [8], have been shown to increase pharyngoesophageal segment opening in patients with a wide variety of underlying etiologies for dysphagia. However, the technique has not been evaluated in patients with a specific diagnosis of cricopharyngeal achalasia. Theoretically, improved thyrohyoid activation as a consequence of this therapy [9] might allow traction forces to help overcome the non-relaxing UES.

Dilation of the CP muscle via tapered bougies or catheter-attached balloons has been reported to be of benefit in patients with cricopharyngeal dysfunction in all age groups. Objective responses to such therapy have not been reported consistently, but improved pharyngoesophageal segment opening has been reported on videofluoroscopy, as have reductions in basal UES pressure [10]. In adults, dilation diameters of 16–20 mm are usually employed. The benefits, in terms of symptomatic response, are usually immediate, although not every patient responds, and some require repeat dilations at varying intervals. Factors predicting response to therapy have not been reported. Potential risks of this approach include perforation and hemorrhage in the pharynx or esophagus, if introduction of the dilator or its introducer is into an unrecognized diverticulum or tight stricture. These risks can be minimized by appropriate videofluoroscopic and/or endoscopic pre-dilation assessment of anatomy, as well as the use of these modalities to guide dilator passage in select cases. An additional benefit of dilation therapy is that it allows concomitant dilation of hitherto unsuspected subtle stenoses or webs in the pharyngoesophageal segment.

Botulinum toxin has also been used to treat cricopharyngeal achalasia. Injections can be via operative rigid laryngoscopy, flexible upper endoscopy, or percutaneous EMG-guided needles. Injections are usually bilateral, unless there is a priori knowledge that a unilateral disorder is present. The dose has not been standardized, and no dose–response studies have been performed. Larger doses have been used in adults than in infants. Potency differs among different manufacturers, so that lower doses are used with Botox (2.5–100 units; Allergan, Irvine, California) than with Dysport (60–300 units; Ipsen, Paris France) [11]. Onset of subjective benefit is usually by day 7, with duration of benefit usually in the range of 3–4 months. Treatments can be repeated. There are no high-quality data supporting objecting beneficial changes in either deglutitive inhibitory pressures on manometry or electrical quiescence on EMG. Use of botulinum toxin response to predict subsequent response to cricopharyngeal myotomy remains controversial. The prevailing experience is that botulinum toxin has better symptomatic response when cricopharyngeal dysfunction occurs in the absence of other disturbances in the swallowing mechanism. Complication rates are low, but there is the risk for spread of the toxin to the muscles of the larynx and pharynx, particularly with large doses. The result could be paradoxical worsening of dysphagia or airway compromise.

Cricopharyngeal myotomy can be performed via either a trans-cervical or endoscopic approach. The risk for complications is higher than with previously described therapies, and includes hematomas, abscesses, fistula, nerve injury, and pneumonia. Depending upon the patient group treated, the overall complication rate may be as high as 10 %. Complete ablation of the UES might seem to predispose patients with significant reflux disease to esophagopharyngeal reflux and aspiration. A small study that included five patients with documented reflux disease showed no increase in postoperative episodes of acid regurgitation into the pharynx [12]. However,

such events were rare preoperatively in this group, and only a 24 h period was studied. It is also unclear if any of these patients were obese, a factor for increasing proximal extent of acid reflux. On the other hand, most studies indicate that myotomy does not completely abolish the UES resting tone recorded on manometry [13]. Outcomes of cricopharyngeal myotomy tend to be poor when significant pharyngeal weakness is also present.

Cricopharyngismus

The normal response of the UES to gastroesophageal reflux of air is a relaxation, which serves to allow venting of air from the upper digestive tract. This "belch reflex" can also be triggered by abrupt distension of the esophageal lumen with air [14]. The duration of this UES relaxation is longer than that observed during deglutition. In part, this may be because action of the thyrohyoid muscle serves to pull the UES open during belching [15]. Because the CP muscle receive higher cortical input, these stereotypic motor responses can be modified. For example, some subjects exhibit occasional "anticipatory" UES relaxations that precede the actual reflux of air into the esophagus [16]. Indeed, when healthy volunteers are asked to refrain from belching during esophageal air distension, they can change the UES relaxation response to one of UES contraction and avoid air venting [17]. In a few subjects examined with concurrent manometry and videofluoroscopy, this author has observed that during such belch blockade the normal anterior excursion of the hyoid is also inhibited.

I have coined the term "cricopharyngismus" for this altered UES response to esophageal air distension. This is analogous to the term anismus, which is used to denote the inappropriate contraction of the anal sphincter during defecation in patients with outlet obstruction constipation. All studies of this phenomenon have been with manometry, rather than direct EMG recordings from the CP muscle. Deglutitive UES relaxation is in the majority reported cases completely normal. Cricopharyngismus might be of utility in situations where the sound of eructation might cause social embarrassment. However, there are two rare situations in which this motor response is associated with troublesome and potentially life-threatening consequences.

Patients with achalasia of the lower esophageal sphincter have been found to have an abnormality of the UES relaxation response to esophageal air distension [18]. This is either a failure to relax or a paradoxical contraction of the UES, at stimulus volumes that are perceived as a need to belch by the patients. Achalasia patients commonly have retained fluid in the esophagus, and disordered contractions in the esophageal body could lead to regurgitation of this fluid into the hypopharynx if the UES does not contract. In fact, the UES has been shown to exhibit repetitive contractions in response to repetitive pressure increases in the esophageal body in achalasia patients [19]. Presumably, an inability to discern whether a pressure increase is going to result in liquid reflux or gas eructation has lead most achalasia patients subconsciously to modify their UES belch reflux, although this is by no means certain.

The problem with this modification for achalasia patients is that rarely it can contribute to acute airway obstruction. In such cases, air swallowing without eructation leads to tense distension of the esophageal lumen. This can lead to tracheal compression. In some cases, the dilated esophageal lumen dissects into a space behind and above the CP, compressing and displacing the larynx anteriorly. Patients present with rapidly progressive respiratory distress, stridor, and respiratory arrest. Examination frequently shows a tense mass in the neck from the distended esophagus. Emergency endotracheal intubation may be necessary. Intubating the esophagus usually results in a massive gush of air and fluid, with resolution of the respiratory distress. When it has been evaluated, the UES belch reflex in achalasia patients with such airway obstruction has been abnormal [20–22].

A less dramatic, but still troublesome, manifestation of cricopharyngismus is chest pain. In this situation, air refluxed up from the stomach rises to the upper esophagus and becomes trapped when the UES does not relax. The resulting esophageal distension results in chest pain severe enough to affect quality of life [23]. There may be an additional component of visceral hypersensitivity, as patients with noncardiac chest pain and an impaired UES relaxation response to air distension are more likely to have their chest pain provoked by esophageal balloon distension [24]. At least one patient with inability to belch but without associated chest pain has been reported [25]. The rare cases reported with this condition have related long-standing inability to belch.

A presumptive diagnosis of the condition can be made on videofluoroscopy following ingestion of gas-forming solutions. Air can be observed to reflux into the upper esophagus and remain there, until cleared by primary or secondary peristalsis (often to immediately reflux again). This gaseous distension reproduces the typical symptoms. Definitive diagnosis is demonstrated by manometry of the UES, showing impaired relaxation of the UES to esophageal air distension, which reproduces the typical pain. Treatment is problematic at this time. Passage of a nasoesophageal tube can vent the trapped gas and relieve the pain acutely, but this is an unacceptable chronic solution for patients. Helpful dietary and lifestyle modifications include avoidance of carbonated beverages and assuming a recumbent position in the immediate postprandial period (to decrease the frequency of the transient lower esophageal sphincter relaxations responsible for most gastroesophageal gas reflux).

Cricopharyngeal Hypertonicity

Essentially all of the data on purported CP muscle hypertonicity have been based on the finding of elevated UES pressures on manometry; there are no studies describing abnormal resting EMG activation. What constitutes abnormal elevation in UES pressure remains controversial because of a lack of standardization in recording technique and variations in normal values across the age spectrum. Moreover, the normal vigorous contractile responses of the CP muscle to multiple different stimuli and changes in cognitive/emotional states require careful control for the presence of these factors before one can conclude that any elevated UES pressure recording reflects the true "resting state" of muscle activity.

Despite the above caveats, some patients undergoing manometric evaluation of cervical symptoms truly seem to have striking elevations of inter-deglutitive UES pressure above the norm. In addition to elevations in the "resting" state, exaggerated responses to changes in intraluminal esophageal pressure can be seen (Fig. 37.3a, b). Deglutitive relaxation can be completely normal. The etiology of these elevated pressures remains largely obscure. In this author's experience, a few subjects undergoing EMG evaluation have had evidence for myotonia or myopathy. Whether hypertonicity could also reflect a response to active inflammation or a form of upper motor neuron syndrome of the CP muscle remains unknown.

There is no consistent set of symptoms or findings that indicate the presence of CP muscle hypertonicity. Some studies in patients with globus sensation have found that a portion of these exhibit either an increased resting UES tone [26], or an exaggerated UES phasic response to respiration [27]. Patients with globus sensation elevate their basal UES pressure in response to acute stress, but no more so than do normal subjects [28]. Such elevation does not reproduce the globus symptom. Again, deglutitive relaxation of the UES has appeared normal. It is possible that the elevated cricopharyngeal tone in some patients with globus simply represents a marker for the presence of another neuropathic disorder, rather than a causative feature of the symptom. While some studies have suggested that cricopharyngeal hypertonicity can cause dysphagia, these have either assumed the presence of hypertonicity based on videofluoroscopic findings and/or have not reliably excluded abnormal deglutitive relaxation as the actual cause for the dysphagia.

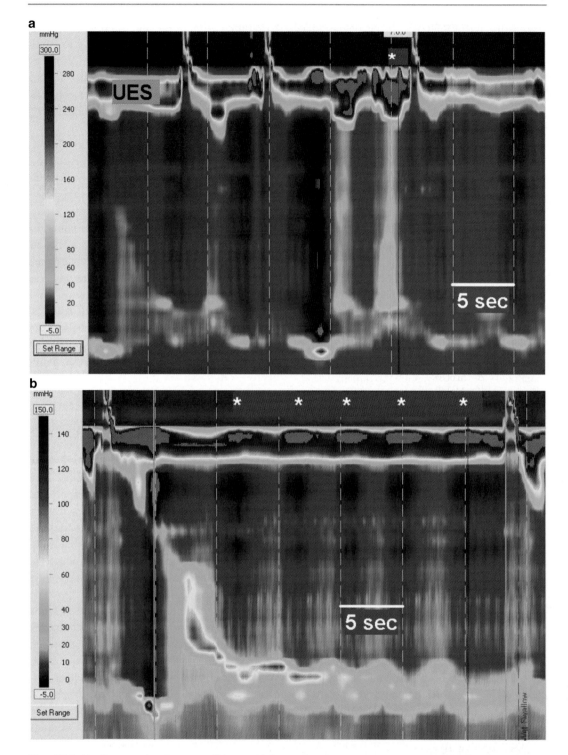

Fig. 37.3 (**a**) Contour plot from a solid-state high-resolution manometry study in a patient with a hypertonic upper esophageal sphincter (UES). Baseline upper esophageal sphincter (UES) pressure exceeds 150 mmHg, but during a tertiary contraction in the esophageal body, pressures increase to over 500 mmHg (*). Deglutitive UES relaxations appear normal. The spontaneous dry swallows observed do not trigger a peristaltic wave in the esophageal body. (**b**) Same patient as in **a**, although patient is recumbent. UES shows striking (up to 300 mmHg) pressure elevations with inspiration (*)

References

1. Knuff DA, Kounev VJ, Lawal A, Hogan WJ, Shaker R, Massey BT. Abnormal UES deglutitive function is improved with water swallows compared to that seen with dry swallows. Dysphagia. 2006;21:297.

2. Halum SL, Merati AL, Kulpa JI, Danielson SK, Jaradeh SS, Toohill RJ. Videofluoroscopic swallow studies in unilateral cricopharyngeal dysfunction. Laryngoscope. 2003;113:981–4.

3. Olsson R, Castell JA, Castell DO, Ekberg O. Solid-state computerized manometry improves diagnostic yield in pharyngeal dysphagia: simultaneous videoradiography and manometry in dysphagia patients with normal barium swallows. Abdom Imaging. 1995;20:230–5.

4. Kounev V, Knuff DA, Lawal A, Hogan WJ, Shaker R, Massey BT. Radiographic swallow studies are insensitive in the detection of upper esophageal sphincter dysfunction. Dysphagia. 2007;22:399.

5. Knuff DA, Hogan WJ, Shaker R, Massey BT. Esophageal motor disturbances are common in patients with UES dysfunction. Dysphagia. 2006;21:314.

6. de Leon A, Thörn SE, Wattwil M. High-resolution solid-state manometry of the upper and lower esophageal sphincters during anesthesia induction: a comparison between obese and non-obese patients. Anesth Analg. 2010;111:149–53.

7. Shemirani NL, Halum SL, Merati AL, Toohill RJ, Jaradeh S. Cricopharyngeal electromyography: patterns of injury based on etiology. Otolaryngol Head Neck Surg. 2007;137:792–7.

8. Shaker R, Easterling C, Kern M, Nitschke T, Massey B, Daniels S, Grande B, Kazandjian M, Kikeman K. Rehabilitation of swallowing by exercise in tube-fed patient with dysphagia secondary to abnormal UES Opening. Gastroenterology. 2002;122:1314–21.

9. Mepani R, Antonik S, Massey B, Kern M, Logemann J, Pauloski B, Rademaker A, Easterling C, Shaker R. Augmentation of deglutitive thyrohyoid muscle shortening by the Shaker exercise. Dysphagia. 2009;24:26–31.

10. Hatlebakk JG, Castell JA, Spiegel J, Paoletti V, Katz PO, Castell DO. Dilatation therapy for dysphagia in patients with upper esophageal sphincter dysfunction–manometric and symptomatic response. Dis Esophagus. 1998;11:254–9.

11. Moerman MB. Cricopharyngeal Botox injection: indications and technique. Curr Opin Otolaryngol Head Neck Surg. 2006;14(6):431–6.

12. Williams RB, Ali GN, Hunt DR, Wallace KL, Cook IJ. Cricopharyngeal myotomy does not increase the risk of esophagopharyngeal acid regurgitation. Am J Gastroenterol. 1999;94:3448–54.

13. Shaw DW, Cook IJ, Jamieson GG, et al. Influence of surgery on deglutitive upper esophageal sphincter mechanics in Zenker's diverticulum. Gut. 1996;38:806–11.

14. Kahrilas PJ, Dodds WJ, Dent J, Wyman JB, Hogan WJ, Arndorfer RC. Upper esophageal sphincter function during belching. Gastroenterology. 1986;91:133–40.

15. Shaker R, Ren J, Kern M, Dodds WJ, Hogan WJ, Li Q. Mechanisms of airway protection and upper esophageal sphincter opening during belching. Am J Physiol. 1992;262(4 Pt 1):G621–8.

16. Pandolfino JE, Ghosh SK, Zhang Q, Han A, Kahrilas PJ. Upper sphincter function during transient lower oesophageal sphincter relaxation (tLOSR); it is mainly about microburps. Neurogastroenterol Motil. 2007;19:203–10.

17. Massey BT, Hogan WJ, Dantas RO, Arndorfer RC, Dodds WJ. Conscious suppression of the upper esophageal sphincter belch reflex in normal volunteers. Gastroenterology. 1990;98:A373.

18. Massey BT, Hogan WJ, Dodds WJ, Dantas RO. Alteration of the upper esophageal sphincter belch reflex in patients with achalasia. Gastroenterology. 1992;103:1574–9.

19. Zhang ZG, Diamant NE. Repetitive contractions of the upper esophageal body and sphincter in achalasia. Dysphagia. 1994;9:12–9.

20. Becker DJ, Castell DO. Acute airway obstruction in achalasia. Possible role of defective belch reflex. Gastroenterology. 1989;97:1323–6.

21. Ali GN, Hunt DR, Jorgensen JO, deCarle DJ, Cook IJ. Esophageal achalasia and coexistent upper esophageal sphincter relaxation disorder presenting with airway obstruction. Gastroenterology. 1995;109:1328–32.

22. Arcos E, Medina C, Mearin F, Larish J, Guarner L, Malagelada JR. Achalasia presenting as acute airway obstruction. Dig Dis Sci. 2000;45:2079–83.

23. Kahrilas PJ, Dodds WJ, Hogan WJ. Dysfunction of the belch reflex. A cause of incapacitating chest pain. Gastroenterology. 1987;93:818–22.

24. Gignoux C, Bost R, Hostein J, Turberg Y, Denis P, Cohard M, Wolf JE, Fournet J. Role of upper esophageal reflex and belch reflex dysfunctions in noncardiac chest pain. Dig Dis Sci. 1993;38:1909–14.

25. Tomizawa M, Kusano M, Aoki T, Ohashi S, Kawamura O, Sekiguchi T, Mori M. A case of inability to belch. J Gastroenterol Hepatol. 2001;16:349–51.

26. Corso MJ, Pursnani KG, Mohiuddin MA, Gideon RM, Castell JA, Katzka DA, Katz PO, Castell DO. Globus sensation is associated with hypertensive upper esophageal sphincter but not with gastroesophageal reflux. Dig Dis Sci. 1998;43:1513–7.

27. Kwiatek MA, Mirza F, Kahrilas PJ, Pandolfino JE. Hyperdynamic upper esophageal sphincter pressure: a manometric observation in patients reporting globus sensation. Am J Gastroenterol. 2009;104:289–98.

28. Cook IJ, Dent J, Collins SM. Upper esophageal sphincter tone and reactivity to stress in patients with a history of globus sensation. Dig Dis Sci. 1989;34:672–6.

UES Opening Muscle Dysfunction

38

Caryn Easterling and Reza Shaker

Abstract

The upper esophageal sphincter (UES) is composed of the cricopharyngeus (CP), the inferior pharyngeal constrictor (IPC), and the most proximal segment of the esophagus and maintains a high pressure zone between pharynx and esophagus. UES opening mechanism during deglutition is multifactorial and includes the combination of neural relaxation of tonically contracted crycopharyngeus muscle, traction forces imparted by the suprahyoid (SH) UES opening muscles, intrabolus pressure generated by the oncoming bolus, and distensibility of the UES musculature [1, 2]. Each of the aforementioned factors involved in UES opening can potentially be modified to compensate for deficiency of others in a compensated state allowing complete pharyngeal clearance; failing to do so results in an uncompensated state, diminished deglutitive UES opening resulting in incomplete pharyngeal clearance, and postdeglutitive residue and potentially postdeglutitive aspiration.

While the end result of this complex mechanism namely UES opening in health and disease has been extensively studied, the relative contribution of each of the components of this mechanism has received less and variable attention. Abnormal UES opening can be classified as *primary*, namely those due to (1) lack of neural relaxation and (2) abnormal UES distensibility, or it can be *secondary* namely due to inadequate traction forces imparted on the sphincter by the contraction of SH muscles. This chapter focuses on the latter topic.

C. Easterling, Ph.D.
Department of Communication Sciences and Disorders,
University of Wisconsin-Milwaukee, 2400 East Hartford
Avenue, Milwaukee, WI 53201-0413, USA

R. Shaker, M.D. (✉)
Division of Gastroenterology and Hepatology,
Digestive Disease Center, Clinical and Translational
Science Institute, Medical College of Wisconsin,
9200 W. Wisconsin Ave, Milwaukee, WI 53226, USA
e-mail: rshaker@mcw.edu

R. Shaker et al. (eds.), *Principles of Deglutition: A Multidisciplinary Text for Swallowing and its Disorders*,
DOI 10.1007/978-1-4614-3794-9_38, © Springer Science+Business Media New York 2013

Keywords

Secondary dysfunction • UES opening • Muscle dysfunction • Diminished UES deglutitive opening diameter • Weakened suprahyoid muscles • UES traction forces

Anatomy and Physiology of UES Opening Muscles

Contribution of the hyoid superior and anterior movement to the opening of UES has been long recognized [1–3]. Significance of this recognition is in the implied role of the SH muscles in the opening of the UES. These UES opening muscles include those located superior and inferior to the hyoid bone. The superior hyoid group includes the geniohyoideus, mylohyoideus, stylohyoideus, hyogolossus, and anterior belly of the digastricus. As indicated by their name, the superior or SH muscles originate in locations superior to the hyoid bone and insert to its superior aspect [4]. As these muscles contract, the hyoid bone moves superiorly and anteriorly [1–3]. The anterior digastric and geniohyoid muscles are innervated by cranial nerves V and XII, while the posterior digastric and stylohyoid muscles are innervated by cranial nerve VII. The muscles inferior to the hyoid include the thyrohyoideus, sternohyoideus, sternothyroideus, and omohyoideus. The thyrohyoideus originates at the thyroid cartilage, the strenohyoideus originates from the clavicle and manubrium, the sternothyroideus originates from the manubrium and upper vertebrae, and the omohyoideus from the scapula. All of these muscles insert at the inferior portion of the hyoid bone [4]. As the inferior muscles contract they pull the hyoid bone and thyroid cartilage inferior and anterior. The action of these muscles located anterior to the UES is primarily to move the hyoid bone. The thyrohyoideus muscle forms the connection between the hyoid and larynx. As the anterior muscles simultaneously contract, the result is movement or excursion of the hyoid bone and larynx in the anterior plane.

Another muscle contributing to deglutitive UES opening is the thyrohyoid muscle. By contracting during swallowing, it locks the thyroid and hyoid together allowing transfer of force induced by contraction of SH muscles to the cricoid cartilage and CP muscle [5]. Studies have shown that thyrohyoid shortening can be augmented by strengthening the thyrohyoid muscles using rehabilitative exercises such as the Shaker Exercise [6].

The relative contribution of these muscles to UES opening during deglutition varies and has not been systematically studied. However it has been shown that SH muscle contraction is modified by oropharyngeal sensory signals induced by the volume of the swallowed bolus. This modification is evidenced by direct relationship of the extent of hyoid excursion with the volume of swallowed bolus [2, 3].

The SH and infrahyoid (IH) muscles are recruited differently during various functions involving the UES [7]. For example, concurrent videofluoroscopic and manometric studies have shown that the hyoid bone exhibits a characteristic movement pattern during belching that is different from its movement during swallowing [8]. The hyoid bone moves clockwise on an anteriorly oriented elongated loop during belching. The longer axis of the loop ranges between 0.3 and 0.8 cm, and its short axis ranges between 0.05 and 0.1 cm. The excursion loop oriented only anteriorly in the majority of study subjects (Fig. 38.1a). The duration of hyoid bone movement during a belch averaged 1.2 ± 0.12 s [3]. The movement duration was significantly shorter than the duration of hyoid bone movement ($2.1 + 0.08$ s) during swallowing ($P < 0.01$). The distinctly different excursion pattern of the hyoid bone suggests that muscles from both the SH and IH muscle groups are involved in the belch reflex, and the direction of the hyoid bone movement is

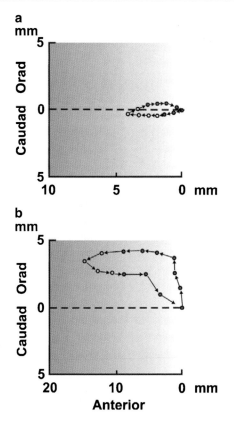

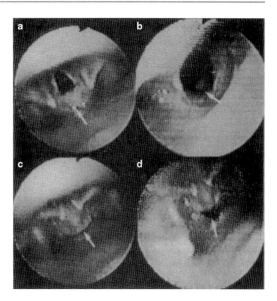

Fig. 38.2 Comparison of UES opening during belching and swallowing. (**a**) Endoscopic view of glottis and hypopharynx at rest. Area of UES opening is shown by arrow; (**b**) oval/round UES opening during swallowing; (**c**) slit-like UES opening during belching; (**d**) triangular UES opening during belching. Although shape of UES opening during belching could vary between slit-like and triangular, its shape during swallowing was oval/round. From Shaker et al. Am J Physiol 1992;262:G621–8 with permission

Fig. 38.1 Direction and orbit of hyoid bone movement during belching (**a**) and swallowing (**b**). *Open circles* indicate UES opening observed by videofluoroscopy (note difference in scales). Although hyoid bone movement during swallowing was invariably upward-forward and counterclockwise, its movement during belching was mainly anterior and clockwise. Magnitude of hyoid bone movement during belching was significantly less than its movement during swallowing ($P<0.01$). From Shaker et al. Am J Physiol 1992;262:G621–8 with permission

determined by the final vector of force that results from the summation of the opposing forces of these contracting muscle groups during belching. In contrast, the hyoid bone movement pattern during swallowing is directed superiorly and anteriorly and follows an alpha-shaped, counter-clockwise loop (Fig. 38.1b). Anterior excursion of hyoid bone during swallowing averaged 1.8 ± 0.9 cm and was significantly more than its excursion of 0.78 ± 0.1 cm during belching [8].

These findings indicate the pivotal role of the SH and IH muscles in UES opening other than during swallowing. They also indicate a modification of the contraction duration, magnitude,

and involvement for different members of a given muscle group depending on the specific function and related sensory input (Fig. 38.2). The sum force vector of SH and IH muscle contractions influences the shape, duration, and magnitude of UES opening. As seen in Fig. 38.1, UES opening occurs at the apogee of hyoid excursion. There is also a direct relationship between the magnitude of anterior excursion of the hyolaryngeal complex and UES opening [2, 3].

The stylopharyngeus, palatopharyngeus, pterygopharyngeus, and other superiorly and posteriorly located pharyngeal muscles make up the posterior UES opening muscles. The actions of these posterior muscles are to elevate and stabilize the posterior wall of the pharynx [4].

UES Relaxation Versus Opening

As stated earlier, successful deglutitive UES opening that results in efficient bolus transport from the pharynx through the UES and into the

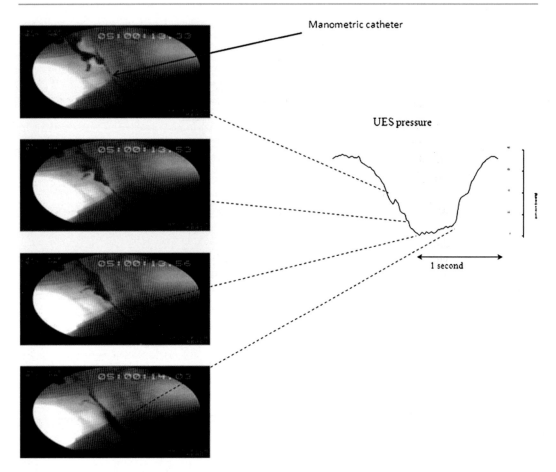

Fig. 38.3 Concurrent manometric and videofluoroscopic recording during a 5 mL barium swallow manometric relaxation is seen as a precipitous drop in pressure demonstrated in the manometric recording on the *right*. Still frames from concurrent fluoroscopic recording are shown on the *left*. Manometric recording catheter with recording sites at 1.5 cm intervals is visible in the pharynx, across the UES, and esophagus. As seen the drop in UES pressure precedes the opening of the sphincter manifested by flow of the barium bolus through the UES. While relaxation of the UES is a neural phenomenon, its opening is due to traction forces imparted on the sphincter by contraction of suprahyoid muscles

esophagus is dependent upon the following four conditions: (a) relaxation of the tonically contracted UES; (b) distraction of the sphincter as a result of the external traction forces generated by supra-hyoid muscles. This external traction results in anterior hyolaryngeal excursion and by virtue of anatomical attachment induces UES opening in anteroposterior plane during swallowing; (c) the distensibility namely the muscle property that allows the UES to stretch and accommodate the bolus passage; and (d) the distending effect of oncoming bolus and its intrabolus pressure.

During swallowing, relaxation of the UES takes place prior to the clinician's visual recognition or the radiographic documentation of the deglutitive opening of the sphincter (Fig. 38.3). Sphincter relaxation occurs during superior laryngeal excursion and occurs before opening by an average of 0.1 s. A precipitous drop in UES tone can be appreciated as a decrease in manometrically measured luminal pressure prior to the arrival of the bolus at the sphincteric segment [2, 5, 9].

Finally, intrabolus pressure namely the pressure within the fluid bolus also contributes to the UES opening. Intrabolus pressure can be measured by a manometric catheter as the bolus covers the pressure sensor. As the bolus traverses the UES, intrabolus pressure is a measure of the force required to push the fluid bolus through the open sphincter and reflects the resistance to trans-sphincteric flow [2, 5, 9].

Diminished UES Deglutitive Opening Diameter in Healthy Elderly Adults: Weakened SH Muscles or UES Traction Forces

Until recently, diminished hyolaryngeal excursion associated with decreased UES opening was mostly considered a consequence of neurologic abnormalities. Combination of advancing age and decreased physical activity can result in weakening of striated muscles. Exercise, specifically, isometric and isokinetic exercise have been shown to reverse sarcopenic changes in striated muscles of the limbs in the elderly. With regular exercise, physiologic change occurs including muscle hypertrophy, an increase in myofibrils and myosin concentration as well as changes in capillary density and an increase in connective tissue. The benefit of strengthening exercise is appreciated as cellular changes, which are then reflected in functional increase in muscular power and strength. Exercising the muscles of swallowing, specifically the SH muscles, is reasonable as they are striated muscles and will benefit from strengthening exercise. Improved strengthening of this muscle group will result in improved traction force and thus improved deglutitive function. This is the basis for the Shaker Exercise.

Alterations in the deglutitive UES opening can occur as an effect of aging [10]. If alterations or changes occur in deglutitive UES opening mechanisms, deglutitive failure or disorders may occur. The traction force although an important opening mechanism, the other three elements described above are primary to the intrinsic qualities of the muscles that make up the sphincter. The traction or distraction forces are important opening mechanisms but are described as secondary because they are extra-sphincteric, that is beyond the direct muscular or neural properties

of the sphincter yet as important to the success or failure of the UES in deglutitive function.

Shaw and colleagues found that deglutitive UES compliance diminished with healthy aging resulting in increased intrabolus pressure and resistance to flow through the sphincter [11]. Disruption or weakening of the SH muscles or traction forces was thought to be the contributing cause of significantly decreased anteroposterior deglutitive UES opening diameter in healthy older adults compared to young adults [7, 10]. In a placebo-controlled study the effect of performance of a head lift exercise, also known as the Shaker Exercise, for 6 weeks was found to increase anterior deglutitive hyoid and laryngeal excursion, resulting in significantly increased anteroposterior deglutitive UES opening diameter in healthy older adults compared to young adults [7].

It was hypothesized that the Shaker Exercise could be rehabilitative in those dysphagic patients with secondary UES failure from weakened SH muscles contributing to diminished traction forces as identified through videofluoroscopic evaluation and characterized by diminished anteroposterior deglutitive UES opening diameter, postdeglutitive residuals, and postdeglutitive aspiration. The initial study found improved anterior hyolaryngeal excursion, decreased incidence of aspiration, and increased anteroposterior UES opening diameter after completion of 6 weeks of Shaker Exercise in a small group of patients with abnormal UES opening, postdeglutitive aspiration, and dependent on nonoral nutritional support [12]. Thus strengthening of the SH muscles was thought to diminish the incidence of postdeglutitive aspiration and postdeglutitive residual and improve anteroposterior deglutitive UES opening diameter.

Although the effectiveness of the Shaker Exercise in increasing UES opening during swallowing was demonstrated through manometric and videofluoroscopic studies in healthy elderly and a group of dysphagic patients, the muscle group strengthened by the exercise had not been confirmed. The preliminary studies, utilizing surface electromyography (sEMG) to evaluate the specific muscles strengthened by exercise, used spectral analysis to measure muscle fatigue of the

UES opening muscles [13–15]. A study by Ferdjallah and colleagues evaluated and quantified the sEMG activities from the SH, IH, and sterno-cleidomastoid (SCM) muscle groups in healthy adult controls during the isometric portion of the Shaker Exercise. The results of the spectral analysis showed that all three muscle groups showed fatigue from the 60 s isometric portion of the exercise indicating muscle strengthening. The SCM showed a higher rate of fatigue than the SH or IH muscle groups, indicating that the SCM may limit exercise as the appreciation of fatigue in the SCM prior to elicitation of fatigue and thus strengthening in the target SH group [16].

Diminished UES Deglutitive Opening Diameter in Dysphagic Patients: Weakened SH Muscles or UES Traction Forces

Volitional augmentation of UES opening has been described using the Mendelsohn Manuever, a maneuver requiring purposeful prolongation of the superior and anterior displacement of the larynx at midswallow. This purposeful prolongation results in increased duration of the anterior–superior hyolaryngeal excursion and thus maintenance of the applied traction forces. The prolongation of traction force to UES function allows for prolonged duration and extent of UES deglutitive opening [17]. The SH muscle strengthening effect of this exercise or maneuver has not been systematically studied or verified.

The Shaker Exercise, a 6-week isometric and isokinetic regimen, has been shown to strengthen the SH and the thyrohyoid muscles resulting in a significant increase in deglutitive anterior laryngeal excursion and anteroposterior deglutitive UES opening diameter in healthy older adults while decreasing the incidence of postdeglutitive aspiration and pharyngeal residual in patients with secondary UES failure due to decreased traction force. The patients included in the studies were able to discontinue feeding tube use after completion of the strengthening exercise [18].

Currently the Shaker Exercise and other rehabilitative exercises are used clinically to rehabilitate the secondary causes of abnormal UES opening, that is, dysfunction of SH UES opening muscles.

References

1. Kahrilas PJ, Dodds WJ, Dent J, Logemann JA, Shaker R. Upper esophageal sphincter function during deglutition. Gastroenterology. 1988;95(1):52–62.
2. Cook IJ, Dodds WJ, Dantas RO, Massey B, Kern M, Lang IM, Brasseur J, Hogan WJ. Opening mechanisms of the upper esophageal sphincter. Am J Physiol. 1989;257:G748–59.
3. Dodds WJ, Man KM, Cook IJ, Kahrilas PJ, Stewart ET, Kern MK. Influence of bolus volume on swallow-induced hyoid movement in normal subjects. Am J Roentgenol. 1988;150:1307–9.
4. Gray H, Goss CM. Anatomy of the human body. Philadelphia: Lea & Febiger; 1968.
5. Cook IJ, Dodds WJ, Dantas RO, Kern MK, Massey BT, Shaker R, et al. Timing of videofluoroscopic, manometric events and bolus transit during the oral and pharyngeal phases of swallowing. Am J Physiol Gastrointest Liver Physiol. 2003;284(6):G933–9.
6. Mepani R, Antonik S, Massey B, Kern M, Logemann J, Pauloski B, Rademaker A, Easterling C, Shaker R. Augmentation of deglutitive thyrohyoid muscle shortening by the Shaker Exercise. Dysphagia. 2009; 24(1):26–31.
7. Shaker R, Kern M, Bardan E, Taylor A, Stewart ET, Hoffman RG, Arndorfer RC, Hofman C, Bonnevier J. Augmentation of deglutitive upper esophageal sphincter opening in the elderly by exercise. Am J Physiol. 1997;272:G1518–22.
8. Kahrilas PJ, Dodds WJ, Dent J, Wyman JB, Hogan WJ, Arndorfer RC. Upper esophageal sphincter function during belching. Gastroenterology. 1986;91:133–40.
9. McConnell FM, Cerendo D, Jackson RT, Guffin Jr TN. Timing of major events of pharyngeal swallowing. Arch Otolaryngol Head Neck Surg. 1988;114:1413–6.
10. Kern M, Shaker R, Arndorfer R, Hofmann C. The effect of aging on the cross sectional area of upper esophageal sphincter (UES) opening during swallowing. Gastroenterology. 1994;106:A613.
11. Shaw DW, Cook IJ, Gabb M, Holloway RH, Simula ME, Panagopoulos V, Dent J. Influence of normal aging on oral-pharyngeal and upper esophageal sphincter function during swallowing. Am J Physiol. 1995;31:G389–96.
12. Easterling C, Kern M, Nitschke T, Grande B, Daniels S, Cullen GM, Massey BT, Shaker R. Effect of a novel exercise on swallow function and biomechanics in tube fed cervical dysphagia patients: a preliminary report. Dysphagia. 1999;14:119.
13. Alfonso M, Ferdjallah M, Shaker R, Wertsch JJ. Electrophysiologic validation of deglutitive UES

opening head lift exercise. Gastroenterology. 1998; 114:G2942.

14. Jurell KC, Shaker R, Mazur A, Haig AJ, Wertsch JJ. Spectral analysis to evaluate hyoid muscles involvement in neck exercise. Muscle Nerve. 1996; 19:1224.

15. Jurell KC, Shaker R, Mazur A, Haig AJ, Wertsch JJ. Effect of exercise on upper esophageal sphincter opening muscles: a spectral analysis. Gastroenterology. 1997;112:A757.

16. Ferdjallah M, Wertsch JJ, Shaker R. Spectral analysis of surface electromyography (EMG) of upper esophageal sphincter opening muscles during head lift exercise. J Rehabil Res Dev. 2000;37:335–40.

17. Kahrilas PJ, Logemann JA, Krugler C, Flanagan E. Volitional augmentation of upper esophageal sphincter opening during swallowing. Am J Physiol. 1991;260:G450–6.

18. Shaker R, Easterling C, Kern M, Nitschke T, Massey B, Daniels S, Grande B, Kazandjian M, Dikeman K. Rehabilitation of swallowing by exercise in tube-fed patients with pharyngeal dysphagia secondary to abnormal UES opening. Gastroenterology. 2002; 122:1314–21.

Part X

Esophageal Phase Dysphagia: Motor Disorders

Achalasia and Ineffective Esophageal Motility

39

Joel E. Richter

Abstract

Achalasia and ineffective esophageal motility (IEM) represent the extreme ends of the spectrum of esophageal motility disorders. Achalasia is characterized by aperistalsis in the body of the esophagus and failure of LES relaxation. Patients present with dysphagia for solids and liquids, bland regurgitation, chest pain, and weight loss. The diagnosis is suggested by the barium esophagram and confirmed by manometry. The goal of therapy is to (1) relieve symptoms, (2) improve esophageal emptying by disrupting the poorly relaxing LES, and (3) prevent the development of megaesophagus. Surgical myotomy and pneumatic dilation are the most effective treatments for disrupting the LES gradient. Botulinum toxin and calcium channel blockers may be useful therapies in older patients or those with severe co-morbid illnesses. Ineffective esophageal peristalsis is characterized by the presence of distal esophageal contractions of very low amplitude (<30 mmHg) and/or non-transmitted contractions. It is the most common motility disorder in GERD patients, probably due to impaired cholinergic stimulation along the esophageal body. The diagnosis is best made with esophageal manometry combined with impedance testing to confirm poor bolus transit. Once established, IEM is not improved by acid-suppressive medications, most prokinetic drugs, or anti-reflux surgery.

Keywords

Achalasia • Pneumatic dilation • Surgical myotomy • Botulinum toxin • Calcium channel blockers • Impedance testing • Ineffective esophageal peristalsis

J.E. Richter, MD (✉)
Division of Digestive Diseases and Joy McCann
Culverhouse Swallowing Center, University of South
Florida, Tampa, FL, USA
e-mail: jrichte1@health.usf.edu

Achalasia is the most recognized motor disorder of the esophagus, and is the only primary motility disorder with an established pathophysiology. The term means "failure to relax," and describes the primary predominant feature of this disorder, a poorly relaxing lower esophageal sphincter (LES) seen in association with aperistalsis of the esophageal body. The first case of achalasia was reported more than 300 years ago by Thomas Willis; where the patient's cardiospasm responded to dilation with a whalebone [1].

Epidemiology and Pathophysiology

Achalasia occurs with equal frequency in men and women. There is no racial predilection. Case studies show an age distribution between birth and the ninth decade, with the peak incidence between 30 and 60 years of age. In children, it can be part of the Triple A syndrome, characterized by achalasia, alacrima, and adrenocorticotropic hormone-resistant adrenal insufficiency. Achalasia is an uncommon disease, but occurs frequently enough to be encountered at least yearly by most gastroenterologists. Esophageal specialists, both gastroenterologists and surgeons, may see ten or more cases a year [2]. The disease prevalence is approximately ten cases per 100,000 population. Its incidence has been fairly stable over the last 50 years at approximately 0.5 cases per 100,000 population per year. The overall life expectancy of patients with achalasia does not differ from those of the general population [3].

The histologic abnormalities in patients with achalasia have been well described at autopsy or from myotomy specimens [4, 5]. The primary region of damage is the esophageal myenteric (Auerbach's) plexus, and includes prominent but patchy inflammatory response, consisting of predominantly CD3- and CD8-positive cytotoxic T lymphocytes, variable numbers of eosinophils and mast cells, loss of ganglion cells, and some degree of myenteric neurofibrosis. Early disease has more of an inflammatory component, with some of the ganglion cells appearing to be intact, while end-stage disease is associated with complete loss of ganglion cells and replacement with myenteric fibrosis [5]. Even during the early inflammatory stages of achalasia, there is a selective loss of postganglionic inhibitory neurons containing nitric oxide and vasoactive intestinal polypeptide. Since postganglionic excitatory neurons are spared, cholinergic stimulation continues unopposed, leading sometimes to high resting LES pressure. The loss of inhibitory input results in abnormal and usually incomplete LES relaxation. This occurs for all stimuli, including electrical field stimulation of muscle strips from achalasia patients, intravenous cholecystokinin, esophageal distension, and gastric distension fail to induce transient LES relaxation in achalasia patients [6]. Aperistalsis is caused by the loss of the latency gradient that permits sequential contractions along the esophageal body, a process mediated by nitric oxide.

Although achalasia is the best characterized of the esophageal motility disorders, its pathogenesis is still not fully elucidated. Available data suggest that hereditary, degenerative, autoimmune, and infectious factors are possible causes—the latter two being the most commonly accepted [7]. The presence of cytotoxic T lymphocytes, IgM antibodies and evidence of complement activation and antibodies against myenteric neurons, especially in patients with specific HLA genotype (DQA1*0103, DQB1*0603 alleles), point toward an autoimmune origin of the myenteric ganglionitis [8]. However, some of these antineuronal antibodies may be seen in healthy patients and patients with GERD, suggesting they may represent an epiphenomenon, and not a causative factor [9]. Although these findings are all very interesting, it still remains obscure why only neurons in the esophagus and LES are destroyed. Furthermore, the exact stimulus initiating this immune response or the antigen targeted remains unidentified. The fact that achalasia is confined to the esophagus and LES has led to the hypotheses that neurotropic viruses, especially viruses with predilection for squamous epithelium, may be involved. However, studies focusing on the presence of viral antibodies in the serum or viral DNA in esophageal tissue show conflicting results [10, 11]. A recent study provided evidence that after HSV-1 infection, the virus persists in the neurons of the esophagus triggering a persistent immune-activation, consisting of infiltration of the ganglia with cytotoxic CD8 + T cells and circulating antineuronal antibodies [12].

Clinical Presentation

The diagnosis of achalasia should be suspected in any patients complaining of dysphagia for solids and liquids with regurgitation of bland food and saliva. The onset of the dysphagia is usually gradual, being described initially as an infrequent "fullness in the chest" or "sticking sensation," but usually occurs daily or with every meal by the time the patient sees a physician. Initially, the dysphagia may be primarily for solids; however, by the time of clinical presentation, nearly all complain of dysphagia for solids and liquids while eating and drinking, especially cold beverages. Various maneuvers, including "power swallows" and carbonated beverages, both of which increase intraesophageal pressure, may be used to improve esophageal emptying. Regurgitation becomes a problem with progression of the disease, especially when the esophagus becomes dilated. Regurgitation of bland, undigested retained foods or accumulated saliva, sometimes misdiagnosed as postnasal phlegm or bronchitis, occur postprandially and at night, often waking the patient from sleep because of coughing and choking. Rarely, aspiration pneumonia is a problem. Chest pain occurs in some patients, primarily at night, and is especially seen in patients with milder disease when the esophagus is minimally dilated. The mechanism of chest pain is unknown, but it is not simply repetitive episodes of simultaneous contractions, causing the esophageal lumen to be occluded. Whereas pneumatic dilation or surgery usually relieves dysphagia and regurgitation, the chest pain in achalasia patients responds much less predictably. Fortunately, the chest pain seems to get better over time, possibly as the esophagus dilates [13]. Heartburn is a frequent complaint in achalasia, despite the fact that achalasia is not associated with increased episodes of acid reflux by pH monitoring. The cause of this symptom is speculative, but probably related to retention of

acid beverages such as carbonated or fruit drinks and, in some cases, the production of lactic acid from retained food in a markedly dilated esophagus. Most achalasia patients have some degree of weight loss at presentation; however, the loss is usually only 5–20 lbs over months to years.

Diagnostic Evaluation

When achalasia is suspected, a barium esophagram with fluoroscopy is the best initial diagnostic test. The esophagus is usually dilated and sometimes tortuous, does not empty, and retained food and saliva produces an air–fluid level at the top of the barium column. The distal esophagus is characterized by a smooth tapering from the closed LES, resembling a bird's beak, and sometimes an epiphrenic diverticulum is noted (Fig. 39.1). Fluoroscopy always shows a lack of peristalsis, replaced by to-and-fro movement in the supine position. We have popularized a modification of the barium esophagram known as the timed barium swallow [14]. The test is individualized for each patient and primarily assesses esophageal emptying of barium in the upright position over 5 min. Tests can be repeated serially after therapy to evaluate esophageal emptying and correlate it with the patients' symptoms (Fig. 39.1).

Esophageal manometry is required to establish the diagnosis of achalasia and must be done in any patient where invasive treatments such as pneumatic dilation or surgical myotomy are planned. Because achalasia only involves the smooth muscles of the esophagus, the manometry abnormalities are confined to the distal two-thirds of the esophagus. All patients have at least two pathognomonic abnormalities: aperistalsis and abnormal LES relaxation. The aperistalsis is usually characterized by low amplitude, simultaneous mirror image (isobaric) waves, due to a common cavity phenomenon. Physiologically, the low amplitude waves (usually <30 mmHg) represent simultaneous fluid movement in a fluid-filled dilated esophagus, rather than true lumen occluding contractions. When pressure waves have a higher amplitude and different morphology, indicating active contractions of

a

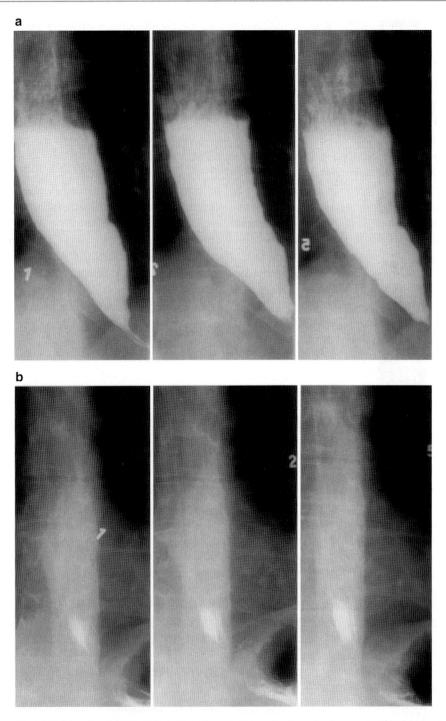

b

Fig. 39.1 Timed barium swallow. Barium is drunk rapidly over 1 min and esophageal emptying evaluated in the upright position over 5 min. A normal subject has all the barium out of the esophagus in 1 min. (**a**) Initial timed barium swallow in a 52-year-old woman with achalasia showing moderate esophageal dilation, bird-beaking, and essentially no emptying over 5 min. (**b**) Using similar amounts of barium to initial study, timed barium swallow was repeated 6 weeks after pneumatic dilation with 3.0 cm Rigiflex balloon. Barium study shows prompt esophageal emptying with decrease in esophageal dilation. This striking improvement paralleled the total resolution of the symptoms of dysphagia and regurgitation. Follow-up symptoms and barium X-rays over the last 7 years show the patient is still doing well

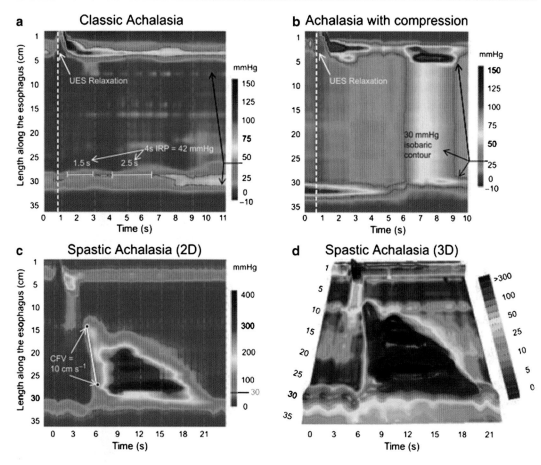

Fig. 39.2 Achalasia subtypes by high-resolution manometry: (**a**) type I (classic achalasia)—there is no significant pressurization within the esophageal body (all dark blue) and impaired LES relaxation (IRP = 42 mmHg); (**b**) type II (achalasia with compression)—water swallows cause rapid pan-esophageal pressurization which may exceed LES pressure, causing the esophagus to empty; (**c**) type III (spastic achalasia)—although this is also associated with rapidly propagated pressurization, the pressurization is attributable to an abnormal lumen obliterating contraction. From J. E. Pandolfino et al. Neurogastroenterol Motil 2009;21:796–806 with permission

the esophageal body, it is called "vigorous" achalasia. Abnormal LES relaxation is seen in all achalasia patients; about 70–80% have absent or incomplete LES relaxation with wet swallows, while the remainder will have complete but shortened LES relaxation (<6 s). LES resting pressure may be elevated in approximately 50% of patients with achalasia. Sometimes, an increase in the esophageal baseline greater than gastric baseline is seen due to retention of food and saliva.

The recent introduction of high-resolution manometry has greatly helped in making the diagnosis of achalasia [15, 16]. It allows a more careful evaluation of LES and esophagogastric junction relaxation using the integrated relaxation pressure (IRP). As reported by the Northwestern group in a series of achalasia patients [15], the traditional LES nadir pressure had a false-negative rate of 48%, while an IRP >15 mmHg was seen in all but 3% of achalasia patients. The group also described three patterns of achalasia: type I (classical achalasia: impaired relaxation with esophageal dilation and negligible esophageal pressurization), type II (pan-esophageal pressurization), and type III (vigorous achalasia with spastic contractions of the distal esophageal segment) [16] (Fig. 39.2).

Although most cases are idiopathic, it should be noted that Chagasic achalasia and pseudoachalasia may lead to a similar picture. Chagas' disease is endemic in Central and South America as a consequence of an infection with the parasite *Trypanosoma cruzi*. Ganglion cells are destroyed throughout the body, resulting in megaesophagus, megaduodenum, megacolon and rectum in addition to cardiac involvement, the leading cause of death in Chagas' patients [18]. Approximately 2–4% of patients suspected with achalasia suffer from pseudoachalasia [19]. In general, patients with pseudoachalasia are older and have a shorter history of dysphagia and marked weight loss. However, this triad tends to have poor specificity [20]. The most common cause of pseudoachalasia is a malignancy infiltrating the gastroesophageal junction. Therefore, all patients with suspected achalasia need a careful upper endoscopy with close examination of the cardia and gastroesophageal junction. If pseudoachalasia is still suspected, endoscopic ultrasound with a small 20 mHz probe or CT scanning of the chest may be helpful.

Although the symptoms of achalasia are relatively classic, and the diagnostic tests, especially barium X-rays and manometry, readily available, there is still a considerable delay between the onset of symptoms and the diagnosis. In one report, patients on average reported symptoms of dysphagia for approximately 5 years and had seen several physicians before the correct diagnosis was made. Interestingly, the frequent delay in the diagnosis was not due to an atypical clinical presentation of the disease, but rather to misinterpretation of typical findings by the physician consulted [21].

Treatment of Achalasia

No treatment can restore muscular activity to the denervated esophagus in achalasia. Esophageal aperistalsis and impaired LES relaxation are rarely, if ever, reversed by any mode of therapy. Therefore, every treatment for achalasia is directed to reducing the pressure gradient across the LES with three goals of (1) relieving patients' symptoms, especially dysphagia and bland regurgitation; (2) improving esophageal emptying by

disrupting the poorly relaxing LES; and (3) preventing the development of megaesophagus.

The disruption of the LES gradient is best accomplished by pneumatic dilation or surgical myotomy and, less effectively, by pharmacologic agents, such as botulinum toxin or calcium channel blockers. Symptoms of regurgitation and dysphagia are the easiest to treat, but chest pain is more unpredictable [13]. Overall, using single or multiple modalities of treatment, over 90% of achalasia patients will do well [22]. However, achalasia is never "cured" and touch-up therapies after pneumatic dilation or Heller myotomies are often needed with higher recurrence rates with longer periods of follow-up. Therefore, I recommend that all achalasia patients be followed up every 1–2 years by a gastroenterologist or surgeon familiar with the disease. In my experience, the timed barium swallow is very helpful in following these patients [23]; however, my colleagues in Europe prefer to do serial measurements of LES pressure [24, 25].

Pneumatic Dilation

Pneumatic dilation aims at disrupting the LES by forceful dilation using air-filled balloons. This procedure has become standardized with the Microvasive Rigiflex balloon system (Boston Scientific Corporation, MA, USA). These noncompliant polyethylene balloons are available in three diameters (3.0, 3.5, and 4.0 cm), on a flexible catheter placed over a guidewire at endoscopy. The catheter within the balloon has radiopaque markers, which can help identify its location at fluoroscopy. Briefly, pneumatic dilation is performed at the time of endoscopy, with the balloon placed over the guidewire and positioned across the LES. Position is confirmed either by fluoroscopy or endoscopy. The actual balloon distention protocol varies across centers (Table 39.1) [26]. Generally the balloon is gradually inflated until the waist, caused by the nonrelaxing LES, is flattened or effaced. The pressure required is usually 7–15 psi of air, held for 15–60 s. Sometimes multiple balloon distensions are done at the same setting. Some investigators

Table 39.1 General techniques for pneumatic dilation using Rigiflex balloon [26]

1. Every patient should be on a liquid diet for several days and fasting at least 12 h before endoscopy. Patients with megaesophagus may require esophageal lavage with a large bore tube.
2. Generally done as an outpatient in the morning. This ensures that appropriate X-rays and clinical observation do not extend late into the evening, especially if surgical complications should occur.
3. Standard conscious sedation and upper endoscopy in the left lateral position.
4. Savary guidewire placed in the stomach and Rigiflex balloon passed over it.
5. The smallest balloon (3.0 cm) is usually used first. In patients with prior failed pneumatic dilations, young patients or after prior Heller myotomy, beginning with a 3.5 cm balloon may be preferred.
6. Accurate placement of the balloon by fluoroscopy with the patient in the supine position. Key is to carefully locate the balloon so the waist caused by the non-relaxing LES impinges on the middle portion. This is usually at or above the level of the diaphragm. In patients after Heller myotomy, the narrowing may be below the diaphragm.
7. Balloon is gradually distended until the waist, caused by the non-relaxing LES is flattened. The pressure required is usually 7–15 psi of air, held for 15–60 s.
8. Patient repositioned in the left lateral position to minimize aspiration and the balloon carefully removed after deflating.
9. Overall post-procedure observation for 4–6 h to exclude perforation and evaluate for chest pain and fever. Patient discharged to home after drinking fluids without difficulty. Patients with pain during this observation period should be sent for gastrograffin followed by barium swallow to exclude esophageal perforation.
10. Outpatient clinic follow-up in 2–4 weeks to assess symptoms and esophageal function, especially emptying. Tests should include upright timed barium swallow and/or esophageal manometry.
11. Persistent symptoms, especially if associated with poor esophageal emptying or an LES pressure above 10 mmHg warrants repeat dilation with the next larger size balloon. This sequence is completed until symptom relief or failure to respond to the 4.0 cm balloon, at which point the patient is usually referred to surgery.

Table 39.2 Long-term efficacy and complications of Rigiflex balloon dilation vs. Heller myotomy for achalasia

	Rigiflex balloon	Laparoscopic myotomy[a]
Number of studies	24	39
Number of patients	1,144	3,086
Excellent/good symptom response (%)	78%	89.3%
Follow-up (months)	37	35
Complications (%)	1.9% (perforation)	15% (gastroesophageal reflux)

[a]Surgical series with over ten patients

only perform one dilation [21], but most use a graded dilation protocol starting with 3.0 cm, followed by 3.5 cm and then 4.0 cm balloon, in subsequent sessions [27]. A few European centers perform serial progressive dilations over several days, until the manometrically measured LES pressure is below 10–15 mmHg [24, 25]. In the United States, the need for further dilations is determined by persistence of symptoms often correlated with esophageal emptying studies at 4- to 6-week intervals after treatment [22, 27]. Pneumatic dilation is now routinely done in outpatient centers, with the patient being observed for up to 6 h, to ensure that no complications have occurred. Some perform Gastrografin followed by barium swallows to exclude perforations; others do not recommend obtaining routine barium X-ray films unless clinically indicated.

Table 39.2 summarizes the good-to-excellent symptom relief with the Rigiflex balloons in 1,144 patients [28]. These 24 studies, with an average follow-up of 37 months, found that the clinical response improves in a graded fashion with increasing size of the balloon diameter—good-to-excellent response in 74%, 86%, and 90% with the 3.0, 3.5, and 4.0 balloons, respectively. Over a third of achalasia patients treated with pneumatic dilation will experience symptom recurrence during a 4- to 6-year period of follow-up [21, 22, 25, 28]. Long-term remission

Table 39.3 Pneumatic dilation: predictors of relapse

Related to patient
- Younger age (<40 years)
- Male gender
- Wide esophagus

Related to procedure
- Single dilation
- Small size balloon (<30 mm)
- Incomplete obliteration of the balloon's waist after pneumatic dilation
- LES pressure >10–15 mmHg
- Poor esophageal emptying on barium swallow post-treatment

Related to manometry
- Type I and III pattern on high-resolution manometry

can be achieved in virtually all of these patients treated by repeated pneumatic dilation according to an "on demand" strategy, based on symptom recurrence [29]. Therefore, in clinical practice, pneumatic dilation is a nonsurgical treatment that will require periodic "touch ups" over the life of the patient. Pneumatic dilation is the most cost-effective method for treating achalasia, when compared to Heller myotomy or botulinum toxin, over a time period of 5–10 years [30, 31].

With the standardization of the Rigiflex balloons, we are beginning to define the risk factors for relapse after pneumatic dilation (Table 39.3). These are mainly young age (<40 years), male gender, single dilation with a 3.0 cm balloon, post-treatment LES pressure >10–15 mmHg, and poor esophageal emptying on timed barium swallow. The effects of age on the success of pneumatic dilation are most reproducible from as far back as 1971, even with the older balloons [32]. For example, Eckhardt et al. [33], using a 4 cm Brown-McHardy dilator, demonstrated a 5-year remission rate of 16% for patients younger than 40 years, compared to 58% for those older than 40 years. Recent studies suggest young men do not do as well as young women with the pneumatic dilation. In a study of 126 patients, Ghoshal et al. [34] found that male gender, but not age, was independently associated with poor outcome after dilation. Another large study from the Cleveland Clinic (106 patients, 51 women) confirmed the importance of age but also found

gender to be equally important [35]. Men, up to age 50 years, did not do well with a single 3.0 cm Rigiflex pneumatic dilation. However, only young women (<35 years of age) did poorly with pneumatic dilation, while older women had sustained relief over at least 5 years with a single pneumatic dilation.

Physiologic studies can also predict the long-term success rate of pneumatic dilation. Eckhardt and colleagues reported that all patients with post-procedure LES pressure <10 mmHg were in remission after 2 years, compared with 71% for pressures between 10 and 20 mmHg and 23% for pressures over 20 mmHg [21]. More recently, the Leuven group observed that 66% of their patients with post-procedure LES pressure <15 mmHg were in symptomatic remission after an average of 6 years [25]. Using the timed barium swallow, we found that patients with complete symptom relief, correlating with marked improvement of esophageal emptying, were more likely to do well at 3 years than those with symptom relief, but poor esophageal emptying (82% vs. 10%, respectively) [23]. A randomized clinical trial of pneumatic dilation vs. surgery found that patients with <50% improvement in the height of the barium column at 1 min post-treatment had a 40% risk of treatment failure during follow-up [36]. Most recently, the Northwestern group [16] observed that patients with type II achalasia pattern (esophageal pressurization) on high-resolution manometry were more likely to respond to any therapy (botulinum toxin 71%, pneumatic dilation 91%, Heller myotomy 100%), compared to type I (56% overall) and type III (29% overall). This was a single-center study and confirmation by other investigators is needed.

The only absolute contraindication to pneumatic dilation is poor cardiopulmonary status or other co-morbid illnesses preventing surgery, should an esophageal perforation occur. Some have suggested that patients with vigorous achalasia, achalasia associated with epiphrenic diverticulum or hiatal hernia, malnutrition, or more than one previous dilation may have an increased risk of perforation. However, a retrospective study of 237 patients found no difference in clinical, endoscopic, manometric, or radiographic characteristics among seven patients who had perforations, compared to the 230 who did not [37]. Pneumatic dilation can be safely done after a failed Heller myotomy, although larger diameter balloons are required (I usually start with a 3.5 cm balloon) and the success rate is not as good [38].

Complications after pneumatic dilation are reported in up to 33% of patients with most complications being minor, including chest pain, aspiration pneumonia, bleeding usually self-limited, transient fever, esophageal mucosal tear without perforation, and esophageal hematoma [28]. Esophageal perforation is the most serious complication after pneumatic dilation, with an overall rate in experienced hands of 1.9% (range 0–16%) [28]. Most perforations occur during the first dilation and the initial size of the balloon may be a factor. For small perforations and deep painful tears, treatment may be conservative with antibiotics and total parenteral nutrition for days to weeks. However, surgical repair through a thoracotomy is best for large symptomatic perforations with extensive soilage of the mediastinum. Severe complications of gastroesophageal reflux disease (esophagitis, peptic stricture, Barrett's esophagus) are rare after pneumatic dilation, but 15–35% of patients have heartburn, responding to proton pump inhibitors [28].

Laparoscopic Heller Myotomy

The first successful surgery for achalasia was performed in 1913, by the German surgeon Ernest Heller [39]. This surgery consisted of an anterior and posterior (double) lower esophageal myotomy through a laparotomy. Subsequently, the operation was modified to a single anterior myotomy performed usually through a left posterior thoracotomy. This operation was the primary surgical treatment for achalasia, until the mid-1990s, with reported good success rate (60–94%) but high postoperative morbidity, making this treatment much less attractive [40]. This dramatically changed with the introduction of the minimally invasive myotomy by Pellegrini and coworkers, in 1992 [41]. Initially performed through the chest, the overall success of the laparoscopic operation through the abdomen is superior to the thorascopic approach. Patients are usually hospitalized for less than 48 h and can return to work within 1–2 weeks. Recent improvements on the operation have included extending the myotomy 2–3 cm onto the proximal stomach to cut the gastric sling fibers, further decreasing LES pressure and improving dysphagia [42]. This more aggressive myotomy accentuates the risk for postoperative gastroesophageal reflux; therefore, the consensus is to add an incomplete fundoplication, either an anterior Dor or posterior Toupet, to prevent this complication [43]. Esophageal myotomy lowers LES pressure more consistently than pneumatic dilation. Depending on the extent of the myotomy onto the cardia, LES pressure is lowered by 55–75% with the remaining residual LES pressure usually less than 10 mmHg [42].

In a recent review of 39 studies including nearly 3,100 patients, the good to excellent symptom relief with laparoscopic myotomy was 89.3% with average follow-up of 35 months [44]. Younger patients, especially men and patients with higher LES pressures, may benefit most from primary surgery. The former may be related to the greater tensile strength of the LES in young men; while the later is postulated to reflect overall less severely damaged esophageal muscle function with better bolus clearance once the obstruction is relieved [45]. Importantly, patients who fail pneumatic dilation or botulinum toxin treatment can be successfully treated with surgical myotomy [35, 45, 46], although some groups suggest a 15–21% lower success rate [47, 48]. Repeated botulinum toxin injections significantly hinder the dissection of the submucosal plane, leading to mucosal perforations in 7–15% of operations [28]. Although these perforations are usually recognized and repaired at the time of the initial operation, some studies suggest a negative effect on long-term results. For example, Portale et al. [46] found the myotomy success rate of 19 patients previously treated with pneumatic dilation was 94% at 5 years, but only 75% for the 26 patients previously treated with botulinum toxin. Long-term studies suggest deterioration of surgical success over 5–11 years. Three groups have recently reported the long-term results of laparo-scopic Heller myotomy (mean follow-up between 5.3 and 11.2 years) in 179 patients [45, 49, 50]. Deterioration over time seems to occur with striking consistency in these multinational studies; 18% required pneumatic dilation, 5% botulinum toxin injection, and 5–10% required repeat myotomy or esophagectomy. Surgical expertise is key, with most complications occurring in the first 50 operations [51]. Surgery is the most costly treatment for achalasia [31]. It may, however, be cost-effective, but only if its effectiveness reliably lasts at least 10 years [31].

Recurrence of dysphagia after myotomy is usually the result of an incomplete myotomy, particularly on the gastric side. These patients may do well with a subsequent pneumatic dilation [45]. Other factors include esophageal scarring possibly due to excessive electrical cautery, obstruction by the fundoplication, megaesophagus, or complications of severe GERD including esophagitis and peptic stricture. The role of a sigmoid megaesophagus (maximum diameter >6–9 cm with horizontal configuration) contributing to the failure of myotomy is controversial. Several series suggest [45, 48] many of these patients will do poorly after surgery with up to 50% having persistent dysphagia. Others report [52, 53] these patients did as well after surgery as those with minimal dilation. Therefore, most recommend initial treatment with a laparoscopic myotomy, reserving esophagectomy for the failures. Nevertheless, 2–5% of patients with a megaesophagus will eventually require an esophagectomy [22].

Surgical complications of laparoscopic Heller myotomy include death (0.1%) and esophageal perforation (7–15%) [28]. The most common long-term problem is chronic GERD and its sequelae, occurring overall in 17% of patients (range 5–55%) [28]. Most of these patients have reflux symptoms; some esophagitis, and rarely Barrett's esophagus and secondary adenocarcinoma of the esophagus have been reported after Heller myotomy. The addition of an incomplete fundoplication decreases, but does not eliminate, the complications of GERD [43]. A recent study by Csendes et al. [54] illustrates the potential for

GERD complications, especially among patients followed for over 10 years. This study reported on 67 patients with Heller myotomy and Dor fundoplication after open laparotomy with a mean follow-up of nearly 16 years (range 6.6–30 years). Overall, 31% of the patients developed GERD, and 55% had abnormal pH studies 20 years after their myotomy. Importantly, nine patients (13%) developed Barrett's esophagus (six short- and three long-segment), with the frequency increasing over time, reaching 30% after 20 years. In this series, poor or failed results were seen in 22.4% of the patients, but only one was due to an incomplete myotomy, with the remaining 14 due to complications of severe GERD. These alarming results may not be translatable to the laparoscopic operation, where the minor dissection of the perihiatal tissue theoretically should reduce the risk of postoperative GERD. However, careful studies will be required to address this concern.

Pneumatic Dilation or Surgical Myotomy?

Ideally, the choice between two treatment options should be based upon prospective, randomized comparative studies. Recently, studies comparing pneumatic dilation with the Rigiflex balloon and laparoscopic Heller myotomy have been reported. These studies are appearing at a critical time, when many gastroenterologists have stopped performing pneumatic dilations and the laparoscopic technique has made Heller myotomy the most favored treatment for achalasia.

A large study from the Cleveland Clinic [35] compared 106 patients treated with Rigiflex balloons by a single gastroenterologist, and 73 patients undergoing primarily laparoscopic Heller myotomy (20 had failed pneumatic dilation and crossed over to surgery) by a single esophageal surgeon. The success of graded pneumatic dilation and myotomy, defined as dysphagia/regurgitation <3 times a week or freedom from alternative treatment, was similar; 96% vs. 89% at 6 months, decreasing to 44% vs. 57% at 6 months. Causes of symptom recurrence were incompletely treated achalasia (96% after pneumatic dilation vs. 64%

after myotomy) and complications of GERD (4% after dilation vs. 36% after surgery).

Another method to address this issue is to investigate large population-based databases comparing outcomes of these two procedures in typical practice settings. This was recently reported by Lopushinsky and Urbach [55] in a retrospective longitudinal study in Ontario, Canada, from July 1991 to December 2002. A total of 1,461 persons aged 18 years or older received treatment for achalasia; 1,181 (80.8%) had pneumatic dilation and 280 (19.2%) had surgical myotomy as their first procedure. The cumulative risk of any subsequent intervention for achalasia (pneumatic dilation, myotomy, or esophagectomy) after 1, 5 and 10 years, respectively, was 36.8%, 56.2% and 63.5% after initial pneumatic dilation treatment, as compared to 16.4%, 30.3% and 37.5% after initial myotomy (hazard risk: 2.37 CI 1.86–3.02, $p = <0.001$). The difference in risk between these two procedures was observed only when repeat pneumatic dilation was recorded as an adverse outcome. Since "on demand" pneumatic dilation is the accepted approach to treating achalasia, this cannot logically be viewed as failure of this treatment modality [29]. Interestingly, the 33% need for subsequent pneumatic dilation and 18% risk of repeat surgery following myotomy were much higher than the current surgery literature suggests, probably defining the more realistic surgical experience in the clinical community.

Fortunately, randomized comparison studies are now available. To date, two small randomized studies have been reported comparing Rigiflex balloon dilation and laparoscopic myotomy. The first (16 pneumatic dilation, 14 Heller myotomy) found no difference in success rates [56]. The second series (26 dilations, 25 surgery), with follow-up for at least 12 months, observed six failures in the dilation group and one with surgery. This difference reached statistical significance ($p = 0.04$) in the per protocol analysis, but not the intention-to-treat analysis ($p = 0.09$) [36]. Most recently, an achalasia trial involving five European countries [57] randomized 94 patients to Rigiflex pneumatic dilation (3.0 and 3.5 cm) and 106 to laparoscopic Heller

myotomy with Dor fundoplication. Patients having recurrent symptoms after pneumatic dilation were allowed to be retreated a maximum of three series of pneumatic dilations. After 2 years of follow-up, both treatments had comparable success rates—92% for pneumatic dilation and 87% for laparoscopic myotomy. Barium swallow emptying and LES pressures were similar for both groups. Four perforations occurred after pneumatic dilations, all in older patients treated initially with a 3.5 cm balloon, compared to 11 perioperatively recognized perforations (1 converted to open operation) during laparoscopic Heller myotomy. Preexisting daily chest pain, the height of barium column after 5 min, and an esophageal width of less than 4 cm before treatment were identified as predictors of treatment failure in Cox regression analysis. These data confirmed that monitoring esophageal emptying after treatment is a helpful tool to predict recurrence and to decide whether further dilation is required [23]. Why a diameter of the esophagus less than 4 cm before treatment is associated with failure is unclear, unless this may be indicative of vigorous achalasia, known to have a worse outcome [16]. Although age was not a predictive factor of clinical success for either treatment, patients younger than age of 40 presented more often with recurrent symptoms requiring re-dilation. This finding seems to support the proposal to preferentially treat younger patients (especially men) with laparoscopic Heller myotomy although longer follow-up is required. This study indicates that both treatments are equally effective.

Pharmacologic Treatments

Smooth Muscle Relaxants

Lower esophageal sphincter pressure can be transiently reduced by smooth muscle relaxants [58]. Nitrates increase the nitric oxide concentration in smooth muscle cells, which subsequently increases cyclic guanosine monophosphate (GMP) levels and results in muscle relaxation. Calcium is necessary for esophageal muscle contractions and its action is blocked by calcium antagonists. Nitrates and calcium channel blockers decrease LES pressure in a dose-dependent manner, with a maximum effect of approximately 50%, thereby temporarily relieving dysphagia. These drugs are taken 15–30 min before meals, the improvement in dysphagia is usually incomplete and short-lived, efficacy decreases with time, and side effects (headache, dizziness, pedal edema) are common. As a result, there is infrequently a place for these drugs in the clinical management of achalasia. The same holds true for sildenafil, a phosphodiesterase inhibitor that reduces the breakdown of cyclic GMP, the second messenger mediating NO-induced relaxation [59].

Botulinum Toxin

Botulinum toxin (Botox) is a potent inhibitor of acetylcholine release from nerve endings [58]. The inactive form is synthesized by the Clostridium botulinum bacteria. Botox cleaves SNAP-25, a cytoplasmic protein involved in the fusion of acetylcholine containing presymptomatic vesicles with the neuronal plasma membrane. Exocytosis of acetylcholine is inhibited and paralysis of the innervated muscle occurs. Botox counteracts the unopposed stimulation of the LES by cholinergic neurons, helping to restore the LES to a lower resting pressure. On average, Botox injections decrease LES pressure by 50%, while partially improving esophageal emptying [58].

Botox is commercially available in a lyophilized powder which should be stored below −5°C. The toxin is gently diluted with 5 mL of preservative-free sterile saline. Bubbles should not be formed during the mixing process, so as not to decrease the toxin's potency. Total dose of 100 units is endoscopically injected through a sclerotherapy needle into the LES in divided 25 unit aliquots, one in each quadrant of the sphincter. Increasing the dose to 200 units does not improve the success rate, but repeated 100 units may improve efficacy. One study reported that patients receiving 100 units of Botox, followed by a second injection of 100 units 30 days later, had an 80% remission rate at 12 months, compared with the 55% rate with the traditional regimen [60].

The drug is contraindicated in patients with allergy to egg proteins. It should be administered cautiously to patients receiving aminoglycosides, because these medications may potentiate the effect of the toxin. The most common side effects of Botox injection is chest pain in 16–25% of patients.

Based on numerous studies, some placebo-controlled, botulinum toxin markedly improves symptoms in approximately 75% of achalasia patients [28]. However, symptoms recur in more than 50% of patients within 6 months, possibly because of regeneration of the affected receptors [60–62]. Of those responding to the first injection of 100 units of Botox, nearly 75% will respond to a second injection, but the response decreases with further injections, probably from antibody production to the foreign proteins. Less than 20% of the patients failing to respond to the initial Botox injection respond to a second injection [63]. Patients older than 60 years of age, and those with vigorous achalasia, are more likely to get a sustained response, up to 1.5–2 years after botulinum toxin injection [61]. Serial injections of botulinum toxin are required to give sustained relief, and comparison studies demonstrate its long-term efficacy is inferior to pneumatic dilation or myotomy [62, 64]. A single vial of Botox costs approximately $500. Serial botulinum toxin injections are more expensive than pneumatic dilation, because of the need for repeated injections. This treatment may have a cost advantage for patients living <2 years [65].

Endoscopic Treatments

The concept of natural orifice transluminal endoscopic surgery has inspired endoscopists and endoscopic surgeons to create less invasive treatment for esophageal achalasia. However, the first endoscopic myotomy, reported in 1980, was done using a modified needle knife to dissect the muscle layer directly through the mucosal layer. Visual control of the movement of the needle tip during the myotomy was impossible, thus perforation or injury to surrounding structures could not be avoided [66]. Almost three decades later,

Pasricha et al. [67] reported, in a pig model, the possibility of endoscopic myotomy through a submucosal tunnel. More recent animal studies compared endoscopic submucosal esophageal myotomy and open myotomy in a pig model [68]. Postoperative LES pressure dropped 50% in the endoscopic group and 69% with the open procedure. After the procedure, the resistance to distension at the esophagogastric junction was similar after both procedures. The key to success for both procedures was cutting the circular fibers at the level of the EGJ, not extending the myotomy proximally on the esophagus.

Inoue et al. [69] recently reported the first clinical experience of peroral endoscopic myotomy in 17 achalasia patients, including five with a sigmoid esophagus. The innovation brought by Inoue's technique consisted of dividing selectively the circular muscle bundles, leaving the outer longitudinal esophageal muscles intact. The endoscopic length of the myotomy reproduced the classical 6-cm esophageal and 2-cm gastric surgical standards. In all cases, significant reduction of resting LES pressure (from mean 52.4 to 19.9 mmHg) was noted and improvement of dysphagia persisted for at least 5 months after initial treatment. No serious complications were encountered with the procedure. One patient developed mild reflux esophagitis, easily treated with proton pump inhibitors.

General Recommendations

Figure 39.3 is a suggested treatment algorithm for treating achalasia based on a recent clinical review from US and European authorities in this

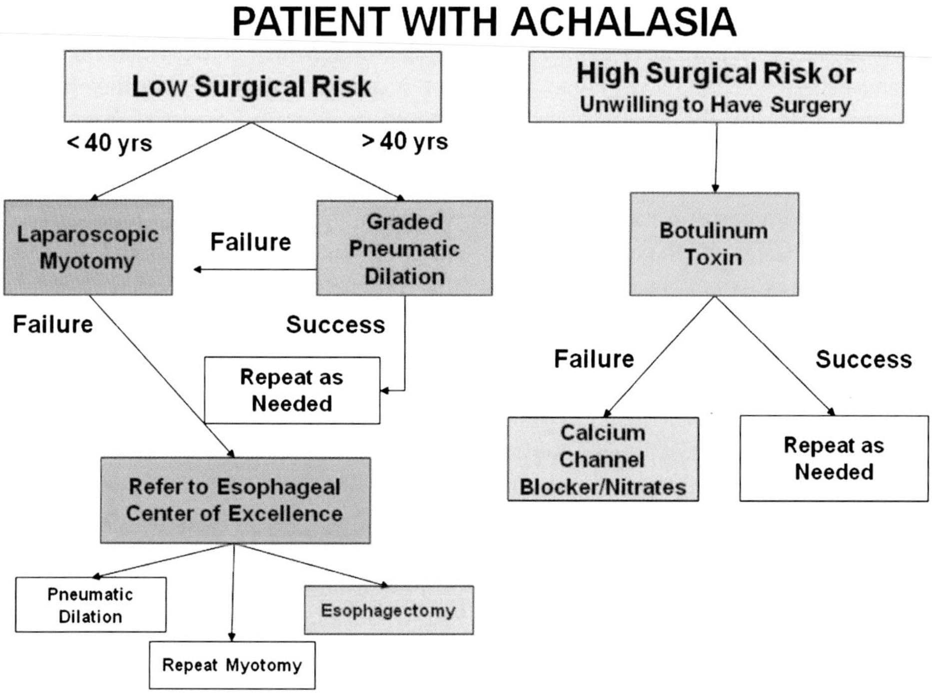

PATIENT WITH ACHALASIA

Fig. 39.3 Suggested algorithm for the treatment of achalasia. Healthy patients with low risk of complications after surgery can be offered potentially definitive therapy with either pneumatic dilation or laparoscopic myotomy. Patients younger than 40 years may preferentially be referred to surgery, as they frequently need more repeat dilations than older subjects. Failures are best referred to Esophageal Centers of Excellence with expertise in pneumatic dilation, repeat myotomy, and esophagectomy. High-risk patients, especially the elderly, are best treated with botulinum toxin injections, or alternately pneumatic dilation, if the latter procedure is done at high volume centers. From J.E. Richter and G.E. Boeckxstaens. Recent advances in clinical practice: Management of achalasia. Gut (in press), published online February 8, 2011, with permission

disease [26]. Healthy patients with achalasia should be given the option of graded pneumatic dilation or laparoscopic Heller myotomy since a review of the literature suggests relatively similar efficacy in the hands of experienced gastroenterologists and surgeons [28]. Pneumatic dilation has the advantage of being an outpatient procedure, with minimal pain, return to work the next day, GERD is an infrequent problem, and can be performed in any age group and during pregnancy. Pneumatic dilation does not hinder the performance of a future myotomy, and all cost analyses find it less expensive than Heller myotomy over 5–10 years. Laparoscopic Heller myotomy has the advantage of being a single procedure, dysphagia relief is longer at the cost of more troubling heartburn, and a myotomy may be more effective treatment than pneumatic dilation in adolescents and young adults, especially men. Myotomy is definitely the treatment of choice in uncooperative patients and patients in whom pseudoachalasia cannot be excluded. In healthy subjects, we do not offer botulinum toxin as an option, because the treatment is not definitive, and the duration of relief short term. On the other hand, botulinum toxin injections are the treatment of choice in patients who are poor surgical candidates and the elderly because it is safe, improves symptoms and generally older patients require retreatment no more frequently than once a year. However, pneumatic dilation is a reasonable alternative in high surgical risk patients if performed in high volume centers with surgical expertise should the rare perforation occur. Initial treatment of uncomplicated achalasia can be done by experienced community physicians and surgeons. Failures, particularly after surgery, should be referred to Esophageal Centers of Excellence with a multi-discipline team experienced with pneumatic dilation, repeat myotomy, and esophagectomy. Nearly 90% of achalasia patients can have near-normal swallowing and good quality of life, but few are "cured" with a single treatment and intermittent "touch up" procedures (especially pneumatic dilation and sometimes repeat myotomy) may be required [22].

The Future

There are still many challenges and questions to be answered regarding achalasia and its treatment. We need to understand the triggers leading to the destruction of the esophageal and LES neurons and possibly how to prevent these insults. If this is due to an autoimmune process, one possible alternative therapeutic approach may be immune-modulating drugs. Animal studies should continue to explore the potential of stem cell transplantation to restore esophageal and LES function. Recent studies of mice suggest that transplantation of neuronal stem cells injected in the pylorus survive and even express NO synthase [70]. Future large, randomized, prospective trials will need to compare laparoscopic Heller myotomy and pneumatic dilation to address the superiority of one technique to the other over a 5- to 10-year period, or to determine which therapies should be reserved for a certain subset of patients. Initial trials should be done in Centers of Excellence with surgeons and gastroenterologists skilled with this disease, but a later comparative study in the community setting would best define where these patients should be initially treated. Finally, the progress of an endoscopic treatment for achalasia warrants a team approach and careful long-term follow-up of symptoms and physiologic studies such as LES pressure and esophageal emptying.

Ineffective Esophageal Motility

Unlike achalasia, ineffective esophageal motility (IEM) is a poorly described motility disorder whose etiology and treatment are not defined. Ineffective esophageal motility evolved from a further refinement of the non-achalasia motility disorders not meeting the criteria for diffuse esophageal spasm, scleroderma, or nutcracker esophagus. The manometric pattern is that of peristaltic failure characterized by the presence of distal esophageal contractions of very low amplitude (<30 mmHg) and/or non-transmitted contractions. The definition of IEM is based on the simultaneous videomanometry studies by Kahrilas et al. [71] who reported that contraction waves in the distal esophagus with amplitudes lower than 30 mmHg were associated with failure of bolus clearance.

Epidemiology and Pathophysiology

Ineffective esophageal motility is the most prominent motility disorder in GERD patients, being diagnosed in 20–50% of patients [72]. It is also reported in 31–53% of patients with aerodigestive disorders associated with GERD [73]. The majority of these patients have between 30% and 70% of their swallows followed by these "ineffective contractions" [74]. IEM was observed in up to 30% of patients with non-obstructive dysphagia unrelated to GERD [75]. These periods of peristaltic failure have been associated with delayed esophageal clearance after reflux [73, 76], extra-esophageal symptoms [77], and dysphagia both before and after anti-reflux surgery [78].

Incomplete data suggest that IEM is due to impaired cholinergic stimulation along the esophageal body, whether a primary motor disorder or secondary to chronic inflammation. Experimental animal studies show that acute acid injury inducing esophagitis is associated with esophageal hypomotility that can disappear after spontaneous mucosal healing [79]. However, among patients with chronic erosive GERD, healing of esophagitis does not predictably improve esophageal dysmotility and patients with non-erosive GERD may have poor peristaltic function, suggesting a primary disorder [80, 81]. Potential factors contributing to this esophageal hypomotility include impaired neuromuscular control, muscle hypertrophy, extensive fibrosis, or inflammatory mediators such as interleukin-6 and platelet activating factor diffusing through the esophageal wall and reducing acetylcholine release from excitatory motor neurons to circular smooth muscle [82, 83].

Diagnostic Evaluation

The classical criteria for IEM, as published by Leite et al. [76], include hypocontraction in the distal esophagus, with at least 30% of wet swallows exhibiting any combination of the following: (1) non-transmitted contractions not propagating throughout the esophagus, and/or (2) low amplitude peristaltic contractions with amplitude <30 mmHg (Fig. 39.4). The functional impact of IEM can be assessed by the combination of esophageal manometry and impedance. In a recent study of 70 patients with IEM, 68% of liquid and 59% of viscous swallows showed normal bolus transit with impedance testing, and almost one-third of patients received an overall diagnosis of normal bolus transit for both liquid and viscous swallows [74]. Thus, the manometric findings must be correlated with esophageal function, reserving the term IEM for patients with severe hypomotility and impaired bolus transit.

Treatment

Prevention of IEM theoretically may be achieved with early aggressive control of GERD. Once established, IEM seems to be unmodified by acid-suppressive medications [80] or anti-reflux surgery [81]. Some studies find no effect of prokinetic therapy [84, 85] on IEM. However, a recent study [86] of seven patients with severe IEM found that bethanechol 50 mg orally reduced by nearly two-thirds the percentage of ineffective liquid swallows by impedance testing. Three patients had normalization of their liquid bolus transit. Another drug, the 5-HT$_1$ agonist sumatriptan, can elicit an increase in amplitude of esophageal contractions and LES pressure in healthy subjects. When given to 16 patients with chest pain and IEM, sumatriptan 6 mg subcutaneous increased the number of primary peristaltic waves. However, the drug had no effect on contraction amplitude, reducing the potential role of this drug as a stimulus to reverse IEM [87]. When surgery is indicated for severe gastroesophageal

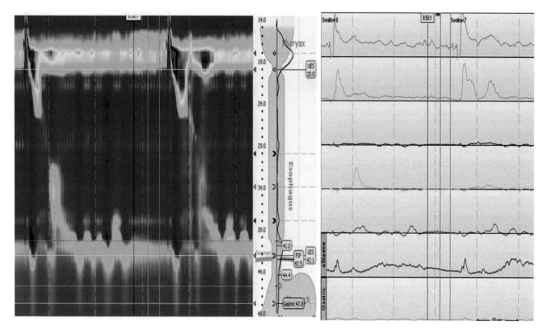

Fig. 39.4 Example of ineffective esophageal peristalsis using high-resolution manometry. On the left is the color contour; on the right the more traditional pressure tracing. The first swallow is peristaltic, but low amplitude (<30 mmHg), while the second swallow is non-transmitted

reflux associated with IEM, partial fundoplication (rather than a Nissen fundoplication) may be preferred to facilitate esophageal emptying and decrease the risk of postoperative dysphagia, but this concept remains controversial [81, 88].

References

1. Willis T. Pharmaceutic rationalis: sive diatriba de medicamentorum; operatimibus in humano corpore. London: Hagae-Comitis; 1674.
2. Mayberry JF. Epidemiology and demographics of achalasia. Gastrointest Endosc Clin North Am. 2001; 11:235–47.
3. Eckhardt VF, Hoischen T, Bernhard G. Life expectancy, complications and causes of death in patients with achalasia: results of a 33-year follow-up investigation. Eur J Gastroenterol Hepatol. 2008;20:956–60.
4. Goldblum JR, Whyte RI, Orringer MB, et al. Achalasia: a morphologic study of 42 resected specimens. Am J Surg Pathol. 1994;18:327–37.
5. Goldblum JR, Rice TW, Richter JE. Histopathologic features in esophagomyotomy specimens from patients with achalasia. Gastroenterology. 1996;111:648–54.
6. Holloway RH, Dodds WJ, Helm JF, et al. Integrity of cholinergic innervation to the lower esophageal sphincter in achalasia. Gastroenterology. 1986;90:924–9.
7. Park W, Vaezi MF. Etiology and pathogenesis of achalasia: the current understanding. Am J Gastroenterol. 2005;100:1401–14.
8. Ruiz-De-Leon A, Mendoza J, De-La-Concha EG, et al. Myenteric antiplexus antibodies and class II HLA in achalasia. Dig Dis Sci. 2002;47:15–9.
9. Moses PL, Ellis LM, Anees MR, et al. Antineuronal antibodies in idiopathic achalasia and gastroesophageal reflux disease. Gut. 2003;52:629–36.
10. Niwamoto H, Okamoto E, Fujmoto J, et al. Are human herpes viruses or measles virus associated with esophageal achalasia? Dig Dis Sci. 1995;40:859–64.
11. Birgissen S, Galinski MS, Goldblum JR, et al. Achalasia is not associated with measles as known herpes or human papilloma viruses. Dig Dis Sci. 1997;42:300–6.
12. Facco M, Brun P, Zaninotto G, et al. T cells in the myenteric plexus of achalasia patients show a skewed TCR repertoire and react to HSV-1 antigens. Am J Gastroenterol. 2008;103:1598–609.
13. Eckardt VF, Stauf B, Bernhard G. Chest pain in achalasia: patient characteristics and clinical course. Gastroenterology. 1999;116:1300–4.
14. DeOliveira JMA, Birgisson S, Doinoff C, et al. Timed-barium swallow: a simple technique for evaluating esophageal emptying in patients with achalasia. Am J Roentgenol. 1997;169:473–9.
15. Ghosh SK, Pandolfino JE, Rice J, et al. Impaired deglutitive ECJ relaxation in clinical manometry: a quantitative analysis of 400 patients and 75 controls.

Am J Physiol Gastrointest Liver Physiol. 2007;293(4):G878–85.

16. Pandolfino JE, Kwiatek MA, Nealis T, et al. Achalasia: a new clinically relevant classification by high resolution manometry. Gastroenterology. 2008;135:1526–33.

17. Pandolfino JE, Fox MR, Bredenoord AJ, Kahrilas PJ. High resolution manometry in clinical practice: utilizing pressure topography to classify oeosophageal motility abnormalities. Neurogastroenterol Motil. 2009;21:796–806.

18. Herbella FAM, Aquino JLB, Stefani-Nokana S, et al. Treatment of achalasia: lessons learned from Chagas' disease. Dis Esophagus. 2008;21:461–7.

19. Gockel I, Eckhard VF, Schmitt T, Junginger T. Pseudoachalasia: a case series and analysis of the literature. Scand J Gastroenterol. 2005;40:378–85.

20. Sandler RS, Bozymski EM, Orlando RC. Failure of clinical criteria to distinguish between primary achalasia and achalasia secondary to tumor. Dig Dis Sci. 1982;27:209–13.

21. Eckhardt VF, Kohne A, Junginger T, et al. Risk factors for diagnostic delay in achalasia. Dig Dis Sci. 1997;42:580–5.

22. Vela MF, Richter JE, Wachsberger D, et al. Complexities of managing achalasia at a tertiary referral center: use of pneumatic dilation, Heller myotomy and botulinum toxin injection. Am J Gastroenterol. 2004;2:389–94.

23. Vaezi MF, Baker MF, Achkar E, Richter JE. Timed barium esophagram: better predictor of long-term success after pneumatic dilation than symptoms assessment. Gut. 2002;50:765–70.

24. Eckardt VF, Aignherr C, Bernhard G. Predictors of outcome in patients with achalasia treated by pneumatic dilation. Gastroenterology. 1992;103:1732–8.

25. Hulselmans M, Vanuytsel T, Degreef T, et al. Long-term outcome of pneumatic dilation in the treatment of achalasia. Clin Gastroenterol Hepatol. 2010;8:30–5.

26. Richter JE, Boeckxstaens GE. Management of achalasia: surgery or pneumatic dilation. Gut. 2011;6:869–76.

27. Kadakia SC, Wong RKH. Graded pneumatic dilation using rigiflex achalasia dilators in patients with primary esophageal achalasia. Am J Gastroenterol. 1993;88:34–8.

28. Richer JE. Update on the management of achalasia: balloons, surgery and drugs. Exp Rev Gastroenterol Hepatol. 2008;2:435–45.

29. Zerbid F, Thetiot V, Richy F, et al. Repeated pneumatic dilations as long-term maintenance therapy for esophageal achalasia. Am J Gastroenterol. 2006;101:692–7.

30. O'Connor JB, Singer ME, Richter JE, et al. The cost-effectiveness of treatment strategies for achalasia. Dig Dis Sci. 2002;47:1516–25.

31. Karanicolas PJ, Smith SE, Gafni A, et al. The cost of laparoscopic myotomy versus pneumatic dilatation for esophageal achalasia. Surg Endosc. 2007;21:1198–206.

32. Vantrappen G, Hellemans J, Deloof W, et al. Treatment of achalasia with pneumatic dilation. Gut. 1971;12:268–75.

33. Eckardt VF, Kanzler G, Westermeier T. Complications and their impact after pneumatic dilation for achalasia: prospective long-term follow-up study. Gastrointest Endosc. 1997;45:349–53.

34. Ghoshal UC, Kumar S, Saraswat VA, et al. Long-term follow-up after pneumatic dilation for achalasia of the cardia: factors associated with treatment failure and recurrence. Am J Gastroenterol. 2004;99:2304–10.

35. Vela M, Richter JE, Khandwala E, et al. The long-term efficacy of pneumatic dilation and Heller myotomy for the treatment of achalasia. Clin Gastroenterol Hepatol. 2006;4:580–7.

36. Kostic S, Kjellin A, Ruth M, et al. Pneumatic dilation or laparoscopic myotomy in the management of newly diagnosed idiopathic achalasia. World J Surg. 2007;31:470–8.

37. Metman EH, Lagasse JP, Alteroche L, et al. Risk factors for immediate complications after progressive pneumatic dilation for achalasia. Am J Gastroenterol. 1999;94:1179–85.

38. Guardino J, Vela M, Connor J, Richter JE. Pneumatic dilation for the treatment of achalasia in untreated patients and patients with failed Heller myotomy. J Clin Gastroenterol. 2004;38:855–60.

39. Heller E. Extramukoese cardinplastik bein chronischen cardiopsasmus mit dilation des oesophagus. Mitt Grenzgeb Med Chir. 1914;27:141–5.

40. Vaezi MF, Richer JE. Current therapies for achalasia comparison and efficacy. J Clin Gastroenterol. 1998;27:21–35.

41. Pelligrini C, Wetter LA, Patti M, et al. Thoracoscopic esophagomyotomy. Initial experience with a new approach for achalasia. Ann Surg. 1992;216:291–6.

42. Oelschlager BK, Chang L, Pellegrini CA. Improved outcomes after extended gastric myotomy for achalasia. Arch Surg. 2003;138:490–5.

43. Richards W, Torquati A, Holzman M, et al. Heller myotomy versus Heller myotomy with Dor fundoplication for achalasia: a prospective randomized double-blind clinical trial. Ann Surg. 2004;240:405–15.

44. Campos GM, Vittinghoff E, Rabl C, et al. Endoscopic and surgical treatments of achalasia. Ann Surg. 2009;249:45–57.

45. Constantini MI, Zanninotta G, Guirroli E, et al. The laparoscopic-Dor operation remains effective treatment for achalasia at a minimum of 6 years follow-up. Surg Endosc. 2005;19:345–51.

46. Portale G, Constantini M, Rizzetto C, et al. Long term outcome of laparoscopic heller-Dor surgery for achalasia: possible detrimental role of previous endoscopic treatment. J Gastrointest Surg. 2005;9:1332–9.

47. Schuchert MJ, Luketich JD, Landreneau RJ, et al. Minimally-invasive esophagomyotomy in 200 consecutive patients: factors influencing postoperative outcome. Ann Thorac Surg. 2008;85:1729–34.

48. Snyder CW, Burton RC, Brown LE, et al. Multiple preoperative endoscopic interventions are associated with worse outcome after laparoscopic Heller myotomy for achalasia. J Gastrointest Surg. 2010;14(4):2095–13.

49. Grockel I, Junginger T, Eckhardt V. Long-term results of conventional myotomy in patients with achalasia: a prospective 20 year analysis. Soc Surg Alimen Tract. 2006;10:1400–8.

50. Bonatti H, Hinder RA, Klocker J, et al. Long-term results of laparoscopic Heller myotomy with partial fundoplication for the treatment of achalasia. Am J Surg. 2005;190:874–8.

51. Sharp KW, Khaitan L, Scholz S, et al. 100 Consecutive minimally invasive Heller myotomies: lessons learned. Ann Surg. 2002;235:631–9.

52. Patti MG, Feo CV, Diener U, et al. Laparoscopic Heller mytomy relieves dysphagia in achalasia when the esophagus is dilated. Surg Endosc. 1999;13:843–6.

53. Mineo TC, Pompeo E. Long-term outcome in Heller myotomy achalasia sigmoid esophagus. J Thorac Cardiovasc Surg. 2004;128:402–7.

54. Csendes A, Braghetto I, Burdiles P, Korn O, et al. Very late results of esophagomyotomy for patients with achalasia. Ann Surg. 2006;243(2):196–203.

55. Lopushinsky SR, Urbach DR. Pneumatic dilation and surgical myotomy for achalasia. J Am Med Assoc. 2006;296:2227–33.

56. Shimi S, Nathanson LK, Cuschieri A. Laparoscopic cardiomyotomy for achalasia. J R Coll Surg Edinb. 1991;36:152–4.

57. Boeckxstaens G, Annese V, Chaussade S, et al. Endoscopic pneumodilation versus laparoscopic Heller myotomy with Dor anti-reflux procedure for idiopathic achalasia. N Engl J Med. 2011;364:1807–16.

58. Hoogerwerf WA, Pasricha PJ. Pharmacologic therapy in treating achalasia. Gastrointest Endosc Clin North Am. 2001;11:311–23.

59. Bortolotti M, Mari C, Lopilato C, et al. Effects of sildenafil on esophageal motility of patients with idiopathic achalasia. Gastroenterology. 2000;118:253–7.

60. Annese V, Bassotti G, Coccia G, et al. A multicenter randomized study of intrasphincteric botulinum toxin in patients with oesophageal achalasia. Gut. 2000;46:597–600.

61. Pasricha PJ, Rai R, Ravich WJ, et al. Botulinum toxin for achalasia: long-term outcome and predictor of response. Gastroenterology. 1996;110:1410–5.

62. Vaezi MJ, Richter JE, Wilcox CM, et al. Botulinum toxin versus pneumatic dilation in the treatment of achalasia: a randomized trial. Gut. 1999;44:231–9.

63. Fishman VM, Parkman HP, Schiano TD, et al. Symptomatic improvement in achalasia after botulinum toxin injection of the lower esophageal sphincter. Am J Gastroenterol. 1996;91:1724–30.

64. Mikaeli J, Fazel A, Montazeri G, et al. Randomized controlled trial comparing botulinum toxin injection to pneumatic dilatation for the treatment of achalasia. Aliment Pharmacol Ther. 2001;15:1389–96.

65. Panaccione R, Gregor JC, Reynolds RPE, et al. Intrasphincteric botulinum toxin versus pneumatic dilatation for achalasia: a cost minimization analysis. Gastrointest Endosc. 1999;50:492–8.

66. Ortega JA, Madureri V, Perez I. Endoscopic myotomy in the treatment of achalasia. Gastrointest Endosc. 1980;26:8–10.

67. Pasricha PJ, Hawari R, Ahmed I, et al. Submucosal endoscopic esophageal myotomy: a novel experimental approach for the treatment of achalasia. Endoscopy. 2007;39:761–4.

68. Perretta S, Dallemagne B, Donnatelli G, et al. Transoral endoscopic esophageal myotomy based on esophageal function testing in a survival porcine model. Gastrointest Endosc. 2011;73:111–6.

69. Inoue H, Minami H, Kobayashi Y, et al. Peroral endoscopic myotomy (POEM) for esophageal achalasia. Endoscopy. 2010;42:265–71.

70. Micci MA, Learish RD, Li H, et al. Neural stem cell expresses RET, produces nitric oxide and survives transplantation in the GI tract. Gastroenterology. 2001;121:7757–66.

71. Kahrilas PJ, Dodds WJ, Hogan WJ. Effect of peristaltic dysfunction on esophageal volume clearance. Gastroenterology. 1988;94:73–80.

72. Kahrilas PJ, Pandolfino JE. Ineffective esophageal peristalsis does not equate to GERD. Am J Gastroenterol. 2003;98:715–7.

73. Diener U, Patti MG, Molena D, et al. Esophageal dysmotility and gastroesophageal reflux disease. J Gastrointest Surg. 2001;5:260–5.

74. Tutuian R, Castell DO. Clarification of the esophageal function defect in patients with manometric ineffective esophageal motility studies using combined impedance-manometry. Clin Gastroenterol Hepatol. 2004;2:230–6.

75. Conchillo M, Nguyen NQ, Sansom M, et al. Multichannel intraluminal impedance monitoring in the evaluation of patients with non-obstructive dysphagia. Am J Gastroenterol. 2005;100:2624–32.

76. Leite LP, Johnson BT, Barrett J, et al. Ineffective esophageal motility: the primary finding in patients with non-specific esophageal motility disorders. Dig Dis Sci. 1997;42:1859–65.

77. Fouad YM, Katz PO, Hatlebakk JG, et al. Ineffective esophageal motility: the most common motility abnormality in patients with GERD-associated respiratory symptoms. Am J Gastroenterol. 1999;94:1464–7.

78. Lund RJ, Wetcher GJ, Raiser F, et al. Laparoscopic toupet for gastroesophageal reflux disease with poor esophageal body motility. J Gastrointest Surg. 1997;1:301–8.

79. Zhang X, Geboes K, Depoortere I, et al. Effect of repeated cycles of acute esophagitis and healing on esophageal peristalsis; time and length. Am J Physiol. 2005;288:G1339–46.

80. Singh P, Adamopoulos A, Taylor RH, et al. Oesophageal motor function before and after healing of oesophagitis. Gut. 1992;33:1590–6.

81. Fibbe C, Layer P, Keller J, et al. Esophageal motility in reflux disease before and after fundoplication: a prospective, randomized, clinical and manometric study. Gastroenterology. 2001;121:5–14.

82. Cao W, Cheng L, Behar J, et al. Proinflammatory cytokines alter/reduce esophageal circular muscle contraction in experimental cat esophagitis. Am J Physiol Gastrointest Liver Physiol. 2004;287: G1131–9.

83. Rieder F, Cheng L, Harnett KM, et al. Gastroesophageal reflux disease-associated esophagitis induces endogenous cytokine production leading to otor abnormalities. Gastroenterology. 2007;132:154–65.

84. Corazziari E, Bontempo I, Anzini F. Effects of cisapride on distal esophageal motility in humans. Dig Dis Sci. 1989;34:1600–5.

85. Grande L, Lacima G, Ros E, et al. Lack of effect of metoclopramide and domperidone on esophageal peristalsis, and esophageal clearance in reflux esophagitis. A randomized, double-blind study. Dig Dis Sci. 1992;37:583–8.

86. Agrawal A, Hila A, Tutuian R, et al. Bethanechol improves smooth muscle function in patients with severe ineffective esophageal motility. J Clin Gastroenterol. 2007;41:366–70.

87. Grossi L, Ciccaglione AF, Marzio L. Effect of the 5-HT$_1$ agonist sumatriptan on oesophageal motor patterns in patients with ineffective oesophageal motility. Neurogastroenterol Motil. 2003;15:9–14.

88. Montenovo M, Tatum RP, Figueredo, et al. Does combined multichannel intraluminal esophageal impedance and manometry predict post-operative dysphagia after laparoscopic nissen fundoplication? Dis Esophagus. 2009;22:656–63.

Esophageal Spasm/Noncardiac Chest Pain Hypertensive Esophageal Peristalsis, (Nutcracker Esophagus) and Hypertensive Lower Esophageal Sphincter

40

Monika A. Kwiatek and John Pandolfino

Abstract

Dysphagia and noncardiac chest pain can be associated with spastic and hypercontractile esophageal motor disorders, provided that structural lesions, inflammation, and gastroesophageal reflux are excluded. Currently one of the best methods used to identify and classify esophageal contractile abnormalities is esophageal manometry. In the last years, manometry has undergone a significant paradigm shift. Combination of solid-state high-resolution manometry with esophageal pressure topography (EPT) provides a seamless dynamic display of esophageal pressure morphology and function, which is subjectively easy to interpret, yet lends itself to more sophisticated analyses and detailed characterization of normal and abnormal esophageal motility. The purpose of this chapter is to provide an overview of pathophysiology underlying the esophageal spasm, spastic achalasia, hypertensive peristalsis, and hypercontractile lower esophageal sphincter, as well as the criteria for their diagnosis based on the features observable on EPT. Together with presenting patient complaint, phenotypes of esophageal motor disorders defined by EPT may help guide the management of spastic and hypercontractile esophageal motor disorders. Additionally, these phenotypes may also refine future clinical trials and improve our understanding of how these motor abnormalities may generate symptoms.

Keywords

Achalasia • Dysphagia • Esophageal hypercontractility • Esophageal pressure topography esophageal spasm • High-resolution manometry • Hypertensive esophageal peristalsis • Hypercontractile lower esophageal sphincter • Non-cardiac chest pain • Nutcracker esophagus

M.A. Kwiatek, PhD • J. Pandolfino, MD, MSCI (✉)
Department of Medicine, Northwestern Memorial
Hospital, Chicago, IL, USA
e-mail: j-pandolfino@northwestern.edu

Introduction

Although abnormal esophageal motility can lead to dysphagia and chest pain, as a general rule, initial diagnostic exclusion of esophageal structural lesions by endoscopy, radiography, histology, or empiric proton pump inhibitor (PPI) trial is required. Achalasia is the best defined esophageal motor disorder associated with dysphagia; however, an association between dysphagia and/or chest pain with other motility disorders such as diffuse esophageal spasm (DES), hypertensive contractile esophagus, or hypercontractile lower esophageal sphincter has also been reported [1]. Spastic disorders are typically defined based on abnormal peristaltic propagation leading to premature contractions or rapid contractions associated with bolus entrapment during swallowing. In contrast, hypercontractile disorders have normal propagation but are associated with exaggerated contractions that may have extremely high contraction amplitudes or prolonged contractions outside of the typical time-dependent programmed deglutitive window. Although these disorders are associated with dysphagia and chest pain, these motor abnormalities are found in patients presenting with GERD and even asymptomatic controls. Thus, it appears that there are distinct phenotypes that directly generate symptoms and other phenotypes that rely on secondary modulators, such as visceral hypersensitivity and hyperawareness.

Esophageal contractile disorders are best indentified and classified with esophageal manometry. Manometric evaluation of the tubular esophagus assesses the integrity, rate of progression, and segmental architecture of the contractile complex, i.e., amplitude, duration, and repetitive nature of contractions. Esophageal motor patterns previously classified with conventional manometry used 3–8 pressure sensors spaced 3–5 cm apart and displayed pressure as tracings along a time continuum. Recent advances in high-resolution manometry hardware, computer processing, and software, however, have shifted the diagnostic paradigm of esophageal disease. HRM provides a greater number of closely spaced high-fidelity pressure sensors, enabling a greatly enhanced display algorithm over simple conventional line tracings. The resultant esophageal pressure topography (EPT) plot provides a seamless dynamic representation of esophageal pressure morphology and function (Fig. 40.1). Its key advantage is in the additional ability to assess pressure profiles along the length of the esophagus (as continuous spatial-pressure variation plots) and, thus, improving both the accuracy and detail of the study compared to the conventional approach. HRM and EPT were initially described experimentally by Clouse in the 1990s [2] and have since become increasingly used in clinical practice. The detailed EPT display format is subjectively easier to interpret, and provides a more accurate and sophisticated characterization of esophageal motility. The purpose of this chapter is to highlight the pathophysiology, classification, and diagnosis of spastic and hypercontractile esophageal motor disorders based on EPT criteria. This review will also describe the management of these disorders; however, details regarding specific therapies will be covered more extensively in Chapters XX.

Esophageal Manometry

Manometric Catheters

Esophageal manometry is a test in which intraluminal pressure sensors, either water perfused or solid state, are positioned axially within the esophagus. The manometric catheter is inserted transnasally and connected to a recording unit (via a hydraulic pump in case of perfused pressure sensors). Whereas conventional technique used catheters with few and widely spaced pressure sensors, the currently available HRM catheters typically consist of 36 solid-state pressure sensors spaced 1 cm apart. The concept of HRM is to employ a sufficient number of pressure sensors within the esophagus such that intraluminal pressure can be monitored as a continuum along the entire length of the esophagus over time. Figure 40.1 superimposes representative conventional manometric and HRM recordings, with the

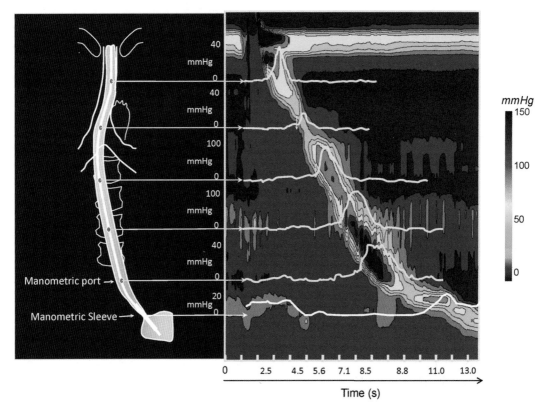

Fig. 40.1 Depiction of normal esophageal motility by conventional manometry (white line tracings) and high-resolution manometry with esophageal pressure topography (EPT). The positions of pressure sensors in the esophagus for the conventional manometry are indicated in the anatomical drawing on the *left* with a sleeve device across the esophagogastric junction (EGJ). On the *right*, the conventional manometry tracings and EPT are overlaid to illustrate how they correspond with each other. The peristaltic wave strips the bolus from the esophagus with the pressure upstroke (conventional) or isobaric contour (EPT) demarcating the bolus/no bolus interface. Note the tremendously enhanced detail provided by EPT, especially in the area of the EGJ

HRM displayed in EPT format. HRM provides sufficient recording length (35 cm) to span from the hypopharynx to the stomach (with several intra-gastric sensors) without the need for a pull-through technique or catheter repositioning once the proper location is established. The pressure sensor/transducer components configured into currently available solid-state HRM manometric catheters consist of either strain gauge transducers or TactArray™ devices (a proprietary transducer technology). The TactArray™ sensors provide 12 separate measurements and will depict the information as an average of the measures while the other configurations utilize a strain gauge within a fluid-filled bead to provide a circumferential estimate of pressure. There are no data to support which sensor is superior; however, normative values and thresholds for diagnosis should not be interchanged between devices as they may be different.

Manometric Protocol

Esophageal manometry is usually performed in the supine position. This position allows the testing of peristaltic function without the effect of gravity on bolus transit and provides a slight stress to elicit peristaltic activity. All currently available normative data for HRM have been established in supine position.

A typical manometry protocol consists of a 30-s basal period in the absence of swallowing followed by ten 5-mL test swallows of water.

The test swallows are separated by at least 20–30 s to reestablish basal activity and avoid having deglutitive inhibition from the prior swallow affect the subsequent swallow [3]. The manometric diagnosis is based on the analysis of the test swallows and focuses on a description of distinct patterns at the esophagogastric junction (EGJ) and along the tubular esophagus. Multiple rapid swallows are sometimes included as a simple assessment of the integrity of deglutitive inhibition, defects of which are thought to be responsible for some spastic motility disorders [4].

Esophageal Pressure Topography Analysis and Classification of Esophageal Disorders

When HRM is coupled with a display of the pressure data as EPT plots, contractility is visualized as a spatial and temporal continuum, with the magnitude of intra-esophageal pressure displayed as graded spectral colors denoting isobaric conditions among the sensors. Figure 40.2 depicts a normal swallow as an EPT plot encompassing both the upper esophageal sphincter (UES) and the EGJ, the timing of deglutitive UES and EGJ relaxation and the contractions of the intervening esophageal body. The normal swallow on EPT is a seamless wave of contraction with no defects or breaks in the isobaric contour set at 20 mmHg. The normal contraction propagates at a velocity below 9 cm/s and does not intersect the EGJ before 4.5 s to allow time for bolus emptying. Additionally, the contraction wavefront will usually have a maximal amplitude less than 240 mmHg and contractile activity within the range of 1,000–5,000 mmHg cm s. The measurements utilized to classify spastic and hypercontractile disorders will be discussed in the following sections.

The algorithm for classifying esophageal motor disorders using EPT is based on a systematic analysis that begins by separating the plot into two functional domains: the EGJ and the esophageal body. Abnormal EGJ pressure morphology or impaired deglutitive EGJ relaxation can profoundly affect pressure topography within the esophageal body. Consequently, the first step

in analyzing esophageal motility should focus on the EGJ (Fig. 40.3) [5]. Consistent with this, a stepwise analysis algorithm first characterizes the location of the EGJ and the pressure morphology, such as presence of hiatus hernia which is seen on EPT as a separation of the EGJ components, lower esophageal sphincter, and the crural diaphragm, in the 30-s basal period without swallowing [6]. Once the location is confirmed and a respiratory inversion is defined to document placement of the catheter into the intra-abdominal space, the adequacy of deglutitive EGJ relaxation is defined. The measurement of EGJ relaxation can be performed using the 4-s integrated relaxation pressure (IRP). IRP is defined as the lowest average pressure for four contiguous or noncontiguous seconds within 10 s after deglutitive UES relaxation (the relaxation window, Fig. 40.2a), and 15 mmHg serves as a cutoff threshold for diagnosing achalasia [7].

Once the EGJ anatomy and deglutitive relaxation are defined, the analysis focuses on the peristaltic integrity of the tubular esophagus with each swallow. With normal EGJ relaxation, the integrity of the 30 mmHg isobaric contour is a key concept in using EPT to characterize peristalsis. The 30 mmHg isobaric contour circumscribes areas on the plot with pressure exceeding 30 mmHg. It is a reliable threshold distinguishing intrabolus pressure from luminal closure, and the minimal, yet still optimal, pressure facilitating bolus clearance. When the EGJ is normal and the 30 mmHg isobaric contour is continuous from the UES to the EGJ, there is virtual certainty of normal bolus transit and clearance. Breaks in the 30 mmHg isobaric contour are indicative of areas along the esophagus with a peristaltic amplitude of less than 30 mmHg and increased likelihood of incomplete bolus clearance (retrograde bolus escape). Based on the degree or length of these defects, swallows are classified as intact, defective, or failed (Table 40.1). It is worth mentioning here that the contractile pattern of each swallow is also examined for an abnormal esophageal pressurization occurring with the contractile activity such as pan-esophageal pressurization that appears in some achalasia cases or pressurization between the contractile front and the EGJ

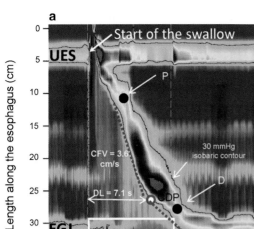
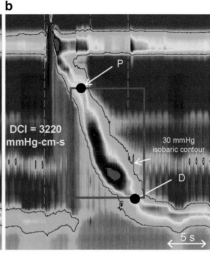
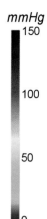

Fig. 40.2 A normal swallow in an esophageal pressure topography (EPT) plot. The two high-pressure zones, visualized before and after the swallow start, denote the upper esophageal sphincter (UES) and the esophagogastric junction (EGJ). The peristaltic contraction ensues after the start of the swallow and propagates in time and space towards the EGJ. Its distal component spans two pressure troughs: a proximal, P, and a distal, D, one. (**a**) First, deglutitive EGJ relaxation is assessed within the EGJ relaxation window (*white box at the EGJ*) that extends for 10 s after the start of the swallow. EGJ relaxation characterized by a 4-s integrated relaxation pressure (IRP), the lowest average pressure for four contiguous or noncontiguous seconds within the relaxation window, of < 15 mmHg is considered normal. Next, the peristalsis is defined using the 30 mmHg isobaric contour (*black line*) which circumscribes areas on

the EPT plot with intraluminal pressure > 30 mmHg. By fitting two tangential lines at the isobaric contour to the initial and terminal portions of the isobaric contour and noting intersection of the lines the contractile deceleration point (CDP, *white dot*) is located. CDP represents the point at which the esophageal peristaltic clearance shifts to the emptying of the phrenic ampulla. Hence, the contractile front velocity (CFV) is based on the tangential line between P and the CDP. A CFV < 9 cm/s defines normal esophageal peristalsis. (**b**) The distal contractile integral (DCI) defines the contractile vigor of the distal esophagus. DCI is calculated by multiplying the length of the esophageal segment between the P and the D troughs, the duration of the contraction, and the mean pressure of the contraction encased within the 20 mmHg isobaric contour (*pink box*). A normal swallow has a DCI between 500 and 5,000 mmHg cm s

indicative of increased intrabolus pressure. This is a unique feature of EPT as these patterns are much more evident in pressure topography compared to the conventional line-tracing format.

Swallows with either intact or small defects in peristalsis are then further characterized by their contractile front velocity (CFV), distal contractile integral (DCI), and distal latency (DL). Given the importance of defining abnormal propagation and contractile vigor in identifying spasmodic or hypertensive contractions, special emphasis will be given to these measurements in the next subsections.

Propagation Velocity

Contractile front velocity (CFV) is measured from the proximal pressure trough to the contractile deceleration point (CDP) defined as the point

in the contractile continuum where the most abrupt deceleration in velocity occurs prior to the contraction reaching the distal pressure trough (Fig. 40.2a). CDP defines a transition from esophageal peristaltic clearance to emptying of the phrenic ampulla, where the mechanism is dominated by re-elongation of the distal esophagus and recoil of the phrenoesophageal ligament rather than peristaltic propagation [8]. CFV is based on the best-fit tangent between the proximal pressure trough and CDP (Fig. 40.2a) with 9 cm/s being the upper limit of normal [5].

Contractile Vigor

The vigor of the distal esophageal contraction is quantified using the distal contractile integral (DCI) (Fig. 40.2b). Conceptually, the DCI

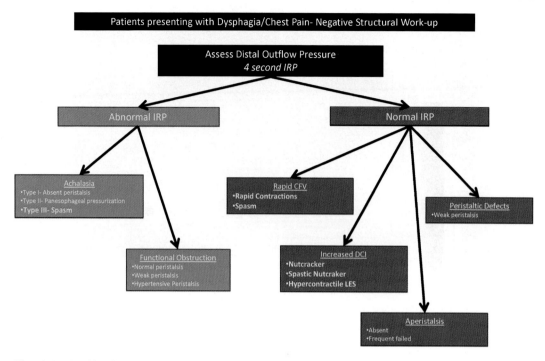

Fig. 40.3 Algorithm for analysis of EPT studies according to the Chicago Classification. Note that motility disorders should be considered as a cause of dysphagia and/or chest pain only after first evaluating for structural disorders, eosinophilic esophagitis, and, where appropriate, cardiac disease. The first branch point is to identify patients meeting criteria for achalasia (elevated IRP and absent peristalsis), which is then subclassified. Patients meeting partial criteria for achalasia or exhibiting swallow-induced contractions with short latency or rapid propagation are then characterized. Note that some of these patients likely have variant forms of achalasia while, at the other extreme, some are probably normal variants. The third branch point in the algorithm is to identify hyper- or hypocontractile conditions. Note that some individuals with high DCI may have slightly elevated values of IRP. (*IRP* integrated relaxation pressure, *CFV* contractile front velocity, *DCI* distal contractile integral, *DL* distal latency)

corresponds to the "volume" of the distal contraction in dimensions of time, length, and amplitude with a value between 500 and 5,000 mmHg cm s considered as normal [9].

Distal Contractile Latency

The esophageal deglutitive response is initiated with the oropharyngeal swallow. However, the subsequent peristaltic contraction in the distal esophagus is preceded by a period of quiescence. Behar and Biancani introduced the concept of latency to quantify this period of quiescence and suggested that contractile latency was substantially reduced in patients with simultaneous contractions than in those with normal peristaltic velocity (Fig. 40.4) [10]. In EPT terms, distal contractile latency (DL) is defined as the duration of the interval between upper esophageal sphinc-

ter relaxation and the CDP, with the lower limit of normal of 4.5 s being similar to that described by Behar and Biancani (Fig. 40.4) [11]. DL measure provides the last step in characterizing each swallow as shown in Table 40.1.

Summarizing the EGJ relaxation, peristaltic integrity, CFV, DCI, and DL characteristics of the ten test swallows form the foundation of diagnosis according to the Chicago Classification (Table 40.2). Figure 40.3 highlights the diagnoses of esophageal hypercontractility.

Other Techniques to Evaluate Esophageal Motility

Historically, fluoroscopy was the first method utilized to assess esophageal motility disorders.

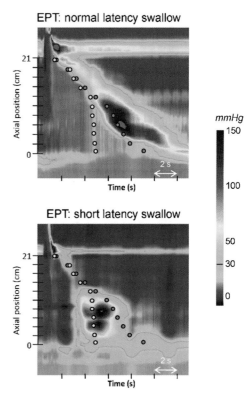

EPT: normal latency swallow

EPT: short latency swallow

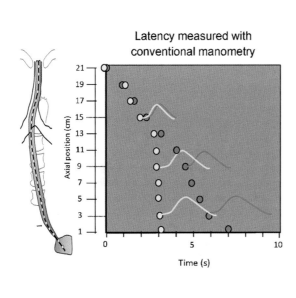

Latency measured with conventional manometry

Fig. 40.4 The concept of reduced distal latency in spasm as described by Behar and Biancani. The left panel shows the latency of propagation for normal controls (*blue circles*) and a patient with spasm (*white circles*) adapted from Behar and Biancani. The latency interval was measured using conventional manometry as the time from onset of contraction at sensor 21 to onset of contraction at sensor 1. The latency interval was determined to be a marker of the inhibitory ganglionic integrity, suggesting that patients with spasm had evidence of reduced latency and premature contraction. In the right panels, the latency interval plots from the conventional manometry study are superimposed on EPT tracings of a swallow with normal latency (*top*) and short latency (*bottom*). In each case, the time and sensor position scales are adjusted to approximate those of the conventional manometry tracing

However, the fluoroscopic assessment of esophageal contractility is indirect because it reflects only the efficiency of bolus transit within the esophagus and across the EGJ, without substantial metrics of their functional role. Despite this limitation, fluoroscopy is still extremely useful in describing anatomical abnormalities prior to esophageal surgery, for assessing the functional outcome after Heller myotomy, and to evaluate post-fundoplication symptoms.

Multichannel intraluminal esophageal impedance monitoring is a relatively new technology developed to monitor bolus transit through the esophagus without radiation exposure. Impedance monitoring is based on the concept that electrical resistance (impedance) between adjacent electrodes in the esophagus will vary depending on whether the electrodes are in contact with luminal contents or only the esophageal mucosa. When bridged by liquid the impedance decreases. By placing several electrode pairs along a probe that is then positioned transnasally within the esophagus, the flow of the swallowed bolus through the esophagus can be monitored by following sequential anterograde drops in impedance. Bolus transit is then characterized as a dichotomous outcome of complete or incomplete. The esophageal function affecting flow can be assessed when impedance is combined with HRM. The role of assessing bolus transit alone in spastic and hypercontractile disorders is unclear.

Table 40.1 Esophageal pressure topography scoring of individual swallows

Integrity of contraction	
Intact contraction	20 mmHg isobaric contour without large or small break
Weak contraction	a) Large break in the 20 mmHg isobaric contour (>5 cm in length) b) Small break in the 20 mmHg isobaric contour (2–5 cm in length)
Failed peristalsis	Minimal (<3 cm) integrity of the 20 mmHg isobaric contour distal to the proximal pressure trough (P) in any swallow
Contraction pattern (for intact or weak peristalsis with small breaks)[a]	
Premature contraction	DL <4.5 s
Hypercontractile	DCI >8,000 mmHg s cm
Rapid contraction	CFV >9 cm/s
Normal contraction	Not achieving any of the above diagnostic criteria
Intrabolus pressure pattern (30 mmHg isobaric contour)	
Pan-esophageal pressurization	Uniform pressurization extending from the UES to the EGJ
Compartmentalized esophageal pressurization	Pressurization extending from the contractile front to a sphincter
EGJ pressurization	Pressurization restricted to zone between the LES and CD in conjunction with hiatus hernia
Normal pressurization	No bolus pressurization >30 mmHg

Modified from Pandolfino et al. [5]
DL Distal latency, *CFV* Contractile Front Velocity, *DCI* Distal Contractile Integral
[a]CFV and DCI are not calculated in failed swallows or weak peristalsis if the defect is greater than 5 cm

Table 40.2 The Chicago classification for diagnosis of esophageal motility abnormalities

Diagnosis	Diagnostic criteria
Achalasia	
Type I achalasia	Classic achalasia: mean IRP > upper limit of normal, 100 % failed peristalsis with absent contractile activity
Type II achalasia	Achalasia with esophageal compression: mean IRP > upper limit of normal, no normal peristalsis, pan-esophageal pressurization with ≥20 % of swallows
Type III achalasia	Mean IRP > upper limit of normal, no normal peristalsis, preserved fragments of distal peristalsis or premature (spastic) contractions with ≥20 % of swallows
EGJ outflow obstruction[a]	Mean IRP > upper limit of normal, some instances of intact peristalsis or weak peristalsis with small breaks such that the criteria for achalasia are not met
Distal esophageal spasm	Normal mean IRP, ≥20 % premature contractions
Hypercontractile esophagus	At least one swallow DCI >8,000 mmHg s cm with single peaked or multi-peaked (jackhammer) contraction
Absent peristalsis	Normal mean IRP, 100 % of swallows with failed peristalsis
Weak peristalsis with large peristaltic defects	Mean IRP <15 mmHg and >20 % swallows with large breaks in the 20 mmHg isobaric contour (>5 cm in length)
Weak peristalsis with small peristaltic defects	Mean IRP <15 mmHg and >30 % swallows with small breaks in the 20 mmHg isobaric contour (2–5 cm in length)
Rapid contractions with normal latency	Rapid contraction with ≥20 % of swallows, DL >4.5 s
Hypertensive peristalsis (nutcracker esophagus)	Mean DCI >5,000 mmHg s cm, but not meeting criteria for hypercontractile esophagus
Frequent failed peristalsis	>30 %, but <10 % of swallows with failed peristalsis
Normal	Not achieving any of the above diagnostic criteria

This classification is not intended to include postsurgical conditions (fundoplication, Lapband, etc.) that may be associated with secondary motility disturbances
[a]May be an achalasia variant

Esophageal Motor Disorders

Pathophysiology

The control of esophageal peristalsis varies along the length of the esophagus. This change coincides with the transition from the striated muscle proximally to smooth muscle distally, with the proximal trough/transition zone being the most overt feature on EPT. There is also a distinct division in neurologic control of the peristaltic sequence. The initiation of the sequence proximally is controlled by direct cholinergic stimulation from motor neurons originating in the Nucleus Ambiguus, which sequentially activate the esophageal muscularis propria [12]. In the distal (smooth muscle) esophagus, including the lower esophageal sphincter (LES), the deglutitive response is more intricate. The efferent motor neurons from the Dorsal Motor Nucleus of the Vagus (DMV) synapse onto the ganglia of the myenteric plexus. Two physiologically distinct populations of DMV preganglionic neurons are identifiable originating from caudal and rostral locations within the DMV. Although both are cholinergic, and neither exhibit sequenced activation, in the esophagus one population synapses onto inhibitory (nitric oxide) myenteric neurons while the other synapses on excitatory (cholinergic) ones [13]. Thereafter, the timing of contraction of the muscularis propria at each esophageal level is dependent on the balance between the effects of inhibitory (hyperpolarizing) and excitatory (depolarizing) myenteric neurons on the membrane potential of the myocytes (Fig. 40.5). The progressive aboral dominance of the inhibitory myenteric neurons results in increasing latency of contraction [13]. The amplitude of contraction at each locus is additionally modulated by both the myocyte number and excitability [14]. The gross effect of these neuromyenteric controls can be easily appreciated on EPT plots through the sequence of esophageal deglutition that starts with UES relaxation, and then proceeds through a well-timed sequence of EGJ relaxation and peristalsis, with the latter varying in velocity and contractile vigor in its proximal-to-distal progression (Fig. 40.2a).

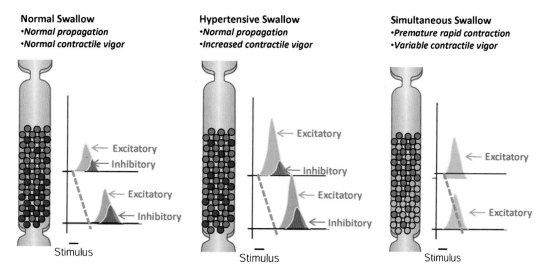

Fig. 40.5 In a normal swallow (*left panel*), the cholinergic excitatory innervation of the distal esophagus decreases gradually aborally (*blue circles*), while the inhibitory innervation increases (*red circles*). As a result, upon stimulation the distal latency increases gradually along the esophagus resulting in the characteristic peristaltic sequence seen on EPT (*green dashed line* represents normal propagation). In the case of a hypertensive swallow (*middle panel*), the inhibitory innervation decreases, but a peristaltic sequence can be still achieved. The absence of inhibition can result in simultaneous contraction (*right panel*) devoid of peristalsis. From J. Crist et al. Proc Natl Acad Sci USA 1984;81(11):3595–9; H. Mashimo and R.K. Goyal. Physiology of esophageal motility. GI motility online; 2006 with permission

Esophageal motility disorders can result from either primary diseases of the musculature or from a disruption in the balance between inhibitory and excitatory innervations. The resultant disruption of the features of the peristaltic sequence can show up as deviations from normal on EPT plots. Early achalasia is characterized by a loss of function by inhibitory myenteric neurons [15] showing on EPT as impaired EGJ relaxation. Hypertensive peristalsis could be associated with muscle hypertrophy, hyperexcitability, or possibly increased activation by excitatory myenteric plexus neurons. Smooth muscle atrophy is observed in the distal esophagus of patients with scleroderma and is associated with aperistalsis [16].

The manometric diagnostic criteria and treatment options designed to address neuromyenteric abnormalities leading to spastic and hypercontractile motility disorders are summarized in Tables 40.1 and 40.2.

Esophageal Spasm

The pathophysiology of diffuse esophageal spasm (DES) involves an impairment of inhibitory mechanisms leading to both premature and rapidly propagated or simultaneous contractions in the distal esophagus. Experimental inhibition of nitric oxide in control subjects induces simultaneous esophageal contraction; hence, the mechanism appears to be related to a reduction in the distal latency of the contraction. In contrast, the administration of nitric oxide donors prolongs the distal latency in patients with DES and decreases the contraction amplitude [17].

Diagnostic Criteria
Although most undiagnosed chest pain is not caused by esophageal spasm, esophageal manometry is often performed in the course of symptom evaluation and rapidly propagated esophageal contractions are frequently reported as indicative of an esophageal spasm [18]. However, these rapid contractions rarely cause chest pain and most experts agree that use of this criterion leads to over-diagnosis of distal esophageal spasm (DES)

[18]. Castell and Spechler proposed modifying the manometric criteria for DES to require (1) simultaneous (rapid) contractions in >10 % of wet swallows and (2) contraction amplitude greater than 30 mmHg [19]. The inclusion of a contractile amplitude threshold in the definition was intended to exclude low-amplitude pressure waves from guiding the diagnosis, but the defining feature of "simultaneous contractions" was retained.

Recently, there has been renewed interest in re-classifying distal esophageal spasm using EPT, as it has become clear that the conventional criteria for defining spasm are not easily applied to EPT. Normal regional variability in contraction velocity and regional boundaries demarcating functional esophageal segments are much more evident in EPT requiring, at the very least, that diagnostic criteria based on propagation velocity to be re-examined [5, 9]. Two recently described tools in EPT analysis that may improve the recognition of spasm are the CDP and DL described in the previous section on manometry. The CDP is the distal esophageal locus at which peristalsis terminates [8]. Consequently, identification of the CDP provides a reliable landmark for measuring peristaltic velocity or CFV. The DL is a related measure in that it times the occurrence of distal peristalsis relative to deglutitive UES relaxation. Together, these EPT measures facilitate objective measurement of peristaltic velocity and a means for quantifying the latency of the distal contraction as a surrogate for the integrity of the neural contractile inhibition [10, 11].

The combination of CFV and DL can be utilized to describe distinct phenotypes of rapid contraction that are likely to be clinically relevant (Fig. 40.6, Table 40.2). Recently, our group reviewed 1,070 consecutive EPT studies to assess the prevalence of rapid contraction and spasm using the criteria in Table 40.1. Of 1,070 evaluable patients, 91 (8.5 %) had a high CFV and/or low DL. Patients with only rapid contractions ($n = 67$) were heterogeneous in diagnosis (weak peristalsis, 38; hypertensive, 5; functional obstruction 7; normal 14) and symptoms with the majority ultimately categorized as weak peristalsis or normal. In contrast, 96 % of the patients with premature contraction had dysphagia and all

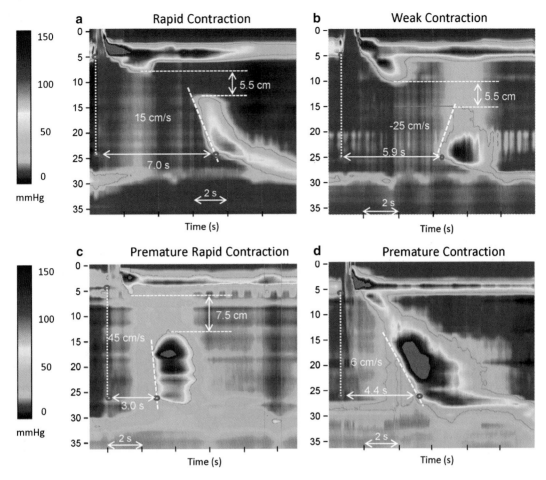

Fig. 40.6 EPT phenotypes of abnormal propagation based on DL and CFV measurements. The most common phenotypes are (**a**) and (**b**) with normal latency and a large defect in the 30 mmHg isobaric contour. The swallow in panel (**a**) with a rapid contraction and a large proximal break fulfills criteria for both weak peristalsis and rapid contraction. Panel (**b**) illustrates the problem with measuring CFV with weak peristalsis and a non-propagating segmental contraction. Although the CDP provides a reasonable temporal endpoint for measuring velocity, the large break eliminates any appropriate proximal landmark resulting in what would be a negative CFV. However, the DL is normal suggesting this to be an artifact of weak peristalsis. The swallow in panel (**c**) is also associated with a large break (7.5 cm), however, it is also associated with short latency (3.0 s) and rapid CFV (45 cm/s) thereby representing a distinct phenotype compared to panels (**a**) and (**b**). The swallow in panel (**d**) is premature (DL = 4.4 s) with a normal CFV (6 cm/s). This swallow is associated with impaired EGJ relaxation and bolus pressurization consistent with functional EGJ obstruction or an achalasia variant

(n = 24, 2.2 % overall) were ultimately managed as having spastic achalasia or DES.

Treatment

The treatment of spastic disorders of the esophagus is dependent on the phenotype that is defined using EPT (Table 40.3) and the presenting complaint. Patients with rapid contraction alone have either weak peristalsis, borderline hypertensive peristalsis, or normal peristalsis with regional segments of rapid contraction and thus, would be unlikely to respond to therapy focused on relaxing smooth muscle. Patients with premature contractions are probably more likely to respond to therapy focused on inducing smooth muscle relaxation similar to the treatment for achalasia. Finally, all patients presenting with chest pain without achalasia or a spastic motor disorder

Table 40.3 Treatment of motility disorders

Treatment	Indications
Pharmacologic	
Nitrates	DES, hypertensive peristalsis, spastic nutcracker (jackhammer)
Phosphodiesterase inhibitors	DES, hypertensive peristalsis, spastic nutcracker (jackhammer)
Calcium channel blockers	DES, hypertensive peristalsis, spastic nutcracker (jackhammer)
Antidepressants: tricyclic antidepressant, serotonine uptake inhibitors	DES, hypertensive peristalsis, spastic nutcracker (jackhammer)
Endoscopic	
Pneumatic dilation	Achalasia (DES?)
Botulinum toxin	Achalasia (DES?)
Surgical	
Heller myotomy	Achalasia
Heller with long myotomy	DES (achalasia type 3?)
Behavioral (hypnotherapy)	DES, hypertensive peristalsis, spastic nutcracker (jackhammer)

associated with reduced DL should undergo a trial of empiric GERD therapy with a PPI.

Pharmacological Treatment

As with achalasia, nitrates and calcium channel blockers have been proposed to treat esophageal spastic motility disorders [20]. However, the efficacy of these treatments in treating chest pain that is thought to be related to spasm is limited. Sildenafil represents a new option to treat spastic motility disorders. It reduces pressure amplitude and propagation velocity in both controls and patients with motility disorders. Preliminary data suggest it to be effective on relieving esophageal symptoms and in improving manometric findings in patients with spastic motility disorders [21, 22].

Patients with rapid contraction and normal DL may respond to therapy focused on reducing visceral sensitivity. Low-dose antidepressants can improve a patient's reaction to pain without objectively improving motility function [23]. The only controlled trial showing efficacy for this strategy was with the anxiolytic, trazadone (serotonin uptake inhibitor), suggesting that reassurance and control of anxiety are

important therapeutic goals [23]. Consistent with that conclusion, success has also have been reported using behavioral modification and biofeedback [24].

Endoscopic Treatment

Although the rationale for dilation is unclear, some success has been reported in treating spastic disorders with dilation. However, an important caveat is that it is completely uncertain as to whether patients who benefitted from pneumatic dilation would not be more properly categorized as spastic achalasia or achalasia with esophageal compression, emphasizing the need for accurate manometric classification.

Botulinum toxin injection is a pathophysiologically attractive approach to treating patients with spastic disorders. Therapeutic trials suggest botulinum toxin can reduce chest pain [25]. The technique has not been standardized in this application with some reports injecting botulinum toxin only at the level of the LES and others also injecting the distal esophagus [25]. No trial has yet compared botulinum toxin injection with other treatments.

Surgical Treatment

Long myotomy extending from the LES proximally onto the esophageal body has been used to treat patients with spastic disorders. The extent of the myotomy may be guided by manometric findings [26]. In an uncontrolled study, surgical treatment seemed more effective than medical treatment [26].

Spastic Achalasia

Apart from improving the sensitivity of manometry in the detection of achalasia, EPT has also defined a clinically relevant sub-classification of achalasia [27]. In its most obvious form, achalasia occurs in the setting of esophageal dilatation with negligible pressurization within the esophagus (type I achalasia, Fig. 40.7a). However, a substantial pressurization within the esophagus can still occur in achalasia. In fact, a very common pattern includes esophageal compression characterized

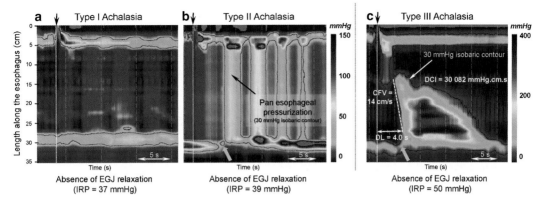

Fig. 40.7 Achalasia subtypes. All three subtypes are characterized by impaired EGJ relaxation (IRP >15 mmHg). (**a**) In type I, there is absent peristalsis and negligible pressurization in the esophageal body, evident by the absence of any area circumscribed by the 30 mmHg isobaric contour (*black line*). (**b**) In type II, the peristalsis is also absent, but pan-esophageal pressurization occurs evident by the banding pattern of the 30 mmHg isobaric contour spanning the length of tubular esophagus. This represents elevated intrabolus pressure and is associated with contraction of the longitudinal muscle and the "shift" of the EGJ orally (*orange arrow*). (**c**) type III is characterized by spastic contractions (rapid contractile front velocity (CFV) and short distal latency (DL)) in the esophageal body, but the pressurization is also attributable to an abnormal lumen obliterating contraction and an associated contraction of the longitudinal muscle "shifting" the EGJ orally

by pan-esophageal pressurization that also coincides with esophageal shortening noticeable by oral shift of the EGJ (type II achalasia, Fig. 40.7b). It is important to not confuse this pattern with spastic achalasia (type III, Fig. 40.7c) as the two subtypes are associated with very different treatment outcomes [27]. Logistic regression analysis found that the presence of pan-esophageal pressurization was a significant predictor of a good treatment response, as opposed to poor predictive treatment response in spastic achalasia. These findings were recently validated in a large series of patients with achalasia reported in an Italian cohort [28]. Adopting these sub-classifications will likely strengthen future prospective studies of treatment efficacy in achalasia. Additionally, these data also support that the type III variant of achalasia may require adjunct therapy focused on the peristaltic abnormality, as this pattern is typically maintained despite effective treatment for the poorly relaxing LES.

Hypertensive Peristalsis

Vigorous esophageal contractions with normal propagation have been reported in association with chest pain [29]. The pathophysiology of hypertensive peristalsis is unclear, but it is believed to be related to either excessive excitation, reactive compensation for increased EGJ obstruction, or myocyte hypertrophy [30]. An additional theory proposed from a study using high-frequency intraluminal ultrasound is of asynchrony between the circular and longitudinal muscularis propria contractions, an anomaly that is reversed with atropine [31, 32]. The ultrasound findings further support the concept that excessive cholinergic drive could be an important pathophysiological component of these conditions.

The conventional manometric definition of hypertensive peristalsis used the term "nutcracker" esophagus, defined by a peak peristaltic amplitude > 180 mmHg over ten swallows using recordings at 3 and 8 cm above the LES [19]. Subsequently, the defining peristaltic amplitude has been debated and more recent work suggests that the threshold should be increased to 260 mmHg, a value that is more likely to be associated with chest pain and dysphagia [29].

The introduction of HRM and EPT has allowed further stratification of hypertensive peristalsis to account for both excessive amplitude and abnormal morphology of the peristaltic contraction. The summary metric for contractile activity, the DCI, with values >5,000 mmHg cm s, but less

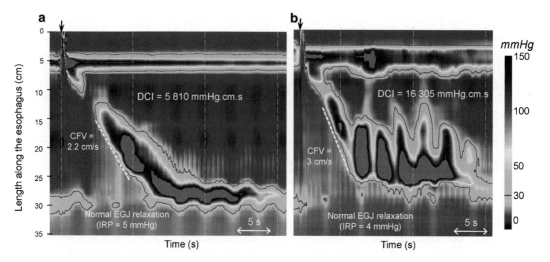

Fig. 40.8 Hypertensive peristalsis and spastic "nut-cracker" ("jackhammer") esophagus. (**a**) Hypertensive contractions are defined by a DCI>5,000 mmHg cm s. This example is associated with a hypercontractile LES, but normal EGJ relaxation. (**b**) An extremely abnormal contraction in a spastic nutcracker patient with repetitive prolonged contractions evoking the action of the jackhammer

than 8,000 mmHg cm s, is found in individuals with hypertensive peristalsis akin to "nutcracker" esophagus in conventional terms (Fig. 40.8a). However, because values in this range are also encountered in normal individuals, they are classified as hypertensive peristalsis to avoid implying a pathological condition. In contrast, DCI values >8,000 mmHg cm s are almost always associated with chest pain and dysphagia. These patients appear to have a more exaggerated pattern of hypercontractility that is repetitive and more akin to a "jackhammer" than a "nutcracker" (Fig. 40.8b). The current version of the Chicago Classification refers to this condition as spastic "nutcracker" (Table 40.2); however, that nomenclature is confusing given the fact that this entity is not associated with a rapid or premature contraction, features consistent with spasmodic contractility. The clinical relevance of "nutcracker" or "jackhammer" esophagus is still unclear. Nonetheless, focusing future trials on patients with a DCI >8,000 mmHg cm s rather than the lower threshold of 5,000 is more likely to identify a homogeneous population potentially amenable to pharmacological treatment focused on reducing contractility.

Pharmacologic Treatment

The same therapeutic options utilized for DES have also been advocated for patients with hypertensive peristalsis. Smooth muscle relaxants such as calcium channel blockers and nitrates have been used for these disorders. Although they reduce peristaltic amplitude, neither has been shown to relieve chest pain or dysphagia in clinical trials. Sildenafil is an appealing alternative due to its profound effect of reducing contraction amplitude and potentially reducing the occurrence of repetitive contractions [33]. Again, any supportive clinical trial data are absent. Finally, botulinum toxin injection in the esophageal muscle with or without endoscopic ultrasound guidance may be an option for patients with refractory symptoms.

Due to a potential overlap of the diagnosis of hypertensive peristalsis with GERD and the observation that many of these patients have coexistent psychological distress, therapy focused on modulating acid secretion, visceral sensitivity, and stress has been attempted. Proton pump inhibitors have been proposed to treat hypertensive peristalsis based on the hypothesis that GERD can induce chest pain and hypertensive peristalsis [34]. Similarly, treatment with low-dose tricyclic anitdepressants may reduce contractions via the anitcholinergic effect and may alter visceral sensitivity.

Hypercontractile LES

The LES is a 2–4 cm segment of smooth muscle that exhibits tonic contraction at rest and is modulated by various afferent stimuli from the oropharynx, esophagus, and stomach, unlike the smooth muscle of the esophageal body that is phasic and relaxed at rest and will only exhibit tone or contraction upon stimulation. Basal tone at the intrinsic LES is a composite of three mechanisms: (1) independent myogenic tone, (2) cholinergic excitatory tone, and (3) nitric oxide derived inhibitory tone. The excitatory and inhibitory influences are important in controlling basal tone and are also important in generating LES relaxation during swallowing. Preganglionic cholinergic nerves arising from the caudal DMN synapse onto the inhibitory myenteric neurons which then effect LES relaxation through NO and VIP neurotransmitters. Preganglionic nerves from the rostral DMN synapse on excitatory myenteric neurons which contain acetylcholine to effect LES contraction. The inhibitory and excitatory myenteric nerves are also modulated by sensory input from the esophagus and stomach thus affecting LES baseline tone. Esophageal distension stimulates the inhibitory pathways often leading to LES relaxation akin to the deglutitive reflex, while phase III of the gastric migrating motor complex can augument the basal tone above the normal expiratory basal pressure range of 10–35 mmHg.

Relaxation of the sphincter secondary to swallowing and subsequent distention of the striated muscle occurs through inhibitory input via a centrally mediated vago-vagal reflex. Relaxation that arises secondary to distention within the esophageal smooth muscle is controlled through the reflexes of the myenteric plexus and, hence, not abolished by vagotomy. Once a stimulus is activated, the LES relaxes for approximately 8–10 s. The LES also exhibits an after-contraction that

lasts approximately 7–10 s and this contraction likely represents a balance between the off-contraction induced by the dissipation of the nitrergic influence and the augmentation of on-contraction induced by the excitatory cholingeric influence.

The hypertensive LES and the hypercontractile LES are usually associated with normal latency and intact propagation and thus, are not a manifestation of impaired inhibition. More likely, these disorders represent an over-activity of the excitatory nerves or an over-activity of the smooth muscle response to excitatory input. Although there is overlap between the two disorders [9], they are distinguished by the extent and timing of the contractile augmentation . The hypertensive LES is defined by a basal expiratory pressure greater than 35 mmHg (Fig. 40.9a), while the hypercontractile LES is defined by the presence of a focus of hypertensive contraction >180 mmHg during the after-contraction. The latter motor disorder has recently been described by EPT using a mean DCI of >5,000 mmHg s cm and defining the location of the contraction within the segment of peristaltic contraction aboral to the distal pressure trough. Given the location and the threshold value of the contraction, this disorder has also been referred to as the "nutcracker LES" (Fig. 40.9b).

The extent to which hypercontractile LES contributes to the symptoms of dysphagia and chest pain cannot be isolated in light of its coexistence with vigorous esophageal contractions (Fig. 40.5a) [29]. Since heartburn can be the most frequent symptom in patients presenting with hypertensive LES [35], gastroesophageal reflux needs to be ruled out before proceeding with further treatment focused on reducing contractile vigor. Case reports suggest that some cases of hypercontractile LES may respond to therapy focused on inducing smooth muscle relaxation with nitrates and calcium channel blockers; however, no controlled trials have been performed to confirm this response. Additionally, some investigators have advocated using botulinum toxin to reduce the presynaptic release of acetylcholine from the myenteric neurons innervating the LES.

a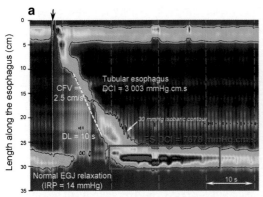

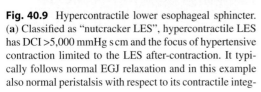

b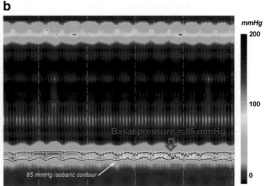

Fig. 40.9 Hypercontractile lower esophageal sphincter. (**a**) Classified as "nutcracker LES", hypercontractile LES has DCI >5,000 mmHg s cm and the focus of hypertensive contraction limited to the LES after-contraction. It typically follows normal EGJ relaxation and in this example also normal peristalsis with respect to its contractile integ- rity, CFV, DCI, and DL. (**b**) Hypertensive LES can be best recognized during the non-deglutitive period by its basal expiratory pressure in excess of 35 mmHg. Similar to hypercontractile LES, patients with hypertensive LES tend to exhibit normal EGJ relaxation and esophageal peristalsis

Conclusion

Spastic and hypercontractile esophageal motility disorders are diagnosed and classified using the gold standard, high-resolution esophageal manometry with esophageal pressure topography display. The major recognized disorders are distal esophageal spasm, spastic achalasia, hypercontractile (jackhammer), hypertensive peristalsis (nutcracker), and the hypercontractile LES. The most common symptoms associated with these conditions are typically dysphagia and chest pain and therapy is typically focused on reducing contractility with smooth muscle relaxants. Patients with borderline abnormalities or phenotypes that more closely resemble weak peristalsis or normal peristalsis should have therapy focused on reducing visceral sensitivity or acid suppression if GERD is a possibility and the presenting symptoms are associated with heartburn, regurgitation, or extra-esophageal complaints, such as cough and hoarseness. Further studies utilizing the improved diagnostic accuracy of HRM are required to improve management of patients with spastic disorders.

Acknowledgments This work was supported in part by R01 DK079902 (JEP) and R01DK56033 (PJK) from the Public Health Service.

References

1. Pandolfino JE, Kahrilas PJ. American Gastroenterological Association medical position statement: clinical use of esophageal manometry. Gastroenterology. 2005;128(1):207–8.
2. Clouse RE, Staiano A, Alrakawi A. Development of a topographic analysis system for manometric studies in the gastrointestinal tract. Gastrointest Endosc. 1998;48(4):395–401.
3. Murray JA, Clouse RE, Conklin JL. Components of the standard oesophageal manometry. Neurogastroenterol Motil. 2003;15(6):591–606.
4. Sifrim D, Janssens J, Vantrappen G. Failing deglutitive inhibition in primary esophageal motility disorders. Gastroenterology. 1994;106(4):875–82.
5. Pandolfino JE, Fox MR, Bredenoord AJ, Kahrilas PJ. High-resolution manometry in clinical practice: utilizing pressure topography to classify oesophageal motility abnormalities. Neurogastroenterol Motil. 2009;21(8):796–806.
6. Pandolfino JE, Kim H, Ghosh SK, Clarke JO, Zhang Q, Kahrilas PJ. High-resolution manometry of the EGJ: an analysis of crural diaphragm function in GERD. Am J Gastroenterol. 2007;102(5):1056–63.
7. Ghosh SK, Pandolfino JE, Rice J, Clarke JO, Kwiatek M, Kahrilas PJ. Impaired deglutitive EGJ relaxation in clinical esophageal manometry: a quantitative analysis of 400 patients and 75 controls. Am J Physiol Gastrointest Liver Physiol. 2007;293(4):G878–85.
8. Pandolfino JE, Leslie E, Luger D, Mitchell B, Kwiatek MA, Kahrilas PJ. The contractile deceleration point: an important physiologic landmark on oesophageal pressure topography. Neurogastroenterol Motil. 2010;22(4):395–400.

9. Pandolfino JE, Ghosh SK, Rice J, Clarke JO, Kwiatek MA, Kahrilas PJ. Classifying esophageal motility by pressure topography characteristics: a study of 400 patients and 75 controls. Am J Gastroenterol. 2008;103(1):27–37.

10. Behar J, Biancani P. Pathogenesis of simultaneous esophageal contractions in patients with motility disorders. Gastroenterology. 1993;105(1):111–8.

11. Roman S, Lin Z, Pandolfino JE, Kahrilas PJ. Distal contraction latency: a measure of propagation velocity optimized for esophageal pressure topography studies. Am J Gastroenterol. 2011;106(3):443–51.

12. Goyal RK, Chaudhury A. Physiology of normal esophageal motility. J Clin Gastroenterol. 2008;42(5):610–9.

13. Crist J, Gidda JS, Goyal RK. Intramural mechanism of esophageal peristalsis: roles of cholinergic and noncholinergic nerves. Proc Natl Acad Sci USA. 1984;81(11):3595–9.

14. Pehlivanov N, Liu J, Kassab GS, Puckett JL, Mittal RK. Relationship between esophageal muscle thickness and intraluminal pressure: an ultrasonographic study. Am J Physiol Gastrointest Liver Physiol. 2001;280(6):G1093–8.

15. Gockel I, Bohl JR, Eckardt VF, Junginger T. Reduction of interstitial cells of cajal (ICC) associated with neuronal nitric oxide synthase (n-NOS) in patients with achalasia. Am J Gastroenterol. 2008;103(4):856–64.

16. Roberts CG, Hummers LK, Ravich WJ, Wigley FM, Hutchins GM. A case–control study of the pathology of oesophageal disease in systemic sclerosis (scleroderma). Gut. 2006;55(12):1697–703.

17. Grubel C, Borovicka J, Schwizer W, Fox M, Hebbard G. Diffuse esophageal spasm. Am J Gastroenterol. 2008;103(2):450–7.

18. Pandolfino JE, Kahrilas PJ. AGA technical review on the clinical use of esophageal manometry. Gastroenterology. 2005;128(1):209–24.

19. Spechler SJ, Castell DO. Classification of oesophageal motility abnormalities. Gut. 2001;49(1):145–51.

20. Baunack AR, Weihrauch TR. Clinical efficacy of nifedipine and other calcium antagonists in patients with primary esophageal motor dysfunctions. Arzneimittelforschung. 1991;41(6):595–602.

21. Eherer AJ, Schwetz I, Hammer HF, et al. Effect of sildenafil on oesophageal motor function in healthy subjects and patients with oesophageal motor disorders. Gut. 2002;50(6):758–64.

22. Agrawal A, Tutuian R, Hila A, Castell DO. Successful use of phosphodiesterase type 5 inhibitors to control symptomatic esophageal hypercontractility: a case report. Dig Dis Sci. 2005;50(11):2059–62.

23. Clouse RE, Lustman PJ, Eckert TC, Ferney DM, Griffith LS. Low-dose trazodone for symptomatic patients with esophageal contraction abnormalities.

A double-blind, placebo-controlled trial. Gastroenterology. 1987;92(4):1027–36.

24. Latimer PR. Biofeedback and self-regulation in the treatment of diffuse esophageal spasm: a single-case study. Biofeedback Self Regul. 1981;6(2):181–9.

25. Storr M, Allescher HD, Rosch T, Born P, Weigert N, Classen M. Treatment of symptomatic diffuse esophageal spasm by endoscopic injections of botulinum toxin: a prospective study with long-term follow-up. Gastrointest Endosc. 2001;54(6):754–9.

26. Patti MG, Pellegrini CA, Arcerito M, Tong J, Mulvihill SJ, Way LW. Comparison of medical and minimally invasive surgical therapy for primary esophageal motility disorders. Arch Surg. 1995;130(6):609–15. discussion 615–606.

27. Pandolfino JE, Kwiatek MA, Nealis T, Bulsiewicz W, Post J, Kahrilas PJ. Achalasia: a new clinically relevant classification by high-resolution manometry. Gastroenterology. 2008;135(5):1526–33.

28. Salvador R, Costantini M, Zaninotto G, et al. The preoperative manometric pattern predicts the outcome of surgical treatment for esophageal achalasia. J Gastrointest Surg. 2010;14(11):1635–45.

29. Agrawal A, Hila A, Tutuian R, Mainie I, Castell DO. Clinical relevance of the nutcracker esophagus: suggested revision of criteria for diagnosis. J Clin Gastroenterol. 2006;40(6):504–9.

30. Dogan I, Puckett JL, Padda BS, Mittal RK. Prevalence of increased esophageal muscle thickness in patients with esophageal symptoms. Am J Gastroenterol. 2007;102(1):137–45.

31. Jung HY, Puckett JL, Bhalla V, et al. Asynchrony between the circular and the longitudinal muscle contraction in patients with nutcracker esophagus. Gastroenterology. 2005;128(5):1179–86.

32. Korsapati H, Bhargava V, Mittal RK. Reversal of asynchrony between circular and longitudinal muscle contraction in nutcracker esophagus by atropine. Gastroenterology. 2008;135(3):796–802.

33. Fox M, Sweis R, Wong T, Anggiansah A. Sildenafil relieves symptoms and normalizes motility in patients with oesophageal spasm: a report of two cases. Neurogastroenterol Motil. 2007;19(10):798–803.

34. Pehlivanov N, Liu J, Mittal RK. Sustained esophageal contraction: a motor correlate of heartburn symptom. Am J Physiol Gastrointest Liver Physiol. 2001;281(3):G743–51.

35. Gockel I, Lord RV, Bremner CG, Crookes PF, Hamrah P, DeMeester TR. The hypertensive lower esophageal sphincter: a motility disorder with manometric features of outflow obstruction. J Gastrointest Surg. 2003;7(5):692–700.

36. Mashimo H, Goyal RK. Physiology of esophageal motility. GI Motility online 2006. Accessed February 10, 2011, 2011.

Benign and Malignant Tumors of the Esophagus

41

Kenneth K. Wang

Abstract

On a global basis, esophageal squamous cell carcinoma (ESCC) is still the leading cancer in the esophagus, and it is ranked as the eighth in incidence and the sixth in mortality among tumors of all sites. However, its incidence varies significantly among different geographic and ethnic subgroups. The Asian Esophageal Cancer Belt includes western and northern China, Mongolia, southern parts of the former Soviet Union, Iran, Iraq, and eastern Turkey. The highest incidence, 700 per 100,000, was reported in Linxian, China. The multifactorial causes for this high incidence are still to be further elucidated, but they likely include cigarette smoking, excessive alcohol use, dietary habit (vitamin deficiency etc.), different food processing, environmental exposure, etc.

Keywords

Autofluorescence imaging (AFI) videoendoscopy • Benign tumors • Confocal laser endomicroscopy (CLE) • Esophagus • Malignant tumors • Narrow band imaging (NBI)

Epidemiology

On a global basis, esophageal squamous cell carcinoma (ESCC) is still the leading cancer in the esophagus, and it is ranked as the eighth in incidence and the sixth in mortality among tumors of all sites [1]. However, its incidence varies significantly among different geographic and ethnic subgroups (Table 41.1) [2, 3]. The Asian Esophageal Cancer Belt includes western and northern China, Mongolia, southern parts of the former Soviet Union, Iran, Iraq, and eastern Turkey. The highest incidence, 700 per 100,000, was reported in Linxian, China [4]. The multifactorial causes for this high incidence are still to be further elucidated, but they likely include cigarette smoking, excessive alcohol use, dietary habit (vitamin deficiency etc.), different food processing, environmental exposure, etc.

K.K. Wang, MD (✉)
Department of Gastroenterology and Hepatology,
Mayo Clinic, Rochester, MN, USA
e-mail: wang.kenneth@mayo.edu

Table 41.1 Incidence of esophageal squamous cancer in selected regions of the world

Region	Locality	Incidence (per 100,000)	
		Male	Female
Asian esophageal cancer belt		>100	>100
China	Yangcheng	135.2	84.4
	Tianjin	16.6	8
India	Kashmir	42.6	27.9
	Bombay	11.4	8.9
	Bangalore	6.6	5.3
Europe			
Northern Europe		<4.0	<2.0
Eastern Europe		<4.0	<2.0
France	Calvados	26.5	–
UK	East Scotland	8.5	4.3
	England and Wales	6.5	3.2
South America			
Uruguay		40	–
Brazil	Porto Alegre	26.3	7.8
North America			
USA	Los Angeles	16.4	4.9
	Washington DC		
	Black	16.9	4.5
	White	4.1	1.7
Africa			
Transkei		37.2	21.1

Source: Ribeiro et al. British Journal of Surgery 1996; 83: 1174–185

The incidence of ESCC in United States has been declining since 1973. This is in line with the decrease of adult cigarette smoking rate from about 42 % in the 1960s to about 20 % currently according to Centers for Disease Control and Prevention (CDC) reports. However, this decline of cigarette smoking has been stalled and caused significant public health concerns as we failed to drop below 12 %, a goal set by *Healthy People 2010*.

Although the esophageal adenocarcinoma has surpassed ESCC since the early 1990s, a high incidence is still seen among urban population and African Americans [1], and patients with certain comorbidities such as achalasia, head and neck cancer, tylosis, etc. (Table 41.4). The incidence among African-American men (16.8 per 100,000) is five times higher than Caucasians (3.0 per 100,000) [5] and the mortality is three times higher. In Western countries, the consumption of tobacco and alcohol could explain more

than 90 % of the ESCC cases [6]. This higher ESCC rate among African Americans parallels with the higher adult cigarette smoking rates. According to Surveillance, Epidemiology, and End Results (SEER) cancer registry data from 1992 to 1998, the ESCC incidence rates for Native American and white Hispanics were not higher than the general population.

Diagnosis

Patients with ESCC may present with dysphagia, weight loss, cough, and GI bleeding (hematemesis and/or melena). But there is no specific physical finding for ESCC, and rarely lymph nodes in the periphery could be appreciated. For cases with metastatic lesions, hepatomegaly could be present (Fig. 41.1).

The followings modalities are commonly used to establish the diagnosis of ESCC.

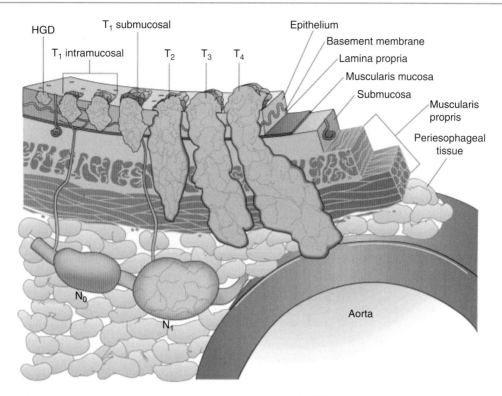

Fig. 41.1 Layers of esophagus and stages of esophageal cancer. From Rice WR: Diagnosis and staging of esophageal carcinoma. From F.G. Pearson et al. Esophageal surgery, 2nd ed. New York: Churchill Livingstone; 2002:687 with permission

1. Esophagogastroduodenoscopy (EGD) with lugol sprays

Lugol solution has been used in medicine since 1985. During EGD exam, lugol solution, approximately 10–20 ml of 1.5 % Lugol iodine solution (but the concentration may vary), is applied through a catheter over the entire esophagus. Since lugol solution contains potassium iodine and iodine, it should be avoided in patients with hyperthyroidism or iodine allergy. Some authors believe that patients with hypopharyngeal tumors are not candidates unless under endotracheal intubation due to concerns of possible laryngeal edema caused by iodine.

The lugol staining pattern is associated with the degree of glycogen within the squamous epithelium [7], and a squamous cell carcinoma does not include glycogen, hence is not stained and a clear identification is feasible. This enables the endoscopist to visualize the dysplastic areas as lugol-voiding lesions

(LVLs). Biopsies could then target at these LVLs to increase the yield. The overall sensitivity is 96–100 % and specificity varies from 40 to 95 %. It could also be used for intraoperative determination of tumor margin to assist the surgical resection.

LVLs could also be of prognostic value. In a study of 227 patients with head and neck squamous cell carcinoma (HNSCC), those with no LVLs did not have metachronous ESCC during median follow-up of 28 months; however, 15 % of those with numerous irregular LVLs lesions developed ESCC [8]. One study examined the nondysplasia epithelium (NDE) from lugol-voiding lesions, and it found 20 % of them had $p53$ hotspot mutation, and 40 % among dysplasia epithelium in contrast to no $p53$ mutations in 103 paired NDE samples with normal Lugol staining. It was also suggested that the chance of finding dysplasia was much higher from a patient with more LVLs than those with fewer ones.

EGD with lugol spray is currently considered as the most effective noninvasive way to diagnose squamous cell dysplasia and ESCC. Other newer methods such as narrow band imaging (NBI) or autofluorescence imaging (AFI) have been compared with lugol spray to assess their accuracy.

2. Narrow band imaging (NBI)

NBI is a novel noninvasive endoscopic approach to visualize the microvasculature on the tissue surface. Compared to WLE, NBI imaging only uses blue light at 415 nm and green light at 540 nm, which gives hemoglobin special absorption characteristics. Thus it provides better visualization of superficial and subsurface vessels that helps the ESCC detection. Often time the ESCC lesion appears reddish, likely due to microvascular proliferation and/or dilation.

In one nonrandomized study of head and neck squamous cell carcinoma (HNSCC) patients, NBI endoscopy with magnification was shown to have very high sensitivity, specificity, accuracy, positive predictive value, and negative predictive value (100 %, 97.5 %, 97.8 %, 83.3 %, and 100 %, respectively) [9]. In another multicenter, prospective, randomized controlled trial with 320 patients, NBI was shown to have 97 % sensitivity for superficial ESCC.

As to high-grade dysplasia, one study showed the intraepithelial papillary capillary loop (IPCL) patterns were very helpful, but the sensitivity and specificity are not satisfactory in contrast to a recent meta-analysis that demonstrated NBI was very sensitive (96 %) and specific (94 %) in detecting high-grade dysplasia (HGD) and intramucosal adenocarcinoma for Barrett's esophagus. It is noteworthy that all studies in this meta-analysis used NBI from a GIFQ240Z scope, an instrument maintains the capabilities of a standard video endoscope, but also affords a continuous range of image magnification adjustment up to X80.

However, NBI is not useful for detecting the depth of esophageal lesions based on current studies.

3. Autofluorescence imaging (AFI) videoendoscopy

When white light from the xenon lamp travels through a special optical filter, only the blue excitation light at 390–470 nm and green reflected light at 540–560 nm penetrate through. Interestingly, the blue excitation light can cause living tissue to emit autofluorescence, which passes through another filter and is then captured by the CCD at the end of the scope. AFI system works by combining autofluorescence (from blue light) and reflectance (from green light) to differentiate the neoplastic lesions (appears purple or magenta) from normal background (green). For the EGD scope that is equipped with AFI, the endoscopist can simply press the AFI button to switch from regular white light endoscopy (WLE) to AFI. However, the flat or depressed ESCC lesions appears to be dark green, which makes it very difficult to distinguish from the green color from normal squamous cell background [10]. Because of this, AFI was considered not as sensitive as narrow band imaging (NBI) for these flat or depressed lesions, making it a less attractive method, despite that AFI had higher ESCC detection rate (79 %) compared to WLE (51 %). A multicenter randomized trial showed that in detecting dysplasia and early cancer from Barrett's mucosa, the sensitivity, specificity, positive predictive value, and negative predictive value for AFI were 42 %, 92 %, 12 %, 98.5 %, respectively. Thus at the current time, AFI is best used as a complementary method and not a screening test due to the low sensitivity.

AFI has been also used in bronchoscopy and colonoscopy for squamous cell carcinoma of the lungs and dysplasia among ulcerative colitis patients in some studies with various results.

4. Confocal laser endomicroscopy (CLE)

CLE is a new technology that allows in vivo examination of histopathology at the cellular and subcellular levels by using cellular and vascular criteria. The term "confocal" refers to the alignment of both illumination and collection systems in the same focal plane. The laser light could be focused at the different layers of the tissue of interest. Then the reflected light from this layer is refocused and allowed to pass back to the lens in the endoscope and to be processed and presented on the monitor. Thus, different depths of the tissue can be examined in vivo, the so-called optical biopsy. Fluorescent contrasts, either intravenously or sprayed topically, can enhance the quality of CLE imaging [11].

In a recent study, CLE provided an in vivo diagnosis in 21 patients who had known ESCC, and the sensitivity and specificity using histology as gold standard were 100 % and 95 %, respectively. It holds promise for determination of the depth of squamous cell esophageal cancer [12]. Another CLE study after Lugol spray and intravenous fluorescein sodium showed the overall accuracy was 95 %, and the sensitivity and specificity were 100 % and 87 %, respectively. Intraobserver agreement was almost perfect (kappa=0.95) and interobserver agreement was substantial (kappa=0.79) [13].

CLE would potentially enable the endoscopist to proceed directly to endoscopic therapy, saving time and avoiding expensive and unnecessary further endoscopies. However, due to the limited tissue infiltration from the blue laser light, CLE may not be the right choice for submucosal lesions.

5. Endoscopic ultrasound (EUS)

After systematic metastatic lesions are ruled out for ESCC patients, EUS could be performed by using either conventional EUS scope or miniprobe sonography (MPS) through the regular endoscope channel. It is considered as the most accurate noninvasive method for T staging and for evaluation of the lymph nodes in the areas around the esophagus. It could also evaluate other organs such as the adrenal glands, pancreas, liver, bile ducts, mediastinal structures, etc. Final needle biopsy (FNA) of the lymph nodes can be done if necessary. However, it is difficult to distinguish T1a and T1b lesions sometimes even with MPS. When a patient has scarring from previous radiation therapy, endoscopic resection, or significant ongoing inflammation, it is also very challenging to provide accurate information. Despite

all of these, the overall T staging accuracy of EUS is 85 %–90 % as compared with 50 %–80 % for CT; the accuracy of regional lymph nodes staging is 70 %–80 % for EUS and 50 %–70 % for CT [14, 15]. However, a recent review showed [16] T-stage from EUS had concordance of only 65 % when compared with pathology specimens obtained by endoscopic mucosal resection (EMR) or surgery.

MPS is a small probe that could safely pass through a tight stricture or narrowing, and it could achieve higher resolution by using higher frequency. The use of MPS can also represent an improvement in the comfort and safety and is highly cost-effective [17]. The drawbacks for MPS are (1) inability to perform real-time ultrasound controlled biopsy; and (2) lower penetration depth due to higher frequency used, which means a decreased ability to assess structures (lymph nodes, etc.) that are further away from the GI tract.

6. Radiology: esophagraphy/CT/PET/MRI

An esophagram with barium swallow could identify a mass lesion for patients with dysphagia. However, this role has been largely supplanted by EGD, which could in addition provide biopsy of suspected tissues. Once high-grade dysplasia or mucosal ESCC are identified, chest CT with or without PET scan could be used to assess systemic involvement. This global evaluation of a patient's metastatic status (M and N staging) should be performed before EUS.

For T staging, EUS is superior to PET scan, which can only be considered when EUS or CT is inadequate. For N staging, EUS can more reliably distinguish the primary tumor from periesophageal lymph nodes based on a review in 2007. In centers with adequate experience, EUS should be the first choice, unless it cannot be performed due to a severe stenosis. For M staging, PET scan has clear advantage for detection of disease beyond the celiac axis; however, it is challenging to differentiate the regional node, N1 node, and the celiac axis M1a node. As to the overall impact on the management, PET scan changed 17 % of patients from curative to palliative, 4 % from palliative to curative, and another 17 % change in treatment modality or delivery based on the results from a study of 68 esophageal cancer patients.

United States Preventive Services Task Force (USPSTF) recommends PET scan to improve the accuracy of M staging for patients who are potential candidates for curative therapy; however, no adequate research examined the value to predict response to neoadjuvant therapy or to evaluate the suspected recurrence.

Recently, the accuracy of diffusion-weighted MR imaging for postoperative nodal recurrence of esophageal squamous cell cancer was found comparable to FDG-PET [18]. The role of MRI needs more investigation to be further defined.

7. Thoracoscopy and laparoscopy

Some surgical centers use these methods for esophageal cancer staging because of the superiority over noninvasive methods. Indeed, an intergroup trial of 107 patients reported that thoracoscopy and laparoscopy could increase the detection rate of positive lymph nodes from 41 % when using noninvasive staging tests (e.g., CT, MRI, EUS) to 56 % by thoracoscopy and laparoscopy, and no major complications or deaths were reported[19–21]. A more recent study in 2002 examined 111 esophageal cancer patients and compared the thoracoscopy and laparoscopy vs. noninvasive methods such as CT, MRI, and/or EUS, and it showed very low concordance ranging from 14 % to 25 % for TMN staging. This paper also pointed out that when compared with the final surgical pathology, a 100 % specificity and positive predictive value were achieved by thoracoscopy and laparoscopy staging in the diagnosis of lymph node metastasis. Although the sensitivity was about 75 % (vs. 45 % from noninvasive tests), the accuracy of thoracoscopy and laparoscopy could reach 90.8 % and 96.4 % in chest and abdomen metastases, respectively; these values were significantly higher than noninvasive staging methods (58 % and 68 %, respectively, for chest and abdomen) [22].

Staging

The typical workup includes CT scan of chest (and abdomen if advanced lesions are suspected), whole body PET (integrated PET-CT is preferred), and endoscopic ultrasound if no metastatic lesions are found, then surgical consult should be offered if it is considered as resectable. The American Joint Committee on Cancer (AJCC) recently released its seventh edition of cancer staging manual (Table 41.2).

Prognostication

The most significant prognostic factor is TNM staging, although emerging biomarkers could also explain some of the variations in survival.

1. TNM staging

An early study in the 1990s showed that early ESCC lesions that did not invade through muscularis mucosa had low lymph node metastasis rate (2–4 %) or vascular invasion (8 %) [23, 24]. Resection of such lesions yielded excellent prognosis with 5-year survival of 90–100 % [25–28]. It was also reported that tumor budding, the isolated cancer cells, or microscopic clusters of undifferentiated cancer cells (usually less than five cancer cells) outside the tumor margin was associated with significantly lower 5-year survival rates [29].

The number of lymph node metastases was found to impact the survival. In a retrospective study of 1,149 ESCC patients, the overall 5-year survival rates for the patients with 0, 1, and ≥2 positive nodes were 59.8, 33.4, and 9.4 %, respectively. And the stage-specific 5-year survival for T2N1M0 and T3N1M0 was significantly higher in the group with one positive lymph node than the group with ≥2 positive nodes (T2N1M0: 41.5 vs. 24.1 %; T3N1M0: 31.2 vs. 6.8 %) [30].

Among the ESCC patients with negative lymph nodes who generally have good 5-year survival, the finding of positive lymphatic invasion was linked to higher risk for hematogenous dissemination [31]. This is the result

Table 41.2 TNM staging of esophageal squamous cell cancer (SCC)

Part-1	
Primary tumor (T)[a]	
TX	Primary tumor cannot be assessed
T0	No evidence of primary tumor
Tis	High-grade dysplasia[b]
T1	Tumor invades lamina propria, muscularis mucosae, or submucosa
T1a	Tumor invades lamina propria or muscularis mucosae
T1b	Tumor invades submucosa
T2	Tumor invades muscularis propria
T3	Tumor invades adventitia
T4	Tumor invades adjacent structures
T4a	Resectable tumor invading pleura, pericardium, or diaphragm
T4b	Unresectable tumor invading adjacent structures, such as aorta, vertebral body, trachea, etc.
Regional lymph nodes (N)[c]	
NX	Regional lymph node(s) cannot be assessed
N0	No regional lymph node metastasis
N1	Metastasis in 1–2 regional lymph nodes
N2	Metastasis in 3–6 regional lymph nodes
N3	Metastasis in seven or more regional lymph nodes
Distant metastasis (M)	
M0	No distant metastasis
M1	Distant metastasis
Part-2	
Histologic grade (G)	
GX	Grade cannot be assessed—stage grouping as G1
G1	Well differentiated
G2	Moderately differentiated
G3	Poorly differentiated
G4	Undifferentiated—stage grouping as G3 squamous

Anatomic stage/prognostic groups

Squamous cell carcinoma[d]

Stage	T	N	M	Grade	Tumor location[e]
0	Tis (HGD)	N0	M0	1, X	Any
IA	T1	N0	M0	1, X	Any
IB	T1	N0	M0	2–3	Any
	T2-3	N0	M0	1, X	Lower, X
IIA	T2-3	N0	M0	1, X	Upper, middle
	T2-3	N0	M0	2–3	Lower, X
IIB	T2-3	N0	M0	2–3	Upper, middle
	T1-2	N1	M0	Any	Any
IIIA	T1-2	N2	M0	Any	Any
	T3	N1	M0	Any	Any
	T4a	N0	M0	Any	Any
IIIB	T3	N2	M0	Any	Any
IIIC	T4a	N1-2	M0	Any	Any

(continued)

Table 41.2 (continued)

	T4b	Any	M0	Any	Any
	Any	N3	M0	Any	Any
IV	Any	Any	M1	Any	Any

Note: cTNM is the clinical classification, pTNM is the pathologic classification
The original source for this material is the AJCC Cancer Staging Manual, Seventh Edition (2010) published by Springer New York
[a]At least maximal dimension of the tumor must be recorded and multiple tumors require the T(m) suffix
[b]High-grade dysplasia (HGD) includes all noninvasive neoplastic epithelia that was formerly called carcinoma in situ, a diagnosis that is no longer used for columnar mucosae anywhere in the gastrointestinal tract
[c]Number must be recorded for total number of regional nodes sampled and total number of reported nodes with metastasis
[d]Or mixed histology including a squamous component or NOS
[e]Location of the primary cancer site is defined by the position of the upper (proximal) edge of the tumor in the esophagus

from a study of 88 consecutive patients with ESCC who underwent three-field lymph node dissection and no positive lymph nodes were found initially. Among those patients who eventually have lymph node invasion, the incidence of lymphatic invasion was higher than vascular invasion (79 % vs. 38 %), suggesting that lymphatic invasion was more commonly seen than vascular invasion. Both lymphatic and vascular invasion were independently associated with poor survival (relative risk of 4.9 and 3.5, respectively).

2. Biomarkers

CIAPIN1 is a downstream effector of the receptor tyrosine kinase-Ras signaling pathway in animal cell lines. The decreased expression of CIAPIN1 was statistically correlated with the lower degree of differentiation, more depth of invasion, and lymph node metastasis among ESCC patients. Consistently, the survival rates of patients with CIAPIN1-negative tumors tended to be statistically lower than those with CIAPIN1-positive tumors. [32]

Higher tumor-specific expression of survivin, a member of the inhibitors of apoptosis gene family, has been found to be a significant marker for poorer survival for ESCC but not esophageal adenocarcinoma. The disease-specific survival rate of patients with low survivin mRNA expression was greater than those with high survivin (43 % vs.12 % at 5 years) [33].

Serum squamous cell carcinoma (SCC) antigen positivity, which indicates the circulating esophageal squamous cancer cells in peripheral blood, was found more often among advanced ESCC, but its prognostic value is limited [34, 35]

Over-expression of CyclinD1, an amino acid frequently expressed in G1 phase of the cell cycle, was thought to play an important role in cell growth and cancer progression. On the other hand, E-Cadherin, the most essential of the Cadherin family which is the backbone of cell to cell adhesion, is also a key molecule in the initial step of cancer cell invasion. Increased CyclinD1 expression and reduced E-Cadherin expression was a significant prognostic factor in patients with esophageal squamous cell carcinoma [36].

Prevention

1. Reduce exposures to risk factors

Carcinogenesis of ESCC is a complex process and no single risk factor can explain the variations of incidence rates among different groups. These potential factors may also exert synergistic impact on each other during this multistep carcinogenesis (Table 41.3).

(a) Tobacco and alcohol

It is undisputable that tobacco and alcohol, acting alone or synergistically, are the significant risks for ESCC. In one study, the significant synergistic impact of cigarette smoking and alcohol drinking on the risk of ESCC was staggering (odds ratio=50). Population attributable risk (PAR), the difference in rate of a condition between an exposed population and an unexposed pop-

Table 41.3 Risks associated with ESCC

Environmental/dietary/ behavior factors	Host factors
Tobacco	Ethnicity (African American)
Alcohol	Head and neck squamous cell carcinoma
Nitrosamines/its precursors (Barbeque)	Tylosis
Hot liquid	Achalasia
Nutritional deficiency	Lichen planus
Caustic injury (lye)	Scleroderma
Radiation	Plummer–Vinson syndrome
Agent orange (case reports)	

ulation, for the ever-smokers who consumed more than 30 alcoholic drinks per week were 56.9 % and 44.9 %, respectively. Tobacco and alcohol use was also associated with higher numbers of dysplasia lesions, and *p53* and *p21* gene mutations were also linked to ESCC during the early stage of the neoplasia evolving process.

The risk varies among different types of smoking (pipe and cigar smoking have higher risk) and alcohol beverage. Interestingly, the polymorphisms in acetaldehyde dehydrogenase 2 (ALDH2), which could cause flushing after alcohol use, was found to be a useful sign identifying individuals susceptible to ESCC development [37].

(b) Achalasia

In Greek achalasia means "do not relax." It is a condition that causes no peristalsis in the distal segment of esophagus where the musculature is mainly smooth muscle and inability to relax the LES (lower esophageal sphincter). This is likely the result of neuron degeneration in the myenteric plexuses from many reasons such as inflammation, infection, infiltration, etc. The annual incidence is approximately 1 case per 100,000, and both genders are equally affected. The features of achalasia include dysphagia for solids and liquid, excessive belching, etc. The diagnosis can be established by symptoms, barium swallow, esophageal manometry, and EGD

exam. The relation between achalasia and esophageal carcinoma was first reported by Fagge in 1872.

Because achalasia patients often have difficulty in swallowing at baseline, clinicians should have low threshold to initiate a new workup plan for ESCC among these patients. Studies have shown that these cases were often diagnosed late and the prognosis was very dismal. However, close endoscopy surveillance does not seem cost-effective, and other modalities such as blind brush cytology still warrant research. Even so the surveillance should be carried out among those who are fit enough to undergo surgical resection if tumors are found.

Regardless of treatment or not, one report showed 8.6 % of achalasia patients could have ESCC in 15–20 years after the onset of symptoms [38]. In another study of 1,062 achalasia patients (9,864 person–year follow-up), 2.3 % had ESCC, a 16-fold increase of cancer risk compared to general population [39]. It is very difficult to determine the true prevalence of ESCC among the achalasia patients, as it varies from 1.7 % to even 20 %. Likely this variation is due to different referral base and length of follow-up. One study showed the mean interval between the diagnosis of achalasia and carcinoma was 5.7 years.

(c) Tylosis

Tylosis (focal non-epidermolytic palmoplantar keratoderma), an autosomal dominant skin disorder with thickening of the skin in the palms and soles, was associated with a high risk of squamous cell carcinoma. It was first described in 1958 in two large Liverpool families. The causative locus, the tylosis esophageal cancer (TOC) gene, has been localized to a small region on chromosome 17q25. Studies on loss of heterozygosity (LOH) have indicated a role for the TOC gene in sporadic squamous cell esophageal cancer and Barrett's adenocarcinoma. About half of tylosis patients may develop ESCC by 45 years old or 95 % by the age of 65 [40, 41].

(d) Scleroderma

Scleroderma is skin thickening and hardening associated with many different medical conditions, and it is called systemic sclerosis when other organs/systems are also involved. Most of these patients have manifestations in GI tract and half of them may be asymptomatic. In the esophagus, it predominantly causes distal esophageal hypomotility and weak lower esophageal sphincter pressure, although the upper sphincter pressure and proximal esophageal motility is normal. And clinically it can present as heartburn, dysphagia, etc. and it is associated with esophagitis, ulceration, strictures, Barrett's esophagus, spontaneous esophageal rupture, esophageal adenocarcinoma, or ESCC. On esophageal manometry, it has distinctive features of low contractility and inability to relax the LES.

Both ESCC and adenocarcinoma of the esophagus were found among up to 70 % of scleroderma patients in an early study in 1979 [42]. However, a more recent review of seven studies showed that the link between scleroderma and cancer was not overwhelming with probably a modest increase in lung cancer [43]. This cancer risk might be much lower among localized scleroderma (morphea) patients.

(e) Head and neck squamous cell carcinoma (HNSCC)

It is well known that some patients with HNSCC could have either synchronous (found around the time of HNSCC diagnosis) or metachronous ESCC (diagnosed during follow-up) [44]. SEER data from 1973 to 1987 showed the incidence of esophageal cancer was about 1.6 % among 21,371 HNSCC patients, a 23 times increase of risk compared to general population [45]. One study showed 5 % of 389 patients were found to have synchronous esophageal squamous cell carcinomas within 1 year after the diagnosis of HNSCC [46]. It also revealed that metachronous ESCC was found more often among

hypopharyngeal cancer patients (about 16 %) than in laryngeal, oropharyngeal, or oral cancer patients. By combining seven studies with a total of 25,834 HNSCC patients, the rough estimate of esophageal cancer is about1.6 %.

Although no societal guideline is available, some authors suggested panendoscopic examination (bronchoscopy, pharyngo-esophagoscopy, and laryngoscopy) in patients with early stage head and neck cancer at the time of diagnosis and then every 6 months for 5 years [47].

(f) Human papillomavirus (HPV)

The relationship between HPV infection and ESCC remains controversial. It was demonstrated in a high-risk population in China, but not in low-risk patients in Europe [48–50].

2. Preventive measures

(a) Screening

Lots of efforts have been made in searching for optimal screening methods. The cytologic detection of ESCC or precursor lesions by using balloon and sponge samplers yielded very low sensitivity [51], although a recent study showed greater than 90 % sensitivity in detecting Barrett's esophagus by using Cytosponge [52]. However, the latter study also utilized trefoil factor 3, an immunostain diagnostic marker for Barrett's esophagus based on the systematic gene expression profiling, which may have enhanced the sensitivity significantly.

(b) Chemoprevention

Isotretinoin is a synthetic retinoid with chemopreventive effect that induces a differentiated state. It could potentially reduce the ESCC rate from 24 % to 4 % among HNSCC patients in a placebo controlled study [53].

Although providing a protective effect on patients with mild esophageal squamous dysplasia after 10-month use, selenomethionine failed to inhibit esophageal squamous carcinogenesis for high-risk subjects based on a randomized, placebo-controlled study,

Table 41.4 Recommendations regarding endoscopy surveillance for ESCC for high-risk patients (American Society for Gastrointestinal Endoscopy)

| Risk factors | EGD surveillance | |
	Starting time	Intervals
Achalasia	Insufficient data for surveillance. If considered, could initiate 15 years after onset of symptoms	Undefined
Tylosis	Age 30 years old	Requires more studies; no more than every 1–3 years
Caustic ingestion	15–20 years after caustic ingestion.	No more than every 1–3 years. Low threshold to evaluate swallowing problems with endoscopy

This table is based on "The role of endoscopy in the surveillance of premalignant conditions of the upper gastrointestinal tract." Gastrointest Endosc 2006; 63:570–80

which also demonstrated that celecoxib had no detectable protective benefit [54].

(c) Surveillance

The American Society for Gastrointestinal Endoscopy (ASGE) recommended surveillance on three high-risk populations: achalasia, caustic ingestion, and tylosis [55] (Table 41.4).

Cancer Management

Generally ESCC patients seek for medical attention when significant symptoms emerge, such as unexplained weight loss and dysphagia, at which time it is highly likely that the disease has spread to the degree that only palliative care could be provided. About 75 % of patients presented with stage III or IV disease. National Comprehensive cancer network (NCCN) provides a very detailed guideline in esophageal cancer management on their website. Based on this guideline and other publications, the current consensus can be summarized as follow:

1. Early ESCC

Although we have many steps to go through to find the optimal screening and surveillance methods, the best strategy is primary prevention. Secondary prevention can identify the high risks and detect the cancer at its early stage. Nowadays, we have much more experience in treating the early stage ESCC or adenocarcinoma.

(a) Endoscopic mucosal resection (EMR)

EMR is a minimal invasive endoscopic procedure to remove the mucosal lesions that are less than 2 cm or piecemeal removal of larger size lesions. Most commonly used techniques can be subdivided as injection-, cap-, and ligation-assisted EMR. Specifically EMR techniques include Injection-assisted EMR, Endocopic Muscoal Resection cap with suction, snare mucosectomy, or Duette Multiband Mucosectomy Kit [56]. An alternative for en bloc resection of a large lesion is ESD (endoscopic submucosal dissection), but its utility in the esophagus is still under investigation as it takes much longer time to perform and has higher complication rates.

About 2–4 % of mucosal ESCC (Tis or T1a) patients have lymph nodes invasion, and a few studies had shown that endoscopic mucosal resection (EMR) is the preferred for this population [57–59]. EUS is performed first before EMR to ensure there are no lymph nodes involved. EMR could be performed for diagnostic and therapeutic purposes. In an experienced hand, it has very low complications such as short-lived chest discomfort and pain, or minor bleeding (<2 g/dl of hemoglobin drop). Other rare complications include perforation and stenosis especially after multiple EMR in one session. The recurrence after EMR varies and it largely depends on the patient selection and whether or not extensive biopsies are performed at the index EGD exam (i.e., is it a true recurrence or a synchronous lesion missed due to sampling error?). One study of 142 mucosal ESCC patients who underwent EMR showed no recurrence of diseases in 9 years of follow-up [57].

The Mayo clinic researchers in Barrett's esophagus unit conducted a study and found that antiplatelet agents can be continued after the procedure to minimize cardiovascular complications among high thromboenbolic risk patients. Based on American Society of Gastroendoscopy (ASGE), the patients who need to continue anticoagulation can be bridged with low-molecular-weight heparin.

Patients with mucosal ESCC who undergo EMR should have endoscopic surveillance every 3 months for 1 year and then annually afterwards.

(b) Photodynamic therapy (PDT)

Since the 1980s PDT has been used for various medical conditions such as cancers (skin cancer, cholangiocarcinoma, esophageal neoplasia) and wet macular degeneration. PDT uses a special agent, such as sodium porfimer (approved in North America) and 5-aminolevulinic acid (5-ALA, used in Europe), either orally or intravenously to sensitize the tumor about 4 h (oral agent) or 24 h (intravenous agent) before photoradiation. Then laser light at 630–635 nm wavelength from a very small fiber through the endoscope channel is applied. This can activate the drug, which in turn interact with oxygen molecule to generate a singlet oxygen state causing cell death [60].

The response rate varies from 50 % to 100 % based on different studies. Severe dysplasia and superficial mucosal cancer (<2 mm in depth) can be completely ablated by 5-ALA-PDT. However, it may not be able to eradicate the early carcinoma thicker than 2 mm in depth. A large retrospective study of 123 patients (104 ESCC, 19 adenocarcinoma) showed no difference in complete response rate and survival rate between (1) PDT alone and PDT plus multimodal treatment groups (with chemoradiation), (2) between the

adenocarcinoma and squamous cell carcinoma groups. PDT-related complications include stenosis (35 %) and cutaneous photosensitization (13 %) [61]. Other side effects may include stricture, fistula, chest pain, nausea, and vomiting; however, the perforation rate was about 1 % which is lower than EMR.

However, although it is simpler to perform, the role of PDT in treatment of esophageal diseases has been limited when other newer and safer methods such as EMR and radiofrequency ablation (RFA) are gaining more popularity.

(c) Other modalities

Although radiofrequency ablation (RFA) has been used widely among Barrett's esophagus patients, the experience is still limited for ESCC. Only one case of ESCC with RFA treatment was reported in 2008. Very scarce experience with cryotherapy or argon plasma coagulation (APC) for ESCC has been reported.

2. Locally advanced ESCC

It is defined as any T stages with local lymph nodes but no evidence of distant disease. The chemotherapy regimen should be individualized based on tumor stage and patients' performance status. Unfortunately most of these regimens have low to median response rate and significant toxic profiles.

In reviewing the studies on chemoradiation and surgery, it is worth noting that: (1) most clinical studies recruited not only ESCC, but also esophageal adenocarcinoma, and some even stomach cancers; (2) some studies were criticized because of overall design (e.g. not randomized), small sample size, enrollment bias, uncontrolled crossover between study arms, underperformance of control arm (thus type I error), etc., so one should interpret the results with precautions; (3) these different regimens may prolong the median survival but usually no more than 12 months (most of them had benefits of 3–9 months compared to best supportive care) at the price of very serious adverse effects; (4) multimodality therapy has better response but more adverse effects; (5) surgery alone or surgery combined with other modalities, but not chemotherapy or radiation therapy (RT) alone, could be potentially curative for the patients with early stage cancer.

(a) Chemotherapy

The most frequently investigated and clinically used regimen includes infusion of cisplatin and 5-Fluorouracil (5-FU) at the first and fourth week of radiation therapy (RT). Its response rate varies from 20 % to 50 %. A randomized phase II study of cisplatin and 5-fluorouracil (5-FU) vs. cisplatin alone in advanced squamous cell esophageal cancer revealed that combined therapy failed to improve the survival time but had significantly more adverse effects such as grade 4 aplasia and septicemia, meningeal hemorrhage, cerebrovascular accident, and ischemia [62]. Actually, cisplatin seems to be the most active agent (response rate of approximately 20 %). But in practice, cisplatin and 5-FU are most commonly used in combination.

Other choices are ECF regimen (epirubicin, cisplatin, and 5-FU), DCF (docetaxel, cisplatin, and 5-FU), MCF (mitomycin, cisplatin, and 5-FU), irinotecan and cisplatin, gemicitabine and cisplatin. The REAL-2 study revealed that capecitabine, an oral agent that converts into 5-FU at tumor tissue, was as effective as 5-FU, and that oxaliplatin was similar to cisplatin but with significantly less grade 3 or 4 neutropenia, alopecia, kidney toxicity, and thromboembolism, but slightly more grade 3 or 4 diarrhea and neuropathy [63].

(b) Radiation therapy

External plus intraluminal radiotherapy was superior to external alone in both local control and long-term survival [64, 65]; however, the complications such as bleeding, fistula, ulcerations, and complication-related mortality were much higher in the combined group. Up to 70 %–80 % patients with dysphagia from the tumor could improve their symptoms [66].

Among postoperative ESCC patients, one retrospective study demonstrated that higher total radiation dose (> 50 Gy) after surgery was associated with fewer locoregional recurrence and better disease-free survival without more serious acute and late complications, but no improvement of overall mortality [67].

However, by randomizing nonsurgical patients with T1 to T4, N0/1, M0 squamous cell carcinoma or adenocarcinoma to receive higher dose RT (64.8 Gy) or standard dose RT (50.4 Gy) while receiving the same 5-FU and cisplatin therapy, INT 0123 study showed that higher dose RT (64.8 Gy) treatment did not yield statistically significant improvement in median survival when compared to 50.4 Gy group (18.1 vs. 13.0 months); and that the locoregional failure was about the same (56 % vs. 52 %). More treatment-related mortality was observed in the higher dose RT group. Thus RT with 50.4 Gy is currently considered as standard dose when combined with chemotherapy.

In summary, the current recommendation is to use 50.4 Gy radiation together with chemotherapy.

(c) Chemoradiation therapy

Chemoradiation therapy is considered more efficacious than alone therapy. For patients with significant cardiopulmonary issues who are not surgical candidates, this could be a potential cure.

A prospective trial in 1992 randomized patients to either the group with combined 5-FU and cisplatin plus 50.0 Gy of radiation therapy or to radiation therapy (RT) alone group (64.0 Gy). The results showed that combined therapy prolonged the median survival from 9 to 12.5 months, and the survival rates at 12 and 24 months were 50 % and 38 % in combined group vs. 33 % and 10 % in RT alone group [68].

In another prospective study, 196 ESCC and adenocarcinoma patients with T1-T3 N0-N1 and M0 staging, Karnofsky score of at least 50, were randomized to

Table 41.5 Resectability of the esophageal cancer

Staging of esophageal cancer	Methods for resection
Tis and T1a tumors (within the mucosa)	Endoscopic mucosal resection
T1b (submucosa)	Esophagectomy
T1–T3 with regional nodal metastases (N1)	Esophagectomy
T4 with involvement in pericardium, pleural, or diaphragm	Esophagectomy
Stage IVa, distal cancer with resectable celiac nodes, but sparing the celiac artery, aorta, or other organs	Esophagectomy
Stage IVa, distal cancer with unresectable celiac nodes; involvement of celiac artery, aorta, or other organs	Unresectable
Stage IVb, unresectable tumor invading other adjacent structures, such as aorta, vertebral body, trachea, etc.	Unresectable

chemotherapy (cisplatin and 5-FU) plus RT (50.0 Gy) vs. RT (64.0 Gy) alone. It showed the 5-year survival for combined therapy was 26 % compared to 0 % from the RT only group. However, due to the serious or even life-threatening adverse effects from the combined treatment, only 68 % the patients completed the whole chemoradiation therapy. [69]

For potentially resectable ESCC of the mid or lower esophagus, the two- or three-stage esophagectomy with two-field dissection or chemoradiotherapy offered similar survival based on results from the prospective randomized trial—CURE study the Chinese University Research Group for Esophageal Cancer (CURE) [70]. The regimen they used was 5-FU 200 mg/m^2/day infusion from day 1 to 42, cisplatin 60 mg/m^2 on days 1 and 22, and total RT of 50–60 Gy.

In summary, chemoradiation therapy is more efficacious than either chemo- or RT alone. For resectable patients, surgery could provide similar benefit as chemoradiotherapy.

(d) Surgery

Cervical and cervicothoracic esophageal carcinoma located at<5 cm from the cricopharyngeus should be treated with definitive chemoradiation rather than surgery [52]. For appropriate candidates, surgical options include trans-hiatal esophagectomy or the Ivor-Lewis procedure (requires thoracotomy and laparotomy) (Table 41.5).

- The acceptable surgical options include [63]:
- Standard Ivor Lewis esophagogastrectomy (laparotomy and right thoracotomy) or minimally invasive Ivor Lewis (laparotomy and limited right thoracotomy)
- Standard McKeown esophagogastrectomy (laparotomy, right thoracotomy, and cervical anastomosis) or minimally invasive McKeon (limited laparotomy, right thoracotomy, and cervical anastomosis)
- Transhiatal esophagogastrectomy (laparotomy and cervical anastomosis)
- Robotic minimally invasive esophagogastrectomy
- Left transthoracic or thoracoabdominal incision with anastomosis in the chest or neck.
- Options for reconstruction after esophagectomy include gastric pull-up, colon interposition, or jejunal interposition.

(e) Surgery with vs. without preoperative therapy (neoadjuvant)

A recent review (2007) regarding the overall efficacy of the neoadjuvant therapy with chemoradiation suggested better curative resection rates and lower locoregional recurrence, but the overall benefit for survival was not clearly demonstrated although some studies revealed such trend. Many of these studies, however, were not optimally designed; study groups were mixed (gastric cancer, esophageal adenocarcinoma, and esophageal squamous cell carcinoma);

sample size was small with inadequate power; and some yielded conflicting results. The multicenter, randomized trial to compare preoperative chemoradiotherapy followed by surgery with surgery alone in patients with stage I and II squamous cell cancer of the esophagus failed to show a difference in the overall survival although it did prolong disease-free survival.

The CROSS trial is a multicenter, randomized phase III, clinical trial which compares neoadjuvant chemoradiotherapy followed by surgery with surgery alone in patients with potentially curable esophageal adenocarcinoma and ESCC with inclusion of 175 patients per arm. The results of this study are still pending.

- The practice guideline from Cancer Care Ontario (http://www.cancercare. on.ca/) recommended the following:
- *Bi-modal regimen:* a published abstract of an individual patient data-based meta-analysis of nine randomized trials (2,102 patients) comparing preoperative chemotherapy followed by surgery (CT + S) to surgery alone demonstrated a 4 % (from 16 to 20 %) absolute overall survival advantage for chemotherapy at 5 years. Based on seven trials (1,849 patients), the disease-free survival (DFS) was 10 % in CT + S group vs. 6 % in surgery alone group. No difference was seen in postoperative death.
- *Tri-modal regimen:* a meta-analysis of 10 randomized trials comparing esophageal adenocarcinoma patients who received preoperative chemoradiotherapy followed by surgery to surgery alone showed a 13 % absolute benefit in survival at 2 years for preoperative chemoradiotherapy.
- Thus, Tri-modal is preferred to bi-modal regimen if preoperative therapy is considered.
- Randomized trials demonstrated no survival benefit for radiation therapy given alone, either preoperatively or postoperatively, compared with surgery alone.

- Randomized trials demonstrated no survival benefit for postoperative chemotherapy compared with surgery alone.
- In summary, based on less-than-optimal studies, neoadjuvant therapy prior to surgery may provide a small benefit in overall survival and is currently recommended.

(f) Surgery with or without postoperative therapy (adjuvant therapy)
Compared to neoadjuvant therapy, fewer studies addressed the issue of adjuvant therapy. One randomized study in 2003 suggested cisplatin and 5-FU adjuvant therapy improved the 5-year disease free survival from 45 % to 55 % ($p = 0.037$) for ESCC patients with stages IIA, IIB, III, or IV due to distant node involvement (M1 lymph node) after surgery.

In 2000, a study randomized 556 patients with either resectable gastric and GE junction adenocarcinoma, to postoperative chemoradiotherapy or surgery alone. Patients in the postoperative chemoradiation arm had a median survival of 36 months and patients in the surgery alone arm had a median survival of 27 months ($p = 0.005$).

A more recent study in 2009 prospectively randomized 151 ESCC patients (stage II–III) to surgery and adjuvant therapy vs. surgery alone, and it showed significant better 5- and 10-year survival rates of 42.3 % and 24.4 % for the group with adjuvant therapy vs. 33.8 % and 12.5 % for the surgery alone group. The local recurrence rates in the combined group and surgery alone group were 14.9 % and 36.4 % ($p < 0.05$).

In summary, based on limited data, adjuvant therapy with chemoradiation may provide some survival benefit when compared to surgery alone.

(g) Target therapy
Since the current therapy has limited response for esophageal cancer patients, target therapy aiming towards certain molecules such as HER-2, VEGFR, is an area with active investigation.

The ToGA trial which included HER-2 positive patients with gastroesophageal and gastric adenocarcinoma demonstrated that 5-FU/cisplatin/trastuzumab was superior to 5-FU/cisplatin with median survival of 13.5 vs. 11.1 months. Besides trastuzumab, other agents used in the targeted therapy include cetuximab, erlotinib, matuzumab, gefitinib (anti-HER2 antibodies), bevacizumab (an anti-VEGFR antibody) are also under investigations.

(h) Herbal agents

A recent Cochrane review was unable to identify a true randomized control trial among the 43 articles regarding herbal use as an adjunct therapy to chemoradiation for esophageal cancer patients. The herbals in these studies were from a large variety of plants and no specific brand or names were listed. This review concluded that we have no solid evidence to support or refute the use of herbal agents among esophageal cancer patients.

3. Metastatic diseases and palliative care

Patients with Eastern Cooperative Oncology Group Performance (ECOG) score of ≥3 could be supported by best care; if ECOG score is ≤2, chemotherapy may be considered. No regimen is considered as standard.

For space-occupying lesions, esophageal stents could be placed to restore esophageal patency, but ESCC within 2 cm of upper esophageal sphincter (EUS) is a contraindication. Sometime dilation with balloon or Savary dilators may be necessary before stent placement. Self-expanding metal stents (SEMS) have been improved continuously over the last decade in its diameter, shape, distal and proximal flanges, and types of coatings; they are preferred over plastic stents for palliative purpose. SEMS could be placed via endoscopy with or without fluoroscopy by gastroenterologists or under fluoroscopy by radiologists. The complications of stents include migration, bleeding, perforation, tumor overgrowth, pressure necrosis, etc., and the rates vary by types of stents and anatomic location of the placement. The placement success rate is 90–97 %.

Percutaneous endoscopic gastrostomy (PEG) can be considered if a patient cannot swallow saliva. If jejunum access is needed, percutaneous endoscopic jejunostomy (PEJ) or PEG tube with jejunum extension can be placed.

If patients have bleeding from the tumor surface, then endoscopy treatment with APC (argon plasma coagulation) or electrocoagulation might be helpful. However, if severe bleeding is from fistualization between tumor and aorta, endoscopy intervention is insufficient and patients suffer from high mortality.

Family Screening

There is no specific recommendation for family screening. However, if the family is exposed to the similar environments or has similar life style as in the index case, screening seems appropriate although no formal recommendation is available.

Case Studies

A 67-year-old Caucasian female has a 22 year history of achalasia and underwent Heller myotomy 12 years previous. She has had progressively worsening heartburn symptoms despite PPI therapy. For a few years she has intermittent vomiting especially when she lies flat. The vomitus may include undigested food from a previous meal. She presented to clinic with progressive dysphagia to solids and was sustained on liquid nutrition supplement and a mechanical soft diet. She also had a 25 lb weight loss that she attributed to poor appetite. She was ambulatory and capable of self-care but unable to carry out work activities.

Q1: what are the possible underlying etiologies for her dysphagia?

In a different scenario, if this lady presented a few days after her Heller myotomy, it is still possible that her symptoms are due to tissue swelling from the surgery, or possible scar formation if it is a few weeks after her operation.

However, in her current situation, she is suffering from the reflux of the food retained in her distal esophagus. It is possible that her achalasia had recurred. Another possible etiology for her dysphagia (the worst-case scenario) is squamous cell carcinoma of the esophagus, or esophageal adenocarcinoma, which could be the reason for her solid food dysphagia.

Q2. What is the next step in her medical care?

One could start with esophagram, but definite diagnostic modality is EGD exam with biopsy. If cancer is found, then PET/CT scans are the next step in this investigation. If negative, then endoscopic ultrasound (EUS) can be performed for T staging.

Q3. What are the treatment options?

It certainly depends on the TMN staging and her performance status. If she has metastatic diseases and space occupying mass that caused her dysphagia, then self-expanding metal stent could provide palliation. Chemotherapy or RT is also an option to reduce the tumor size.

If it is locally advanced disease, then neoadjuvant chemotherapy with ECF regimen (Epirubicin, Cisplatin, and 5-FU) with radiation therapy followed by esophagectomy could be offered.

If it is only a mucosal lesion (which is highly unlikely given her dysphagia), endoscopic mucosal resection (EMR) could be a potential cure.

Key Patient Consent Issue

Consent for EGD/EUS/EMR/Stent

Mr. (or Mrs) X, we will perform upper endoscopy exam under sedation with ultrasonic view of your esophageal lesion and surrounding lymph nodes. If it is a shallow lesion, we may perform a procedure to resect it. It may cause some bleeding where the resection takes place, but the vast majority of patients will stop the oozing spontaneously without intervention, otherwise, cautery, coagulation, hemoclip, etc. can be utilized to stop the bleeding. Other significant, but fortunately very rare complications are infection or perforation.

If your lesion in the esophagus is occupying the lumen, we could place a metal stent over it to relieve the trouble with swallowing. The risks include bleeding, stent migration, tumor tissue growth into the stent causing obstruction, or necrosis and even perforation.

Discussion for Some Chemotherapy Regimens

The adverse effects could be serious from some of the agents. For example, oxaliplatin plus capecitabine regimen could cause leukopenia (50.0 %), nausea and vomiting (51.6 %), diarrhea (50.0 %), stomatitis (39.1 %), polyneuropathy (37.5 %), and hand-foot syndrome (37.5 %) [71]. We will closely monitor you and terminate your treatment if you are not able to tolerate it.

References

1. Jemal A, Murray T, Ward E, Samuels A, Tiwari RC, Ghafoor A, et al. Cancer statistics. Cancer J Clin. 2005;55:10–30.
2. Mahboubi E, Kmet J, Cook PJ, Day NE, Ghadirian P, Salmasizadeh S. Oesophageal cancer studies in the Caspian Littoral of Iran: the Caspian cancer registry. Br J Cancer. 1973;28:197–214.
3. Zheng S, Vuitton L, Sheyhidin I, Vuitton DA, Zhang Y, Lu X. Northwestern China: a place to learn more on oesophageal cancer. Part one: behavioural and environmental risk factors. Eur J Gastroenterol Hepatol. 2010;22(8):917–25.
4. Cradock VM. Cancer of the esophagus. New York: Cambridge University Press; 1993.
5. Blot WJ, Devesa SS, Kneller RW, et al. Rising incidence of adenocarcinoma of the esophagus and gastric cardia. J Am Med Assoc. 1991;265:1287–9.
6. Brown LM, Hoover R, Silverman D, Baris D, Hayes R, Swanson GM, Schoenberg J, Greenberg R, Liff J, Schwartz A, Dosemeci M, Pottern L, Fraumeni Jr JF. Excess incidence of squamous cell esophageal cancer among US Black men: role of social class and other risk factors. Am J Epidemiol. 2001;153:114–22.
7. Mori M, Adachi Y, Matsushima T, Matsuda H, Kuwano H, Sugimachi K. Lugol staining pattern and histology of esophageal lesions. Am J Gastroenterol. 1993;88:701–5.
8. Muto M, Hironaka S, Nakane M, Boku N, Ohtsu A, Yoshida S. Association of multiple Lugol-voiding lesions with synchronous and metachronous esophageal squamous cell carcinoma in patients with head and neck cancer. Gastrointest Endosc. 2002; 56(4):517–21.
9. Nonaka S, Saito Y, Oda I, Kozu T, Saito D. Narrow-band imaging endoscopy with magnification is useful

for detecting metachronous superficial pharyngeal cancer in patients with esophageal squamous cell carcinoma. J Gastroenterol Hepatol. 2010;25(2):264–9.

10. Yoshida Y, Goda K, Tajiri H, Urashima M, Yoshimura N, Kato T. Assessment of novel endoscopic techniques for visualizing superficial esophageal squamous cell carcinoma: autofluorescence and narrow-band imaging. Dis Esophagus. 2009;22(5):439–46. Epub 2009 Jan 23.

11. ASGE Technology Committee, Kantsevoy SV, Adler DG, Conway JD, Diehl DL, Farraye FA, Kaul V, Kethu SR, Kwon RS, Mamula P, Rodriguez SA, Tierney WM. Confocal laser endomicroscopy. Gastrointest Endosc. 2009;70(2):197–200.

12. Iguchi Y, Niwa Y, Miyahara R, Nakamura M, Banno K, Nagaya T, Nagasaka T, Watanabe O, Ando T, Kawashima H, Ohmiya N, Itoh A, Hirooka Y, Goto H. Pilot study on endomicroscopy for determination of the depth of squamous cell esophageal cancer in vivo. J Gastroenterol Hepatol. 2009;24(11):1733–9. Epub 2009 Sep 25.

13. Pech O, Rabenstein T, Manner H, Petrone MC, Pohl J, Vieth M, Stolte M, Ell C. Confocal laser endomicroscopy for in vivo diagnosis of early squamous cell carcinoma in the esophagus. Clin Gastroenterol Hepatol. 2008;6(1):89–94.

14. Ziegler K, Sanft C, Zeitz M, et al. Evaluation of endosonography in TN staging of oesophageal cancer. Gut. 1991;32(1):16–20.

15. Tio TL, Coene PP, den Hartog Jager FC, et al. Preoperative TNM classification of esophageal carcinoma by endosonography. Hepatogastroenterology. 1990;37(4):376–81.

16. Young PE, Gentry AB, Acosta RD, Greenwald BD, Riddle M. Systematic review, endoscopic ultrasound does not accurately stage early adenocarcinoma or high-grade dysplasia of the esophagus. Clin Gastroenterol Hepatol. 2010;8(12):1037–41.

17. Menzel J, Hoepffner N, Nottberg H, et al. Preoperative staging of esophageal carcinoma: miniprobe sonography versus conventional endoscopic ultrasound in a prospective histopathologically verified study. Endoscopy. 1999;31:291–7.

18. Shuto K, Saito H, Ohira G, Natsume T, Kono T, Tohma T, Sato A, Ota T, Akutsu Y, Aoyagi T, Matsubara H. Diffusion-weighted MR imaging for postoperative nodal recurrence of esophageal squamous cell cancer in comparison with FDG-PET. Gan To Kagaku Ryoho. 2009;36(12):2468–70.

19. Bonavina L, Incarbone R, Lattuada E. Preoperative laparoscopy in management of patients with carcinoma of the esophagus and of the esophagogastric junction. J Surg Oncol. 1997;65(3):171–4.

20. Sugarbaker DJ, Jaklitsch MT, Liptay MJ. Thoracoscopic staging and surgical therapy for esophageal cancer. Chest. 1995;107(6 Suppl):218S–23. Pubmed Abstract.

21. Luketich JD, Schauer P, Landreneau R. Minimally invasive surgical staging is superior to endoscopic ultrasound in detecting lymph node metastases in esophageal cancer. J Thorac Cardiovasc Surg. 1997;114(5):817–21. discussion 821–3.

22. Krasna MJ, Jiao X, Mao YS, Sonett J, Gamliel Z, Kwong K, Burrows W, Flowers JL, Greenwald B, White C. Thoracoscopy/laparoscopy in the staging of esophageal cancer: Maryland experience. Surg Laparosc Endosc Percutan Tech. 2002;12(4):213–8.

23. Endo M, Kawano T. Detection and classification of early squamous cell esophageal cancer. Dis Esophagus. 1997;10(3):155–8.

24. Endo M, Kawano T. Analysis of 1125 cases of early esophageal carcinoma in Japan. Dig Endosc. 1991;4:71–6.

25. Moghissi K. Surgical resection for stage I cancer of the oesophagus and cardia. Br J Surg. 1992;79:935–7.

26. DeMeester T, Stein HJ. Surgical therapy for cancer of the esophagus and cardia. In: Castell DO, editor. The esophagus. Boston: Little, Brown; 1992. p. 299–341.

27. Nabeya K, Hanaoka T, Li S, Myumura T. What is ideal treatment for early esophageal cancer? Endoscopy. 1993;25:670–1.

28. Sugimachi K, Ikebe M, Kitamura K, et al. Long term results of esophagectomy for early esophageal carcinoma. Hepatogastroenterology. 1993;40:203–6.

29. Koike M, Kodera Y, Itoh Y, Nakayama G, Fujiwara M, Hamajima N, Nakao A. Multivariate analysis of the pathologic features of esophageal squamous cell cancer: tumor budding is a significant independent prognostic factor. Ann Surg Oncol. 2008;15(7):1977–82. Epub 2008 Apr 12.

30. Zhang HL, Chen LQ, Liu RL, Shi YT, He M, Meng XL, Bai SX, Ping YM. The number of lymph node metastases influences survival and International Union against cancer tumor-node-metastasis classification for esophageal squamous cell carcinoma. Dis Esophagus. 2010;23(1):53–8. Epub 2009 Apr 15.

31. Shahabi M, Noori Daloii MR, Langan JE, Rowbottom L, Jahanzad E, Khoshbin E, Taghikhani M, Field JK, Risk JM. An investigation of the tylosis with oesophageal cancer (TOC) locus in Iranian patients with oesophageal squamous cell carcinoma. Int J Oncol. 2004;25(2):389–95.

32. Zheng X, Zhao Y, Wang X, Li Y, Wang R, Jiang Y, Gong T, Li M, Sun L, Hong L, Li X, Liang J, Luo G, Jin B, Yang J, Zhang H, Fan D. Decreased expression of CIAPIN1 is correlated with poor prognosis in patients with esophageal squamous cell carcinoma. Dig Dis Sci. 2010;55(12):3408–14.

33. Rosato A, Pivetta M, Parenti A, Iaderosa GA, Zoso A, Milan G, Mandruzzato S, Del Bianco P, Ruol A, Zaninotto G, Zanovello P. Survivin in esophageal cancer: an accurate prognostic marker for squamous cell carcinoma but not adenocarcinoma. Int J Cancer. 2006;119(7):1717–22.

34. Kosugi S, Nishimaki T, Kanda T, Nakagawa S, Ohashi M, Hatakeyama K. Clinical significance of serum carcinoembryonic antigen, carbohydrate antigen 19-9, and squamous cell carcinoma antigen levels in esophageal cancer patients. World J Surg. 2004;28(7):680–5. Epub 2004 Jun 4.

35. von Brevern M, Hollstein MC, Risk JM, Garde J, Bennett WP, Harris CC, Muehlbauer KR, Field JK.

Detection of circulating oesophageal squamous cancer cells oesophageal tumors in the tylosis oesophageal cancer (TOC) gene region of chromosome 17q. Br J Surg. 2004;91(8):1055–60.

36. Research Committee on Malignancy of Esophageal Cancer, Japanese Society for Esophageal Diseases. Prognostic significance of CyclinD1 and E-Cadherin in patients with esophageal squamous cell carcinoma: multiinstitutional retrospective analysis. J Am Coll Surg. 2001;192(6):708–18.

37. Morita M, Kumashiro R, Kubo N, Nakashima Y, Yoshida R, Yoshinaga K, Saeki H, Emi Y, Kakeji Y, Sakaguchi Y, Toh Y, Maehara Y. Alcohol drinking, cigarette smoking, and the development of squamous cell carcinoma of the esophagus: epidemiology, clinical findings, and prevention. Int J Clin Oncol. 2010;15(2):126–34.

38. Messmann H. Squamous cell cancer of the oesophagus. Best Pract Res Clin Gastroenterol. 2001;15(2):249–65.

39. Sandler RS, Nyren O, Ekbom A, et al. The risk of esophageal cancer in patients with achalasia. A population-based study. J Am Med Assoc. 1995;274:1359–62.

40. Marger RS, Marger D. Carcinoma of the esophagus and tylosis. A lethal genetic combination. Cancer. 1993;72:17–9.

41. Maillefer RH, Greydanus MP. To B or not to B: it tylosis B truly benign? Two North American genealogies. Am J Gastroenterol. 1999;94:829–34.

42. Whitaker JA, Bishop R. Scleroderma with carcinoma of the esophagus case report. Am J Gastroenterol. 1979;71:496–500.

43. Pearson JE, Silman AJ. Risk of cancer in patients with scleroderma. Ann Rheum Dis. 2003;62(8):697–9.

44. Li Z, Seah TE, Tang P, Ilankovan V. Incidence of second primary tumours in patients with squamous cell carcinoma of the tongue. Br J Oral Maxillofac Surg. 2011;49(1):50–2.

45. Day G, Blot W. Second primary tumors in patients with oral cancer. Cancer. 1992;70:1,14–19.

46. Su YY, Fang FM, Chuang HC, Luo SD, Chien CY. Detection of metachronous esophageal squamous carcinoma in patients with head and neck cancer with use of transnasal esophagoscopy. Head Neck. 2010;32(6):780–5.

47. Sauterau D. Screening for early esophageal cancer: whom and how? Endoscopy. 1999;31:325–8.

48. Chang F, Syrjanen S, Shen Q, et al. Human papillomavirus involvement in esophageal carcinogenesis in the high-incidence area of China. A study of 700 cases by screening and type-specific in situ hybridization. Scand J Gastroenterol. 2000;35:123–30.

49. Lagergren J, Wang Z, Bergstrom R, et al. Human papillomavirus infection and esophageal cancer: a nationwide seroepidemiologic case-control study in Sweden. J Natl Cancer Inst. 1999;91:156–62.

50. Talamini G, Capelli P, Zamboni G, et al. Alcohol, smoking and papillomavirus infection as risk factors for esophageal squamous-cell papilloma and esophageal squamous-cell carcinoma in Italy. Int J Cancer. 2000;86:874–8.

51. Roth MJ, Liu SF, Dawsey SM, Zhou B, Copeland C, Wang GQ, Solomon D, Baker SG, Giffen CA, Taylor PR. Cytologic detection of esophageal squamous cell carcinoma and precursor lesions using balloon and sponge samplers in asymptomatic adults in Linxian, China. Cancer. 1997;80(11):2047–59.

52. Kadri SR, Lao-Sirieix P, O'Donovan M, Debiram I, Das M, Blazeby JM, Emery J, Boussioutas A, Morris H, Walter FM, Pharoah P, Hardwick RH, Fitzgerald RC. Acceptability and accuracy of a non-endoscopic screening test for Barrett's oesophagus in primary care: cohort study. Br Med J. 2010;341:c4372.

53. Hong WK, Lippman SM, Itri LM, et al. Prevention of second primary tumors with isotretinoin in squamous-cell carcinoma of the head and neck. N Engl J Med. 1990;323:795–801.

54. Limburg PJ, Wei W, Ahnen DJ, Qiao Y, Hawk ET, Wang G, Giffen CA, Wang G, Roth MJ, Lu N, Korn EL, Ma Y, Caldwell KL, Dong Z, Taylor PR, Dawsey SM. Randomized, placebo-controlled, esophageal squamous cell cancer chemoprevention trial of selenomethionine and celecoxib. Gastroenterology. 2005;129(3):863–73.

55. American Society for Gastrointestinal Endoscopy. The role of endoscopy in the surveillance of premalignant conditions of the upper gastrointestinal tract. Gastrointest Endosc. 2006;63:570–80.

56. Soehendra N, Binmoeller KF, Bohnacker S, et al. Endoscopic snare mucosectomy in the esophagus without any additional equipment: a simple technique for resection of at early cancer. Endoscopy. 1997;29:380–3.

57. Inoue H, Tani M, Nagai K, et al. Treatment of esophageal and gastric tumors. Endoscopy. 1999;31:47–55.

58. Takeshita K, Tani M, Inoue H, et al. Endoscopic treatment of early oesophageal or gastric cancer. Gut. 1997;40:123–7.

59. Giovannini M, Bernardini D, Moutardier V, et al. Endoscopic mucosal resection (EMR): results and prognostic factors in 21 patients. Endoscopy. 1999;31:698–701.

60. Wang KK, Lutzke L, Borkenhagen L, Westra W, Song MW, Prasad G, Buttar NS. Photodynamic therapy for Barrett's esophagus: does light still have a role? Endoscopy. 2008;40(12):1021–9.

61. Sibille A, Lambert R, Souquet JC, et al. Long-term survival after photodynamic therapy for esophageal cancer. Gastroenterology. 1995;108:337–44.

62. Bleiberg H, Conroy T, Paillot B, Lacave AJ, Blijham G, Jacob JH, Bedenne L, Namer M, De Besi P, Gay F, Collette L, Sahmoud T. Randomised phase II study of cisplatin and 5-fluorouracil (5-FU) versus cisplatin alone in advanced squamous cell oesophageal cancer. Eur J Cancer. 1997;33(8):1216–20.

63. Wei X, Chen Z, Yang X, Wu T. Chinese herbal medicines for esophageal cancer. National comprehensive cancer network guidelines in Oncology, v.2.2010. Cochrane Database Syst Rev. 2009 7;(4):CD004520 http://www.nccn.org/professionals/physician_gls/PDF/esophageal.pdf.

64. Okawa T, Tanaka M, Kita-Okawa M, et al. Superficial esophageal cancer: multicenter analysis of results of

definitive radiation therapy in Japan. Radiology. 1995;196:271–4.

65. Smith TJ, Ryan LM, Douglass Jr HO, et al. Combined chemoradiotherapy vs. radiotherapy alone for early stage squamous cell carcinoma of the esophagus: a study of the Eastern Cooperative Oncology Group. Int J Radiat Oncol Biol Phys. 1998;42:269–76.

66. Casciato D. Manual of clinical oncology. 5th ed. Philadelphia: Lippincott Williams Wilkins; 2004. p. 188–9.

67. Moon S, Kim H, Chie E, Kim J, Park C. Positive impact of radiation dose on disease free survival and locoregional control in postoperative radiotherapy for squamous cell carcinoma of esophagus. Dis Esophagus. 2009;22(4):298–304.

68. Herskovic A, Martz K, Al-Sarraf M, Leichman L, Brindle J, Vaitkevicius V, Cooper J, Byhardt R, Davis L, Emami B. Combined chemotherapy and radiotherapy compared with radiotherapy alone in patients with cancer of the esophagus. N Engl J Med. 1992;326(24):1593–8.

69. Cooper JS, Guo MD, Herskovic A, Macdonald JS, Martenson Jr JA, Al-Sarraf M, Byhardt R, Russell AH, Beitler JJ, Spencer S, Asbell SO, Graham MV, Leichman LL. Chemoradiotherapy of locally advanced esophageal cancer: long-term follow-up of a prospective randomized trial (RTOG 85-01). Radiation Therapy Oncology Group. J Am Med Assoc. 1999;281(17):1623–7.

70. Chiu PW, Chan AC, Leung SF, Leong HT, Kwong KH, Li MK, Au-Yeung AC, Chung SC, Ng EK. Multicenter prospective randomized trial comparing standard esophagectomy with chemoradiotherapy for treatment of squamous esophageal cancer: early results from the Chinese University Research Group for Esophageal Cancer (CURE). J Gastrointest Surg. 2005;9(6):794–802.

71. Qin TJ, An GL, Zhao XH, Tian F, Li XH, Lian JW, Pan BR, Gu SZ. Combined treatment of oxaliplatin and capecitabine in patients with metastatic esophageal squamous cell cancer. World J Gastroenterol. 2009;15(7):871–6.

Strictures, Rings, Webs (Peptic, Caustic, Radiation, Anastomotic)

42

Eric Johnson, Eric Gaumnitz, and Mark Reichelderfer

Abstract

Mechanical dysphagia has many possible etiologies, though all commonly share the process of narrowing the lumen of the esophagus with subsequent delay in passage of solid foods. Benign strictures, webs, and rings are among the most common causes of mechanical obstruction of the esophagus.

Keywords

Anastomotic • Caustic • Esophageal structural abnormalities • Peptic • Radiation • Rings • Strictures • Web

Introduction

Mechanical dysphagia has many possible etiologies, though all commonly share the process of narrowing the lumen of the esophagus with subsequent delay in passage of solid foods. Benign strictures, webs, and rings are among the most common causes of mechanical obstruction of the esophagus.

Peptic Stricture

Definition

A peptic esophageal stricture is a narrowing of the esophagus, typically at the squamocolumnar junction, related to acid exposure from gastroesophageal reflux disease (GERD). These strictures typically have a smooth mucosal surface and are usually less than 1 cm in length, although longer strictures, up to 8 cm, are occasionally seen [1].

Prevalence

Peptic stricture accounts for between 70% and 80% of all benign esophageal strictures (anastomotic and caustic strictures making up the majority of the remainder) [1]. Peptic strictures occur, by definition, in patients with GERD.

E. Johnson, MD • E. Gaumnitz, MD
• M. Reichelderfer, MD (✉)
Division of Gastroenterology and Hepatology,
University of Wisconsin School of Medicine
and Public Health, Madison, WI, USA
e-mail: mxr@medicine.wisc.edu

R. Shaker et al. (eds.), *Principles of Deglutition: A Multidisciplinary Text for Swallowing and its Disorders*, 599
DOI 10.1007/978-1-4614-3794-9_42, © Springer Science+Business Media New York 2013

About 10–20% of the patients with untreated reflux esophagitis will develop a peptic esophageal stricture, and the incidence increases with age and duration of reflux disease [2]. There are several risk factors associated with the development of peptic strictures, primarily due to increased risk for GERD. Caucasians are approximately ten times more likely to develop peptic strictures than African Americans or Asians [3]. Hiatal hernias are another important risk factor for the development of strictures. While hiatal hernias are found in about 10–15% of the general population, the incidence increases to 63% in patients with esophagitis on endoscopy and up to 85% of the patients with peptic strictures [4]. Other conditions predisposing to peptic strictures include scleroderma, Zollinger–Ellison syndrome, NSAID use, and prolonged nasogastric intubation [5–8].

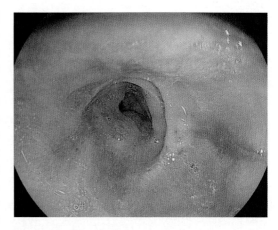

Fig. 42.1 Peptic stricture—typical stricture associated with active erosive reflux esophagitis

Pathophysiology

Peptic strictures form when stomach acid refluxes into the esophagus and damages the esophageal wall. This injury causes an inflammatory process leading to the deposition of connective tissue and, eventually, fibrosis. It is believed that nonerosive esophagitis, erosive esophagitis, and esophageal peptic strictures are all processes on the spectrum of GERD-related complications [1]. In the initial stages of injury, esophageal narrowing is primarily from edema and muscle spasm, and therefore reversible with acid suppression [9]. After more prolonged injury, the fibrosis extends into the submucosa and muscle, and damages the intrinsic nervous system. The narrowing becomes irreversible as the esophageal wall thickens, shortens, and becomes noncompliant from advanced fibrosis [10].

Diagnosis

The most common presenting symptom of peptic esophageal strictures is dysphagia. Dysphagia is typically first noticed with solid foods, but can progress to liquids. Symptoms of dysphagia are more common once the stricture has narrowed the lumen of the esophagus to less than 13 mm,

although some studies suggest the degree of esophagitis is nearly as important as the degree of stricturing for the development of dysphagia [9]. Patients with benign strictures often alter their diets to more soft foods to be able to meet their caloric needs and thus tend not to lose weight, and may not even complain of dysphagia if the softer foods they eat no longer cause symptoms. Significant weight loss should prompt the physician to search for alternative diagnoses such as esophageal carcinoma or achalasia. As discussed earlier, GERD is necessary to develop a peptic stricture. A history of heartburn symptoms is present in over 75% of the patients with peptic strictures [11]. Patients may also present with chest pain related to esophagitis, esophageal spasm, or food impaction.

When a stricture is suspected based on history, the diagnosis is confirmed with the use of upper endoscopy or a barium esophagram (Fig. 42.1). Each of these tests has advantages, and in practice, both are often used to complement each other. Several studies show that the barium esophagram is a more sensitive test for peptic strictures than endoscopy, approaching 100% in strictures less than 9 mm in diameter and 90% for strictures greater than 10 mm [12]. Barium esophagram also has the advantage of being non-invasive, and being able to evaluate the length of the stricture. Radiographic techniques can also incorporate swallowed food in an attempt to duplicate the patient's symptoms and identify functional obstruction. Though not quite as sensitive for subtle strictures, endoscopy is essential to evaluate all esophageal strictures. Esophagoscopy provides viewing of the mucosa itself, allowing for the diagnosis of esophagitis, Barrett's esophagus, or carcinoma. There are varying reports on whether chronic peptic strictures are associated with increased frequency of Barrett's esophagus [13, 14]. Biopsies can be taken from the stricture if Barrett's or carcinoma is suspected. A peptic stricture should appear as a smooth narrowing in the distal esophagus at the squamocolumnar junction, sometimes extending more proximally. Air insufflation will not expand a true peptic stricture. The other major advantage of endoscopy for evaluation of a stricture is the ability to provide therapeutic dilation, if necessary. Other modalities that may be helpful in the evaluation of a suspected peptic stricture include esophageal manometry (if one suspects a motility disorder), ambulatory pH monitoring, and a serum gastrin level to rule out Zollinger–Ellison syndrome if the patients have refractory strictures.

Management (Medical Management, Endoscopic Management in Next Chapter)

The management of peptic strictures is multifaceted and includes lifestyle modifications to reduce acid reflux, acid-suppression medications, esophageal dilation with or without intralesional steroid injection, and occasionally surgical intervention.

Lifestyle modifications to reduce acid reflux include elevating the head of the bed, avoidance of meals for 2–3 h before sleeping, eating smaller meals, weight reduction in obese patients, and reducing alcohol intake. Patients with known strictures also must adjust the way they eat in order to avoid food impactions. Patients should cut food into small pieces, chew thoroughly, and avoid eating hurriedly. A careful review of medications should also be done to ensure avoidance of drugs that can cause pill esophagitis.

Medical management for peptic strictures has improved dramatically since the advent of proton pump inhibitors. The majority of peptic esophageal strictures occur in the setting of longstanding reflux esophagitis, and as stated earlier, the degree

of reflux may be as important as luminal diameter in the degree of dysphagia reported by the patient. Marks et al. treated patients with peptic strictures and concurrent esophagitis and showed that regardless of the drug therapy, patients with healed esophagitis at 3 and 6 months were more likely to be dysphagia free and required fewer dilations [15]. Treatment of peptic strictures using H-2 blockers is not effective in reducing the frequency of dilation [16, 17]. However, more potent acid-suppressive regimens using proton pump inhibitors have proven to be effective. Several studies have compared proton pump inhibitors to either placebo or to H-2 blockers and have shown a significant decrease in frequency of dilations and improvement in dysphagia with the use of proton pump inhibitors [15, 18, 19].

Dilation is the mainstay of treatment for benign esophageal strictures. For simple esophageal strictures (<2 cm in length, straight, with a diameter that allows passage of an endoscope), either bougie or balloon dilation can be used [20]. For most patients, 1–3 dilations are required to relieve symptoms, with an additional 25% requiring repeat dilations [21]. Predictors of early recurrence include a narrower stricture diameter, persistence of heartburn after dilation, and the presence of hiatal hernia [22]. For patients who have developed recurrent stricture after dilation, endoscopic intralesional corticosteroid injection has been used in an attempt to reduce recurrence of the stricture. Several small, nonrandomized studies have shown that this technique is effective in reducing the need for repeat dilation and increasing the average time to repeat dilation [23–25]. One randomized, blinded trial has been published which showed that 60% of the patients treated with sham injections needed repeat dilations in the first year compared with 13% of the patients in the steroid group [26]. Incisional therapy and stent placement are two other management options that have been used in some cases of anastomotic, caustic, or malignant strictures with varying success, but their use in peptic strictures has not been well studied.

Surgical therapy for peptic strictures is indicated in patients who fail medical therapy or are not candidates for maximal medical therapy.

Patients with strictures that are refractory to medical treatment require evaluation for complicating factors such as a motility disorder, pill-induced esophagitis, or Zollinger–Ellison syndrome. If antireflux surgery is deemed necessary, the experience of the surgeon is an important factor in the success of the procedure [27]. While several small studies have described successful treatment of recurrent peptic strictures using antireflux surgery, a larger, randomized trial showed no significant difference between the fundoplication group and the medical therapy group in terms of frequency of treatment of esophageal strictures [28]. The most radical therapy for refractory peptic strictures is the resection of the entire esophagus. Esophagectomy is typically reserved for those patients that have features of an irreversibly damaged esophagus such as the inability to dilate the stricture, rapid recurrence of a stricture after dilation, and evidence of aperistalsis on manometry [1].

Caustic Injury and Stricture

Definition

Caustic injury to the esophagus occurs with ingestion of either acid or alkali with stricture arising as a consequence of esophageal injury (Fig. 42.2).

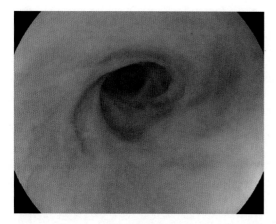

Fig. 42.2 Lye stricture—chronic stricture with scoring in adult due to accidental lye ingestion as a child

Incidence

Most caustic injury occurs in children with the vast majority being due to accidental ingestion of cleaning products. In 2006, 11,964 injuries due to cleaning products were reported to the National Electronic Injury Surveillance System with 68% of these being ingestions [29]. Fortunately, there was a documented decrease in incidence from 1990 when there were 22,141 injuries reported, although this remains a major public health problem. Most injuries were in children 1–3 years old and more in boys (60%) than girls. Most ingestions in adults occur as a result of attempted suicide [30, 31].

Pathophysiology

The organ sustaining the most damage following ingestion is usually the esophagus with the stomach and small intestine also being affected in some patients. The degree of damage is dependent on the agent, volume ingested, and contact time. In a rabbit in vitro model, injury to lye (sodium hydroxide) was dependent on the pH of the preparation, requiring a pH of greater than 11.5 for injury [32]. Damage was time and pH dependent, with increasing injury causing epithelial permeability and then liquefaction necrosis. Both allow deeper penetration of alkali in the esophageal wall and thereby deeper injury including full-thickness injury and perforation. Contact time and concentration of caustic soda was similarly found to affect the degree of injury in an in vivo rat model, with necrosis produced in as little as 10 min [33].

Acid can cause as severe an injury, even though it has been thought to not do so as it seemed to cause a more superficial injury with coagulation necrosis rather than liquefaction [34]. For example, in a recent series with a high incidence of glacial acetic acid ingestion, severe injuries were more common with acid than alkali (at least grade 2 injury was present in 60 of 85 acid patients as opposed to 46 of 94 alkali patients) [30].

Diagnosis

Neither the absence of lip or oropharyngeal burns nor the absence of symptoms excludes esophageal injury. Endoscopy is therefore recommended as an early intervention to assess esophageal injury, once the airway has been evaluated and the patient resuscitated. However, this recommendation is based on clinical experience and not prospective trials, and remains somewhat controversial in patients without burns or symptoms [35]. The local Poison Control Center should be contacted for further recommendations concerning the specific ingested agent.

A variety of endoscopic scoring systems have been proposed with one system using grade I for superficial injury with erythema or edema, grade II for transmucosal injury with superficial ulcers either focal (IIa) or diffuse or circumferential (IIb), and grade III for transmural injury with deep ulcers and necrosis (divided by some into focal—IIIa and extensive—IIIb) [36, 37]. Endoscopic severity correlates well with outcome. In a recent review of 273 adults, stricture incidence was 0% in grade I injury, 4% and 9% in grades IIa and b, and 28% and 54% in grades IIIa and b (including gastric strictures) with an overall stricture rate of 24% [38]. In addition, grade 3b predicted prolonged hospital stay, ICU admission, and both GI and systemic complications. Likewise, in 50 children, 5 of 10 patients with grade II injury (using an equivalent scale) developed strictures as compared to none of the 17 patients with grade I injury [39]. Of note, six children in this series had significant esophageal injury in the absence of oropharyngeal burns.

Management

Management is supportive with airway management and resuscitation. Prevention of vomiting and aspiration is crucial. A nasogastric tube can be placed in the event of significant esophageal injury. Patients with severe injury should be followed closely for perforation with serial imaging.

Steroids have been used to treat caustic injury and to try to prevent complications including stricture. However, a recent systematic review analyzed 13 identified studies with 328 total patients with grade II injury [36]. Although heterogeneity prevented formal metaanalysis, there was no benefit to steroid treatment in terms of stricture prevention, as 30 of 244 (12%) patients receiving steroids developed stricture as opposed to 16 of 84 (19%) not so treated.

Once a stricture has developed, the main therapy is dilation with bougies or balloons. Refractory strictures remain a problem with success of dilation reported as low as 50% [31] and as high as 94%.

A feared late complication of caustic esophageal injury is squamous cell carcinoma, reported in 15 patients from Finland with cancer diagnosis occurring 22–81 years after the ingestion [40]. The ASGE guidelines therefore recommend endoscopic surveillance every 1–3 years beginning 15–20 years after injury [41].

Radiation Strictures

Definition

Stricturing remains the most common and problematic chronic injury to the esophagus related to radiation therapy. Radiation damage to the esophagus is more frequently described in the era of multimodality treatment for mediastinal malignancies, lung, breast, and head and neck cancers. Radiation injury of the esophagus occurs as a collateral effect of radiation treatment and is variable in presentation depending on tumor site, extent of the radiation field, amount of radiation, and if combined with chemotherapy. Damage to the esophagus may occur as both acute and late injury; stricture formation has ranged from 1 to 60 months post radiation (median, 6 months). The most common clinical presentation is dysphagia or odynophagia. Early effects of radiation to the esophagus may include disruption of normal motility patterns in addition to mild mucosal damage. Some patients are susceptible to the more severe spectrum of esophageal involvement with the development of ulceration, strictures, total obliteration, or perforation [42–44]. Studies have not shown a direct relation between the common acute esophagitis and the uncommon late effects such as stricturing [45].

Head and neck cancers are frequently associated with significant oropharyngeal dysphagia and nasal regurgitation. Dysphagia in a head and neck cancer patient is multifactoral and may be independent of radiation therapy but directly related to the extent of surgical resection, incisional scarring, or nerve and muscle function disruption. Additional factors that predispose HNCC patients are the field of radiation, dose and schedule of radiation, and whether chemotherapy was employed [46]. The hypopharynx seems to be more susceptible to radiation damage due to the close proximity of mucosal membranes and risk for subsequent circumferential scarring.

Prevalence

The prevalence and severity of radiation strictures depend on the location of the primary tumor, the amount of radiation applied, and the concurrent use of chemotherapy [43, 47]. Additional predisposing factors include hypopharyngeal tumor location, twice daily dosing of radiation, female gender [48], nutritional status, and concurrent esophageal infection. With combined modality therapy, stricture rates from 21 to 37% have been reported in head and neck cancers [48, 49] and typically involve the proximal esophagus and upper esophageal sphincter. Radiation strictures in the mid- and distal esophagus from lung or mediastinal malignancies are similarly more common, more severe, and occur at lower radiation doses when combined as chemoradiotherapy. Combination therapy is felt to enhance the therapeutic effects of radiation, but potentiates the tissue to be more susceptible to collateral damage. Newman et al. reported dysphagia in up to 17% of the patients treated with combination chemoradiotherapy [50]. Lee et al. found that 21% of the patients with head and neck cancers treated with chemoradiotherapy developed symptomatic

radiation strictures [48]. Radiotherapy alone is uncommonly associated with esophageal strictures: 2–3% for strictures after a 60-Gy dose [42, 51]. Historically, minimal changes to the esophagus occur at doses less than 30 Gy. Thus, it has been accepted that a dose of <60 Gy is a dose level corresponding to a low number of complications [49]. Alternatively, esophageal strictures related to chemotherapy alone are quite rare.

Confounding factors that cause dysphagia in patients with head and neck cancers include surgical alteration of the laryngopharynx and healing scar. Other indirect effects of radiation that contribute to dysphagia would include radiation-induced xerostomia and percutaneous gastric feeding tubes. Gastric tubes are commonly placed prior to radiation treatment but may add to the risk of stricture formation because they indirectly contribute to inactivity of the pharyngeal and esophageal musculature [52].

Pathophysiology

Superficial erosions are the earliest sign of mucosal toxicity and typically occur several weeks after initiation of radiation. Simple erosions will generally resolve within a month following last dose of radiation. After several months of higher dose radiation or concurrent chemotherapy, fibrosis develops and the esophagus strictures. Late effects of radiation may include dense strictures that occur years after last radiation dose. Fistulas and perforation may occur late, likely due to radiation vasculitis, ischemia, and transmural inflammation. Reports of squamous cell carcinomas following radiation esophagitis have been noted.

Diagnosis

Diagnosis of radiation injury to the esophagus is made early with endoscopy (Fig. 42.3). Endoscopy is the most sensitive test for the early findings of erythema and erosions that occur during the acute phase of esophageal damage. Endoscopy additionally lends an opportunity for therapeutic options in addition to diagnosis. If strictures or

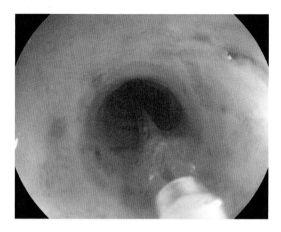

Fig. 42.3 Radiation stricture—upper esophageal stricture with scoring due to radiation for cancer

fistulas are suspected, then radiologic contrast studies are best to assess perforation, determine fistulas, or characterize strictures. CT scan can also be used to assess for perforation, identify regional fistulization, and visualize extrinsic mediastinal structures.

Treatment

Treatment of early esophageal damage of radiation has shown some limited benefit from indomethacin and aspirin, likely through inhibition of the cyclooxygenase enzymes. No benefit from H2-blocker therapy or proton pump inhibitors has been shown to date. The majority of benign esophageal strictures are effectively treated with endoscopic therapy [7]. Endoscopic dilation of radiation strictures remains the best treatment option, especially if the strictures are of relatively short length, straight, and are easily traversed with the endoscope. Dilation may be used in combination with injection of corticosteroids for more refractory strictures. Refractory lesions may also be amenable to electrocautery incisions or endoscopic scissors, which may reduce the refractoriness and recurrence [23]. Complete esophageal obstruction typically precludes antegrade endoscopic dilation, but can be treated with a rendezvous procedure. The rendezvous procedure simultaneously combines direct antegrade endoscopy and retrograde endoscopy via a gastrostomy

in order to visualize the stricture from both sides and provide transillumination in order to accurately dissect and recannulate the lumen [53].

Stenting for benign esophageal strictures due to radiation may be considered, but durable results from temporary stent placement have been disappointing. Esophageal stenting for radiation strictures have resulted in less than 50% of the patients having stricture resolution. Both self-expanding metal stents and more recently, self-expanding plastic stents, have been tried. Radiation strictures considered for stenting would include longer, tortuous, or smaller diameter that are refractory to standard treatment [54]. More favorable outcomes have been recently reported with self-expanding stents after placement and upon subsequent removal [55]. Rarely, patients have required surgical resection of the esophagus and gastric pull up with pharyngeal reconstruction [49].

Anastomotic Stricture

Definition

An anastomotic stricture occurs at a surgical anastomosis following resection or bypass of an abnormal segment of the GI tract. The most common surgical procedure resulting in a stricture affecting swallowing is esophagectomy for esophageal cancer (Fig. 42.4), with stricture a major source of morbidity in these patients [38, 56].

Incidence

Esophageal cancer is the most rapidly increasing GI malignancy, with an estimated 16,640 new cases in 2010 and 14,500 deaths [57]. Up to 50% of cancer patients present with locoregional disease and undergo esophagectomy either with or without chemoradiation [58]. The reported incidence of stricture after esophagectomy has been highly variable and depends on the definition of significant stricture, with stricture measurement being problematic. Inability to pass a standard 9–10 mm endoscope has been used by some

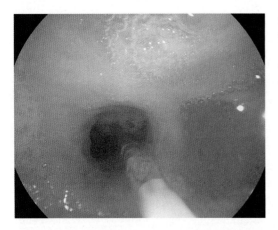

Fig. 42.4 Anastomotic stricture—stricture followed transhiatal esophagectomy for esophageal cancer

authors, which will underreport strictures over 10 mm in size, while others rely on surrogates such as the development of dysphagia (which can occur in the absence of stricture) or performance of dilation, which will over report strictures [56]. It is therefore not surprising that a recent systematic review found that eight randomized controlled trials reported a wide range of stricture incidence, occurring in 0–37% of the patients [59]. However, the incidence is significant in most series, with one representative recent large series (which defined stricture by the presence of dysphagia requiring dilation) finding that 253 (42%) patients developed a stricture with 55 of these being refractory (needing more than ten dilations for symptom relief) [60]. Thus, anastomotic stricture is a common complication of esophagectomy.

Strictures also occur in other conditions requiring esophageal anastomosis with a classic example being reestablishment of esophageal continuity in children presenting with esophageal atresia. Two recent large series found strictures requiring dilation in 8% of 101 and 37% of 62 such children [61, 62].

Pathophysiology

Surgical technique has been carefully studied in an attempt to reduce stricture incidence. A systematic review examined randomized trials of hand-sewn versus stapled transthoracic anastomosis and found no difference in stricture rate [59]. In addition, there was no difference between cervical and thoracic anastomosis in these series [59, 63]. The size of stapler used for anastomosis has also been evaluated with a recent study of 194 patients finding no difference between small 23–25 mm and large 28–33 mm EEA staplers [64]. The use of a colon conduit has been reported to cause less anastomotic strictures [60, 65], but is declining in usage. Surgical technique is in evolution with minimally invasive transhiatal thoracoscopic/laparoscopic esophagectomy (MIE) in rapid development. A recent metaanalysis analyzed eight trials comparing MIE to open esophagectomy and found an increase in stricture rate [66], suggesting that stricture incidence may increase as MIE is more widely adopted.

Conduit ischemia and anastomotic leakage are well-recognized risk factors for stricture development. For example, in 363 patients followed for more than a month in a recent series, 9% developed ischemia and 11% had a leak [65]. Eighty patients were found to have a stricture defined as inability to pass a 9 mm endoscope with both ischemia and leak being associated with stricture formation (10 strictures occurring in 21 patients with ischemia, 13 of 28 patients with leak, and 5 of 10 with both, although 52 of 80 stricture patients had neither) [65]. Likewise, anastomosis leakage was associated with subsequent strictures in a large series of 607 patients, as well as cardiovascular disease (via the mechanism of ischemia presumably) [60]. In this series, the development of refractory strictures was predicted independently by leakage, chemoradiation, and stricture development within 90 days [60]. Conduit ischemia is not surprising in this setting as the gastric tube is supplied exclusively by the right gastroepiploic artery.

Acid might also play a role in stricture formation with prevention possible in some patients by prevention of acid reflux postoperatively. A randomized, controlled trial of 80 patients found strictures in 5 of 39 (13%) patients receiving twice daily PPI therapy as compared to 18 of 40 (45%) who did not [67]. PPI therapy successfully reduced acid exposure in both the gastric tube as well as the esophageal segment above the anastomosis (although the latter in the supine position only).

Diagnosis

The presence of a stricture is suggested by the development of dysphagia and confirmed by endoscopy. Dysphagia can be caused by tortuous postoperative anatomy or abnormal swallowing mechanics in the absence of stricture [56] and thus always requires endoscopic evaluation prior to instituting therapy [58]. Late stricture development (more than 1 year) is suggestive of cancer recurrence and should be evaluated accordingly.

Management

Stricture dilation with either wire-guided Savary dilators or through- the-endoscopic low compliance balloons is the current standard of care, and is associated with a high success rate. Of 244 patients requiring dilation in one series, dilation was successful in 83% defined as the ability to eat solids (11% were excluded by dying before symptomatic relief was achieved) [60]. Success rates of 93% and 77% have also been reported [58, 65]. Some authors have used Maloney dilators and then taught patients to self-dilate [38], although this technique is not in widespread use.

In part because dilation failures still occur and in part because some patients require frequent repeat dilations, newer techniques are in development including electrocautery incision of the stricture with a polypectomy snare or needle-knife [68, 69]. Because of a negative recent randomized trial suggesting that incision and Savary dilation are equivalent, the addition of balloon dilation to incision therapy or additional cautery with argon plasma coagulation has been suggested [68, 70, 71].

Esophageal Rings

Definition

Esophageal rings are smooth, thin (<4 mm axial length) mucosal structures that compromise the esophageal lumen at the gastro-esophageal junction and are composed of squamous mucosa

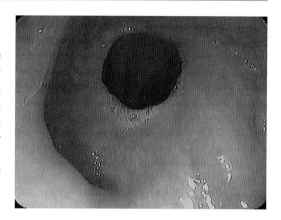

Fig. 42.5 Schatzki's ring—ring at gastroesophageal junction

above and columnar epithelium below (Fig. 42.5) [72]. The ring described above is a B ring, also known as a Schatzki ring. There is no muscular component to mucosal esophageal rings and thus the caliber of the lumen does not change during peristalsis. Another, less common, esophageal ring characterized by muscular hypertrophy and located in the body of the esophagus is called the A ring. This hypertrophied muscle is located approximately 2 cm above the gastroesophageal junction, is covered with squamous epithelium on both sides, and can change in diameter with peristalsis [73].

Prevalence

Lower esophageal rings are seen in up to 14% of routine barium examinations, but symptomatic rings account for only about 0.5% of these studies, meaning that these rings are considered to be normal structures in many people [74]. A Schatzki ring is responsible for about 26% of all patients with esophageal dysphagia [75]. The muscular A-ring rarely causes any symptoms.

Pathophysiology

The cause of lower esophageal rings is unclear. Almost all cases of Schatzki ring occur in patients with hiatal hernias, and some studies have shown an association with GERD and the development of esophageal rings [76, 77], but evidence from other research would contradict this observation [78, 79]. Interestingly, the presence of a Schatzki ring is associated with a lower incidence of Barrett's esophagus [80], but do not protect against acid reflux [81]. In recent years, the emergence of eosinophilic esophagitis, often with concentric rings, as a prominent cause of dysphagia has led many researchers to evaluate the link between eosinophilic esophagitis and lower esophageal rings. This association was first described in the pediatric population by Nurko et al. in 2004, when nearly 50% of the patients with a Schatzki ring met histologic criteria for eosinophilic esophagitis. While lower esophageal rings can certainly be present in eosinophilic esophagitis, biopsy studies have shown a marked difference between mucosal biopsy specimens of patients with eosinophilic esophagitis compared with patients with a ring [82].

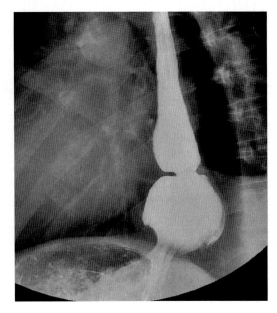

Fig. 42.6 Schatzki's ring—esophagram showing typical ring at gastroesophageal junction

Diagnosis

Patients with a symptomatic ring typically present with solid food dysphagia. Patients frequently report symptoms located in the neck, followed by the sternal notch, and then the mid-chest [83]. A ring narrowing the esophageal lumen to less than 13 mm almost always causes symptoms, while rings over 20 mm rarely present with dysphagia. While patients usually have intermittent symptoms for months or even years, their first presentation to a healthcare provider may be with food impaction. The classic presentation is dysphagia after eating meat, the so-called "steakhouse syndrome," but breads and other dry foods are also common offenders.

The diagnosis can be made with a barium esophagram (Fig. 42.6), which has up to a 95% sensitivity in symptomatic patients with a lower esophageal ring if performed properly [84]. In the same study, upper endoscopy was shown to be less accurate with a detection rate of 58%, although the yield of endoscopy depends on the size of the scope used, the diameter of the ring, and the experience of the endoscopist. If upper

endoscopy is performed and is negative in a patient with solid food dysphagia, it should be followed with a barium study of the lower esophagus. Manometry offers little in this clinical setting and was unable to differentiate patients with lower esophageal rings from controls [85].

Management

The treatment of Schatzki ring has classically involved dilation with bougie or balloon dilators, and both seem to have similar efficacy [86]. In contrast to peptic strictures, the goal of dilation in lower esophageal rings is to fracture, as opposed to merely stretching, the ring. The safety of abrupt and aggressive dilation is well established and most series report no complications to the procedure. The exception to this rule may be when the Schatzki ring is associated with eosinophilic esophagitis, where the safety of dilation is still controversial. Several studies have shown an increased risk of perforation in dilation performed in eosinophilic esophagitis patients, while other studies have refuted this claim [87–89]. If eosinophilic esophagitis is suspected, dilation should be delayed and biopsies should be taken. If biopsies confirm this diagnosis, medical management can be pursued instead of dilation.

Unfortunately, while most patients initially improve after dilation, many studies have shown that recurrence of the ring is common, with 68% of the patients being symptom free at 1 year post-dilation and only 11% being symptom free at 5 years postdilation [90]. In another study of 61 patients with symptomatic Schatzki rings, 63% developed recurrent dysphagia in the 75-month follow-up after initial successful dilation [91]. Risk factors for recurrence of the ring have not been identified, although studies have shown that initial diameter of the ring did not predict the need for repeat dilation [90, 91]. The presence of GERD has been shown to correlate in some studies, but no association was found in others. Given this uncertainty, it seems reasonable to treat patients with lower esophageal rings and reflux esophagitis with acid suppression therapy, despite the lack of evidence that such treatment decreases the need for dilation [92].

All patients with rings treated with dilation should be told to monitor for symptoms and advised that recurrence is likely, and that dilation may need to be repeated if dysphagia returns. Patients should also be reminded of lifestyle modifications to reduce the incidence of food impaction such as chewing thoroughly, cutting food into small pieces, and eating slowly.

Esophageal Webs

Definition

Esophageal webs are thin, eccentric, superficial structures of the esophageal mucosa that effectively narrow the lumen (Fig. 42.7). Webs are less often circumferential membranous structures. They are most commonly found in the proximal esophagus on the anterior wall of the postcricoid region, though they may be found throughout the esophagus. Most esophageal webs are asymptomatic; however, if symptoms are attributed to an esophageal web, then a proximal location is more likely. Proximal webs are often referred to as "cervical webs" and may present with extraesophageal

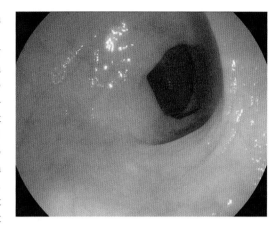

Fig. 42.7 Web—cervical web

symptoms of nasal reflux and oropharyngeal regurgitation in addition to classic esophageal dysphagia. Distal esophageal webs can cause a pattern of intermittent dysphagia ("steak house syndrome") with problem foods and pills.

Prevalence

Given the frequent asymptomatic nature, the true prevalence of esophageal webs is unknown and may be as high as 5–15% of dysphagic patients [93]. A radiographic investigation of 1134 dysphagic patients revealed 7.5% of patients had esophageal webs. Esophageal mucosal webs may be more frequently noticed as endoscopists are more aware of eosinophilic esophagitis, which can present with both rings and webs on imaging studies.

Pathophysiology

Esophageal webs may be divided into congenital or acquired causes. Congenital webs are assumed to be present from childhood through adulthood and attributed to a defect in the development of the squamous mucosa during embryonic stages. A described congenital triad of findings has been known as Plummer–Vinson or Paterson–Brown–Kelly syndrome which includes: dysphagia, glossitis, and iron deficiency anemia with the findings of esophageal webs on imaging studies. Genetic and nutritional factors are likely to play a role. The syndrome tends to occur in the fifth and sixth decades with a 3:1 male-to-female ratio. There is an increased risk for esophageal squamous cell cancer associated with this syndrome.

Acquired mucosal webs are the consequence of mucosal damage and subsequent healing and repair of the mucosa. Caustic exposures of the esophageal mucosa that have been cited include: acid reflux, caustic ingestion, chemo and radiotherapy, pill esophagitis, and infection. There has been association with other chronic conditions such as thyroid disease, Zenker's diverticuli, graft vs. host disease, pemphigoid and epidermolysis bullosa, psoriasis, and eosinophilic esophagitis. Gastric inlet patches in the proximal esophagus have also been associated with esophageal web formation [94].

Esophageal webs are composed of connective tissue within both the mucosal and submucosal layers. The overlying squamous epithelium is endoscopically normal. Microscopic appearance of webs may be completely normal but may also include inflammatory cells in the subepithelial tissue. There is no involvement of and beyond the muscularis mucosa as is seen with the more dense lesions of esophageal strictures.

Diagnosis

Most mucosal webs are diagnosed incidentally during endoscopy due to the increased volume of these procedures performed as the initial imaging study for esophageal symptoms. Webs may be missed on endoscopy as highly proximal esophageal lesions may be disrupted during endoscopic intubation of the esophagus and thus not detected upon with drawing of the endoscope. Barium swallow study remains a more sensitive imaging method to detect webs in patients who clinically report dysphagia, especially when a predominance of oropharyngeal symptoms is present (Fig. 42.8). Videoradiography is helpful in fully characterizing these lesions as anatomic views from two different vantage points are employed.

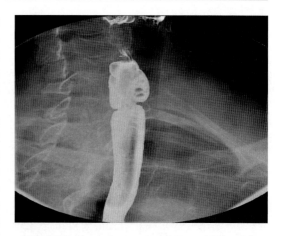

Fig. 42.8 Cervical web—esophagram

Treatment

Most esophageal webs are asymptomatic and subsequently do not require therapy. Mild symptoms may be amenable to simple adjustment of eating habits including cutting and biting foods into small pieces and then followed by slow, purposeful chewing and swallowing. If there is notable dysphagia, then endoscopic dilation either with Savary wire-guided bougie or "through the scope" balloon dilators is reasonable. Unlike distal esophageal rings where a single large bore bougie dilation is recommended, more gentle and gradual dilation of webs is prudent as these can be related to active inflammatory changes and tend to be more fragile to dilation [95]. There has been an association with several of the secondary causes of webs and an increased occurrence of esophageal perforation. Newer endoscopic therapies to disrupt the webs have been described; YAG laser therapy has been used successfully in some patients to open the esophageal lumen. Rarely aggressive surgical intervention is required, including esophagectomy for refractory and extensively involved esophageal mucosa.

Preventative therapy is best directed at symptomatic patients who have a likely secondary factor to explain mucosal damage such that treatment can be directed appropriately towards a specific factor. Patients with suspected reflux disease should be treated with acid suppression therapy and instigate antireflux measures. If eosinophilic esophagitis is possible, then biopsy diagnosis must be made and treatment with topical steroids prescribed.

Key Points

- Peptic strictures occur in the setting of GERD, and most frequently present with dysphagia.
- Medical management with proton pump inhibitors and esophageal dilation will typically improve dysphagia symptoms.
- Radiation strictures are more common if radiation was given in combination with chemotherapy.
- Esophageal rings are thin mucosal folds in the distal esophagus that partially occlude the lumen, typically presenting with solid food dysphagia. Barium esophagram or endoscopy are the diagnostic tests of choice.
- Esophageal webs are often asymptomatic, but more likely to be symptomatic the more proximally located in the esophagus.
- Secondary causes of esophageal mucosal inflammation should be addressed when treating esophageal webs.
- The incidence of anastomotic strictures is increased in patients with anastomotic leaks or conduit ischemia.
- Caustic strictures can occur from either acid or alkaline ingestion.
- Endoscopic dilation remains the primary mode of treatment for esophageal stricture.

References

1. Richter JE. Peptic strictures of the esophagus. Gastroenterol Clin North Am. 1999;28(4):875–91.
2. Richter JE. Long-term management of gastroesophageal reflux disease and its complications. Am J Gastroenterol. 1997;92(4 Suppl):30S–4. discussion 34 S–35 S.
3. El-Serag HB, Sonnenberg A. Associations between different forms of gastro-oesophageal reflux disease. Gut. 1997;41(5):594–9.
4. Berstad A, Weberg R, Froyshov Larsen I, Hoel B, Hauer-Jensen M. Relationship of hiatus hernia to reflux oesophagitis. A prospective study of coincidence, using endoscopy. Scand J Gastroenterol. 1986;21(1):55–8.
5. Buchin PJ, Spiro HM. Therapy of esophageal stricture: a review of 84 patients. J Clin Gastroenterol. 1981;3(2): 121–8.
6. El-Serag HB, Sonnenberg A. Association of esophagitis and esophageal strictures with diseases treated with nonsteroidal anti-inflammatory drugs. Am J Gastroenterol. 1997;92(1):52–6.
7. Marks RD, Richter JE. Peptic strictures of the esophagus. Am J Gastroenterol. 1993;88(8):1160–73.
8. Miller LS, Vinayek R, Frucht H, Gardner JD, Jensen RT, Maton PN. Reflux esophagitis in patients with Zollinger–Ellison syndrome. Gastroenterology. 1990; 98(2):341–6.
9. Dakkak M, Hoare RC, Maslin SC, Bennett JR. Oesophagitis is as important as oesophageal stricture diameter in determining dysphagia. Gut. 1993;34(2): 152–5.
10. Jeyasingham K. What is the histology of an esophageal stricture before and after dilatation? The esophageal mucosa. Amersterdam: Elsevier; 1994. p. 335.
11. Patterson DJ, Graham DY, Smith JL, et al. Natural history of benign esophageal stricture treated by dilatation. Gastroenterology. 1983;85(2):346–50.
12. Ott DJ, Gelfand DW, Lane TG, Wu WC. Radiologic detection and spectrum of appearances of peptic esophageal strictures. J Clin Gastroenterol. 1982;4(1): 11–5.
13. Spechler SJ, Sperber H, Doos WG, Schimmel EM. The prevalence of Barrett's esophagus in patients with chronic peptic esophageal strictures. Dig Dis Sci. 1983;28(9):769–74.
14. Kim SL, Wo JM, Hunter JG, Davis LP, Waring JP. The prevalence of intestinal metaplasia in patients with and without peptic strictures. Am J Gastroenterol. 1998;93(1):53–5.
15. Marks RD, Richter JE, Rizzo J, et al. Omeprazole versus H2-receptor antagonists in treating patients with peptic stricture and esophagitis. Gastroenterology. 1994;106(4):907–15.
16. Ferguson R, Dronfield MW, Atkinson M. Cimetidine in treatment of reflux oesophagitis with peptic stricture. Br Med J. 1979;2(6188):472–4.
17. Spechler SJ. Comparison of medical and surgical therapy for complicated gastroesophageal reflux disease in veterans. The department of Veterans Affairs Gastroesophageal Reflux Disease Study Group. N Engl J Med. 1992;326(12):786–92.
18. Smith PM, Kerr GD, Cockel R, et al. A comparison of omeprazole and ranitidine in the prevention of recurrence of benign esophageal stricture. Restore Investigator Group. Gastroenterology. 1994;107(5): 1312–8.
19. Silvis SE, Farahmand M, Johnson JA, Ansel HJ, Ho SB. A randomized blinded comparison of omeprazole and ranitidine in the treatment of chronic esophageal stricture secondary to acid peptic esophagitis. Gastrointest Endosc. 1996;43(3):216–21.
20. Siersema PD. Treatment options for esophageal strictures. Nat Clin Pract Gastroenterol Hepatol. 2008;5(3): 142–52.

21. Pereira-Lima JC, Ramires RP, Zamin Jr I, Cassal AP, Marroni CA, Mattos AA. Endoscopic dilation of benign esophageal strictures: report on 1043 procedures. Am J Gastroenterol. 1999;94(6):1497–501.
22. Said A, Brust DJ, Gaumnitz EA, Reichelderfer M. Predictors of early recurrence of benign esophageal strictures. Am J Gastroenterol. 2003;98(6):1252–6.
23. Zein NN, Greseth JM, Perrault J. Endoscopic intralesional steroid injections in the management of refractory esophageal strictures. Gastrointest Endosc. 1995;41(6):596–8.
24. Kochhar R, Ray JD, Sriram PV, Kumar S, Singh K. Intralesional steroids augment the effects of endoscopic dilation in corrosive esophageal strictures. Gastrointest Endosc. 1999;49(4 Pt 1):509–13.
25. Altintas E, Kacar S, Tunc B, et al. Intralesional steroid injection in benign esophageal strictures resistant to bougie dilation. J Gastroenterol Hepatol. 2004;19(12): 1388–91.
26. Ramage Jr JI, Rumalla A, Baron TH, et al. A prospective, randomized, double-blind, placebo-controlled trial of endoscopic steroid injection therapy for recalcitrant esophageal peptic strictures. Am J Gastroenterol. 2005;100(11):2419–25.
27. Salminen P, Hiekkanen H, Laine S, Ovaska J. Surgeons' experience with laparoscopic fundoplication after the early personal experience: does it have an impact on the outcome? Surg Endosc. 2007;21(8): 1377–82.
28. Spechler SJ, Lee E, Ahnen D, et al. Long-term outcome of medical and surgical therapies for gastroesophageal reflux disease: follow-up of a randomized controlled trial. J Am Med Assoc. 2001;285(18): 2331–8.
29. McKenzie LB, Ahir N, Stolz U, Nelson NG. Household cleaning product-related injuries treated in US emergency departments in 1990–2006. Pediatrics. 2010;126(3):509–16.
30. Poley JW, Steyerberg EW, Kuipers EJ, et al. Ingestion of acid and alkaline agents: outcome and prognostic value of early upper endoscopy. Gastrointest Endosc. 2004;60(3):372–7.
31. Cheng HT, Cheng CL, Lin CH, et al. Caustic ingestion in adults: the role of endoscopic classification in predicting outcome. BMC Gastroenterol. 2008;8:31.
32. Atug O, Dobrucali A, Orlando RC. Critical pH level of lye (NaOH) for esophageal injury. Dig Dis Sci. 2009;54(5):980–7.
33. Mattos GM, Lopes DD, Mamede RC, Ricz H, Mello-Filho FV, Neto JB. Effects of time of contact and concentration of caustic agent on generation of injuries. Laryngoscope. 2006;116(3):456–60.
34. Zargar SA, Kochhar R, Nagi B, Mehta S, Mehta SK. Ingestion of corrosive acids. Spectrum of injury to upper gastrointestinal tract and natural history. Gastroenterology. 1989;97(3):702–7.
35. Gupta SK, Croffie JM, Fitzgerald JF. Is esophagogastroduodenoscopy necessary in all caustic ingestions? J Pediatr Gastroenterol Nutr. 2001;32(1):50–3.
36. Fulton JA, Hoffman RS. Steroids in second degree caustic burns of the esophagus: a systematic pooled

analysis of fifty years of human data: 1956–2006. Clin Toxicol. 2007;45(4):402–8.
37. Zargar SA, Kochhar R, Mehta S, Mehta SK. The role of fiberoptic endoscopy in the management of corrosive ingestion and modified endoscopic classification of burns. Gastrointest Endosc. 1991;37(2):165–9.
38. Chang AC, Orringer MB. Management of the cervical esophagogastric anastomotic stricture. Semin Thorac Cardiovasc Surg. 2007;19(1):66–71.
39. Riffat F, Cheng A. Pediatric caustic ingestion: 50 consecutive cases and a review of the literature. Dis Esophagus. 2009;22(1):89–94.
40. Isolauri J, Markkula H. Lye ingestion and carcinoma of the esophagus. Acta Chir Scand. 1989;155(4–5): 269–71.
41. Hirota WK, Zuckerman MJ, Adler DG, et al. ASGE guideline: the role of endoscopy in the surveillance of premalignant conditions of the upper GI tract. Gastrointest Endosc. 2006;63(4):570–80.
42. Goldstein HM, Rogers LF, Fletcher GH, Dodd GD. Radiological manifestations of radiation-induced injury to the normal upper gastrointestinal tract. Radiology. 1975;117(1):135–40.
43. Lepke RA, Libshitz HI. Radiation-induced injury of the esophagus. Radiology. 1983;148(2):375–8.
44. Collazzo LA, Levine MS, Rubesin SE, Laufer I. Acute radiation esophagitis: radiographic findings. AJR Am J Roentgenol. 1997;169(4):1067–70.
45. Silvain C, Barrioz T, Besson I, et al. Treatment and long-term outcome of chronic radiation esophagitis after radiation therapy for head and neck tumors. A report of 13 cases. Dig Dis Sci. 1993;38(5):927–31.
46. Eisbruch A, Lyden T, Bradford CR, et al. Objective assessment of swallowing dysfunction and aspiration after radiation concurrent with chemotherapy for head-and-neck cancer. Int J Radiat Oncol Biol Phys. 2002;53(1):23–8.
47. Chabora BM, Hopfan S, Wittes R. Esophageal complications in the treatment of oat cell carcinoma with combined irradiation and chemotherapy. Radiology. 1977;123(1):185–7.
48. Lee WT, Akst LM, Adelstein DJ, et al. Risk factors for hypopharyngeal/upper esophageal stricture formation after concurrent chemoradiation. Head Neck. 2006;28(9):808–12.
49. Laurell G, Kraepelien T, Mavroidis P, et al. Stricture of the proximal esophagus in head and neck carcinoma patients after radiotherapy. Cancer. 2003;97(7): 1693–700.
50. Newman LA, Vieira F, Schwiezer V, et al. Eating and weight changes following chemoradiation therapy for advanced head and neck cancer. Arch Otolaryngol Head Neck Surg. 1998;124(5):589–92.
51. Roswit B. Complications of radiation therapy: the alimentary tract. Semin Roentgenol. 1974;9(1):51–63.
52. Mekhail TM, Adelstein DJ, Rybicki LA, Larto MA, Saxton JP, Lavertu P. Enteral nutrition during the treatment of head and neck carcinoma: is a percutaneous endoscopic gastrostomy tube preferable to a nasogastric tube? Cancer. 2001;91(9):1785–90.

53. Dellon ES, Cullen NR, Madanick RD, et al. Outcomes of a combined antegrade and retrograde approach for dilatation of radiation-induced esophageal strictures (with video). Gastrointest Endosc. 2010;71(7): 1122–9.

54. Siersema PD. Stenting for benign esophageal strictures. Endoscopy. 2009;41(4):363–73.

55. Oh YS, Kochman ML, Ahmad NA, Ginsberg GG. Clinical outcomes after self-expanding plastic stent placement for refractory benign esophageal strictures. Dig Dis Sci. 2010;55(5):1344–8.

56. Rice TW. Anastomotic stricture complicating esophagectomy. Thorac Surg Clin. 2006;16(1): 63–73.

57. American Cancer Society Statistics. 2010.

58. Williams VA, Watson TJ, Zhovtis S, et al. Endoscopic and symptomatic assessment of anastomotic strictures following esophagectomy and cervical esophagogastrostomy. Surg Endosc. 2008;22(6):1470–6.

59. Kim RH, Takabe K. Methods of esophagogastric anastomoses following esophagectomy for cancer: a systematic review. J Surg Oncol. 2010;101(6): 527–33.

60. van Heijl M, Gooszen JA, Fockens P, Busch OR, van Lanschot JJ, van Berge Henegouwen MI. Risk factors for development of benign cervical strictures after esophagectomy. Ann Surg. 2010;251(6):1064–9.

61. Sistonen SJ, Koivusalo A, Nieminen U, et al. Esophageal morbidity and function in adults with repaired esophageal atresia with tracheoesophageal fistula: a population-based long-term follow-up. Ann Surg. 2010;251(6):1167–73.

62. Serhal L, Gottrand F, Sfeir R, et al. Anastomotic stricture after surgical repair of esophageal atresia: frequency, risk factors, and efficacy of esophageal bougie dilatations. J Pediatr Surg. 2010;45(7):1459–62.

63. Walther B, Johansson J, Johnsson F, Von Holstein CS, Zilling T. Cervical or thoracic anastomosis after esophageal resection and gastric tube reconstruction: a prospective randomized trial comparing sutured neck anastomosis with stapled intrathoracic anastomosis. Ann Surg. 2003;238(6):803–12. discussion 812–804.

64. Yendamuri S, Gutierrez L, Oni A, et al. Does circular stapled esophagogastric anastomotic size affect the incidence of postoperative strictures? J Surg Res. 2011;165(1):1–4.

65. Briel JW, Tamhankar AP, Hagen JA, et al. Prevalence and risk factors for ischemia, leak, and stricture of esophageal anastomosis: Gastric pull-up versus colon interposition. J Am Coll Surg. 2004;198(4):536–41. discussion 541–532.

66. Sgourakis G, Gockel I, Radtke A, et al. Minimally invasive versus open esophagectomy: meta-analysis of outcomes. Dig Dis Sci. 2010;55(11):3031–40.

67. Johansson J, Oberg S, Wenner J, et al. Impact of proton pump inhibitors on benign anastomotic stricture formations after esophagectomy and gastric tube reconstruction: results from a randomized clinical trial. Ann Surg. 2009;250(5):667–73.

68. Simmons DT, Baron TH. Electroincision of refractory esophagogastric anastomotic strictures. Dis Esophagus. 2006;19(5):410–4.

69. Lee TH, Lee SH, Park JY, et al. Primary incisional therapy with a modified method for patients with benign anastomotic esophageal stricture. Gastrointest Endosc. 2009;69(6):1029–33.

70. Hordijk ML, van Hooft JE, Hansen BE, Fockens P, Kuipers EJ. A randomized comparison of electrocautery incision with Savary bougienage for relief of anastomotic gastroesophageal strictures. Gastrointest Endosc. 2009;70(5):849–55.

71. Schubert D, Kuhn R, Lippert H, Pross M. Endoscopic treatment of benign gastrointestinal anastomotic strictures using argon plasma coagulation in combination with diathermy. Surg Endosc. 2003;17(10):1579–82.

72. Schatzki R. The lower esophageal ring long term follow-up of symptomatic and asymptomatic rings. Am J Roentgenol Radium Ther Nucl Med. 1963;90: 805–10.

73. Pharyngeal and esophageal diverticula, rings, and webs. Nature Publishing Group; 2006.

74. DeVault KR. Lower esophageal (Schatzki's) ring: pathogenesis, diagnosis and therapy. Dig Dis. 1996;14(5): 323–9.

75. Schatzki R, Gary JE. The lower esophageal ring. Am J Roentgenol Radium Ther Nucl Med. 1956;75(2): 246–61.

76. Marshall JB, Kretschmar JM, Diaz-Arias AA. Gastroesophageal reflux as a pathogenic factor in the development of symptomatic lower esophageal rings. Arch Intern Med. 1990;150(8):1669–72.

77. Chen YM, Gelfand DW, Ott DJ, Munitz HA. Natural progression of the lower esophageal mucosal ring. Gastrointest Radiol. 1987;12(2):93–8.

78. Jamieson J, Hinder RA, DeMeester TR, Litchfield D, Barlow A, Bailey Jr RT. Analysis of thirty-two patients with Schatzki's ring. Am J Surg. 1989;158(6):563–6.

79. Goyal RK, Bauer JL, Spiro HM. The nature and location of lower esophageal ring. N Engl J Med. 1971;284(21):1175–80.

80. Mitre MC, Katzka DA, Brensinger CM, Lewis JD, Mitre RJ, Ginsberg GG. Schatzki ring and Barrett's esophagus: do they occur together? Dig Dis Sci. 2004;49(5):770–3.

81. Winters 3rd GR, Maydonovitch CL, Wong RK. Schatzki's rings do not protect against acid reflux and may decrease esophageal acid clearance. Dig Dis Sci. 2003;48(2):299–302.

82. Gonsalves N, Policarpio-Nicolas M, Zhang Q, Rao MS, Hirano I. Histopathologic variability and endoscopic correlates in adults with eosinophilic esophagitis. Gastrointest Endosc. 2006;64(3):313–9.

83. Smith DF, Ott DJ, Gelfand DW, Chen MY. Lower esophageal mucosal ring: correlation of referred symptoms with radiographic findings using a marshmallow bolus. AJR Am J Roentgenol. 1998;171(5): 1361–5.

84. Ott DJ, Chen YM, Wu WC, Gelfand DW, Munitz HA. Radiographic and endoscopic sensitivity in detecting

lower esophageal mucosal ring. AJR Am J Roentgenol. 1986;147(2):261–5.

85. Rohl L, Aksglaede K, Funch-Jensen P, Thommesen P. Esophageal rings and strictures. Manometric characteristics in patients with food impaction. Acta Radiol. 2000;41(3):275–9.

86. Scolapio JS, Pasha TM, Gostout CJ, et al. A randomized prospective study comparing rigid to balloon dilators for benign esophageal strictures and rings. Gastrointest Endosc. 1999;50(1):13–7.

87. Kaplan M, Mutlu EA, Jakate S, Bruninga K, Losurdo J, Keshavarzian A. Endoscopy in eosinophilic esophagitis: "feline" esophagus and perforation risk. Clin Gastroenterol Hepatol. 2003;1(6): 433–7.

88. Jung KW, Gundersen N, Kopacova J, et al. Occurrence of and risk factors for complications after endoscopic dilation in eosinophilic esophagitis. Gastrointest Endosc. 2011;73(1):15–21.

89. Jacobs Jr JW, Spechler SJ. A systematic review of the risk of perforation during esophageal dilation for patients with eosinophilic esophagitis. Dig Dis Sci. 2010;55(6):1512–5.

90. Eckardt VF, Kanzler G, Willems D. Single dilation of symptomatic Schatzki rings. A prospective evaluation of its effectiveness. Dig Dis Sci. 1992;37(4):577–82.

91. Groskreutz JL, Kim CH. Schatzki's ring: long-term results following dilation. Gastrointest Endosc. 1990;36(5):479–81.

92. Spechler SJ. AGA technical review on treatment of patients with dysphagia caused by benign disorders of the distal esophagus. Gastroenterology. 1999;117(1): 233–54.

93. Webb WA, McDaniel L, Jones L. Endoscopic evaluation of dysphagia in two hundred and ninety-three patients with benign disease. Surg Gynecol Obstet. 1984;158(2):152–6.

94. Buse PE, Zuckerman GR, Balfe DM. Cervical esophageal web associated with a patch of heterotopic gastric mucosa. Abdom Imaging. 1993;18(3):227–8.

95. Lindgren S. Endoscopic dilatation and surgical myectomy of symptomatic cervical esophageal webs. Dysphagia. 1991;6(4):235–8.

Esophageal Foreign Bodies: Food Impaction and Foreign Bodies

43

Ian C. Grimes and Patrick R. Pfau

Abstract

Esophageal foreign bodies and food bolus impactions occur frequently and are a common endoscopic emergency. Though the vast majority of gastrointestinal bodies do not result in serious clinical sequelae or mortality, it has been estimated that 1,500–2,750 patients die annually in the United States because of the ingestion of foreign bodies. More recent studies have suggested the mortality from GI foreign bodies to be significantly lower, with no deaths reported in over 850 adults and one death in approximately 2,200 children with a GI foreign body. As a result of the frequency of this problem and the rare but possible negative consequences, it is important to understand the patients at risk for food impactions and ingestion of foreign bodies, the best method for a prompt diagnosis, and the correct management with avoidance of unwanted complications.

Keywords

Foreign body • Food impaction • Stricture • Ingestion • Retrieval • Endoscopy

Epidemiology

True foreign bodies may be the result of either unintentional or intentional ingestion. The most common patient group that unintentionally ingests foreign bodies is children. Eighty percent of foreign body ingestions occur in children with most occurring between the ages of 6 months and 3 years [1, 2]. Pediatric ingestions are almost always accidental, due to the child's natural oral curiosity [3]. The most common items ingested by children are coins but also frequently include small toys, crayons, buttons, pins, jewels, nails, pins, and disk batteries [3–7].

In adults common risk factors include impaired tactile sensation, compromised judgment, and occupational hazards. Patients with impaired oral tactile sensation may ingest a foreign body during swallowing because of their dentures or dental work [8, 9] and are at high risk of ingesting one's

I.C. Grimes, MD • P.R. Pfau, MD (✉)
Division of Gastroenterology and Hepatology,
University of Wisconsin School of Medicine
and Public Health, 1685 Highland Avenue,
Suite 400, Madison, WI 53705, USA
e-mail: prp@medicine.wisc.edu

R. Shaker et al. (eds.), *Principles of Deglutition: A Multidisciplinary Text for Swallowing and its Disorders*,
DOI 10.1007/978-1-4614-3794-9_43, © Springer Science+Business Media New York 2013

own dentures [10]. Additionally, patients with compromised judgment or senses such as the very elderly, demented, or intoxicated are more likely to ingest a foreign body. Accidental coin ingestion has been encountered in young college students secondary to a popular drinking game "Quarters" where a quarter may inadvertently be swallowed and become lodged in the esophagus [11]. A third patient group at a higher risk of accidental foreign body ingestion is based on occupational hazards associated with roofers, tailors, carpenters, or seamstresses. These patients have an increased rate of foreign body ingestion due to accidental swallowing of nails or needles placed in the mouth during work.

Intentional ingestion of foreign bodies is frequent in psychiatric patients or prisoners [12, 13] (Fig. 43.1). These patients ingest foreign bodies for a secondary gain and often have a history of previous foreign body ingestion, ingest multiple objects, and often ingest the most complex objects.

Esophageal food impaction is a much more common problem than true esophageal foreign body ingestion with an estimated annual incidence of 13–16 episodes per 100,000 people [14]. The majority (75–100%) of patients who present with a food impaction have some type of predisposing esophageal pathology [14–18] (Fig. 43.2). The most commonly observed abnormalities associated with food impaction are Schatzki's rings or peptic strictures and with increasing frequency eosinophilic esophagitis [19]. Less commonly found as the predisposing cause are webs, extrinsic compression, surgical anastomoses, fundoplication wraps, and bariatric gastroplasties [20]. Esophageal cancer rarely presents with acute food bolus impaction but should be considered if history is supportive [21, 22]. Motility disorders such as achalasia, diffuse esophageal spasm, and nutcracker esophagus are infrequent causes of food impactions [23].

Food impactions most commonly occur in adults starting in their fourth or fifth decade of life but are becoming more prevalent in young adults due to the increasing incidence of eosinophilic esophagitis. The type of food impacted correlates with cultural and regional dietary habits.

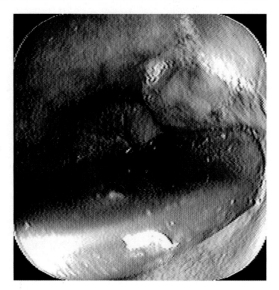

Fig. 43.1 Endoscopic photo of an eye glass lens impacted in the esophagus of a psychiatric inpatient

In the United States meat such as hot dogs, pork, beef, and chicken is the most common while in Asian countries and coastal areas fish and fish bones are the most common food to result in impaction [24–26].

Pathophysiology and Pathogenesis

The majority, 80–90%, of ingested foreign bodies and food bolus impactions will pass spontaneously without clinical sequelae [27]. However, 10–20% of GI foreign bodies will require endoscopic intervention [15, 21, 28]. Therefore, it is important to understand how ingested foreign bodies can result in significant disease and which patients are more likely to ingest complex foreign bodies, and in which parts of the GI tract foreign bodies are most likely to cause damage. This will ensure appropriate use of endoscopic intervention.

The most common complications related to foreign bodies are obstruction and perforation which can occur in any area of the GI tract where there is narrowing, angulation, anatomic sphincters, or previous surgery [29]. The posterior hypopharynx is the first area of the GI tract in which a foreign body may become lodged,

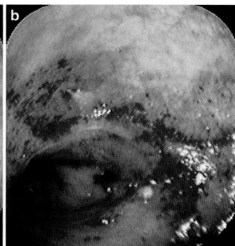

Fig. 43.2 (**a**) Endoscopic photo of a patient that presented with acute dysphagia and chest pain during dinner. Endoscopy revealed a mixture of duck and peas that were successfully passed into the stomach with the push technique. (**b**) Same patient after clearance of food with esophagus showing a distal peptic stricture which led to the food impaction

particularly small sharp objects such as needles, chicken, or fish bones [30, 31].

In the esophagus there are four areas of physical narrowing where a food bolus or foreign body is likely to impact. These include the upper esophageal sphincter, the level of the aortic arch, the crossing of the main stem bronchus, and the lower esophageal sphincter/gastroesophageal junction. All of these areas have been shown to be the areas of true luminal narrowing with diameters of 23 mm or less in the adult patient [32]. Independent of the physiologic areas of narrowing the majority of food boluses are associated with esophageal pathology including rings, webs, diverticuli, and peptic strictures [33]. Multiple esophageal rings associated with eosinophilic esophagitis lead to esophageal food impaction at much greater incidence in young adults [19, 34]. Uncommonly, esophageal motor disturbances such as achalasia, diffuse esophageal spasm, or segmental variations in peristalsis may contribute to food and foreign body impactions [35–38].

Foreign bodies and food impactions in the esophagus generally have the highest incidence of complications with the rate of complication being directly proportional to the time the object spends in the esophagus. Esophageal foreign bodies may lead to perforation, abscess, mediastinitis, pneumothorax, fistula formation, and cardiac tamponade [39, 40].

Among patients presenting with symptoms related to a foreign body, the perforation rate has been estimated to be as high as 5% overall and up to 35% for sharp and pointed objects [21, 41]. Esophageal perforation is the most frequent cause of significant morbidity and mortality [39]. The risk of perforation of the esophagus increases dramatically when foreign bodies or food boluses are left impacted in the esophagus for greater than 24 h. Other reported complications secondary to esophageal foreign bodies, including those that have been reported to lead to fatalities, are gastrointestinal bleeding, aortoenteric fistulae, aspiration, abscess formation, and true rarities such as perforation of the heart and lead and zinc toxicity [42–48].

Clinical Features

History and Physical Examination

For communicative adults a history of ingestion including timing, type of foreign body ingested, and onset of symptoms is usually reliable. History is particularly reliable for food impactions as patients are almost always symptomatic and can detail the exact onset of symptoms. Small sharp objects or fish bones often present with a foreign body sensation or odynophagia in the posterior pharynx or cervical esophagus. This can occur even if the foreign body has passed to the stomach because of a small esophageal mucosal laceration. Esophageal obstruction, partial or complete, almost always results in symptoms such as substernal chest pain, dysphagia, gagging, vomiting, or a sensation of choking [49]. More complete obstruction can lead to drooling and the inability to handle oral secretions.

The type of symptoms may aid in determining whether an esophageal foreign body is still present and where in the esophagus it may be located. If the patient presents with dysphagia, dysphonia, or odynophagia there is almost an 80% chance that a foreign body or food impaction will be present. If the symptom is only retrosternal pain or pharyngeal discomfort less than 50% of patients will have an identifiable esophageal foreign object [50]. The patient may be able to successfully localize the object in the posterior pharynx or at the level of the cricopharyngeal muscle. However, for objects located more distally in the esophagus and into the stomach, patient localization becomes poor with an accuracy of 30–40% in the esophagus and almost 0% in the stomach [51, 52].

The history and symptoms for true foreign bodies are often less reliable than food impaction because true foreign bodies are often ingested by children, mentally impaired adults, or adults who have ingested the foreign body for secondary gain. With esophageal foreign bodies, 20–38% of children will be asymptomatic [51, 53]. Further, in children and non-communicative adults there may be no history of a foreign body ingestion from the patient or the caregiver in up to 40% of cases [54], necessitating a high degree of suspicion. Symptoms are more subtle and include drooling, poor feeding, blood-stained saliva, or a failure to thrive [54, 55]. Respiratory compromise may occur with aspiration or a proximally located esophageal foreign body that compresses the trachea causing wheezing and stridor [54, 56].

Past medical history is important in regard to previous episodes of either food impaction or foreign body ingestion. Previous food impaction or a previous need for esophageal dilation makes recurrent episodes more likely. A history of allergies (asthma, allergic rhinitis, urticaria, hay fever, atopic dermatitis, food or medicine allergy) may be a clue that the patient has eosinophilic esophagitis [57]. Patients with previous true foreign body ingestion are often patients who are multiple ingestors that are more likely to ingest multiple objects and complex objects.

Physical exam and laboratory data will aid little in determining the presence or location of a foreign body, but is important to detect potential ingestion-related complications, and possible underlying causes. Determination of airway and level of consciousness is crucial before any endoscopic or non-endoscopic intervention. Lung examination should be performed to detect the presence of wheezing or aspiration. Esophageal or oropharyngeal perforation may result in swelling, erythema, or crepitus of the neck or chest region. Laboratory data usually add little to what is already known. Peripheral eosinophilia is present in only 50% of patients with eosinophilic esophagitis [58].

Diagnosis

For suspected true foreign bodies diagnostic evaluation should begin with plain film radiographs. Patients with suspected foreign body ingestion should undergo anteroposterior and lateral radiographs of the chest and abdomen to help determine the presence, type, and location of a foreign body [41] (Fig. 43.3). Anteroposterior and lateral neck and chest films are suggested if there is a suspicion of a foreign body in the esophagus vs. the trachea or if there is a foreign object that may be obscured by overlying spine [54, 59] (Fig. 43.3). Plain films also aid in detecting complications such as aspiration, abdominal free air, or subcutaneous emphysema [49, 60].

Radiographic studies are more controversial in children. Since history is often poor from children, mouth-to-anus screening films have been

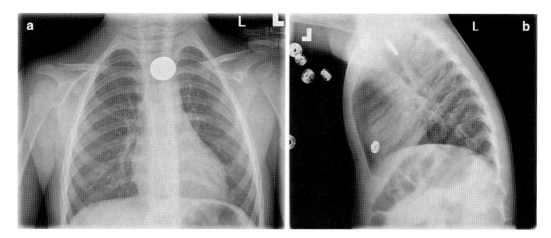

Fig. 43.3 (**a, b**) Posterior–anterior and lateral chest X-ray of a young child with a coin impacted in the upper esophagus

advocated in suspected foreign body ingestions [41]. Others have suggested a more directed approach or non-radiographic methods in determining the presence and location of foreign bodies in children [61]. To limit radiation handheld metal detectors have been used with a sensitivity of >95% for the detection and localization of metallic foreign bodies [62].

Plain films are satisfactory in some true foreign bodies and occasionally in food ingestions with larger bones. However, smaller bones or thin metal objects are not readily seen and many objects including plastic, wood, and glass are not radiopaque [4]. False-negative rates with plain films are as high as 47% and false-positive rates close to 20% in the investigation of foreign bodies [50, 63]. False-negative rates for food impactions have been reported as high as 87% [64]. Further, 35% of films read by a non-radiologist for the presence of foreign bodies have been found to be misread [65].

Generally, it is accepted that barium studies should not be performed in the evaluation of gastrointestinal foreign bodies. If aspiration occurs the hypertonic contrast agents used can cause acute pulmonary edema [66]. Barium evaluation can delay a necessary therapeutic endoscopic procedure by interfering with endoscopic visualization and complicating removal of a foreign body [67].

Advanced imaging such as computed tomography (CT) or magnetic resonance imaging (MRI) may be used in unusual or difficult to diagnose cases and may aid in detecting soft-tissue inflammation or the presence of an abscess. Three-dimensional computed tomography has been used to diagnose foreign bodies not seen with other imaging and may aid in detecting complications of foreign body ingestion such as perforation or abscess prior to the use of endoscopy. MRI may have a role in demonstrating soft-tissue peri-esophageal pathology [54, 68, 69]. MRI should never be performed prior to plain films being obtained to rule out an occult metal ingestion.

Endoscopy provides the most accurate diagnostic modality in suspected foreign body ingestions and food impactions. Any patient with persistent symptoms and a continued clinical suspicion of a gastrointestinal foreign body should undergo an upper endoscopy even after negative or unrevealing radiographic evaluation [70]. This approach ensures the correct diagnosis of food impactions, non-radiopaque, and radiopaque objects that are obscured by overlying bony structures [29].

Endoscopy is the best method to detect underlying pathology such as esophageal strictures or rings that contribute to a food impaction or foreign body that would not pass readily through the GI tract. Endoscopy can also closely examine the gastrointestinal mucosa to assess for laceration or damage that may contribute to continuing symptoms after a foreign body has spontaneously passed. Foremost, diagnostic endoscopy is directly linked to when endoscopy will be used for therapy—treatment or extraction of a known or suspected foreign body. Diagnostic endoscopy is contraindicated when there is physical exam or radiographic evidence of a bowel perforation anywhere in the esophagus.

Treatment

Seventy-five to ninety percent of foreign bodies pass through the GI tract spontaneously without complication [15, 71]. Two recent studies have emphasized conservative management with 86–97% of foreign bodies passing spontaneously with minimal complications [72, 73]. Importantly, esophageal foreign bodies were excluded from the above studies and generally conservative management or just observing esophageal foreign bodies to see if they pass with time is not accepted therapy.

A number of medical therapies for esophageal foreign bodies or food impactions have been studied as primary treatment or in conjunction with endoscopic therapy. The most frequently used medication is glucagon, a smooth muscle relaxant which significantly reduces lower esophageal sphincter pressure [74]. Doses of 0.25–1.0 mg in a single or divided dose are acceptable doses when attempting to treat esophageal foreign bodies or food impactions with glucagon. Glucagon has reported successes of 12–58% in treating esophageal food impactions [75–77], but may be less successful in meat food impactions [78]. A randomized trial, however, found glucagon no better than placebo in treating children with coins lodged in the esophagus [79]. Glucagon is generally safe but may result in nausea, abdominal distension, and rarely vomiting. Glucagon is less likely to work with a fixed obstruction present. Further glucagon does not provide definitive examination and treatment of coexisting esophageal pathology as will flexible endoscopy. Glucagon may however help when used with endoscopy by lowering lower esophageal sphincter pressure and facilitating the endoscope pushing

a food impaction into the stomach [80]. Given the safety of glucagon and ease of use it is worthwhile to give the majority of patients a trial of glucagon before endoscopy is attempted. If the patient has relief of symptoms and is able to handle fluids this can be considered a successful treatment.

Nitroglycerin and nifedipine are other smooth muscle relaxants that have been anecdotally described as promoting passage of esophageal impactions into the stomach but should be avoided due to low efficacy and high number of side effects [41]. Medical methods that have been described but should be avoided are gas-forming agents, emetics, and papain meat tenderizer. Gas-forming agents combined with a smooth muscle relaxant have been reported to have success rates of almost 70% in clearing esophageal foreign bodies into the stomach [81]. However, esophageal rupture and perforation have occurred with these agents, particularly if there is a fixed obstruction or the foreign body has been present for greater than 6 h [82, 83]. Papain, a meat tenderizer, used for the treatment of food impaction and emetics are two methods which should never be used because of the risk of esophageal necrosis, perforation, and aspiration [33, 84, 85].

The radiologic literature has multiple descriptions of methods to remove esophageal foreign bodies under fluoroscopic guidance, particularly in the pediatric population. Reported methods include extraction with Foley balloon catheters, suction catheters, wire baskets, or a magnetic catheter to extract ferromagnetic metal objects [60, 86]. The largest experience has been with Foley catheters where the catheter is passed either nasally or orally into the esophagus and past the foreign body. The balloon is then inflated and withdrawn to deliver the foreign body to the oropharynx where it can be retrieved. Though high success rates have been reported, the major drawback is loss of control of the foreign body, particularly at the level of the upper esophageal sphincter and laryngopharynx. In addition, radiology methods can be challenging or impossible to perform on objects that are radiopaque and cannot be seen on fluoroscopy. Complications reported include nosebleeds, dislodgment of the

Table 43.1 Equipment for treatment and removal of gastrointestinal foreign bodies and food impactions

Endoscopes	Overtubes	Accessory equipment
1) Flexible endoscope	1) Standard esophageal overtube	1) Retrieval net
2) Rigid endoscope	2) 45–60 cm foreign body overtube	2) Alligator or rat tooth forceps
3) Laryngoscope		3) Dormia basket
4) Kelly or McGill forceps		4) Polypectomy snare
		5) Three-pronged grabber
		6) Magnetic extractor
		7) Steigmann–Goff variceal ligator cap
		8) Latex protector hood

foreign body in the nose, laryngospasm, vomiting, and of largest concern aspiration with resultant airway obstruction and even death [87, 88]. As radiologic methods do not match the efficacy or safety of endoscopy few indications exist for their use. Radiologic methods to remove foreign bodies or food impactions should be limited to when endoscopy is not available or cannot be available within 12–24 h.

Flexible endoscopy has clearly become the diagnostic and therapeutic method of choice in both true gastrointestinal foreign bodies and food boluses in both the pediatric and adult population. This is based upon multiple, large series using endoscopy for the treatment of gastrointestinal foreign bodies with success rates greater than 95% and associated morbidity and mortality reported at 0% in most studies but always less than 5% [5, 14–17, 67, 89–92]. Though treatment failures are rare, predictors of endoscopic failure and complications include intentional ingestion, ingestion of multiple complex foreign bodies, and lack of patient cooperation [41].

The indication and timing for intervention with endoscopy is important. Generally, if a patient is symptomatic, intervention is required. For esophageal foreign bodies this includes patients with odynophagia, dysphagia, vomiting, inability to handle secretions, drooling, chest pain, or the sensation of a present foreign body. If the patient is not overtly symptomatic or cannot accurately give a history concerning their symptoms, the location (esophageal vs. already passed to the stomach) and characteristics of the foreign body define the need for intervention.

As a general rule all esophageal foreign bodies and food impactions require intervention in an urgent or emergent fashion. No foreign body should be allowed to remain lodged in the esophagus greater than 24 h and generally should be assessed and treated within 6–12 h of presentation. The time a foreign body is present in the esophagus is directly related to an increase in complications [93, 94].

Prior to initiating endoscopic therapy for foreign bodies and food boluses, proper procedure, equipment, and patient preparation will increase the success rate while maintaining a low complication rate. The endoscopist should be aware of the type of foreign bodies that may be encountered in that particular patient and the safest method to remove these objects. Prior to endoscopy it may be beneficial to perform a "dry run" on a similar object ex vivo [15]. This allows proper retrieval device selection and will make the extraction safer and easier.

Endoscopes, endoscopic retrieval devices, and accessory equipment available to assist in the removal of foreign bodies and food impactions are listed in Table 43.1. Prior to an attempt at removing complex foreign bodies an endoscopy suite should be equipped with a minimum of a rat tooth forceps, polypectomy snares, Dormier baskets, and retrieval nets [27, 95].

Standard size overtubes that extend past the upper esophageal sphincter and overtubes of length 45–60 cm that extend past the lower esophageal sphincter should be available. An overtube provides airway protection, allows frequent passes of the endoscope, and protects the mucosa from superficial and deep lacerations

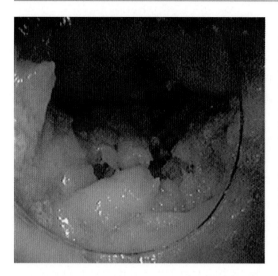

Fig. 43.4 Endoscopic photo of a clear overtube with food impaction just distal. Patient with esophageal cancer ate a bowl of chicken noodle soup which could not be pushed into the stomach. An overtube that went through the upper esophageal sphincter and covered the airway allowed multiple passes of the endoscope facilitating removal of the food impaction

flexible endoscopes particularly in screening for the presence of esophageal foreign bodies. However, nasoendoscopes have limited therapeutic use in the removal of an esophageal foreign body [101]. Laryngoscopes with the aid of a Kelly or McGill forceps should be available and may help in the removal of small, sharp objects at the hypopharynx.

Intravenous conscious sedation will provide enough needed sedation in the majority of adult patients with foreign bodies or food impactions. General anesthesia with endotracheal intubation in certain patients is preferred as it provides complete control over the airway and the patient. General anesthesia should be used in the majority of pediatric patients and should be considered in uncooperative patients, patients who are difficult to sedate, and patients with multiple or complex foreign bodies in whom removal will take an extended period of time or have failed previous extraction.

Finally, an ex vivo study has shown that success and speed of foreign body retrieval is directly related to endoscopist experience [96]. For complex foreign bodies the most experienced endoscopist at an institution should attempt endoscopic retrieval. If concern exists about experience with foreign body retrieval or a lack of necessary endoscopic equipment and accessories, the patient should be transferred to a tertiary care center for successful treatment and extraction of the foreign body.

[96] (Fig. 43.4). The longer overtube can aid in removing sharp objects and objects that cannot be pulled retrogradely through the lower esophageal sphincter. The longer overtube may be used in esophageal bodies that need to be pushed into the stomach first before retrieval. A latex protector hood that can be simply attached to the end of the endoscope also helps prevent mucosal trauma in retrieval of sharp objects when overtubes are not available or when objects cannot easily be pulled through an overtube [97, 98].

The flexible endoscope is the preferred endoscopic method for treating foreign bodies and food impactions because of the high success rate, low complication rate, availability, patient comfort, affordability, and lack of need for general anesthesia [30, 99]. Rigid esophagoscopy has equal efficacy to flexible endoscopy in the treatment of esophageal foreign bodies. Rigid endoscopes require the use of general anesthesia and may be particularly effective for larger objects in the proximal esophagus that are unable to easily pass retrograde through the upper esophageal sphincter [100]. Flexible nasoendoscopes have been suggested as an alternative to standard

Food Bolus Impaction

Esophageal food bolus impaction is the most common "foreign body" in adults that can cause symptoms and require endoscopic intervention. In the United States the most common impacted foods are meat products including beef, chicken, pork, and hot dogs [20, 21]. Food impaction may occur in association with alcohol ingestion during which the patient may not chew food as carefully, leading to the terms, "Steakhouse Syndrome" and "Backyard Barbecue Syndrome." In Asia and coastal areas the most common food foreign bodies are fish bones. Fish bones rarely cause food impaction but cause symptoms because of the sharp and pointed ends of bones that either impact into the esophageal mucosa or cause mucosal tears.

Food boluses may pass spontaneously, thus endoscopic intervention needs to be based on symptoms. If there is evidence of near or complete obstruction with the patient unable to handle their secretions, salivating, or drooling, endoscopy should be performed on an urgent basis. If the patient has the sensation of the food bolus passing either spontaneously or after pre-endoscopy glucagon a gentle trial of fluids then solids may be sufficient, and endoscopy can be avoided. However, if there is any concern that the food bolus remains, endoscopy should be performed as all esophageal food impactions should be removed in 24 h due to increased complications with ideal removal in the first 6–12 h after the onset of symptoms [27, 102, 103]. Further, endoscopy is indicated because of the high esophageal-related pathology associated with food impactions. Lack of appropriate follow-up has been shown to be a predictor for recurrent food impactions [104].

The accepted first endoscopic method used for the treatment of esophageal food impactions is the "push technique" with success rates over 90% and minimal complications [17]. This technique entails gently pushing the esophageal food bolus into the stomach with the endoscope. Prior to pushing the food bolus into the stomach an attempt should be made to steer the endoscope around the impaction and into the stomach. This allows assessment of the nature and degree of any obstructive esophageal pathology beyond the food bolus. Generally, if an endoscope can be advanced around a food bolus and past any obstruction into the stomach the push technique will be successful. After steering around the food bolus the endoscope is pulled back proximal to the food impaction and the food is gently pushed forward. This is aided by esophageal muscle relaxation induced by sedation, expansion of the esophageal lumen with endoscopic air-insufflation and intravenous glucagon if it has been given [41].

Even if the endoscope cannot be initially maneuvered around the impaction a trial of gently pushing the food bolus can be safely attempted. However, forcefully pushing the endoscope or blindly advancing dilators or retrieval devices past the food bolus is not recommended because of the high percentage of patients with esophageal pathology [27, 41]. This may result in mucosal tears or rarely perforation of the esophagus. For larger food impactions, particularly meats such as chicken or beef that can be broken apart, the push technique can be performed after breaking the meat into smaller pieces with a forceps or snare and then pushing the smaller pieces into the stomach.

With the increasing prevalence of eosinophilic esophagitis extra care should be taken pushing food through the esophagus blindly due to the potential increased chance of perforation and mucosal tears [105]. Particular care should be used in using rigid endoscopes if eosinophillic esophagitis is suspected with perforation rates reported as high as 20% [106]. However, more recent studies have suggested that food impaction in patients with eosinophilic esophagitis can be treated effectively and safely with the push method and still should be considered the first attempted endoscopic therapy of food impactions [19].

Certain cases of food impactions cannot be safely pushed into the stomach and must be retrieved with the endoscope via the mouth. An overtube is useful to protect the airway and allow multiple passes of the endoscope. This is particularly useful in meat impactions such as pork or chicken in which the food will shred and break into multiple pieces before it can be completely removed. Standard endoscopic grasping forceps, snares, and baskets used under direct visualization can be employed alone or together. The Roth retrieval net can be particularly useful in managing food impactions as the food bolus can be contained completely within the net avoiding the use of an overtube and minimizing the risk of aspiration [107]. For well-impacted food boluses the use of a Steigmann–Goff endoscopic ligator with the bands removed can be used to suction up large pieces of food that can be removed via the mouth [108, 109].

Sharp Objects

Sharp and pointed objects account for a third of all perforations caused by GI foreign bodies and if untreated up to 15–35% of sharp/pointed foreign bodies may lead to a gastrointestinal complication. Sharp objects, particularly tooth-picks and animal bones, are the most likely to cause a perforation leading to the need for surgi-cal management [110]. Bones, toothpicks, and dental bridgework are the most common inadver-tently swallowed sharp foreign bodies. More complex and varied pointed objects such as razor blades, pins, needles, nails, writing instruments, and metal wires are seen in patients with psychi-atric illnesses or incarcerated patients. Sharp objects are often the most difficult esophageal foreign bodies to remove and may have higher complication rates associated with their removal.

Sharp objects in the esophagus should be addressed in an emergent fashion with an attempt to remove the object within 6–12 h after inges-tion. When removing sharp ingested foreign bodies Chevalier Jackson's axiom should be remembered; "advancing points puncture, trail-ing points do not" [111]. When removing sharp objects, the foreign body should be grasped in a position so that the sharp or pointed end trails distally to the endoscope thus lowering the chance of a significant procedure related perforation or mucosal trauma during extraction. This is espe-cially important in retrieving sharp objects from the esophagus. If the sharp side of the object is facing towards the upper esophagus (cranial) the object should not be grabbed and pulled retro-grade as the sharp point of the object can tear the mucosa or even perforate the esophagus. In such sharp objects, the foreign body can be gently pushed into the stomach. Once in the stomach the foreign body can be rotated and grasped on the blunt end of the object. With the blunt end facing upwards and being the advancing end the object can then usually be safely removed with minimal trauma.

Polypectomy snares and foreign body retrieval forceps such as a rat tooth or alligator forceps are the most commonly used devices for removing sharp foreign bodies with the most endoscopic control. If the size and shape of the foreign body prohibits easy withdrawal of the object an over-tube, either standard or foreign body overtube (45–60 cm) should be used to protect the esopha-gus, airway, and oropharynx [98]. An alternative is a soft latex protector hood that provides mucosal protection. The hood is simply placed or tied to the end of the endoscope with suture and folded back upon itself to obtain endoscopic visualization. After the foreign body is grasped, as it is pulled through the lower or upper esopha-geal sphincter the hood flips over the end of the endoscope and the tightly grasped foreign body which is protected within the hood.

Coins, Button Batteries, and Magnets

Coins are the most common and button batteries one of the most dangerous foreign bodies in chil-dren. Coins in the esophagus that are not promptly removed can result in pressure necrosis of the esophageal wall with possible perforation or fistulaization. In children prior to attempted endoscopic removal, airway protection should be provided via general anesthesia with endotra-cheal intubation. In adults small coins will usually pass through the esophagus and do not need to be treated but larger coins such as quarters may become lodged. In older children or adults particularly those who have the coin in the distal third of the esophagus a short period of observa-tion of 8–16 h or less may be acceptable to see if the coin passes spontaneously into the stomach and a procedure can be avoided [112]. For an adult, an overtube can be used for airway pro-tection if the coin can be pulled through it. Pinch biopsy forceps should be avoided because greater control is provided with a rat tooth forceps or a basket. The preferred retrieval device for coins is a retrieval net which allows easy snaring of the coin and additionally protects the airway as the coin is pulled past the larynx [96] (Fig. 43.5). Retrieval with a net can be performed by directly snaring the coin in the esophagus and then pull-ing out the endoscope, net, and coin in toto. Alternatively if there is no resistance, the coin can be gently pushed into the stomach and then

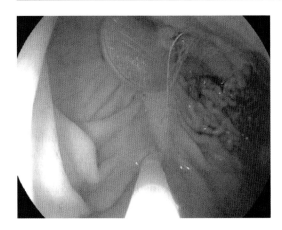

Fig. 43.5 Coin in the stomach of an infant. The coin was impacted in the esophagus. It was gently pushed into the stomach and then removed with a retrieval net

more easily snared and retrieved by the net and subsequently removed via the mouth. Bougieage has been suggested as a safe and relatively affective way to push the coin out of the esophagus and into the stomach when endoscopy is not readily available but should be avoided in centers with flexible endoscopy due to lack of control and possible complications [113].

Button batteries are of special concern because they may contain an alkaline solution that can rapidly cause a liquefaction necrosis of esophageal tissue resulting in perforation or fistula formation. Ten percent of ingested button batteries become symptomatic, with children less than 5 years of age being the most common victims [114]. The incidence of button battery ingestion and severe complications from ingestion has continued to rise with the increased number of devices that use button batteries [115]. The mechanism of injury can be caused by direct corrosive action, low-voltage burns, and pressure necrosis [15]. Thus any clinical suspicion or radiographic evidence of a disk battery localized in the esophagus should lead to emergent endoscopy.

In the retrieval of button disk batteries it is crucial to protect the airway with endotracheal tube intubation in children or an overtube in adults or older children. Traditionally the button battery had a high endoscopic failure rate of up to 60% of cases because its shape and contour made it difficult to grasp [116]. The use of the Roth retrieval net has solved this problem making retrieval of button batteries successful in almost all cases. The battery can be retrieved from the esophagus or pushed into the stomach and retrieved. One in the stomach and beyond button batteries rarely cause problems but case reports exist of damage even outside the esophagus re-iterating the need for all button batteries to be removed in the shortest time possible [117, 118].

Ingested magnets within the reach of the endoscope should also be removed on an urgent basis. Single magnets rarely will cause symptoms. However, the concern exists if multiple magnets are ingested it is unable to be discerned how many magnets were ingested or if magnets were ingested with other metal objects. This can lead to attraction between magnets to each other and possible subsequent pressure necrosis, fistula formation, and bowel perforation [119, 120]. This will rarely occur in the esophagus proper, but if a magnet is present in the esophagus and it is known or unclear if the patient ingested other magnets or metal objects, removal from the esophagus is recommended before it passes into the rest of the GI tract. Removal can be performed with rat tooth forceps, retrieval nets, or wire baskets. Using metal retrieval devices that attract the magnet may also make it easier to remove the magnets.

Long Objects

Objects longer than approximately 5–10 cm may have difficulty passing through the lower esophageal sphincter thus impacting the esophagus and often are difficult to remove through the upper esophageal sphincter. Objects of concern are toothbrushes, spoons/forks, and pens/pencils. The objects can easily be grasped with a snare or basket. The object must be grabbed at the end of the object to allow retrograde removal through the lower esophageal sphincter, esophagus, and upper esophageal sphincter. Grasping the object near the center will orient the object in a horizontal plane prohibiting pulling the long object through the lower esophageal sphincter or the esophagus.

24. Lim CT, Quah RF, Loh LE. A prospective study of ingested foreign bodies in Singapore. Arch Otolaryngol Head Neck Surg. 1994;120:96–101.

25. Ngan JHL, Fok PJ, Lai ECS, et al. A prospective study on fish bone ingestion: experience of 358 patients. Ann Surg. 1990;211:459–62.

26. Lin HH, Lee SC, Chu HC, et al. Emergency endoscopic management of dietary foreign bodies in the esophagus. Am J Emerg Med. 2007;25:662–5.

27. Eisen GM, Baron TH, Dominitz JA, et al. Guideline for the management of ingested foreign bodies. Gastrointest Endosc. 2002;55:802–6.

28. Nandi P, Ong GB. Foreign body of the esophagus: review of 2394 cases. Br J Surg. 1978;65:5–9.

29. Ginsberg GG. Management of ingested foreign objects and food bolus impactions. Gastrointest Endosc. 1995;41:33–8.

30. Stack LB, Munter DW. Foreign bodies in the gastrointestinal tract. Emerg Med Clin North Am. 1996;14:493–521.

31. O'Flynn P, Simp R. Fish bones and other foreign bodies. Clin Otolaryngol. 1993;18:231–3.

32. Bloom RR, Nakano PH, Gray SW, et al. Foreign bodies of the gastrointestinal tract. Am Surg. 1986;10:618–21.

33. Lyons MF, Tsuchida AM. Foreign bodies of the gastrointestinal tract. Med Clin North Am. 1993;77: 1101–14.

34. Desai TK, Stecevic V, Chang CH, et al. Association of eosinophillic inflammation with esophageal food impaction in adults. Gastrointest Endosc. 2005;61:795–801.

35. Rohl L, Aksglaede K, Funch-Jensen P, Thommesen P. Esophageal rings and strictures: manometric characteristics in patients with food impaction. Acta Radiol. 2000;41:275–9.

36. McCord GS, Staiano A, Clouse RE. Achalasia, diffuse spasm, and non-specific motor disorders. Baillieres Clin Gastroenterol. 1991;5:307–35.

37. Tibbling L, Bjorkhoel A, Jansson E, et al. Effect of spasmolytic drugs on esophageal foreign bodies. Dysphagia. 1995;10:126–7.

38. Stein HJ, Schwizer W, DeMeester TR, et al. Foreign body entrapment in the esophagus of healthy subjects—a manometric and scintigraphic study. Dysphagia. 1992;7:220–5.

39. Brady P. Esophageal foreign bodies. Gastroenterol Clin North Am. 1991;20:691–701.

40. Scher R, Tegtmeyer C, McLean W. Vascular injury following foreign body perforation of the esophagus. Review of the literature and report of a case. Ann Otol Rhinol Laryngol. 1990;99:698.

41. Pfau PR, Ginsberg GG, Foreign bodies and bezoars. In: Fordtran JS, Schleiseinger MH, editors. Gastrointestinal and liver disease. Pathophysiology/ diagnosis/management. Philadelphia, PA: WB Saunders; 2002. p. 386–98.

42. Jiraki K. Aortoesophageal conduit due to a foreign body. Am J Forensic Med Pathol. 1996;17:347–8.

43. Simic MA, Budakov BM. Fatal upper esophageal hemorrhage caused by a previously ingested chicken bone: case report. Am J Forensic Med Pathol. 1998;19:166–8.

44. Spitz L, Kimber C, Nguyen K, et al. Perforation of the heart by a swallowed open safety-pin in an infant. J R Coll Surg Edinb. 1998;43:114–6.

45. Drnovsek V, Fontanez-Garcia D, Wakabayashi MN, et al. Gastrointestinal case of the day. Pyogenic liver abscess caused by perforation by a swallowed wooden toothpick. Radiographics. 1999;19:820–2.

46. Sevastos N, Rafailidis P, Kolokotronis K, et al. Primary aortojejunal fistula due to a foreign body: a rare cause of gastrointestinal bleeding. Eur J Gastroenterol Hepatol. 2002;14:797–800.

47. McNutt TK, Chambers-Emerson J, Dethlefsen M, et al. Bite the bullet: lead poisoning after ingestion of 206 lead bullets. Vet Hum Toxicol. 2001;43:288–9.

48. Bennett DR, Baird CJ, Chan KM, et al. Zinc toxicity following massive coin ingestion. Am J Forensic Med Pathol. 1997;18:148–53.

49. Taylor RB. Esophageal foreign bodies. Emerg Clin Med North Am. 1987;5:301–11.

50. Herranz-Gonzalez J, Martinez-Vidal J, Garcia-Sarandeses A, et al. Esophageal foreign bodies in adults. Otolaryngol Head Neck Surg. 1991;105: 649–54.

51. Connolly AA, Birchall M, Walsh-Waring GP, et al. Ingested foreign bodies: patient guided localization is a useful clinical tool. Clin Otolaryngol. 1992;17: 520–4.

52. Lee J. Bezoars and foreign bodies of the stomach. Gastrointest Endosc Clin N Am. 1996;6:605–19.

53. Binder L, Anderson WA. Pediatric gastrointestinal foreign body ingestions. Ann Emerg Med. 1984;13:112–7.

54. Muniz AE, Joffe MD. Foreign bodies, ingested and inhaled. JAAPA. 1999;12:23–46.

55. Choudhurg CR, Bricknell MC, MacIver D. Oesophageal foreign body, an unusual cause of respiratory symptoms in a three week old baby. J Laryngol Otol. 1992;106:556–7.

56. Yoshida C, Peura D. Foreign bodies in the esophagus. In: Castell D, editor. The esophagus. Boston, MA: Little Brown; 1995. p. 379–94.

57. Roy-Ghanta S, Larosa DF, Katzka DA. Atopic characteristics of adult patients with eosinophilic esophagitis. Clin Gastroenterol Hepatol. 2008;6:531–5.

58. Straumann A, Spichtin HP, et al. Natural history of primary eosinophilic esophagitis: a follow-up of 30 adult patients for up to 11.5 years. Gastroenterology. 2003;125:1660–9.

59. Webb WA, Taylor MB. Foreign bodies of the upper gastrointestinal tract. In: Taylor MB, editor. Gastrointestinal emergencies. 2nd ed. Philadelphia, PA: Lippincott Williams & Wilkins; 1996. p. 204–16.

60. Shaffer HA, de Lange EE. Gastrointestinal foreign bodies and strictures: radiologic interventions. Curr Probl Diagn Radiol. 1994;23:205–49.

61. Bassett KE, Schunk JE, Logan L. Localizing ingested coins with a metal detector. Am J Emerg Med. 1999;17:338–41.

62. Gooden EA, Forte V, Papsin B. J Otolaryngol. 2000;29:218–20.

63. Hodge D, Tecklenburg F, Fleischer G. Coin ingestion: does every child need a radiograph? Ann Emerg Med. 1985;14:443–6.

64. Wu WT, Chiu CT, Kuo CJ, et al. Endoscopic management of suspected esophageal foreign body in adults. Dis Esophagus. 2011;24:131–7.

65. Jones NS, Lannigan FJ, Salama NY. Foreign bodies in the throat: a prospective study of 388 cases. J Laryngol Otol. 1991;105:104–8.

66. Mosca S. Management and endoscopic techniques in cases of ingestion of foreign bodies. Endoscopy. 2000;32:232–3.

67. Mosca S, Manes G, Martino L, et al. Endoscopic management of foreign bodies in the upper gastrointestinal tract: report on a series of 414 adult patients. Endoscopy. 2001;33:692–6.

68. Takada M, Kashiwagi R, Sakane M, et al. 3D-CT Diagnosis for ingested foreign bodies. Am J Emerg Med. 2000;18:192–3.

69. Silva RG, Ahluwaiia JP. Asymptomatic esophageal perforation after foreign body ingestion. Gastrointest Endosc. 2005;61:615–9.

70. Ciriza C, Garcia L, Suarez P, et al. What predictive parameters best indicate the need for emergent gastrointestinal endoscopy after foreign body ingestion? J Clin Gastroenterol. 2000;31:23–8.

71. Velitchkov NG, Grigorov GI, Losanoff JE, et al. Ingested foreign bodies of the gastrointestinal tract. Retrospective analysis of 542 cases. World J Surg. 1996;20:1001–5.

72. Kurkciyan I, Frossard M, Kettenbach J, et al. Conservative management of foreign bodies in the gastrointestinal tract. Z Gastroenterol. 1996;34: 173–7.

73. Weiland ST, Schurr MJ. Conservative management of ingested foreign bodies. J Gastrointest Surg. 2002;6:496–500.

74. Colon V, Grade A, Pullman G, et al. Effect of doses of glucagon used to treat food impaction on esophageal motor function of normal subjects. Dysphagia. 1999;14:27–30.

75. Ferrucci JT, Long LA. Radiologic treatment of esophageal food impaction using intravenous glucagon. Radiology. 1977;125:25–8.

76. Trenker SW, Maglinte DT, Lehman G, et al. Esophageal food impaction: treatment with glucagon. Radiology. 1983;149:401–3.

77. Al-Haddad M, Ward EM. Glucagon for the relief of esophageal food impaction: does it really work? Dig Dis Sci. 2006;51:1930–3.

78. Sodeman TC, Harewood GC, Baron TH. Assessment of the predictors of response to glucagon in the setting of acute esophageal food bolus impaction. Dysphagia. 2004;19:18–21.

79. Mehta D, Attia M, Quintana E, et al. Glucagon use for esophageal coin dislodgment in children: a prospective double-blind, placebo-controlled trial. Acad Emerg Med. 2001;8:200–3.

80. Alaradi O, Bartholomew M, Barkin JS. Upper endoscopy and glucagon: a new technique in the management of acute esophageal food impaction. Am J Gastroenterol. 2001;96:912–3.

81. Robbins MI, Shortsleeve MJ. Treatment of acute esophageal food impaction with glucagon, an effervescent agent, and water. AJR Am J Roentgenol. 1994;162:325–8.

82. Kaszar-Seibert DJ, Korn WT, Bindman DJ, et al. Treatment of acute esophageal food impaction with a combination of glucagon, effervescent agent, and water. AJR Am J Roentgenol. 1990;154:533–4.

83. Smith JC, Janower ML, Geiger AH. Use of glucagon and gas-forming agents in acute esophageal food impaction. Radiology. 1986;159:567–8.

84. Maini S, Rudralingam M, Zeitoun H, et al. Aspiration pneumonitis following papain enzyme treatment for oesophageal meat imapaction. J Laryngol Otol. 2001;115:585–6.

85. Litovitz T, Scmitz BF. Ingestion of cylindrical and button batteries: an analysis of 2382 cases. Pediatrics. 1992;89:747–57.

86. Paulson EK, Jaffe RB. Metallic foreign bodies in the stomach: fluoroscopic removal with a magnetic orogastric tube. Radiology. 1990;174:191–4.

87. Hawkins DB. Removal of blunt foreign bodies from the esophagus. Ann Otol Rhinol Laryngol. 1990;99:935–40.

88. Schunk JE, Harrison AM, Corneli HM, et al. Fluoroscopic foley catheter removal of esophageal foreign bodies in children: experience with 415 cases. Pediatrics. 1994;94:709–14.

89. Blair SR, Graeber GM, Cruzzavala JL, et al. Current management of esophageal impactions. Chest. 1993;104:1205–9.

90. Thapa BR, Singh K, Dilawari JB. Endoscopic removal of foreign bodies from the gastrointestinal tract. Indian Pediatr. 1993;30:1105–10.

91. Khurana AK, Saraya A, Jain N, et al. Management of foreign bodies of the upper gastrointestinal tract. Trop Gastroenterol. 1998;19:32–3.

92. Conway WC, Sugawa C, Ono H, et al. Upper GI foreign body: an adult urban emergency hospital experience. Surg Endosc. 2007;21:455–60.

93. Bonadio WA, Emslander H, Milner D, et al. Esophageal mucosal changes in children with an acutely ingested coin lodged in the esophagus. Pediatr Emerg Care. 1994;10:333–4.

94. Chaikhouni A, Kratz JM, Crawford MA. Foreign bodies of the esophagus. Am Surg. 1985;51:173–9.

95. Nelson DB, Bosco JJ, Curtis WO, et al. Endoscopic retrieval devices. Gastrointest Endosc. 1999; 50: 932–934.

96. Faigel DO, Stotland BR, Kochman ML, et al. Device choice and experience level in endoscopic foreign

the incidence of dysphagia in proportion to the thickness of the plates themselves [3, 4].

Several investigators have reviewed the natural history of dysphagia after anterior cervical surgery and found that the dysphagia tends to be most severe early on, likely as a result of swelling. It slowly resolves over 1–3 months, but some patients continue to describe some level of dysphagia years after surgery. In a prospective study of 221 patients after anterior cervical surgery, Bazaz described the change in dysphagia over time. The group reported an overall incidence of dysphagia of 50 % at 1 month, 32 % at 2 months, and 18 % at 6 months. The incidence of moderate-to-severe dysphagia at 6 months was 5 % [5]. Lee et al., found a dysphagia rate of 13.6 % in a cohort of 310 patients followed 2 years after surgery [3].

One confounding factor in this population of patients is the seemingly high incidence of preoperative dysphagia. One group studied patients undergoing anterior cervical surgery preoperatively with video fluoroscopic swallowing evaluations. They found 48 % of patients had objective findings of swallowing dysfunction, but none had subjective symptoms of difficulties with swallowing. Thus, careful preoperative evaluation may predict the likelihood of developing prolonged postoperative dysphagia [6].

Early and progressively worsening dysphagia should be evaluated with barium studies and perhaps CT scan to rule out the presence of hematoma formation or retropharyngeal abscess from inadvertent esophageal perforation or deep space infections. Other correctable causes of dysphagia in this population include stricture formation from fibrosis related to plates, or unrecognized self-limited infections. Recurrent laryngeal nerve injuries have been reported and tend to present more with hoarse voice than with dysphagia. Concurrent presentation of voice changes and dysphagia imply injury to the main trunk of the vagus—most likely only in high cervical surgery [7].

Thyroid surgery for benign or malignant disease is a common procedure that exposes patients to the risk of recurrent laryngeal and superior laryngeal nerve injury. The most common reason for litigation after thyroid surgery is injury of the recurrent laryngeal nerve and its attendant effect on the character of a patient's voice [8]. Not as well recognized or reported are the long-term effects on swallowing function. As with anterior cervical surgery, some degree of early postoperative dysphagia related to tissue swelling has been reported to approach 15 % in patients with no nerve injury, and as high as 30 % in patients with unilateral nerve injury [9, 10].

A confounding factor is the preoperative presence of dysphagia in patients who undergo thyroidectomy. This is as a result of a mechanical obstruction by an enlarged gland or tumor, invasion of tumor into the neural or esophageal structures, or as a result of preoperative radiation therapy to the tumor bed. There is a paucity of literature to provide an accurate estimate of the incidence of preoperative dysphagia; however, given the cervical surgery literature it is likely significant. There have been two prospective studies looking at baseline dysphagia in patients with thyroid disease. Lombardi and colleagues used a quality of life questionnaire to identify dysphagia in 52 of 110 patients preoperatively. One week after surgery 73.6 % of these patients had worse dysphagia, but at 3 months their swallowing returned to preoperative baseline, and at 1 year it had improved significantly in all but 20 % [11].

A second study by Greenblatt and colleagues also used a validated quality of life tool (SWAL-QOL) to investigate pre- and postoperative dysphagia. The SWAL-QOL instrument measures the impact of dysphagia on several different dimensions of function and produces a range of scores from 0 (very poor QOL) to 100 (perfect). In this study, 116 patients completed the quality of life instrument preoperatively with the mean score of the group reflecting, "imperfect swallowing." The physical domain, which encompassed symptoms such as food sticking, choking when eating, or drinking, was 81.2 preoperatively. The patients were scored again 1 year after surgery and at this point had a statistically significant improvement to 87.1 ($p < 0.0001$). The group did not report any data on early dysphagia following surgery, which is a limit of the study, but certainly by 1-year post-procedure the patient's swallowing QOL was better than at baseline [12].

Evaluation of these patients should begin with understanding the operative details. For cervical disk surgery these details include the surgical approach, the number of levels fused, and the use of plating. For thyroid surgery they include the extent of surgery (total vs. partial thyroidectomy), evidence of recurrent laryngeal nerve injury, and the use of radiation. A modified barium swallow will illuminate swallowing dysfunction and may also elucidate the impact of the cervical plates on swallowing function. It will identify stricture formation and aspiration related to disordered swallowing mechanisms. Indirect laryngoscopy to evaluate for laryngeal nerve injury is indicated if changes in the patients' voice occur in conjunction with dysphagia.

Therapeutic interventions in this group of patients tend to be supportive in the first few months unless early dysphagia is secondary to hematomas or abscess. Long-term dysphagia is managed by supportive functional therapy with the help of speech pathologists. Unfortunately, the literature is sparse regarding the impact of functional therapies on postoperative dysphagia. Endoscopic dilation of strictures, and Botulinum toxin injection for some motor dysfunctions are also options [10, 11].

Foregut Surgery

The explosion of minimally invasive procedures in the late 1980s began with Dr. Eric Muhe's reports of the first video-laparoscopic cholecystectomies [13]. The improvement in recovery and decrease in overall patient morbidity inspired many groups to direct the new techniques at other surgical pathology. Dallemagne reported the first laparoscopic fundoplication, followed shortly thereafter by the first reported laparoscopic bariatric procedures [14]. As the eagerness of both patients and surgeons grew for the benefits of minimally invasive procedures, many patients began seeking out surgery for common problems such as gastroesophageal reflux and obesity. Unfortunately, the sharp increase in demand for

surgery coupled with a fledgling experience in laparoscopic surgery created a perfect storm for postoperative complications.

Fundoplication

Rudolph Nissen first described *trans*-abdominal fundoplication for GERD in 1958 [15]. The goal of the operation was to buttress the LES by wrapping the gastric fundus around the lower esophagus, and in doing so also create a longer intra-abdominal esophagus. The length of esophagus wrapped with fundus at that time was nearly 5 cm long, which offered complete resolution of GERD, but at the cost of often significant, disabling dysphagia from obstruction of the esophageal outlet. The modern versions of the fundoplication offer shorter, looser, and even partial wrapping of the esophagus, which significantly reduce the incidence and severity of dysphagia.

Dysphagia after fundoplication is common in the first 2–8 weeks after surgery, with half of those who undergo surgery reporting some level of dysphagia. As swelling of the hiatus, esophagus, and stomach resolves, so should the symptoms. Dietary modification to a full liquid diet for 1–2 weeks postoperatively is often used to avert severe symptoms from solids traversing the swollen and wrapped esophagus [16, 17]. Swelling should resolve within the first month after surgery and, if present, should not be severe. If symptoms persist beyond 8 weeks or are severe at any point, then further evaluation is warranted (Table 44.1).

The greatest risk factor for postoperative dysphagia is the presence of preoperative dysphagia, and thus evaluation should begin with the patient's preoperative symptoms [18]. Dysphagia can be caused by primary motor disorders of the esophagus, impairment of motility related to significant acid exposure and esophagitis, or stricture formation. Postoperatively, patients can have significant gastroesophageal reflux if the operation was not successful in restoring the integrity of the LES, either from a poorly constructed fundoplication or dehiscence of the hiatal closure.

Table 44.1 Causes of dysphagia following fundoplication

Location	Technical reasons	Inherent disease
Esophagus	Too loose a wrap with recurrent esophagitis	Preoperative peptic stricture Achalasia Scleroderma Eosinophilic esophagitis
Hiatus/chest	Too tight a cruroplasty, inflammatory reaction from mesh, failure of repair with herniation of wrap, paraesophageal component	
Stomach/fundus	Too tight a wrap, wrap includes greater curvature (twisted), wrap slipped onto stomach, too long a wrap	Gastroparesis

Understanding dysphagia after fundoplication should begin with understanding several operative details. The ideal fundoplication loosely encircles the distal intra-abdominal esophagus for a length of 2–2.5 cm if complete (Nissen) or up to 3 cm if partial (Toupet wrap). Closure of the hiatus should also be loose enough to allow the easy passage of food boluses, but snug enough to contribute to the anti-reflux barrier (ARB). Frequently, surgeons use a bougie to calibrate both the tightness of the wrap and hiatal closure. The use of a bougie reduces the incidence of postoperative dysphagia [19].

The details of hiatal closure are also important as the use of nonabsorbable mesh to reinforce this closure has become more popular and is a well-known contributor to dysphagia both in the early and late postoperative periods. More recently, the use of bio-absorbable mesh appears to produce less associated dysphagia and significantly less risk of erosion, and in some trials a significant decrease in recurrence of hiatal hernias in the early postoperative period [20, 21].

Postoperative evaluation of dysphagia begins with either endoscopy or barium study. Barium studies are most helpful if performed by an experienced radiologist and with the use of either a 13 mm barium tablets, or barium soaked cookie or marshmallow. These help illustrate the location of obstruction to varied consistencies of food. Additionally, barium studies can show the presence of a hiatal hernia and suggest a twisted or slipped wrap. Additionally, some understanding of the disordered esophageal motor function like esophageal spasm, esophageal dilation, or achalasia can be obtained. High-resolution esophageal manometry is also useful in identifying esophageal outlet obstruction from a too tight fundoplication (Fig. 44.1). It is the method of choice for identifying disorders of esophageal motor function.

If there is evidence of obstruction to flow across the GEJ, then endoscopic evaluation is important to determine the cause of this obstruction. If UGI does not suggest a slipped, recurrent, or twisted wrap, then the culprit could be a wrap that is too tight or too long. If obstruction is present then a trial at dilation is reasonable as up to 67 % of patients will derive some improvement, many (75 %) after only one dilation [16, 17]. The degree of dilation is variable and can be guided by knowing the size of bougie, if any, used at the time of surgery to calibrate the fundoplication or hiatal closure.

If the UGI suggests abnormal orientation of the wrap, then endoscopy will be important in evaluating the construction of the wrap itself. Fundoplications have characteristic views on retroflexed evaluation [22]. The two most common fundoplications are the 360° Nissen fundoplication and the 270° posterior partial Toupe fundoplication. The presence of a hiatal hernia on UGI should be investigated endoscopically to exclude the presence of a paraesophageal hernia component that is compressing the distal esophagus and causing dysphagia. The presence of a double-chambered stomach can occur with a slipped fundoplication or a twisted wrap. A slipped fundoplication usually occurs when the length of the esophagus was misjudged and the fundus is wrapped around the proximal stomach, or the wrap itself slips onto the stomach due to a combination of downward pressure exerted by the diaphragm and a retracting, foreshortened

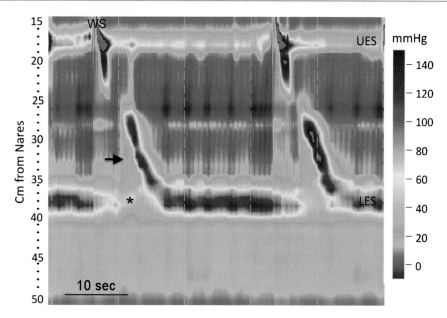

Fig. 44.1 Tight Nissen fundoplication. This is a high-resolution esophageal manometry from a patient with dysphagia after Nissen fundoplication. In these recordings pressure is depicted as color (*color bar* on the right), sensor position from the nares is on the *left*, and time is on the *x*-axis. With wet swallows (WS) there is normal function of the upper esophageal sphincter (UES) and striated muscle esophagus. The typical features of a tight fundoplication are failed or incomplete LES relaxation (*asterisk*) and elevated intrabolus pressure (*arrow*) as the bolus is being pushed ahead of the peristaltic contraction against an obstructed GE junction

esophagus. Obstruction to flow of this type may lead to dilation of the proximal stomach pouch. A twisted wrap occurs because the wrap is formed between the distal greater curvature and fundus, instead of fundus to fundus. All three of these conditions usually require reoperation, albeit with less favorable results than a primary fundoplication. Dilation of the wrap in these conditions has not shown itself to be of any benefit.

An uncommon, but certainly described, cause of post-fundoplication dysphagia is preoperatively unrecognized motility disorder. Achalasia can be an insidious disease that may present early with heartburn that responds partially to proton pump inhibitor therapy. Patients may have evidence of esophagitis on endoscopic biopsy suggesting reflux as an etiology. When achalasia is not identified preoperatively with esophageal manometry, fundoplication will produce a progressively worsening, and often-severe dysphagia [23]. Making the diagnosis of achalasia after fundoplication can become quite challenging, because fundoplication alone can increase the resting pressure and residual (relaxation) pressure of the LES. In this situation, the diagnosis of achalasia rests upon the absence of esophageal peristalsis. If the too tight fundoplication is unattended, a form of pseudoachalasia with failure of esophageal peristalsis and LES relaxation may ensue. Normal esophageal motor function may not return when the fundoplication is taken down.

Bariatric Surgery

The popularity of weight loss surgery has grown significantly over the last 10 years in parallel with the epidemic of obesity that has swept across the United States. It is estimated that 34 % of the American population is obese, while another 5 % is considered morbidly obese, and thus qualify for weight loss surgery. By comparison only 1.5 % of Americans who qualify pursue weight loss surgery, but that still resulted in 220,000 operations in 2008 [24–26].

In the United States there are four frequently performed laparoscopic operations (in order of frequency): Roux en Y Gastric Bypass (GBP), Adjustable Gastric Band (AGB), Sleeve Gastrectomy (SG), and Biliopancreatic Diversion with Duodenal Switch (BPD-DS). These surgeries are performed laparoscopically in over 95 % of centers. All of the operations share restriction, or shrinking capacitance of the stomach, as a common mechanism of action.

Difficult deglutition after weight loss surgery is a function of the type of surgery performed, and can be difficult to elicit as a complaint, as patients often perceive some dysphagia as expected and a positive contributor to weight loss. Similar to other foregut surgery, all weight loss surgeries produce swelling which resolves over a period of 1–3 months. During this period of time patients can expect to have occasional dysphagia usually related to eating behaviors such as eating too large a portion or eating too rapidly.

All weight loss surgeries have in common one mechanism of action: restriction of the amount of food that one can consume. GBP also adds malabsorption as one of its principal components. GBP converts a 1.5 L capacity stomach to a small pouch that can contain 30–50 mL at first. Over time this volume increases but should rarely exceed 100–150 mL. The pouch is connected to a roux limb, which allows foodstuffs to bypass gastric juices as well as all the absorption that occurs in the proximal jejunum and duodenum. Most bariatric surgeons construct a 100–150 cm roux limb, which allows for union of the gastric juices with the food well distal to the gastric pouch.

Sleeve gastrectomy is a relatively new weight loss surgery during which a long thin gastric sleeve is created along the lesser curvature by resecting the fundus, body, and a portion of the antrum. In doing so, a 70–120 mL pouch remains, which includes at least a portion of the antral mill apparatus, as well as the pylorus.

The AGB is quickly becoming the most frequently performed weight loss procedure in the United States. It creates a small gastric pouch in the proximal stomach by wrapping a band around the upper stomach, 2–3 cm below the gastroe-sophageal junction to form a 30 mL pouch. Along the inside of the band there is a soft-walled balloon that is inflated to narrow the stomal diameter between the upper pouch and distal stomach. By inflating the balloon and increasing resistance to passage of solid food, the small gastric pouch can stretch and provide a sense of satiety. As patients lose weight, the stoma created by the band's balloon will usually increase in diameter—and thus patient's portion sizes will increase. The patients can then have fluid added to the balloon to again narrow the stoma, decrease portion sizes and thus continue weight loss.

A popular operation in the 1970s and 1980s was the vertical banded gastroplasty. Although rarely performed currently, these patients frequently present with complaints of dysphasia and reflux. The vertical banded gastroplasty formed a small gastric pouch by creating a staple line parallel to the lesser curvature. This staple line was not divided early on, but because of problems with staple line dehiscence it eventually became a standard practice to divide the stomach. Wrapping either mesh or a silastic ring around the outlet further restricted the outflow from this pouch.

Because of the inherently restrictive nature of weight-loss surgeries many patients can be expected to present, at least transiently, with restriction-associated dysphagia. It is important to know which procedure was performed and subsequently to understand the timeline of the dysphagia onset. For instance was dysphagia felt immediately following the operation, or has it worsened after more recent interventions such as filling of the band's balloon or ingestion of new medications. To understand the etiology of dysphagia it is best to understand the nuances that create dysphasia with each operation.

Gastric Bypass

GBP can create dysphagia based on difficulties in emptying the esophagus, emptying the gastric pouch, or propelling food past the jejuno-jejunostomy. Difficulty emptying the esophagus can be due to an undiagnosed primary esophageal disease, but more commonly is secondary and related to the development of a hiatal hernia with diaphragmatic compression of the pouch outlet. Although rarely reported, this phenomenon is important to diagnose.

In morbidly obese patients, the phreno-esophageal fat pad can obscure the hiatus, making it difficult to visualize a hiatal hernia at the time of the primary operation. Subsequently, as the patient loses significant weight, the fat in and around the hiatus shrinks and allows development of a sliding hiatal hernia. Frequently, these patients present after significant weight loss with severe reflux disease and esophagitis associated with dysphagia or odynophagia [25, 26]. Repair of this hernia frequently relieves the symptoms and in ideal situations is combined with an anti-reflux procedure such as a Hill or Belsey repair done transthoracically.

Difficulty emptying the gastric pouch should be investigated, particularly if it occurs more than 6 weeks after the operation. The differential diagnosis for dysphagia occurring greater than 6 weeks after GBP includes strictures with associated marginal ulcers related to roux limb ischemia, overproduction of acid, foreign body reaction, tobacco use, or NSAID use.

The anastomosis between the gastric pouch and small intestine is calibrated to be between 11 and 14 mm in diameter. This small diameter anastomosis places this junction at risk for stricture formation, which is reported in between 13 and 52 % of patients undergoing endoscopy for UGI symptoms after GBP [27–29]. Dysphagia along with regurgitation is the typical symptom of patients presenting with stricture formation; however, in one study only 39 % of patients with dysphagia were found to have stomal stenosis, and the rest had only marginal ulcers. In this same study, over half of the patients with stenosis also had an associated marginal ulcer [27]. Most stenosis- or ulcer-associated dysphagia occurs within the first 6 months after surgery, frequently between 6 and 18 weeks. Dysphagia related to strictures is improved after a single dilation in one half to two-thirds of patients.

Because strictures frequently result from over production of acid, the presence of a gastro-gastric fistula should be investigated. These usually appear endoscopically as hyperemic area associated with the lateral staple line of the pouch. They can be difficult to identify endoscopically and frequently are more easily appreciated on barium studies. There have been descriptions of closure of these fistulae by endoscopic means, but with variable results [30].

An important modification of GBP is the fixed ring or mesh reinforced gastric outlet variant. The concept that a fixed stoma diameter may help maintain long-term weight loss led to wrapping of proline or marlex mesh of a fixed diameter around the gastric outlet of pouches. Unfortunately, mesh has a tendency to shrink over time, patients may present years later with dysphagia and regurgitation from a very narrow gastric outlet. Furthermore, in some patients the mesh actually erodes into the lumen of the bowel, which is often mistaken for ulcer formation early in its migration. In an attempt to minimize these untoward effects of mesh, some surgeons began placing silastic rings instead of mesh. Sometimes referred to as the Fobi pouch, this operation was popularized in the late 1990s. Unfortunately, many patients still reported worsening dysphagia over time, but there was significantly less erosion and luminal migration with the ring. The ring however is capable of slipping distally, thereby occluding egress of foodstuffs from the pouch. Patients who present with these issues frequently require revisional surgery to either divide or remove the mesh or ring. Occasionally complete reconstruction of the gastrojejunostomy is required. A few centers are now endoscopically addressing the ring type erosions and slippages with no need for further surgery [30–33].

A rare contributor to dysphagia after GBP can be aberrant emptying of the roux limb. Stricture of the distal anastomosis of the roux limb is rarely reported and can be challenging to diagnose. Upper GI contrast studies that do not include a small bowel follow thru often miss dilation and stasis of the roux limb or stasis of fluid above the jejuno-jejunostomy. Once identified, this stricture can be dealt with by endoscopic dilation or surgical revision.

Surgical disorientation can lead to errors in construction of the roux limb. This phenomenon

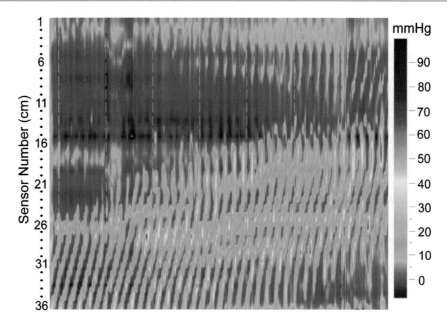

Fig. 44.2 Reversed Roux limb. This high-resolution manometry was obtained from the roux limb of a gastric bypass patient complaining of dysphagia, postprandial regurgitation, and profound weight loss. It demonstrates retrograde propagation of both the phase III of the migrating myoelectrical complex, and its individual peristaltic contractions. This is the manometric pattern of a reversed roux limb

entitled, "Roux-en-O" is the inadvertent anastomosis of the segment of bowel originating from the distal stomach to the gastric pouch. The segment of bowel is placed in an anti-peristaltic orientation, so patients present with severe dysphagia and frequently with bilious emesis. Frequently, UGI studies appear normal but careful and prolonged fluoroscopy may identify retrograde peristalsis of the contrast column. Intubation of the limb with high-resolution manometry can also identify retrograde peristalsis (Fig. 44.2). Frequently these patients undergo multiple revisional operations with no improvement if the diagnosis is not made [34, 35].

Adjustable Gastric Banding

The AGB is quickly becoming the most popular bariatric surgery in the United States [36]. There are currently two band manufactures in the United States with a total of seven different designs that have been implanted since FDA approval in 2003. The original designs incorporated low volume, high-pressure balloons within their bands, so

called: 9.5 mm, 10.5 mm and Vanguard Bands (Allergan, Santa Barbara, CA). These lower volume bands had a narrower range at which they would provide resistance and not dysphagia. More recent iterations are created to accept higher volumes of saline at lower pressures, allowing a greater range of operation—AP-Standard, AP-Large (Allergan), and Realize and Realize-C Bands (Ethicon Endosurgery Cinncinati, OH).

Given that the sole mechanism of action of bands is impediment to flow of foodstuffs, it is commonly associated with difficulty in deglutition, which is not always pathologic. Dysphagia is often most pronounced after filling of the band's balloon, but is transient as minor swelling associated with the balloon fill resolves over a period of 24–48 h. Less commonly, persistent difficulties in deglutition occur as a result of slippage of the band or chronic overfilling of the band (Fig. 44.3). This may lead to esophageal dilation with or without esophageal dysmotility.

Band slippage occurs in 2–6 % of patients with AGBs. Slippage is the asymmetric migration

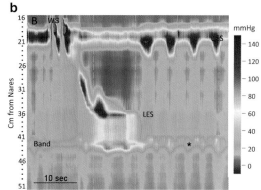

Fig. 44.3 Obstructing lap band. These are high-resolution esophageal manometries from patients with dysphagia after laparoscopic gastric band. In (**a**), pressures produced by diaphragmatic contraction with inspiration (*asterisk*) and the LES are located at the same position (43–44 cm from the nares), so there is no hiatal hernia. Another high-pressure zone about 8 cm below the GE junction is caused by the AGB. Notice that there is pressurization of the gastric pouch following the WS, suggest-

ing an outlet obstruction. Also there is feeble peristalsis only in the proximal smooth muscle esophagus and failure in the distal smooth muscle esophagus. This is an indication that the esophagus is failing. In (**b**), the LES is hypotensive and located at about 36 cm from the nares. The diaphragm (*asterisk*) and band are located at about 7 cm below the GE junction, indicating a hiatal hernia. Again the WS produces pressurization of the hernia pouch

of distal stomach above the band, causing tissue cluttering at the stoma, which leads to outflow obstruction. It can occur gradually and at first can result in the loss of the sense of restriction as the pouch enlarges. Subsequently, patients develop de novo or worsening GERD, as well as dilation of the esophagus. As the stomal outlet narrows further, patients may experience sensations of chest pressure or pain, as well as regurgitation of clear sputum. Acute slippage results not only in these symptoms, but can also lead to acute ischemia of the stomach with associated acute pain and hematemesis. Acute slippage requires emergency removal of band fluid and usually surgical intervention. Slippage is prevented by plication of the fundus over the band to anchor the distal stomach in place.

Esophageal dilation, after gastric banding, is becoming a more frequently recognized complication the early incidence of which is estimated from 6 to 15 %, and has been reported as high as 68 % in longer-term studies (Fig. 44.4). The incidence of esophageal dilation is least common in patients younger than 25 and more common in patients older than 50 [37–39]. Preoperative

manometric findings do not appear to predict the development of this phenomenon; patients with abnormal manometry have been studied after band placement and have not had dilation. Conversely, patients with normal preoperative manometry seem to make up the large percentage of patients who develop postoperative dilation [37, 40].

Defining esophageal dilation is a difficult task, as there are no authoritative studies defining normal esophageal diameter. Demaria, as a part of the original FDA band trial, defined esophageal dilation as an increase in diameter of 30 % above baseline, and reported a 71 % dilation rate among 25 patients studied. Dargent reviewed the phenomenon in a series of 1,232 and reported a dilation rate of 0.6 % but provided no size criteria for his diagnosis [41]. Milone's retrospective study on 440 AGB patients defined a diameter greater than 35 mm as dilation "based on discussion with the radiologists" at their institution (Table 44.2) [37]. On the basis of this definition, a long-term study showed that of 167 patients in whom bands were placed, 108 had some degree of dilation with radiographically defined abnormal motility ranging from mild to severe. The study incorperated a

esophageal mucosa. In addition, a direct toxic mechanism is plausible as NSAIDs are weak acidic molecules with pKa values of 4–5, which facilitates diffusion into the mucosa in the setting of an acidic pH in the distal esophagus [74].

The use of aspirin and NSAIDs (including over-the-counter prescription) is associated with esophageal strictures [75, 76]. In addition, perforation and bronchoesophageal fistula have been reported [27, 30, 77]. NSAID ulcers are typically large, shallow, discrete mid-esophageal ulcers with normal intervening mucosa. Histological findings are nonspecific with isolated mucosal erosions and ulcers commonly seen [78]. Nonspecific or reflux esophagitis may be seen. Basal cell hyperplasia may be absent as cell proliferation is inhibited by the prostaglandin inhibitors [79].

Potassium Chloride

Potassium chloride (KCl) tablets may cause ulcers and strictures throughout the GI tract [80]. DEI is mediated by a local high concentration of dissolved KCl that results in local hyperosmolality leading to tissue desiccation and vascular injury [13]. Toxicity is reported more commonly with slow-release wax matrix formulation but this may be a reflection of its more widespread prescription compared to the microencapsulated preparation [6].

KCl-mediated injury is usually reported in association with left atrial enlargement or cardiac surgery though this may be confounded by the high prevalence of cardiac disease in patients on KCl treatment [81, 82]. Prior cardiac surgery may result in entrapment of the esophagus between the aorta and the vertebral column [83]. The esophagus may be fixed in position by adhesions that may predispose to pill retention.

KCl has often been associated with severe and lethal complications including strictures, perforation into the left atrium, bronchial artery, aorta, and mediastinum [84–89]. In contrast to the sudden onset of chest pain with other culprit medications, DEI mediated by KCl presents with progressive dysphagia often in the absence of significant pain [30]. The relative absence of pain may account for the progression to strictures before medical attention is sought.

Iron

Iron is associated with corrosive injury of the upper GI tract [90, 91]. Iron deposition occurs relatively frequently with crystalline iron deposition found in 0.9 % of one series of upper GI biopsies though case reports of clinically manifested DEI are uncommon [20, 92, 93]. Differentiating primary iron-associated mucosal injury from iron deposition in a preexisting lesion may be challenging as concomitant conditions that could have caused the underlying condition may be found in about half of these patients. Biopsies reveal luminal crystalline iron deposition adjacent to the surface epithelium or admixed with luminal fibroinflammatory exudates. Iron deposition in the lamina propria, either covered by an intact epithelium, subjacent to small superficial erosions, or admixed with granulation tissue may be seen. Iron-containing thrombi in mucosal blood vessels are infrequent findings. An exuberant reactive proliferation of fibroblasts and epithelial tissues near esophageal ulcers containing iron may occasionally mimic malignancy [78].

Quinidine

Quinidine has been associated with DEI and stricture formation either when ingested alone or together with KCl [6]. The presence of a profuse exudate with nodularity may be mistaken for malignancy [18, 29].

Chemotherapeutic Agents

Dactinomycin, bleomycin, cytarabine, daunorubicin and 5-fluorouracil, vincristine and methotrexate, and other chemotherapy regimens have been associated with esophagitis usually in the setting of concomitant oral mucositis. These are mostly self-limiting though they may persist for months after cessation of treatment [94]. In addition, oral methotrexate (MTX) has been implicated in a single case of ulcerative esophagitis in an adolescent with Crohn's disease that resolved upon discontinuation of MTX [95]. Dysphagia from delayed

diaphragmatic compression of the pouch outlet. Although rarely reported, this phenomenon is important to diagnose.

In morbidly obese patients, the phreno-esophageal fat pad can obscure the hiatus, making it difficult to visualize a hiatal hernia at the time of the primary operation. Subsequently, as the patient loses significant weight, the fat in and around the hiatus shrinks and allows development of a sliding hiatal hernia. Frequently, these patients present after significant weight loss with severe reflux disease and esophagitis associated with dysphagia or odynophagia [25, 26]. Repair of this hernia frequently relieves the symptoms and in ideal situations is combined with an anti-reflux procedure such as a Hill or Belsey repair done transthoracically.

Difficulty emptying the gastric pouch should be investigated, particularly if it occurs more than 6 weeks after the operation. The differential diagnosis for dysphagia occurring greater than 6 weeks after GBP includes strictures with associated marginal ulcers related to roux limb ischemia, overproduction of acid, foreign body reaction, tobacco use, or NSAID use.

The anastomosis between the gastric pouch and small intestine is calibrated to be between 11 and 14 mm in diameter. This small diameter anastomosis places this junction at risk for stricture formation, which is reported in between 13 and 52 % of patients undergoing endoscopy for UGI symptoms after GBP [27–29]. Dysphagia along with regurgitation is the typical symptom of patients presenting with stricture formation; however, in one study only 39 % of patients with dysphagia were found to have stomal stenosis, and the rest had only marginal ulcers. In this same study, over half of the patients with stenosis also had an associated marginal ulcer [27]. Most stenosis- or ulcer-associated dysphagia occurs within the first 6 months after surgery, frequently between 6 and 18 weeks. Dysphagia related to strictures is improved after a single dilation in one half to two-thirds of patients.

Because strictures frequently result from over production of acid, the presence of a gastro-gastric fistula should be investigated. These usually appear endoscopically as hyperemic area associated with the lateral staple line of the pouch. They can be difficult to identify endoscopically and frequently are more easily appreciated on barium studies. There have been descriptions of closure of these fistulae by endoscopic means, but with variable results [30].

An important modification of GBP is the fixed ring or mesh reinforced gastric outlet variant. The concept that a fixed stoma diameter may help maintain long-term weight loss led to wrapping of proline or marlex mesh of a fixed diameter around the gastric outlet of pouches. Unfortunately, mesh has a tendency to shrink over time, patients may present years later with dysphagia and regurgitation from a very narrow gastric outlet. Furthermore, in some patients the mesh actually erodes into the lumen of the bowel, which is often mistaken for ulcer formation early in its migration. In an attempt to minimize these untoward effects of mesh, some surgeons began placing silastic rings instead of mesh. Sometimes referred to as the Fobi pouch, this operation was popularized in the late 1990s. Unfortunately, many patients still reported worsening dysphagia over time, but there was significantly less erosion and luminal migration with the ring. The ring however is capable of slipping distally, thereby occluding egress of foodstuffs from the pouch. Patients who present with these issues frequently require revisional surgery to either divide or remove the mesh or ring. Occasionally complete reconstruction of the gastrojejunostomy is required. A few centers are now endoscopically addressing the ring type erosions and slippages with no need for further surgery [30–33].

A rare contributor to dysphagia after GBP can be aberrant emptying of the roux limb. Stricture of the distal anastomosis of the roux limb is rarely reported and can be challenging to diagnose. Upper GI contrast studies that do not include a small bowel follow thru often miss dilation and stasis of the roux limb or stasis of fluid above the jejuno-jejunostomy. Once identified, this stricture can be dealt with by endoscopic dilation or surgical revision.

Surgical disorientation can lead to errors in construction of the roux limb. This phenomenon

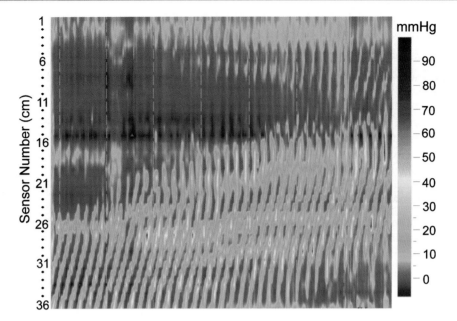

Fig. 44.2 Reversed Roux limb. This high-resolution manometry was obtained from the roux limb of a gastric bypass patient complaining of dysphagia, postprandial regurgitation, and profound weight loss. It demonstrates retrograde propagation of both the phase III of the migrating myoelectrical complex, and its individual peristaltic contractions. This is the manometric pattern of a reversed roux limb

entitled, "Roux-en-O" is the inadvertent anastomosis of the segment of bowel originating from the distal stomach to the gastric pouch. The segment of bowel is placed in an anti-peristaltic orientation, so patients present with severe dysphagia and frequently with bilious emesis. Frequently, UGI studies appear normal but careful and prolonged fluoroscopy may identify retrograde peristalsis of the contrast column. Intubation of the limb with high-resolution manometry can also identify retrograde peristalsis (Fig. 44.2). Frequently these patients undergo multiple revisional operations with no improvement if the diagnosis is not made [34, 35].

Adjustable Gastric Banding

The AGB is quickly becoming the most popular bariatric surgery in the United States [36]. There are currently two band manufactures in the United States with a total of seven different designs that have been implanted since FDA approval in 2003. The original designs incorporated low volume, high-pressure balloons within their bands, so

called: 9.5 mm, 10.5 mm and Vanguard Bands (Allergan, Santa Barbara, CA). These lower volume bands had a narrower range at which they would provide resistance and not dysphagia. More recent iterations are created to accept higher volumes of saline at lower pressures, allowing a greater range of operation—AP-Standard, AP-Large (Allergan), and Realize and Realize-C Bands (Ethicon Endosurgery Cinncinati, OH).

Given that the sole mechanism of action of bands is impediment to flow of foodstuffs, it is commonly associated with difficulty in deglutition, which is not always pathologic. Dysphagia is often most pronounced after filling of the band's balloon, but is transient as minor swelling associated with the balloon fill resolves over a period of 24–48 h. Less commonly, persistent difficulties in deglutition occur as a result of slippage of the band or chronic overfilling of the band (Fig. 44.3). This may lead to esophageal dilation with or without esophageal dysmotility.

Band slippage occurs in 2–6 % of patients with AGBs. Slippage is the asymmetric migration

a

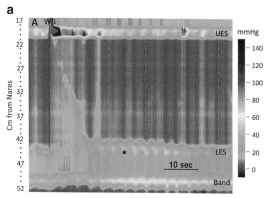

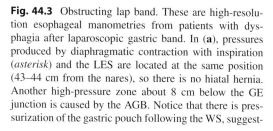

b

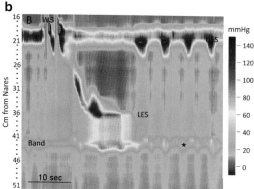

Fig. 44.3 Obstructing lap band. These are high-resolution esophageal manometries from patients with dysphagia after laparoscopic gastric band. In (**a**), pressures produced by diaphragmatic contraction with inspiration (*asterisk*) and the LES are located at the same position (43–44 cm from the nares), so there is no hiatal hernia. Another high-pressure zone about 8 cm below the GE junction is caused by the AGB. Notice that there is pressurization of the gastric pouch following the WS, suggesting an outlet obstruction. Also there is feeble peristalsis only in the proximal smooth muscle esophagus and failure in the distal smooth muscle esophagus. This is an indication that the esophagus is failing. In (**b**), the LES is hypotensive and located at about 36 cm from the nares. The diaphragm (*asterisk*) and band are located at about 7 cm below the GE junction, indicating a hiatal hernia. Again the WS produces pressurization of the hernia pouch

of distal stomach above the band, causing tissue cluttering at the stoma, which leads to outflow obstruction. It can occur gradually and at first can result in the loss of the sense of restriction as the pouch enlarges. Subsequently, patients develop de novo or worsening GERD, as well as dilation of the esophagus. As the stomal outlet narrows further, patients may experience sensations of chest pressure or pain, as well as regurgitation of clear sputum. Acute slippage results not only in these symptoms, but can also lead to acute ischemia of the stomach with associated acute pain and hematemesis. Acute slippage requires emergency removal of band fluid and usually surgical intervention. Slippage is prevented by plication of the fundus over the band to anchor the distal stomach in place.

Esophageal dilation, after gastric banding, is becoming a more frequently recognized complication the early incidence of which is estimated from 6 to 15 %, and has been reported as high as 68 % in longer-term studies (Fig. 44.4). The incidence of esophageal dilation is least common in patients younger than 25 and more common in patients older than 50 [37–39]. Preoperative manometric findings do not appear to predict the development of this phenomenon; patients with abnormal manometry have been studied after band placement and have not had dilation. Conversely, patients with normal preoperative manometry seem to make up the large percentage of patients who develop postoperative dilation [37, 40].

Defining esophageal dilation is a difficult task, as there are no authoritative studies defining normal esophageal diameter. Demaria, as a part of the original FDA band trial, defined esophageal dilation as an increase in diameter of 30 % above baseline, and reported a 71 % dilation rate among 25 patients studied. Dargent reviewed the phenomenon in a series of 1,232 and reported a dilation rate of 0.6 % but provided no size criteria for his diagnosis [41]. Milone's retrospective study on 440 AGB patients defined a diameter greater than 35 mm as dilation "based on discussion with the radiologists" at their institution (Table 44.2) [37]. On the basis of this definition, a long-term study showed that of 167 patients in whom bands were placed, 108 had some degree of dilation with radiographically defined abnormal motility ranging from mild to severe. The study incorporated a

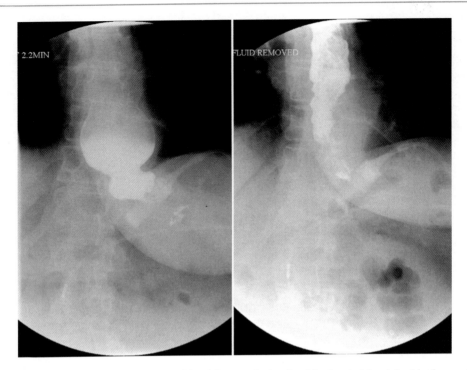

Fig. 44.4 Radiographic evidence of obstructed band. In (**a**) there is high-grade obstruction at the level of the band with little contrast passing into the stomach. The esophagus is dilated. In (**b**), there is again high-grade obstruction at the band and food materials retained in the esophagus. There are also tertiary contractions in the smooth muscle esophagus, suggesting a spastic motor disorder

Table 44.2 Grading of esophageal dysfunction after adjustable gastric band [41]

Grade of dilation	Esophogram findings	Intervention
I	Dilation (>35 mm) with delay in emptying of esophagus	Frequent evaluations, if symptoms are present or arise temporary removal of fluid from band
II	Dilated, hypercontractile esophagus (tertiary waves) with poor emptying	Temporary removal of fluid from band
III	Significant dilation of esophagus with anterior/posterior pouch slippage	Removal of fluid from band until resolution of dilation. If persistence of symptoms despite fluid removal evaluate for band revision/removal
IV	Massively dilated esophagus with failure of resolution of dilation after fluid removal from band	Removal of band. No clear recommendations on conversion to gastric bypass or sleeve gastrectomy based on paucity of data on outcomes of esophagus

classification system developed by Dargent to stratify the impact of AGB on motility, and determine the therapy that should be employed to improve esophageal motor dysfunction. Most esophageal dilation was resolved with complete removal of fluid from the balloon. However, 5.5 % of patients had megaesophagus and pseudoachalasia despite prolonged deflation of the band. In these patients the band had to be removed for resolution of dilation and return of normal esophageal function [42]. To avoid weight regain in some of these patients, there is growing experience in conversion of AGB to either GBP or sleeve gastrectomy. The published literature is very small but seems to indicate a resolution of esophageal dilation with both procedures [43, 44].

Esophageal dilation in the absence of slippage is likely a consequence of a chronically overfilled band. In this overfilled state the band fails to act as an adjustable band, but acts more like a fixed obstruction.

Prior studies have shown mixed results in terms of the effects of the band on the LES: decreased or no change in resting LES pressure and impaired LES relaxation are reported. Burton attempted to establish what normal manometric pressures should be in patients whose band is filled to an ideal volume at which there are no symptoms and expected weight loss. He compared 20 AGB patients to 20 preoperative patients with normal esophageal motility. He examined esophageal function at ideal fill volumes (expected weight loss and no symptoms), 20 % below (under fill) and 20 % above (overfill) ideal fill volumes. He found that the mean intra-luminal pressure at the level of the band was 26.9 mmHg when ideally filled, dropped to 2.72 mmHg when under filled, and rose sharply to 68 mmHg when overfield. The LES relaxed normally in all of the subjects, although patients with AGBs seemed to have slightly lower resting LES pressures. At ideal fill volumes and under filled volumes peristalsis was comparable to controls. Esophageal peristalsis was disrupted with on overfilled AGB (50 % normal swallows vs. 70–80 % in controls and those with ideal inflation). The major motor abnormality was hypertensive contractions [45]. This study implies a range of intra-luminal pressures at which ideal fill volumes might exist and above which esophageal dysfunction may begin.

Sleeve Gastrectomy

Sleeve gastrectomy creates a long, narrow gastric conduit parallel to the lesser curvature. Sleeve size is calibrated by dividing the stomach along a bougie, which sits against the lesser curvature, while leaving 5–6 cm of antrum intact. The diameter of bougie used varies from 32 to 60 Fr. Studies looking at the mechanics of this pouch revealed that there is a significantly lower compliance when compared to the native stomach, and thus the sleeve reaches a higher pressure at a lower volume [46]. One clinical effect of the low compliance system is frequent complaints of difficulty swallowing in the first 4–8 weeks postoperatively. In addition, construction of the narrow sleeve disrupts the claps/sling fiber interactions at the lower esophageal sphincter, potentially affecting its function [47]. De novo GERD has been reported in up to 21 % of patients followed for 5 years after sleeve gastrectomy [48]. Additionally, the creation of a very narrow sleeve can cause transient but significant regurgitation or dysphagia in up to 30 % of patients [47].

Dysphagia after sleeve gastrectomy is not well understood due to the relatively little outcome data available to date. Several authors report severe swelling leading to an inability to tolerate ingestion of anything but thin liquids. Severe dysphagia, even within the first days postoperatively, should be evaluated by upper GI X-rays with water-soluble contrast in an attempt to identify surgically correctable abnormalities. If severe mucosal edema is the etiology for dysphagia, then intolerance to liquids has typically resolved with I.V. hydration and time [49]. Dysphagia occurring within the first 6 weeks after surgery, particularly following normal progression to solid foods, may be associated with a stenosis. Upper GI contrast studies help define areas of narrowing, slow passage or frank obstruction, and aid in directing therapy (Fig. 44.5). Endoscopic identification of strictures and their dilation has been reported, but unlike strictures seen after GBP, these frequently require more than one dilation [50]. Long strictures do not usually respond to dilation therapy; authors have reported seromyotomy, stricturoplasties as well as conversions to roux y GBP [51].

A cause of dysphagia unique to sleeve gastrectomy is the functional obstruction. Functional obstruction can be caused by a kink in the thin gastric tube at the level of the incisura, narrowing where gastric tube is stapled or over sewn too narrowly, and spiraling of the staple line, i.e., more anterior stomach is removed in relation to posterior stomach creating an axial rotation. These defects often require intervention. Their diagnosis is suggested by UGI contrast studies. There are often only subtly abnormal endoscopic findings because insufflation of gas can temporarily dilate the area and allow passage of the scope.

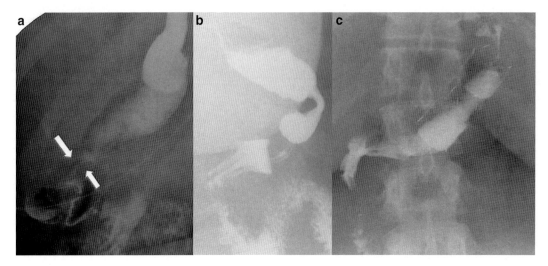

Fig. 44.5 Narrowed gastric sleeve. (**a**) The subtle narrowing identified by an early UGI following a sleeve gastrectomy. The lumen was too narrow at the incisura (*arrows*). (**b**) The same patient 2 months postoperatively. There is a definite narrowing and stenosis at the site of narrowing seen 2 months previously. They reported heartburn and regurgitation that was not responsive to PPI. (**c**) A stent across the narrowed area. This improved the regurgitation, but the heartburn persisted

The evaluation of a postbariatric surgery patient who presents with dysphasia should begin with understanding the operation that was performed. Obtaining either an operative report or discussing with the surgeon the conduct of the procedure is important. The postoperative dysphagia work up should begin with either an endoscopy or upper GI contrast studies, and may be supplemented by manometry. Postoperative dypshagia while common is usually transient, should not be persistent, and can frequently be treated nonoperatively.

References

1. Frempong-Boadu A, Houten JK, Osborn B, Opulencia J, Kells L, Guida DD, Le Roux PD. Swallowing and speech dysfunction in patients undergoing anterior cervical discectomy and fusion: a prospective, objective preoperative and postoperative assessment. J Spinal Disord Tech. 2002;15:362–8.
2. Tervonen H, Niemela M, Lauri ER, Back L, Juvas A, Rasanen P, Roine RP, Sintonen H, Salmi T, Vilkman SE, Aaltonen LM. Dysphonia and dysphagia after anterior cervical decompression. J Neurosurg Spine. 2007;7: 124–30.
3. Lee MJ, Bazaz R, Furey CG, Yoo J. Influence of anterior cervical plate design on dysphagia: a 2-year prospective longitudinal follow-up study. J Spinal Disord Tech. 2005;18:406–9.
4. Rihn JA, Kane J, Albert TJ, Vaccaro AR, et al. What is the incidence and severity of dysphagia after anterior cervical surgery? Clin Orthop Relat Res. 2011;469: 658–65.
5. Bazaz R, Lee MJ, Yoo JU. Incidence of dysphagia after anterior cervical spine surgery: a prospective study. Spine (Phila Pa 1976). 2002;27:2453–8.
6. Boadu A, Houten JK, Osborn B, Opulencia J, Kells L, Guida DD, Le Roux PD. Swallowing and speech dysfunction in patients undergoing anterior cervical discectomy and fusion: a prospective, objective preoperative and postoperative assessment. J Spinal Disord Tech. 2002;15:362–8.
7. Winslow C, Meyers AD. Otolaryngologic complications of the anterior approach to the cervical spine. Am J Otolatyngol. 1999;20(1):16–27.
8. Rosato L, Carlevato MT, De Toma G, Avenia N. Recurrent laryngeal nerve damage and phonetic modifications after total thyroidectomy: surgical malpractice only or predictable sequence? World J Surg. 2005;29:780–4.
9. Pereira JA, Girvent M, Sancho JJ, Parada C, Sitges-Serra A. Prevalence of long-term upper aero- digestive symptoms after uncomplicated bilateral thyroidectomy. Surgery. 2003;133(3):318–22.
10. Bou-Malhab F, Hans S, Perie S, Laccourreye O, Brasnu D. Swallowing disorders in unilateral recurrent laryngeal nerve paralysis. Ann Otolaryngol Chir Cervicofac. 2000;117:26–33.
11. Lombardi CP, Raffaelli M, De Crea C, et al. Long-term outcome of functional post-thyroidectomy voice

and swallowing symptoms. Surgery. 2009;146(6): 1174–81.

12. Greenblatt DY, Sippel R, Leverson G, Frydman J, Schaefer S, Chen H. Thyroid resection improves perception of swallowing function in patients with thyroid disease. World J Surg. 2009;33:255–60.

13. Litynski GS. Erich Mühe and the rejection of laparoscopic cholecystectomy (1985): a surgeon ahead of his time. JSLS. 1998;2(4):341–6.

14. Dallemagne B, Weerts JM, Jehaes C, Markiewicz S, Lombard R. Laparoscopic Nissen fundoplication: preliminary report. Surg Laparosc Endosc. 1991;1(3):138–43.

15. Nissen R. Eine einfacheoperation zur beeinflussung der refluxeosophagitis. Schweiz Med Wochenschr. 1956;86:590–2.

16. Wo JM, Trus TL, Richardson WS, et al. Evaluation and management of postfundoplication dysphagia. Am J Gastroenterol. 1996;91:2318–22.

17. Malhi-Chowla N, Gorecki P, Bammer T, et al. Dilation after fundoplication: timing, frequency, indications and outcome. Gastrointest Endosc. 2002;55:219–23.

18. Herron DM, Swanström LL, Ramzi N, Hansen PD. Factors predictive of dysphagia after laparoscopic nissen fundoplication. Surg Endosc. 1999;13:1180.

19. Patterson EJ, Herron DM, Hansen PD, Ramzi N, Standage BA, Swanström LL. Effect of an esophageal bougie on the incidence of dysphagia following nissen fundoplication. Arch Surg. 2000;135(9): 1055–61.

20. Zehetner J, DeMeester SR, Ayazi S, Kildaya P, Augustin F, Hagen JA, Lipham JC, Sohn HJ, DeMeester TR. Laparoscopic versus open repair of paraesophageal hernia: the second decade. J Am Coll Surg. 2011;212(5):813–20.

21. Horgan S, Pohl D, Bogetti D, et al. Failed antireflux surgery. What have we learned from reoperations? Arch Surg. 1999;134:809–17.

22. Jobe BA, Kahrilas PJ, Vernon AH, Sandone C, Gopal DV, Swanstrom LL, Aye RW, Hill LD, Hunter JG. Endoscopic appraisal of the gastroesophageal valve after antireflux surgery. Am J Gastroenterol. 2004;99:233–43.

23. Castell DO. Esophageal manometry prior to antireflux surgery: required, preferred, or even needed? Gastroenterology. 2001;121:214–6.

24. Buchwald H, Oien DM. Metabolic/bariatric surgery Worldwide 2008. Obes Surg. 2009;19:1605–11.

25. Poulose BK, Holzman MD, Zhu Y, Smalley W, Richards WO, Wright JK, Melvin W, Griffin MR. National variations in morbid obesity and bariatric surgery use. J Am Coll of Surg. 2005;201(1):77–84.

26. Chen RH, Lautz D, Gilbert RJ, Bueno R. Antireflux operation for gastroesophageal reflux after Roux-en-Y gastric bypass for obesity. Ann Thorac Surg. 2005;80:1938–40.

27. Huang CS, Forse RA, Jacobson BC, Farraye FA. Endoscopic findings and their clinical correlations in patients with symptoms after gastric bypass surgery. Gastrointest Endosc. 2003;58(6):859–66.

28. Lee JK, Jacques VD, Morton JM, Curet MJ, Banerjee S. Endoscopy is accurate, safe, and effective in the assessment and management of complications following gastric bypass surgery. Am J Gastroenterol. 2009;104(3):575–82.

29. Wilson JA, Romagnuolo J, Byrne TK, Morgan K, Wilson FA. Predictors of endoscopic findings after Roux-en-Y gastric bypass. Am J Gastroenterol. 2006;101(10):2194–9.

30. Campos JM, Evangelista LF, Ferraz AA, Galvao Neto MP, De Moura EG, Sakai P, Ferraz EM. Treatment of ring slippage after gastric bypass: long-term results after endoscopic dilation with an achalasia balloon (with videos). Gastrointest Endosc. 2010;72(1):44–9.

31. Neto MP, Ramos AC, Campos JM, Murakami AH, Falcao M, Moura EH, Evangelista LF, Escalona A, Zundel N. Endoscopic removal of eroded adjustable gastric band: lessons learned after 5 years and 78 cases. Surg Obes Relat Dis. 2010;6(4):423–7.

32. Chen Yi, Mei SG, Tam W, Nind G, Singh R. Endoscopic removal of migrating silastic band after vertical banding gastroplasty. Endoscopy. 2010;42 Suppl 2:E253.

33. Blero D, Eisendrath P, Vandermeeren A, Closset J, Mehdi A, Le Moine O, Deviere J. Endoscopic removal of dysfunctioning bands or rings after restrictive bariatric procedures. Gastrointest Endosc. 2010;71(3):468–74.

34. Nelson LG, Sarr MG, Murr MM. Errant and unrecognized antiperistaltic Roux limb construction during Roux-en-y gastric bypass for clinically significant obesity. Surg Obes Relat Dis. 2006;2(5):523–7.

35. Mitchell MT, Gasparaitis AE, Alverdy JC. Imaging findings in Roux-en-O and other misconstructions: rare but serious complications of Roux-en-Y gastric bypass surgery. AJR Am J Roentgenol. 2008;190(2): 367–73.

36. Buchwald H, Oien DM. Metabolic/bariatric surgery Worldwide 2008. Obes Surg. 2009;19(12):1605–11.

37. Milone L, Daud A, Durak E, Olivero Rivera L, Schrope B, Inabnet WB, et al. Esophageal dilation after laparoscopic adjustable gastric banding. Surg Endosc. 2008;22:1482–6.

38. Mittermair R, Aigner F, Obermuller S. High complication rate after Swedish adjustable gastric banding in younger patients 25 years. Obes Surg. 2009;19: 446–50.

39. Mittermair RP, Aigner F, Obermuller S. Results and complications after Swedish adjustable gastric banding in older patients. Obes Surg. 2008;18:1558–62.

40. Lew JI, Daud A, DiGorgio MF, Olivero-Rivera L, David DG, Bessler M. Preoperative esophageal manometry and outcome of laparoscopic adjustable silicone gastric banding. Surg Endosc. 2006;20: 1242–7.

41. Dargent J. Esophageal dilatation after laparoscopic adjustable gastric banding: definition and strategy. Obes Surg. 2005;15:843–8.

42. Naef M, Mouton W, Naef U, et al. Esophageal dysmotility disorders after laparoscopic gastric banding—an

underestimated complication. Ann Surg. 2011;253(2): 285–90.

43. Arias IE, Radulescu M, Stiegeler R, Singh JP, Martinez P, Ramirez A, Szomstein S, Rosenthal R. Diagnosis and treatment of megaesophagus after adjustable gastric banding for morbid obesity. Surg Obes Relat Dis. 2009;5(2):156–9.

44. Rodgers AM. Improvement of esophageal dysmotility after conversion from gastric banding to gastric bypass. Surg Obes Relat Dis. 2010;6:681–3.

45. Burton PR, Brown W, Laurie C, et al. The effect of laparoscopic adjustable gastric bands on esophageal motility and the gastroesophageal junction: analysis using high-resolution video manometry. Obes Surg. 2009;19(online):905–14.

46. Yehoshua RT, Eidelman LA, Stein M, et al. Laparoscopic sleeve gastrectomy—volume and pressure assessment. Obes Surg. 2008;18:1083–8.

47. Braghetto I, Lanzarini E, Korn O, Valladares H, Molina JC, Henriquez A. Manometric changes of the lower esophageal sphincter after sleeve gastrectomy in obese patients. Obes Surg. 2010;20:357–62.

48. Himpens J, Dapri G, Cadiere G. A prospective randomized study between laparoscopic gastric banding and laparoscopic isolated sleeve gastrectomy: results after 1 and 3 years. Obes Surg. 2006;16: 1450–6.

49. Acholonu E, McBean E, Court I, et al. Safety and short-term out- comes of laparoscopic sleeve gastrectomy as a revisional approach for failed laparoscopic adjustable gastric banding in the treatment of morbid obesity. Obes Surg. 2009;19:1612–6.

50. Zundel N, Hernandez JD, Galvao Neto M, Campos J. Strictures after laparoscopic sleeve gastrectomy. Surg laparosc Endosc Percutan Tech. 2010;20(3): 154–8.

51. Dapri G, Cadiere GB, Himpens J. Laparoscopic seromyotomy for long stenosis after sleeve gastrectomy with or without duodenal switch. Obes Surg. 2009;19:495–9.

Drug-Induced Esophageal Injury

45

Vikneswaran Namasivayam and Joseph A. Murray

Abstract

Medication-induced esophageal injury is a relatively uncommon diagnosis in comparison to the millions of prescription and over-the-counter medication consumed annually. Though only a few classes of drugs account for the large majority of reported cases, over 100 medications have been implicated, though mainly in isolated case reports. The condition is probably underrecognized as the clinical presentation may be mistakenly ascribed to other conditions such as gastroesophageal reflux disease. Yet, the importance of this condition lies in the fact that it is an iatrogenic condition that can be cured in most instances with prompt recognition and discontinuation of the offending agent. Awareness of the factors that increase the risk for drug-induced esophageal injury (DEI) may allow for prevention in the first place.

Keywords

Drug-induced esophageal injury • Bisphosphonates • NSAIDs • Mycophenolate mofetil • Chemotherapeutic agents • Quinidine

Abbreviations

DEI	Drug-induced esophageal injury
GI	Gastrointestinal
HSV	Herpes simplex virus
KCl	Potassium chloride
LES	Lower esophageal sphincter
MMF	Mycophenolate mofetil
MTX	Methotrexate
NSAIDs	Nonsteroidal anti-inflammatory drugs

V. Namasivayam, MBBS, MRCP
Department of Gastroenterology and Hepatology,
Singapore General Hospital,
Singapore, Singapore

J.A. Murray, MD (✉)
Division of Gastroenterology and Hepatology,
Mayo Clinic, Rochester, MN, USA
e-mail: murray.joseph@mayo.edu

Introduction

Medication-induced esophageal injury is a relatively uncommon diagnosis in comparison to the millions of prescription and over-the-counter medication consumed annually. Though only a few classes of drugs account for the large majority of reported cases, over 100 medications have been implicated, though mainly in isolated case reports. The condition is probably under-recognized as the clinical presentation may be mistakenly ascribed to other conditions such as gastroesophageal reflux disease. Yet, the importance of this condition lies in the fact that it is an iatrogenic condition that can be cured in most instances with prompt recognition and discontinuation of the offending agent. Awareness of the factors that increase the risk for drug-induced esophageal injury (DEI) may allow for prevention in the first place.

Drugs may induce esophageal injury through local effects of the ingested drug or systemic effects. The latter would include gastroesophageal reflux induced by medications that relax the lower esophageal sphincter (LES), mucositis from chemotherapy, and infectious esophagitis resulting from immunosuppressive medication. This chapter focuses on drug-induced injury mediated by local effects on the mucosa.

Epidemiology

Reports of DEI date back to 1970 and over 1,000 cases implicating more than 100 drugs have been reported in peer-reviewed literature [1]. There is, however, a paucity of data on the incidence with studies largely confined to case series that are biased by reporting of newly implicated drugs, unusual complications, and clustering of cases. A Swedish study from the 1970s estimates the incidence of DEI at four cases per 100,000 population per year [2]. This is probably an underestimate as DEI is under-recognized and may be confused with alternative diagnoses such as cardiorespiratory illness or reflux especially in the setting of atypical symptoms. Furthermore, this study predates the advent of bisphosphonates and the increasing trend towards polypharmacy that would favor a higher current estimate. Nonetheless, DEI remains a relatively uncommon occurrence in comparison to the numerous pills prescribed each year.

DEI may occur at any age. A female preponderance has been suggested in DEI with a literature

review citing a mean age of over 41 years. This in all likelihood reflects the epidemiology of the underlying indication for the medication rather than a propensity for DEI per se. Quinidine affects patients at a mean age of 60 years versus 30 years where oral antibiotics are implicated [3]. Advanced age, female gender, diabetes, and ischemic heart disease have been associated with DEI [4]. The elderly seem to be at particular risk for DEI. This may be due to a combination of increased rates of polypharmacy, decreased awareness, cardiomegaly causing esophageal compression, esophageal dysmotility, and decreased saliva production partly related to anticholinergic medication use seen in the elderly.

Pathophysiology

The mechanism of injury in DEI is postulated to be prolonged contact of the injurious contents of the medications with the esophageal mucosa. There are several lines of evidence favoring local injury as the underlying mechanism. The onset of symptoms is often preceded by sensation of tablet sticking in the esophagus and a history of improper ingestion of medication may be volunteered. The typical esophageal lesion in DEI is a sharply demarcated ulcer which may correspond to the site of pill holdup. Endoscopy and biopsy of the site of injury may occasionally reveal pill fragments. Furthermore, the ulcer is usually located at sites of either anatomical or pathological narrowing of the esophageal lumen which are regions of relative stasis (Fig. 45.1). The site of injury is at the level of the aortic arch in 75 % of cases [3]. This corresponds to the aortic indentation of the esophageal lumen as well as the manometric transition zone with a nadir in the amplitude of esophageal peristalsis where the skeletal and smooth muscles overlap. Experimental studies have suggested that the distal esophagus above the GE junction is the commonest site of pill holdup rather than the mid-esophagus. But, in practice, DEI in the distal esophagus is probably under-recognized and often ascribed to reflux. Pathological narrowing of the esophagus may occur in either intrinsic

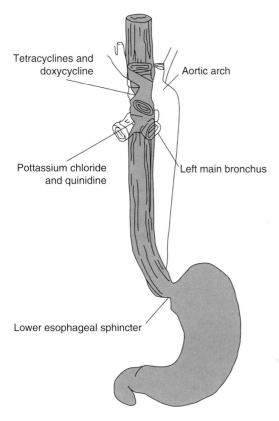

Tetracyclines and doxycycline

Aortic arch

Pottassium chloride and quinidine

Left main bronchus

Lower esophageal sphincter

Fig. 45.1 Sites of esophageal ulceration due to disordered anatomy. From A.S. Arora and J.A. Murray. Curr Gastroenterol Rep 2000;2:224–9 with permission

esophageal diseases or extrinsic esophageal compression from an enlarged left atrium or mediastinal lymphadenopathy. Though underlying motility disorders may conceivably contribute to medication holdup, there is a paucity of data to support a predisposition towards DEI in esophageal motility disorders [5]. This may be partly accounted for by increased attention paid towards swallowing by patients with underlying esophageal dysmotility that may mitigate the risk of medication holdup. Experiments have reproduced lesions by keeping pills in contact with the esophageal mucosa in animals and buccal mucosa of human volunteers thus lending credence to the notion of a local caustic injury accounting for DEI [6]. The role of direct pill to mucosa contact is further supported by the fact that, at least in the case of tetracycline, there is no data to show DEI results from the use of its parenteral formulation

or ingestion of its liquid formulation. In the case of the latter, the caustic potential might possibly be diluted by saliva.

The occurrence of DEI is influenced by both patient-related factors as well as medication-related factors. This may be deduced from the following observations. DEI occurs as a relatively rare complication of several commonly prescribed medications implying that the medication per se may be an insufficient factor in causing DEI. Conversely, DEI occurs frequently without an underlying motility disorder and indeed, esophageal dysmotility has not been convincingly demonstrated to be a risk factor for DEI.

Several medication-related factors have been implicated in causing mucosal damage. The size, shape, and physical character may influence the likelihood of pill retention. Large pills are less likely to be cleared from the esophagus than smaller one. Round tablets are retained more often than oval ones [7, 8]. Capsules are cleared from the esophagus within 15 s if taken with water in an upright position by an otherwise healthy individual. Gelatin capsules become sticky when dissolved in an inadequate amount of liquid and may become lodged in the esophagus even with repeated swallows thus increasing the mucosal contact time. Doxycycline capsules remain in the esophagus thrice as long as the tablet preparation [9]. Sustained-release formulations have been implicated in pill retention as well [10].

Of greater importance are the pill-taking practices of the patient. Supine posture is associated with a prolonged esophageal transit and pill retention despite size or shape [11]. Likewise a larger volume of ingested liquid is associated with a shortened esophageal transit time. Sleeping immediately after pill ingestion may predispose to DEI due to the elimination of the effect of gravity on pill clearance and the reduction in saliva production and deglutitive episodes during sleep. However, DEI may occur in the absence of these factors as pill retention in the esophagus has been described in asymptomatic volunteers consuming pills with water in the upright position [12].

Delayed transit per se is insufficient for causing DEI. The caustic potential of the pill is also dependent on the contents of the pill and is reflected in the heterogeneity of mechanisms of injury that have been documented. Certain drugs have a low pH (pH < 3) when dissolved in solution that could cause ulcers. These would include doxycycline, tetracycline, clindamycin, ferrous sulfate, ascorbic acid, and emepronium bromide. In contrast, phenytoin gives rise to a caustic alkaline solution (pH > 10). Potassium chloride (KCl) gives rise to a near neutral solution that is hyperosmotic and causes tissue desiccation. NSAIDs may cause DEI by disrupting the cytoprotective barrier of the esophageal mucosa [12, 13].

Clinical Approach

The diagnosis of DEI is self-evident in a patient who presents with an abrupt onset of odynophagia following the ingestion of pills known to cause DEI, usually in the absence of any chronic esophageal symptoms. The patient may volunteer a history of the ingested pill lodging in the retrosternal region prior to the onset of odynophagia, ingesting the pill with minimal water or taking the pills immediately before going to bed. In these instances, a clinical diagnosis may be made confidently without recourse to further investigation. In addition to odynophagia, the patients may experience chest pain or dysphagia. These symptoms typically progress within days and resolve within a few weeks. Further investigation may be pursued if the presentation is atypical, symptoms are persistent despite cessation of the offending medication or complications, such as bleeding, occur.

Upper GI endoscopy is the most sensitive investigation with abnormal findings seen in virtually 100 % of cases and it helps to rule out an alternative etiology [14] (Fig. 45.2). Barium esophagram is thought to be inferior to endoscopy in this regard though there are no comparative studies. Esophagram may better delineate extrinsic compression as a contributor to DEI in selected instances. Endoscopy reveals one or several discrete ulcers with normal intervening mucosa. These are typically located in the mid-esophagus which corresponds to an area of relative luminal narrowing due to bronchial or aortic indentation. On occasion, remnants of the culprit medication may be identified in the ulcer.

DEI accounted for 23 % of all esophageal ulcers in one series [15]. Apart from ulcers and erosions, esophagitis with exudates and thickening of the esophageal wall may be seen with bisphosphonates [16, 17]. Strictures have been described [12]. DEI may also give rise to nodules that mimic esophageal tumors [18]. Biopsies yield nonspecific findings that are usually that of an ulcer. Iron may give rise to erosive injury and brown-black crystalline material overlying the eroded epithelium that may be highlighted with iron stains [19, 20]. Nonetheless biopsies may occasionally be useful in excluding an infectious etiology or malignancy.

Several conditions may give rise to a similar presentation. Herpes simplex (HSV) esophagitis may present with mid-esophageal ulcers. However, HSV ulcers tend to be multiple and somewhat more widespread. HSV esophagitis typically occurs in immunocompromised patients especially in the transplant setting [21, 22]. HSV esophagitis has been described in healthy immunocompetent individuals, but these patients often present with a febrile prodrome that precedes the onset of odynophagia [23, 24]. Crohn's disease may rarely involve the esophagus but is generally associated with Crohn's disease affecting other parts of the gastrointestinal tract [25, 26]. Ulcers resulting from nasogastric intubation may be inferred from the clinical history. Carcinomatous lesions usually give rise to a more protracted history and may be differentiated from DEI by biopsy. Ulcers arising in a Barrett's esophagus may give rise to a similar appearance. Esophageal foreign bodies may present with an acute history, but the endoscopy is diagnostic in this instance.

Complications from DEI are rare but strictures, hemorrhage from ulceration, esophageal perforation, and esophageal-respiratory fistula may occur [12, 27]. Esophageal strictures are typically caused by NSAIDs. The formation of multiple esophageal septa from potassium-induced esophagitis has been reported [28]. In the absence of strictures, symptoms typically resolve within 2–3 weeks and radiological findings may resolve in 7–10 days [29].

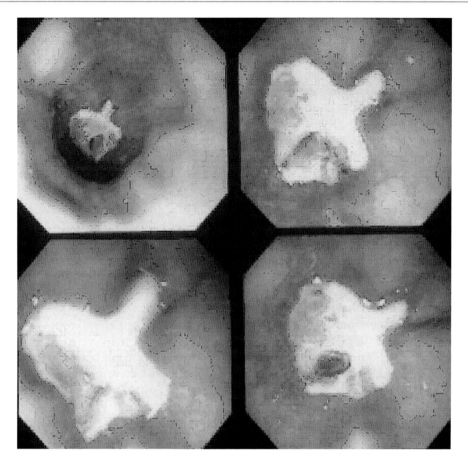

Fig. 45.2 Esophageal ulcer (photo courtesy of Dr. Jeff Alexander, Mayo Clinic)

Prevention and Treatment

There is no specific treatment for DEI. Management is supportive and largely centered on discontinuation of the offending drug. This may be a challenge in patients with a compelling indication for continued use of the culprit drug in the absence of an effective alternative. Occasionally, parenteral hydration and alimentation are required. Viscous lidocaine may be used for local anesthesia. Occasionally opioids may be needed. Sucralfate suspension has been used to coat the ulcerated mucosa. Antisecretory medication to treat concomitant reflux is often prescribed, but there is little rationale for its use unless the patient also has GERD. Strictures are dilated endoscopically.

The risk of recurrent injury with reintroduction of the offending medication has not been ascertained. It is also unclear if the risk of recurrence with rechallenge could be mitigated with adequate precautions on medication ingestion. Nonetheless, patients should be advised to swallow medication with at least 8 oz of clear liquid and remain upright for half hour after medication intake as is recommended for oral bisphosphonates. There is also limited data to guide the use of these medications in the setting of esophageal dysmotility. Treatment decisions should be carefully individualized after consideration of risk–benefits and alternative treatment options.

DEI from Specific Medication Groups

There are several classes of medication that have been associated with drug-related esophageal injury.

Antibiotics and Antivirals

Antibiotics account for more than half the reported cases of DEI. While most of these are due to tetracycline and in particular, doxycycline, many other classes of antibiotics, including penicillin, rifampin, and clindamycin, have also been implicated in case reports [30–37]. The epidemiology of the reported patients largely reflects the underlying indication for the culprit drug with tetracycline-induced DEI being described in young males and females who use it for treating acne, dental, or malaria prophylaxis [38–40]. The actual risk of DEI from doxycycline, however, has been reported to be low even with long-term usage [41]. This propensity for DEI is a reflection of the widespread use of antibiotics in general rather than a propensity for esophageal injury per se. Tetracycline gives rise to a local acid burn. The corrosive action of doxycycline may relate to its accumulation within the basal layer of the squamous epithelium [42, 43]. The patient usually complains of odynophagia and retrosternal pain, but dysphagia has been reported in over half of patients in one series despite the absence of significant strictures [44]. The endoscopic findings are that of superficial ulceration in the mid-esophagus with normal surrounding mucosa (Fig. 45.3). Given the superficial nature of the injury, hemorrhage and strictures are rare. Symptoms resolve in 2–7 days after cessation of the culprit medication though some patients may take up to 6 weeks. Endoscopic findings resolve within 3–4 weeks [39, 45].

Antiviral agents have also been implicated in pill esophagitis, especially antiretroviral drugs such as zalcitabine, zidovudine, and nelfinavir [46–48]. Infectious causes for the esophagitis should be actively sought and excluded in these patients especially in patients with low CD4 counts before the esophagitis is ascribed to medication use.

Bisphosphonates

Bisphosphonates are inhibitors of osteoclast-mediated bone resorption that are effective in the treatment of osteoporosis, Paget disease, and

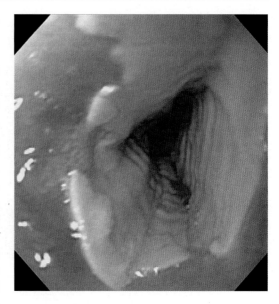

Fig. 45.3 Tetracycline esophagitis (photo courtesy of Dr. David Katzka, Mayo Clinic)

hypercalcemia of malignancy [49–51]. These have been associated with the development of esophagitis with the largest amount of data available for alendronate. A postmarketing analysis of over 475,000 patients on alendronate revealed 199 esophageal adverse events with 51 experiencing esophagitis or esophageal ulceration [17]. These largely occurred in patients who had not complied with product instructions on consuming adequate liquids and remaining upright though esophagitis may occur even with strict compliance to instructions on medication intake. Hemorrhage and esophageal stricture were each reported in only two patients. Esophageal perforation has been reported with the use of alendronate [52]. Most of the adverse effects were reported soon after commencing treatment. Pamidronate, etidronate and, to a lesser extent, risedronate and ibandronate have been implicated as well [53–57]. It appears to be less frequent with weekly or monthly administration; however, a temporal association between esophageal symptoms and the taking of the pill should alert the clinician to a potential role that the medication could be causing the patient symptoms.

Despite the reports of DEI, the overall risk appears to be small in relation to the large number of prescriptions. In contrast to postmarketing reports, clinical trials have largely failed to demonstrate an increased risk for both daily and weekly administrations [58, 59]. This may reflect the enforced compliance to proper medication use that occurs in a trial setting as well as the exclusion of patients with preexisting upper GI disease in some of the trials [60]. A pooled analysis of nine clinical trials with over 10,000 patients on daily risedronate showed no increased risk of adverse GI events. The rate of upper GI adverse events per 100 patient-years was 20 in the risedronate group compared to 19.2 in the placebo group ($p=0.3$). This study included a high proportion of patients with preexisting GI disease and use of antisecretory medications and NSAIDs [56]. Concerns of an increased upper GI risk with the concomitant use of alendronate and NSAID raised by some studies have not been borne out [61]. Daily and weekly risedronate in patients with high prevalence of NSAID users was not associated with an increased risk of upper GI events in a pooled analysis of over 2,400 patients [62]. Trials looking at extended dosing intervals of bisphosphonates to improve compliance have not demonstrated a statistically significant reduction in adverse GI event with monthly or weekly dosing as opposed to daily dosing [63–65].

The causticity of bisphosphonates appears to be mediated locally. Clinically relevant concentrations of alendronate and risedronate suppress the growth of normal human epidermal keratinocytes by inhibiting farnesyl diphosphate synthase [66]. The corrosive effect of alendronate is potentiated by an acidic pH [67]. This situation may conceivably arise in vivo when the pill-containing esophagus bathes in physiological reflux of gastric acid. Alternatively, reflux following dissolution of the pill in gastric acid may plausibly account for the esophagitis. Of note, severe ulcerative esophagitis involving 10 cm of the esophagus has been reported with alendronate which may be more in keeping with the latter explanation [17]. The attenuation of injury with proper pill-taking practices would, however, favor the former as the more likely mechanism. It is unclear what the role of underlying gastroesophageal reflux disease in influencing the risk of DEI with bisphosphonates. The relatively lower rates of DEI reported with risedronate may be partly related to the rapid esophageal transit of the risedronate tablet that minimizes contact with the esophageal mucosa [68].

Patients present with dysphagia, odynophagia, or chest pain. A history of noncompliance to proper medication intake (i.e., ingestion in the upright position with 8 oz of liquid and remaining upright for half hour) may be elicited. Endoscopy reveals circumscribed erosions and ulcerations that may be covered with a thick leukofibrinous exudate that resembles a pseudomembrane [16]. The histological findings are nonspecific. Biopsy of the ulcer shows an inflammatory exudate with granulation tissue. Polarizable crystalline foreign material with adjacent multinucleate giant cells is seen. Adjacent squamous tissue shows active inflammation with enlarged hyperchromatic nuclei [69]. Management focuses on cessation of the offending medication. The use of antisecretory medication in this setting is largely anecdotal.

NSAIDs

NSAIDs are among the most commonly prescribed drugs in the world and may affect the entire gastrointestinal tract. Reports of esophageal injury are fewer than gastric complications with NSAID-induced esophageal injury occurring in only a small fraction of all NSAID users. Most NSAIDs have been implicated in esophageal injury with aspirin, naproxen, indomethacin, and ibuprofen accounting for the majority of cases, perhaps more a reflection of their more frequent usage in general [30]. However, NSAIDs appear to be disproportionately associated with a risk of bleeding in comparison to DEI from other drugs. Aspirin and NSAIDs are also associated with an increase in the risk of reflux symptoms as well as esophagitis and esophageal ulcers [70, 71]. The underlying mechanism is unclear though NSAIDs may increase the duration of acid exposure [72]. Aspirin also renders the esophageal mucosa more permeable to acid and pepsin [73]. Aspirin and NSAIDs may exert their ulcerogenic effects by reducing the cytoprotective effects of prostaglandins on the esophageal mucosa. In addition, a direct toxic mechanism is plausible as NSAIDs are weak acidic molecules with pKa values of 4–5, which facilitates diffusion into the mucosa in the setting of an acidic pH in the distal esophagus [74].

The use of aspirin and NSAIDs (including over-the-counter prescription) is associated with esophageal strictures [75, 76]. In addition, perforation and bronchoesophageal fistula have been reported [27, 30, 77]. NSAID ulcers are typically large, shallow, discrete mid-esophageal ulcers with normal intervening mucosa. Histological findings are nonspecific with isolated mucosal erosions and ulcers commonly seen [78]. Nonspecific or reflux esophagitis may be seen. Basal cell hyperplasia may be absent as cell proliferation is inhibited by the prostaglandin inhibitors [79].

Potassium Chloride

Potassium chloride (KCl) tablets may cause ulcers and strictures throughout the GI tract [80]. DEI is mediated by a local high concentration of dissolved KCl that results in local hyperosmolality leading to tissue desiccation and vascular injury [13]. Toxicity is reported more commonly with slow-release wax matrix formulation but this may be a reflection of its more widespread prescription compared to the microencapsulated preparation [6].

KCl-mediated injury is usually reported in association with left atrial enlargement or cardiac surgery though this may be confounded by the high prevalence of cardiac disease in patients on KCl treatment [81, 82]. Prior cardiac surgery may result in entrapment of the esophagus between the aorta and the vertebral column [83]. The esophagus may be fixed in position by adhesions that may predispose to pill retention.

KCl has often been associated with severe and lethal complications including strictures, perforation into the left atrium, bronchial artery, aorta, and mediastinum [84–89]. In contrast to the sudden onset of chest pain with other culprit medications, DEI mediated by KCl presents with progressive dysphagia often in the absence of significant pain [30]. The relative absence of pain may account for the progression to strictures before medical attention is sought.

Iron

Iron is associated with corrosive injury of the upper GI tract [90, 91]. Iron deposition occurs relatively frequently with crystalline iron deposition found in 0.9 % of one series of upper GI biopsies though case reports of clinically manifested DEI are uncommon [20, 92, 93]. Differentiating primary iron-associated mucosal injury from iron deposition in a preexisting lesion may be challenging as concomitant conditions that could have caused the underlying condition may be found in about half of these patients. Biopsies reveal luminal crystalline iron deposition adjacent to the surface epithelium or admixed with luminal fibroinflammatory exudates. Iron deposition in the lamina propria, either covered by an intact epithelium, subjacent to small superficial erosions, or admixed with granulation tissue may be seen. Iron-containing thrombi in mucosal blood vessels are infrequent findings. An exuberant reactive proliferation of fibroblasts and epithelial tissues near esophageal ulcers containing iron may occasionally mimic malignancy [78].

Quinidine

Quinidine has been associated with DEI and stricture formation either when ingested alone or together with KCl [6]. The presence of a profuse exudate with nodularity may be mistaken for malignancy [18, 29].

Chemotherapeutic Agents

Dactinomycin, bleomycin, cytarabine, daunorubicin and 5-fluorouracil, vincristine and methotrexate, and other chemotherapy regimens have been associated with esophagitis usually in the setting of concomitant oral mucositis. These are mostly self-limiting though they may persist for months after cessation of treatment [94]. In addition, oral methotrexate (MTX) has been implicated in a single case of ulcerative esophagitis in an adolescent with Crohn's disease that resolved upon discontinuation of MTX [95]. Dysphagia from delayed esophageal transit has been reported with vincristine in the absence of mucosal abnormalities. The findings were reversible with discontinuation [96, 97]. This may possibly be due to neurotoxicity resulting from vincristine-mediated disruption of microtubule function in the neuronal axons. Esophagitis has also been reported in patients with gastrointestinal stromal tumor treated with imatinib [98]. Esophageal strictures have been reported following chemotherapy for acute lymphoblastic leukemia. Of note, none of the four cases had received radiotherapy but all had either esophageal or systemic candidiasis [99]. Concurrent chemotherapy and thoracic radiotherapy also increases the risk of esophageal toxicity [100].

Mycophenolate Mofetil

MMF is an immunosuppressive drug used in solid organ transplantation. While diarrhea is a well-recognized adverse effect, ulcerative esophagitis has also been described [101]. Increased apoptosis on biopsies resembling graft-versus-host disease has been described as a finding indicative of MMF-related gastrointestinal injury but the utility of this finding in the esophagus is less well established [102].

Others

Several other medications have been implicated in DEI, mainly in isolated case reports. These would include alprenolol, emepronium bromide, captopril, phenobarbital, serratiopeptidase, pancreatic enzyme supplements, cyproterone acetate and ethinylestradiol, and mexiletine [36, 103–109].

Homeopathic pills have also been implicated in DEI that occurs in the absence of underlying esophageal disease [110].

Summary

In conclusion, drug-induced esophagitis is painful and, while infrequent, may be an under-recognized disorder. It can largely be prevented by careful attention to the timing and mode of swallowing of medications. The chemical and physical properties of medications may be quite important in determining the likelihood of impaction, and a few medications, such as bisphosphonates, may be particularly prone to cause esophageal injury. It is important to suspect drug-induced esophagitis when patients present with particularly severe esophagitis or esophagitis recalcitrant to treatment for gastroesophageal reflux.

References

1. Pemberton J. Oesophageal obstruction and ulceration caused by oral potassium therapy. Br Heart J. 1970;32(2):267–8.
2. Carlborg B, Kumlien A, Olsson H. Drug-induced esophageal strictures. Lakartidningen. 1978;75(49):4609–11.
3. Zografos GN, Georgiadou D, Thomas D, Kaltsas G, Digalakis M. Drug-induced esophagitis. Dis Esophagus. 2009;22(8):633–7.
4. Abid S, Mumtaz K, Jafri W, Hamid S, Abbas Z, Shah HA, et al. Pill-induced esophageal injury: endoscopic features and clinical outcomes. Endoscopy. 2005;37(8):740–4.
5. Walta DC, Giddens JD, Johnson LF, Kelley JL, Waugh DF. Localized proximal esophagitis secondary to ascorbic acid ingestion and esophageal motor disorder. Gastroenterology. 1976;70(5 PT.1):766–9.
6. Kikendall JW. Pill-induced esophageal injury. Gastroenterol Clin North Am. 1991;20(4):835–46.
7. Channer KS, Virjee JP. The effect of size and shape of tablets on their esophageal transit. J Clin Pharmacol. 1986;26(2):141–6.
8. Channer KS, Virjee J. Effect of posture and drink volume on the swallowing of capsules. Br Med J (Clin Res Ed). 1982;285(6356):1702.
9. Carlborg B, Densert O. Esophageal lesions caused by orally administered drugs. An experimental study in the cat. Eur Surg Res. 1980;12(4):270–82.
10. McCord GS, Clouse RE. Pill-induced esophageal strictures: clinical features and risk factors for development. Am J Med. 1990;88(5):512–8.
11. Evans KT, Roberts GM. Where do all the tablets go? Lancet. 1976;2(7997):1237–9.
12. Bonavina L, DeMeester TR, McChesney L, Schwizer W, Albertucci M, Bailey RT. Drug-induced esophageal strictures. Ann Surg. 1987;206(2):173–83.
13. Boley SJ, Allen AC, Schultz L, Schwartz S. Potassium-induced lesions of the small bowel. I. Clinical aspects. J Am Med Assoc. 1965;193:997–1000.
14. Kikendall JW, Friedman AC, Oyewole MA, Fleischer D, Johnson LF. Pill-induced esophageal injury. Case reports and review of the medical literature. Dig Dis Sci. 1983;28(2):174–82.
15. Higuchi D, Sugawa C, Shah SH, Tokioka S, Lucas CE. Etiology, treatment, and outcome of esophageal

ulcers: a 10-year experience in an urban emergency hospital. J Gastrointest Surg. 2003;7(7):836–42.

16. Ribeiro A, DeVault KR, Wolfe 3rd JT, Stark ME. Alendronate-associated esophagitis: endoscopic and pathologic features. Gastrointest Endosc. 1998;47(6):525–8.

17. de Groen PC, Lubbe DF, Hirsch LJ, Daifotis A, Stephenson W, Freedholm D, et al. Esophagitis associated with the use of alendronate. N Engl J Med. 1996;335(14):1016–21.

18. Wong RK, Kikendall JW, Dachman AH. Quinaglute-induced esophagitis mimicking an esophageal mass. Ann Intern Med. 1986;105(1):62–3.

19. Haig A, Driman DK. Iron-induced mucosal injury to the upper gastrointestinal tract. Histopathology. 2006;48(7):808–12.

20. Abraham SC, Yardley JH, Wu TT. Erosive injury to the upper gastrointestinal tract in patients receiving iron medication: an underrecognized entity. Am J Surg Pathol. 1999;23(10):1241–7.

21. McBane RD, Gross Jr JB. Herpes esophagitis: clinical syndrome, endoscopic appearance, and diagnosis in 23 patients. Gastrointest Endosc. 1991;37(6):600–3.

22. McDonald GB, Sharma P, Hackman RC, Meyers JD, Thomas ED. Esophageal infections in immunosuppressed patients after marrow transplantation. Gastroenterology. 1985;88(5 Pt 1):1111–7.

23. Ramanathan J, Rammouni M, Baran Jr J, Khatib R. Herpes simplex virus esophagitis in the immunocompetent host: an overview. Am J Gastroenterol. 2000;95(9):2171–6.

24. Canalejo Castrillero E, Garcia Duran F, Cabello N, Garcia MJ. Herpes esophagitis in healthy adults and adolescents: report of 3 cases and review of the literature. Medicine (Baltimore). 2010;89(4):204–10.

25. Howden FM, Mills LR, Rubin JW. Crohn's disease of the esophagus. Am Surg. 1994;60(9):656–60.

26. Naranjo-Rodriguez A, Solorzano-Peck G, Lopez-Rubio F, Calanas-Continente A, Galvez-Calderon C, Gonzalez-Galilea A, et al. Isolated oesophageal involvement of Crohn's disease. Eur J Gastroenterol Hepatol. 2003;15(10):1123–6.

27. Singh NP, Rizk JG. Oesophageal perforation following ingestion of over-the-counter ibuprofen capsules. J Laryngol Otol. 2008;122(8):864–6.

28. McCullough RW, Afzal ZA, Saifuddin TN, Alba LM, Khan AH. Pill-induced esophagitis complicated by multiple esophageal septa. Gastrointest Endosc. 2004;59(1):150–2.

29. Creteur V, Laufer I, Kressel HY, Caroline DF, Goren RA, Evers KA, et al. Drug-induced esophagitis detected by double-contrast radiography. Radiology. 1983;147(2):365–8.

30. Kikendall JW. Pill-induced esophageal injury. In: Castell DO, Richter JE, editors. The esophagus. 4th ed. Philadelphia: Lippincott Williams & Wilkins; 2004. p. 572.

31. Sutton DR, Gosnold JK. Oesophageal ulceration due to clindamycin. Br Med J. 1977;1(6076):1598.

32. Agha FP, Wilson JA, Nostrand TT. Medication-induced esophagitis. Gastrointest Radiol. 1986;11(1):7–11.

33. Buyukberber M, Demirci F, Savas MC, Kis C, Gulsen MT, Koruk M. Pill esophagitis caused by telithromycin: a case report. Turk J Gastroenterol. 2006;17(2):113–5.

34. Smith SJ, Lee AJ, Maddix DS, Chow AW. Pill-induced esophagitis caused by oral rifampin. Ann Pharmacother. 1999;33(1):27–31.

35. Akyuz U, Erzin Y, Yalniz FF, Senkal IV, Ekici ID, Pata C. Severe odynophagia in a patient developing after azithromycin intake: a case report. Cases J. 2010;3:48.

36. Ovartlarnporn B, Kulwichit W, Hiranniramol S. Medication-induced esophageal injury: report of 17 cases with endoscopic documentation. Am J Gastroenterol. 1991;86(6):748–50.

37. Chang TT, Nedorost ST. Esophagitis due to tetracycline and its derivatives in dermatology patients. J Drugs Dermatol. 2006;5(3):247–9.

38. Morris TJ, Davis TP. Doxycycline-induced esophageal ulceration in the U.S. Military service. Mil Med. 2000;165(4):316–9.

39. Kadayifci A, Gulsen MT, Koruk M, Savas MC. Doxycycline-induced pill esophagitis. Dis Esophagus. 2004;17(2):168–71.

40. Segelnick SL, Weinberg MA. Recognizing doxycycline-induced esophageal ulcers in dental practice: a case report and review. J Am Dent Assoc. 2008;139(5):581–5.

41. Donta ST, Engel Jr CC, Collins JF, Baseman JB, Dever LL, Taylor T, et al. Benefits and harms of doxycycline treatment for Gulf War veterans' illnesses: a randomized, double-blind, placebo-controlled trial. Ann Intern Med. 2004;141(2):85–94.

42. Fraser GM, Odes HS, Krugliak P. Severe localised esophagitis due to doxycycline. Endoscopy. 1987;19(2):86.

43. Leong RW, Chan FK. Drug-induced side effects affecting the gastrointestinal tract. Expert Opin Drug Saf. 2006;5(4):585–92.

44. Al-Mofarreh MA, Al Mofleh IA. Esophageal ulceration complicating doxycycline therapy. World J Gastroenterol. 2003;9(3):609–11.

45. Tankurt IE, Akbaylar H, Yenicerioglu Y, Simsek I, Gonen O. Severe, long-lasting symptoms from doxycycline-induced esophageal injury. Endoscopy. 1995;27(8):626.

46. Edwards P, Turner J, Gold J, Cooper DA. Esophageal ulceration induced by zidovudine. Ann Intern Med. 1990;112(1):65–6.

47. Hutter D, Akgun S, Ramamoorthy R, Dever LL. Medication bezoar and esophagitis in a patient with HIV infection receiving combination antiretroviral therapy. Am J Med. 2000;108(8):684–5.

48. Indorf AS, Pegram PS. Esophageal ulceration related to zalcitabine (ddC). Ann Intern Med. 1992;117(2):133–4.

49. Liberman UA, Weiss SR, Broll J, Minne HW, Quan H, Bell NH, et al. Effect of oral alendronate on bone mineral density and the incidence of fractures in postmenopausal osteoporosis. The alendronate phase III osteoporosis treatment study group. N Engl J Med. 1995;333(22):1437–43.

50. Reid IR, Nicholson GC, Weinstein RS, Hosking DJ, Cundy T, Kotowicz MA, et al. Biochemical and radiologic improvement in Paget's disease of bone treated with alendronate: a randomized, placebo-controlled trial. Am J Med. 1996;101(4):341–8.

51. Saunders Y, Ross JR, Broadley KE, Edmonds PM, Patel S. Systematic review of bisphosphonates for hypercalcaemia of malignancy. Palliat Med. 2004;18(5):418–31.

52. Famularo G, De Simone C. Fatal esophageal perforation with alendronate. Am J Gastroenterol. 2001;96(11):3212–3.

53. Macedo G, Azevedo F, Ribeiro T. Ulcerative esophagitis caused by etidronate. Gastrointest Endosc. 2001;53(2):250–1.

54. Lufkin EG, Argueta R, Whitaker MD, Cameron AL, Wong VH, Egan KS, et al. Pamidronate: an unrecognized problem in gastrointestinal tolerability. Osteoporos Int. 1994;4(6):320–2.

55. Lanza FL, Rack MF, Li Z, Krajewski SA, Blank MA. Placebo-controlled, randomized, evaluator-blinded endoscopy study of risedronate vs. Aspirin in healthy postmenopausal women. Aliment Pharmacol Ther. 2000;14(12):1663–70.

56. Taggart H, Bolognese MA, Lindsay R, Ettinger MP, Mulder H, Josse RG, et al. Upper gastrointestinal tract safety of risedronate: a pooled analysis of 9 clinical trials. Mayo Clin Proc. 2002;77(3):262–70.

57. Chesnut IC, Skag A, Christiansen C, Recker R, Stakkestad JA, Hoiseth A, et al. Effects of oral ibandronate administered daily or intermittently on fracture risk in postmenopausal osteoporosis. J Bone Miner Res. 2004;19(8):1241–9.

58. Black DM, Cummings SR, Karpf DB, Cauley JA, Thompson DE, Nevitt MC, et al. Randomised trial of effect of alendronate on risk of fracture in women with existing vertebral fractures. Fracture intervention trial research group. Lancet. 1996;348(9041):1535–41.

59. Lanza F, Sahba B, Schwartz H, Winograd S, Torosis J, Quan H, et al. The upper GI safety and tolerability of oral alendronate at a dose of 70 milligrams once weekly: a placebo-controlled endoscopy study. Am J Gastroenterol. 2002;97(1):58–64.

60. Bauer DC, Black D, Ensrud K, Thompson D, Hochberg M, Nevitt M, et al. Upper gastrointestinal tract safety profile of alendronate: the fracture intervention trial. Arch Intern Med. 2000;160(4):517–25.

61. Ettinger B, Pressman A, Schein J. Clinic visits and hospital admissions for care of acid-related upper gastrointestinal disorders in women using alendronate for osteoporosis. Am J Manag Care. 1998;4(10):1377–82.

62. Adami S, Pavelka K, Cline GA, Hosterman MA, Barton IP, Cohen SB, et al. Upper gastrointestinal tract safety of daily oral risedronate in patients taking NSAIDs: a randomized, double-blind, placebo-controlled trial. Mayo Clin Proc. 2005;80(10):1278–85.

63. Schnitzer T, Bone HG, Crepaldi G, Adami S, McClung M, Kiel D, et al. Therapeutic equivalence of alendronate 70 mg once-weekly and alendronate 10 mg daily in the treatment of osteoporosis. Alendronate once-weekly study group. Aging (Milano). 2000;12(1):1–12.

64. Harris ST, Watts NB, Li Z, Chines AA, Hanley DA, Brown JP. Two-year efficacy and tolerability of risedronate once a week for the treatment of women with postmenopausal osteoporosis. Curr Med Res Opin. 2004;20(5):757–64.

65. Reginster JY, Adami S, Lakatos P, Greenwald M, Stepan JJ, Silverman SL, et al. Efficacy and tolerability of once-monthly oral ibandronate in postmenopausal osteoporosis: 2 year results from the MOBILE study. Ann Rheum Dis. 2006;65(5):654–61.

66. Reszka AA, Halasy-Nagy J, Rodan GA. Nitrogen-bisphosphonates block retinoblastoma phosphorylation and cell growth by inhibiting the cholesterol biosynthetic pathway in a keratinocyte model for esophageal irritation. Mol Pharmacol. 2001;59(2):193–202.

67. Dobrucali A, Tobey NA, Awayda MS, Argote C, Abdulnour-Nakhoul S, Shao W, et al. Physiological and morphological effects of alendronate on rabbit esophageal epithelium. Am J Physiol Gastrointest Liver Physiol. 2002;283(3):G576–86.

68. Perkins AC, Wilson CG, Frier M, Blackshaw PE, Juan D, Dansereau RJ, et al. Oesophageal transit, disintegration and gastric emptying of a film-coated risedronate placebo tablet in gastro-oesophageal reflux disease and normal control subjects. Aliment Pharmacol Ther. 2001;15(1):115–21.

69. Abraham SC, Cruz-Correa M, Lee LA, Yardley JH, Wu TT. Alendronate-associated esophageal injury: pathologic and endoscopic features. Mod Pathol. 1999;12(12):1152–7.

70. Ruszniewski P, Soufflet C, Barthelemy P. Nonsteroidal anti-inflammatory drug use as a risk factor for gastro-oesophageal reflux disease: an observational study. Aliment Pharmacol Ther. 2008;28(9):1134–9.

71. Lanas A, Hirschowitz BI. Significant role of aspirin use in patients with esophagitis. J Clin Gastroenterol. 1991;13(6):622–7.

72. Cryer B, Spechler S. Effects of nonsteroidal anti-inflammatory drugs (NSAIDs) on acid reflux in patients with gastroesophageal reflux disease (GERD). Gastroenterology. 2000;4 Suppl 2:A862.

73. Lanas AI, Sousa FL, Ortego J, Esteva F, Blas JM, Soria J, et al. Aspirin renders the oesophageal mucosa more permeable to acid and pepsin. Eur J Gastroenterol Hepatol. 1995;7(11):1065–72.

74. Jaspersen D. Drug-induced oesophageal disorders: pathogenesis, incidence, prevention and management. Drug Saf. 2000;22(3):237–49.

75. Kim SL, Hunter JG, Wo JM, Davis LP, Waring JP. NSAIDs, aspirin, and esophageal strictures: are

over-the-counter medications harmful to the esophagus? J Clin Gastroenterol. 1999;29(1):32–4.

76. Heller SR, Fellows IW, Ogilvie AL, Atkinson M. Non-steroidal anti-inflammatory drugs and benign oesophageal stricture. Br Med J (Clin Res Ed). 1982;285(6336):167–8.

77. McAndrew NA, Greenway MW. Medication-induced oesophageal injury leading to broncho-oesophageal fistula. Postgrad Med J. 1999;75(884):379–81.

78. Chen Z, Scudiere JR, Montgomery E. Medication-induced upper gastrointestinal tract injury. J Clin Pathol. 2009;62(2):113–9.

79. Noffsinger AE. Update on esophagitis: controversial and underdiagnosed causes. Arch Pathol Lab Med. 2009;133(7):1087–95.

80. Lee FD. Drug-related pathological lesions of the intestinal tract. Histopathology. 1994;25(4):303–8.

81. Chesshyre MH, Braimbridge MV. Dysphagia due to left atrial enlargement after mitral Starr valve replacement. Br Heart J. 1971;33(5):799–802.

82. Boyce Jr HW. Dysphagia after open heart surgery. Hosp Pract (Off Ed). 1985;20(9):40. 43, 47 passim.

83. Whitney B, Croxon R. Dysphagia caused by cardiac enlargement. Clin Radiol. 1972;23(2):147–52.

84. McCall AJ. Letter: slow-k ulceration of oesophagus with aneurysmal left atrium. Br Med J. 1975;3(5977): 230–1.

85. Henry JG, Shinner JJ, Martino JH, Cimino LE. Fatal esophageal and bronchial artery ulceration caused by solid potassium chloride. Pediatr Cardiol. 1983;4(3): 251–2.

86. Sumithran E, Lim KH, Chiam HL. Atrio-oesophageal fistula complicating mitral valve disease. Br Med J. 1979;2(6204):1552–3.

87. Rosenthal T, Adar R, Militianu J, Deutsch V. Esophageal ulceration and oral potassium chloride ingestion. Chest. 1974;65(4):463–5.

88. Learmonth I, Weaver PC. Letter: potassium stricture of the upper alimentary tract. Lancet. 1976;1(7953): 251–2.

89. Peters JL. Benign oesophageal stricture following oral potassium chloride therapy. Br J Surg. 1976;63(9): 698–9.

90. Tenenbein M, Littman C, Stimpson RE. Gastrointestinal pathology in adult iron overdose. J Toxicol Clin Toxicol. 1990;28(3):311–20.

91. Abbarah TR, Fredell JE, Ellenz GB. Ulceration by oral ferrous sulfate. J Am Med Assoc. 1976;236(20):2320.

92. Areia M, Gradiz R, Souto P, Camacho E, Silva MR, Almeida N, et al. Iron-induced esophageal ulceration. Endoscopy. 2007;39 Suppl 1:E326.

93. Zhang ST, Wong WM, Hu WH, Trendell-Smith NJ, Wong BC. Esophageal injury as a result of ingestion of iron tablets. J Gastroenterol Hepatol. 2003;18(4):466–7.

94. McGuire DB, Johnson J, Migliorati C. Promulgation of guidelines for mucositis management: educating health care professionals and patients. Support Care Cancer. 2006;14(6):548–57.

95. Batres LA, Gabriel CA, Tsou VM. Methotrexate-induced esophagitis in a child with Crohn disease. J Pediatr Gastroenterol Nutr. 2003;37(4):514–6.

96. Wang WS, Chiou TJ, Liu JH, Fan FS, Yen CC, Chen PM. Vincristine-induced dysphagia suggesting esophageal motor dysfunction: a case report. Jpn J Clin Oncol. 2000;30(11):515–8.

97. Chisholm RC, Curry SB. Vincristine-induced dysphagia. South Med J. 1978;71(11):1364–5.

98. Saponara M, Di Battista M, Lolli C, Pantaleo MA, Azzaroli F, Santini D, et al. Severe esophagitis in a patient with gastrointestinal stromal tumor treated with imatinib. Endoscopy. 2009;41 Suppl 2:E67–8.

99. Kelly K, Storey L, OS M, Butler K, McDermott M, Corbally M, et al. Esophageal strictures during treatment for acute lymphoblastic leukemia. J Pediatr Hematol Oncol. 2010;32(2):124–7.

100. Werner-Wasik M. Treatment-related esophagitis. Semin Oncol. 2005;32(2 Suppl 3):S60–6.

101. Parfitt JR, Jayakumar S, Driman DK. Mycophenolate mofetil-related gastrointestinal mucosal injury: variable injury patterns, including graft-versus-host disease-like changes. Am J Surg Pathol. 2008;32(9):1367–72.

102. Nguyen T, Park JY, Scudiere JR, Montgomery E. Mycophenolic acid (cellcept and myofortic) induced injury of the upper GI tract. Am J Surg Pathol. 2009;33(9):1355–63.

103. Olovson SG, Havu N, Regardh CG, Sandberg A. Oesophageal ulcerations and plasma levels of different alprenolol salts: potential implications for the clinic. Acta Pharmacol Toxicol (Copenh). 1986;58(1):55–60.

104. Kavin H. Oesophageal ulceration due to emepronium bromide. Lancet. 1977;1(8008):424–5.

105. Stiris MG, Oyen D. Oesophagitis caused by oral ingestion of aptin (alprenolol chloride) durettes. Eur J Radiol. 1982;2(1):38–40.

106. Al Mahdy H, Boswell GV. Captopril-induced oesophagitis. Eur J Clin Pharmacol. 1988;34(1):95.

107. Walsh J, Kneafsey DV. Phenobarbitone induced oesophagitis: a case report. Ir Med J. 1980; 73(10):399.

108. Gulsen MT, Buyukberber NM, Karaca M, Kadayifci A. Cyproterone acetate and ethinylestradiol-induced pill oesophagitis: a case report. Int J Clin Pract Suppl. 2005;147:79–81.

109. Adler JB, Goldberg RI. Mexiletine-induced pill esophagitis. Am J Gastroenterol. 1990;85(5): 629–30.

110. Corleto VD, D'Alonzo L, Zykaj E, Carnuccio A, Chiesara F, Pagnini C, et al. A case of oesophageal ulcer developed after taking homeopathic pill in a young woman. World J Gastroenterol. 2007;13(14):2132–4.

111. Arora AS, Murray JA. Iatrogenic esophagitis. Curr Gastroenterol Rep. 2000;2:224–9.

Infectious Esophagitis

46

Vikneswaran Namasivayam and Joseph A. Murray

Abstract

Infectious esophagitis is relatively rare in an immunocompetent host. The presence of an esophageal infection is usually indicative of an impairment of either local or systemic defense mechanisms that normally act to prevent the colonization of a digestive organ that has a relatively transient contact with swallowed microbes. The spectrum of esophageal infections has changed over the past few decades. Esophageal infections were rare before the advent of acquired immune deficiency syndrome (AIDS) and posttransplant immunosuppressive treatment regimens with case reports largely confined to autopsy series. The explosion in opportunistic esophageal infections heralded by human immunodeficiency virus (HIV) and medication treatment-induced immunosuppression has been largely reversed by the efficacy of highly active retroviral therapy (HAART) in treating HIV and refinements in immunosuppressive therapy and transplant management in general [1–3]. Nevertheless, socioeconomic barriers to widespread availability of HAART, a lack of compliance, and continued use of immunosuppressive therapy in a variety of diseases will likely perpetuate the morbidity from esophageal infections.

Keywords

Infectious esophagitis • Fungal esophagitis • Candidal infection • HIV infection • Herpes simplex virus (HSV) • Esophagitis • Actinomyces

V. Namasivayam, MBBS, MRCP
Department of Gastroenterology
and Hepatology, Singapore General Hospital,
Singapore, Singapore

J.A. Murray, MD (✉)
Division of Gastroenterology and Hepatology,
Mayo Clinic, Rochester, MN, USA
e-mail: murray.joseph@mayo.edu

R. Shaker et al. (eds.), *Principles of Deglutition: A Multidisciplinary Text for Swallowing and its Disorders*,   657
DOI 10.1007/978-1-4614-3794-9_46, © Springer Science+Business Media New York 2013

Abbreviations

AIDS	Acquired immune deficiency syndrome
CMV	Cytomegalovirus
HAART	Highly active retroviral therapy
HIV	Human immunodeficiency virus
HSV	Herpes simplex virus
PCR	Polymerase chain reaction
TB	Tuberculosis
VZV	Varicella-zoster virus

Introduction

Infectious esophagitis is relatively rare in an immunocompetent host. The presence of an esophageal infection is usually indicative of an impairment of either local or systemic defense mechanisms that normally act to prevent the colonization of a digestive organ that has a relatively transient contact with swallowed microbes. The spectrum of esophageal infections has changed over the past few decades. Esophageal infections were rare before the advent of acquired immune deficiency syndrome (AIDS) and post-transplant immunosuppressive treatment regimens with case reports largely confined to autopsy series. The explosion in opportunistic esophageal infections heralded by human immunodeficiency virus (HIV) and medication treatment-induced immunosuppression has been largely reversed by the efficacy of highly active retroviral therapy (HAART) in treating HIV and refinements in immunosuppressive therapy and transplant management in general [1–3]. Nevertheless, socioeconomic barriers to widespread availability of HAART, a lack of compliance, and continued use of immunosuppressive therapy in a variety of diseases will likely perpetuate the morbidity from esophageal infections.

Predisposing Factors

Though immunosuppression in general can result in infectious esophagitis, infections are most likely to occur in patients with HIV infection, malignancies especially during chemotherapy, and hematological stem cell transplantation [4]. The risk of opportunistic esophageal infections in HIV is related to the CD4 count with patients noncompliant to HAART more likely to be infected [5]. Chemotherapy and radiation may predispose to esophageal infections due to the immunosuppression as well as the direct cytotoxic effects on the mucosal barrier. Hematological malignancies are more likely to be associated with infectious esophagitis than solid tumors, though the risk is attenuated with routine antimicrobial prophylaxis [6]. The risk of esophageal infections in bone marrow transplantation is higher in allogeneic than autologous transplants.

In the immunocompetent individual, impaired esophageal clearance of swallowed organisms may foster a permissive environment for the development of esophageal infections. These would include impaired saliva production, altered esophageal motility contributing to stasis, and gastric hypochlorhydria. Injury to the esophageal mucosa either from inflammation or endoscopic procedures may facilitate infection in certain instances (see below). Individuals with diabetes mellitus, alcoholism, and adrenal insufficiency may be predisposed to infectious esophagitis through mechanisms that are yet to be fully elucidated.

General Considerations

The clinical approach to evaluating a suspected esophageal infection is guided by the presence of any underlying immune-compromise, the presenting symptoms, and the physical findings. Candida is generally the commonest esophageal infection and has been described in immunocompromised patients as well as immunocompetent individuals. The presence of oral thrush on physical examination may suggest esophageal candidiasis, though this is not invariable. The absolute CD4 count stratifies the risk of an opportunistic infection in HIV and coinfections may occur, especially with profound immunosuppression. Dysphagia and odynophagia are the commonest presenting symptoms, though on occasion constitutional complaints may dominate the clinical presentation. Odynophagia is usually indicative of underlying esophageal ulceration which mandates endoscopy with biopsies as the identification of a specific pathogen facilitates targeted therapy. Endoscopic brushings with cytological evaluation may be useful in specific instances such as herpes simplex and candidal infections. Though esophageal infections are uncommon in an immunocompetent individual, the spectrum of infections is different. In particular, most cases of herpes simplex esophagitis occur in immunocompetent individuals [7].

A key diagnostic challenge in esophageal infections is ascertaining the role of an isolated microorganism in disease causation as many purported pathogens are commensals that may be found even in healthy individuals. Colonization of the oral cavity facilitates colonization of the esophagus following deglutition. Hence diagnosis of infection requires corroborative endoscopic and histological findings. The use of viral culture and polymerase chain reaction (PCR) may increase the diagnostic yield but often at the expense of specificity partly due to contamination from latently infected cells. Serologic testing has little role in the evaluation of esophageal infection.

Fungal Esophagitis

Candidal Infection

Candidal infections are the commonest cause of infectious esophagitis and the esophagus is the commonest site of gastrointestinal infection after the oropharynx [8]. Candida is a commensal organism found in the oral, gastrointestinal, and vaginal flora and is a ubiquitous organism in the environment. Gastrointestinal disease occurs in patients colonized with Candida who are predisposed to an overgrowth of their indigenous flora as a result of perturbed commensal flora, illness, or local reduction in host resistance. Clinically predisposing factors would include immunodeficiency, diabetes mellitus, adrenal insufficiency, steroid use, alcoholism, and antibiotic use, but Candidal esophagitis may occur in the absence of predisposing factors [9, 10]. Nevertheless, even

in immunocompetent hosts, an underlying mechanism should be sought. These would include esophageal diseases associated with stasis of luminal contents such as achalasia and systemic sclerosis with esophageal involvement [11]. The use of acid-suppressive medication has been implicated as a risk factor for Candidal esophagitis in systemic sclerosis [12]. The use of inhaled steroids for respiratory diseases may cause esophageal candidiasis in otherwise healthy adults [13, 14]. Advanced age may predispose to esophageal candidiasis. Typical manifestations, such as dysphagia and concomitant oral thrush, are often absent and Candidal esophagitis is associated with a poor 1-year survival in the elderly. Candidal superinfection has also been reported in esophageal intramural pseudodiverticulosis [15]. Chronic mucocutaneous candidiasis is a rare condition characterized by chronic onychomycosis and mucocutaneous Candidal infection. This disease results from multiple immune defects with the end result of chronic Candidal infection at anatomic sites where it normally resides as a commensal. This syndrome may be associated with a thymoma or autoimmune polyendocrine syndrome type 1 [16, 17].

Invasive candidiasis, manifesting predominantly as candidemia, is the commonest fungal infection in solid organ transplants, with liver and pancreas transplants reporting the highest rates of candidal infections in general [18]. Corresponding data for esophageal candidiasis is generally lacking. Esophageal candidiasis has been reported in approximately 15% of kidney and combined kidney–pancreas transplants [19]. The use of alentuzumab, a humanized monoclonal antibody directed against C [20] D52, has been associated with esophageal candidiasis [21]. While *Candida albicans* remains the commonest pathogens in invasive candidiasis, there is a shift toward non-*albicans* species, especially *Candida glabrata* which is less susceptible to fluconazole [22]. Likewise, the introduction of antifungal prophylaxis has reduced the morbidity and mortality of invasive candidiasis in hematopoietic stem cell transplantation, but there is an increasing incidence of infection with azole-resistant Candida species [23, 24]. Whether this holds true for esophageal candidiasis in particular is unclear.

Candida in HIV Infection

The prevalence of Candidal esophagitis in AIDS patients has fallen dramatically as a result of the advent of HAART, while the number of patients with conditions not unique to AIDS, such as gastroesophageal reflux disease, has increased. The prevalence of opportunistic infections in symptomatic HIV patients undergoing endoscopy has decreased from 69% to 13% from 1995 to 1998, with an 80% reduction in patients diagnosed with esophageal candidiasis or cytomegalovirus (CMV) infection [25]. Patients with esophageal opportunistic infections tend to be noncompliant to medication, have lower CD4 counts, and had similar pathogens compared to those on HAART with normal endoscopies [5]. Nevertheless, Candida continues to be, by far, the commonest esophageal infection in HIV patients in both Western and Asian populations [26] and often coexists with other diseases in this setting. Although Candidal esophagitis largely occurs in patients with AIDS, it has also been described in primary HIV infection resulting from transient immunosuppression [27]. Most cases of esophageal candidiasis are caused by *C. albicans* either alone or in mixed infection, though symptomatic infections with *C. glabrata* and *Candida krusei* alone have also been described [28, 29].

Clinical Features

Patients generally present with painful swallowing. Patients may experience dysphagia and chest pain or may even be asymptomatic. Severe odynophagia, however, is uncharacteristic of Candida and should prompt evaluation for ulcerative esophagitis. Constitutional findings including fever and, occasionally, epigastric pain may occur. The presence of oropharyngeal candidiasis and dysphagia is predictive of esophageal candidiasis. Most patients (70%) with esophageal candidiasis will have oropharyngeal thrush [30, 31]. However, the absence of oral thrush does not exclude esophageal candidiasis. Esophageal candidiasis may rarely result in the development of bleeding, perforation, stricture, and fistula formation with pulmonary abscess, but these are rare [32–35].

A specific etiological diagnosis is established by endoscopy with or without biopsy or cytological brushings. Endoscopy reveals the presence of characteristic confluent yellow-white plaques overlying and adherent to an erythematous mucosa. The presence of ulceration is unusual and should prompt further evaluation for an alternative etiology. Endoscopic findings without biopsy have been reported to have a sensitivity and specificity of 100% and 83%, respectively, for a diagnosis of candidal esophagitis. The severity of endoscopic findings may be graded into four grades from tiny exudates less than 2 mm to confluent pseudomembranes that narrow the esophageal lumen [36]. The endoscopic grade of severity however does not correlate well with the CD4 count in HIV patients [37].

The histological diagnosis of Candidal esophagitis requires the demonstration of invasive hyphae and budding yeast as the mere presence of topical yeast may be ascribed to swallowed orocutaneous Candida from thrush. Colonization of the esophagus by Candida may occur in approximately 20% of a healthy adult population [38]. Brushings may be obtained and stained with Gomori silver or periodic acid-Schiff stains. Fungal culture is not performed routinely as it is generally not useful except in defining the species and drug sensitivities, especially in treatment-resistant cases.

Given the preponderance of Candidal esophagitis in HIV infection, an empirical trial of fluconazole for HIV patients with presumed candidiasis (for example, with oropharyngeal thrush) has been recommended by some experts as an alternative to endoscopic examination, deferring endoscopy for those with persistent symptoms [39]. This strategy seems to be safe, efficacious, and cost-effective. Most patients with esophageal candidiasis will have resolution of symptoms within 7 days after commencement of treatment with fluconazole [40]. Persistent symptoms beyond this period should be evaluated with endoscopic examination.

Management

Expert consensus guidelines recommend systemic antifungal therapy for esophageal candidiasis. Oral fluconazole 200–400 mg (3–6 mg/kg) daily for 14–21 days is recommended. If oral therapy cannot be tolerated, intravenous fluconazole 400 mg daily, amphotericin B, or an echinocandin, such as caspofungin, micafungin, or anidulafungin may be used [39]. A diagnostic trial of antifungal therapy is appropriate before diagnostic examination. Posaconazole is efficacious in 74% of patients with refractory esophageal candidiasis. Voriconazole has efficacy similar to that of fluconazole but is associated with a higher rate of adverse events [41]. The echinocandins are associated with higher rate of relapses than with fluconazole [42].

Recurrent infections occur in patients with immunosuppression, especially those with AIDS. Long-term suppressive therapy with thrice weekly fluconazole is effective in preventing recurrences [43]. HAART treatment is recommended in patients with AIDS to reduce recurrent infections.

Other Fungal Infections

Aspergillus, Blastomyces, Cryptococcus, and Histoplasma species may infect the esophagus [44, 45]. Unlike Candida, these are not commensals and are acquired by significantly immune-compromised individuals from the environment. Aspergillus infection occurs as a result of contiguous spread from mediastinal infection [46–49]. Blastomyces and Histoplasma infect the esophagus from a concomitant pulmonary infection or from disseminated infection [50]. Mediastinal fibrosis with esophageal obstruction and esophageal fistula may occur with histoplasmosis [51, 52]. Primary infection of the esophagus is very unusual and has been described in immunocompromised patients [53].

Viral Esophagitis

Cytomegalovirus Esophagitis

The rise in the morbidity of Cytomegalovirus (CMV) infection has largely paralleled the advent of AIDS and transplant-related immunosuppression. Gastrointestinal CMV infection has been associated with AIDS, organ transplantation, and less commonly, malignancy and end-stage renal failure requiring dialysis. Although CMV is the most commonly identified pathogen in AIDS, it is less often found in the esophagus than Candida with which it may coexist. The esophagus is nonetheless the second commonest site of gastrointestinal involvement by CMV after the colon. CMV esophagitis occurs primarily in patients with severe T-cell impairment characterized by a CD4 count below 50 cell/µL in AIDS patients. The risk of CMV infection is low in those on HAART therapy and the occurrence of CMV while on HAART may be indicative of noncompliance to treatment [5]. A recent series reported CMV infection in only 10 of 124 upper gastrointestinal endoscopies in HIV patients [54].

CMV disease in solid organ transplant tends to have a predilection for the organ transplanted. Disease rates are higher in pancreas and heart–lung transplants compared to kidney transplants, with seronegative recipients from a CMV seropositive organ donor being at highest risk [55]. The use of antiviral prophylaxis has reduced the incidence of CMV infection, but delayed onset disease is increasingly recognized especially after discontinuation of prophylaxis [56]. Gastrointestinal CMV was the commonest site of involvement in one series with over half reporting upper gastrointestinal disease [57].

Gastrointestinal CMV disease is rare in malignancy, being reported in 0.02% of cancer patients in one series [58]. It typically occurs in patients who either have a hematological malignancy or have additional immunosuppression from AIDS or hematopoietic stem cell transplantation. It is more common in allogeneic than autologous hematopoietic stem cell transplantation (incidence of 608 versus 58 per 100,000 patients). The esophagus is involved in 17% of cancer patients with CMV disease. Predictors of mortality include AIDS, disseminated CMV disease, and absolute lymphocyte counts below 1,000 cells/µL.

Patients with CMV esophagitis clinically present with dysphagia, odynophagia, or nonspecific symptoms such as nausea, vomiting, abdominal pain, anorexia, and fever that reflect multiorgan or systemic involvement. Thrombocytopenia and leucopenia may be present but are not invariable. Endoscopy may reveal variable findings from esophageal erosions to deep ulcers located in the mid or distal esophagus with a halo of edema. In the setting of hematopooietic stem cell transplantation, they may be macroscopically confused with graft-versus-host disease. The ulcers may, on occasion, appear similar to herpetic ulcers and idiopathic ulcers associated with HIV infection. Stricture formation is relatively uncommon despite the occurrence of deep ulceration in CMV. These may occur either during active CMV infection, following successful antiviral treatment, or even in the absence of ulceration [59, 60]. Total luminal obliteration may rarely occur [61]. Acute esophageal necrosis ("black esophagus") has been reported from CMV infection in a renal transplant patient [62]. Patients with gastrointestinal CMV infection may have concurrent CMV retinitis and formal ophthalmological assessment is advised as ocular CMV can rapidly threaten sight.

Diagnosis Requires a Combination of Histology and Demonstration of CMV in Tissue Specimens. The histological hallmark of CMV is the presence of cytomegalic cells on hematoxylin and eosin staining of mucosal biopsy. The infected cells are enlarged and contain Cowdry type A intranuclear inclusions with a surrounding halo ("owl's eye" inclusions). Hematoxylin and eosin staining has comparable sensitivity and specificity to immunohistochemical staining with monoclonal antibodies but at a lower cost [63]. Endothelial cells are the primary target for CMV infection. It has been postulated that CMV infection of the endothelial cells in the lamina propria capillaries cause ischemia with ensuing epithelial injury and ulceration. Since CMV has a predilection for fibroblasts and not squamous epithelial cells, biopsies should be obtained from the base of ulcers. Brushings from ulcers are less likely to yield diagnostic information in CMV for the same reason.

The use of CMV DNA PCR on mucosal biopsy specimens increases the detection of CMV, but only a fraction of these patients have typical histological changes [64]. This increased yield with PCR may be due to contamination from latently infected cells. Likewise, the late CMV antigen (pp 65) assay has 89–100% sensitivity for CMV viremia but are not predictive for CMV disease [65, 66]. Conversely, CMV disease as detected on histology may be present even in the absence of CMV detection in the blood. Testing for CMV antibody is of limited utility except when it is negative, because most infections are the result of reactivation of latent infection rather than primary infection.

Management

IV ganciclovir is the treatment of choice for CMV disease. Valganciclovir is the oral precursor to ganciclovir and has been shown to be noninferior to IV ganciclovir for treating CMV in certain solid organ transplantation recipients [67]. However, IV ganciclovir is preferred in patients who do not tolerate oral treatment and those with life-threatening CMV disease. The use of foscarnet has been limited by its nephrotoxicity. The role of maintenance treatment is not well defined though guidelines for secondary prophylaxis in the presence of increased risk of CMV recurrence have been proposed [68]. Reduction in immunosuppression should be individualized but considered in transplant recipients with CMV disease.

Herpes Simplex Virus Esophagitis

Herpes simplex virus (HSV) esophagitis is an opportunistic infection that affects patients with transplantation, HIV infection, malignancy, burns, and immunosuppressive therapy. Most infections in immunocompromised patients probably represent viral reactivation as these patients have higher baseline seroprevalence rates.

Although the esophagus is the most frequent site of gastrointestinal involvement, HSV esophagitis is uncommon. Autopsy series report a prevalence of 0.5–1.8% of HSV esophagitis [69, 70]. The vast majority of documented cases are due to HSV-1, though HSV-2 esophagitis from heterosexual orogential contact in an immunocompetent patient has been described [71]. HSV esophagitis is most frequently described in solid organ and bone marrow transplant recipients [4, 72, 73]. It has also been reported in the setting of acute rejection [74]. In contrast to transplant recipients, it is less commonly described in HIV patients, accounting for only 3–5% of esophagitis in HIV patients [75–77].

HSV has rarely been described in immunocompetent individuals as a self-limiting illness that typically occurs as a primary infection affecting young adults. A male predilection is seen in patients younger than 40 years [7].

Clinical Features

Symptoms are similar in both immunocompetent and immunocompromised patients. HSV in the immunocompetent is characterized by the acute onset of odynophagia, in 60–76% of patients, retrosternal chest pain or heartburn [7, 78]. This may be associated with fever and systemic manifestations. Concurrent oral lesions have only been reported in a minority of patients and herpetic skin lesions are uncommon. Symptoms may be more severe in immunocompromised patients with bleeding, perforation, tracheoesophageal fistula, and necrotizing esophagitis having been reported [79–83].

The distal esophagus is the commonest site of involvement, though extensive contiguous esophageal involvement is often seen. The entire esophagus may be involved in 15% of patients [78]. Vesicles which are the earliest manifestations are rarely seen. These coalesce to form ulcers often with normal intervening mucosa. Multiple esophageal ulcers are the commonest endoscopic finding seen in 59–86% of HSV patients, but these are nonspecific [7, 78]. The presence of ulceration on endoscopy is only attributable to HSV in 1–9% of patients [75, 84]. The ulcers are usually small and discrete or occasionally confluent. The ulcers are "volcano-like" in appearance in contrast to CMV ulcers which are linear or longitudinal and deeper. In addition to ulcers, friable mucosa and white exudates are commonly seen on endoscopy in HSV esophagitis.

The diagnosis is usually based on a combination of histological findings and viral isolation.

Biopsies from the edge of the ulcers provide the highest diagnostic yield as the base of the ulcers often lack epithelial cells. The presence of eosinophilic intranuclear inclusions (Cowdry type A inclusion bodies), multinucleated giant cells, and ballooning degeneration of epithelial cells is diagnostic. These findings, however, may also be seen in other viral infections such as those caused by CMV and VZV. However, CMV and VZV infections of the esophagus are unusual in immunocompetent individuals [85]. HSV isolation in the absence of histological findings is of questionable significance as it may represent asymptomatic viral shedding. Serology is of limited value because of the high seroprevalence in the healthy adult population, though seroconversion may be useful in a suspected primary HSV infection.

Management

The management strategy is determined by the patient's underlying immune status. Acyclovir for 14–21 days has been advocated in the treatment of immunocompromised individuals with the use of intravenous preparations in those unable to swallow. Acyclovir resistance in HSV may result from mutations in the thymidine kinase gene of HSV [86]. In contrast to immunocompromised patients, HSV esophagitis in the immunocompetent is an indolent but usually self-limiting disease. The value of treatment with acyclovir is uncertain [7]. While case reports suggest therapeutic benefit in hastening illness resolution, the relative rarity of the condition precludes any randomized controlled trials, and spontaneous resolution usually occurs within 1–2 weeks. A search should be made for any underlying immunosuppressive illness in patients presenting with HSV esophagitis.

Varicella-Zoster Virus

VZV is rarely associated with esophagitis in severely immunocompromised patients. The typical cutaneous vesicular eruptions are usually present when esophagitis occurs. Esophageal

VZV may be a harbinger of disseminated VZV. The endoscopic appearance may be variable with vesicles and ulcers seen [87]. Esophago-bronchial fistula has been reported to occur in VZV infection in an AIDS patient [88]. Biopsies reveal ballooning degeneration, multinucleated giant cells, and intranuclear inclusion bodies similar to HSV, and viral culture is needed to distinguish the two viruses. Though VZV esophagitis is self-limited in immunocompetent patients, it is typically treated with acyclovir for routine and foscarnet for resistant cases.

Ebstein–Barr Virus

Esophageal ulcerations have been very rarely reported in Ebstein–Barr virus infection in both immunocompetent and immunocompromised patients. The ulcers are deep, linear, and involve the mid-esophagus. Koilocytosis, epithelial thickening, and cell multinucleation are seen on biopsy. The number of patients is too small to draw any firm conclusion on treatment indications [89]. Ebstein–Barr virus associated post-transplant lymphoproliferative disease involving the esophagus has been described in the solid organ transplant setting [90].

Human Papilloma Virus

Human papilloma virus has been isolated in <40% of patient with squamous papilloma [91]. These are rare, benign lesions found in the mid-esophagus and are mostly asymptomatic [92]. Treatment usually consists of endoscopic resection of the lesion.

Human Immunodeficiency Virus

Idiopathic ulcers may account for 40% of esophageal ulcers in HIV infection [75]. These usually occur in AIDS with CD4 count below 100 or during the acute seroconversion syndrome that is characterized by a self-limited infectious mononucleosis-like illness [93]. These ulcers are typically multiple small well-demarcated ulcers surrounded by normal appearing mucosa that may cause odynophagia. These typically heal within 2 weeks. Large esophageal ulcers may also develop in patients with AIDS resembling CMV ulcers but with no identifiable microorganisms on histology, culture, or immunohistochemistry. The exact mechanism is not known but is unlikely to be due to HIV infection of the squamous epithelium [94]. Diagnosis is made by excluding infective organisms. Systemic and intralesional steroids and thalidomide have been used for treatment, though CMV and HSV must be excluded before steroids are exhibited [95, 96]. Misoprostol suspended in viscous lidocaine and antiretroviral have also been used for treatment [97].

Bacterial Esophagitis

Bacterial infection is a rare cause of esophagitis. It has been described in hematologic malignancies with neutropenia, bone marrow transplant patients, diabetic ketoacidosis, and steroid therapy [98, 99]. It is usually polymicrobial and derived from oral flora such as *Streptococcus viridians,* staphylococci, and Bacillus spp. The diagnosis is made by demonstrating bacterial clusters on Gram stain with evidence of subepithelial bacterial invasion on endoscopic biopsies [100]. Treatment is with broad-spectrum antibiotics.

Esophageal Tuberculosis

Esophageal tuberculosis (TB) is rare even in countries endemic for TB. It constituted only 0.5% of all patients presenting with persistent dysphagia in a series from India [101]. Conversely esophageal lesions were only found in 0.14% of TB patients in an autopsy series of over 18,000 patients [102]. Most cases are secondary to either contiguous spread from tuberculous involvement of the mediastinum, lungs, larynx, or spine or hematogenous spread from miliary TB. Primary infection of the esophagus is even rarer. The mid-esophagus is commonly involved at the level of the carina due to contiguous spread from a tuberculous lymph node [103]. A linear mid-esophageal ulcer with smooth edges and a necrotic base is typically seen. The surrounding mucosa may be normal. A hypertrophic pseudotumor may be mistaken for malignancy which may also coexist. These findings may be associated with strictures or fistula [104]. The patients may complain of dysphagia from esophageal involvement by TB, esophageal compression from adjacent tubercular lymph nodes or from mediastinal fibrosis. Cough while eating may indicate the development of a tracheoesophageal fistula. Bleeding from an aorto-esophageal fistula has also been described [105]. Diagnosis is confirmed by demonstrating acid-fast bacilli and caseating granulomas on histology. The detection of typical caseating granuloma on endoscopy specimens may be low (25–61%) as the granulomas are located in the submucosal layer [106]. Hence recourse to multiple, deep biopsies repeat endoscopic procedures or even surgical biopsies may be required. The presence of granulomas per se may be nonspecific, especially in a non-endemic population and could be ascribed to other granulomatous conditions such as Crohn's disease, sarcoidosis, syphilis, and fungal infections. The identification of acid-fast bacilli may be lower in extra-pulmonary disease. Mycobacterial culture takes 6–8 weeks to become positive. PCR assays for TB may allow for a rapid diagnosis to be made, thus facilitating institution of treatment while awaiting results of cultures and antimicrobial sensitivities. Tuberculin skin testing and quantiferon gold assays are commonly used to detect tuberculosis, but are not entirely sensitive for the disease. A prolonged course of multidrug anti-mycobacterial treatment is warranted and this is often associated with healing of fistula [104].

Actinomyces

Actinomyces has rarely been reported to infect the esophagus in both immuncompetent and immunocompromised patients [107, 108]. While it is a known commensal of the oral flora, infections have been reported, often in the setting of an antecedent infectious or an inflammatory process or an endoscopic procedure, such as dilatation, that disrupts the esophageal mucosa [109]. Infections may coexist with Candida [110]. Patients present with dysphagia or odynophagia, with endoscopy documenting the presence of an esophageal ulcer [108, 111]. Fistulization may occur. The diagnosis is typically made upon demonstration of sulfur granules on biopsy. Little data exist regarding treatment, though anecdotal success has been documented with high-dose penicillin [112].

Treponema Pallidum

Tertiary syphilis affecting the esophagus is an extremely rare occurrence of historical interest. Interestingly, the AIDS pandemic has not resulted in increased reports of syphilitic esophagitis. Tertiary gumma, fibrotic ulcers, and strictures of the proximal esophagus have been reported in the remote past [113, 114].

Protozoal Infections

Trypanosoma Cruzi

Trypanosoma cruzi may infect the myenteric plexus of the esophagus, giving rise to Chagas disease in endemic regions of South America. Esophageal manifestations may occur decades after the acute infection. The disease is clinically, radiologically, and manometrically similar to achalasia but differences have been described. The lower esophageal sphincter pressure is lower than normal patients in Chagas disease unlike idiopathic achalasia where it is elevated [115]. This is a reflection of the damage to both excitatory and inhibitory innervations in Chagas disease unlike idiopathic achalasia where the excitatory innervation is preserved. Treatment modalities are similar to that of achalasia and focus on palliative measures to reduce lower esophageal sphincter pressures and improve symptoms [116].

Table 46.1 Organisms implicated in infectious esophagitis

Fungal	Candida
	Actinomyces
	Aspergillus
	Blastomyces
	Cryptococcus
	Histoplasma
Viral	Cytomegalovirus
	Herpes Simplex
	Varicella-zoster
	Ebstein–Barr
	Human Papilloma virus
	HIV
Bacterial	Polymicrobial
	Mycobacterium tuberculosis
Protozoal	*Trypanosoma cruzi*
	Leishmania

Leishmaniasis

Visceral leishmaniasis may rarely involve the esophagus. The reported cases have been described in HIV-infected patients and often occur as a coinfection with other opportunistic infections [117, 118]. Diffuse erythematous mucosa with extensive ulceration may be seen on endoscopy. *Leishmania amastigotes* are identified on biopsy of the esophageal ulcers [119]. (Table 46.1).

References

1. Raufman JP. Declining gastrointestinal opportunistic infections in HIV-infected persons: a triumph of science and a challenge for our HAARTs and minds. Am J Gastroenterol. 2005;100(7):1455–8.
2. Mocroft A, Oancea C, van Lunzen J, Vanhems P, Banhegyi D, Chiesi A, et al. Decline in esophageal candidiasis and use of antimycotics in European patients with HIV. Am J Gastroenterol. 2005;100(7):1446–54.
3. Gooley TA, Chien JW, Pergam SA, Hingorani S, Sorror ML, Boeckh M, et al. Reduced mortality after allogeneic hematopoietic-cell transplantation. N Engl J Med. 2010;363(22):2091–101.
4. McDonald GB, Sharma P, Hackman RC, Meyers JD, Thomas ED. Esophageal infections in immunosuppressed patients after marrow transplantation. Gastroenterology. 1985;88(5 Pt 1):1111–7.
5. Monkemuller KE, Lazenby AJ, Lee DH, Loudon R, Wilcox CM. Occurrence of gastrointestinal opportunistic disorders in AIDS despite the use of highly active antiretroviral therapy. Dig Dis Sci. 2005;50(2):230–4.
6. Eid AJ, Razonable RR. New developments in the management of cytomegalovirus infection after solid organ transplantation. Drugs. 2010;70(8):965–81.
7. Ramanathan J, Rammouni M, Baran Jr J, Khatib R. Herpes simplex virus esophagitis in the immunocompetent host: an overview. Am J Gastroenterol. 2000;95(9):2171–6.
8. Scott BB, Jenkins D. Gastro-oesophageal candidiasis. Gut. 1982;23(2):137–9.
9. Baehr PH, McDonald GB. Esophageal infections: risk factors, presentation, diagnosis, and treatment. Gastroenterology. 1994;106(2):509–32.
10. Badarinarayanan G, Gowrisankar R, Muthulakshmi K. Esophageal candidiasis in non-immune suppressed patients in a semi-urban town, southern India. Mycopathologia. 2000;149(1):1–4.
11. Kjellin AP, Ost AE, Pope 2nd CE. Histology of esophageal mucosa from patients with achalasia. Dis Esophagus. 2005;18(4):257–61.
12. Hendel L, Svejgaard E, Walsoe I, Kieffer M, Stenderup A. Esophageal candidosis in progressive systemic sclerosis: occurrence, significance, and treatment with fluconazole. Scand J Gastroenterol. 1988;23(10):1182–6.
13. Aun MV, Ribeiro MR, Costa Garcia CL, Agondi RC, Kalil J, Giavina-Bianchi P. Esophageal candidiasis– an adverse effect of inhaled corticosteroids therapy. J Asthma. 2009;46(4):399–401.
14. Kanda N, Yasuba H, Takahashi T, Mizuhara Y, Yamazaki S, Imada Y, et al. Prevalence of esophageal candidiasis among patients treated with inhaled fluticasone propionate. Am J Gastroenterol. 2003;98(10):2146–8.
15. Koyama S, Watanabe M, Iijima T. Esophageal intramural pseudodiverticulosis (diffuse type). J Gastroenterol. 2002;37(8):644–8.
16. Kirkpatrick CH. Chronic mucocutaneous candidiasis. J Am Acad Dermatol. 1994;31(3 Pt 2):S14–7.
17. Ahonen P, Myllarniemi S, Sipila I, Perheentupa J. Clinical variation of autoimmune polyendocrinopathy-candidiasis-ectodermal dystrophy (APECED) in a series of 68 patients. N Engl J Med. 1990;322(26):1829–36.
18. Fishman JA. Infection in solid-organ transplant recipients. N Engl J Med. 2007;357(25):2601–14.
19. Veroux M, Macarone M, Fiamingo P, Cappello D, Gagliano M, Di Mare M, et al. Caspofungin in the treatment of azole-refractory esophageal candidiasis in kidney transplant recipients. Transplant Proc. 2006;38(4):1037–9.
20. Bodey GP, Mardani M, Hanna HA, Boktour M, Abbas J, Girgawy E, et al. The epidemiology of *Candida glabrata* and *Candida albicans* fungemia

in immunocompromised patients with cancer. Am J Med. 2002;112(5):380–5.

21. Peleg AY, Husain S, Kwak EJ, Silveira FP, Ndirangu M, Tran J, et al. Opportunistic infections in 547 organ transplant recipients receiving alemtuzumab, a humanized monoclonal CD-52 antibody. Clin Infect Dis. 2007;44(2):204–12.

22. Pfaller MA, Diekema DJ. Epidemiology of invasive candidiasis: a persistent public health problem. Clin Microbiol Rev. 2007;20(1):133–63.

23. Goodman JL, Winston DJ, Greenfield RA, Chandrasekar PH, Fox B, Kaizer H, et al. A controlled trial of fluconazole to prevent fungal infections in patients undergoing bone marrow transplantation. N Engl J Med. 1992;326(13):845–51.

24. Slavin MA, Osborne B, Adams R, Levenstein MJ, Schoch HG, Feldman AR, et al. Efficacy and safety of fluconazole prophylaxis for fungal infections after marrow transplantation–a prospective, randomized, double-blind study. J Infect Dis. 1995;171(6):1545–52.

25. Monkemuller KE, Call SA, Lazenby AJ, Wilcox CM. Declining prevalence of opportunistic gastrointestinal disease in the era of combination antiretroviral therapy. Am J Gastroenterol. 2000;95(2):457–62.

26. Chong VH, Lim CC. Human immunodeficiency virus and endoscopy: Experience of a general hospital in Singapore. J Gastroenterol Hepatol. 2005;20(5):722–6.

27. Kassutto S, Rosenberg ES. Primary HIV type 1 infection. Clin Infect Dis. 2004;38(10):1447–53.

28. Sangeorzan JA, Bradley SF, He X, Zarins LT, Ridenour GL, Tiballi RN, et al. Epidemiology of oral candidiasis in HIV-infected patients: colonization, infection, treatment, and emergence of fluconazole resistance. Am J Med. 1994;97(4):339–46.

29. Phillips P, Zemcov J, Mahmood W, Montaner JS, Craib K, Clarke AM. Itraconazole cyclodextrin solution for fluconazole-refractory oropharyngeal candidiasis in AIDS: correlation of clinical response with in vitro susceptibility. AIDS. 1996;10(12):1369–76.

30. Wilcox CM, Straub RF, Clark WS. Prospective evaluation of oropharyngeal findings in human immunodeficiency virus-infected patients with esophageal ulceration. Am J Gastroenterol. 1995;90(11):1938–41.

31. Tavitian A, Raufman JP, Rosenthal LE. Oral candidiasis as a marker for esophageal candidiasis in the acquired immunodeficiency syndrome. Ann Intern Med. 1986;104(1):54–5.

32. Tran HA, Vincent JM, Slavin MA, Grigg A. Esophageal perforation secondary to angio-invasive Candida glabrata following hemopoietic stem cell transplantation. Clin Microbiol Infect. 2003;9(12):1215–8.

33. Hyun JJ, Chun HJ, Keum B, Seo YS, Kim YS, Jeen YT, et al. Candida esophagitis complicated by

esophageal stricture. Endoscopy. 2010;42 Suppl 2:E180–1.

34. Kim BW, Cho SH, Rha SE, Choi H, Choi KY, Cha SB, et al. Esophagomediastinal fistula and esophageal stricture as a complication of esophageal candidiasis: a case report. Gastrointest Endosc. 2000;52(6):772–5.

35. Kanzaki R, Yano M, Takachi K, Ishiguro S, Motoori M, Kishi K, et al. Candida esophagitis complicated by an esophago-airway fistula: report of a case. Surg Today. 2009;39(11):972–8.

36. Kodsi BE, Wickremesinghe C, Kozinn PJ, Iswara K, Goldberg PK. Candida esophagitis: a prospective study of 27 cases. Gastroenterology. 1976;71(5):715–9.

37. Werneck-Silva A, Prado I. The relationship between immunological status and severity of endoscopic lesions in candida esophagitis is not perfect in HIV-infected patients. Gastrointest Endosc. 2007;65(5):AB148.

38. Andersen LI, Frederiksen HJ, Appleyard M. Prevalence of esophageal Candida colonization in a Danish population: special reference to esophageal symptoms, benign esophageal disorders, and pulmonary disease. J Infect Dis. 1992;165(2):389–92.

39. Pappas PG, Kauffman CA, Andes D, Benjamin Jr DK, Calandra TF, Edwards Jr JE, et al. Clinical practice guidelines for the management of candidiasis: 2009 update by the Infectious Diseases Society of America. Clin Infect Dis. 2009;48(5):503–35.

40. Wilcox CM, Alexander LN, Clark WS, Thompson 3rd SE. Fluconazole compared with endoscopy for human immunodeficiency virus-infected patients with esophageal symptoms. Gastroenterology. 1996;110(6):1803–9.

41. Ally R, Schurmann D, Kreisel W, Carosi G, Aguirrebengoa K, Dupont B, et al. A randomized, double-blind, double-dummy, multicenter trial of voriconazole and fluconazole in the treatment of esophageal candidiasis in immunocompromised patients. Clin Infect Dis. 2001;33(9):1447–54.

42. Villanueva A, Gotuzzo E, Arathoon EG, Noriega LM, Kartsonis NA, Lupinacci RJ, et al. A randomized double-blind study of caspofungin versus fluconazole for the treatment of esophageal candidiasis. Am J Med. 2002;113(4):294–9.

43. Goldman M, Cloud GA, Wade KD, Reboli AC, Fichtenbaum CJ, Hafner R, et al. A randomized study of the use of fluconazole in continuous versus episodic therapy in patients with advanced HIV infection and a history of oropharyngeal candidiasis: AIDS Clinical Trials Group Study 323/Mycoses Study Group Study 40. Clin Infect Dis. 2005;41(10):1473–80.

44. Jacobs DH, Macher AM, Handler R, Bennett JE, Collen MJ, Gallin JI. Esophageal cryptococcosis in a patient with the hyperimmunoglobulin E-recurrent infection (Job's) syndrome. Gastroenterology. 1984;87(1):201–3.

45. McKenzie R, Khakoo R. Blastomycosis of the esophagus presenting with gastrointestinal bleeding. Gastroenterology. 1985;88(5 Pt 1):1271–3.

46. Alioglu B, Avci Z, Canan O, Ozcay F, Demirhan B, Ozbek N. Invasive esophageal aspergillosis associated with acute myelogenous leukemia: successful therapy with combination caspofungin and liposomal amphotericin B. Pediatr Hematol Oncol. 2007;24(1):63–8.

47. Akyol Erikci A, Ozyurt M, Terekeci H, Ozturk A, Karabudak O, Oncu K. Oesophageal aspergillosis in a case of acute lymphoblastic leukaemia successfully treated with caspofungin alone due to liposomal amphotericin B induced severe hepatotoxicity. Mycoses. 2009;52(1):84–6.

48. Choi JH, Yoo JH, Chung IJ, Kim DW, Han CW, Shin WS, et al. Esophageal aspergillosis after bone marrow transplant. Bone Marrow Transplant. 1997;19(3):293–4.

49. Chionh F, Herbert KE, Seymour JF, Prince HM, Wolf M, Zimet A, et al. Ante-mortem diagnosis of localized invasive esophageal aspergillosis in a patient with acute myeloid leukemia. Leuk Lymphoma. 2005;46(4):603–5.

50. Marshall JB, Singh R, Demmy TL, Bickel JT, Everett ED. Mediastinal histoplasmosis presenting with esophageal involvement and dysphagia: case study. Dysphagia. 1995;10(1):53–8.

51. Coss KC, Wheat LJ, Conces Jr DJ, Brashear RE, Hull MT. Esophageal fistula complicating mediastinal histoplasmosis. Response to amphotericin. Br Am J Med. 1987;83(2):343–6.

52. Gilliland MD, Scott LD, Walker WE. Esophageal obstruction caused by mediastinal histoplasmosis: beneficial results of operation. Surgery. 1984;95(1):59–62.

53. Fucci JC, Nightengale ML. Primary esophageal histoplasmosis. Am J Gastroenterol. 1997;92(3):530–1.

54. Huppmann AR, Orenstein JM. Opportunistic disorders of the gastrointestinal tract in the age of highly active antiretroviral therapy. Hum Pathol. 2010;41(12):1777–87.

55. Baroco AL, Oldfield EC. Gastrointestinal cytomegalovirus disease in the immunocompromised patient. Curr Gastroenterol Rep. 2008;10(4):409–16.

56. Arthurs SK, Eid AJ, Pedersen RA, Kremers WK, Cosio FG, Patel R, et al. Delayed-onset primary cytomegalovirus disease and the risk of allograft failure and mortality after kidney transplantation. Clin Infect Dis. 2008;46(6):840–6.

57. Fica A, Cervera C, Perez N, Marcos MA, Ramirez J, Linares L, et al. Immunohistochemically proven cytomegalovirus end-organ disease in solid organ transplant patients: clinical features and usefulness of conventional diagnostic tests. Transplant Infect Dis. 2007;9(3):203–10.

58. Torres HA, Kontoyiannis DP, Bodey GP, Adachi JA, Luna MA, Tarrand JJ, et al. Gastrointestinal cytomegalovirus disease in patients with cancer: a two decade experience in a tertiary care cancer center. Eur J Cancer. 2005;41(15):2268–79.

59. Wilcox CM. Esophageal strictures complicating ulcerative esophagitis in patients with AIDS. Am J Gastroenterol. 1999;94(2):339–43.

60. Goodgame RW, Ross PG, Kim HS, Hook AG, Sutton FM. Esophageal stricture after cytomegalovirus ulcer treated with ganciclovir. J Clin Gastroenterol. 1991;13(6):678–81.

61. Sheth A, Boktor M, Diamond K, Lavu K, Sangster G. Complete esophageal obliteration secondary to cytomegalovirus in AIDS patient. Dis Esophagus. 2010;23(6):E32–4.

62. Trappe R, Pohl H, Forberger A, Schindler R, Reinke P. Acute esophageal necrosis (black esophagus) in the renal transplant recipient: manifestation of primary cytomegalovirus infection. Transplant Infect Dis. 2007;9(1):42–5.

63. Monkemuller KE, Bussian AH, Lazenby AJ, Wilcox CM. Special histologic stains are rarely beneficial for the evaluation of HIV-related gastrointestinal infections. Am J Clin Pathol. 2000;114(3):387–94.

64. Peter A, Telkes G, Varga M, Sarvary E, Kovalszky I. Endoscopic diagnosis of cytomegalovirus infection of upper gastrointestinal tract in solid organ transplant recipients: Hungarian single-center experience. Clin Transplant. 2004;18(5):580–4.

65. Rowshani AT, Bemelman FJ, van Leeuwen EM, van Lier RA, ten Berge IJ. Clinical and immunologic aspects of cytomegalovirus infection in solid organ transplant recipients. Transplantation. 2005;79(4):381–6.

66. Koskinen PK, Nieminen MS, Mattila SP, Hayry PJ, Lautenschlager IT. The correlation between symptomatic CMV infection and CMV antigenemia in heart allograft recipients. Transplantation. 1993;55(3):547–51.

67. Asberg A, Humar A, Rollag H, Jardine AG, Mouas H, Pescovitz MD, et al. Oral valganciclovir is noninferior to intravenous ganciclovir for the treatment of cytomegalovirus disease in solid organ transplant recipients. Am J Transplant. 2007;7(9):2106–13.

68. Kotton CN, Kumar D, Caliendo AM, Asberg A, Chou S, Snydman DR, et al. International consensus guidelines on the management of cytomegalovirus in solid organ transplantation. Transplantation. 2010;89(7):779–95.

69. Itoh T, Takahashi T, Kusaka K, Kawaura K, Nakagawa Y, Yamakawa J, et al. Herpes simplex esophagitis from 1307 autopsy cases. J Gastroenterol Hepatol. 2003;18(12):1407–11.

70. Nash G, Ross JS. Herpetic esophagitis. A common cause of esophageal ulceration. Hum Pathol. 1974;5(3):339–45.

71. Wishingrad M. Sexually transmitted esophagitis: primary herpes simplex virus type 2 infection in a healthy man. Gastrointest Endosc. 1999;50(6):845–6.

72. McBane RD, Gross Jr JB. Herpes esophagitis: clinical syndrome, endoscopic appearance, and diagnosis in 23 patients. Gastrointest Endosc. 1991;37(6):600–3.

73. Eisen HJ, Kobashigawa J, Keogh A, Bourge R, Renlund D, Mentzer R, et al. Three-year results of a randomized, double-blind, controlled trial of mycophenolate mofetil versus azathioprine in cardiac transplant recipients. J Heart Lung Transplant. 2005;24(5):517–25.

74. Mosimann F, Cuenoud PF, Steinhauslin F, Wauters JP. Herpes simplex esophagitis after renal transplantation. Transplant Int. 1994;7(2):79–82.

75. Wilcox CM, Schwartz DA, Clark WS. Esophageal ulceration in human immunodeficiency virus infection. Causes, response to therapy, and long-term outcome. Ann Intern Med. 1995;123(2): 143–9.

76. Bini EJ, Micale PL, Weinshel EH. Natural history of HIV-associated esophageal disease in the era of protease inhibitor therapy. Dig Dis Sci. 2000;45(7): 1301–7.

77. Bonacini M, Young T, Laine L. The causes of esophageal symptoms in human immunodeficiency virus infection. A prospective study of 110 patients. Arch Intern Med. 1991;151(8):1567–72.

78. Canalejo Castrillero E, Garcia Duran F, Cabello N, Garcia Martinez J. Herpes esophagitis in healthy adults and adolescents: report of 3 cases and review of the literature. Medicine (Baltimore). 2010; 89(4):204–10.

79. Dieckhaus KD, Hill DR. Boerhaave's syndrome due to herpes simplex virus type 1 esophagitis in a patient with AIDS. Clin Infect Dis. 1998;26(5):1244–5.

80. Cirillo NW, Lyon DT, Schuller AM. Tracheoesophageal fistula complicating herpes esophagitis in AIDS. Am J Gastroenterol. 1993;88(4):587–9.

81. Nagri S, Hwang R, Anand S, Kurz J. Herpes simplex esophagitis presenting as acute necrotizing esophagitis ("black esophagus") in an immunocompetent patient. Endoscopy. 2007;39 Suppl 1:E169.

82. Cattan P, Cuillerier E, Cellier C, Carnot F, Landi B, Dusoleil A, et al. Black esophagus associated with herpes esophagitis. Gastrointest Endosc. 1999;49(1): 105–7.

83. Gurvits GE, Robilotti JG. Isolated proximal black esophagus: etiology and the role of tissue biopsy. Gastrointest Endosc. 2010;71(3):658.

84. Higuchi D, Sugawa C, Shah SH, Tokioka S, Lucas CE. Etiology, treatment, and outcome of esophageal ulcers: a 10-year experience in an urban emergency hospital. J Gastrointest Surg. 2003;7(7):836–42.

85. Lavery EA, Coyle WJ. Herpes simplex virus and the alimentary tract. Curr Gastroenterol Rep. 2008;10(4): 417–23.

86. Frobert E, Ooka T, Cortay JC, Lina B, Thouvenot D, Morfin F. Herpes simplex virus thymidine kinase mutations associated with resistance to acyclovir: a site-directed mutagenesis study. Antimicrob Agents Chemother. 2005;49(3):1055–9.

87. Gill RA, Gebhard RL, Dozeman RL, Sumner HW. Shingles esophagitis: endoscopic diagnosis in two patients. Gastrointest Endosc. 1984;30(1):26–7.

88. Moretti F, Uberti-Foppa C, Quiros-Roldan E, Fanti L, Lillo F, Lazzarin A. Oesophagobronchial fistula caused by varicella zoster virus in a patient with AIDS: a unique case. J Clin Pathol. 2002;55(5): 397–8.

89. Kitchen VS, Helbert M, Francis ND, Logan RP, Lewis FA, Boylston AW, et al. Epstein-Barr virus associated oesophageal ulcers in AIDS. Gut. 1990;31(11):1223–5.

90. Kranz B, Vester U, Becker J, Woltering T, Wingen AM, Paul A, et al. Unusual manifestation of post-transplant lymphoproliferative disorder in the esophagus. Transplant Proc. 2006;38(3):693–6.

91. Neumann H, Kuester D, Monkemuller K. Atypical esophagitis. Gastroenterology. 2009;137(3):790. 1188.

92. Mosca S, Manes G, Monaco R, Bellomo PF, Bottino V, Balzano A. Squamous papilloma of the esophagus: long-term follow up. J Gastroenterol Hepatol. 2001;16(8):857–61.

93. Smith PD, Eisner MS, Manischewitz JF, Gill VJ, Masur H, Fox CF. Esophageal disease in AIDS is associated with pathologic processes rather than mucosal human immunodeficiency virus type 1. J Infect Dis. 1993;167(3):547–52.

94. Wilcox CM, Zaki SR, Coffield LM, Greer PW, Schwartz DA. Evaluation of idiopathic esophageal ulceration for human immunodeficiency virus. Mod Pathol. 1995;8(5):568–72.

95. Kotler DP, Reka S, Orenstein JM, Fox CH. Chronic idiopathic esophageal ulceration in the acquired immunodeficiency syndrome. Characterization and treatment with corticosteroids. J Clin Gastroenterol. 1992;15(4):284–90.

96. Alexander LN, Wilcox CM. A prospective trial of thalidomide for the treatment of HIV-associated idiopathic esophageal ulcers. AIDS Res Hum Retroviruses. 1997;13(4):301–4.

97. Adeoti AG, Vega KJ, Dajani EZ, Trotman BW, Kloser PC. Idiopathic esophageal ulceration in acquired immunodeficiency syndrome: successful treatment with misoprostol and viscous lidocaine. Am J Gastroenterol. 1998;93(11):2069–74.

98. Richert SM, Orchard JL. Bacterial esophagitis associated with CD4+ T-lymphocytopenia without HIV infection. Possible role of corticosteroid treatment. Dig Dis Sci. 1995;40(1):183–5.

99. Ezzell Jr JH, Bremer J, Adamec TA. Bacterial esophagitis: an often forgotten cause of odynophagia. Am J Gastroenterol. 1990;85(3):296–8.

100. Walsh TJ, Belitsos NJ, Hamilton SR. Bacterial esophagitis in immunocompromised patients. Arch Intern Med. 1986;146(7):1345–8.

101. Jain SK, Jain S, Jain M, Yaduvanshi A. Esophageal tuberculosis: is it so rare? Report of 12 cases and review of the literature. Am J Gastroenterol. 2002;97(2):287–91.

102. Carr D, Spain D. Tuberculosis in a carcinoma of the esophagus. Annu Rev Tubercul. 1942;46:346–9.

103. Park JH, Kim SU, Sohn JW, Chung IK, Jung MK, Jeon SW, et al. Endoscopic findings and clinical features of esophageal tuberculosis. Scand J Gastroenterol. 2010;45(11):1269–72.

104. Devarbhavi HC, Alvares JF, Radhikadevi M. Esophageal tuberculosis associated with esophagotracheal or esophagomediastinal fistula: report of 10 cases. Gastrointest Endosc. 2003;57(4):588–92.

105. O'Leary M, Nollet DJ, Blomberg DJ. Rupture of a tuberculous pseudoaneurysm of the innominate artery into the trachea and esophagus: report of a case and review of the literature. Hum Pathol. 1977;8(4):458–67.

106. Welzel TM, Kawan T, Bohle W, Richter GM, Bosse A, Zoller WG. An unusual cause of dysphagia: esophageal tuberculosis. J Gastrointestin Liver Dis. 2010;19(3):321–4.

107. Yagi T, Fujino H, Hirai M, Inoue T, Sako M, Teshima H, et al. Esophageal actinomycosis after allogeneic peripheral blood stem cell transplantation for extranodal natural killer/T cell lymphoma, nasal type. Bone Marrow Transplant. 2003;32(4):451–3.

108. Chou FT, Cheng KS, Chiang IP. Esophageal actinomycosis. Adv Ther. 2006;23(4):623–6.

109. Murchan EM, Redelman-Sidi G, Patel M, Dimaio C, Seo SK. Esophageal actinomycosis in a fifty-three-year-old man with HIV: case report and review of the literature. AIDS Patient Care STDS. 2010;24(2):73–8.

110. Arora AK, Nord J, Olofinlade O, Javors B. Esophageal actinomycosis: a case report and review of the literature. Dysphagia. 2003;18(1):27–31.

111. Lee SA, Palmer GW, Cooney EL. Esophageal actinomycosis in a patient with AIDS. Yale J Biol Med. 2001;74(6):383–9.

112. Sudhakar SS, Ross JJ. Short-term treatment of actinomycosis: two cases and a review. Clin Infect Dis. 2004;38(3):444–7.

113. Hudson TR, Head JR. Syphilis of the esophagus. J Thorac Surg. 1950;20(2):216–21.

114. Stone J, Friedberg SA. Obstructive syphilitic esophagitis. J Am Med Assoc. 1961;177(10):711.

115. Padovan W, Godoy RA, Dantas RO, Meneghelli UG, Oliveira RB, Troncon LE. Lower oesophageal sphincter response to pentagastrin in chagasic patients with megaoesophagus and megacolon. Gut. 1980;21(2):85–90.

116. Matsuda NM, Miller SM, Evora PR. The chronic gastrointestinal manifestations of Chagas disease. Clinics (Sao Paulo). 2009;64(12):1219–24.

117. Gutierrez-Macias A, Alonso-Alonso JJ, Aguirre-Errasti C. Esophageal leishmaniasis in a patient infected with the human immunodeficiency virus. Clin Infect Dis. 1995;21(1):229–30.

118. Laguna F, Garcia-Samaniego J, Soriano V, Valencia E, Redondo C, Alonso MJ, et al. Gastrointestinal leishmaniasis in human immunodeficiency virus-infected patients: report of five cases and review. Clin Infect Dis. 1994;19(1):48–53.

119. Villanueva JL, Torre-Cisneros J, Jurado R, Villar A, Montero M, Lopez F, et al. Leishmania esophagitis in an AIDS patient: an unusual form of visceral leishmaniasis. Am J Gastroenterol. 1994;89(2):273–5.

Eosinophilic Esophagitis

47

Sameer Dhalla and Ikuo Hirano

Abstract

Eosinophilic esophagitis (EoE) is a relatively recently recognized, esophageal disorder with symptoms that are dominated in adults by dysphagia. Based on a 2011 consensus recommendation by a working group of adult and pediatric gastroenterologists, allergists, and pathologists, EoE has been conceptually defined as a chronic, immune/antigen-mediated disease characterized clinically by symptoms related to esophageal dysfunction and histologically by eosinophil-predominant inflammation [1]. Once viewed as an esoteric diagnosis, EoE has emerged over the past two decades as an important consideration in the evaluation of abnormal deglutition and foregut symptoms in both children and adults. Studies over the past few years have demonstrated that EoE is now a leading cause of esophageal dysphagia amongst adult patients, second only to gastroesophageal reflux disease (GERD). The disease has significant impact on patients quality of life and important complications of esophageal strictures, food impaction, and esophageal perforation.

The pathogenesis of EoE involves both environmental and genetic factors with evidence supporting a primary role for food antigens inciting the inflammatory response. Medical therapy with topical corticosteroids, dietary therapies incorporating elimination of specific food antigens and esophageal dilation are highly effective.

Keywords

Eosinophilic esophagitis • Gastroesophageal reflux disease • Dysphagia • Secondary causes of esophageal eosinophilia • Initial therapy for EoE

S. Dhalla, MD, MHS
Division of Gastroenterology and Hepatology,
Johns Hopkins Hospital, Baltimore, MD, USA
e-mail: sdhalla1@jhmi.edu

I. Hirano, MD (✉)
Division of Gastroenterology, Northwestern University
Feinberg School of Medicine, Chicago, IL, USA
e-mail: i-hirano@northwestern.edu

R. Shaker et al. (eds.), *Principles of Deglutition: A Multidisciplinary Text for Swallowing and its Disorders*,
DOI 10.1007/978-1-4614-3794-9_47, © Springer Science+Business Media New York 2013

Abbreviations

APT	Atopy patch testing
EoE	Eosinophilic esophagitis
eos/hpf	Eosinophils/high-power field
GERD	Gastroesophageal reflux disease
PP	Proton pump inhibitor
SPED	Six food elimination diet
SPT	Skin prick testing

Introduction/Definition

Eosinophilic esophagitis (EoE) is a relatively recently recognized, esophageal disorder with symptoms that are dominated in adults by dysphagia. Based on a 2011 consensus recommendation by a working group of adult and pediatric gastroenterologists, allergists, and pathologists, EoE has been conceptually defined as a chronic, immune/antigen-mediated disease characterized clinically by symptoms related to esophageal dysfunction and histologically by eosinophil-predominant inflammation [1]. Once viewed as an esoteric diagnosis, EoE has emerged over the past two decades as an important consideration in the evaluation of abnormal deglutition and foregut symptoms in both children and adults. Studies over the past few years have demonstrated that EoE is now a leading cause of esophageal dysphagia amongst adult patients, second only to gastroesophageal reflux disease (GERD). The disease has significant impact on patient's quality of life and important complications of esophageal strictures, food impaction, and esophageal perforation.

Incidence and Prevalence

EoE has been reported in all continents except Africa and can affect patients of all ages, from infants to octogenarians. The largest case series have originated from western, industrialized countries. Patient cohorts from around the world have uniformly identified a male predominance of over 70%. While the typical patient is Caucasian, other ethnic groups including Asian, Hispanic, and African-American patients have been reported. A number of epidemiologic studies have shown that the incidence and prevalence of eosinophilic esophagitis are significantly higher today than when it was first described in 1978 [2, 3]. An analysis of an adult cohort from Olmsted County, Minnesota, USA, showed that the incidence of EoE increased from 0.35 cases per 100,000 person years during 1991–1995, up to 9.45 cases per 100,000 person-years during 2001–2005. The prevalence in this group was 55.0 patients per 1,000,000 persons as of January 1, 2006 [4]. In a demographically stable adult cohort in Olten County, Switzerland, the incidence increased from two cases in 1989 to six cases per 100,000 person-years in 2009. The prevalence increased from 2 to 35 patients per 100,000 persons over this same time period [5, 6].

This same trend is seen in a pediatric cohort from Hamilton County, Ohio, USA. The incidence of EoE increased from 9 to 12 annual cases per 100,000 persons between 1999 and 2003; prevalence grew from 10 to 43 patients per 100,000 persons over this time [7]. Fewer than 3% of the 315 diagnosed pediatric cases in Hamilton County occurred prior to 2000, suggesting a relatively recent rise in annual incidence. The incidence and prevalence reported in the aforementioned studies and others [3] exceed well-recognized inflammatory gastrointestinal disorders such as Crohn's disease [8].

The rapid rise in observed incidence could be explained by increases in disease recognition reflected in changes in clinical practice over time. Since the early 1990s, there have been more upper endoscopies performed as well as greater esophageal biopsy acquisitions by clinicians aware of EoE [9]. Increased awareness of the disease is evidenced by the rapid rise in the number of publications by investigators as well as allergy and gastroenterology societies [1, 10]. On the other hand, if one considers that the prevalence of other atopic illnesses such as asthma is on the rise [11], a true rise in the prevalence of EoE is likely. Supporting the contention that EoE is truly a new disease is the observation that the ringed esophagus, a characteristic feature of eosinophilic esophagitis, was first reported in small case series in the past 30 years in spite of the fact that both barium studies and endoscopy have been around for decades prior. Interestingly, early reports attributed the ringed esophagus to a manifestation of congenital esophageal stenosis or GERD.

Pathophysiology

The pathway leading to esophageal eosinophilia and dysfunction is a subject of active investigation. Eosinophils are normally found in small

Table 47.1 Secondary causes of esophageal eosinophilia

Gastrointestinal diseases	GERD
	Achalasia
	Celiac disease
	Crohn's disease
Autoimmune diseases	Connective tissue disease
	Vasculitis
	Bullous skin disorders
Treatment-related conditions	Graft-versus-host disease
	Drug hypersensitivity
Infection	Parasitic infection
	Fungal infection
	HIV-associated esophageal ulcers
Eosinophilic disorders	Hypereosinophilic syndrome
	Eosinophilic gastroenteritis

numbers in the lamina propria throughout the GI tract but are normally absent within the esophageal mucosa, where their presence points to a diverse group of disease states including EoE, GERD, eosinophilic gastroenteritis, inflammatory bowel disease, drug hypersensitivity, fungal/parasitic infection, drug hypersensitivity, or the hypereosinophilic syndrome [1] (Table 47.1). The histopathology of EoE characteristically incorporates dense eosinophilic infiltration within the squamous epithelium with associated histologic changes that include eosinophil microabscess formation, basal cell hyperplasia, rete peg elongation, and dilated intercellular spaces [12] (Fig. 47.1). The environmental and genetic factors that induce this brisk eosinophil migration and degranulation are central to understanding the pathogenesis of EoE.

Non-EoE related food allergy is estimated to affect 6% of children and 3.7% of adults in the US population [13]. Up to 90% of EoE children and adults have evidence of hypersensitivity to a food or aeroallergen based on IgE testing, while only a small subset have a history of food-associated anaphylaxis [13, 14]. These observations suggest that the immunopathogenesis of EoE may involve multiple inflammatory pathways. The most convincing evidence for the role of food hypersensitivity in EoE is the pediatric and

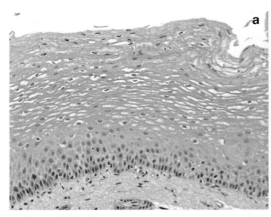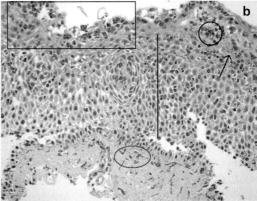

Fig. 47.1 Histologic features of EoE. (**a**) Normal esophageal mucosa. (**b**) Histopathology of eosinophilic esophagitis. Characteristic features include dense eosinophilic infiltrate with superficial layering (*rectangle*), basal zone hyperplasia (*vertical line*), extracellular eosinophilic granules (*arrow*), eosinophilic microabscess (*black oval*), and lamina propria fibrosis (*red oval*). Images courtesy Elizabeth Montgomery, M.D

adult studies showing symptomatic and histologic resolution with removal of common dietary antigens and relapse with re-introduction of specific foods [14–16].

Aeroallergens are also implicated in human observational studies showing higher rates of diagnosis in peak aeroallergen spring/summer months [17, 18] and in mouse model studies showing that inhalation of aeroallergens such as *Aspergillus fumigatus* can induce esophageal eosinophilia [19]. In a separate study, initial epicutaneous antigen exposure potentiated esophageal inflammation by aeroallergen exposure [20]. These findings in animals indicate that sensitization pathways could occur in human EoE and antigen-presenting cells (APCs) may play an important role in the pathogenesis [13].

The overabundant esophageal accumulation of eosinophils and mast cells follows allergen sensitization. Unlike eosinophils, mast cells are normally found in small numbers in the esophagus but are found in larger numbers and in an activated state in EoE [21, 22]. Mast-cell-related gene expression is increased in EoE and suppressed after removal of causative dietary allergens [23]. This complicated process is attributed in part to a local Type-2 T cell-mediated immune response, which leads to the activation of B-lymphocytes that produce immunoglobins while promoting the growth, recruitment, and activation of eosinophils. Interleukin-5 (IL-5)—a cytokine produced by CD4+ Type-2 Helper T-cells (T_h2) and mast cells—is a key mediator of the latter effect. Esophageal biopsy samples of EoE patients have a marked overexpression of IL-5 in as well as an overabundance of T_h2 and mast cells [24]. In IL-5 gene-deficient knockout mice, EoE could not be induced as it could in wild-type mice. Mice with overabundant IL-5 expression through transgenic splicing demonstrated brisk trafficking of eosinophils to the esophagus [19, 25]. This inflammatory milieu is similarly seen in the affected tissues of other atopic diseases such as allergic rhinitis and asthma [26] and shows the central role of IL-5. Recent studies have demonstrated improvement in the eosinophilic inflammation in both children and adults with EoE following therapy with

specific antibodies directed at IL-5 [27–29]. Furthermore, it supports the theory that EoE is a local manifestation of a systemic atopic diathesis that may affect multiple organs [30].

In addition to IL-5, eotaxin-3 is another important eosinophil chemoattractant found in high levels in the affected esophagus. Eotaxin-3 is one of a family of molecules—which also includes MIP-1, RANTES, MCP-2, MCP-3, MCP-4, eotaxin-1, eotaxin-2—that selectively binds the CCR3 receptor on the eosinophil surface. CCR3 is a specific and abundant eosinophil surface receptor; binding to its ligands induces a potent chemotaxis and activation of eosinophils [31–33]. An important study by Blanchard et al. [34] showed that eotaxin-3 was highly expressed in the esophageal epithelium of EoE patients and that eotaxin-3 protein and mRNA strongly correlated with levels of tissue eosinophilia and mastocytosis. Furthermore, using a gene microarray study technique, they showed that Eotaxin-3 was the most highly induced gene among EoE patients relative to controls. Lastly, a single nucleotide polymorphism (SNP) in the eotaxin-3 gene was associated with disease susceptibility. This study not only shows a potential causative role of eotaxin-3 in the pathogenesis of EoE, but also begins to clarify its inherited component. In a study of eotaxin-3-knockout mice, the level of esophageal eosinophilia was reduced by a factor of 15 compared to wild-type mice following experimental induction of EoE [19, 25].

Polymorphisms in the gene encoding the cytokine thymic stromal lymphopoietin (TSLP) on chromosome 5q22 have been found to be associated with EoE in a genome-wide association study [35]. These polymorphisms lead to TSLP overexpression and an exaggerated T_h2 immune response. TSLP overexpression has already been identified in the pathogenesis of other atopic diseases such as asthma, atopic dermatitis, and food allergies in both patients and murine models [36–38]. In a recent study, Siracusa et al. [39] demonstrated that TSLP overexpression promotes systemic basophilia and an exaggerated Th2 response in a subset of patients with EoE. Esophageal tissue samples in these patients showed basophils in an activated state not seen in wild-type TSLP populations. Along with eotaxin-3, TSLP may be an important genetic mediator of the EoE phenotype.

The morphological changes that lead to esophageal dysfunction in EoE are not merely a result of eosinophil and mast cell accumulation into the mucosal layers, but also due to the products of their activation [40]. This is a distinct feature in EoE compared to other causes of esophageal eosinophilia. Activated eosinophils release granules that contain major basic protein (MBP)-1 and -2, eosinophilic cationic protein (ECP), eosinophil-derived neurotoxin (EDN), and eosinophil peroxidase (EPO) [41, 42]. MBP, EPO, and ECP are cytotoxic to epithelium. MBP also can cause smooth muscle dysfunction [43], degranulation of mast cells [41], and epithelial hyperplasia [44]. EDN promotes the T_h2 response described earlier [45]. Activated mast cells release granules of tryptase, a protease with many downstream tissue-remodeling effects [46]. Eosinophils and mast cells produce lipid mediators that alter smooth muscle function, vascular permeability, and mucus production. They also express leukotrienes that recruit other inflammatory cells [13].

These inflammatory conditions promote specific fibrostenotic structural changes in the affected esophagus. In the epithelium of the EoE patient, squamous papillary hyperplasia [47] and hyperplasia of the epithelial basal zone (to >20% of the total epithelial thickness) are commonly seen, as are increased numbers of esophageal blood vessels compared to both GERD and healthy controls. These blood vessels tend to have an "activated" endothelium, suggesting their presence is a response to local inflammation. The endothelium surface expresses VCAM-1, whose function includes eosinophil adhesion and tissue transmigration [48]. It is in the first subepithelial layer—the lamina propria—where many profibrotic events that distinguish EoE from other forms of esophagitis may occur. Studies have shown that increased collagen deposition in the lamina propria (LP) leads to subepithelial fibrosis in 57–90% of children with EoE but very uncommonly in controls or GERD subjects [49, 50]. Subepithelial fibrosis was correlated with eosinophil degranulation (measured by BMP release)

but not eosinophil count itself. Aceves et al. [48, 49] demonstrated that only EoE patients (compared to GERD and normal controls) had an increased expression of the profibrotic cytokine $TGF\beta_1$ and its downstream mediator, phosphorylated SMAD2/3. The source of $TGF\beta_1$ and p-SMAD2/3 included eosinophils in the epithelium and LP. An activating C509T mutation in the promoter region of the $TGF\beta_1$ gene seen in some EoE patients was associated with persistence of subepithelial fibrosis even after topical steroid therapy. This gene has also been implicated in airway remodeling in asthma [51, 52] and again highlights the shared mechanisms between these two related diseases.

These microscopic findings have macroscopic consequences. Endosonography of untreated EoE patients versus healthy controls has shown an increased overall mucosal thickness without a difference in epithelial thickness [24, 27, 28, 53]. Using a functional luminal imaging probe (EndoFLIP®), esophageal distensibility was diminished in 33 EoE patients as compared to 15 controls [54]. Diffuse esophageal luminal narrowing in a condition known as small-caliber esophagus [55] along with focal strictures [56, 57] is seen in patients with EoE (Fig. 47.2) and responsible for prominent symptoms such as dysphagia and food impaction.

Clinical Evaluation

EoE is a clinicopathologic disease that is characterized by symptoms of esophageal dysfunction and histologically by eosinophil-predominant inflammation [1]. One or more biopsy specimens are required to demonstrate 15 or greater eosinophils/high power field (hpf). The disease is isolated to the esophagus as esophageal eosinophilia may be present in eosinophilic gastroenteritis. Other causes of secondary esophageal eosinophilia need be excluded (Table 47.1).

Onset commonly occurs in the first decade of childhood or in the third or fourth decade of adulthood [58]. In children, typical symptoms are abdominal pain, nausea/vomiting, chest pain, reflux symptoms, and feeding intolerance [59]. In

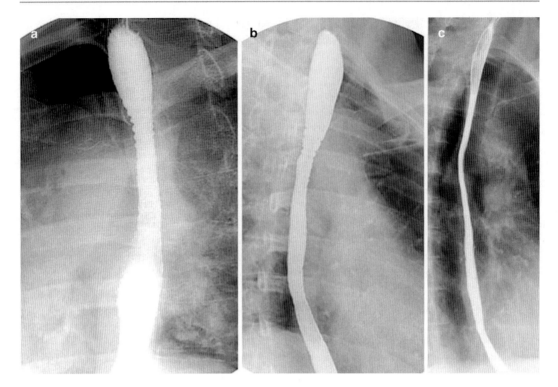

Fig. 47.2 Features of eosinophilic esophagitis on barium esophagram. (**a**) Proximal esophageal stricture with multiple rings causing an appearance of "trachealization." (**b**) Narrow caliber esophagus with ring deformity in the proximal esophagus. (**c**) Narrow caliber esophagus with high-grade stenosis of the entire esophagus (**a**) A normal barium esophagram with peristalsis, (**b**) Eosinophilic esophagitis with fixed concentric rings and focal strictures, and (**c**) Narrow-caliber esophagus. Courtesy Dr. Ikuo Hirano

adults, typical symptoms are dysphagia, food impaction, and less commonly reflux symptoms [1]. Clinicopathological severity is highly variable; some patients present with rare episodes of minor dysphagia, while other patients suffer from repeated food impaction, food avoidance, and weight loss [60]. Atopic disorders (e.g., food allergies, asthma, allergic rhinitis, and/or atopic dermatitis) are found in 70–90% of EoE patients [13, 61, 62]. Familial clustering is demonstrated by studies showing that siblings of EoE patients are significantly more likely than the general population to also be diagnosed [63] and that approximately 6–10% of first-degree relatives of EoE patients have a history of biopsy-proven EoE or dysphagia requiring endoscopic dilatation [64]. In both animal and human studies, this familial clustering has been attributed to a combination of shared environmental exposures [19] and inherited genetic susceptibility [34].

There is no single test or finding that is pathognomonic for EoE; the diagnosis requires a careful history and histological assessment [1]. EoE should be considered in young children with persistent GERD-like symptoms, including feeding problems, and in older children and adults with GERD-like symptoms, especially in those with dysphagia or esophageal food impaction [65]. The history should include characterization of esophageal and upper-gastrointestinal symptoms, atopic symptoms, and family histories of allergy and dysphagia [66]. Dietary modification including prolonged meal times, increased liquid ingestion during meal times, and food avoidance may reflect coping strategies used by patients to adapt to a chronic dysphagia.

The differences in presenting symptoms between children and adults are of importance. In a 10-year retrospective case series of 381 pediatric eosinophilic esophagitis from a single referral center, Liacouras et al. [67] found that 312 (82%) presented with GERD symptoms and only 69 (18%) presented with dysphagia. In the GERD-type symptom subgroup, 70% of patients presented with vomiting or regurgitation and 61% had heartburn or epigastric pain. In the dysphagia group, only 24 patients had esophageal luminal narrowing. Conversely, in an adult study of 74 patients diagnosed with EoE, the most common presenting symptom was dysphagia (90%), food impaction (55%), heartburn (31%), and abdominal pain (4%) [68]. Compared to children, adults are more prone to mechanically obstructive symptoms on presentation. This difference in symptom presentation may reflect difficulties in symptom reporting by young children or progression of disease from esophageal inflammation to fibrostenotic complications.

The physical examination of the patient is often unhelpful because EoE patients typically lack systemic findings [66]. The examination of the lungs, skin, and nares may provide helpful clues when signs of atopy are present. Furthermore, the presence of oral or cutaneous pathology may point to a secondary cause of esophageal eosinophilia such as bullous skin disease, infectious pharyngitis/esophagitis, or a connective tissue disorder. Currently available noninvasive biomarkers are of limited utility in diagnosing or following EoE. Peripheral blood eosinophilia is seen in up to 50% of adults and children and may track with disease activity [47, 68–70]. However, due to the limited sensitivity and specificity in the presence of other atopic disorders in EoE patients, the clinical utility of peripheral eosinophilia is not reliable. Increased serum immunoglobulin E (IgE) levels, positive skin prick test, and positive radioallergosorbent can be found in 40–73% of patients [71]. The presence of these laboratory findings can be suggestive of EoE, but lack sensitivity and specificity to be diagnostic on their own [66].

Endoscopic and Manometric Evaluation

Esophagogastroduodenoscopy (EGD) is an important tool in the evaluation of EoE. Careful endoscopic examination should include assessment of all segments of the esophagus for vascular pattern, surface contour, and lumen diameter. Endoscopy serves an important role in the exclusion of disease states associated with esophageal eosinophilia including bullous pemphigus, infectious esophagitis, neoplasia, and achalasia. Characteristic esophageal mucosal changes detected on endoscopy in patients with EoE include fixed rings, longitudinal furrows, exudates, and loss of vascular markings (Fig. 47.3). The loss of the fine submucosal vascular pattern, referred to as mucosal edema or pallor, is thought to be the consequence of cellular infiltration and mucosal thickening. Straumann et al. [72] found a loss of vascularity in 28 out of 30 EoE patients (93.3%). A series of 74 adults with EoE described the prevalence of esophageal abnormalities on endoscopy as follows: fixed rings (81%), longitudinal furrows (74%), exudates (15%), and stricture (31%) [73]. A normal appearance of the esophageal mucosa has been reported in up to 30% of pediatric and adult series but this lower sensitivity may reflect variability in reporting methods and a lack of consistent definition of the criteria for evaluation of the esophageal features of EoE.

The sensitivities of these endoscopic findings have been evaluated. Prasad et al. [74] performed an EGD with biopsy on 376 adults with dysphagia and compared the endoscopic findings to the histologic finding of esophageal eosinophilia. The sensitivity of stricture was 50% while rings, furrows, and exudates were 38% sensitive. When patients with dysphagia and no endoscopic findings were biopsied, 10% were found to have EoE. In a similar study of all patients referred for upper endoscopy, not just those with dysphagia, esophageal rings were 52%, furrows 48%, strictures 28%, and plaques 20% sensitive in predicting esophageal eosinophilia [75]. If any single esophageal abnormality was present, the sensitivity for endoscopy was 72%. Higher sensitivities for esophageal findings in adults

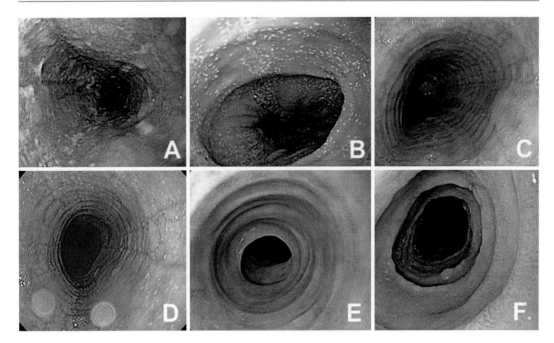

Fig. 47.3 Features of eosinophilic esophagitis on upper endoscopy. (**a**) Mucosal exudates (plaques) with loss of vascular markings (edema). (**b**) Punctate white exudates in the distal esophagus with a focal distal esophageal ring-like stricture and loss of vascular markings. (**c**) Subtle mucosal rings and longitudinal furrows. (**d**) Subtle mucosal rings, longitudinal furrows, diffuse mucosal exudates, and loss of vascular markings. (**e**) Distinct mucosal rings with a proximal ring-like structure that did not permit passage of an adult, diagnostic upper endoscope. (**f**) Distinct mucosal rings with loss of vascular markings

with EoE exceeding 90% have been reported in adult series utilizing observations from investigators with greater experience in EoE [27, 28, 76]. However, in light of the significant proportion of patients lacking characteristic esophageal features and varied experience of clinicians, mucosal biopsies should be obtained in all patients with suspected EoE regardless of the appearance on endoscopy.

A system for classifying and grading the endoscopically identified, esophageal features of EoE has been proposed [77] (Table 47.2). The establishment of uniform nomenclature facilitates communication between clinicians and different medical centers as well as comparisons in clinical studies. Grading the features should allow improved characterization of disease, as esophageal remodeling is an important determinant of disease complications that is not well evaluated by mucosal histology.

Whether specific esophageal motility disturbances exist with higher prevalence in EoE is controversial. In one study, ineffective peristalsis was seen in 5/6 (83.3%) with EoE versus 10/32 (31.2%) patients without it. This same study failed to identify any significant differences in LES pressurization, the presence of esophageal spasm, or esophageal body pressurization [78]. Bassett et al. [79] found that the prevalence of nonspecific esophageal motor disorder (NSEMD) had similar prevalence in EoE (10%) as historical GERD controls. Studies using augmented techniques such as 24-h ambulatory manometry [80] and high-resolution manometry [81] have identified higher rates of ineffective peristalsis and abnormal bolus pressurization, respectively. In light of these variable results, current guidelines state that esophageal manometry does not offer clear clinical benefit in the diagnostic workup of EoE [1]. Further research is needed in this area.

Table 47.2 Proposed classification and grading system for the endoscopic assessment of the esophageal features of eosinophilic esophagitis (Moy et al. [77])

Major features
Fixed rings (also referred to concentric rings, corrugated esophagus, corrugated rings, ringed esophagus, trachealization)
Grade 0: none
Grade 1: mild-subtle circumferential ridges
Grade 2: moderate-distinct rings that do not impair passage of a standard diagnostic adult endoscope (outer diameter 8–9.5 mm)
Grade 3: severe-distinct rings that do not permit passage of a diagnostic endoscope
Exudates (also referred to as white spots, plaques)
Grade 0: none
Grade 1: mild-lesions involving less than 10% of the esophageal surface area
Grade 2: severe-lesions involving greater than 10% of the esophageal surface area
Furrows (also referred to as vertical lines, longitudinal furrows)
Grade 0: Absent
Grade 1: mild-vertical lines present without visible depth
Grade 2: severe-vertical lines with mucosal depth (indentation)
Edema (also referred to as decreased vascular markings, mucosal pallor)
Grade 0: absent. distinct vascularity present
Grade 1: loss of clarity or absence of vascular markings
Stricture
Grade 0: absent
Grade 1: present
Minor features
Crepe paper esophagus (mucosal fragility or laceration upon passage of diagnostic endoscope but not after esophageal dilation)
Grade 0: absent
Grade 1: present
Narrow caliber esophagus (reduced luminal diameter of the majority of the tubular esophagus)
Grade 0: absent
Grade 1: present

Histopathology

The esophageal eosinophilia that characterizes EoE is patchy and best assessed with multiple biopsy samples from different locations within the esophagus. Two to four mucosal biopsy specimens of the proximal and distal esophagus are recommended [1, 73]. Sampling of the proximal esophagus is thought to help discriminate EoE from GERD, but this has not been subjected to adequate study [82]. When clinically indicated by symptoms or endoscopic findings, patients should have biopsies taken from the stomach and duodenum to exclude secondary causes of esophageal eosinophilia such as celiac disease and eosinophilic gastroenteritis [1]. The typical histologic features of EoE include a high peak eosinophil count ($\geq$15 eos/hpf), eosinophil microabscesses, superficial layering of eosinophils, extracellular eosinophil granules, basal cell hyperplasia, dilated intercellular spaces, rete peg elongation, subepithelial lamina propria fibrosis, and increases in other cell types such as lymphocytes [1] (Fig. 47.1).

Eosinophilic Esophagitis and GERD

The distinction between GERD and EoE has important clinical, pathophysiologic, and therapeutic implications. Studies from the eighties identified esophageal eosinophilia in both children and adults as a diagnostic criterion for GERD [83, 84]. The presence of esophageal eosinophilia correlated with abnormal esophageal acid exposure. In most cases, the eosinophils numbered less than ten per microscopic high power field (hpf) and were concentrated in the distal esophagus [12]. In the early 1990s, two adult case series first described EoE as a entity distinct from GERD [85, 86]. The presentation of dysphagia and food impaction in atopic individuals with endoscopic findings of esophageal rings and longitudinal furrows was distinct from the heartburn, regurgitation, and erosive esophagitis that typified GERD. The degree of esophageal eosinophilic infiltration of the squamous epithelium in EoE exceeded that typically seen in GERD. Furthermore, these first EoE series included patients with normal pH testing or failed response to proton pump inhibitor (PPI) therapy. The distinction between EoE and GERD was supported in a retrospective pediatric study that found an inverse correlation between the degree of esophageal eosinophilia and reflux severity determined by pH testing [87]. Abnormal reflux testing was more likely in children with ≤5 eos/hpf and uncommon in those with >20 eos/hpf. Another pediatric study characterized esophageal eosinophilia as a predictor of poor symptom response to reflux therapy [88].

The notion that EoE and GERD were separate entities was furthered by investigations of allergic cell mediators and biomarkers. Histologic detection of mast cells and tissue expression of eotaxin-3 and eosinophil peroxidase were significantly greater in EoE compared with GERD [12, 21, 34, 42]. Genome-wide microarray analysis detected an mRNA transcript signature involving 1% of the human genome in EoE that was distinct from chronic esophagitis (presumably related to GERD) [34]. These observations led to the concept that detection of elevated esophageal eosinophilia was indicative of an "allergic," non-GERD esophagitis.

Over the past decade, it has become evident that esophageal eosinophilia does not exclude the presence of GERD. Twenty-five percent to 50% of pediatric and adult EoE patients have evidence of increased distal esophageal acid exposure on pH monitoring [69, 89, 90]. Additional studies have demonstrated the presence of distal esophageal erosions in patients with symptoms and histologic evidence of EoE. The presence of objective GERD diagnostic parameters did not implicate GERD as the cause of the esophageal eosinophilia since these series identified patients who had failed therapeutic trials of PPI. Instead, the data supported the coexistence of EoE and GERD. The intersection between the entities is not only reasonable but expected given the high prevalence of GERD in the general population.

The concept that patients with suspected EoE might have GERD originated in a case series of three patients with symptoms, endoscopic features, and histopathology consistent with EoE who responded to PPI [91]. Two recent, retrospective pediatric studies involving 79 children with EoE reported a 39% response to PPI therapy, with response defined by <5 eos/hpf [92, 93]. A prospective study examined the response to PPI therapy amongst 35 adults with esophageal eosinophilia defined by >15 eos/hpf [94]. Seventy-five percent of the patients with esophageal eosinophilia responded to an 8-week course of rabeprazole 20-mg BID, with response defined by achieving <5 eos/hpf. Furthermore, a subgroup of esophageal eosinophilia patients with a symptom profile (dysphagia or food impaction) and endoscopic findings (rings, furrows) characteristic for EoE had a 50% response to the PPI trial.

The high response rate of esophageal eosinophilia to PPI seemingly supports the original supposition that esophageal eosinophilia is a manifestation of GERD. The delineation between GERD and EoE is, however, not straightforward [95]. Symptom or histologic response to PPI should not necessarily define GERD in the context of patients with suspected EoE. Acid reflux may cause or exacerbate an allergic inflammatory response by a variety of postulated mechanisms that include (1) acid increases eosinophil viability [96], (2) esophageal acid exposure induces the release of mast cell mediators [97], and (3) GERD is associated with dilated intercellular spaces in the squamous epithelium that might allow penetration of allergens. Furthermore, PPI therapy may have anti-inflammatory effects beyond acid suppression [98].

The differentiation between GERD and EoE has important implications in terms of patient management. One of the earliest studies on EoE reported a cohort of children with esophageal eosinophilia who were diagnosed with GERD deemed refractory to medical therapy, the majority of whom underwent fundoplication without improvement [99]. The children were subsequently shown to respond symptomatically and histologically to an elemental diet. EoE should be considered in patients with "refractory reflux" prior to consideration of anti-reflux surgery. While this scenario is more commonly encountered in pediatrics, prospective adult studies have detected EoE in 1–4% of patients with reflux symptoms failing PPI therapy [100, 101]. On the other hand, committing patients with suspected EoE to long-term steroid or elimination diet therapy who might otherwise respond to PPI is also important. The safety profile of PPI is established while the long-term physical and psychosocial implications of topical steroids and dietary intervention are unknown. The utility of bio-markers and reflux diagnostic testing with pH studies is being investigated. An empiric thera-peutic trial of PPI therapy in suspected EoE patients is a practical approach until better means of distinguishing GERD from EoE become avail-able [60]. Patients demonstrating a symptom and histologic response to the PPI trial are classified as having "PPI-responsive esophageal eosino-philia" and may have either GERD or a PPI-responsive form of eosinophilic esophagitis. On the other hand, patients with persistent symptoms and eosinophilic inflammation meet the 2011 consensus recommendation definition of EoE. Uncertainty exists regarding patients with partial response to PPI therapy or who demonstrate clin-ical but not histologic response to PPI therapy. Combinations of PPI therapy with primary ther-apy directed at EoE may be appropriate in such circumstances.

Natural History

Prospective data pertaining to the natural history and the long-term prognosis of EoE is inherently limited given its relatively recent recognition as a distinct clinicopathologic entity [85, 102]. Much of what we know about the natural history is gleaned from retrospective cohort studies, case series, and placebo groups in controlled trials [103–105].

Straumann et al. [47] has provided the longest period of prospective follow-up in a study that followed 30 adult patients for a mean of 7.2 years. This study and others [86] describe a disease that is chronic, characterized by years of persistent dysphagia in adults. Further evidence of chronic-ity is suggested by studies that identify a high rate of relapse following medical treatment. In an Australian therapeutic trial of topical corticoster-oids, 14 of 19 patients (74%) experienced relapse 3 months after cessation of the drug [89]. This finding has also been observed in a 10-year retro-spective cohort of children [67].

Patients can experience fluctuations in disease activity independent of treatment. Among 11 children receiving placebo in a topical steroid trial, one (9%) achieved spontaneous histologic remission and three (27%) achieved resolution of symptoms over a 3-month study period [106]. This fluctuation may represent the nature of EoE itself or the influence of seasonal aeroallergens [107, 108], which has been implicated in basic science studies described earlier.

The variability in EoE activity also extends to the observation that some patients outgrow the disease with or without persistent fibrostenotic sequelae and others follow an unrelenting inflammatory progression leading to complica-tions if left untreated. That said, the concern for progression of EoE to extra-esophageal diseases such as the hypereosinophilic syndrome or eosinophilic gastrointestinal disorders (EGID) has not been supported by the literature [103].

Complications

Impaired Quality of Life

Beyond symptoms of dysphagia, there is an adverse psychosocial impact when the personal and social pleasure attached to eating and drink-ing is compromised. Important indicators of dis-ease burden include food avoidance and dietary modification, prolongation of meal times, and avoidance of social dining, anxiety, uncertainty, or emotional reactions to disease. Addressing these concerns, a disease-specific quality of life instru-ment has been developed and validated [109].

Esophageal Stricture

A high rate of focal strictures has been identified in adults with EoE, seen both radiographically and endoscopically [68, 102, 110] (Figs. 47.2 and 47.3). As described before, adults tend to form focal strictures more readily than children for unknown reasons that may be related to disease duration or differences in the pathogenesis in dif-ferent age groups [67, 68]. The endoscopic appearance of these focal strictures may appear as a solitary ring, a short ringed segment or focally tapered segment. Long-segment narrowing of the esophagus, known as small-caliber esophagus is generally best identified on a barium esophogram [55, 111].

Food Bolus Impaction

Food bolus impaction is a common, serious, and costly complication associated with EoE, often necessitating urgent endoscopy in an emergency room setting. Desai et al. demonstrated that 17 of 31 patients (60%) referred for workup of food impaction received the diagnosis of eosinophilic esophagitis. Complications of esophageal tears and Boerhaave's syndrome have been reported in the setting of food impaction in EoE.

Esophageal Perforation

Three cases of spontaneous esophageal rupture not associated with esophageal dilation have been reported in the literature [104, 105, 112, 113]. Two occurred in the context of nausea and vomiting from a presumed GI infection, and the third occurred in the setting of aggressive retching caused by an impacted food bolus. All patients had preexisting dysphagia and were managed surgically. Esophageal perforation in the setting of diagnostic endoscopy and esophageal dilation is discussed later.

Malignancy Risk

The concern that EoE might predispose to a malignancy is based on three, indirect observations: (1) chronic inflammatory conditions of the GI tract such as inflammatory bowel disease, GERD, and chronic atrophic gastritis can predispose to cancer, (2) certain chronic eosinophilic disorders are associated with T-cell clones that predispose the patient to lymphoproliferative disorders, and (3) the risk of concurrent GERD in a subset of patients with EoE may be an independent risk factor for esophageal cancer. In a cohort of 200 adult EoE patients followed in Olten County, Switzerland for a period of up to 17 years,

no malignant tumor or dysplasia was diagnosed in the esophagus [103–105]. In a prospective case series of 30 adults from the same investigators, none developed a premalignant condition or cancer at a mean 7.2-year follow-up period [47]. Isolated case reports and small series have identified Barrett's esophagus in patients with EoE. However, it remains unproven whether the Barrett's is causally related to the diagnosis of EoE in these patients or that the prevalence of Barrett's in these cohorts is any higher than the general population.

Therapy

In the relatively short time since the recognition of EoE as a distinct entity, studies have identified a number of effective medical, dietary, and endoscopic therapies in both children and adults with EoE (Table 47.3). The goals of therapy of EoE include not only alleviation of presenting symptoms but also prevention of disease recurrence, improvement in quality of life, and prevention of complications. Uncertainty exists regarding the most pertinent endpoints of treatment of EoE. Symptoms are a commonly tracked clinical outcome. The interpretation of symptom improvement is problematic as patients may modify their diets to minimize ingestion of foods that are difficult to swallow whereas others have sporadic symptoms that may not manifest during a short follow-up period. Some patients alter their eating habits by means of meticulous mastication and prolonged meal times. While such alterations may result in a patient reporting minimal dysphagia, a substantial reduction in quality of life may result from adverse effects on social interaction and meal enjoyment [114].

In existing studies, response is determined by a reduction in esophageal eosinophilia. However, the appropriate degree of reduction is uncertain and different target endpoints have been used including <15, <10, or <5 eosinophils per high power field (eos/hpf). Other markers of tissue injury such as eosinophil degranulation proteins, basal cell hyperplasia, or subepithelial fibrosis may be as important as the actual number of

Table 47.3 Treatment options for eosinophilic esophagitis

Treatment	Advantages	Disadvantages
Medications		
Topical steroids	Ease of administration	Candidiasis
Fluticasone	High degree of efficacy in randomized controlled trials	Recurrent disease after cessation
Budesonide	High degree of effectiveness in uncontrolled studies	
High degree of effectiveness in randomized trials	High degree of efficacy in randomized controlled trials	Toxicities of systemic steroid
	Ease of administration	Recurrent disease after cessation
Antihistamines	Ease of administration	Limited data to support effectiveness
Leukotriene antagonist	Symptom improvement in uncontrolled studies	High doses may be needed for effect
		No change in esophageal eosinophilia
		Side effects of nausea and myalgias
Immunomodulator	Steroid sparing agent	Immunosuppression
		Side effects
		Limited data to support effectiveness
Anti-TNF therapy	Rationale based on increased tissue expression of TNF	No clinical improvement in a small, uncontrolled trial
Anti-IL-5 therapy	Rationale based on role of IL-5	Conflicting data to support efficacy in systemic eosinophilic disorders
Cromolyn sodium	Rationale based on asthma model	Limited pediatric data does not support effectiveness
Diet		
Elemental	High degree of effectiveness	Poor palatability
	Simplified diet	Requires prolonged period of food reintroduction
	Avoidance of long-term use of medications	Repeated EGD and biopsies to identify allergen
Directed elimination	High degree of effectiveness	Skin prick test with poor predictive value
	Theoretical advantage of more selective diet	Atopy patch testing not standardized or widely available
	Avoidance of long-term use of medications	Repeated EGD and biopsies to identify allergen
Empiric elimination	High degree of effectiveness	Repeated EGD and biopsy to identify causative food
	Avoidance of long-term use of medications	High degree of vigilance to avoid contamination
Dilation		
	High degree of effectiveness	Reports of esophageal laceration causing significant pain and infrequent hospitalization
	Prolonged symptom response without medications	Infrequent reports of esophageal perforation

eosinophils [48, 49]. Furthermore, studies have demonstrated that esophageal eosinophilia can extend to involve the submucosa as well as muscularis layers, regions that are not routinely sampled by esophageal mucosal biopsies [53, 115]. Finally, structural alterations in the esophagus may not necessarily reverse with treatment directed at esophageal inflammation. Endoscopic esophageal mucosal changes, radiographic presence of esophageal strictures, and alterations in esophageal mural distensibility are important consequences of EoE that may serve as objective outcomes [54].

The majority of the published therapeutic studies to date have focused on therapeutic outcomes of symptoms and esophageal eosinophilia. When comparing existing treatment studies, differences in patient selection, definition of therapeutic response, and duration of treatment are important parameters that may explain heterogeneity in results. Validation of EoE dysphagia scoring instruments and an EoE activity index combining clinical with endoscopic and histologic parameters are under way and should offer a standardized assessment of patient response to therapy for clinical studies.

Initial Therapy for EoE

For adults, topical steroids are the most commonly used treatment given the ease of administration and published data supporting their efficacy and safety. Several prospective uncontrolled studies and six randomized controlled trials have evaluated the effectiveness and efficacy of steroids, respectively [27, 28, 76, 89, 106, 116, 117, 130, 131]. With the exception of one study, the adult trials with topical steroids have consistently demonstrated marked, significant clinical and histologic improvement after therapy administered from 15 days to 3 months. Histologic response rates defined by less than 6 eos/hpf were achieved in recent studies in over 70% of patients. Endoscopic signs of rings, furrows, and strictures visibly improve but may not completely resolve [116]. Significant variability in the degree of response to topical steroids has been observed. Interestingly, in pediatric studies, allergic individuals identified by reactivity on skin testing and taller subjects demonstrated lower response rates [76, 106]. The data suggest that the efficacy of topical steroids may be affected by the dose of steroid as well as degree of underlying atopy. The mode of administration through swallowed aerosolized particles or viscous liquid preparations may affect the delivery and contact time of the steroid with the esophageal mucosal surface. Based on pediatric data, the efficacy of topical and systemic steroids appears comparable [117]. Compliance with prolonged therapy has been a concern as the symptomatic benefits are not immediate and tend to last for prolonged periods after cessation.

Limitations of topical steroids include disease recurrence in 90% following cessation and uncertainty regarding long-term safety [67]. A proportion of patients have limited responsiveness to topical steroids perhaps owing to drug delivery, intrinsic steroid resistance, or an underlying strong allergic predisposition. Whether such patients would respond to higher doses of topical steroids, therapy directed at allergic environmental triggers, or systemic steroids has yet to be determined. The primary side effect of topical steroids has been oropharyngeal or esophageal candidiasis. A prospective study in children administered fluticasone at doses of 220–440 mcg QID found esophageal candidiasis in 15% of patients, although the patients did not report symptoms attributable to the infection [117]. Potential concerns for steroid side effects such as adrenal insufficiency or osteoporosis have not been reported. Pharyngeal irritation is more commonly reported with aerosolized steroid and may be related to contact irritation by the propellant.

Systemic corticosteroids were one of the first treatment options reported for EoE. Retrospective studies have demonstrated their effectiveness in inducing symptomatic and histologic remission. Nevertheless, prolonged systemic corticosteroids use is associated with well-known toxicities. A pediatric study randomized 80 patients to therapy with either topical fluticasone 220–440 mcg four times a day or oral prednisone 1 mg/kg twice a day [117]. Posttreatment tissue eosinophilia was similarly reduced to <5 eos/hpf in 67% and 78% of the fluticasone and prednisone groups, respectively. Adverse effects were seen in 40% of the prednisone group including Cushingoid features and weight gain whereas 15% of the fluticasone group developed esophageal candidiasis that was asymptomatic.

Montelukast is a leukotriene D4 receptor antagonist. Attwood et al. [118] used doses of montelukast, up to 100 mg/day, in eight adult patients with median follow-up of 14 months. Symptom improvement was found in seven patients. Six patients noted recurrence of symptoms in less than 3 weeks after discontinuing therapy. Montelukast did not change the density of eosinophils although this may not be relevant given the mechanism of this agent. In a separate pediatric study, however, biopsies from patients with EoE did not show a significant increase in leukotrienes compared with control, calling into question the rationale for use of a leukotriene antagonist [119]. Side effects including nausea, headache, and myalgia may limit the use of montelukast in some patients with EoE.

Analogous to their use in inflammatory bowel disease, biologic therapy offers potential therapy as disease modifying agents. Translational research studies have identified key immune mediators in the pathogenesis of EoE that include IL-5, TNF-a, IL-13, and IgE. Given the efficacy of interleukin (IL)-5 in other eosinophilic disorders, it has been postulated that anti-IL-5 antibody may be an efficacious therapeutic option for EoE. Mepolizumab is a fully humanized monoclonal IgG antibody that selectively binds and inactivates IL-5. Stein et al. [120] demonstrated that mepolizumab effectively reduced peripheral blood eosinophilia by ninefold and the number of circulating CCR3+ cells in four patients with EoE. Maximal esophageal eosinophil counts fell from 153 to 28 eos/hpf with 4 weeks of therapy. Patients reported improvement in quality of life and symptoms. There were no reported serious adverse effects of mepolizumab. A second randomized, controlled study included 11 patients with EoE who were unresponsive or dependent on systemic corticosteroid therapy. Mepolizumab was administered for 4 weeks. There was a statistically significant decrease in both peripheral and esophageal eosinophilia; however, no patient achieved histologic remission (<5 eos/hpf) and symptom benefit was modest. Further studies to determine the role of anti-IL-5 therapy in EoE are ongoing. Anti-IgE therapy has also been proposed in patients with EoE. In an open label trial, nine adults with eosinophilic gastroenteritis, of whom seven also had EoE, were put on omalizumab. While there was a significant decrease in symptoms, IgE levels, and peripheral eosinophilia, increased esophageal eosinophilia was noted [121]. Recent studies have shown the increased expression of tumor necrosis factor (TNF) in patients with EoE. Thus, the use of TNF alpha monoclonal antibody, infliximab, to induce remission in EoE may be a potential therapeutic option. An open label pilot study of three patients treated with two doses of infliximab 5 mg/kg at weeks 4 and 6 was not able to demonstrate an improvement in symptoms, esophageal eosinophilia, or tissue expression of TNF alpha [104]. More data on the use of biologic therapy as monotherapy or in combination with existing therapies are needed.

Available data support the effectiveness of dietary therapy in adults with EoE although the majority of studies have been from pediatric centers. The three dietary approaches used in children include elemental diet, allergy testing directed elimination diet, and empiric elimination diet [15, 67, 122]. In 1995, Kelly and Sampson introduced the concept of food antigen elimination as primary therapy for EoE. Ten children with symptoms of GERD and esophageal eosinophilia who failed conventional reflux therapies were placed on an elemental, amino acid based formula for 6 weeks. Complete symptom resolution was seen in 80% of patients with marked reduction in esophageal eosinophilia [99]. The effectiveness of elemental diet was confirmed in larger retrospective trials. Liacouras et al. reported significant clinical and histologic improvement in 97% of 164 children who were fed an amino acid based formula (Neocate 1+, SHS North America, Gaithersburg, MD; Elecare, Ross Pediatrics, Abbott Laboratories, Abbott Park, IL) [67, 123]. Eosinophils were reduced from 39 eos/hpf pre-therapy to 1 eos/hpf after treatment. Because of the formula's unpleasant taste, 80% of patients were fed by nasogastric (NG) tube. While elemental diet remains the "gold standard" dietary approach, the difficulties with administration and compliance limit its use in practice.

Kagalwalla and Li introduced the six-food elimination diet (SFED) as a means of avoiding the problems with the elemental diet [122]. SFED empirically eliminated the six most common food allergies: milk protein, soy, peanut/tree nuts, egg, wheat, and seafood. This approach allows the patient to continue to consume a variety of foods such as chicken, beef, pork, rice, fruits, and vegetables. In the initial study of 35 children who underwent the SFED, 74% had significant histologic improvement (<10 eos/hpf) after 6 weeks of treatment. Overall, esophageal eosinophilia was reduced from 80 to 14 eos/hpf. Patients who achieved histologic resolution of EoE on SFED subsequently underwent stepwise reintroduction of the eliminated foods into the diet. A recent prospective study of adults applied the empiric elimination of common food allergens for 6 weeks followed by systematic food reintroduction [16]. Histologic response rates defined by less than 10 eos/hpf were achieved in 65%. Symptom improvement in dysphagia occurred in almost every patient with demonstrable improvement in endoscopic abnormalities. Milk and wheat were the most common food triggers identified. Based on the response to food reintroduction testing amongst responders, skin prick testing for food allergens led to both false-negative and false-positive results in the majority of patients.

Although pediatric series describe hundreds of EoE patients treated effectively with diet, none of the studies have been randomized controlled trials. It is important to emphasize that the goal of dietary therapy is not only achieving symptomatic and histologic disease remission but moreover the identification of specific food allergens. In some instances, patients may prefer the dietary approach as a non-pharmacologic intervention to eliminate environmental triggers to their disease. The dietary approach requires a highly motivated patient willing to avoid common food groups for a defined period of time with vigilance regarding dietary contamination. The success is optimized by close supervision by a dietician with experience in food allergy.

Disadvantages of elimination diet therapies include the potential impact on patient quality of life during the initial elimination phase of the diet as well as long-term selective elimination of specific food. Currently, the reintroduction phase incorporates symptom assessment combined with periodic endoscopic surveillance for esophageal eosinophilia. The performance of multiple EGD with biopsies is associated with both time and expense for patients. The accuracy of following only symptom rather than symptom and histologic recurrence upon food reintroduction has not been determined. A noninvasive biomarker of disease activity would greatly improve the acceptance of the dietary therapy of EoE. Moreover, an allergy assay that accurately predicts causative food allergens would clearly be ideal. The long-term effectiveness of dietary elimination and eventual ability to reintroduce identified food triggers are the subject of ongoing investigations.

Esophageal dilation was one of the first therapies used for adult patients with EoE. Early reports of complications related to esophageal dilation in EoE included not only chest pain but also perforation generated trepidation amongst gastroenterologists. Of the 84 adult patients reported prior to 2008 who underwent dilation, 5% experienced an esophageal perforation and 7% were hospitalized for chest pain [124]. Further compounding this concern were early reports of esophageal tears and perforations from food impactions and diagnostic endoscopies, suggesting susceptibility towards esophageal mural fragility in EoE [125]. Such findings led to a consensus statement publication that recommended that medical or dietary therapy for EoE is attempted prior to the performance of esophageal dilation [65].

Three recent retrospective studies from adult centers reported complication rates for sequelae of perforation or pain requiring hospitalization that were considerably lower than that of initial reports [126–128]. Only three perforations were reported amongst 404 patients undergoing 839 esophageal dilations. Incorporating the newer studies, the perforation rate for dilation is 0.8% and chest pain in 5%. Furthermore, the perforations were partial ruptures and many determined by extravasation of air and not contrast or gastric contents. Major bleeding defined by need for endoscopic hemostasis or blood product transfusion was reported in only one patient. None of the reported perforations required surgical intervention. A very high degree of patients' acceptance for primary therapy with esophageal dilation was reported in a post-dilation survey [128]. An important factor that may have influenced the higher complication rates in earlier reports has to do with disease awareness. Many of the initial reports of esophageal perforation occurred in patients in whom EoE was not initially recognized and prior to publications describing the dangers of esophageal dilation. As such, the greater safety reported in the studies by more recent series may reflect the adoption of a more conservative approach by gastroenterologists aware of the potential hazards of dilation in EoE.

In spite of the greater safety margin reported in these recent studies of esophageal dilation, the role of dilation as a primary therapy of EoE is still controversial and should be individualized until more data are available. Dilation can provide immediate and long-lasting relief of dysphagia in patients with high-grade esophageal strictures. EoE in adults affects otherwise healthy, young to middle-aged patients who, if given the option, might prefer periodic dilation to chronic use of a medication or an elimination diet. On the other hand, monotherapy with dilation does not improve the underlying inflammatory process responsible for stricture development. In the absence of high-grade esophageal stenosis, a trial of medical or dietary therapy prior to performance of esophageal dilation is reasonable.

At this time, there is no prospective data to guide the decision for selecting the most appropriate initial therapy for patients with EoE. The available data supports the use of topical steroids, diet, or dilation as effective means of managing the dysphagia that dominates the clinical presentation in adults. The only randomized, controlled trials performed to date establish the efficacy of topical steroids but the ability of steroids to reverse esophageal structural alterations remains poorly defined. A stepwise approach is suggested whereby patients are initially placed on a trial of PPI therapy. PPI unresponsive patients are offered therapy with either diet or steroids, with selected patients undergoing esophageal dilation. Patients who are unresponsive to initial therapy can be switched to an alternative therapy. The role for initial combination therapy, other than dilation with topical steroids, has not been evaluated.

Maintenance Therapy

Maintenance therapy is an important consideration for EoE patients since the majority develops recurrent symptoms and histopathology upon cessation of therapy with either steroid or dietary elimination. As there is limited data to suggest that EoE is a progressive disorder that leads to increased esophageal stricturing over time, long-term therapeutic strategies are currently individualized. For patients with mild and intermittent dysphagia without significant strictures or food impaction, intermittent on-demand topical steroids may be appropriate assuming that the patient is reliable and has clinical follow-up. For patients with severe dysphagia, repeated food impaction and high-grade esophageal strictures at presentation and who respond to initial medical therapy, maintenance therapy seems reasonable. Lowering the dosage of topical steroids below that used to induce clinical remission is a consideration but a recent study that attempted this strategy noted a significant reduction in treatment efficacy [129]. Maintenance with nonsteroid medications such as antihistamines, immunomodulators, or leukotriene antagonists has been reported in very small retrospective case series. Finally, the prolonged relief of dysphagia reported after esophageal dilation needs to be considered given the inconvenience and potential side effects of long-term medical or dietary therapy.

Conclusion

Over the past 20 years, EoE, a chronic, immune-mediated disease affecting esophageal structure and function, has emerged as a leading cause of dysphagia. It is histologically characterized by a dense mucosal eosinophilic infiltration with fibrostenosis. The relationship between EoE and GERD is complex and poorly understood. Highly effective therapies include topical steroids, food allergen avoidance, and esophageal dilation as well as promising novel biologic therapies. Further research is needed on the pathogenesis, natural history, and targeted therapies for this important and growing entity.

References

1. Liacouras CA, Furuta GT, et al. Eosinophilic esophagitis: updated consensus recommendations for children and adults. J Allergy Clin Immunol. 2011;128(1):3–20.
2. Landres RT, Kuster GG, et al. Eosinophilic esophagitis in a patient with vigorous achalasia. Gastroenterology. 1978;74(6):1298–301.
3. Cherian S, Smith NM, et al. Rapidly increasing prevalence of eosinophilic oesophagitis in Western Australia. Arch Dis Child. 2006;91(12):1000–4.
4. Prasad GA, Alexander JA, et al. Epidemiology of eosinophilic esophagitis over three decades in Olmsted county, Minnesota. Clin Gastroenterol Hepatol. 2009;7(10):1055–61.
5. Straumann A, Simon HU. Eosinophilic esophagitis: escalating epidemiology? J Allergy Clin Immunol. 2005;115(2):418–9.
6. Hruz P, Straumann A, et al. Escalating incidence of eosinophilic esophagitis: A 20-year prospective, population-based study in Olten County, Switzerland. J Allergy Clin Immunol. 2011;128(6):1349–50.
7. Noel RJ, Putnam PE, et al. Clinical and immunopathologic effects of swallowed fluticasone for eosinophilic esophagitis. Clin Gastroenterol Hepatol. 2004;2(7):568–75.
8. Kugathasan S, Judd RH, et al. Epidemiologic and clinical characteristics of children with newly diagnosed inflammatory bowel disease in Wisconsin: a statewide population-based study. J Pediatr. 2003;143(4):525–31.
9. Hassall E. Esophageal biopsy in children—essential, valuable, or a waste of time? It all depends. J Pediatr Gastroenterol Nutr. 2005;41 Suppl 1:S24–7.
10. Nielsen RG, Husby S. Eosinophilic oesophagitis: epidemiology, clinical aspects, and association to allergy. J Pediatr Gastroenterol Nutr. 2007;45(3):281–9.
11. Asher MI, Montefort S, et al. Worldwide time trends in the prevalence of symptoms of asthma, allergic rhinoconjunctivitis, and eczema in childhood: ISAAC phases One and three repeat multicountry cross-sectional surveys. Lancet. 2006;368(9537):733–43.
12. Odze RD. Pathology of eosinophilic esophagitis: what the clinician needs to know. Am J Gastroenterol. 2009;104(2):485–90.
13. Mishra A. Mechanism of eosinophilic esophagitis. Immunol Allergy Clin North Am. 2009;29(1):29–40. viii.
14. Spergel JM. Eosinophilic esophagitis in adults and children: evidence for a food allergy component in many patients. Curr Opin Allergy Clin Immunol. 2007;7(3):274–8.
15. Spergel JM, Andrews T, et al. Treatment of eosinophilic esophagitis with specific food elimination diet directed by a combination of skin prick and patch tests. Ann Allergy Asthma Immunol. 2005;95(4):336–43.
16. Gonsalves N, Yang GY, et al. Elimination diet effectively treats eosinophilic esophagitis in adults; food reintroduction identifies causative factors. Gastroenterology. 2012; 142(7):1451–1459.
17. Almansa C, Krishna M, et al. Seasonal distribution in newly diagnosed cases of eosinophilic esophagitis in adults. Am J Gastroenterol. 2009;104(4):828–33.
18. Moawad FJ, Veerappan GR, et al. Correlation between eosinophilic oesophagitis and aeroallergens. Aliment Pharmacol Ther. 2010;31(4):509–15.
19. Mishra A, Hogan SP, et al. An etiological role for aeroallergens and eosinophils in experimental esophagitis. J Clin Invest. 2001;107(1):83–90.
20. Akei HS, Mishra A, et al. Epicutaneous antigen exposure primes for experimental eosinophilic esophagitis in mice. Gastroenterology. 2005;129(3):985–94.
21. Kirsch R, Bokhary R, et al. Activated mucosal mast cells differentiate eosinophilic (allergic) esophagitis from gastroesophageal reflux disease. J Pediatr Gastroenterol Nutr. 2007;44(1):20–6.
22. Dellon ES, Chen X, et al. Tryptase staining of mast cells may differentiate eosinophilic esophagitis from gastroesophageal reflux disease. Am J Gastroenterol. 2011;106(2):264–71.
23. Hsu Blatman KS, Gonsalves N, et al. Expression of mast cell-associated genes is upregulated in adult eosinophilic esophagitis and responds to steroid or dietary therapy. J Allergy Clin Immunol. 2011;127(5):1307–8.
24. Straumann A, Bauer M, et al. Idiopathic eosinophilic esophagitis is associated with a T(H)2-type allergic inflammatory response. J Allergy Clin Immunol. 2001;108(6):954–61.
25. Mishra A, Hogan SP, et al. IL-5 promotes eosinophil trafficking to the esophagus. J Immunol. 2002;168(5):2464–9.
26. Shen HH, Ochkur SI, et al. A causative relationship exists between eosinophils and the development of allergic pulmonary pathologies in the mouse. J Immunol. 2003;170(6):3296–305.
27. Straumann A, Conus S, et al. Budesonide is effective in adolescent and adult patients with active eosinophilic Esophagitis. Gastroenterology. 2010;139(5):1526–37.
28. Straumann A, Conus S, et al. Anti-interleukin-5 antibody treatment (mepolizumab) in active eosinophilic oesophagitis: a randomised, placebo-controlled, double-blind trial. Gut. 2010;59(1):21–30.
29. Spergel JM, Rothenberg ME, et al. Reslizumab in children and adolescents with eosinophilic esophagitis: results of a double-blind, randomized, placebo-controlled study. J Allergy Clin Immunol. 2012;129(2):456–63.
30. Mishra A, Rothenberg ME. Intratracheal IL-13 induces eosinophilic esophagitis by an IL-5, eotaxin-1, and STAT6-dependent mechanism. Gastroenterology. 2003;125(5):1419–27.
31. Elsner J, Hochstetter R, et al. Human eotaxin represents a potent activator of the respiratory burst of human eosinophils. Eur J Immunol. 1996;26(8):1919–25.
32. Forssmann U, Uguccioni M, et al. Eotaxin-2, a novel CC chemokine that is selective for the chemokine

receptor CCR3, and acts like eotaxin on human eosinophil and basophil leukocytes. J Exp Med. 1997;185(12):2171–6.

33. Kitaura M, Suzuki N, et al. Molecular cloning of a novel human CC chemokine (eotaxin-3) that is a functional ligand of CC chemokine receptor 3. J Biol Chem. 1999;274(39):27975–80.

34. Blanchard C, Wang N, et al. Eotaxin-3 and a uniquely conserved gene-expression profile in eosinophilic esophagitis. J Clin Invest. 2006;116(2):536–47.

35. Rothenberg ME, JSpergel JM, et al. Common variants at 5q22 associate with pediatric eosinophilic esophagitis. Nat Genet. 2010;42(4):289–91.

36. Al-Shami A, Spolski R, et al. A role for thymic stromal lymphopoietin in CD4(+) T cell development. J Exp Med. 2004;200(2):159–68.

37. Ying S, O'Connor B, et al. Thymic stromal lymphopoietin expression is increased in asthmatic airways and correlates with expression of Th2-attracting chemokines and disease severity. J Immunol. 2005;174(12):8183–90.

38. Mou Z, Xia J, et al. Overexpression of thymic stromal lymphopoietin in allergic rhinitis. Acta Otolaryngol. 2009;129(3):297–301.

39. Siracusa MC, Saenz SA, et al. TSLP promotes interleukin-3-independent basophil haematopoiesis and type 2 inflammation. Nature. 2011;477(7363):229–33.

40. Mueller S, Aigner T, et al. Eosinophil infiltration and degranulation in oesophageal mucosa from adult patients with eosinophilic oesophagitis: a retrospective and comparative study on pathological biopsy. J Clin Pathol. 2006;59(11):1175–80.

41. Rothenberg ME, Hogan SP. The eosinophil. Annu Rev Immunol. 2006;24:147–74.

42. Protheroe C, Woodruff SA, et al. A novel histologic scoring system to evaluate mucosal biopsies from patients with eosinophilic esophagitis. Clin Gastroenterol Hepatol. 2009;7(7):749–55. e711.

43. Jacoby DB, Gleich GJ, et al. Human eosinophil major basic protein is an endogenous allosteric antagonist at the inhibitory muscarinic M2 receptor. J Clin Invest. 1993;91(4):1314–8.

44. Mulder DJ, Pacheco I, et al. FGF9-Induced proliferative response to eosinophilic inflammation in oesophagitis. Gut. 2009;58(2):166–73.

45. Yang D, Chen Q, et al. Eosinophil-derived neurotoxin acts as an alarmin to activate the TLR2-MyD88 signal pathway in dendritic cells and enhances Th2 immune responses. J Exp Med. 2008;205(1):79–90.

46. Sommerhoff CP. Mast cell tryptases and airway remodeling. Am J Respir Crit Care Med. 2001;164(10 Pt 2):S52–8.

47. Straumann A, Spichtin HP, et al. Natural history of primary eosinophilic esophagitis: a follow-up of 30 adult patients for up to 11.5 years. Gastroenterology. 2003;125(6):1660–9.

48. Aceves SS, Newbury RO, et al. Esophageal remodeling in pediatric eosinophilic esophagitis. J Allergy Clin Immunol. 2007;119(1):206–12.

49. Aceves SS, Newbury RO, et al. Distinguishing eosinophilic esophagitis in pediatric patients: clinical, endoscopic, and histologic features of an emerging disorder. J Clin Gastroenterol. 2007;41(3):252–6.

50. Chehade M, Sampson HA, et al. Esophageal subepithelial fibrosis in children with eosinophilic esophagitis. J Pediatr Gastroenterol Nutr. 2007;45(3):319–28.

51. Silverman ES, Palmer LJ, et al. Transforming growth factor-beta1 promoter polymorphism C-509T is associated with asthma. Am J Respir Crit Care Med. 2004;169(2):214–9.

52. Ueda T, Niimi A, et al. TGFB1 promoter polymorphism C-509T and pathophysiology of asthma. J Allergy Clin Immunol. 2008;121(3):659–64.

53. Fox VL, Nurko S, et al. High-resolution EUS in children with eosinophilic "allergic" esophagitis. Gastrointest Endosc. 2003;57(1):30–6.

54. Kwiatek MA, Hirano I, et al. Mechanical properties of the esophagus in eosinophilic esophagitis. Gastroenterology. 2011;140(1):82–90.

55. Vasilopoulos S, Murphy P, et al. The small-caliber esophagus: an unappreciated cause of dysphagia for solids in patients with eosinophilic esophagitis. Gastrointest Endosc. 2002;55(1):99–106.

56. Schoepfer AM, Schossmann JG, et al. Esophageal strictures in adult eosinophilic esophagitis: dilation is an effective and safe alternative after failure of topical corticosteroids. Endoscopy. 2008;40(2):161–4.

57. Robles-Medranda C, Villard F, et al. Severe dysphagia in children with eosinophilic esophagitis and esophageal stricture: an indication for balloon dilation? J Pediatr Gastroenterol Nutr. 2010;50(5):516–20.

58. Chehade M, Sampson HA. Epidemiology and etiology of eosinophilic esophagitis. Gastrointest Endosc Clin N Am. 2008;18(1):33–44. viii.

59. Franciosi JP, Liacouras CA. Eosinophilic esophagitis. Immunol Allergy Clin North Am. 2009;29(1):19–27. viii.

60. Garrean C, Hirano I. Eosinophilic esophagitis: pathophysiology and optimal management. Curr Gastroenterol Rep. 2009;11(3):175–81.

61. Spergel JM, Beausoleil JL, et al. The use of skin prick tests and patch tests to identify causative foods in eosinophilic esophagitis. J Allergy Clin Immunol. 2002;109(2):363–8.

62. Simon D, Marti H, et al. Eosinophilic esophagitis is frequently associated with IgE-mediated allergic airway diseases. J Allergy Clin Immunol. 2005;115(5):1090–2.

63. Rothenberg ME. Biology and treatment of eosinophilic esophagitis. Gastroenterology. 2009;137(4):1238–49.

64. Noel RJ, Putnam PE, et al. Eosinophilic esophagitis. N Engl J Med. 2004;351(9):940–1.

65. Furuta GT, Liacouras CA, et al. Eosinophilic esophagitis in children and adults: a systematic review and consensus recommendations for diagnosis and treatment. Gastroenterology. 2007;133(4):1342–63.

66. Straumann A. Clinical evaluation of the adult who has eosinophilic esophagitis. Immunol Allergy Clin North Am. 2009;29(1):11–8. vii.

67. Liacouras CA, Spergel JM, et al. Eosinophilic esophagitis: a 10-year experience in 381 children. Clin Gastroenterol Hepatol. 2005;3(12):1198–206.
68. Croese J, Fairley SK, et al. Clinical and endoscopic features of eosinophilic esophagitis in adults. Gastrointest Endosc. 2003;58(4):516–22.
69. Teitelbaum JE, Fox VL, et al. Eosinophilic esophagitis in children: immunopathological analysis and response to fluticasone propionate. Gastroenterology. 2002;122(5):1216–25.
70. Arora AS, Perrault J, et al. Topical corticosteroid treatment of dysphagia due to eosinophilic esophagitis in adults. Mayo Clin Proc. 2003;78(7):830–5.
71. Arora AS, Yamazaki K. Eosinophilic esophagitis: asthma of the esophagus? Clin Gastroenterol Hepatol. 2004;2(7):523–30.
72. Straumann A, Spichtin HP, et al. Eosinophilic esophagitis: red on microscopy, white on endoscopy. Digestion. 2004;70(2):109–16.
73. Gonsalves N, Policarpio-Nicolas M, et al. Histopathologic variability and endoscopic correlates in adults with eosinophilic esophagitis. Gastrointest Endosc. 2006;64(3):313–9.
74. Prasad GA, Talley NJ, et al. Prevalence and predictive factors of eosinophilic esophagitis in patients presenting with dysphagia: a prospective study. Am J Gastroenterol. 2007;102(12):2627–32.
75. Veerappan GR, Perry JL, et al. Prevalence of eosinophilic esophagitis in an adult population undergoing upper endoscopy: a prospective study. Clin Gastroenterol Hepatol. 2009;7(4):420–6. 426 e421-422.
76. Dohil R, Newbury R, et al. Oral viscous Budesonide is effective in children with eosinophilic esophagitis in a randomized, placebo-controlled trial. Gastroenterology. 2010;139(2):418–29.
77. Hirano I, Moy N, et al. Endoscopic assessment of the oesophageal features of eosinophilic oesophagitis: validation of a novel classification and grading system. Gut 2012. PMID 22619364.
78. Garcia-Compean D, Gonzalez Gonzalez JA. Prevalence of eosinophilic esophagitis in patients with refractory gastroesophageal reflux disease symptoms. A prospective study. Dig Liver Dis. 2011;43(3):204–8.
79. Bassett J, Maydonovitch C, et al. Prevalence of esophageal dysmotility in a cohort of patients with esophageal biopsies consistent with eosinophilic esophagitis. Dis Esophagus. 2009;22(6):543–8.
80. Nurko S, Rosen R, et al. Esophageal dysmotility in children with eosinophilic esophagitis: a study using prolonged esophageal manometry. Am J Gastroenterol. 2009;104(12):3050–7.
81. Roman S, Hirano I, et al. Manometric features of eosinophilic esophagitis in esophageal pressure topography. Neurogastroenterol Motil. 2011;23(3):208–14. e111.
82. Lee S, de Boer WB, et al. More than just counting eosinophils: proximal oesophageal involvement and subepithelial sclerosis are major diagnostic criteria for eosinophilic oesophagitis. J Clin Pathol. 2010; 63(7):644–7.
83. Winter HS, Madara JL, et al. Intraepithelial eosinophils: a new diagnostic criterion for reflux esophagitis. Gastroenterology. 1982;83(4):818–23.
84. Brown LF, Goldman H, et al. Intraepithelial eosinophils in endoscopic biopsies of adults with reflux esophagitis. Am J Surg Pathol. 1984;8(12):899–905.
85. Attwood SE, Smyrk TC, et al. Esophageal eosinophilia with dysphagia. A distinct clinicopathologic syndrome. Dig Dis Sci. 1993;38(1):109–16.
86. Straumann A, Spichtin HP, et al. Idiopathic eosinophilic esophagitis: a frequently overlooked disease with typical clinical aspects and discrete endoscopic findings. Schweiz Med Wochenschr. 1994;124(33):1419–29.
87. Steiner SJ, Gupta SK, et al. Correlation between number of eosinophils and reflux index on same day esophageal biopsy and 24 hour esophageal pH monitoring. Am J Gastroenterol. 2004;99(5):801–5.
88. Ruchelli E, Wenner W, et al. Severity of esophageal eosinophilia predicts response to conventional gastroesophageal reflux therapy. Pediatr Dev Pathol. 1999;2(1):15–8.
89. Remedios M, Campbell C, et al. Eosinophilic esophagitis in adults: clinical, endoscopic, histologic findings, and response to treatment with fluticasone propionate. Gastrointest Endosc. 2006;63(1):3–12.
90. Shah A, Kagalwalla AF, et al. Histopathologic variability in children with eosinophilic esophagitis. Am J Gastroenterol. 2009;104(3):716–21.
91. Ngo P, Furuta GT, et al. Eosinophils in the esophagus—peptic or allergic eosinophilic esophagitis? Case series of three patients with esophageal eosinophilia. Am J Gastroenterol. 2006;101(7):1666–70.
92. Dranove JE, Horn DS, et al. Predictors of response to proton pump inhibitor therapy among children with significant esophageal eosinophilia. J Pediatr. 2009;154(1):96–100.
93. Sayej WN, Patel R, et al. Treatment with high-dose proton pump inhibitors helps distinguish eosinophilic esophagitis from noneosinophilic esophagitis. J Pediatr Gastroenterol Nutr. 2009;49(4):393–9.
94. Molina-Infante J, Zamorano J. Acid-suppressive therapy and eosinophilic esophagitis: friends or foes? Am J Gastroenterol. 2010;105(3):699–700.
95. Spechler SJ, Genta RM, et al. Thoughts on the complex relationship between gastroesophageal reflux disease and eosinophilic esophagitis. Am J Gastroenterol. 2007;102(6):1301–6.
96. Kottyan LC, Collier AR, et al. Eosinophil viability is increased by acidic pH in a cAMP- and GPR65-dependent manner. Blood. 2009;114(13):2774–82.
97. Paterson WG. Role of mast cell-derived mediators in acid-induced shortening of the esophagus. Am J Physiol. 1998;274(2 Pt 1):G385–8.
98. Zhang X, Cheng E, et al. In esophageal squamous epithelial cell lines from patients with eosinophilic esophagitis (EoE), omeprazole blocks the stimulated secretion of eotaxin-3: a potential anti-inflammatory effect of omeprazole in EoE that is independent of acid inhibition. Gastroenterology. 2010;138(5):S122. 877.

99. Kelly KJ, Lazenby AJ, et al. Eosinophilic esophagitis attributed to gastroesophageal reflux: improvement with an amino acid-based formula. Gastroenterology. 1995;109(5):1503–12.

100. Garcia-Compean D, Gonzalez Gonzalez JA, et al. Prevalence of eosinophilic esophagitis in patients with refractory gastroesophageal reflux disease symptoms: A prospective study. Dig Liver Dis. 2011;43(3):204–8.

101. Poh CH, Gasiorowska A, et al. Upper GI tract findings in patients with heartburn in whom proton pump inhibitor treatment failed versus those not receiving antireflux treatment. Gastrointest Endosc. 2010;71(1):28–34.

102. Vitellas KM, Bennett WF, et al. Idiopathic eosinophilic esophagitis. Radiology. 1993;186(3):789–93.

103. Straumann A. The natural history and complications of eosinophilic esophagitis. Gastrointest Endosc Clin N Am. 2008;18(1):99–118. ix.

104. Straumann A, Bussmann C, et al. Anti-TNF-alpha (infliximab) therapy for severe adult eosinophilic esophagitis. J Allergy Clin Immunol. 2008;122(2): 425–7.

105. Straumann A, Bussmann C, et al. Eosinophilic esophagitis: analysis of food impaction and perforation in 251 adolescent and adult patients. Clin Gastroenterol Hepatol. 2008;6(5):598–600.

106. Konikoff MR, Noel RJ, et al. A randomized, double-blind, placebo-controlled trial of fluticasone propionate for pediatric eosinophilic esophagitis. Gastroenterology. 2006;131(5):1381–91.

107. Fogg MI, Ruchelli E, et al. Pollen and eosinophilic esophagitis. J Allergy Clin Immunol. 2003;112(4): 796–7.

108. Wang FY, Gupta SK, et al. Is there a seasonal variation in the incidence or intensity of allergic eosinophilic esophagitis in newly diagnosed children? J Clin Gastroenterol. 2007;41(5):451–3.

109. Taft TH, Kern E, et al. The adult eosinophilic oesophagitis quality of life questionnaire: a new measure of health-related quality of life. Aliment Pharmacol Ther. 2011;34(7):790–8.

110. Khan S, Orenstein SR, et al. Eosinophilic esophagitis: strictures, impactions, dysphagia. Dig Dis Sci. 2003;48(1):22–9.

111. Vasilopoulos S, Shaker R. Defiant dysphagia: small-caliber esophagus and refractory benign esophageal strictures. Curr Gastroenterol Rep. 2001;3(3): 225–30.

112. Riou PJ, Nicholson AG, et al. Esophageal rupture in a patient with idiopathic eosinophilic esophagitis. Ann Thorac Surg. 1996;62(6):1854–6.

113. Cohen MS, Kaufman AB, et al. An audit of endoscopic complications in adult eosinophilic esophagitis. Clin Gastroenterol Hepatol. 2007;5(10):1149–53.

114. Kern E, Taft T, et al. Patient reported outcomes in adults with eosinophilic esophagitis. Gastroenterology. 2010;138(5):S175. S1081.

115. Stevoff C, Rao S, et al. EUS and histopathologic correlates in eosinophilic esophagitis. Gastrointest Endosc. 2001;54(3):373–7.

116. Lucendo AJ, Pascual-Turrion JM, et al. Endoscopic, bioptic, and manometric findings in eosinophilic esophagitis before and after steroid therapy: a case series. Endoscopy. 2007;39(9):765–71.

117. Schaefer ET, Fitzgerald JF, et al. Comparison of oral prednisone and topical fluticasone in the treatment of eosinophilic esophagitis: a randomized trial in children. Clin Gastroenterol Hepatol. 2008;6(2): 165–73.

118. Attwood SE, Lewis CJ, et al. Eosinophilic oesophagitis: a novel treatment using montelukast. Gut. 2003;52(2):181–5.

119. Gupta SK, Peters-Golden M, et al. Cysteinyl leukotriene levels in esophageal mucosal biopsies of children with eosinophilic inflammation: are they all the same? Am J Gastroenterol. 2006;101(5):1125–8.

120. Stein ML, Collins MH, et al. Anti-IL-5 (mepolizumab) therapy for eosinophilic esophagitis. J Allergy Clin Immunol. 2006;118(6):1312–9.

121. Foroughi S, Foster B, et al. Anti-IgE treatment of eosinophil-associated gastrointestinal disorders. J Allergy Clin Immunol. 2007;120(3):594–601.

122. Kagalwalla AF, Sentongo TA, et al. Effect of six-food elimination diet on clinical and histologic outcomes in eosinophilic esophagitis. Clin Gastroenterol Hepatol. 2006;4(9):1097–102.

123. Spergel J, Rothenberg ME, et al. Eliminating eosinophilic esophagitis. Clin Immunol. 2005; 115(2):131–2.

124. Hirano I. Dilation in eosinophilic esophagitis: to do or not to do? Gastrointest Endosc. 2010;71(4):713–4.

125. Straumann A, Rossi L, et al. Fragility of the esophageal mucosa: a pathognomonic endoscopic sign of primary eosinophilic esophagitis? Gastrointest Endosc. 2003;57(3):407–12.

126. Dellon ES, Gibbs WB, et al. Esophageal dilation in eosinophilic esophagitis: safety and predictors of clinical response and complications. Gastrointest Endosc. 2010;71(4):706–12.

127. Fiocca R, Mastracci L, et al. Long-term outcome of microscopic esophagitis in chronic GERD patients treated with esomeprazole or laparoscopic antireflux surgery in the LOTUS trial. Am J Gastroenterol. 2010;105(5):1015–23.

128. Schoepfer AM, Gonsalves N, et al. Esophageal dilation in eosinophilic esophagitis: effectiveness, safety, and impact on the underlying inflammation. Am J Gastroenterol. 2010;105(5):1062–70.

129. Straumann A, Conus S, et al. Long-term Budesonide maintenance treatment is partially effective for patients with eosinophilic esophagitis. Clin Gastroenterol Hepatol. 2011;9(5):400–9.

130. Alexander JA, Jung KW et al. Swallowed Fluticasone Improves Histologic but Not Symptomatic Response of Adults With Eosinophilic Esophagitis. Clin Gastroenterol Hepatol. 2012. PMID 22475741.

131. Peterson KA, Thomas KL, et al. Comparison of esomeprazole to aerosolized, swallowed fluticasone for eosinophilic esophagitis. Dig Dis Sci. 2010;55(5): 1313–9.

Gastroesophageal Reflux Disease

48

Denis M. McCarthy

Abstract

Gastroesophageal reflux, when excessive, causes a variety of injuries to the esophagus and adjacent organs: only local injuries to esophagus (gastroesophageal reflux disease—GERD), and their consequences are dealt with here. Discussed is the definition of GERD, diagnosis, epidemiology, pathogenesis, natural history, risk factors, management, complications, and how various facets of the disease give rise to disordered deglutition. In dealing with all aspects of GERD, a major emphasis is placed on prevention or reversal of severe disease, key to which is good medical management, not only by pharmacologic therapy, but also by providing the patient with education and insight into anatomical, functional, and lifestyle aspects of their disease, and how any specific adverse risk factors in their particular case can be minimized or abolished. The roles of neuromuscular abnormalities, transient lower sphincter relaxations, hypotensive sphincters, and hiatus hernia, in exposing the esophagus to impaired clearance of a noxious refluxate, with consequent mucosal injury, are summarized. Beyond these, and potentially increasing tissue injury, are numerous additional risk factors, comorbid conditions, and adverse effects of a number of drugs commonly used in treating other illnesses. Existing drug therapies for GERD (antacids, histamine antagonists, proton pump inhibitors, sucralfate) are examined in detail, and emerging pharmacotherapies are briefly reviewed. Endoscopic and surgical therapies are examined elsewhere in this volume.

D.M. McCarthy, MD, PhD (✉)
Division of Gastroenterology and Hepatology,
Department of Medicine, University of New Mexico
Health Sciences Center, 2211 Lomas Blvd. NE,
Albuquerque, NM 87131, USA
e-mail: denis.mccarthy2@va.gov;
dmccarthy@salud.unm.edu

R. Shaker et al. (eds.), *Principles of Deglutition: A Multidisciplinary Text for Swallowing and its Disorders*,
DOI 10.1007/978-1-4614-3794-9_48, © Springer Science+Business Media New York 2013

Keywords

Gastroesophageal reflux disease (GERD) • Neuromuscular abnormalities • Impaired esophageal clearance • Histamine H2-receptor antagonists (H2RAs) • Alginic acid/alginates • Rebound hypersecretion (RH)

Introduction

Gastroesophageal reflux (GER) is the effortless retrograde passage of gastric contents into the esophagus, a frequently occurring normal physiologic process that occurs daily in everybody, generally without causing symptoms. However, under a variety of different circumstances described later, GER may become pathological and give rise to gastroesophageal reflux disease (GERD), causing chronic symptoms or varying degrees of injury to the various tissue components of the esophagus and adjacent structures. GERD may manifest solely as symptoms, such as heartburn or regurgitation, or may be accompanied by a variety of observable changes in the structure or function of the esophagus that may interfere with the organ's normal physiologic task, the process of deglutition or swallowing. This process achieves the transfer of the ingested and masticated contents of the pharynx to the digestive and mixing reservoir of the stomach. Strictly speaking, GERD in many cases involves additional organs, because the refluxed gastric contents frequently contain substances refluxed from the duodenum, including pancreatic, biliary, and intestinal secretions. In like manner, GERD may extend beyond the esophagus causing injury to the larynx, lung, pharynx, and adjacent organs. However, this chapter mainly pertains to the ways in which GERD may interfere with deglutition.

For over a century, investigators have sought to understand the process of reflux, and various mechanisms have been postulated as the sole or main cause. In retrospect many of these postulates have merit, but no single pathogenic mechanism can be accepted as explaining GER in all cases. In the past 20 years, it has become apparent that multiple pathogenic factors operate in many cases and that, even in an individual case, different factors may be dominant at different times or stages of the disease. This chapter will try to cover the disease broadly, in the full realization that the factors operating in the individual may be unique to that case. On the other hand, some causes of reflux and some failures of defenses against it are of much more general importance.

Definition

An operational definition of GERD as *"a condition which develops when the reflux of stomach contents causes troublesome symptoms and/or complications,"* known as the "Montreal Definition," has gained wide acceptance by interested parties, including the American Gastroenterological Association [1, 2]. However, despite its popularity, the definition lacks any quantitative dimensions that help epidemiologists or research scholars to measure accurately the incidence, prevalence, or severity of the disease. The principal symptoms of GERD are heartburn and regurgitation, both of which may also occur in normal subjects, associated with overeating or other dietary indiscretions. Such occasional occurrence of symptoms does not rise to the level of a disease and should not be used to justify prescribing powerful, expensive drugs, often used long term, when sensible adjustments to behavior or lifestyle could avoid the symptoms. Personally, I favor a clinical definition, such as *"GERD is the occurrence of heartburn or regurgitation once or more daily, for at least 3 months."* Others might argue for a frequency of *"twice per week,"* or even *"weekly"* instead of *"daily,"* but most would agree that, in order to accept such patient complaints as a disease, they should be chronic. A basic clinical definition should be based on symptoms and not on complications that occur only in a minority of those with the disease. Findings at endoscopy, on X-ray, pH-metry, biopsy, or other modality can be used to classify the disease or measure its severity, but are not needed for diagnosis in most cases. I accept that such a definition underestimates the true prevalence of the disease, which in some cases may give rise to other less typical presenting symptoms, including epigastric pain, pharyngeal burning, regurgitation of gastric contents, acidic or bitter taste in the mouth, atypical chest pain, dysphagia, or rarely odynophagia. Occasionally the disease may present with extra-esophageal complications or with a condition such as anemia that on investigation proves due to esophageal disease, but such presentations are much less common. Any definition of GERD is ultimately arbitrary, frustrating attempts to measure its impact or accurately assess the effects of therapy. However, there is danger that an overly liberal or loose definition, such as the Montreal definition may lead to excesses in drug therapy, diagnostic procedures, public anxiety, and hence costs of care, for a disease that in most cases can be readily controlled and has a good outcome.

Diagnosis

The essential requirement for diagnosis of GERD is the demonstration of gastric contents in the esophagus. This is usually achieved indirectly by recording intra-esophageal changes in pH showing the presence of acid, changes in bilirubin absorbance showing the presence of duodenal contents, or changes in electrical impedance showing the cephalad migration of liquid or gas from distal to more proximal esophagus. Endoscopy does not establish the presence or absence of reflux but, either by visually documenting esophagitis or its complications, or by obtaining mucosal biopsies for microscopy, endoscopy is important in establishing the severity of the disease. Because GERD is frequently associated with disorders of motility, this aspect of a patient's symptoms is evaluated by manometric recording of intra-luminal pressures, with changes over time in various anatomical regions. These techniques are described in detail in Volume II.

Epidemiology

Over the past century, but especially in the past 30 years, there has been major evolution in our understanding, recognition, classification, and management of GERD [3]. Earlier attempts to describe the epidemiology [4–7] suffered from the lack of an exact definition of the condition, of a gold standard for its diagnosis, and from longstanding confusion about the relationship between GERD and hiatus hernia. Early studies equated the prevalence of GERD with that of the cardinal symptoms heartburn and regurgitation, although these symptoms may be absent in 65% of patients with esophagitis and in most patients with Barrett's esophagus (BE) [5]. With growing recognition of non-erosive esophagitis, it is now established that endoscopic appearances of the mucosa are normal in up to 75% of patients with GERD symptoms [8]. Heartburn, often but not necessarily associated with regurgitation, is very common, occurring in about 20% of the US population weekly, with regurgitation alone occurring in about 2% [9]. The exact prevalence of chronic or sustained heartburn (as defined earlier) has not been studied, but is probably about 10–20% in western countries and 1–5% in Asia. Only a minority of patients with occasional symptoms has a serious chronic disease. However, among the 20% with at least weekly heartburn in the USA, 79% had nocturnal heartburn: among these 65% suffered both day and night, with the night time heartburn being rated as more troubling in over half the subjects [10].

In prevalence studies of whole populations, 4–7% have daily symptoms and 2–3% esophagitis [11]. In contrast, among selected patients referred for upper gastrointestinal endoscopy, about 20% have esophagitis, most of it mild. Two population-based studies from Scandinavia showed no significant effect of age on the *prevalence* of reflux esophagitis, but among patients with GERD, the *severity* of esophagitis and related complications increases with age [12–14], as do hospitalizations for esophagitis, esophageal ulcer, and esophageal stricture [15]. At the same time, due to diminished organ sensitivity, the prevalence and severity of heartburn may decrease and mask the presence of severe esophagitis [13]. Aging is thus associated with more severe patterns of acid reflux, esophagitis, and related conditions, but these are less reliably associated with typical symptoms: this leaves some uncertainty about prevalence in the elderly [14].

In a large US study of the distribution of all forms of GERD, esophagitis, esophageal ulcer, stricture, hiatus hernia (HH), and pyrosis (heartburn) were found clustered in the same patient population, with older age, male sex, and white ethnicity being risk factors for the most severe types [16]. Heartburn, often milder and sometimes functional, was common in women. Data on the incidence of the disease are scarce and somewhat contradictory [6], but incidence rates of new cases of esophagitis in northern European countries are between 4.5 and 120 cases per 100,000 of population per year [6, 11]: mortality attributable to GERD is negligible [7]. So many reservations surround interpretation of data on the prevalence and incidence of GERD, that while perhaps 10% of the population are significantly affected, all estimates are at best crude and changing.

All forms of GERD and its complications exhibit numerous temporal, geographic, and demographic variations. Prevalence is highest in developed countries but comparatively lower in developing countries in Africa and Asia, though rising rapidly in Japan. In the USA, all forms of GERD occur more in Caucasians than in African Americans or Native Americans. Worldwide, all variants and complications of the disease seem to be on the increase, including adenocarcinoma of the esophagus, which is now surpassing gastric cancer in Ireland and the UK. While this increase in GERD is incompletely understood, three risk factors at least are suggested as contributing to the time trends, namely eradication of *Helicobacter pylori* (*H. pylori*) infection [17], dietary changes [18], and obesity [19].

The prevalence of *H. pylori* infection, and associated gastritis, is rapidly decreasing in many countries due to both improved socioeconomic conditions and to pharmacological eradication. *H. pylori*-attributable gastritis, in some cases lowers acid secretion and diminishes gastric acidity. Conversely, disappearance of infection increases gastric acidity and in many cases that of GE refluxate. Increased acidity stresses mucosal defenses, may increase the incidence of GERD, esophagitis, and rarely in other complications, including BE and adenocarcinoma [17]. The risks of these complications occurring may be higher in obese subjects and in those with hiatus hernia.

In major surveys in both the USA and Asia, certain dietary patterns are linked to the occurrence of reflux, GERD, and adenocarcinomas of both the esophagus and gastric cardia, with diets high in food derived from animals, particularly fats, associated with increasing the risks [18, 20]. Diets with foods derived from plants are associated with much lower risks. In addition to these qualitative differences in diet, quantitative increases in certain dietary components, particularly fats and refined sugars, are associated with increased caloric intake and, combined with diminishing physical activity, are leading to an epidemic of obesity, in all age groups, in many regions of the world. In individuals, becoming obese is accompanied by the development of GERD, the severity increasing with increasing body mass index (BMI) [20, 21]. The mechanisms by which obesity affects reflux and clearance are numerous, with adverse consequences exacerbated in the presence of hiatus hernia [22]. The impact of rising prevalence of obesity on all aspects of GERD is clearly discernible in population studies from many areas of the world.

Pathogenesis

The etiology of reflux, either as a cause of GERD symptoms or of mucosal disease, is not fully understood, but broad outlines of the problem are known [23, 24]. Mucosal injury develops when the noxious effects of gastric refluxate (acidity, composition, and potency) persist in the esophageal lumen for a time sufficient to overcome the defense mechanisms of the organ (luminal clearance, pH restitution, and mucosal resistance). Most of what we know suggests that its causes arise from disordered neuromuscular function, primarily in the lower esophageal sphincter (LES) but also in the esophageal body. The possibility that the disease arises primarily as a defect in

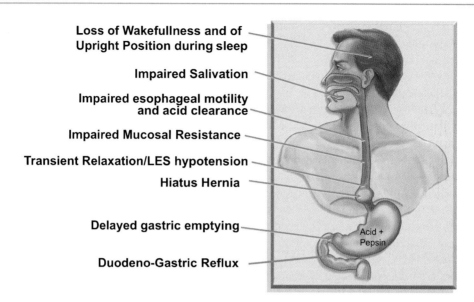

Loss of Wakefullness and of Upright Position during sleep

Impaired Salivation

Impaired esophageal motility and acid clearance

Impaired Mucosal Resistance

Transient Relaxation/LES hypotension

Hiatus Hernia

Delayed gastric emptying

Duodeno-Gastric Reflux

Acid + Pepsin

Fig. 48.1 Protective mechanisms include production of bicarbonate and saliva, which neutralize refluxed acid, and esophageal clearance (caused by gravity and peristalsis), which minimizes the contact time between acid and the esophageal mucosa following a reflux event [2]

esophageal mucosal resistance or motility in some cases cannot be disregarded [25]: a plausible but unproven hypothesis is that "a primary defect in LES function or tissue resistance is responsible for initiation of the disease, and that its chronicity and severity are determined by the type and number of coexistent or subsequently acquired (secondary) defects over time" [23]. For the most part, the disease is best thought of as multifactorial in etiology due to the interaction of a number of different factors, any one of which may be primarily important in an individual patient. These are shown in Fig. 48.1. Many of these are exacerbated by sleep or recumbency.

Neuromuscular Abnormalities

Incompetence of the LES arises in three different ways, as a result of (a) hypotensive LES, (b) transient lower esophageal sphincter relaxations (TLESRs), and (c) anatomic abnormalities associated with hiatus hernia [26]. About 20% of patients have LES incompetence due to decreased sphincter pressure (neuromuscular tone), to increased intra-abdominal pressure (often reversible with pregnancy, obesity, or ascites), or to

defective anatomy (LES < 2 cm long). However, most symptomatic patients have a normal LES pressure (LESP), but experience TLESRs. These are brief episodes of sphincter relaxation, unrelated to swallowing or peristalsis, but reflexly evoked in response to postprandial or other gastric distension, especially with fatty meals that release cholecystokinin. They are mediated by the vagus nerve and thought to facilitate belching, but eructation of gas may be accompanied by reflux of gastric contents. Although they also occur commonly in normal subjects, in GERD patients a higher percentage of TLESRs are accompanied by reflux. In addition to reflux resulting from the above causes, injury may be greatly exacerbated by another neuromuscular factor, impaired, ineffective, or absent peristalsis, resulting in delay in clearance of refluxate from esophagus, as described later.

Transient Lower Esophageal Sphincter Relaxations

While the LES may relax for up to 10 s to allow the passage of a food bolus, it is normally maintained closed in a state of tonic contraction, at a pressure of 5–30 mmHg above intragastric pressure. This is the main barrier to GE reflux. Competence of the sphincter is regulated by two components, the actual intrinsic sphincter in the muscle of the esophageal wall and an extrinsic sphincter formed by the crura of the diaphragm [27]. The normal regulation is complex, but the diaphragmatic component is of key importance. In normals, actions of both component are closely coordinated in space and time: overall sphincteric tone must adjust to inspiration (when intra-thoracic pressure becomes negative), body position, abdominal pressure, and gastric distension, and be actively relaxed to permit vomiting and swallowing.

TLESRs are brief episodes of relaxation that occur in response to gastric distension via stimulation of vagal sensory and motor nerves. They occur in normal subjects and in those with GERD, last from 10 to 35 s, and may or may not result in reflux. They are strongly associated with reflux when it occurs. In both normal patients and those with GERD, the majority of reflux episodes occur during TLESRs: the frequency of reflux-associated TLESRs is increased in those with GERD. They do not occur during sleep.

Whether or not the reflux occurring in the setting of TLESRs results in GERD may depend primarily on the adequacy of the esophageal response, i.e., the adequacy of the secondary peristalsis needed to achieve rapid clearance of the noxious material from the esophagus. At endoscopy, TLESRs are more frequently associated with non-erosive esophageal disease (NERD), although microscopically dilated intercellular spaces (DIS), the most sensitive morphological indicators of mucosal injury, are also visible in NERD, as they are in more severe esophagitis [28, 29]. TLESRs are less commonly seen in association with hiatus hernia or severe or complicated esophagitis, but the presence of HH increases the probability that a TLESR will lead to reflux. Although the contribution to GERD of delayed gastric emptying remains somewhat controversial, it is believed that at least in many cases, accentuated postprandial fundal relaxation may provoke abnormal food retention, increase proximal gastric distension, and trigger an increase in the number of TLESRs and reflux [30]. TLESRs are considered the commonest cause of GERD, much of it occurring postprandially, in daytime, in the upright position, and often associated with mild-to-moderate disease or NERD, despite causing symptoms that may be difficult to control.

Hypotensive LES

When LESP is low or absent ("patulous sphincter"), reflux into the esophagus occurs readily when gastric pressure is even slightly higher than intra-thoracic pressure, or there may even be "free reflux," with contents moving up and down the esophagus with little provocation or in response to swallowing or any kind of abdominal straining. However, very low or absent LESPs may also be seen in the presence of a hiatus hernia (below). Esophageal mucosal injury is generally more severe in patients who have subnormal resting LESP, i.e., impaired intrinsic muscle contractility. Studies in man have indicated a strong correlation between the prevalence of peristaltic dysfunction and the severity of esophagitis, but (using older manometric techniques) did not find a correlation between the occurrence of peristaltic dysfunction and hypotensive LESP [25]. This argues against the probability that the hypotonic sphincter pressures were the consequences of esophagitis, primarily due to impaired peristalsis as may occur in NERD. Experimental injury to the cat esophagus (in the absence of hiatus hernia) leads to a reduction in LESP, reversible on lesion healing. However, in man healing of esophagitis with omeprazole, in patients with low LESP, has very rarely restored esophageal motility to normal [31]. Thus, the cause of hypotonic sphincter remains unclear but it is associated with an increase risk of GER, especially when hiatus hernia is present.

Hiatus Hernia

Hiatus hernia (HH) refers to a group of disorders that result from disruption of the attachments to the diaphragm of the lower end of the esophagus where it passes into the abdomen. This loss of anchorage of the organ allows varying amounts of the esophagus and stomach (and occasionally other organs) to herniate up into the chest, in many cases impairing LES function. There are two main types of hernia, the commonest "sliding" variety accounting for 95% of cases, and the more rare "paraesophageal" hernias for the remainder [23–27]. These anomalies, particularly the "sliding" type, are common, increase with age, and occur in about 50% of subjects in Western countries by age 50 years. They probably arise from lifelong wear and tear on the ligamentous attachments of the organ due to respiration, pregnancy, heavy lifting, defecation, and all causes of increased abdominal pressure. Also hypothesized is that repeated reflux of acid into the esophagus causes repeated contraction of the longitudinal muscle of the organ, pulling it into the chest, gradually losing its anchorage within the abdominal cavity.

Hiatus hernia, most commonly the "sliding" type, can increase reflux in several ways. These may include reducing LES competence, "trapping" of contents above the diaphragm with occasional retrograde propulsion, and impairing (delaying) clearance of refluxed material from the esophagus. The larger the hernia is, the wider the hiatus and the more likely the development of incompetence of the crural component of the sphincter. A critically important feature of HH is that it also leads to spatial separation of the intrinsic and extrinsic sphincters and impairment of the normal temporal coordination of their actions. With cephalad displacement due to HH, the LES also becomes deprived of the synchronized re-enforcing contraction of the extrinsic crural sphincter, the main barrier against reflux. In this setting, minor increases in intra-abdominal pressure easily overcome the diminished resistance of the LES to reflux. With inspiration and increased negative intra-thoracic pressure, contraction of the diaphragm may cause fluid trapped above the diaphragm to escape upwards into the esophagus, past a hypotonic intrinsic LES, and also overwhelming ineffectual peristaltic waves that do not fully occlude the lumen. Reflux is greatest in

the absence of gravitational drainage, in the supine position, and during sleep. In patients with HH, some episodes of reflux may be provoked by TLESRs but, with persistent poor LES tone, most episodes occur in their absence.

Most patients with a hiatus hernia do not have GERD, but most patients with severe erosive esophagitis have a hiatus hernia, especially if complications are present such as an esophageal stricture or Barrett's esophagus. The reason for this is unclear [24].

Increase in volume of reflux and mucosal contact time leads to the development of severe esophagitis and its complications, esophageal ulcers, strictures, and Barrett's esophagus (BE): these are almost invariably associated with HH and rarely occur in its absence. In a study of 644 GERD patients subjected to endoscopy, followed by esophageal manometry and 24-h pH monitoring, the single strongest predictor of severe erosive esophagitis was the presence of a hiatus hernia [32]. Overall, it appears that the combination of HH and a hypotonic LES is associated with severe disease, independent of the occurrence of TLESRs.

Impaired Esophageal Clearance

If some physiologic reflux occurs in a normal subject, the content elicits a secondary peristaltic wave that returns >90% of the refluxate volume to the stomach, without reaching the subject's awareness. If gastric contents are acidic, the surface of the esophagus may temporarily remain at an acidic pH, even though the volume of acid remaining is small. "Restitution" of the pH to normal is achieved by a series of swallows of saliva, containing enough bicarbonate to buffer residual mucosa-adherent acid. If salivation is impaired by disease or effects of drugs, pH restitution may be delayed, although esophageal glands can also secrete small amounts of neutralizing buffer. Thus, normal clearance involves adequate salivation, swallowing, peristalsis, and esophageal glandular secretion, and is helped by the upright position. Clearance is impaired by sleep, which abolishes salivation and peristalsis, greatly delaying clearance [33]. These defense mechanisms are reactivated by adequate arousal, but exacerbated by sedative or hypnotic drugs. Various kinds of dysmotility contribute to impaired clearance, including the presence of weak (low amplitude) peristalsis, peristalsis that fails to propagate adequately, tertiary contractions that fail to propel contents, and occasionally segmental or diffuse esophageal contractions. The rate of occurrence of esophageal motility disorders is closely correlated with the prevalence of severe esophagitis [34].

Diminished clearance is seen in about 50% of patients with severe GERD, especially in the presence of hiatus hernia which appears to be associated with the most severe delays. Delayed clearance prolongs exposure of the mucosa to topical injury and appears more important to the development of esophagitis than the frequency of episodes of reflux, often of small volume and short duration. But the temporal duration of the episode does not appear to be the sole factor determining the severity of GERD. Both the occurrence of extra-esophageal symptoms and the patient's perception of reflux appear to depend on the proximal extent to which refluxate reaches up into the esophagus. This suggests the existence of spatial summation of the symptom stimulus, perhaps accounting partly for the symptoms in NERD patients with normal acid exposure [35].

Refluxate

Most injury to the mucosa results from direct or indirect action of acid, acting either alone or modifying effects of other components of the refluxate [36]. Although it is customary to talk of GER as if the refluxate is solely of gastric origin, studies using intra-esophageal combined pH and bilirubin absorbance monitoring have shown that acid reflux and duodeno-gastro-esophageal-reflux (DGER) occur simultaneously during most episodes [37]. Although acidity and peptic activity are of key importance, the refluxate also contains many other substances (derived from intestinal, biliary, and pancreatic secretions and products such as lysolecithin) whose individual effects on

esophageal mucosa, and their pH dependence, are not well characterized. Tissue injury is accelerated by both pepsin and conjugated bile salts. A pH < 4.0 seems to characterize refluxate closely associated with causing GERD, as assessed by the occurrence either of symptoms or esophagitis. The lower the pH of the refluxate, the higher the peptic activity, and the longer it takes for esophageal pH to return to normal, although the correlation between severity of symptoms and that of esophagitis is poor. At pH > 4.0 the enzyme pepsin is largely inactivated, greatly reducing reflux damage to the esophagus. While the duration of exposure of the mucosa at pH < 4.0 is a major predictor of GERD severity, in a minority of cases, particularly those treated with acid suppressants, persistent symptoms such as regurgitation or heartburn, presumably due to other components, also occur when refluxate pH is only weakly acidic or neutral [35, 38]. In various types of studies that monitor changes in luminal pH or impedance over 24-h, there is poor correlation between such changes and the occurrence of symptoms: symptoms occur without recorded changes and recorded changes also occur without symptoms, implying that the factors responsible for symptoms have not been completely identified. At the present time the volume being refluxed is unmeasurable.

Tissue Resistance

In subjects with normal clearance, GER causes contact between refluxate and esophageal mucosa for 1–2 h/day. The epithelium of the normal esophagus resists injury from this exposure. However, compared to the rest of the GI tract, lined with well-defended columnar epithelium rich in tight junctions, the esophageal squamous epithelium lacks surface mucus-secreting cells and the mucus coat needed to create adequate pH or other chemical gradients between lumen and cell surface. The few human electron microscopic studies performed show a paucity of tight junctions: intercellular spaces, bounded by desmosomes, mainly contain a glycoconjugate matrix substance that partly restricts diffusion of acid, but also appears to be acid soluble. Solubilization of this matrix allows the formation of fluid-filled DIS that increase permeability and offer little resistance to entry of noxious molecules into deeper layers of the tissue [39]. There these substances elicit responses from sensory and motor neurons, giving rise to symptoms and dysmotility; from inflammatory cells giving rise to esophagitis; from mesothelial/connective tissue cells, e.g., fibroblasts, supporting healing and repair at the cost of variable degrees of scarring; and finally from stem cells in the basal layers of the epithelium, where they stimulate proliferation, metaplasia, dysplasia, and carcinogenesis. Tissue resistance is comparatively weak and, in the absence of adequate clearance, easily overcome, thus causing inflammation and complications.

Complications

The basic failure of the epithelium to resist penetration by noxious molecules is manifested at first by the appearance of DIS in microscopic biopsies, followed in turn by increased proliferation of the basal epithelium, progressive increases in visible inflammation on microscopy and, finally, inflammation visible at endoscopy in 20–30% of cases. From initially nonspecific features, one or more small breaks in the mucosa may worsen progressively through more severe changes, as described in the Los Angeles classification [40]. The ultimate complications include focal and circumferential ulcers, "peptic" strictures, Barrett's esophagus (BE) and, very rarely esophageal adenocarcinoma that, in about 50% of cases, arises in the setting of BE. Less than 5% of GERD patients ever develop ulcers or strictures, even among those with erosive esophagitis. However, in one series, on measuring 24-h pH among those with complications, the mean percentage time that pH was < 4.0 was 26.2%, compared to 11.3% in those with esophagitis alone [41]. This was mainly attributable to increased acid reflux in the nocturnal period (midnight to 8 a.m.), 35.6% in those with complications compared to 5.2% in those without [41]. Related to this, the mean duration of

nocturnal reflux periods (15.4 min) was significantly longer in those with complications than in those without (2.1 min, $p < 0.001$), suggesting that impaired clearance was the main cause of complications.

There is no clear pattern of progression between successive grades of disease severity that predicts the development of complications. In most but not all patients, the most severe grade of disease they will develop appears to be diagnosed close to the onset of their disease [7]. Alternatively, without any antecedent history of esophagitis, the patient may present with iron deficiency anemia or with recurrent hemorrhage from an esophageal ulcer: a similar ulcer might be encountered in a patient presenting with odynophagia (painful swallowing). At endoscopy, diffuse or patchy erosive esophagitis may be found around an ulcer, or the ulcers may present acutely with bleeding or perforation. There is a strong association between ulcer and benign stricture [16], strictures (believed to arise from circumferential ulcers) tending to occur at slightly later ages. The classical presentation of a stricture is the development of progressive dysphagia but strictures may also be encountered by chance at endoscopy. However, the epidemiology of GERD is changing and other pathogenic factors may also impact on the development of complications, especially the use of aspirin and nonsteroidal anti-inflammatory drugs (NSAIDs).

Nonsteroidal Anti-Inflammatory Drugs

Aspirin (ASA) and the majority of NSAIDs are weakly acidic compounds, which at normal esophageal pH (7.0) are ionized. Because of this, they have little tendency to diffuse across the lipid membrane of the cell and reach the subcellular organs, e.g., lysosomes or mitochondria, where they can cause damage. However, in the presence of reflux (relatively common), with low intra-esophageal pH, drug ionization ceases and the compounds become highly lipid soluble. They can then readily enter epithelial cells, where they become ionized at the neutral pH, and are trapped inside the cells in high concentrations.

Hence, NSAIDs are believed to do little damage in the absence of reflux, but are quite injurious to the mucosa in its presence [42]. To what extent small amounts of reflux in patients with normal clearance cause injury is uncertain. NSAIDs are believed to injure cells by inhibiting the enzyme cyclooxygenase, thus impairing both cytoprotection and platelet function. The latter effect may cause bleeding from any preexisting GI lesion, e.g., an ulcer, but injury to the mucosa does not usually occur. In esophageal cells, arachadonic acid is primarily metabolized via the lipoxygenase pathway, with very little involvement of either cyclooxygenase or prostaglandins in physiologic functions.

In the inflamed esophagus, prostaglandins, e.g., PGE_2, derived from inflammatory cells are markedly elevated. These have pro-inflammatory effects, lower LESP, and in animal experiments increase the injurious effects of exogenous acid and pepsin, so that NSAIDs usually reduce inflammation. In large, case–control studies, both patients and controls on long-term NSAIDs have less heartburn, and show significantly reduced prevalence of esophagitis and esophageal cancer: it seems that systemic effects of NSAIDs are protective in most subjects. However, in the presence of more severe esophagitis, and in many comorbid conditions associated with long-term NSAID or ASA use, there is an associated high incidence of esophageal ulcers, ulcer bleeding, and strictures [43]. It therefore appears that with delayed transit, esophageal injury by ASA/NSAID is mainly a local effect, i.e., an interaction of both acid-peptic and topical effects that can result in either a focal "pill esophagitis" with scarring, or in more diffuse injury from mucosal exposure to aspirin or NSAID, undissociated at acid pH. Both drug and gastric juices contribute to the injury. All aspects of NSAID injury are greatly increased in those with hiatus hernia. Other factors that also increase the risks of therapy include preexisting GERD, co-therapy with prednisone, drinking alcohol, certain types of drug formulation, body position (recumbency), comorbid disease, e.g., scleroderma, esophageal dysmotility, and old age.

Other Risk Factors

There are numerous factors which increase the risks of both GER and GERD. These can be summarized under two main headings, i.e., factors that incite or exacerbate regurgitation and comorbid diseases known to be associated with GERD.

Factors That May Exacerbate Heartburn or Regurgitation

These are summarized in Table 48.1 and [7, 42, 44]. While all of the above agents have been reported by variable numbers of patients on occasion, none of them causes a problem all the time. Patients with a low LESP should be advised that they should where possible avoid exposure to anything that brings on or exacerbates their symptoms, including peppermint and chocolate. Except for long-term use of adrenergic agonists, theophylline, progesterone, and possibly anticholinergics, none of the medications that lower LESP are likely to play any significant role in pathogenesis of esophagitis or its complications, but may be relevant to symptom management. Progesterone is believed to be important in the heartburn of pregnancy and in symptoms due to hormone replacement therapy in women after menopause, a time when the severity of GERD symptoms usually diminishes.

Comorbid Conditions Clinically Associated with GERD

For a variety of reasons, numerous other diseases are associated with an increased prevalence of various types of GERD, either because of the nature of the disease or a consequence of its treatment. These conditions are summarized in Table 48.2. In general, management of associated GERD simply adds to the overall burden of patient care, but the conditions are not entirely independent. For example, optimal management of diabetes, obesity, or Zollinger–Ellison syndrome may lead to major improvement or remission in GERD symptoms, and adequate treatment of GERD may lead to the relief of laryngitis, hoarseness, or postsurgical morbidity. Weight loss is discussed under Lifestyle measures.

Table 48.1 Factors reported as occasionally provoking heartburn or regurgitation*

Increased intra-abdominal pressure	Use of listed drugs that reduce the lower esophageal sphincter pressure
Bending over, wearing tight belts, corsets or garments, lifting heavy objects, straining or contraction of abdominal muscles, gastric distension by food or drink, by delayed gastric emptying or by increased gastric secretions, pregnancy, ascites, or gross obesity	Anticholinergic drugs including tricyclic antidepressants, and some antihistamines, alpha-adrenergic antagonists, benzodiazepines, beta-adrenergic agonists, benzodiazepines, calcium channel blockers, nitrates, dopamine, theophylline, prostaglandins, lidocaine, narcotics, progesterone, and other related hormones
Ingestion of certain food	Miscellaneous
Onions, peppers, chiles, tomatoes, peppermint, chocolate, fatty meals, orange and other citrus juices, sodas and carbonated drinks, beer or ale (from gastric distension not alcohol effect), caffeine, caffeinated beverages, white wines. Some red wines may be protective	Business or vacation travel, week of long hours at work or work deadlines, stressful day (work, home, or family), anxiety and depression, recumbence, lying down

*The large number of references from which these data are drawn is principally: Sonnenberg and El Serag [7], McCarthy [42], Olivera et al. [44]

Table 48.2 GERD-associated condition

Mechanism	
Diabetes obesity	Delayed gastric emptying, various types, increased intra-abdominal pressure, and sleep apnea causing negative intra-thoracic pressure at night with reflux
Zollinger–Ellison syndrome	Reflux of highly acidic gastric contents
Mental retardation in childhood	Mechanism unknown, possibly genetic factors
Coronary artery disease	Use of nitrates and calcium channel-blockers: selection bias for chest pain
Laryngitis, hoarseness	Irritation by refluxate from esophagus
Chronic obstructive pulmonary disease	Common factor (smoking) delays gastric emptying, weakens lower esophageal sphincter (LES), allows reflux
Duodenal ulcer	Endoscopy may cause detection bias
Hiatus hernia	Weakens LES, facilitates reflux
Systemic sclerosis, CRST variant	Weakens LES tone and peristalsis, causing failure of esophageal clearance
Sicca syndrome	Lack of saliva leads to impaired restoration of pH after GER
Rheumatoid arthritis	GERD exacerbated by NSAID use
Degenerative joint disease	GERD exacerbated by NSAID use
Pregnancy	Increased intra-abdominal pressure with LES weakened due to hormonal factors
Achalasia	Myotomy may damage sphincter as may dilation
Nissen fundoplication	Requiring postoperative dilation
Postsurgical states following esophageal, gastric, and obesity operations	Vagotomy and reflux of duodeno-gastric both followed by gastritis and esophagitis
Surgery or trauma requiring prolonged use of a nasogatric tube	Presence of NG tube facilitates prolonged presence of gastric contents

Most data modified from Sonnenberg and El Serag [7, 43]

Natural History

On this aspect of the disease, definitive evidence is scarce. Although existing publications have been competently reviewed [18], the studies are largely retrospective, observational, and not standardized enough for confident conclusions to be drawn. Despite these limitations, the consensus is that in most cases GERD does not progress to disease much more serious than that described at endoscopy early in its course, although symptoms may change. From a review of published literature, from 0 to 30% of cases progress from NERD to mild esophagitis, and from 1 to 22% progress

Table 48.3 Drugs causing topical mucosal injury: may exacerbate mucosal injury in GERD patients

Alprenolol, ascorbic acid, aspirin, analgesic combinations
Antibiotics: many reported but especially doxycycline, tetracycline, penicillins, lincomycin, clindamycin, tinidazole
Bisphosphonates: alendronate and risidronate
Captopril, cromolyn, chloral hydrate, emempropium bromide, estramustin phosphate, ferrous sulfate and other iron salts, isoretinoin
Nonsteroidal anti-inflammatory drugs
Potassium chloride—nonliquid preparations, quinidine gluconate or sulfate, theophylline and derivatives, valproic acid, and over 70 less commonly used drugs

These drugs may also injure the esophageal mucosa in normal subjects, but are likely to cause more serious injury when their presence in the esophagus is prolonged by the presence of strictures or dysmotility due to GERD [42]

from mild esophagitis to moderate or severe esophagitis [45]. In at least one-third of cases, the disease regresses or disappears: the majority of cases remain uncomplicated. Currently in progress, a prospective European study (PROGERD) of a cohort of 3,894 patients is planned to run for at least 5 years. A preliminary report of results obtained over a 2-year period supports the estimates given earlier [46]. This careful prospective study indicated that Barrett's esophagus appeared to develop de novo in 5.8% of those with LA grade C/D esophagitis, in 1.4% of those with LA Grade A/B, and in 0.5% of those with NERD [46]. Reports of transitions from NERD to erosive disease, or of de novo development of BE, may be somewhat inflated by failure to note the presence of minor abnormalities at the first endoscopy. Development of BE is rare unless present on initial assessment.

In an early retrospective study of 3,880 cases of erosive esophagitis studied over a 12-year period [47], only 1.21% developed strictures; cases were on average 9 years older, frequently had HH, and 75% had at least one other possibly provocative factor (e.g., using NSAIDs). Some of the drugs in common use that can lead to esophageal ulcer or stricture, or exacerbate existing lesions are given in Table 48.3. In a study of discharge diagnoses in a large database, esophageal stricture and esophageal ulcer were strongly associated [15]. Esophagitis, esophageal ulcer, and esophageal stricture all showed age-related rise in hospitalization, especially stricture. This probably reflects increasing severity of disease with age although, as pointed out by the authors, it could reflect the impact of other factors associated with age, such as decreased salivation or peristalsis, or increased acid secretion. As in other studies, the later onset of these complications is thought to reflect the longer time it takes to progress to stricture, but stricture occurs only in a small number (5–8%) of cases [16, 47]: recurrence is reduced by maintenance pharmacotherapy.

Esophagitis and its complications are all interrelated. In a very large retrospective study of 194,527 US veterans with various types of GERD, followed between 1981 and 1994, any type of GERD was ten times more likely to be found in a patient with another type of GERD than without [16]. Omitting symptomatic disease, the relationships found between the four major types of GERD are shown by permission in Fig. 48.2. In addition, the authors later reported on 29,500 patients with erosive esophagitis but without ulcers or strictures, and followed them over a 4-year time period (range 1–12 years): not one of these patients subsequently developed an ulcer or a stricture. In striking contrast, among a comparison group of 5,100 esophagitis patients who had an ulcer of stricture on initial presentation, over 80% were repeatedly diagnosed with the same complications during follow-up [48]. Whether the risks of extra-esophageal complications increase with disease duration has not been investigated. Remaining uncertainties, about the natural history of GERD, as it effects infants, children, and adults, and particularly as it evolves in underdeveloped countries [49], need ongoing well-designed prospective studies.

Impact of GERD on Deglutition

GERD is one of the most common causes of difficulty in swallowing, i.e., of the symptom of dysphagia. This symptom arises from a sensation that may or may not be accompanied by a definable impairment of the swallowing process. Dysphagia should not be confused with odynophagia, painful swallowing. This usually arises from inflammation

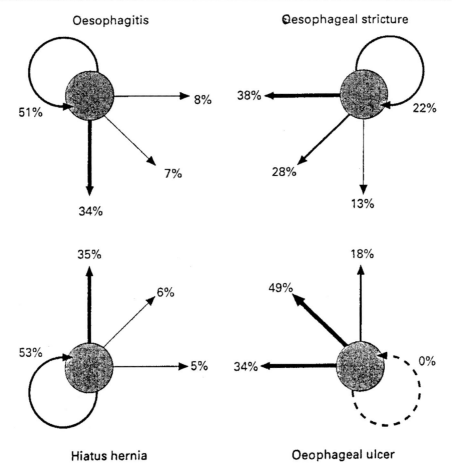

Fig. 48.2 Comorbid associations between four forms of GORD, each *arrow* representing one association. The percentage describes the fraction of patients with one form of GORD (where the *arrow* starts) who also suffer from a second form (to which the *arrow points*). The *circular arrows* represent patients who have one form of GORD as their sole presentation. From H.B. El Serag and A. Sonnenberg. Gut 1997;41:594–9 with permission

due to viral or fungal infections, pill injury or radiation, and is uncommon in GERD. In some cases, both symptoms may occur in the presence of esophageal ulceration, regardless of cause: ulceration can be a complication of GERD. Neither should dysphagia, difficulty in swallowing, be confused with a "Globus" sensation, a persistent non-painful feeling of having "a lump in the throat" unrelated to swallowing and in the absence of any radiologically demonstrable mechanical or anatomical abnormality.

Dysphagia in GERD

Dysphagia may occur in GERD through a variety of mechanisms. The symptom, a sensation, may arise from the presence of a stricture; from esophageal dysmotility of various kinds; from the presence of a ring or obstruction following surgical operations, e.g., fundoplication; or from esophageal hypersensitivity associated with inflammation. It may also rarely be associated with odynophagia.

Stricture

The term is usually applied to a lesion that narrows the lumen to a diameter that impedes the passage of swallowed material from the mouth to the stomach. In most cases the consequent dysphagia is progressive, initially present just for solids, but later for both solids and liquids, ultimately leading to weight loss. As a stricture narrows, heartburn and regurgitation usually diminish as reflux becomes restricted, but may still be presenting symptoms. Most strictures are benign: they vary in diameter, including some that cause total occlusion of the lumen. In length they range from a few millimeters to many centimeters. They are usually accompanied by esophagitis in adjacent mucosa, and biopsies (indicated in all cases) usually reveal the presence of inflammation, edema, and submucosal fibrosis. However, the differential diagnosis at endoscopy, as to their cause, includes carcinoma, rings, extrinsic masses, or muscular spasms, and anywhere in the esophagus biopsies of lesions may reveal the presence of Barrett's esophagus. In those with GERD, strictures evolve slowly, may be associated with HH, and are commoner in the elderly. Once present, they may be exacerbated by use of medications that cause "Pill Esophagitis," including NSAIDs and the medications listed in Table 48.3 [42]. While most strictures respond to one or more dilations at endoscopy, over time they tend to recur. The rate of recurrence appears reduced by long-term therapy with proton pump inhibitors (PPIs) [50]. In a very large study of data from over a million cases in the UK general practice research database from 1994 to 2000, the incidence of esophageal stricture was 1.1 per 10,000 patient years, rising markedly with age [51]; the recurrence rate was 11.1 per 100 patient years but with long-term PPI use the Relative Risk fell to 0.6 (95% CI: 0.3, 1.1). [51]. Rarely strictures are so severe as to require surgical resection or other complex operative procedures.

Esophageal (Schatzki) Rings

A Schatzki or "B ring" is classically a thin, circumferential, diaphragm-like, mucosal ring usually located at the squamo-columnar junction, whose pathogenesis is controversial [52]. Viewed by Schatzki as a congenital diaphragm which, once dilated, never recurred, the location of mild strictures seen in GERD often appears to be identical, and one study showed similar rings in 62% of patients who had ingested medications known to cause "Pill Esophagitis." Symptoms associated with these rings occur only intermittently, e.g., when swallowing a large piece of meat inadequately chewed: the rings or the dysphagia rarely progress. Dysphagia predictably occurs in patients with a luminal diameter of < 13 mm, but may vary with the size of bolus. The diagnosis may be confirmed radiographically by a Barium Swallow, employing barium tablets or barium-impregnated marshmallows of graded sizes. The ring is also visible at esophagoscopy. Patients usually do well after the first dilation with a 54–60 F dilator. However, if GERD symptoms are present and long-standing or previous dilation has been performed, repeat dilations should be gradual and more cautious, as for inflammatory strictures that may suddenly rupture with excessive stretching.

Postoperative Strictures

Surgical procedures, e.g., Nissen or Toupet fundoplication done to treat GERD, may cause a stricture if the wrap is too loose (reflux not abolished). Other operations, e.g., Heller myotomy for Achalasia followed by severe reflux, esophagitis and stricture, or the sequelae of photodynamic, radiofrequency ablation, or mucosal resection therapy of Barrett's esophagus, may also require repeated dilation, the contributions of reflux to these being uncertain.

Dysmotility

GERD, but especially erosive esophagitis, may be associated with a number of motility disorders, all of which interfere with the normal peristalsis that is so important to esophageal clearance, a critical part of the organ's defenses against reflux. Associated abnormalities include diminished amplitude and force of contraction, poor propagation of the peristaltic wave, intermittent tertiary contractions, and other nonspecific changes. The diagnosis of these is much more frequent when test swallows are performed with applesauce instead of water [53]. These disorders of motility may lead to difficulty in swallowing, the severity of which may in some cases be correlated with the severity of erosive esophagitis. In the absence of a stricture, dysphagia usually resolves with improvement in esophagitis.

More recently an entity "ineffective esophageal motility" (IEM) has been defined by the presence of distal esophageal contraction amplitudes of < 30 mmHg or non-transmitted contractions, in >30% of wet swallows [54]. Hypotensive LES and erosive esophagitis are significantly more prevalent in IEM patients than in non-IEM patients, but the relationship of IEM to GERD remains uncertain. The prevalence of IEM is usually associated with abnormal acid exposure, regardless of the presence of defective LES, HH, or esophagitis [55]. Although IEM-associated reflux is mainly acidic, it has been seen in a minority of those with nonacidic reflux. Although IEM is the most frequently observed abnormality in GERD, it may be insufficient as the sole determinant of mucosal injury, and it remains uncertain as to whether it is a primary cause of GERD or a consequence of the disorder. It has also been suggested that there are different manometric subtypes of the disease; patients in the subset featuring a majority of low amplitude simultaneous contractions (LASC) experienced less heartburn (prevalence 26%), but more dysphagia (57%) than those in the subset featuring low amplitude propagated contractions (LAP: heartburn 70%, dysphagia, 24%) or in controls [56]. This may be particularly relevant to GERD patients with dysphagia but no luminal obstruction. Additional evidence that IEM may be a heterogeneous condition comes from ultrasonic measurements of esophageal wall thickness in various esophageal diseases [57, 58]. While many questions remain, IEM may be an integral and even primary part of GERD, regardless of mucosal injury. Effects of specific drug therapies have not been described.

Esophageal Hypersensitivity

While it has been customary to suggest that mucosal inflammation may cause increased patient awareness of the passage of a bolus, in the absence of luminal obstruction or disordered motility, this suggestion is not well supported by experimental data. The role of visceral hypersensitivity as a cause of chest pain is a separate issue. Cases of dysphagia due to hypersensitivity have not been carefully studied for the presence of subtle indicators of the presence of disease, e.g., DIS, IEM, or ultrasonically detected changes in the muscular wall, etc., but lowered pain threshold in responses to distension, or altered compliance of the esophagus, have not been documented in patients with dysphagia. However, recent studies using combined manometry-impedance techniques, performed in healthy volunteers and GERD patients, with and without IEM, showed no association between perception by the subject and either luminal pressures or impedance in any group [59]. This disparity led to the suggestion that "increased bolus passage perception in patients without mechanical obstruction might be due to esophageal hypersensitivity." This remains an area of uncertainty.

Management of GERD

Selection of Therapy

Management of GERD consists primarily of rapidly relieving the main symptoms, heartburn, and effortless regurgitation. Nausea is uncommon in GERD, though it may occasionally occur, especially in the mornings, in those with nocturnal reflux. Complaints of vomiting or retching, accompanied by contraction of the abdominal muscles, should raise suspicion of the presence of gastric or more distal disease, even if heartburn and regurgitation are also present. Use of antiemetic or prokinetic drugs to treat undiagnosed dyspeptic symptoms should be avoided.

Over-the-Counter Remedies

For those with occasional heartburn, patient self-medication with over-the-counter (OTC) drugs is widespread. Chief among the remedies used are antacid preparations containing aluminum or magnesium hydroxides, calcium carbonate, "milk of magnesia," or sodium bicarbonate—also sold as "bread soda," "baking soda," or "baking powder"—all of which can be used in moderation when heartburn is infrequent. However, if these are used very frequently or in excessive doses over a long period, and especially if combined with excessive intake of calcium carbonate, milk, or vitamin D, treatment can induce "milk-alkali syndrome," with metabolic alkalosis, kidney stones, and other side effects. This outcome is now rarely encountered except in those who are also taking daily calcium salts for osteoporosis or other bone diseases. Proprietary antacids, also containing aspirin, should be avoided. Antacids are a valuable adjunct for breakthrough symptoms that occur during acid-suppressive therapy with antihistaminic H_2-receptor antagonists or PPIs; unlike the latter drugs, they do not inhibit activation of PPIs.

Lifestyle Modifications

In previous sections, various risk factors that cause or exacerbate GERD have been identified. It appears axiomatic that avoidance of these should be part of any comprehensive strategy to treat GERD. Similarly, treatment of any comorbid condition associated with an increased prevalence or severity of GERD should be optimized. The quality of evidence available from studies on effects of changing lifestyle on GERD symptoms or esophagitis is confounded by comorbid illnesses, medication use, or study design. Although an industry-sponsored symposium concluded that use of lifestyle measures was not justified in endoscopy-negative reflux disease or reflux esophagitis [60], this opinion has been challenged by both experts and experienced practitioners [61]. What follows is a brief discussion of the roles of lifestyle factors, as presently prescribed by many physicians.

Certain Foods, including chocolate, alcohol (notably wines and beer), carbonated beverages, peppermint, onions, garlic, citrus and other fruit juices, tomato products, spicy foods, and rice cakes, have all been reported to cause reflux symptoms, accompanied by a variety of physiological effects that may or may not relate to symptoms. However, evidence from prospective studies that avoidance of any of these actually reduces the symptoms or severity of disease is either weak or absent [62–64].

Other Measures, shown in numerous studies to reduce esophageal acid exposure, include: using blocks or wedges to elevate the head of the bed 8–10″, sleeping on the left side, decreasing fat intake, ceasing smoking, avoiding recumbency for 3 h postprandially, walking after meals, chewing gum, and avoiding weight lifting or other heavy exercise [62–64]. For these also, evidence of clinical benefit is weak. This is not to say that such alterations are ineffective: it has just been hard to study them as isolated variables. Widely prescribed by practitioners, they may account for much of the 30–40% placebo response rates of symptom relief seen in clinical trials. Among them, elevation of the head of the bed 8–10″ is the most widely used: some patients with very severe nocturnal symptoms even resort to sleeping in recliners or cardiac chairs.

Obesity, in discussing the epidemiology of GERD, mention has been made of association of the rising prevalence of GERD with a worldwide epidemic of obesity, the prevalence rate of GERD being closely associated with BMI. [19]. Effects on symptoms have been harder to define, but there is growing evidence that weight reduction may be a major factor in the overall management of GERD, both in prevention and treatment. Various types of bariatric surgery have led to disappearance of heartburn and regurgitation, but since the surgical operations generally reduce or abolish acid secretion, and also divert all duodenal contents away from the stomach, the ensuing symptom relief cannot be attributed solely to weight loss. In two studies, nonsurgical weight reduction has led to improvement in pH profiles,

LESP, and symptoms, especially regurgitation [65, 66], but another study failed to show benefit [67]. A large prospective cohort study in women showed that a 40% reduction in the risk of GERD symptoms for a reduction in BMI of > 3.5 kg/m^2 [21]. Most recently, in a careful prospective study of 213 obese patients (mean weight 100 kg), followed in a formal weight loss regimen for 12 months, the following changes occurred [68]. At 6 months there were significant reductions in mean weight, proportion of patients with GERD, and mean GERD scores compared to baseline. At the 12-month follow-up visit, changes were still present, but between 6 and 12 months there were increases in mean weight (86.1–89.3 kg), proportion of patients with GERD (16–22%), and mean GERD score (0.72–1.34) (all $p < 0.01$). This is the first prospective study to show a clear temporal relationship between body weight and GERD symptoms [68]. Although these findings are promising, further large, prospective, randomized studies (controlled for comorbidity) are warranted, before the benefit of weight loss alone is unequivocally established. Nonetheless, advising dietary (caloric) restriction is wise in most cases, since long-term therapy with PPIs may cause weight gain. At present, only weight reduction and elevation of the head of the bed are widely regarded as supported by reasonably strong evidence of therapeutic gain. In general, lifestyle measures should be regarded as useful adjuncts to any drug therapy in GERD, but are likely to have their greatest impact (even cure) in those with mild-to-moderate disease.

Histamine H$_2$-Receptor Antagonists

These include cimetidine, ranitidine, famotidine, and nizatidine. These can be used as nonprescription or prescription compounds, on a treatment schedule or as needed, and either as single agents or combined with antacids. For occasional use, the combination is popular: the onset of relief from the antacid, which neutralizes existing acid, is fast, but the relief does not last long. Slower acting by comparison, histamine H$_2$-receptor antagonists (H$_2$RAs) have a much longer duration of action

and block secretion of additional acid. Treatment with H$_2$RAs provides satisfactory control of symptoms in over 70% of cases, and is relatively inexpensive, especially when the cost of a doctor visit is avoided. For those with chronic symptoms who require scheduled regular use of drugs, twice daily use of ranitidine in appropriate dosage (150–300 mg bid) is a popular choice, because in addition to inhibiting acid secretion, ranitidine inhibits cholinesterase, increases cholinergic tone, achieving an increase in LESP and a modest acceleration of gastric emptying [69]. This is a useful benefit in those in whom gastric emptying is somewhat delayed due to sustained hyperglycemia or to co-therapy with opiates, calcium channel blockers, anticholinergics, and other drugs. A similar benefit attends the use of the more expensive but shorter acting nizatidine, but not cimetidine or famotidine. Since H$_2$RAs, unlike the PPIs, are much less affected by incorrect timing of administration, they are very useful in many patients unable to cope with a careful disciplined use of drug or many drugs. Furthermore, they can be administered orally or through feeding tubes, in rapidly bioavailable, liquid forms and in a variety of challenging situations, thus avoiding the high costs of intravenous infusions. For the minority of patients with severe symptoms or severe erosive esophagitis, esophageal ulcers, or strictures, H$_2$RA are considerably less effective than PPIs, especially in the length of time taken to bring symptoms under satisfactory control and are generally not used. However, H$_2$RA are well suited to most patients followed in primary care and are quite effective in over 50% of patients seen in subspecialty clinics, even in those poorly controlled on PPIs.

Administered intravenously, tolerance to HRAs, with associated tachyphylaxis, can develop rapidly, a point of importance in hospitalized patients with upper GI bleeding or hypersecretory disorders, but this tolerance has not been shown to be important clinically either in preventing stress-related mucosal disease or in long-term oral use in treating acid-peptic disorders. In a 1-year maintenance trial comparing ranitidine 150 mg bid against pantoprazole 20 mg qd, no tolerance to or lack of efficacy of ranitidine was apparent [70]. H$_2$RA use is relatively free from the rebound hypersecretion (RH) that follows PPI use and is therefore easier to discontinue, a point of importance in intermittent users. H$_2$RAs are also more effective than PPIs in inhibiting nocturnal acid secretion, but when combined, tolerance to H$_2$RAs may develop in some subjects, diminishing their effects: this issue is poorly studied. Most GERD is mild or moderate and tends to be overtreated, with insufficient emphasis on ensuring the patient modifies their lifestyle.

Alginic Acid/Alginates

A popular consumer, OTC product called Gaviscon™ contains a naturally occurring seaweed compound (alginate) and two antacids. When exposed to gastric acid the ingredients react to form a "raft" or mobile layer of a light but highly viscous gel that floats (because of trapped CO_2 bubbles) on top of any gastric contents. In the erect subject, this raft abolishes the postprandial "acid pocket" that floats at the top of the gastric contents and physically prevents reflux of acidic gastric contents into the esophagus [71]. Available as tablet or liquid preparations, the latter are more popular because of rapidity of relief of symptoms. Gaviscon™ has not been shown to heal erosive esophagitis and is therefore unsuited to use as a sole agent in the treatment of severe disease. However, it is devoid of systemic effects, relieves symptoms, and is therefore a popular choice for use in pregnancy. It may also be helpful in patients with a patulous or hypotonic sphincter, a large hiatus hernia, or as an adjunct to PPI therapy when symptoms persist despite adequate dosage. It is popular in primary care or as an OTC drug.

Sucralfate

Sucralfate is a mucosal protective agent that binds to inflamed tissue and various biologic molecules, e.g., as EGF, and some ingredients of gastric refluxate, e.g., pepsin, trypsin, or bile acids. It stimulates release of somatostatin from antral D-cells. Its mode of action is not precisely known

and little studied, for which reason it is rarely used by gastroenterologists [72]. Depending on pH, it binds to many drugs, potentially inhibiting their absorption, and its effect on the bioavailability of PPIs has not been established: conversely in the absence of acid (caused by the action of a PPI) sucralfate should be unionized and inactive. Despite these uncertainties, sucralfate as sole therapy may be an option in mild-to-moderate disease and appears to be safe in pregnancy. There have been three non-placebo controlled trials in erosive esophagitis, in which sucralfate was rated equally good as alginate, cimetidine, and ranitidine, though estimates of efficacy varied widely [73]. In similar studies which included a placebo arm, healing occurred in an average of 39% of cases, but 95% confidence intervals ranged from 3.6 to 74.8% and were not significantly different from placebo [73]. There is little evidence to support using sucralfate to treat GERD, and recent concerns that aluminum acts as a Th2 adjuvant, enhancing the risk of developing mucosal allergic disorders (possibly eosinophilic esophagitis), may add to current reluctance to use the drug [74].

H$^+$/K$^+$-Adenosine Triphosphatase Inhibitors ("Proton Pump Inhibitors")

This is the class of drugs most widely used to treat GERD. In all major analyses and scholarly reviews, there is strong evidence that, in the acute treatment of GERD, PPIs are statistically significantly superior to H$_2$-receptor antagonists (H$_2$RAs), which in turn are significantly superior to placebo [75]. These two classes of drugs form the backbone of therapy: no other classes enjoy major prescription use or carry similarly strong evidence of efficacy or safety.

Available PPIs

Five major PPIs, marketed in a total of 18 formulations, enjoy FDA approval for use in five indicated conditions. These data are summarized in Table 48.4 [76]. Only two of these indications

Table 48.4 Proton-pump inhibitors and their US Food and Drug Administration-approved indications [76]

Active ingredient	Trade name	Dosage form	Duodenal or gastric ulcer	GERD	Erosive esophagitis maintenance	Erosive esophagitis treatment	NSAID-induced ulcer
Omeprazole	Prilosec®	Oral capsule	X	XX	X	XX	X
		Oral suspension	X	XX	X	XX	X
	Losec® (Canada)	Oral capsule	X	X	–	–	X
	Prilosec OTC®a	Oral tablet	–	Xa	–	–	–
Omeprazole/ sodium bicarbonate	Zegerid®a	Oral suspension	–	X	X	X	–
		Oral capsule	X	X	X	X	–
		Oral chewable tablet	X	X	X	X	–
Lansoprazole	Prevacid®	Oral capsule	X	XX	X	XX	X
		Oral suspension	X	XX	X	XX	X
		Oral tablet	X	X	X	XX	X
	Prevacid FasTab® (Canada)	Oral tablet	X	XX	–	XX	X
Pantoprazole	Protonix®	Oral tablet	–	–	X	X	–
		Oral suspension	–	–	X	X	–
	Pantoloc® (Canada)	Oral tablet	X	X	–	–	X
Rabeprazole	Aciphex®	Oral tablet	Xb	XXc	X	X	–
	Pariet® (Canada)	Oral tablet	X	X	–	–	–
Esomeprazole	Nexium®	Oral capsule	–	XX	X	X	X
		Oral suspension	–	XX	X	X	X

GERD gastroesophageal reflux disease, *NSAID* nonsteroidal anti-inflammatory drug, *X* adults, *XX* pediatrics and adults

aNot available in Canada. Indication=treatment of frequent heartburn (>2 times weekly). Heartburn is listed as the only "use" for Prilosec OTC per product labeling description

bDuodenal ulcers only

cFor patients 12 years and over

concern us here, namely GERD (symptomatic relief) and erosive esophagitis (including complications). Several PPIs are available as OTC compounds and enjoy wide use by consumers, at lower cost but without medical supervision. Happily, the drugs are generally safe, well tolerated, associated with only trivial incidences of minor side effects, except perhaps for small percentages of rare complications in long-term users.

PPI Use

The principal orally used drugs are omeprazole, the s-isomer esomeprazole, lansoprazole, pantoprazole, and rabeprazole. A more rapidly acting compound "Zegrid" combines non-enteric-coated omeprazole powder with 1,680 mg of sodium bicarbonate (460 mg of sodium) but, while this does work rapidly, it delivers a large sodium load, a hazard in many common disease states. As ingested, all PPIs are acid-sensitive, inactive pro-drugs, released in the duodenum and carried by the bloodstream to the gastric mucosa [73]. There, during acid secretion, they are taken up by parietal cells, concentrated in secretory vesicles and canaliculi, and protonated by H^+. Following this they bind to adenosine triphosphatase [Adenosine Triphosphatase (ATPase), the "proton pump"]. The sodium bicarbonate in Zegerid stimulates gastrin release and gastric emptying, accelerates both the bioavailability and the activation of omeprazole, and results in faster onset of action. All PPIs arrest acid secretion only by actively secreting pumps, but do so regardless of the stimulus. For maximal efficacy, PPIs should be taken 30–60 min before eating a meal that stimulates acid secretion (preferably containing protein), so that drug concentrations in plasma are high when pump activation by acid secretion begins. True pharmacologic refractoriness or resistance to PPIs is extremely rare.

Choice of Therapy

All PPIs were originally formulated for once-daily use as a morning dose. However, as described earlier, for optimum responses, PPIs must be taken as instructed, and failure to do so is associated with poor symptom control. A morning dose works best in those with predominantly daytime symptoms. However, skipping or consuming a protein-free breakfast may render PPI therapy ineffective; improper timing of dose or poor patient comprehension of instructions also limit efficacy. In the face of such difficulties, use of an H_2-RA twice daily often proves more effective in patients with mild or moderate symptoms and is much less dependent on strict adherence to instructions. For many once-a-day users, taking their PPI dose before the evening meal is preferable, especially if nocturnal symptoms, erosive esophagitis, or hiatus hernia is present: some such cases may require twice daily therapy. Prior or simultaneous exposure to drugs that inhibit acid secretion greatly impairs activation of any PPI pro-drug and should therefore be avoided. Interfering drugs include H_2RAs, misoprostol, octreotide, anticholinergics, and cannabis. A bedtime dose of an H_2RA, given hours after the PPI, may not prevent activation of a morning dose of PPI, but large doses should be avoided: the practice is controversial. Supplementary small doses of antacid are both effective and preferable in relieving nocturnal breakthrough symptoms occurring during PPI therapy. Failure by physicians to spend time educating the patient, on the need for careful timing and most effective use of the drugs as described, is a common reason for poor response to therapy.

Dose of Drug

The effects of PPIs are somewhat dose dependent, although marketed (40 mg) doses of the newer drugs, e.g., pantoprazole, esomeprazole, and Zegrid™, have close to maximal efficacy: there is no convincing evidence that doses >40 mg/day are accompanied by additional clinical benefit. Among these specific PPIs, 20 mg doses have lesser effects. The term "twice daily PPI" applies to standard doses of omeprazole (20 mg), rabeprazole (20 mg), and probably lansoprazole (30 mg), but not to the 40 mg doses of the newer drugs. Drug trials that compare efficacies of unequal doses of different drugs are scientifically biased and should not guide therapy. In clinical trials, all of the drugs in standard doses heal erosive esophagitis in about 90% of cases but relieve symptoms in only ~75% of cases [73]. This failure of PPIs, to relieve symptoms as effectively as they heal esophagitis, probably arises from including in symptom trials some patients who complain of heartburn in whom reflux has not been demonstrated. Esophagitis-free patients whose symptoms do not respond to PPI, probably have what is now defined, under Rome III criteria, as "functional heartburn" (FH), i.e., burning retrosternal discomfort or pain in the absence of any evidence of GER or motility disorder [77]. Patients with esophageal hypersensitivity to acid (positive Bernstein tests) are excluded from FH, but not those with functional bowel disorders or those with visceral hypersensitivity to mechanical and other nonacidic stimuli in any organ. The apparent efficacy of PPIs to control GERD is lower in a clinical practice setting, particularly in controlling symptoms. This is due not to failure of drugs to act. It is partly attributable to FH, but is also due to widespread failure by physicians to fully understand the actions of the drugs and to educate patients carefully about how to use them [78]. A physician's first response to patient claims of poor effectiveness should be careful patient education and retrial of the normal dose. Only after the normal dose taken correctly fails, should a PPI dose be increased to b.i.d. The second dose is to be taken before the evening meal and not at bedtime. For patients whose symptoms are principally nocturnal, taking 40 mg before the evening meal may be better than taking 20 mg bid. For those with prominent day time symptoms, taking 40 mg in the morning, before breakfast, may best achieve symptom control.

Patterns of Therapy

There are a number of approaches to acute or short-term treatment, consisting of "step-up" therapy, where PPI therapy is reserved for those not responding to full doses of H_2RA taken bid, and "step-down" therapy, where initially PPIs are used but gradually replaced by H_2RAs or antac-

ids, as symptoms are controlled. Step-down therapy is more commonly employed initially for cases with severe symptoms or known severe or complicated esophagitis. Regardless of how treatment is begun, gradual reduction to the lowest effective dose PPI, or better still H_2RA, should be attempted in all cases, with the aim of stopping long-term use of drug whenever possible. For moderately severe disease, step-up and step-down therapies both work to about the same extent, equivalent to submaximal doses of HRAs [79]. The treatments control over two-thirds of patients, compared to a slightly higher number of similar cases treated successfully with "step-in" therapy when patients are treated with PPI throughout the period. How to end therapy is not well established, because of a general failure by doctors to recognize and manage the problem of "rebound hypersecretion" that accompanies the use of PPIs [80, 81], and lack of published, validated information on how best to stop the drug.

Rebound Hypersecretion

Administration of a PPI, by maintaining suppression of acid secretion, over time leads to dose-dependent elevation in serum gastrin, which in turn leads to hyperplasia of the parietal cell mass in the stomach. This increases acid secretory capacity. This Rebound Hypersecretion (RH) is not observable during PPI therapy, but is manifested within a few days when the drug is stopped abruptly [78, 79]. Affected patients experience a temporary increase in both acid secretion and related symptoms for at least the first week off drug, during which time an increase in symptoms may be interpreted as a failed response to therapy. The drug may be then hastily restarted, when symptomatic therapy for a brief period might have sufficed, or when tapering the dose of PPI over a period of weeks or longer, instead of stopping it abruptly, might have avoided the problem. RH has also been observed following H_2RA therapy but was milder and symptoms lasted only 2 days [82]. However, in studies of patients on PPIs for longer periods, the hypersecretion lasted at least 8 but <26 weeks [83]. In 50–75% of patients, the rebound effect is not recognized, and it may be diminished or absent in those with coexistent active gastritis due to *H. pylori* infection. On the other hand, normal volunteers given PPI therapy for a month develop de novo dyspeptic symptoms in 25–44% of cases when the drug is stopped [82]. Finally, PPI dependence and risk of RH appear to increase with duration of therapy, probably correlated with the progressive increase in parietal cell mass. The clinical importance of RH is currently uncertain, but likely to be of considerable importance, and demands prompt investigation.

Step-Down Therapy and Cessation of Therapy

There is no generally accepted way of stopping PPI therapy, and what little information exists comes largely from "step-down" studies. These studies show that patients with symptoms controlled on twice daily PPI can sustain reducing their dose to once daily, in 80% of cases, without developing symptoms [84]. A separate study showed that a gradual step down from PPI therapy, aiming to stop drug in those whose symptoms did not exacerbate, was successful in getting 58% of subjects off all PPIs, with about half the remainder off all drugs [85]. Since gastrin causes histamine release, patients may develop some tolerance to histamine as a result of PPI-induced hypergastrinemia and temporarily lessening the efficacy of H_2RAs, so that it may be prudent to step down from PPI to a relatively high dose of H_2RA (e.g., ranitidine 300 mg bid or famotidine 20 mg bid), later reducing this dose gradually. However, most patients with strictures will need a PPI indefinitely. Interest in funding trials that lessen drug consumption is minimal, so how PPIs should be reduced or stopped remains poorly studied.

Chronic or Long-Term Management: Maintenance Therapy

For those who have chronic symptoms or more severe disease, indefinite maintenance therapy (MT) is indicated. PPIs are clearly more effective than H_2RAs or placebo [86, 87], but are not needed in all cases. The lowest dose of drug needed to control symptoms or maintain healing should be employed. Varying with how the initial therapy is terminated and the success of lifestyle modifications during initial treatment, between 30% and 80% of GERD patients in practice receive maintenance therapy. Maintenance therapy is generally required for those with Barrett's esophagus, severe esophagitis, or strictures. In a study in Denmark, 2.1% of all patients in primary care were receiving long-term PPI care, with valid indications for therapy identified in only 27% of cases [88]. US figures are hard to come by, because of large, nonprescription OTC sales of drug, but are believed to be considerably higher.

Occasional Problems

PPIs alone do not achieve rapid relief of symptoms and are not well suited to being used "as needed" (prn). For relief of mild or intermittent symptoms they are less effective than antacids or HRAs. For patients who get occasional periods of more severe symptoms, and particularly for those who cannot easily afford expensive treatments, several other patterns of use have emerged. These include both "intermittent therapy (IT)" and "on-demand therapy (ODT)" which differ in key respects.

Intermittent Therapy

While often proposed this approach has been little studied. The idea is that if symptoms recur, given their slow onset of action, PPIs should be used for a defined period of time, before stopping: periods of 3–28 days have been proposed but not established, largely because of greater popularity of "on demand" therapy [89].

On-Demand Therapy

The basic concept of ODT is that the patient should decide when to start and when to end therapy, during an acute recurrence of symptoms. Having said this, formal *trials* of the effectiveness of ODT introduce a number of other variables that do not systematically apply in ordinary use, such as: limiting the number of tablets to one per day; asking patients to continue for 24 h after the last symptom; allowing "rescue antacids" that, in ODT, have efficacy not accounted for in trial comparisons; using numerous PPIs, or full or half the standard doses of a particular PPI, etc. A detailed review of the topic is beyond this brief summary but discussed elsewhere [89]. From various observations it is apparent that many patients choose and prefer ODT to continuous therapy. From over 20 trials with PPIs, the following conclusions are generally accepted. In ODT, the use of full or if preferred half doses of the originally effective dose of PPI may be confidently supported in managing (1) patients without erosive disease at endoscopy or (2) in empirically treating all those who have not had endoscopy, accepting that ODT will work fairly well, but not quite as well as continuous therapy with the same dose of the same PPI [90, 91]. Among the marketed PPIs, while all have enjoyed use in ODT, both pharmacokinetic properties and results of trials indicate that rabeprazole may be best suited to this use [92, 93]. Most ODT users are happy with this empowering, much less costly, and physician-independent approach, and elect to continue with it. In the specified types of patients, it enjoys greater patient acceptance than formal "step-up," "step-down," or continuous therapy: these kinds of patients account for upwards of 75% of all GERD patients seen in practice. ODT should not be attempted in those with severe erosive esophagitis (Los Angeles Grades C or D; Savary-Miller Grades 3 or 4) or in those with complications (ulcers, strictures, or Barrett's esophagus). Using ODT in cases with mild erosive disease has yielded mixed results and remains controversial [91]. In most patients using PPIs long term, it is recommended that stepping down, tapering, or stopping therapy should be attempted regularly: success in cases without a verified indication for therapy is unknown. Patients, in whom medical therapy as described earlier fails, should be referred to centers with special expertise in esophageal diseases that offer a variety of endoscopic and surgical approaches to treatment, but this need is uncommon.

New and Emerging Therapies

Given the high prevalence of GERD and apparent limitations of currently available therapy, there is a considerable amount of ongoing research directed at developing new therapies for the disease. These can be divided into five different approaches, aimed at modifying different aspects of pathogenesis. They are (1) acid-suppressive agents, (2) prokinetics, (3) anti-reflux drugs, (4) visceral pain modulators, and (5) mucosal protectants, in approximately that order.

Acid-Suppressive Therapies

Beyond marketed PPIs, many new formulations of existing PPIs, and a number of novel PPIs, are in various stages of development, the main focus being on the development of compounds with longer durations of action, many with PPIs released in such ways as to maximize their inhibitory effects on nocturnal acid secretion [94]. The most promising of these, still undergoing trials, is tenatoprazole, a new chemical entity devoid of the benzimidazole ring found in all other PPIs, and possessing a half-life of almost 9 h, and the longest duration of action to date. However, acid released at night may not have been first secreted at night but rather may represent re-release from sleep-associated cholinergic drive, of acid that had returned to intracellular vesicles as previous secretion ceased. Hence, there may be an inherent need for development of a compound drug, which combines a PPI with an acid neutralizing, or anticholinergic, or other type of pharmacologic agent, whose target is not the proton pump. This search continues. A Zegrid-like drug without excessive sodium would be attractive. Also under scrutiny are potassium-competitive acid blockers (P-cabs) that target the K^+-binding region of the H^+/K^+-ATPase, acting rapidly from within the lumen, and not requiring systemic absorption. P-cabs are excellent inhibitors of acid secretion, but early members of the class blocked potassium channels in other organs and have proved toxic: other P-cabs are under investigation. Finally, in the area of purely acid inhibiting drugs, a number of PPI–H_2RA combination drugs are under examination, but this approach is tempered by growing evidence that tachyphylaxis to the H_2RA component may develop rapidly: finding the correct doses to be combined, so as to inhibit nocturnal acid secretion despite development of tolerance, yet not impair PPI activation is challenging. A variation on the straightforward PPI is the NO-PPI: here the idea is to combine a PPI with an NO-releasing donor that would add mucosal protection by a gradually released NO to the acid-suppressive effect of a PPI. Initial PPI-NO compounds modifying lansoprazole and rabeprazole are undergoing preliminary testing.

Prokinetics

This term includes drugs that possess one or more of the following actions: increasing esophageal peristalsis (aiding clearance and limiting the proximal extent of penetration by refluxate); raising LES tone (reducing reflux); and increasing gastric emptying and/or intestinal peristalsis (reducing both gastric volume and the load of noxious substances refluxed into the stomach). A drug that would stimulate all of these actions would be of great interest. However, bethanechol, metoclopramide, cisapride, domperidone, tegaserod, procalupride, renzapride, benzamide, and itopride, and macrolide molecules [erythromycin, azithromycin, mitemcinal (GM-611), AB-229] have all been tested for clinical efficacy, but none have proved useful in GERD [95]. The first three, at effective doses, risk unacceptably serious side effects, and the other drugs have shown only unpredictable efficacy. However, the macrolide antibiotics, and more particularly the motilin agonists derived from them, have shown the greatest promise, and various new derivatives of these molecules are being actively studied [96]. The use of earlier motilin agonists was

attended by rapid development of tachyphylaxis, limiting their use. At present, given the absence of any effective safe prokinetic on the market, this is an area of very active research. In all likelihood, use of an effective prokinetic if available would be as an adjunct to PPI therapy, another "combination therapy."

Anti-reflux Agents

Reflux mainly occurs during TLESRs, not only contributing to frequent heartburn in those with NERD, but also contributing to regurgitation of weakly acidic and nonacidic refluxate in those in whom acidity has been suppressed by PPI therapy but who still have symptoms. As reviewed, TLESRs are reflex events mediated through central connections of the vagus nerve that convey efferent inhibitory traffic to the LES. The $GABA_B$ receptors mediating inhibition, and other receptors on the same neurons, can all be inactivated by an assortment of molecules including various GABA receptor agonists, glutamate antagonists, metabotropic glutamate receptor agonists or antagonists, and cannabinoids [95]. Some $GABA_B$ agonists also act at peripheral sites, the location of which is uncertain, achieving the same effects as they do when they act centrally. In addition, peripheral triggering of TLESRs can be inhibited by various cholecystokinin-A and nitric oxide synthase inhibitors. The search for a strong inhibitor of TLESRs, devoid of unwelcome central side effects, ranges over this whole group of molecules involved in inhibiting signals to inhibitory neurons. The first GABA agonist studied was baclofen, which dose dependently reduced esophageal acid exposure, nonacid exposure, and duodeno-gastric reflux and also improved GERD symptoms, both in NERD patients and in those with hiatus hernia. However, it has a short half-life requiring administration t.i.d. and, at clinically useful doses, causes too many CNS side effects. Arbaclofen, an isomeric R-baclofen prodrug, is better tolerated but not yet proven effective. Another of these compounds is lesogaberan, a peripherally restricted GABA agonist, superior to baclofen, thus far devoid of CNS side effects, and is currently being assessed in relieving GERD symptoms in human trials. These drugs or related derivatives that inhibit LES relaxation might be used as sole treatments in patients with NERD. More likely, if approved they may be used as adjuncts to PPI therapy ("combination therapy") in those whose symptoms are not controlled well by PPIs, despite reduction in acid secretion. They may also help those with hiatus hernias and severe erosive esophagitis, in whom TLESRs can be troublesome. Glutamate is the natural agonist involved in the vagal reflex that triggers TLESRs. Glutamate itself, and probably aspartate, bind to several metabotropic glutamate receptors (mGluRs) structurally related to $GABA_B$ receptors. Antagonists to one of these, mGluR5, are potent inhibitors of TLESRs. Antagonists to mGluR5, together with cannabinoid CB1 agonists that similarly inhibit TLESRs, are also being studied for efficacy, side effect profiles, and possible toxicity. Like drugs of the baclofen family, mGluR5 antagonists and cannabinoids may also be candidates for "combined therapy." This area is rapidly evolving and likely to change.

Visceral Pain Modulators

The precise contributions of visceral hypersensitivity and related disorders to various types of chest pains, including those due to functional heartburn (Rome 111 criteria), NERD, and residual symptoms not relieved on PPI therapy, are not clearly known at this time, though under active investigation [93]. In the meantime, a variety of pain modulators (in doses lower than those which alter mood) are being used, often empirically, in those with persistent symptoms. These drugs include: tricyclic antidepressants, trazodone, and selective serotonin or noradrenaline re-uptake inhibitors (SSRIs, SNRIs), all of which have enjoyed limited success, especially in those without evidence of reflux on endoscopy, 24-h multichannel intra-luminal impedance-pH monitoring (MII-pH), or biopsy. Although these appear to be the drugs of choice for functional heartburn, in ordinary clinical practice no clear guidelines have emerged for choosing either the patient or the therapy.

Mucosal Protection

Unlike the columnar epithelial lining most of the GI tract and Barrett's esophagus, the squamous columnar epithelium lining most of the esophagus is relatively "leaky" and unable to withstand prolonged contact with acid. Remaining uncertain is how much improved mucosal protection against reflux will, on its own, contribute to managing GERD. Increases in lumenal bicarbonate, from increasing salivation or from increasing the output of submucosal esophageal glands, are unlikely to control more than mild disease. Although the "mucosal protectant" drug sucralfate has been enjoying minor use for almost 30 years, its use, except perhaps in nonacid reflux, cannot be recommended. In the absence of prospective randomized controlled clinical trials, and clarification of how it works at near-neutral pH (during PPI therapy), mucosal protective therapy has no role.

Management of Dysphagia in GERD

In the first instance, all patients with GERD need standard medical therapy. However, it should now be apparent that relieving dysphagia in GERD first involves determining if a fixed luminal obstruction is present, such as a benign or malignant stricture or a Schatzki ring. This can best be answered by a variety of types of barium-radiographic techniques or by esophagoscopy. These investigations are generally complementary, the radiographic techniques providing information on the location, diameter, extent, and possibly pathologic nature of any anatomical abnormality. In addition, in many cases, fluoroscopy provides information on disturbances of motility or propulsion. Endoscopy, on the other hand, provides a much better appraisal of the mucosal surface, allows biopsy and pathological examinations of any suspicious lesions, and hence provides a definitive diagnosis of infection or cancer if present. Any nonmalignant causes of obstruction can be dealt with endoscopically, with gradual dilation of strictures using a variety of dilators or balloons, discussed elsewhere in more detail [97]. Following dilation of inflammatory strictures due to reflux, the patient should be placed on long-term mainte-nance therapy with a proton-pump inhibitor drug, with the maintenance dose being identical to the treatment dose. Some may be managed by opera-tive dilation and surgical fundoplication [48]. In those with severe and long-standing strictures, in order to avoid problems of drug bioavailablity, administration of a PPI may necessitate the use of commercially available solutions or suspensions of the drugs (Table 48.4) [76, 98]. However, home-made suspensions using broken-up capsules of PPI should be avoided, as the acid-labile drug may not survive passage through the stomach. Patients should also be warned about the dangers of aspi-rin, NSAIDs, and all the other drugs listed in Table 48.3, and followed at regular intervals. The rate of recurrence of strictures is reduced by long-term therapy with PPIs [50, 51] or by surgical fun-doplication [48]. Rarely, strictures are so severe as to require surgical resection or other complex operative procedures.

When there is no mechanical obstruction, the investigation of the dysphagia should include pH, manometric, and (where available) endoscopic ultrasonic studies of the esophageal wall, making every effort to understand the mechanics of the dysphagia in each particular case. Cases with no mechanical obstruction are generally approached by initiating good medical management of GERD by the measures described. Following effective acid-suppressive and anti-reflux therapy, most GERD-associated dysphagia resolves, but in some cases higher than routine doses of PPI may be required. In rare cases, placement of a feeding gas-trostomy or jejunostomy may be indicated, when poor patient health, nutrition, and comorbid disease add excessive risk to other approaches to therapy.

Management of dysphagia in the patient with GERD presents a long-term challenge to effec-tive care by an experienced physician, conversant with all aspects of the disease.

References

1. Vakil N, van Zanten SV, Kahrilas P, Dent J, Jones R. The Montreal definition and classification of gastroe-sophageal reflux disease: a global evidence-based con-sensus. Am J Gastroenterol. 2006;101(8):1900–20.

2. Hiltz SW, Members of AGA Institute Medical Position Panel. Medical position statement on the management of gastroesophageal reflux disease. Gastroenterology. 2008;135:1383–91.

3. Dent J. Review article: from 1906 to 2006—a century of major evolution of understanding of gastro-oesoph-ageal reflux disease. Aliment Pharmacol Ther. 2006;24(9):1269–81.

4. Wienbeck M, Barnert J. Epidemiology of reflux dis-ease and reflux esophagitis. Scand J Gastroenterol Suppl. 1989;156:7–13.

5. Spechler SJ. Epidemiology and natural history of gastro-oesophageal reflux disease. Digestion. 1992;51 Suppl 1:24–9.

6. Ollyo J-B, Monier P, Fontolliet C, Savary M. The natural history, prevalence and incidence of reflux oesophagitis. Gullet. 1993;3(Suppl):3–10.

7. Sonnenberg A, El Serag HB. Epidemiology of gas-troesophageal reflux disease. In: Buchlr MW, Frei E, Klaiber CH, Krahenbuhl L, editors. Gastroesophageal reflux disease (GERD): back to surgery? progress in surgery, vol. 23. Basel: Karger; 1997. p. 20–36.

8. Tack J, Fass R. Review article: approaches to endo-scopic-negative reflux disease: part of the GERD spectrum or a unique acid-related disorder? Aliment Pharmacol Ther. 2004;19 Suppl 1:28–34.

9. Locke III GR, Talley NJ, Fett SL, Zinsmeister AR, Melton III LJ. Prevalence and clinical spectrum of gastroesophageal reflux: a population-based study in Olmsted County, Minnesota. Gastroenterology. 1997;112(5):1448–56.

10. Shaker R, Castell DO, Schoenfeld PS, Spechler SJ. Nighttime heartburn is an under-appreciated clinical problem that impacts sleep and daytime function: the results of a Gallup survey conducted on behalf of the American Gastroenterological Association. Am J Gastroenterol. 2003;98(7):1487–93.

11. Sonnenberg A, El Serag HB. Clinical epidemiology and natural history of gastroesophageal reflux disease. Yale J Biol Med. 1999;72(2–3):81–92.

12. Zhu H, Pace F, Sangaletti O, Bianchi PG. Features of symptomatic gastroesophageal reflux in elderly patients. Scand J Gastroenterol. 1993;28(3):235–8.

13. Johnson DA, Fennerty MB. Heartburn severity under-estimates erosive esophagitis severity in elderly patients with gastroesophageal reflux disease. Gastroenterology. 2004;126:660–4.

14. Becher A, Dent J. Systematic review: ageing and gas-tro-oesophageal reflux disease symptoms, oesopha-geal function and reflux oesophagitis. Aliment Pharmacol Ther. 2011;33(4):442–54.

15. Sonnenberg A, Massey BT, Jacobsen SJ. Hospital dis-charges resulting from esophagitis among Medicare beneficiaries. Dig Dis Sci. 1994;39(1):183–8.

16. El Serag HB, Sonnenberg A. Associations between different forms of gastro-esophageal reflux disease. Gut. 1997;41:594–9.

17. El Serag HB, Sonnenberg A. Opposing time trends of peptic ulcer and reflux disease. Gut. 1998;43(3):327–33.

18. Mayne ST, Navarro SA. Diet, obesity and reflux in the etiology of adenocarcinomas of the esophagus and gastric cardia in humans. J Nutr. 2002;132(11 Suppl):3467S–70.

19. Anand G, Katz PO. Gastroesophageal reflux disease and obesity. Gastroenterol Clin North Am. 2010;39(1):39–46.

20. El Serag HB, Satia JA, Rabeneck L. Dietary intake and the risk of gastro-oesophageal reflux disease: a cross sectional study in volunteers. Gut. 2005;54(1):11–7.

21. Jacobson BC, Somers SC, Fuchs CS, Kelly CP, Camargo Jr CA. Body-mass index and symptoms of gastroesophageal reflux in women. N Engl J Med. 2006;354(22):2340–8.

22. Fornari F, Madalosso CA, Farre R, Gurski RR, Thiesen V, Callegari-Jacques SM. The role of gastro-oesophageal pressure gradient and sliding hiatal hernia on pathological gastro-oesophageal reflux in severely obese patients. Eur J Gastroenterol Hepatol. 2010;22(4):404–11.

23. Orlando RC. Reflux esophagitis. In: Yamada T, editor. Textbook of gastroenterology. 3rd ed. Philladelphia, PA: Lippincott Williams & Wilkins; 1999. p. 1235–63.

24. Kahrilas PJ. GERD pathogenesis, pathophysiology and clinical manifestations. Cleve Clin J Med. 2003;70 Suppl 5:S4–19.

25. Kahrilas PJ, Dodds WJ, Hogan WJ, Kern M, Arndorfer RC, Reece A. Esophageal peristaltic dysfunction in peptic esophagitis. Gastroenterology. 1986;91(4):897–904.

26. Kahrilas P, Spiess A. Hiatus hernia. In: Castell DO, Richter JE, editors. The esophagus. 3rd ed. Philladelphia, PA: Lippincott Williams & Wilkins; 1999. p. 381–96.

27. Mittal RK. Pathophysiology of gastroesophageal reflux disease. In: Castell DO, Richter JE, editors. The esophagus. Philladelphia, PA: Lippincott Williams & Wilkins; 1999. p. 397–408.

28. De Hertogh G, Ectors N, Van Eyken P, Geboes K. Review article: the nature of oesophageal injury in gastro-oesophageal reflux disease. Aliment Pharmacol Ther. 2006;24 Suppl 2:17–26.

29. Caviglia R, Ribolsi M, Maggiano N, Gabbrielli AM, Emerenziani S, Guarino MP, et al. Dilated intercellular spaces of esophageal epithelium in nonerosive reflux disease patients with physiological esophageal acid exposure. Am J Gastroenterol. 2005;100(3): 543–8.

30. Emerenziani S, Sifrim D. Gastroesophageal reflux and gastric emptying: an update. Curr GERD Rep. 2007;1:77–83. also available at: http://www.current-reports.com.

31. Marshall JB, Gerhardt DC. Improvement in esophageal motor dysfunction with treatment of reflux esophagitis: a report of two cases. Am J Gastroenterol. 1982;77(6):351–4.

32. Avidan B, Sonnenberg A, Schnell TG, Sontag SJ. Acid reflux is a poor predictor for severity of erosive reflux esophagitis. Dig Dis Sci. 2002;47(11): 2565–73.

33. Orr WC. Review article: sleep-related gastro-oesophageal reflux as a distinct clinical entity. Aliment Pharmacol Ther. 2010;31(1):47–56.

34. Kahrilas PJ. Gastroesophageal reflux disease and its complications. In: Feldman M, Scharschmidt BF, Sleisenger MH, editors. Sleisenger & Fordtran's gastrointesinal and liver disease. 6th ed. Philadelphia, PA: WB Saunders; 1998. p. 498–517.

35. Ang D, Sifrim D, Tack J. Mechanisms of heartburn. Nat Clin Pract Gastroenterol Hepatol. 2008;5(7): 383–92.

36. McCarthy DM. Acid and the esophagus. Yale J Biol Med. 1999;72(2–3):125–31.

37. Vaezi MF, Richter JE. Contribution of acid and duodenogastro-oesophageal reflux to oesophageal mucosal injury and symptoms in partial gastrectomy patients [see comment]. Gut. 1997;41(3):297–302.

38. Vela MF, Camacho-Lobato L, Srinivasan R, Tutuian R, Katz PO, Castell DO. Simultaneous intraesophageal impedance and pH measurement of acid and nonacid gastroesophageal reflux: effect of omeprazole. Gastroenterology. 2001;120(7):1599–606.

39. Orlando RC. The integrity of the esophageal mucosa. Balance between offensive and defensive mechanisms. Best Pract Res Clin Gastroenterol. 2010;24(6):873–82.

40. Lundell LR, Dent J, Bennett JR, Blum AL, Armstrong D, Galmiche JP, et al. Endoscopic assessment of oesophagitis: clinical and functional correlates and further validation of the Los Angeles classification. Gut. 1999;45(2):172–80.

41. Robertson D, Aldersley M, Shepherd H, Smith CL. Patterns of acid reflux in complicated oesophagitis. Gut. 1987;28(11):1484–8.

42. McCarthy DM. Do drugs or bugs cause GERD? J Clin Gastroenterol. 2007;41 Suppl 2:S59–63.

43. El Serag HB, Sonnenberg A. Association of esophagitis and esophageal strictures with diseases treated with nonsteroidal anti-inflammatory drugs. Am J Gastroenterol. 1997;92(1):52–6.

44. Oliveria SA, Christos PJ, Talley NJ, Dannenberg AJ. Heartburn risk factors, knowledge, and prevention strategies: a population-based survey of individuals with heartburn. Arch Intern Med. 1999;159(14):1592–8.

45. Fullard M, Kang JY, Neild P, Poullis A, Maxwell JD. Systematic review: does gastro-oesophageal reflux disease progress? Aliment Pharmacol Ther. 2006;24(1):33–45.

46. Labenz J, Nocon M, Lind T, Leodolter A, Jaspersen D, Meyer-Sabellek W, et al. Prospective follow-up data from the ProGERD study suggest that GERD is not a categorial disease. Am J Gastroenterol. 2006;101(11):2457–62.

47. Ben Rejeb M, Bouche O, Zeitoun P. Study of 47 consecutive patients with peptic esophageal stricture compared with 3880 cases of reflux esophagitis. Dig Dis Sci. 1992;37(5):733–6.

48. El Serag HB, Sonnenberg A. Outcome of erosive reflux esophagitis after Nissen fundoplication. Am J Gastroenterol. 1999;94(7):1771–6.

49. Vakil N. Disease definition, clinical manifestations, epidemiology and natural history of GERD. Best Pract Res Clin Gastroenterol. 2010;24(6):759–64.

50. El Serag HB, Lau M. Temporal trends in new and recurrent oesophageal strictures in a Medicare population. Aliment Pharmacol Ther. 2007;25(10):1223–9.

51. Ruigomez A, Garcia Rodriguez LA, Wallander MA, Johansson S, Eklund S. Esophageal stricture: incidence, treatment patterns, and recurrence rate. Am J Gastroenterol. 2006;101(12):2685–92.

52. Vasuveda R. Schatzki Ring. http://www.emedicine. medscape.com/article/182647-overview.

53. Basseri B, Pimentel M, Shaye OA, Low K, Soffer EE, Conklin JL. Apple sauce improves detection of esophageal motor dysfunction during high-resolution manometry evaluation of dysphagia. Dig Dis Sci. 2011;56(6):1723–8.

54. Lee KJ, Kim JH, Cho SW. Prevalence of ineffective esophageal motility and its relevance to symptoms and esophageal acid exposure in Korean patients referred for foregut symptoms. Digestion. 2006;73(2–3):171–7.

55. de Miranda Gomes Jr PR, AR Pereira da Rosa, Sakae T, Simic AP, Ricachenevsky GR. Correlation between pathological distal esophageal acid exposure and ineffective esophageal motility. Acta Chir Iugosl. 2010;57(2):37–43.

56. Haack HG, Hansen RD, Malcolm A, Kellow JE. Ineffective oesophageal motility: manometric subsets exhibit different symptom profiles. World J Gastroenterol. 2008;14(23):3719–24.

57. Kim JH, Rhee PL, Son HJ, Song KJ, Kim JJ, Rhee JC. Is all ineffective esophageal motility the same? A clinical and high-frequency intraluminal US study. Gastrointest Endosc. 2008;68(3):422–31.

58. Sifrim D, Blondeau K, Mantilla L. Utility of non-endoscopic investigations in the practical management of oesophageal disorders. Best Pract Res Clin Gastroenterol. 2009;23(3):369–86.

59. Lazarescu A, Karamanolis G, Aprile L, De Oliveira RB, Dantas R, Sifrim D. Perception of dysphagia: lack of correlation with objective measurements of esophageal function. Neurogastroenterol Motil. 2010;22(12):1292–7.

60. Dent J, Brun J, Fendrick AM, et al. An evidence based appraisal of reflux disease management—the Genval workshop report. Gut. 1999;44 Suppl 2:S1–16.

61. Kang JY. Lifestyle measures and reflux. Aliment Pharmacol Ther. 2000;14(8):1103.

62. Meining A, Classen M. The role of diet and lifestyle measures in the pathogenesis and treatment of gastroesophageal reflux disease. Am J Gastroenterol. 2000;95(10):2692–7.

63. DeVault KR, Castell DO. Updated guidelines for the diagnosis and treatment of gastroesophageal reflux disease. Am J Gastroenterol. 2005;100(1):190–200.

64. Kaltenbach T, Crockett S, Gerson LB. Are lifestyle measures effective in patients with gastroesophageal reflux disease? An evidence-based approach. Arch Intern Med. 2006;166(9):965–71.

65. Fraser-Moodie CA. Weight loss has an independent beneficial effect on symptoms of gastroesophageal reflux in patients who are overweight. Scand J Gastroenterol. 1999;34(4):337–40.

66. Mathus-Vliegen EM, van Weeren M, van Eerten PV. Los function and obesity: the impact of untreated obesity, weight loss, and chronic gastric balloon distension. Digestion. 2003;68(2–3):161–8.

67. Kjellin A, Ramel S, Rossner S, Thor K. Gastroesophageal reflux in obese patients is not reduced by weight reduction. Scand J Gastroenterol. 1996;31(11):1047–51.

68. Singh M, Gupta N, Lee J, Gaddam S, et al. Temporal effects of weight change on gastroesophageal reflux disease (GERD) in obese subjects: a large prospective study. Gastroenterology. 2011;40 Suppl 1:S189–90.

69. Bertaccini G, Coruzzi G. Cholinergic-like effects of the new histamine H2-receptor antagonist ranitidine. Agents Actions. 1982;12(1–2):168–71.

70. Kovacs TOG, DeVault K, Metz D, Sasen S, Miska D, Bochenek W, et al. Pantoprazole prevents relapse of healed erosive esophagitis more effectively than ranitidine in gastroesophageal reflux disease patients. Am J Gastroenterol. 1999;94:2590.

71. Kwiatek MA, Roman S, Fareeduddin A, Pandolfino JE, Kahrilas PJ. An alginate-antacid formulation (Gaviscon Double Action Liquid) can eliminate or displace the post-prandial "acid pocket" in symptomatic GERD patients. Aliment Pharmacol Ther. 2011;34(1):59–66.

72. McCarthy DM. Sucralfate. N Engl J Med. 1991; 325(14):1017–25.

73. Maton PN. Profile and assessment of GERD pharmacotherapy. Cleve Clin J Med. 2003;70 Suppl 5: S51–70.

74. Brunner R, Wallmann J, Szalai K, Karagiannis P, Altmeppen H, Riemer AB, et al. Aluminium per se and in the anti-acid drug sucralfate promotes sensitization via the oral route. Allergy. 2009;64(6):890–7.

75. Chiba N, De Gara CJ, Wilkinson JM, Hunt RH. Speed of healing and symptom relief in grade II to IV gastroesophageal reflux disease: a meta-analysis. Gastroenterology. 1997;112(6):1798–810.

76. McDonagh MS, Carson S, Thakurta S. Drug class Review. Proton Pump Inhibitor update #5 < http:// www.ohsu.edu/drugeffectivness/reports/final.cfm. > PPI:1-121.

77. Galmiche JP, Clouse RE, Balint A, Cook IJ, Kahrilas PJ, Paterson WG, et al. Functional esophageal disorders. Gastroenterology. 2006;130(5):1459–65.

78. Barrison AF, Jarboe LA, Weinberg BM, Nimmagadda K, Sullivan LM, Wolfe MM. Patterns of proton pump inhibitor use in clinical practice. Am J Med. 2001;111(6):469–73.

79. Howden CW, Henning JM, Huang B, Lukasik N, Freston JW. Management of heartburn in a large, randomized, community-based study: comparison of

four therapeutic strategies. Am J Gastroenterol. 2001; 96(6):1704–10.

80. Reimer C, Sondergaard B, Hilsted L, Bytzer P. Proton-pump inhibitor therapy induces acid-related symptoms in healthy volunteers after withdrawal of therapy. Gastroenterology. 2009;137(1):80–7. 87.

81. Niklasson A, Lindstrom L, Simren M, Lindberg G, Bjornsson E. Dyspeptic symptom development after discontinuation of a proton pump inhibitor: a double-blind placebo-controlled trial. Am J Gastroenterol. 2010;105(7):1531–7.

82. Smith AD, Gillen D, Cochran KM, El Omar E, McColl KE. Dyspepsia on withdrawal of ranitidine in previously asymptomatic volunteers. Am J Gastroenterol. 1999;94(5):1209–13.

83. McCarthy DM. Adverse effects of proton pump inhibitor drugs: clues and conclusions. Curr Opin Gastroenterol. 2010;26(6):624–31.

84. Inadomi JM, McIntyre L, Bernard L, Fendrick AM. Step-down from multiple- to single-dose proton pump inhibitors (PPIs): a prospective study of patients with heartburn or acid regurgitation completely relieved with PPIs. Am J Gastroenterol. 2003;98(9):1940–4.

85. Inadomi JM, Jamal R, Murata GH, Hoffman RM, Lavezo LA, Vigil JM, et al. Step-down management of gastroesophageal reflux disease. Gastroenterology. 2001;121(5):1095–100.

86. Vakil NB, Shaker R, Johnson DA, Kovacs T, Baerg RD, Hwang C, et al. The new proton pump inhibitor esomeprazole is effective as a maintenance therapy in GERD patients with healed erosive oesophagitis: a 6-month, randomized, double-blind, placebo-controlled study of efficacy and safety. Aliment Pharmacol Ther. 2001;15(7):927–35.

87. Metz DC, Bochenek WJ. Pantoprazole maintenance therapy prevents relapse of erosive oesophagitis. Aliment Pharmacol Ther. 2003;17(1):155–64.

88. Reimer C, Bytzer P. Clinical trial: long-term use of proton pump inhibitors in primary care patients - a

cross sectional analysis of 901 patients. Aliment Pharmacol Ther. 2009;30(7):725–32.

89. Metz DC, Inadomi JM, Howden CW, van Zanten SJ, Bytzer P. On-demand therapy for gastroesophageal reflux disease. Am J Gastroenterol. 2007;102(3): 642–53.

90. Leodolter A, Penagini R. On-demand therapy is a valid strategy in GERD patients: pros and cons. Dig Dis. 2007;25(3):175–8.

91. Pace F, Tonini M, Pallotta S, Molteni P, Porro GB. Systematic review: maintenance treatment of gastro-oesophageal reflux disease with proton pump inhibitors taken 'on-demand'. Aliment Pharmacol Ther. 2007;26(2):195–204.

92. Pace F, Pallotta S, Casalini S, Porro GB. A review of rabeprazole in the treatment of acid-related diseases. Ther Clin Risk Manag. 2007;3(3):363–79.

93. Morgan DG, O'Mahony MF, O'Mahony WF, Roy J, Camacho F, Dinniwell J, et al. Maintenance treatment of gastroesophageal reflux disease: an evaluation of continuous and on-demand therapy with rabeprazole 20 mg. Can J Gastroenterol. 2007;21(12): 820–6.

94. Scarpignato C, Hunt RH. Proton pump inhibitors: the beginning of the end or the end of the beginning? Curr Opin Pharmacol. 2008;8(6):677–84.

95. Armstrong D, Sifrim D. New pharmacologic approaches in gastroesophageal reflux disease. Gastroenterol Clin North Am. 2010;39(3):393–418.

96. Liu Y, Chen Y, Zheng H, et al. 9-Dihydroerythromycins as non-antibiotic motilin receptor agonists. Bioorg Med Chem Lett. 2010;20(19):5658–61.

97. Bansal A, Kahrilas PJ, Marquardt GH. Treatment of GERD complications (Barrett's, peptic stricture) and extra-oesophageal syndromes. Best Pract Res Clin Gastroenterol. 2010;24(6):961–8.

98. Howden CW. Management of acid-related disorders in patients with dysphagia. Am J Med. 2004;117(Suppl 5A):44S–8.

Barrett's Esophagus

49

Stuart Jon Spechler

Abstract

Barrett's esophagus is the condition in which a metaplastic columnar mucosa that predisposes to cancer development replaces the stratified squamous mucosa that normally lines the distal esophagus. The condition develops as a complication of chronic gastroesophageal reflux disease (GERD), which is often severe in patients who have long segments of Barrett's metaplasia extending up the esophagus. Barrett's esophagus is a major risk factors for esophageal adenocarcinoma, a tumor whose frequency has increased more than six-fold over the past several decades. Because of this cancer risk, patients with Barrett's esophagus are advised to have regular endoscopic surveillance with esophageal biopsy sampling to detect dysplasia, the precursor of invasive adenocarcinoma. Until recently, patients with high-grade dysplasia in Barrett's esophagus were treated with esophagectomy. Today, most patients with high-grade dysplasia can be treated successfully with endoscopic eradication therapy. This chapter discusses the diagnosis, epidemiology, pathogenesis and management of Barrett's esophagus.

Keywords

Barrett's esophagus • Dysplasia • Esophagectomy • Gastroesophageal reflux disease (GERD) • Predicting neoplastic progression

Barrett's esophagus is the condition in which a metaplastic columnar mucosa that predisposes to cancer development replaces the stratified squamous mucosa that normally lines the distal esophagus [1]. Metaplasia is the process in which one adult cell type replaces another. The columnar metaplasia of Barrett's esophagus appears to be caused by chronic gastroesophageal reflux disease (GERD), which both damages the native esophageal squamous mucosa and provides an abnormal luminal environment that results in mucosal healing through columnar metaplasia rather than through the regeneration of more

S.J. Spechler, MD (✉)
Division of Gastroenterology, Dallas VA
Medical Center, Berta M. and Cecil O. Patterson
Chair in Gastroenterology, UT Southwestern
Medical Center at Dallas, Dallas, TX, USA
e-mail: sjspechler@aol.com

R. Shaker et al. (eds.), *Principles of Deglutition: A Multidisciplinary Text for Swallowing and its Disorders*,
DOI 10.1007/978-1-4614-3794-9_49, © Springer Science+Business Media New York 2013

squamous cells. Patients with Barrett's esophagus frequently have symptomatic GERD, but Barrett's metaplasia itself causes no symptoms. The condition has clinical importance primarily because it is a risk factor for esophageal adenocarcinoma, a tumor whose frequency has increased more than sixfold in the United States over the past several decades [2].

Diagnosis

The diagnosis of Barrett's esophagus requires an endoscopic examination with procurement of esophageal biopsy specimens [3]. The diagnosis is considered when the endoscopist recognizes that columnar epithelium lines the distal esophagus. The diagnosis is established when biopsy specimens of that epithelium show columnar metaplasia. To recognize columnar epithelium lining the distal esophagus, the endoscopist first must identify the gastroesophageal junction (GEJ), the line at which the esophagus ends and the stomach begins. Non-endoscopists sometimes are surprised to learn that the GEJ cannot be localized with great precision. For endoscopic purposes, the level of the GEJ is usually defined as the most proximal extent of the gastric folds when the esophagus and stomach are partially distended. Columnar epithelium has a reddish-pink color and velvet-like texture that can be distinguished readily from the pale and glossy esophageal squamous epithelium (Fig. 49.1). If columnar epithelium extends above the most proximal extent of the gastric folds, then there is a columnar-lined segment of esophagus. If biopsy specimens of that columnar-lined esophagus reveal a metaplastic epithelium, then that patient has Barrett's esophagus.

The histological finding of an intestinal-type epithelium with goblet cells (which has been called intestinal metaplasia, specialized intestinal metaplasia or specialized columnar epithelium) has come to be considered virtually a *sine qua non* for the diagnosis of Barrett's esophagus [4]. For the past 20 years, most published studies on Barrett's esophagus have used intestinal metaplasia as a requisite diagnostic criterion. Recently,

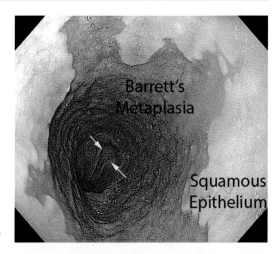

Fig. 49.1 Endoscopic photograph of long-segment Barrett's esophagus. The *arrows* mark the proximal extent of the gastric folds, which is the location of the gastroesophageal junction. Note that Barrett's metaplasia extends well above the GEJ to line the distal esophagus. The *reddish-pink color* and velvet-like texture of Barrett's epithelium contrasts sharply with the pale and glossy appearance of the esophageal squamous epithelium

however, some authorities have argued that gastric cardia-type epithelium, comprising mucus-secreting cells without goblet cells, is also a metaplastic epithelium [5]. Cardia-type epithelium can have intestinal-type histochemical features, and can exhibit genetic and epigenetic abnormalities that might predispose to malignancy. Therefore, some authorities contend that the finding of cardia-type epithelium in the esophagus also should be considered Barrett's esophagus [6]. Although this debate remains unresolved, a recent technical review published by the American Gastroenterological Association recommends that the term "Barrett's esophagus" presently should be used only for patients who have intestinal metaplasia in the esophagus [7].

Before 1994, Barrett's esophagus was recognized primarily in patients with severe GERD who had long segments of columnar epithelium extending well up the esophagus. In 1994, Spechler et al. reported that short segments of intestinal metaplasia could be found frequently in the distal esophagus of consecutive patients seen in a general endoscopy unit, many of whom had no endoscopic signs or symptoms of GERD [8].

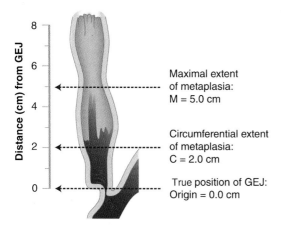

Fig. 49.2 Cartoon depicting the Prague C and M criteria. Note that a circumferential segment of Barrett's metaplasia extends 2 cm above the gastroesophageal junction (GEJ), and that the maximal extent of metaplasia reaches a level 5 cm above the GEJ. This is denoted C2M5. From P. Sharma et al. Gastroenterology 2006;131:1392–9 with permission

Since then, Barrett's esophagus has been categorized as long-segment (when the metaplastic epithelium extends at least 3 cm above the GEJ) or short-segment (when there is less than 3 cm of metaplastic epithelium lining the esophagus) [9]. More recently, the "Prague C and M criteria" were proposed as a system for describing Barrett's esophagus endoscopically. The Prague system identifies both the circumferential extent (C) and the maximum extent (M) of Barrett's metaplasia (Fig. 49.2) [10]. The cancer risk in Barrett's esophagus appears to vary directly with the extent of the metaplastic lining (i.e., the greater the extent of metaplasia, the greater the cancer risk), and GERD tends to be more severe in patients with long-segment Barrett's esophagus. However, the clinical value of the proposed classification systems has not been established and, presently, patients with any extent of Barrett's metaplasia are managed similarly.

Epidemiology

Although Barrett's esophagus has been described in virtually all ethnic groups, the condition has a predilection for whites, and is uncommon in black and Asian populations [11]. Men are affected approximately twice as often as women. Barrett's esophagus is rare in children younger than 10 years of age [12], and the condition typically is discovered during endoscopic examinations performed for GERD symptoms in patients in the sixth and later decades of life. Nevertheless, it is unclear precisely when the condition develops in most patients. Among adult patients who have endoscopic examinations because of GERD symptoms, long-segment Barrett's esophagus can be found in approximately 3%, whereas 10–20% have short-segment Barrett's esophagus [13]. In the general adult population of Western countries, the prevalence of Barrett's esophagus (predominantly short-segment) appears to be between 1.6% and 6.8% [14, 15].

Published estimates on the annual incidence of cancer in series of patients with long-segment Barrett's esophagus have ranged from 0.2 to 2.9%. In 2000, Shaheen reported that many of those reports suffered from publication bias that exaggerated the cancer risk [16]. Over the decade following that publication, it became widely accepted that the risk of cancer for the general population of patients with Barrett's esophagus was approximately 0.5% per year [17]. Recent data suggest that even that estimate may be too high, however, especially for patients who have short-segment Barrett's esophagus without dysplasia. For such patients, the annual cancer risk may be less than 0.3% per year [18]. Although the difference between an annual risk of 0.5% and 0.3% may seem trivial, it can have substantial impact on patient management recommendations [19].

The epidemiology of esophageal adenocarcinoma mirrors that of its precursor condition, Barrett's esophagus. Esophageal adenocarcinoma affects white men predominantly and GERD is strongly associated with the tumor [11, 20]. However, up to 40% of patients with esophageal adenocarcinoma describe no antecedent history of GERD symptoms [20, 21]. Obesity, especially with central adiposity, predisposes to both Barrett's esophagus and esophageal adenocarcinoma [20, 22]. It has been suggested that the rising frequency of obesity in the United States has contributed to the parallel rise in the frequency of esophageal adenocarcinoma. Central adiposity may contribute to carcinogenesis in the esophagus indirectly (by increasing intra-abdominal pressure, which predisposes to GERD and its complications) or directly (by elevating serum levels of pro-proliferative hormones such as insulin-like growth factor-1 and leptin, and by decreasing levels of anti-proliferative hormones such as adiponectin) [23].

It has been suggested that the declining frequency of gastric infection with *Helicobacter pylori* in Western populations might contribute to the rising frequency of esophageal adenocarcinoma. This theory holds that *H. pylori*, which had infected the large majority of the world's population for millennia before the twentieth century (when the frequency of infection in developed countries began to decline) protected against GERD and its complications by causing a gastritis that decreased gastric acid production [24, 25]. Other factors proposed to protect against the development of esophageal adenocarcinoma include the use of aspirin and other nonsteroidal anti-inflammatory drugs (NSAIDs), and the consumption of a diet high in fruits and vegetables [25]. Although cigarette smoking and alcohol consumption are strong risk factors for squamous cell carcinoma of the esophagus, cigarette smoking only modestly increases the risk for esophageal adenocarcinoma and alcohol does not appear to affect it at all [25].

Pathogenesis of Barrett's Esophagus

GERD is strongly associated with Barrett's esophagus, and it is widely accepted that GERD is a key factor in the pathogenesis of Barrett's metaplasia. Patients with long-segment Barrett's esophagus often have severe, symptomatic GERD with reflux esophagitis, weak lower esophageal sphincters and other physiological abnormalities associated with gastroesophageal reflux [26]. In contrast, patients with short-segment Barrett's esophagus frequently have no symptoms or endoscopic signs of GERD [14]. Nevertheless, there are data to suggest that gastroesophageal reflux is responsible for the development of both short- and long-segment Barrett's esophagus.

At the GEJ after meals, a luminal pocket of acid accumulates that escapes the buffering effects of ingested food [27]. This postprandial acid pocket affects the most proximal stomach and can extend above the squamo-columnar junction (the Z-line) into the distal esophagus. In a study in which a pH electrode was fastened to the distal esophagus of healthy volunteers at a level 5 mm above the Z-line, acid was detected in the region for more than 10% of a 24-h monitoring period [28]. Potential consequences of this protracted acid exposure at the GEJ include not only acid-peptic injury, but also exposure to high concentrations of nitric oxide (NO) generated from dietary nitrate (NO_3^-) in green, leafy vegetables.

Most ingested nitrate is absorbed by the small intestine and excreted unchanged in the urine, but approximately 25% is concentrated by the salivary glands and secreted into the mouth where bacteria on the tongue reduce the recycled nitrate to nitrite (NO_2^-). When swallowed nitrite encounters acidic gastric juice, the nitrite is converted rapidly to nitric oxide (NO), a highly reactive and toxic molecule. After nitrate ingestion, high levels of NO can be found at the GEJ [29]. Thus, the GEJ is exposed repeatedly to NO, acid, and pepsin. Such exposures undoubtedly contribute to the inflammation and metaplasia frequently noted at the GEJ, even in otherwise apparently healthy individuals [30].

The progenitor cells that give rise to Barrett's metaplasia are not known. One popular hypothesis holds that metaplasia results when GERD-induced mucosal damage exposes multipotential stem cells in the basal layers of the squamous epithelium to gastric juice, which stimulates their abnormal differentiation into columnar cells. Genes that have been implicated in this metaplasia include Cdx genes, which normally mediate the differentiation of intestinal epithelial cells, and bone morphogenetic protein (BMP)-4, which also is involved in columnar cell differentiation [31]. Reflux esophagitis can upregulate the expression of these genes by the squamous epithelium, and exposure to acid and bile salts has been shown to induce CDX2 mRNA and protein expression in esophageal squamous cell lines from patients with Barrett's esophagus, but not from GERD patients without Barrett's esophagus [32].

Other proposed candidates for Barrett's progenitor cells include stem cells in the ducts of the esophageal submucosal glands and circulating bone marrow stem cells [33]. Recently, it has been proposed that Barrett's metaplasia develops, not from squamous stem cells, but rather from a population of embryonic, columnar-progenitor cells that persist at the GEJ [34]. According to this hypothesis, competitive interactions with esophageal squamous cells normally prevent the proliferation of the embryonic columnar-progenitor cells. When GERD damages the squamous epithelium at the GEJ, the competitive restraints are removed, and the embryonic cells proliferate and give rise to Barrett's metaplasia.

Biomarkers for Predicting Neoplastic Progression of Barrett's Esophagus

To become malignant, cells must acquire the ability to provide their own growth signals, to avoid growth inhibitory signals, to resist apoptosis, to replicate indefinitely, to sustain angiogenesis, to invade adjacent structures, and to metastasize [35]. Metaplastic Barrett's epithelial cells gain these abilities by acquiring a series of genetic and epigenetic alterations. Conceptually, it is useful to classify the many alterations that have been described in Barrett's esophagus according to the major physiological cancer attributes that the alterations endow. For example, the expression of oncogenes (e.g., cyclin D1, K-ras), growth factors [e.g., transforming growth factor (TGF)-a], and growth factor receptors [e.g., epidermal growth factor receptor (EGFR)] all enable Barrett's cells to provide their own growth signals [25]. The ability to avoid growth inhibitory signals can be acquired by inactivating tumor suppressor genes (e.g., p53 and p16) through the processes of mutation, loss of heterozygosity and gene promoter methylation, and inactivation of p53 also enables cells to resist apoptosis [25]. Reactivation

of the enzyme telomerase enables cells to synthesize telomeres needed for cell division and, thereby, to replicate without limit [25]. Angionesis can be sustained by the secretion of angiogenic factors such as vascular endothelial growth factor (VEGF) [25]. The abilities to invade and metastasize can be achieved through the disruption of cell adhesion proteins (e.g., cadherins and catenins) and through the secretion of enzymes that degrade the extracellular matrix such as matrix metalloproteases (MMPs) [25].

During the process of acquiring the genetic alterations described above, Barrett's epithelial cells typically develop abnormalities in DNA content due to gains and losses in different segments of chromosomes. This condition of abnormal DNA content is called aneuploidy, which can be detected by flow cytometry and by fluorescence in situ hybridization (FISH). Aneuploidy has been proposed as a biomarker for neoplastic progression in Barrett's esophagus, as have a number of the genetic alterations discussed in the preceding paragraph [36]. Although there has been much interest in developing useful, predictive biomarkers for Barrett's esophagus, and some studies have had promising preliminary results, the clinical utility of these biomarkers remains unclear. In its recent medical position statement on the management of Barrett's esophagus, the American Gastroenterological Association (AGA) recommends against the use of molecular biomarkers as a method of risk stratification for patients with Barrett's esophagus at this time [37].

Dysplasia in Barrett's Esophagus

Before Barrett's cancers develop, the genetic and epigenetic alterations that endow cells with the growth advantages described above may cause histological changes in the tissue that pathologists recognize as dysplasia. Those changes involve cytological and architectural abnormalities including nuclear alterations (e.g., enlargement, pleomorphism, hyperchromatism, stratification, atypical mitoses), loss of cytoplasmic maturation, and crowding of tubules and villiform surfaces. These histological abnormalities suggest that the tissue is neoplastic and, to emphasize this point, some pathologists prefer to use the term "intraepithelial neoplasia" rather than "dysplasia" [38].

Dysplasia is categorized as low-grade or high-grade depending on the degree of histological abnormalities. Tissue that is reacting to inflammatory injury can exhibit histological features virtually indistinguishable from low-grade dysplasia, and interobserver agreement among pathologists for the diagnosis of low-grade dysplasia may be less than 50%. For high-grade dysplasia, interobserver agreement is approximately 85%, but there can be substantial disagreement in distinguishing high-grade dysplasia (in which neoplastic cells remain confined within the basement membrane of the epithelial layer) from intramucosal carcinoma (in which neoplastic cells penetrate the basement membrane to involve the lamina propria) [39].

Endoscopists traditionally have used a 4-quadrant biopsy sampling system (the "Seattle biopsy protocol") to find dysplasia in Barrett's esophagus [40]. This system was designed to optimize the identification of a lesion that was assumed to be randomly distributed and to cause no visible abnormalities. More recent data suggest that dysplasia frequently is associated with visible abnormalities (e.g., ulcerations, nodules, mucosal and vascular irregularities), although some of those abnormalities may be subtle and easily overlooked [41]. Nevertheless, biopsy sampling error remains a problem for any sampling system in Barrett's esophagus, and it is clear that areas of dysplasia and even cancer can be missed by adherence to the Seattle biopsy protocol. In older series of patients who had esophagectomies because endoscopic biopsy sampling revealed high-grade dysplasia in Barrett's esophagus, a number of studies found that invasive cancer was present in 30–40% of the resected specimens [42]. A recent, critical review of those reports suggests that 13% is a more accurate estimate of the frequency of invasive cancer in this situation and, when a careful endoscopic examination excludes all visible lesions, the frequency of finding invasive cancer at esophagectomy is only approximately 3% [43].

The recent development of high-resolution white light endoscopy has improved the endoscopic recognition of dysplasia in Barrett's esophagus. High-resolution endoscopes, which use a charge coupled device (CCD) comprising 600,000–1,000,000 pixels, can be combined with magnification devices to enlarge the video image up to 150-fold. When displayed on high-definition televisions, these systems provide exquisite detail of the mucosal surface, and they are more sensitive than conventional endoscopy for detecting dysplasia in Barrett's esophagus [7]. Researchers have studied a number of alternative endoscopic techniques for recognizing dysplasia including chromoendoscopy, autofluorescence endoscopy, narrow band imaging, optical coherence tomography, Raman detection methods, and confocal laser endomicroscopy [44]. Presently, it is not clear that any of these techniques add important clinical information beyond that which can be gleaned from a careful inspection of Barrett's esophagus with high-resolution white light endoscopy.

One recent study suggests that patients who have non-neoplastic Barrett's esophagus develop low-grade dysplasia at the rate of 4.3% per year, and high-grade dysplasia at the rate of 0.9% per year [45]. Relatively few studies have focused on the natural history of dysplasia in Barrett's esophagus, and there are wide variations among reported estimates on cancer risk for patients with dysplasia. The incidence of cancer for patients with low-grade dysplasia is especially poorly defined. Some studies have found a cancer risk no greater than that for the general population of patients with Barrett's esophagus, while others have observed cancer rates approaching those for patients with high-grade dysplasia [7]. For patients with high-grade dysplasia, the rate of cancer development appears to be approximately 6–8% per year [38].

Management of Patients with Barrett's Esophagus

There are three major aspects in the management of patients with Barrett's esophagus: (1) Treatment of the associated GERD, (2) Endoscopic surveil-

cough do not have typical symptoms of GERD. One study found that only 63% of patients with reflux-associated cough exhibit classic reflux symptoms. These patients were more likely to exhibit cough in the upright position, during daytime hours, upon arising from a supine position, during phonation, and also often had symptoms associated with eating [10].

The common tests used to diagnose typical GERD have lacked efficacy in the diagnosis of reflux-associated cough. In one study of 45 patients suffering from cough thought secondary to chronic reflux, only 15% had endoscopy-proven esophagitis [11]. The role of 24 h esophageal pH monitoring has also shown limitations. Although the sensitivity of pH monitoring has been reported as high as 90%, the specificity of this test has been quite low [12–17]. Paterson and Murat combined pH monitoring with manometry and found that only 1% of the total cough episodes in patients were associated with hypopharyngeal reflux events [18].

Recent studies have attempted to assess for a temporal relationship between reflux events on pH or impedance monitoring and cough episodes. Sifrim and colleagues studied ambulatory pressure–pH–impedance monitoring with cough and determined that although the majority of cough events were not associated with reflux episodes directly, 31% of patients did cough within 2 min of a reflux episode [19]. Blondeau and colleagues found that of 100 patients with suspected reflux-associated cough, 23% had a significant correlation between coughing spells and reflux during impedance/pH monitoring [20]. Given the lack of outcome studies the clinical relevance of these prevalence studies should not be overstated.

The treatment of patients with suspected reflux-associated cough has also been well studied. Vaezi and Richter found that treatment with omeprazole for acid suppression showed complete resolution of symptoms within 2 months in 10 of 11 patients with GER-associated cough [12]. Another study found that 56% of patients with typical GERD symptoms in addition to cough or hoarseness had resolution of cough symptoms on omeprazole [13]. Although these studies and others have shown that GER-associated cough appears to respond to acid suppressive therapy, other studies have not supported this finding [14]. Some studies suggest that other etiologies of cough (including nonacid reflux) should be pursued among patients unresponsive to aggressive acid suppression.

Nonacid reflux as an etiology of chronic cough has gained recent increased attention. Impedance monitoring is playing an important role in the detection of both acid and nonacid refluxate. Most impedance monitoring studies have shown no increase in reflux events with patients with chronic cough compared to normal controls [20, 62, 63, 66]. However, Patterson and colleagues suggested that patients who have positive symptom association probability (SAP) on impedance may have a higher number of reflux episodes crossing the upper esophageal sphincter compared to SAP-negative patients [15]. A novel study by Smith et al. [16] employing 24-h ambulatory acoustic cough monitoring with simultaneous impedance/pH monitoring in 71 patients with chronic cough has recently raised the importance of neural sensitization and the self-perpetuating cycle which maintains patients' cough episodes. In this study, the authors reported that patients with chronic cough had no greater esophageal exposure to reflux, they were no more likely to have erosive esophagitis but they did have more sensitive cough reflex. Their findings of lack of association between degree and proximal extent of reflux and chronic cough further highlight the complexity of chronic cough etiology and the need for in-depth studies reexamining our current diagnostic tools for this condition.

The evaluation of GER-associated chronic cough should begin with assessment of other causes of chronic cough, including postnasal drip syndrome and asthma. Once the contributions of these conditions have been dismissed, an empiric trial of acid suppression with twice-daily proton pump inhibitor (PPI) therapy for 2–3 months may help identify those in whom GER may be an important contributing factor; however, in most patients a multidisciplinary approach is needed since chronic cough in most patients is multifactorial. The role of diagnostic testing with impedance/pH monitoring or symptom association analyses is unknown at this time, although there may be clinical value to normal test findings in those with continued symptoms despite PPI therapy.

Laryngopharyngeal Reflux

Laryngopharyngeal reflux (LPR) is a term commonly used by ear, nose, and throat (ENT) specialists to describe the GER that reaches the anatomical structures above the upper esophageal sphincter such as the laryngeal or pharyngeal mucosa [17]. Other commonly employed terminology includes reflux laryngitis or GER-related laryngitis. As controversial as the terminology defining the disease might appear, it pales in comparison to identifying who actually has the disease and in whom it is over- or incorrectly diagnosed. For the sake of simplicity we will employ the term LPR to refer to a disease state in which patients have throat symptoms "felt to be" GER-related. Presenting symptoms of suspected LPR may include chronic cough, sore throat, throat clearing, hoarseness, and globus sensation to name a few. LPR is among the extraesophageal syndromes of reflux disease with varying symptom presentations, with many who may not report concomitant presence of classical symptoms of reflux such as heartburn. This results in added complexity to diagnosing true GER-related findings and symptoms in patients with suspected extraesophageal reflux.

The two predominant pathophysiologic mechanisms for LPR are direct and indirect laryngeal exposure to gastric contents. Direct exposure is due to acid, pepsin, and bile acid exposure to laryngopharyngeal mucosa. Protective structures to prevent the former are the GI junctional structures including the lower and upper esophageal sphincters, peristaltic actions of the esophagus, acid neutralization by saliva, protective airway reflexes including the esophagoglottal closure and the cough reflexes, and mucociliary clearance. Animal studies have also documented injurious potential in laryngeal lesions for both gastric and duodenal agents [25, 26]. The indirect mechanism is thought to be due to interactions of refluxate with structures distal to the larynx,

evoking a vagally mediated response of bronchoconstriction [21]. There are some suggestions that the defense mechanisms differ between the esophagus and the laryngopharynx. The esophagus has greater resistance to exposure to acid. One of the carbonic anhydrase isoenzymes, CA III, is noted to exhibit increased expression in esophageal mucosa in response to reflux, while the larynx has decreased CA III levels after exposure to chronic reflux. The response of esophageal mucosa to acid and pepsin is often reversible, while laryngeal tissue can often exhibit irreversible damage [27, 28].

Two tests commonly used in the diagnosis of LPR include 24-h pH monitoring and laryngoscopy. As the initial test performed by our ENT colleagues in patients with chronic throat symptoms, laryngoscopy is sensitive but not specific enough to diagnose GER-related LPR [17]. Normal laryngeal tissue has sharply demarcated landmarks with glistening mucosa with minimal or no laryngeal edema (Fig. 50.2) unlike abnormal laryngeal findings (Fig. 50.3). The epithelium of the larynx is thin and is not adapted to accommodating injury from acid and pepsin [27]. Several laryngeal signs are attributed to GERD, including edema, erythema, pseudosulcus, ventricular obliteration, and postcricoid hyperplasia [17]. However, many such laryngeal findings

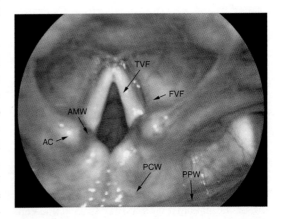

Fig. 50.2 Normal laryngeal tissue. *TVF* true vocal fold, *FVF* false vocal fold, *AMW* arytenoid medial wall, *AC* arytenoid complex, *PCW* posterior cricoid wall, *PPW* posterior pharyngeal wall. From M.F. Vaezi et al. Clin Gastroenterol Hepatol 2003;1(5):333–44 with permission from Elsevier

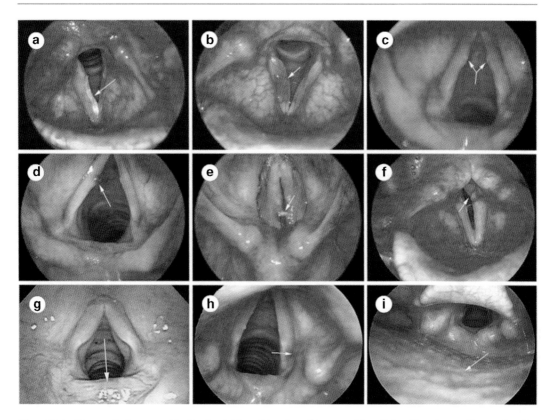

Fig. 50.3 Abnormal larynx. (**a**) Leukoplakia; (**b**) Reinke's edema; (**c**) bilateral true vocal cord nodules; (**d**) true vocal fold hemorrhagic polyp; (**e**) true vocal fold erythema; (**f**) vocal fold granuloma; (**g**) interarytenoid bar; (**h**) arytenoid medial wall erythema; (**i**) posterior pharyngeal wall cobble stoning. From M.F. Vaezi et al. Clin Gastroenterol Hepatol 2003;1(5):333–44 with permission from Elsevier

may be the result of irritants such as smoking and environmental allergens [29]. Abnormal laryngeal signs are more likely to be suspected with flexible laryngoscopy as opposed to rigid laryngoscopy in the same individual, indicating that flexible laryngoscopy may be more sensitive and less specific for detecting laryngeal irritation [22]. Given the poor specificity of laryngoscopy in diagnosing GER-related laryngeal changes, it is not surprising that many are incorrectly diagnosed as having LPR who may not have reflux disease at all. However, one study showed that lesions of the vocal fold might represent more specific signs for LPR, exhibiting 91% specificity and 88% response to treatment with PPIs [23].

When compared to physical exam findings, dual pH-probe monitoring is reported to have superior sensitivity and specificity [26]. A meta-analysis of 16 studies involving a total of 793 subjects who underwent 24-h pH monitoring (529 patients with LPR, 264 controls) showed that the number of pharyngeal reflux events for the control group and for LPR patients differed significantly ($p < 0.0001$). However, the clinical utility of prolonged esophageal or pharyngeal pH monitoring should be scrutinized. Approximately 50–80% of patients with suspected GER have abnormal acid exposure, irrespective of pH probe placement [17]. The sensitivity of proximal esophageal and hypopharyngeal pH monitoring is suboptimal at only 40–50% [24, 30]. In addition, Park et al. demonstrated that pre-therapy demographics, presenting symptoms, pH monitoring, and esophageal manometry were not predictive of 4 month treatment outcome in patients referred for suspected LPR [23]. Overall, pH testing is valuable to suggest the presence or absence of reflux, but it does not suggest a causal link and given its low sensitivity it cannot be viewed as the gold standard in diagnosing LPR in patients referred for evaluation.

Given the poor sensitivity and specificity of diagnostic tests, empiric treatment of suspected GER laryngitis using PPIs is common [17]. Most trials have utilized twice-daily PPIs for 3–4 months [17, 31]. The primary reason for this unapproved high-dose acid suppression is based on pH monitoring data indicating that the chances of normalizing exposure of the esophagus to acid in patients with chronic cough, laryngeal symptoms, or asthma are 99% with a twice-daily PPI [32]. A prospective cohort study (uncontrolled and open-label) assessed optimal PPI dose in patients with LPR, and indicated that twice-daily PPI is more effective than daily PPI in achieving clinical symptom response in patients with suspected LPR [23]. Unfortunately, the enthusiasm of treatment response in uncontrolled studies is dampened by the overall undifferentiated response in controlled studies (Table 50.1). This is most likely due to the overdiagnosis of LPR based on nonspecific laryngeal signs that overpopulate the clinical trials resulting in reduced study power to find a significant clinical benefit to PPI over placebo.

A number of uncontrolled observational studies have suggested efficacy of anti-reflux surgery in patients with LPR. However, studies suggest that the role of fundoplication is best delineated in those who have a positive symptom response to PPI therapy and caution should be exercised in referring patients who do not respond to aggressive acid suppression, especially those with extraesophageal complaints [46, 66, 68, 69]. Swoger et al. [46] evaluated surgical response rate in a group of patients with LPR unresponsive to aggressive PPI therapy. They studied 72 patients with symptoms consistent with LPR and treated them with 4 months of twice-daily PPI therapy. Twenty-five patients had <50% improvement despite maximal medical therapy. Ten of these patients underwent surgical fundoplication, while 15 remained on medical therapy alone. In the surgical group, one patient (10%) reported improvement in laryngeal symptoms at 1 year postoperatively. These studies suggest conserva-

tive nonsurgical approach in those with poor symptomatic response to PPI therapy.

Asthma and GERD

Patients with asthma have a higher prevalence of comorbid GERD than would be expected in the general population. Twenty-four hour pH assessment has shown that asthmatics have significant GERD in up to 80% of patients [47]. Although the majority of asthmatics with comorbid GERD have symptoms of reflux, approximately 40% of patients do not have typical reflux symptoms [48]. Symptoms that can be associated with asthma, including cough and chest pain, are often associated with GERD as well and this overlap can make it more challenging to assess for reflux-related symptoms. The two leading theories to explain the pathophysiologic relationship between GERD and asthma include bronchospasm due to aspiration of gastric contents, and a reflex arc by which acid stimulates sensory afferent nerves in the distal esophagus that trigger a vagally mediated response of bronchospasm [42].

Kiljander and colleagues studied the effect of asthma control in patients with documented GERD by 24-h pH monitoring and found that patients who received PPI therapy did not benefit in asthma control compared to placebo [43]. Later study by Sontag and colleagues evaluated the effects of fundoplication, ranitidine, and placebo on asthma symptoms in patients who had both asthma and GERD [44]. In this population, 75% of post-fundoplication patients noted improvement in nocturnal symptoms compared to 9.2% of those treated with pharmacotherapy alone and 4.2% of control patients. A subsequent controlled trial suggested a therapeutic benefit of PPIs in asthmatics with both nocturnal respiratory and GERD symptoms but no benefit in those without nocturnal symptoms [45]. Littner and colleagues found that patients with asthma and GERD symptoms treated with acid suppressive therapy did have an improvement in asthma-related quality of life and a reduction in asthma exacerbations but did not alter daily symptoms [49]. Most recently, the American Lung

extraesophageal symptoms including asthma, chronic cough, or laryngitis.

- Diagnostic testing should be reserved for those patients unresponsive to therapy. Most recent studies suggest that ambulatory impedance/pH monitoring may be most likely to help exclude reflux as the cause for persistent symptoms.
- Recent randomized placebo-controlled studies in chronic laryngitis, cough, and asthma have been disappointing in showing benefit from acid suppressive therapy.
- We are currently limited in our diagnostic ability to identify the subgroup of patients who might respond to acid suppressive therapy. Further outcome studies are needed to better understand the role of acid or nonacid reflux in patients with extraesophageal symptoms.

References

1. Vakil N, van Zanten SV, Kahrilas P, Dent J, Jones R. The Montreal definition and classification of gastroesophageal reflux disease: a global evidence-based consensus. Am J Gastroenterol. 2006;101(8):1900–20. quiz 1943.
2. Kahrilas PJ, Shaheen NJ, Vaezi MF. American gastroenterological association institute technical review on the management of gastroesophageal reflux disease. Gastroenterology. 2008;135(4):1392–413. 1413 e1391–1395.
3. Kahrilas PJ, Shaheen NJ, Vaezi MF, et al. American gastroenterological association medical position statement on the management of gastroesophageal reflux disease. Gastroenterology. 2008;135(4):1383–91. 1391 e1381–1385.
4. Kavitt RT, Vaezi MF. Gastroesophageal reflux laryngitis. In: Castell DO, Richter JE, editors. The esophagus. 5th ed. Oxford: Wiley-Blackwell; 2011.
5. Frye JW, Vaezi MF. Extraesophageal GERD. Gastroenterol Clin North Am. 2008;37(4):845–58. ix.
6. Moore JM, Vaezi MF. Extraesophageal manifestations of gastroesophageal reflux disease: real or imagined? Curr Opin Gastroenterol. 2010;26(4):389–94.
7. Jacob P, Kahrilas PJ, Herzon G. Proximal esophageal pH-metry in patients with 'reflux laryngitis'. Gastroenterology. 1991;100(2):305–10.
8. Ing AJ, Ngu MC, Breslin AB. Pathogenesis of chronic persistent cough associated with gastroesophageal reflux. Am J Respir Crit Care Med. 1994;149(1):160–7.
9. Smith J, Woodcock A, Houghton L. New developments in reflux-associated cough. Lung. 2010;188 Suppl 1:S81–6.
10. Everett CF, Morice AH. Clinical history in gastroesophageal cough. Respir Med. 2007;101(2):345–8.
11. Baldi F, Cappiello R, Cavoli C, Ghersi S, Torresan F, Roda E. Proton pump inhibitor treatment of patients with gastroesophageal reflux-related chronic cough: a comparison between two different daily doses of lansoprazole. World J Gastroenterol. 2006;12(1):82–8.
12. Vaezi MF, Richter JE. Twenty-four-hour ambulatory esophageal pH monitoring in the diagnosis of acid reflux-related chronic cough. South Med J. 1997;90(3):305–11.
13. Waring JP, Lacayo L, Hunter J, Katz E, Suwak B. Chronic cough and hoarseness in patients with severe gastroesophageal reflux disease. Diagnosis and response to therapy. Dig Dis Sci. 1995;40(5):1093–7.
14. Chang AB, Lasserson TJ, Kiljander TO, Connor FL, Gaffney JT, Garske LA. Systematic review and meta-analysis of randomised controlled trials of gastro-oesophageal reflux interventions for chronic cough associated with gastro-oesophageal reflux. Br Med J. 2006;332(7532):11–7.
15. Patterson N, Mainie I, Rafferty G, et al. Nonacid reflux episodes reaching the pharynx are important factors associated with cough. J Clin Gastroenterol. 2009;43(5):414–9.
16. Smith JA, Decalmer S, Kelsall A, et al. Acoustic cough-reflux associations in chronic cough: potential triggers and mechanisms. Gastroenterology. 2010;139(3):754–62.
17. Vaezi MF, Hicks DM, Abelson TI, Richter JE. Laryngeal signs and symptoms and gastroesophageal reflux disease (GERD): a critical assessment of cause and effect association. Clin Gastroenterol Hepatol. 2003;1(5):333–44.
18. Paterson WG, Murat BW. Combined ambulatory esophageal manometry and dual-probe pH-metry in evaluation of patients with chronic unexplained cough. Dig Dis Sci. 1994;39(5):1117–25.
19. Sifrim D, Dupont L, Blondeau K, Zhang X, Tack J, Janssens J. Weakly acidic reflux in patients with chronic unexplained cough during 24 hour pressure, pH, and impedance monitoring. Gut. 2005;54(4):449–54.
20. Blondeau K, Dupont LJ, Mertens V, Tack J, Sifrim D. Improved diagnosis of gastro-oesophageal reflux in patients with unexplained chronic cough. Aliment Pharmacol Ther. 2007;25(6):723–32.
21. Hanson DG, Jiang JJ. Diagnosis and management of chronic laryngitis associated with reflux. Am J Med. 2000;108((Suppl 4a)):112S–9.
22. Milstein CF, Charbel S, Hicks DM, Abelson TI, Richter JE, Vaezi MF. Prevalence of laryngeal irritation signs associated with reflux in asymptomatic volunteers: impact of endoscopic technique (rigid vs. Flexible laryngoscope). Laryngoscope. 2005;115(12):2256–61.
23. Park W, Hicks DM, Khandwala F, et al. Laryngopharyngeal reflux: prospective cohort study evaluating optimal dose of proton-pump inhibitor therapy and pretherapy predictors of response. Laryngoscope. 2005;115(7):1230–8.

24. Vaezi MF, Schroeder PL, Richter JE. Reproducibility of proximal probe pH parameters in 24-hour ambulatory esophageal pH monitoring. Am J Gastroenterol. 1997;92(5):825–9.

25. Adhami T, Goldblum JR, Richter JE, Vaezi MF. The role of gastric and duodenal agents in laryngeal injury: an experimental canine model. Am J Gastroenterol. 2004;99(11):2098–106.

26. Koufman JA. The otolaryngologic manifestations of gastroesophageal reflux disease (GERD): a clinical investigation of 225 patients using ambulatory 24-hour pH monitoring and an experimental investigation of the role of acid and pepsin in the development of laryngeal injury. Laryngoscope. 1991;101(4 Pt 2 Suppl 53):1–78.

27. Axford SE, Sharp N, Ross PE, et al. Cell biology of laryngeal epithelial defenses in health and disease: preliminary studies. Ann Otol Rhinol Laryngol. 2001; 110(12):1099–108.

28. Johnston N, Bulmer D, Gill GA, et al. Cell biology of laryngeal epithelial defenses in health and disease: further studies. Ann Otol Rhinol Laryngol. 2003;112(6):481–91.

29. Hicks DM, Ours TM, Abelson TI, Vaezi MF, Richter JE. The prevalence of hypopharynx findings associated with gastroesophageal reflux in normal volunteers. J Voice. 2002;16(4):564–79.

30. Shaker R, Bardan E, Gu C, Kern M, Torrico L, Toohill R. Intrapharyngeal distribution of gastric acid refluxate. Laryngoscope. 2003;113(7):1182–91.

31. Field SK, Sutherland LR. Does medical antireflux therapy improve asthma in asthmatics with gastroesophageal reflux?: a critical review of the literature. Chest. 1998;114(1):275–83.

32. Charbel S, Khandwala F, Vaezi MF. The role of esophageal pH monitoring in symptomatic patients on PPI therapy. Am J Gastroenterol. 2005;100(2):283–9.

33. Havas T, Huang S, Levy M, et al. Posterior pharyngolaryngitis: double-blind randomised placebo-controlled trial of proton pump inhibitor therapy. Aust J Otolaryngol. 1999;3:243.

34. Noordzij JP, Khidr A, Evans BA, et al. Evaluation of omeprazole in the treatment of reflux laryngitis: a prospective, placebo-controlled, randomized, double-blind study. Laryngoscope. 2001;111(12):2147–51.

35. El-Serag HB, Lee P, Buchner A, Inadomi JM, Gavin M, McCarthy DM. Lansoprazole treatment of patients with chronic idiopathic laryngitis: a placebo-controlled trial. Am J Gastroenterol. 2001;96(4):979–83.

36. Eherer AJ, Habermann W, Hammer HF, Kiesler K, Friedrich G, Krejs GJ. Effect of pantoprazole on the course of reflux-associated laryngitis: a placebo-controlled double-blind crossover study. Scand J Gastroenterol. 2003;38(5):462–7.

37. Steward DL, Wilson KM, Kelly DH, et al. Proton pump inhibitor therapy for chronic laryngopharyngitis: a randomized placebo-control trial. Otolaryngol Head Neck Surg. 2004;131(4):342–50.

38. Wo JM, Koopman J, Harrell SP, Parker K, Winstead W, Lentsch E. Double-blind, placebo-controlled trial with single-dose pantoprazole for laryngopharyngeal reflux. Am J Gastroenterol. 2006;101(9):1972–8. quiz 2169.

39. Vaezi MF, Richter JE, Stasney CR, et al. Treatment of chronic posterior laryngitis with esomeprazole. Laryngoscope. 2006;116(2):254–60.

40. Reichel O, Dressel H, Wiederanders K, Issing WJ. Double-blind, placebo-controlled trial with esomeprazole for symptoms and signs associated with laryngopharyngeal reflux. Otolaryngol Head Neck Surg. 2008;139(3):414–20.

41. Lam PKY, Ng ML, Cheung TK, et al. Rabeprazole is effective in treating laryngopharyngeal reflux in a randomized placebo-controlled trial. Clin Gastroenterol Hepatol. 2010;8(9):770–6.

42. Gastal OL, Castell JA, Castell DO. Frequency and site of gastroesophageal reflux in patients with chest symptoms. Studies using proximal and distal pH monitoring. Chest. 1994;106(6):1793–6.

43. Kiljander TO, Salomaa ER, Hietanen EK, Terho EO. Gastroesophageal reflux in asthmatics: A double-blind, placebo-controlled crossover study with omeprazole. Chest. 1999;116(5):1257–64.

44. Sontag SJ, O'Connell S, Khandelwal S, et al. Asthmatics with gastroesophageal reflux: long term results of a randomized trial of medical and surgical antireflux therapies. Am J Gastroenterol. 2003;98(5):987–99.

45. Kiljander TO, Harding SM, Field SK, et al. Effects of esomeprazole 40 mg twice daily on asthma: a randomized placebo-controlled trial. Am J Respir Crit Care Med. 2006;173(10):1091–7.

46. Swoger J, Ponsky J, Hicks DM, et al. Surgical fundoplication in laryngopharyngeal reflux unresponsive to aggressive acid suppression: a controlled study. Clin Gastroenterol Hepatol. 2006;4(4):433–41.

47. Parsons JP, Mastronarde JG. Gastroesophageal reflux disease and asthma. Curr Opin Pulm Med. 2010;16(1): 60–3.

48. Mastronarde JG, Anthonisen NR, Castro M, et al. Efficacy of esomeprazole for treatment of poorly controlled asthma. N Engl J Med. 2009;360(15):1487–99.

49. Littner MR, Leung FW, Ballard 2nd ED, Huang B, Samra NK. Effects of 24 weeks of lansoprazole therapy on asthma symptoms, exacerbations, quality of life, and pulmonary function in adult asthmatic patients with acid reflux symptoms. Chest. 2005;128(3):1128–35.

50. Kamal A, Vaezi MF. Diagnosis and initial management of gastroesophageal complications. Best Pract Res Clin Gastroenterol. 2010;24(6):799–820.

51. Richter JE. Peptic strictures of the esophagus. Gastroenterol Clin North Am. 1999;28(4):875–91.

52. El-Serag HB, Lau M. Temporal trends in new and recurrent oesophageal strictures in a Medicare population. Aliment Pharmacol Ther. 2007;25(10):1223–9.

53. Marks RD, Richter JE. Peptic strictures of the esophagus. Am J Gastroenterol. 1993;88(8):1160–73.

54. Marks RD, Richter JE, Rizzo J, et al. Omeprazole versus H2-receptor antagonists in treating patients with peptic stricture and esophagitis. Gastroenterology. 1994;106(4):907–15.

55. Schembre DB. Recent advances in the use of stens for esophageal disease. Gastrointest Endosc Clin N Am. 2010;20(1):103–21.

56. Vakil NB, Traxler B, Levine D. Dysphagia in patients with erosive esophagitis: prevalence, severity, and response to proton pump inhibitor treatment. Clin Gastroenterol Hepatol. 2004;2(8):665–8.

57. Triadafilopoulos G. Nonobstructive dysphagia in reflux esophagitis. Am J Gastroenterol. 1989;84(6):614–8.

58. Lew RJ, Kochman ML. A review of endoscopic methods of esophageal dilation. J Clin Gastroenterol. 2002;35(2):117–26.

59. Saeed ZA, Winchester CB, Ferro PS, Michaletz PA, Schwartz JT, Graham DY. Prospective randomized comparison of polyvinyl bougies and through-the-scope balloons for dilation of peptic strictures of the esophagus. Gastrointest Endosc. 1995;41(3):189–95.

60. Locke 3rd GR, Talley NJ, Fett SL, Zinsmeister AR, Melton 3rd LJ. Prevalence and clinical spectrum of gastroesophageal reflux: a population-based study in Olmsted county, Minnesota. Gastroenterology. 1997; 112(5):1448–56.

61. el-Serag HB, Sonnenberg A. Comorbid occurrence of laryngeal or pulmonary disease with esophagitis in United States military veterans. Gastroenterology. 1997;113(3):755–60.

62. Shay S, Tutuian R, Sifrim D, et al. Twenty-four hour ambulatory simultaneous impedance and pH monitoring: a multicenter report of normal values from 60 healthy volunteers. Am J Gastroenterol. 2004;99(6):1037–43.

63. Zerbib F, des Varannes SB, Roman S, et al. Normal values and day-to-day variability of 24-h ambulatory oesophageal impedance-pH monitoring in a Belgian-French cohort of healthy subjects. Aliment Pharmacol Ther. 2005;22(10):1011–21.

64. Ferguson DD. Evaluation and management of benign esophageal strictures. Dis Esophagus. 2005;18(6): 359–64.

65. Hirano I, Richter JE. ACG practice guidelines: esophageal reflux testing. Am J Gastroenterol. 2007;102(3): 668–85.

66. Tutuian R, Mainie I, Agrawal A, Adams D, Castell DO. Nonacid reflux in patients with chronic cough on acid-suppressive therapy. Chest. 2006;130(2):386–91.

67. Wright RC, Rhodes KP. Improvement of laryngopharyngeal reflux symptoms after laparoscopic hill repair. Am J Surg. 2003;185(5):455–61.

68. Salminen P, Sala E, Koskenvuo J, Karvonen J, Ovaska J. Reflux laryngitis: a feasible indication for laparoscopic antireflux surgery? Surg Laparosc Endosc Percutan Tech. 2007;17(2):73–8.

69. Mainie I, Tutuian R, Agrawal A, Adams D, Castell DO. Combined multichannel intraluminal impedance-pH monitoring to select patients with persistent gastro-oesophageal reflux for laparoscopic Nissen fundoplication. Br J Surg. 2006;93(12):1483–7. vi.

70. Ruigomez A, Garcia Rodriguez LA, Wallander MA, Johansson S, Eklund S. Esophageal stricture: incidence, treatment patterns, and recurrence rate. Am J Gastroenterol. 2006;101(12):2685–92.

71. Spechler SJ. Clinical manifestations and esophageal complications of GERD. Am J Med Sci. 2003;326(5): 279–84.

72. Scolapio JS, Pasha TM, Gostout CJ, et al. A randomized prospective study comparing rigid to balloon dilators for benign esophageal strictures and rings. Gastrointest Endosc. 1999;50(1):13–7.

73. Cox JG, Winter RK, Maslin SC, et al. Balloon or bougie for dilatation of benign esophageal stricture? Dig Dis Sci. 1994;39(4):776–81.

74. Hernandez LV, Jacobson JW, Harris MS. Comparison among the perforation rates of Maloney, balloon, and savary dilation of esophageal strictures. Gastrointest Endosc. 2000;51(4 Pt 1):460–2.

75. Karnak I, Tanyel FC, Buyukpamukcu N, Hicsonmez A. Esophageal perforations encountered during the dilation of caustic esophageal strictures. J Cardiovasc Surg. 1998;39(3):373–7.

76. Mandelstam P, Sugawa C, Silvis SE, Nebel OT, Rogers BH. Complications associated with esophagogastroduodenoscopy and with esophageal dilation. Gastrointest Endosc. 1976;23(1):16–9.

77. Silvis SE, Nebel O, Rogers G, Sugawa C, Mandelstam P. Endoscopic complications. Results of the 1974 American society for gastrointestinal endoscopy survey. J Am Med Assoc. 1976;235(9):928–30.

78. Farup PG, Modalsli B, Tholfsen JK. Long-term treatment with 300 mg ranitidine once daily after dilatation of peptic oesophageal strictures. Scand J Gastroenterol. 1992;27(7):594–8.

79. Ferguson R, Dronfield MW, Atkinson M. Cimetidine in treatment of reflux oesophagitis with peptic stricture. Br Med J. 1979;2(6188):472–4.

80. Starlinger M, Appel WH, Schemper M, Schiessel R. Long-term treatment of peptic esophageal stenosis with dilatation and cimetidine: factors influencing clinical result. European surgical research. Eur Surg Res. 1985;17(4):207–14.

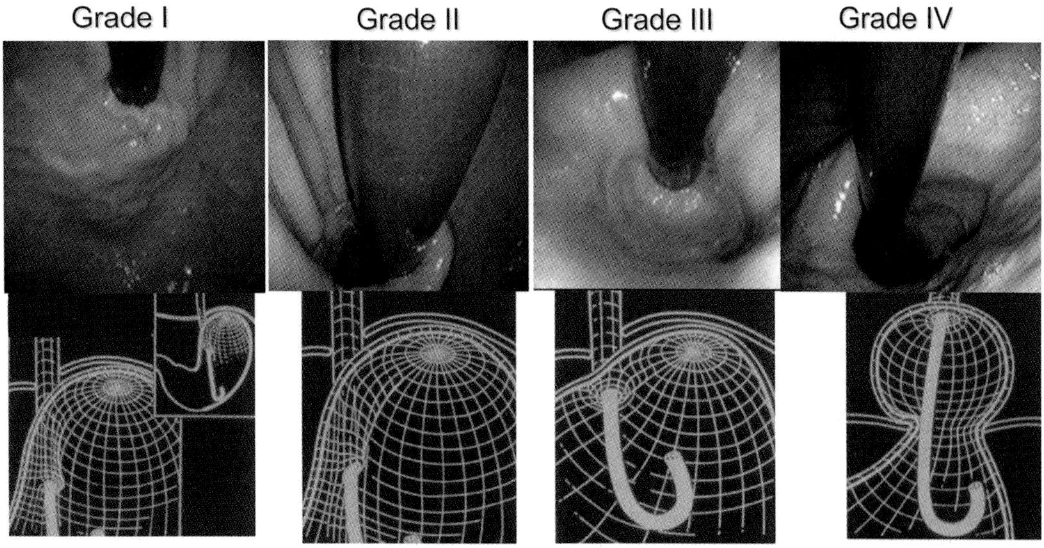

Grade I   Grade II   Grade III   Grade IV

Fig. 51.5 Endoscopic appearance and corresponding three-dimensional representation of the progressive anatomic disruption of the gastroesophageal junction as occurs with the development of a type I hiatus hernia. In the grade I configuration, a ridge of muscular tissue is closely approximated to the shaft of the retroflexed endoscope. With a grade II configuration the ridge of tissue is slightly less well defined and there has been slight orad displacement of the squamocolumnar junction along with widening of the angle of His. In the grade III appearance the ridge of tissue at the gastric entryway is barely present and there is often incomplete luminal closure around the endoscope. Note, however, that this is not a hiatal hernia because the SCJ is not displaced axially in the endoscopic photograph. With grade IV deformity, no muscular ridge is present at the gastric entry. The gastroesophageal area stays open all the time, and squamous epithelium of the distal esophagus can be seen from the retroflexed endoscopic view. A hiatus hernia is always present with grade IV deformity. From L.D. Hill et al. Contemp Surg 1994;44:1 with permission

insufflation of the stomach that might exaggerate the apparent size of the hernia. The variability in endoscopic interpretation of signs consistent with reflux (including hiatus hernia) was recently the subject of an experiment in which 120 endoscopists were asked to interpret the identical 2-min video of an upper endoscopy. Half of the participants were given a patient history consistent with reflux and the other half a patient history of epigastric pain; 42% of the group given the reflux history reported endoscopic findings consistent with reflux as opposed to only 12% given a history of epigastric pain [31].

Another approach to the endoscopic grading of sliding hiatus hernia is to assess the appearance of the EGJ from a retroflexed position and to incorporate an assessment of hiatal integrity along with the assessment of axial displacement. The progression from normal anatomy to type I hernia was well illustrated in an analysis of "flap valve" integrity as a predictor of reflux symptoms (Fig. 51.5) [33]. That analysis concluded that both reflux symptoms and EGJ competence (assessed in a postmortem experiment) were directly correlated to flap valve grade. Note that in Fig. 51.5, only the grade IV flap valve constitutes a sliding hiatal hernia as the SCJ is still at or below the level of the hiatus in types I, II, and III. Differentiating among these types depends on a subjective assessment of cardia integrity, the reproducibility of which has yet to be demonstrated. An attempt at objectifying that assessment utilized image analysis software to quantify the circumference of the gastric cardia using the size of the endoscope traversing the EGJ in the same image as a reference to correct for magnification [34]. That analysis of 273 endoscopies found a direct relationship between the magnitude of the cardia circumference as viewed in retroflexion and the presence (and severity) of GERD.

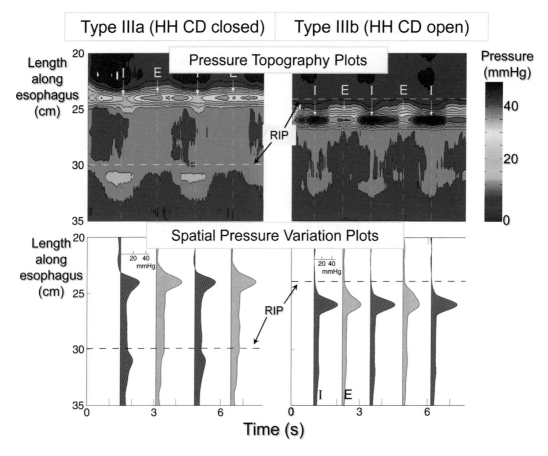

Fig. 51.7 EGJ type IIIa was defined when LES–CD separation was >2 cm at inspiration. This is the high-resolution manometry signature of hiatus hernia. Two subtypes were discernible, IIIa and IIIb, with the distinction being that the respiratory inversion point was proximal to the CD with IIIa and proximal to the LES in IIIb. The shift in respiratory inversion point is likely indicative of a grossly patulous hiatus, open throughout the respiratory cycle. Minimal EGJ pressure increase reflecting CD contraction is observed during inspiration with either type. From J.E. Pandolfino et al. Am J Gastroenterol 2007;102:1056–63 with permission

hernia by detecting intermediate grades of EGJ disruption. It also offers a means for prolonged observation permitting the assessment of intermittent herniation in some individuals [36]. Using high-resolution manometry with topographic plotting, three major subtypes of EGJ pressure morphology are demonstrable (Figs. 51.6 and 51.7): type I with the CD completely superimposed on the LES, type II with 1–2 cm separation between the two, and type III with greater than 2 cm separation. In a recent analysis, it was noted that EGJ type III was rarely found in asymptomatic controls or functional heartburn patients but

was a frequent finding in GERD patients demonstrating the clinical significance to this diagnostic approach [37].

Clinical Presentations of Hiatus Hernia

Hiatus hernia is a frequent condition which may or may not be symptomatic. It was listed as primary or secondary hospitalization cause in 142 of 10,000 inpatients in the US between 2003 and 2006 [38]. Sliding hernia may be associated with gastro-esophageal reflux symptoms or dysphagia.

Grade I   Grade II   Grade III   Grade IV

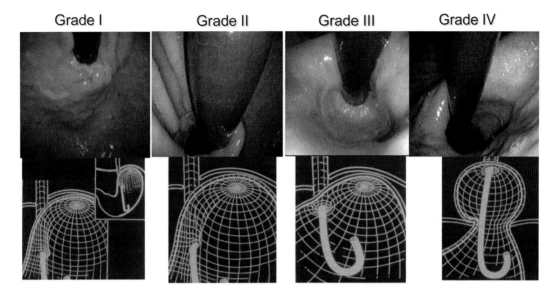

Fig. 51.5 Endoscopic appearance and corresponding three-dimensional representation of the progressive anatomic disruption of the gastroesophageal junction as occurs with the development of a type I hiatus hernia. In the grade I configuration, a ridge of muscular tissue is closely approximated to the shaft of the retroflexed endoscope. With a grade II configuration the ridge of tissue is slightly less well defined and there has been slight orad displacement of the squamocolumnar junction along with widening of the angle of His. In the grade III appearance the ridge of tissue at the gastric entryway is barely present and there is often incomplete luminal closure around the endoscope. Note, however, that this is not a hiatal hernia because the SCJ is not displaced axially in the endoscopic photograph. With grade IV deformity, no muscular ridge is present at the gastric entry. The gastroesophageal area stays open all the time, and squamous epithelium of the distal esophagus can be seen from the retroflexed endoscopic view. A hiatus hernia is always present with grade IV deformity. From L.D. Hill et al. Contemp Surg 1994;44:1 with permission

insufflation of the stomach that might exaggerate the apparent size of the hernia. The variability in endoscopic interpretation of signs consistent with reflux (including hiatus hernia) was recently the subject of an experiment in which 120 endoscopists were asked to interpret the identical 2-min video of an upper endoscopy. Half of the participants were given a patient history consistent with reflux and the other half a patient history of epigastric pain; 42% of the group given the reflux history reported endoscopic findings consistent with reflux as opposed to only 12% given a history of epigastric pain [31].

Another approach to the endoscopic grading of sliding hiatus hernia is to assess the appearance of the EGJ from a retroflexed position and to incorporate an assessment of hiatal integrity along with the assessment of axial displacement. The progression from normal anatomy to type I hernia was well illustrated in an analysis of "flap valve" integrity as a predictor of reflux symptoms (Fig. 51.5) [33]. That analysis concluded that both reflux symptoms and EGJ competence (assessed in a postmortem experiment) were directly correlated to flap valve grade. Note that in Fig. 51.5, only the grade IV flap valve constitutes a sliding hiatal hernia as the SCJ is still at or below the level of the hiatus in types I, II, and III. Differentiating among these types depends on a subjective assessment of cardia integrity, the reproducibility of which has yet to be demonstrated. An attempt at objectifying that assessment utilized image analysis software to quantify the circumference of the gastric cardia using the size of the endoscope traversing the EGJ in the same image as a reference to correct for magnification [34]. That analysis of 273 endoscopies found a direct relationship between the magnitude of the cardia circumference as viewed in retroflexion and the presence (and severity) of GERD.

In summary, there has been little study of the sensitivity or reproducibility of the endoscopic grading and measurement of sliding hiatus hernia. What information does exist suggests that endoscopy suffers from similar limitations to barium swallow radiography but is probably even more subjective because of additional confounding factors. Bits of recent data suggest that endoscopy may provide valuable information regarding the appearance of the EGJ during retroflexed imaging, but this requires further study. Thus in practical terms, unless a strict protocol for measurement is tightly adhered to, the identification of type I hernias less than 3 cm in size with endoscopy is unreliable. Furthermore because of a lack of standardization in the convention when the size measurement of a type I hernia is taken with respect to entry, exit, and the extent of gastric distention, the magnitude of the size estimate has an inherent 2 cm error.

High-Resolution Manometry

Manometric landmarks of the EGJ are different than either endoscopic or radiographic landmarks. The most notable features are (1) that intragastric pressure is greater than intraesophageal pressure, especially during inspiration, (2) that the high pressure zone of the EGJ has both tonic (LES) and phasic (CD) components, and (3) that respiration causes both intraluminal pressure changes and relative movement between pressure sensors and structural components of the EGJ. Thus, as one withdraws a catheter across the EGJ from the stomach, inspiration is associated with pressure augmentation when below the diaphragm and a fall in pressure when above it. The location at which this shift is referred to as the pressure inversion point and, in the simplest case, this is the level of the CD. However, great variability exists among individuals in (1) the magnitude of LES pressure, (2) the magnitude of pressure augmentation associated with CD contraction, (3) the magnitude of difference between intragastric and intraesophageal pressure, and, most importantly, (4) axial separation between the LES and the

CD. Hence, an inspiratory decrease in pressure can be indicative of a supradiaphragmatic location or it can result from movement within a high pressure zone from a locus of higher pressure to a locus of lower pressure. Thus, the pressure inversion point, an essential landmark in the definition of a sliding hiatal hernia, can mean more than one thing and is an inherently unreliable measurement.

By utilizing many closely spaced manometric pressure sensors and interpolating between adjacent sensors, high-resolution manometry with topographic plotting methods depicts the axial pressure profile of the EGJ in real time. Evident in Fig. 51.6, this facilitates the localization and quantification of the CD contraction within the EGJ [35]. In the normal individual (type I) the CD effect is directly superimposed on the LES resulting in substantial pressure augmentation during respiration, the extremes of which are illustrated in the spatial pressure variation plots in the lower panels of Fig. 51.6. One even appreciates that the LES and CD are tethered together by the downward displacement of the EGJ high pressure zone with inspiration.

The right panels of Fig. 51.6 illustrate an example of low-grade disruption of the EGJ (type II) such that there is quantifiable separation between the CD and the LES, but the magnitude of this separation is insufficient to constitute a sliding hernia because the pressure minimum between peaks (lower panel) remains above gastric pressure and luminal closure is maintained along the entire length from above the LES to below the CD. Of all of the methods for assessing sliding hiatus hernia, high-resolution manometry is the only one capable of reliably detecting this condition, the intermediate stage between normal and overt sliding hiatus hernia.

Progressive disruption of the EGJ results in further separation of the CD and LES and an overt sliding hiatus hernia (Fig. 51.7). When this separation exceeds about 2 cm, the pressure minimum between peaks in the spatial pressure variation plots (lower panels) is at or below gastric pressure. Also note the laxity of the fixation between the LES and the diaphragm. No longer does the LES pressure band exhibit downward

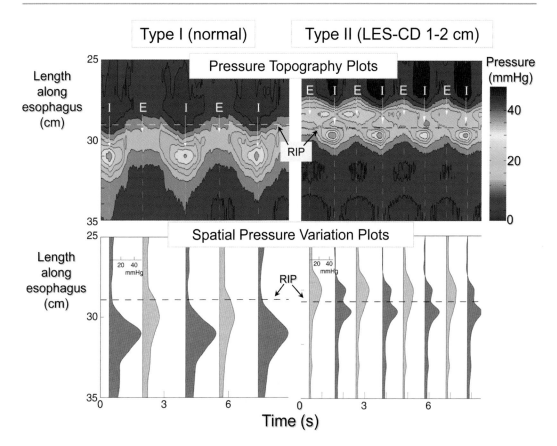

Fig. 51.6 High-resolution manometry examples of EGJ pressure morphology subtypes primarily distinguished by the extent of lower esophageal sphincter–crural diaphragm (LES–CD) separation. The upper plot in each panel is a pressure topography representation of the pressure changes spanning from the distal esophagus, across the EGJ, and into the proximal stomach during several respiratory cycles. The pressure scale is shown at the right. The lower plots illustrate a series of spatial pressure variation plots at the instants of peak inspiration (*dark gray*) and expiration (*light gray*) corresponding to the times marked I and E on the upper panels with pressure magnitude on the *x*-axis and axial location along the *y*-axis. The location of the respiratory inversion point (RIP) is shown by the horizontal dashed line. Type I is characterized by complete overlap of the CD and the LES with a single pressure peak in the spatial pressure variation plots during both inspiration and expiration. The RIP lies at the proximal margin of the EGJ. Type II is characterized by minimal, but discernible, LES–CD separation making for a double peaked spatial pressure variation plot, but the nadir pressure between the peaks was still greater than gastric pressure. The RIP is within the EGJ at the proximal margin of the CD. From J.E. Pandolfino et al. Am J Gastroenterol 2007;102:1056–63 with permission

displacement with inspiration. The distinction between a type IIIa and type IIIb hernia is in the position of the respiratory inversion point (RIP). The RIP was defined as the axial position along the EGJ at which the inspiratory EGJ pressure became less than the expiratory EGJ pressure. Conceptually, this is the position at which the external EGJ environment switches from intra-abdominal to intra-mediastinal pressure. With type IIIa this is still at the proximal boundary of the CD whereas with a type IIIb hernia, the hiatus is so patulous as to never seal off the hernia pouch from the stomach with consequent migration of the RIP to the proximal margin of the LES.

In summary, high-resolution manometry objectifies the assessment of sliding hiatus hernia. For the first time, it offers a means to complete the continuum from normal to overt sliding

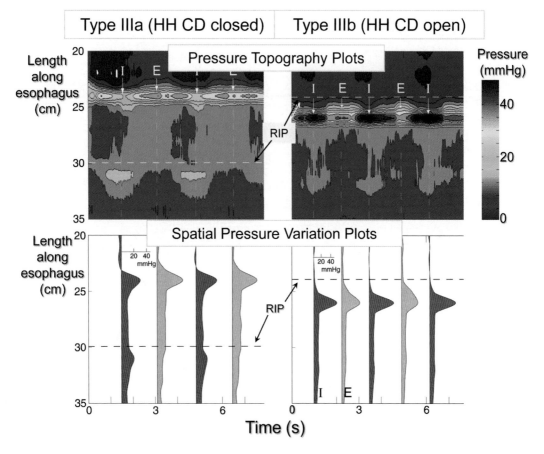

Fig. 51.7 EGJ type IIIa was defined when LES–CD separation was >2 cm at inspiration. This is the high-resolution manometry signature of hiatus hernia. Two subtypes were discernible, IIIa and IIIb, with the distinction being that the respiratory inversion point was proximal to the CD with IIIa and proximal to the LES in IIIb. The shift in respiratory inversion point is likely indicative of a grossly patulous hiatus, open throughout the respiratory cycle. Minimal EGJ pressure increase reflecting CD contraction is observed during inspiration with either type. From J.E. Pandolfino et al. Am J Gastroenterol 2007;102:1056–63 with permission

hernia by detecting intermediate grades of EGJ disruption. It also offers a means for prolonged observation permitting the assessment of intermittent herniation in some individuals [36]. Using high-resolution manometry with topographic plotting, three major subtypes of EGJ pressure morphology are demonstrable (Figs. 51.6 and 51.7): type I with the CD completely superimposed on the LES, type II with 1–2 cm separation between the two, and type III with greater than 2 cm separation. In a recent analysis, it was noted that EGJ type III was rarely found in asymptomatic controls or functional heartburn patients but was a frequent finding in GERD patients demonstrating the clinical significance to this diagnostic approach [37].

Clinical Presentations of Hiatus Hernia

Hiatus hernia is a frequent condition which may or may not be symptomatic. It was listed as primary or secondary hospitalization cause in 142 of 10,000 inpatients in the US between 2003 and 2006 [38]. Sliding hernia may be associated with gastro-esophageal reflux symptoms or dysphagia.

Paraesophageal hernias are either asymptomatic or associated with vague, intermittent symptoms. When present, symptoms are generally related to ischemia or either partial or complete obstruction. The most common symptoms are epigastric or substernal pain, postprandial fullness, substernal fullness, nausea, and retching. Hiatal hernia is also responsible for bleeding and chronic iron deficiency anemia [39]. Gastrointestinal bleeding is a consequence of Cameron lesions. [40]. These linear gastric ulcers or erosions occur on the gastric mucosal folds traversing the diaphragm in patients with large hiatal hernia.

Gastro-Esophageal Reflux Disease

Hiatal hernia may promote reflux by numerous mechanisms. The antireflux barrier is altered by the separation of the LES and the CD. The widening of the esophageal hiatus also impairs the CD's ability to function as a sphincter. Acidic gastric juice is contained in the hiatal sac and may then reflux into the esophagus. Finally the position of the acid pocket is modified by the presence of hiatal hernia and may promote acid reflux.

Anatomical separation of the LES and the CD leads to an altered pressure profile and impaired antireflux barrier function of the EGJ [5]. Thus, the pressure decreases at the level of the EGJ along with the length of functional EGJ. Bredenoord et al. observed that in patients with a small hiatal hernia spatial dissociation of the LES and CD occurred intermittently and that spatial dissociation correlated in time with increased acid reflux [36]. Hiatal hernia size is the dominant determinant of esophagitis presence and severity in GERD [41]. Increasing the size of the hernia is associated with increasing esophageal acid exposure and prolonged acid clearance time [42].

Mechanical properties of EGJ are also modified by the presence of hiatal hernia. In some patients with hiatal hernia dilation of the crural aperture may result in increased EGJ compliance and wider opening diameter during relaxation [13]. This change of EGJ compliance increases the

risk of having liquid reflux and may contribute to the increased acid exposure observed in patients with hiatal hernia [43].

The hiatal sac can also function as a reservoir of potential refluxate. During periods of low sphincter pressure ingested liquid can re-reflux from the hiatal sac into the esophagus [44, 45]. Indeed low LES pressure, impaired clearance, and accumulation of gastric contents in the hiatal sac facilitate reflux during swallow-induced LES relaxation.

Finally the position of acid pocket may also play a role in the genesis of acid reflux in patients with hiatal hernia. Indeed, the presence of hiatal hernia determines the position of the acid pocket. Beaumont et al. showed that the acid pocket extended continuously above the diaphragm in 40% of patients with large hiatal hernia (>3 cm) and migrated intermittently above the diaphragm in the remainder [46]. At the opposite extreme the acid pocket was located immediately distal to the SCJ in healthy volunteers and patients with small hiatal hernia. In the same study acid reflux during a transient LES relaxation occurred more often in patients with a hiatal hernia especially in those with large hiatal hernia and the risk of having acid reflux was mainly determined by the position of the acid pocket above the diaphragm.

Dysphagia

The role of paraesophageal hernia in the genesis of dysphagia is easy to understand. The stomach herniated through the hiatus may exert compression of the distal esophagus and thus cause an extrinsic mechanical obstruction. Sliding hiatus hernia may also promote dysphagia. In some patients barium swallow shows stasis of contrast in the hiatal sac which reflects impaired clearance. As previously mentioned (Fig. 51.2) esophageal shortening and recoil of phrenoesophageal ligament during the swallowing sequence are impaired in patients with hiatal hernia. The recoil of the phrenoesophageal ligament is important for emptying of the distal esophagus [47] and its impairment in case of hiatus hernia may explain dysphagia.

26. Smith AB, Dickerman RD, McGuire CS, East JW, McConathy WJ, Pearson HF. Pressure-overload-induced sliding hiatal hernia in power athletes. J Clin Gastroenterol. 1999;28:352–4.

27. Eren S, Ciris F. Diaphragmatic hernia: diagnostic approaches with review of the literature. Eur J Radiol. 2005;54:448–59.

28. Karpelowsky JS, Wieselthaler N, Rode H. Primary paraesophageal hernia in children. J Pediatr Surg. 2006;41:1588–93.

29. Ott DJ, Gelfand DW, Chen YM, Wu WC, Munitz HA. Predictive relationship of hiatal hernia to reflux esophagitis. Gastrointest Radiol. 1985;10:317–20.

30. Stilson WL, Sanders I, Gardiner GA, Gorman HC, Lodge DF. Hiatal hernia and gastroesophageal reflux. A clinicoradiological analysis of more than 1,000 cases. Radiology. 1969;93:1323–7.

31. Bytzer P. Information bias in endoscopic assessment. Am J Gastroenterol. 2007;102:1585–7.

32. Hill LD, Kraemer SJ, Aye RW. Laparoscopic hill repair. Contemp Surg. 1994;44:1.

33. Hill LD, Kozarek RA, Kraemer SJ, Aye RW, Mercer CD, Low DE, Pope 2nd CE. The gastroesophageal flap valve: in vitro and in vivo observations. Gastrointest Endosc. 1996;44:541–7.

34. Seltman AK, Kahrilas PJ, Chang EY, Mori M, Hunter JG, Jobe BA. Endoscopic measurement of cardia circumference as an indicator of GERD. Gastrointest Endosc. 2006;63:22–31.

35. Pandolfino JE, Kim H, Ghosh SK, Clarke JO, Zhang Q, Kahrilas PJ. High-resolution manometry of the EGJ: an analysis of crural diaphragm function in GERD. Am J Gastroenterol. 2007;102:1056–63.

36. Bredenoord AJ, Weusten BL, Timmer R, Smout AJ. Intermittent spatial separation of diaphragm and lower esophageal sphincter favors acidic and weakly acidic reflux. Gastroenterology. 2006;130:334–40.

37. Kahrilas PJ, Kim HC, Pandolfino JE. Approaches to the diagnosis and grading of hiatal hernia. Best Pract Res Clin Gastroenterol. 2008;22:601–16.

38. Thukkani N, Sonnenberg A. The influence of environmental risk factors in hospitalization for gastro-oesophageal reflux disease-related diagnoses in the United States. Aliment Pharmacol Ther. 2010;31: 852–61.

39. Annibale B, Capurso G, Chistolini A, D'Ambra G, DiGiulio E, Monarca B, DelleFave G. Gastrointestinal causes of refractory iron deficiency anemia in patients without gastrointestinal symptoms. Am J Med. 2001;111:439–45.

40. Maganty K, Smith RL. Cameron lesions: unusual cause of gastrointestinal bleeding and anemia. Digestion. 2008;77:214–7.

41. Jones MP, Sloan SS, Rabine JC, Ebert CC, Huang CF, Kahrilas PJ. Hiatal hernia size is the dominant determinant of esophagitis presence and severity in gastroesophageal reflux disease. Am J Gastroenterol. 2001;96:1711–7.

42. Jones MP, Sloan SS, Jovanovic B, Kahrilas PJ. Impaired egress rather than increased access: an important independent predictor of erosive oeso-phagitis. Neurogastroenterol Motil. 2002;14:625–31.

43. Pandolfino JE, Shi G, Curry J, Joehl RJ, Brasseur JG, Kahrilas PJ. Esophagogastric junction distensibility: a factor contributing to sphincter incompetence. Am J Physiol Gastrointest Liver Physiol. 2002;282: G1052–8.

44. Mittal RK, Lange RC, McCallum RW. Identification and mechanism of delayed esophageal acid clearance in subjects with hiatus hernia. Gastroenterology. 1987;92:130–5.

45. Sloan S, Kahrilas PJ. Impairment of esophageal emptying with hiatal hernia. Gastroenterology. 1991;100:596–605.

46. Beaumont H, Bennink RJ, de Jong J, Boeckxstaens GE. The position of the acid pocket as a major risk factor for acidic reflux in healthy subjects and patients with GORD. Gut. 2010;59:441–51.

47. Lin S, Brasseur JG, Pouderoux P, Kahrilas PJ. The phrenic ampulla: distal esophagus or potential hiatal hernia? Am J Physiol. 1995;268:G320–7.

48. Scherer JR, Kwiatek MA, Soper NJ, Pandolfino JE, Kahrilas PJ. Functional esophagogastric junction obstruction with intact peristalsis: a heterogeneous syndrome sometimes akin to achalasia. J Gastrointest Surg. 2009;13:2219–25.

49. Pandolfino JE, Kwiatek MA, Ho K, Scherer JR, Kahrilas PJ. Unique features of esophagogastric junction pressure topography in hiatus hernia patients with dysphagia. Surgery. 2010;147:57–64.

Part XII

Eating Disorders

is a very rare swallowing condition but could be very traumatic for the patient and result in a decreased quality of life.

Terminology

Several different terms have been used to describe this swallowing condition with a suspected psychogenic origin, for example *choking phobia* [1–3], *globus hystericus* [4–7], *hysterical dysphagia* [8, 9], *phagophobia* [10], and *pseudodysphagia* [11].

Symptoms

Symptoms found to be associated with psychogenic dysphagia were difficulty in initiating the swallow and avoidance of swallowing specific food, fluids, or pills resulting in malnutrition, and weight loss [4, 5, 8, 10, 12, 13]. However, the most obvious and also most frequently noted symptom in a swallowing condition of psychogenic origin was fear of swallowing, because swallowing was associated with fear of choking incidents. Other common symptoms in patients with this condition are complaints of globus, general difficulties in swallowing, and breathing problems [10, 11]. Finkenbine and Miehle [4] described globus as both a manifestation of a physiological disorder and of psychiatric illness. Bradley and Narula [11] described the sensation of a "lump" or "fullness" localized to the throat in association with globus hystericus, hysterical dysphagia, or pseudodysphagia. The condition could be a form of conversion disorder and is described as a:

> 'primary globus pharyngeus' when there was no evident cause, or 'secondary globus pharyngeus' when the etiology was detectable. (p. 689)

Abnormal oral behaviors (e.g., repeated deviant tongue movements) and a feeling of throat pressure may be other possible symptoms associated with a dysphagia with psychogenic origin.

Patients with psychogenic dysphagia may suffer from anxiety and depression, as an unconscious process in which psychological conflicts and anxiety would be transformed into somatic symptoms. There are also speculations that psychogenic dysphagia should be considered a *conversion disorder*. Other theories suggested that persons suffering from psychological conflicts could, as an attempt to reduce unacceptable emotional responses, instead convert them into more acceptable physical manifestations [4, 14].

Nicholson et al. [15] in 2010 note that psychogenic dysphagia is a problematic diagnosis as the psychological mechanism and presentation differs from the conscious simulation. In a case study by Okada et al. [16] six children with phagophobia have been analyzed according to psycho-pathology and current treatment. Their results indicated that evaluation of premorbid personality is crucial to the prognosis. The authors point out the importance to clarify the disorder according to psycho-pathology and describe two different types: (1) post-traumatic type and (2) gain-from-illness type, this clarification is of importance to be able to provide the right treatment. In an older study from 1935 Kanner and colleagues [17] discussed that dysphagia may be a primary conversion disorder. An example is a 12-year-old boy who developed dysphagia to solid foods due to physical abuse from his father for eating improperly. At the Diagnostic Center of Imaging and Functional Medicine at Malmö University Hospital, Malmö, Sweden, we encountered similar cases. An anecdotal case was a middle aged woman who presented with fear of initiating the pharyngeal swallow. She also presented an abnormal oral phase of swallowing during the Videofluoroscopic examination (VFSE). When she was a child a strict grandmother forced her to always empty her plate. When she visited her grandmother she always had great fear, especially when she had to eat together with her. Later in life, when she was exposed to stress she described that it was impossible for her to eat and swallow normally. After the VFSE she was offered dysphagia therapy involving eating sessions by the dysphagia clinician and began therapy. During the same period of time she also had psychological therapy.

Esophageal function may be influence by psychological factors. In 1883, Kronecker and

Meltzer [18] described that esophageal contractions could be a result from psychological stress. It has been suggested that, in some cases, the oral and the esophageal phases of swallowing may react to emotional distress and psychological symptoms. That is, the esophagus may react with non-propulsive contractions not only due to emotional tension, but also in some cases due to cold or hot food probably due to increased swallowing stimulation. Also, stimuli not related to ingestion such as intense short sounds may influence esophageal contraction and are likely to form part of the defense reaction of a healthy organism [6].

Prevalence of Psychogenic Dysphagia

Prevalence of psychogenic dysphagia is not well studied and is variably reported whether conditions such as globus are included in this diagnosis. Malcolmson et al. [19] reported that of the 231 patients diagnosed with globus hystericus, only 20 % were found to have a negative clinical and radiological evaluation.

At our swallowing clinic, at the Diagnostic Center of Imaging and Functional Medicine, Malmö University Hospital, Malmö, Sweden, we have completed 1,844 VFSE studies during the years 2002–2009, and psychogenic dysphagia was diagnosed in 22 cases (0 01 %). The most common swallowing signs and symptoms noticed during the VFSE were as follows.

Fear of swallowing	10/22
Globus complaints	5/22
Oral abnormalities (such as multiple tongue movements with difficulties in propelling the bolus posteriorly to pass the base of the tongue and initiating the pharyngeal swallow) (this was noticed during the VFSE and the evaluation of the patients was not completed)	6/22
Problems in initiating the pharyngeal swallow. (The patient experienced a feeling of being unable to swallow. However at videofluoroscopy we could document a normal pharyngeal swallow.)	8/22
Experienced difficulties in swallowing specific consistencies	11/22
Normal pharyngeal swallow function	22/22

We found that our patients often experienced more than one swallowing symptom. In a patient with suspected esophageal dysfunction or complaint of globus that we could find no pharyngeal dysfunction, recommendations were given to the referring physician to go on with further examinations, for example, to contact either an otolaryngologist or a gastroenterologist.

Thompson and Heaton [20] found 45 % of young and middle aged people have been estimated to suffer from symptoms of globus, often in combination with strong emotion. Another study reported that the symptom of choking phobia was more frequent in females (two-thirds of cases) and had a high comorbidity with anxiety disorders. Different life-events such as a divorce, disease in the family, or unemployment, as well as traumatic eating antecedents, were also frequently present [2].

In 1995, Korkina and Marilov [21] studied 612 patients with different psychosomatic gastrointestinal disorders. In 70 % of these cases, patient relatives also had psychosomatic diseases, suggesting the possible influence of genetic and environmental factors in this condition. In a report from the Johns Hopkins Swallowing Center in Baltimore, USA, Ravich et al. found that 13 % of the referred patients had a psychogenic dysphagia or globus hystericus [5]. They reevaluated 23 patients with the diagnoses of psychogenic dysphagia. The results from that study showed that more than half of these patients were subsequently found to have an underlying physical explanation for their swallowing problems [5]. Pharyngeal dysfunction, structural obstruction, or esophageal dysmotility were found in 15 of 23 (65 %) of these patients. Therefore, diagnosis of psychogenic dysphagia should be made with caution and after organic causes are ruled out. When any changes or progression of symptoms are reported, a careful reevaluation should promptly be performed.

Evaluation

A thorough swallowing evaluation is necessary in a patient with suspected psychogenic dysphagia. It is important to mention that a diagnosis of

following meals and never during sleep. Usually ruminators are unable to control rumination events, with no warning or nausea prior to an event. Nausea symptoms are typically related to or lead to increased autonomic arousal, which then increases the likelihood of rumination. However, a subset of school-aged ruminators are able to regurgitate and reswallow upon request. They may think of rumination as an innocent amusement that they control, like someone who can wiggle their ears.

Physiology

Rumination is considered an exaggeration of the belch reflex [10]. In adults with rumination syndrome, there is an increase in conscious perception with balloon inflation in the stomach and a decrease in lower esophageal sphincter pressure accompanied by proximal gastric distension compared to controls, but there was no data about the rumination event [11]. Presumably, as the voluntary muscles of the abdominal wall and diaphragm contract, the lower esophageal sphincter relaxes and gastric contents move from the higher pressure in the stomach to the lower pressure in the chest and pharynx [12]. In some patients, rumination is under conscious control. In those patients, rumination may be a learned, voluntary relaxation of the diaphragmatic crura.

Standard esophageal or antroduodenal manometry provides convincing diagnostic evidence for patients who refuse to believe the clinician's symptom-based diagnosis. Rumination events are characterized by brief simultaneous increases in pressure in all recording sites, called "r-waves" or "rumination waves." In contrast, true vomiting is characterized by powerful, long duration retrograde contractions from the small bowel through the stomach and up the esophagus. Moreover, the vomiting reflex involves coordinated, violent contractions of respiratory, pharyngeal, and abdominal skeletal muscle, while rumination does not [13].

Differential Diagnosis

Naïve rumination patients typically present with the primary symptom of "vomiting." With every history of vomiting, the clinician clarified if the vomiting was violent or effortless. If the historian is unable to decide, then the clinician may ask the patient to act out what happens. If the patient hesitates, the clinician should demonstrate the difference [14].

Clinicians unfamiliar with rumination may call the symptoms "gastroesophageal reflux." However, there is no heartburn, chest pain, or endoscopic disease associated with rumination. Rumination syndrome does not respond to medical treatment for gastroesophageal reflux.

In a small number of cases, rumination may be the presenting symptom of bulimia nervosa. In such patients it is more effective to target treatment of the eating disorder rather than rumination. Up to 20% of bulimic subjects ruminated [15], and 17% of female ruminators had a history of bulimia [15].

Complications

Children, particularly adolescents, are at risk for adjustment problems and psychosocial complications related to rumination. Social complications are common. School-aged children are often sent home from school for "vomiting" in the classroom, and may stay home from school for weeks or months due to rumination that is neither diagnosed nor treated correctly. Mismanagement of rumination results in unnecessary procedures and emotional distress, as each test returns normal but the patient continues to suffer. Less commonly, students are sent home because of a belching noise that accompanies each rumination event, disrupting class. Adolescents may skip lunch or skip school to avoid the embarrassment associated with rumination. Some students ruminate during athletic activities, limiting their participation. Adults and adolescents may treat themselves by reducing their meal size and number, resulting in weight loss.

Gathering a complete biopsychosocial history is helpful in establishing whether there is medical and/or psychosocial comorbidity and it is an important step in treating patients with rumination. Many ruminators have comorbid psychological symptoms, most often related to anxiety, which increase autonomic arousal and likely contribute to rumination symptoms. Rumination syndrome may coexist with social anxiety, resulting in a person who cannot leave the house because of "vomiting" [10]. About a third of adult patients have a comorbid psychological diagnosis. An anxiety disorder is frequently associated with poor adjustment, including sleep disturbance and inability to attend school or work.

Excessive utilization of medical resources puts the patient at unnecessary risk and increases medical costs. Rumination syndrome is a symptom-based diagnosis. When recognized, it is a diagnosis that is made on the first clinical visit and treated promptly. When rumination goes unrecognized, there are multiple and repeated unhelpful laboratory tests and procedures and radiological studies that may occur. Each negative test increases anxiety for the patient and family, who become fearful that something rare and serious is being missed. This increase in anxiety, and autonomic arousal, may in turn increase symptoms.

Occasionally patients do not accept a diagnosis of rumination syndrome, but insist that there is a digestive disease. When a patient demands a test before accepting the diagnosis, antroduodenal manometry can be utilized to demonstrate the "R-wave," the manometric correlate of the rumination event.

Dental erosions are common, affecting between 2 and 5% of the population. Dental erosions are defined as loss of tooth enamel by a chemical process that does not involve bacteria, compared to caries which involve tooth damage due to bacteria. When teeth are exposed to acid for a prolonged time, dissolution of tooth surface occurs, resulting in loss of tooth substance, pain, and fracture. Dental erosions can be permanent, disfiguring, and disabling. Therefore, if enamel demineralization is detected early, before changes become irreversible, modification in behavior, diet, and medication can be instituted so that the enamel framework can be remineralized.

Vomiting, regurgitation, gastroesophageal reflux disease, and rumination are all intrinsic sources of oral acid. There are several extrinsic sources of acid including diet and medication. Dental erosions are prominent in patients with rumination syndrome. However there have been no prospective studies confirming this link.

Treatment

Most otherwise healthy children and adults who ruminate are eager to rid themselves of the problem. The most important treatment is a behavioral intervention, teaching diaphragmatic breathing. A clinician, often a psychologist, teaches the patient habit reversal techniques to counteract the physiological response that occurs during rumination. Habit reversal via diaphragmatic breathing has been shown to be an effective treatment for rumination among both children [16, 17] and adults [18]. Diaphragmatic breathing achieves abdominal wall distention providing an incompatible response to rumination. The patient is asked to practice diaphragmatic breathing at home for 10 minutes two or three times a day with the stomach empty until the patient becomes comfortable with the technique. Then the patient is asked to do diaphragmatic breathing during and after meals. If the patient is doing the breathing correctly, they will not ruminate. This technique is also useful in achieving heightened relaxation, thus reducing autonomic arousal and gut sensitivity. Additional relaxation skills (e.g., imagery, muscle relaxation) and biofeedback can also help increase physiological control.

No medication is indicated for rumination, although treatment of any underlying psychological disorder may be helpful.

Some adolescents with rumination symptoms present with weight loss and prolonged school absence due to food restriction. Those severely affected by rumination benefited from a rehabilitation hospitalization. Inpatient treatment included habit reversal protocols, such as awareness training (e.g. daily log of symptoms and antecedents), aversive pairing (e.g. reswallow emesis), and an incompatible response (e.g. diaphragmatic breathing). Strategies for self-regulating autonomic arousal and distraction were taught and encouraged. Biofeedback was used to practice diaphragmatic breathing and increase awareness of abdominal muscle contractions during rumination episodes. Oral intake was increased via a habituation protocol, slowly decreasing meal duration and increasing the amount of food throughout the hospital stay [21].

Taste

Gustatory stimulation as a compensatory approach may feasibly influence swallowing biomechanics via two mechanisms. Enhancement of taste may operate purely at bulbar levels to provide greater excitability to the nucleus tractus solitarius for elicitation of a swallowing response. Additionally, as with smell, the presentation of a gustatory sensory stimulus may reasonably act on cortical preparatory mechanisms underlying swallowing.

Early research focused primarily on the application of a sour bolus [14]. Other research has followed this trend, but has expanded to compare and contrast sour with other classes of taste including sweet, bitter and salty [4], or to differentially evaluate taste relative to temperature. Across early studies, taste modification has been documented to produce a reduction in the timing features of swallowing.

More recent research has evaluated the differential effects of a cold stimulus and a sour bolus [15]. Reduced pharyngeal transit time (PTT) was reported in 30 post-stroke patients during intake of a combined 5-ml sour/cold paste bolus as compared to no taste, sour or cold stimuli independently. However, the median PTT of 1.58 s remains considerably longer than the accepted normal duration of ≤1 s.

Pelletier and Lawless [16] employed mixture suppression, adding a taste to another that will mask it to some degree, in a study of the effect of a sweet-masked sour bolus, compared to water and sour citric boluses in 11 nursing home patients. All had acquired neurogenic dysphagia, with aspiration or penetration, and six had dementia. Endoscopic evaluation of swallowing suggested that sour citric bolus significantly reduced aspiration and penetration as compared to water or sweet–sour mix bolus. Additionally, the sour citric bolus increased frequency of swallowing, which may be important in clearance of any residual. The mixing of a sweet taste with a sour one appeared to have no effect on hastening the pharyngeal swallow response but the levels of citric acid were different in the two flavoured conditions. If a minimum taste enhancement level

should prove necessary to produce biomechanical change this needs to be determined in order to create equivalent conditions. It may also be the case that intensities of taste enhancement require adjustment based upon a person's age as taste thresholds increase with advancing years [17].

As a subsequent quantitative measure of biomechanics, Pelletier and Dhanaraj [18] evaluated taste effects on lingual pressure generation. Results from their study of ten healthy young adults revealed that moderate concentrations of sweet, salty and sour tastes in water elicited significantly higher lingual swallowing pressure than water alone. However, higher concentrations did not result in further increases in pressure. It is unclear if the absence of a 'dose' effect is related to the specific concentrations applied in the study or if no further physiologic benefit is gained from increasing concentrations of stimuli once a threshold of change is reached.

The influence of taste on swallowing has been examined using not only biomechanical imaging but also EMG to further explore timing modifications. Intramuscular EMG was used by Palmer et al. [19] to measure activity of the mylohyoid, anterior belly of digastric and geniohyoid muscles during 3-ml water and 3-ml sour lemon bolus swallows. Their eight healthy participants were reported to exhibit stronger muscle contraction and a shorter time for activation onset of all three muscles with the sour bolus when compared to water bolus. However, no significant differences were found for onset of swallowing or muscle activity patterns or duration.

Sciortino et al. [20] conducted a small study of sour taste effects in seven young and seven older healthy adults. Sour taste and cold applied to the faucial pillars produced a significantly faster initiation of swallowing compared to the no-stimulation condition, as measured using sEMG. However, where a second swallow was recorded, the effect had been lost. This suggests that sensory activation of the faucial pillars is short term. In another sEMG study, Ding et al. [21] evaluated the effects of sweet, salty and sour tastes on the timing of pharyngeal swallow in a group of 20 healthy older and 20 healthy younger adults. All taste stimuli significantly reduced the time until

limited. Clinicians should remain mindful of the likelihood that consistency changes in particular can be unacceptable, especially over longer time periods, and that undesirable side effects, such as dehydration may ensue. Further evaluation of the effectiveness of bolus modification strategies using standard measures and considering both immediate and long-term outcomes will benefit clinical decision-making.

Postural Techniques

Several postural techniques have been described as a means of altering oral pharyngeal anatomy with the goal of directing the bolus toward more efficient transfer to the oesophageal inlet. The most common of these include chin tuck, head rotation and neck extension.

Chin Tuck

Chin tuck posturing was initially described in the 1980s and became the subject of considerable biomechanical research in the ensuing years [1, 41–43]. Hypothesised effects of the technique include: widening of the vallecular space to allow greater capacity for holding pre-swallow spillage and so prevent pre-swallow aspiration; a narrowing of the distance between the base of tongue (BOT) and posterior pharyngeal wall (PPW) to increase pressure on the bolus for descent and thereby lessen post-swallow residual and a narrowing of the space between the epiglottis and PPW to improve airway protection and reduce aspiration during the swallow [44]. It has been most often clinically prescribed for patients with a delayed pharyngeal swallow, pre-swallow pooling or post-swallow residual. However as with many of our intervention techniques, conflicting research data and within-patient variability demand that clinicians evaluate this posture carefully using instrumental assessment before patient application.

The Logemann et al. [33] and Robbins et al. [37] studies outlined in the previous section investigated the relative effectiveness of thin liquids taken with chin tuck posturing in inhibiting

aspiration in the short term, and inhibiting the development of pneumonia and other medical morbidities in the long term, when compared to thickening liquids. Chin tuck posturing was less effective for reducing aspiration in the short term [33], but more effective for inhibiting the development of adverse health consequences in the long term. However, it is difficult to make assumptions about the specific value of chin tuck posturing as this technique was methodologically linked to thin liquids and was not systematically assessed in isolation.

Lewin and colleagues [44] sought to evaluate the influence of chin tuck posturing in 21 patients with esophagectomy and aspiration. They report that in 81% of their cohort, this posture inhibited aspiration. However, this appeared to be achieved at different bolus consistencies for different participants thus making it difficult to determine if benefit was derived from the posture itself, the bolus consistency, or a combination of both.

Other researchers have evaluated the influence of chin tuck posturing on pressure generation. A recent investigation by Hori and colleagues [45] found that this technique resulted in increased lingual pressure with a 5-ml water swallow for healthy adults compared to dry and 15-ml water bolus swallows. Although closer approximation of BOT to PPW has been postulated to exert increased downward pressure on a bolus, Bülow et al. [46] found that the chin tuck in healthy adults resulted in decreased pharyngeal contraction pressure as manometrically measured. They speculate that as the chin extends forward and down, and distance diminishes, the pharyngeal constrictor muscles slacken and may therefore less effectively clear the bolus from the pharynx and through the UES. Therefore, although aspiration from post-swallow residual may be eliminated due to improved epiglottic laryngeal closure, the posture may negatively impact the ability to clear larger boluses from the pharynx.

Although chin tuck is a technique widely applied in dysphagia management, questions have been raised about the patient's ability to achieve the desired posture. Nagaya et al. [47] found that only 8% of patients with Parkinson's disease were able to attain the chin tuck position. Given that delayed swallow is a commonly observed difficulty in this clinical population, any compromise to the effectiveness of chin tuck posturing as a management method is of concern.

Head Rotation

Rotating the head to the weaker side is clinically recommended for patients with unilateral sensory or motor impairment as a means to direct the bolus down the unaffected, and therefore more efficient, side for pharyngeal transport. As with chin tuck posturing, this technique was the focus of research in the late 1980s [48] and 1990s [49, 50], but has not been subjected to scrutiny since that time with the exception of two studies.

Tsukamoto [51] reported on a single patient with unilateral pharyngeal paralysis in order to clarify our understanding of the role of head rotation. Using videofluoroscopy and CT, he identified that although head rotation does indeed close off the hemipharynx on the side of rotation, the closure occurs at the level of the hyoid bone, well above the pyriform sinuses. Therefore, while head rotation will direct the bolus down the opposite widened side of the pharynx and primarily into that pyriform sinus, there is potential for bolus accumulation in the hemiparetic pyriform cavity. While this study highlights that an assumption of complete pyriform sinus closure on one side should not be made, it requires testing of greater numbers of patients to discover whether the findings are unique or universal.

In a significantly larger study, Ertekin and colleagues [52] evaluated EMG activity of patients with neurogenic dysphagia and healthy controls performing water swallowing with a variety of postural techniques. Using a novel measurement of 'dysphagia limit', (the volume of bolus that a person can empty from the oral cavity in one swallow), based solely on EMG measures, these researchers identified that their outcome measure did not change significantly with most of the trialled postures. However, dysphagia limit in the patient population improved significantly in 67% of those with unilateral lower cranial lesions when the head was rotated toward the affected side. In patients with bilateral symptoms, a significant improvement occurred in 50% of patients using chin-tuck posture, but in the chin-up position, 55% of the patients experienced a significant compromise in swallowing. Data from this study are difficult to interpret given the novel outcome measure and lack of other biomechanical correlations. However, the study does raise the question of whether research on healthy controls is a viable indicator of treatment effect in the patient population.

Most recently, McCulloch et al. [53] used high-resolution manometry to investigate the effects of head turn and chin tuck on pressures throughout the pharynx. Healthy participants swallowed 5-ml water boluses presented via syringe. No differences were detected between the conditions for velopharyngeal pressures. Maximum tongue base pressure was highest in the neutral head position. UES pressure pre-swallowing was lower with head turn compared to neutral position, but post-swallow was lower with chin tuck posturing than neutral position. Increases in pharyngeal pressure were not reported for any technique.

Conclusion

Categorical evidence to support use of compensatory strategies in the dysphagic population is, at best, sparse. Much of what is used in clinical practice has come about from historic assumption and trial and error attempts. It is only now that randomised control trials, comparing normal and disordered populations are beginning to appear, whereas earlier work was predominantly carried out on small numbers of healthy adults. It is often assumed that in order to theorise and test interventions for dysphagia, there must be a solid body of evidence surrounding normal swallowing physiology from which disordered swallowing can be understood. However, not all studies support this presumption. Many of the small-scale trials have failed to employ standard methodologies, producing results which are not easily interpreted in the context of other work. However, larger trials are not without fault; substantial variability inherent in swallowing behaviour renders identification of significant results difficult at best. Difficulties of heterogeneous participant groups, and conversely, homogenous groups that are too small for generalising results, need to be considered in future research. Control groups are also required although this may require careful ethical consideration.

While compensatory techniques are by their nature a transient solution only, clinicians should bear in mind that these may be used over many years and whilst physiology may change little over time, cognition levels and general aging will affect swallowing action. A strategy that was initially considered to be successful in improving swallowing biomechanics does require regular follow-up to ensure continued effectiveness. Research studies have yet to determine the long-term effects of compensatory strategies. Finally, as has been mentioned throughout this chapter, individual variation in swallowing is extensive and patients must continue to be evaluated on a sole basis to ensure the best options for their treatment are selected.

Key Points

- Compensatory techniques remain the prime management option for certain patient populations.
- Compensatory techniques have traditionally been aimed at bringing about immediate change in swallowing biomechanics; however, new research suggests some areas may provide longer term rehabilitative benefits for swallowing function.
- Brain imaging studies suggest that thermal tactile and flavour compensatory approaches stimulate cortical areas connected with swallowing behaviours and may have potential to elicit permanent change.
- Current research focussed on combined smell and taste (flavour) stimulation may offer new possibilities for immediate adaptation of swallowing biomechanics combined with rehabilitative benefits.
- Outcome data for studies of carbonation is inconclusive but further evaluation of this

technique may offer clinicians an easily applied compensatory strategy.
- Although widely applied in clinical practice, chin tuck posturing has little evidence to support its efficacy in isolation. Clinicians are obliged to evaluate this and other techniques with instrumental assessment prior to patient application.
- Research into compensatory strategies has traditionally been hampered by small sample sizes, minimal investigation using patient populations, lack of control groups in randomised control trials and non-standardised methodology that disallows direct comparison of results.

References

1. Logemann JA. Evaluation and treatment of swallowing disorders. San Diego, CA: College-Hill; 1983.
2. Ali GN, Laundl TM, Wallace KL, deCarle DJ, Cook IJS. Influence of cold stimulation on the normal pharyngeal swallow response. Dysphagia. 1996;11:2–8.
3. Bove M, Mansson I, Eliasson I. Thermal oral-pharyngeal stimulation and elicitation of swallowing. Acta Otolaryngol. 1998;118:728–31.
4. Kaatzke-McDonald MN, Post E, Davis PJ. The effects of cold, touch, and chemical stimulation of the anterior faucial pillar on human swallowing. Dysphagia. 1996;11:198–206.
5. Rosenbek JC, Roecker EB, Wood JL, Robbins J. Thermal application reduces the duration of stage transition in dysphagia after stroke. Dysphagia. 1996;11:225–33.
6. Rosenbek JC, Robbins J, Willford WO, Kirk G, Schiltz A, Sowell TW, et al. Comparing treatment intensities of tactile-thermal application. Dysphagia. 1998;13:1–9.
7. Bisch EM, Logemann JA, Rademaker AW, Kahrilas PJ, Lazarus CL. Pharyngeal effects of bolus volume, viscosity, and temperature in patients with dysphagia resulting from neurologic impairment and in normal subjects. J Speech Hear Res. 1994;37:1041–9.
8. Regan J, Walshe M, Oliver Tobin W. Immediate effects of thermal-tactile stimulation on timing of swallow in idiopathic Parkinson's disease. Dysphagia. 2010;25:207–15.
9. Miyaoka Y, Haishima K, Takagi M, Haishima H, Asari J, Yamada Y. Influences of thermal and gustatory characteristics on sensory and motor aspects of swallowing. Dysphagia. 2006;21(1):38–48.
10. Teismann IK, Steinstrater O, Warnecke T, Suntrup S, Ringelstein EB, Pantev C, Dziewas R. Tactile thermal oral stimulation increases the cortical representation of swallowing. BMC Neurosci. 2009;10:76.

11. Lowell SY, Poletto CJ, Knorr-Chung BR, Reynolds RC, Simonyan K, Ludlow CJ. Sensory stimulation activates both motor and sensory components of the swallowing system. Neuroimage. 2008;42:285–95.
12. Ebihara T, Ebihara S, Maruyama M, Kobayashi M, Itou A, Arai H, Sasaki H. A randomized trial of olfactory stimulation using black pepper oil in older people with swallowing dysfunction. J Am Geriatr Soc. 2006;54(9):1401–6.
13. Munakata M, Kobayashi K, Niisato-Nezu J, Tanaka S, Kakisaka Y, Ebihara T, Ebihara S, Haginoya K, Tsuchiya S, Onuma A. Olfactory stimulation using black pepper oil facilitates oral feeding in pediatric patients receiving long-term enteral nutrition. Tohoku J Exp Med. 2008;214(4):327–32.
14. Logemann JA, Pauloski BR, Colangelo L, Lazarus C, Fujiu M, Kahrilas P. Effects of a sour bolus on oropharyngeal swallowing measures in patients with neurogenic dysphagia. J Speech Hear Res. 1995;38:556–63.
15. Cola PC, Gatto AR, Silva RG, Spadotto AA, Schlep AO, Henry MACA. The influence of sour taste and cold temperature in pharyngeal transit duration in patients with stroke. Arq Gastroenterol. 2010;47(1):18–21.
16. Pelletier CA, Lawless HT. Effect of citric acid and citric acid–sucrose mixtures on swallowing in neurogenic oropharyngeal dysphagia. Dysphagia. 2003;18:231–41.
17. Ekberg O, Feinberg MJ. Altered swallowing function in elderly patients without dysphagia: radiologic findings in 56 cases. AJR Am J Roentgenol. 1991;156(6):1181–4.
18. Pelletier CA, Dhanaraj GE. The effect of taste and palatability on lingual swallowing pressure. Dysphagia. 2006;21(1):121–8.
19. Palmer PM, McCulloch TM, Jaffe D, Neel AT. Effects of a sour bolus on the intramuscular electromyographic (EMG) activity of muscles in the submental region. Dysphagia. 2005;20(3):210–7.
20. Sciortino KF, Liss JM, Case JL, Gerritsen KGM, Katz RC. Effects of mechanical, cold, gustatory, and combined stimulation to the human anterior faucial pillars. Dysphagia. 2003;18:16–26.
21. Ding R, Logemann JA, Larson CR, Rademaker AW. The effects of taste and consistency on swallow physiology in younger and older healthy individuals: a surface electromyographic study. J Speech Lang Hear Res. 2003;46(4):977–89.
22. Leow LP, Huckabee ML, Sharma S, Tooley TP. The influence of taste on swallowingapnea, oral preparation time, and duration and amplitude of submental muscle contraction. Chem Senses. 2007;32(2):119–28.
23. Abdul Wahab N, Jones RD, Huckabee ML. Effects of olfactory and gustatory stimuli on neural excitability for swallowing. Physiol Behav. 2010;101(5):568–75.
24. Abdul Wahab N, Jones RD, Huckabee M-L. Effects of olfactory and gustatory stimuli on the biomechanics of swallowing. Physiol Behav. 2011;102(5):485–90.
25. Babaei A, Kern M, Antonik S, Mepani R, Douglas Ward B, Li S, Hyde J, Shaker R. Enhancing effects of flavored nutritive stimuli on cortical swallowing network activity. Am J Physiol Gastrointest Liver Physiol. 2010;299:G422–9.
26. Bülow M, Olsson R, Ekberg O. Videoradiographic analysis of how carbonated thin liquids and thickened liquids affect the physiology of swallowing in subjects with aspiration on thin liquids. Acta Radiol. 2003;44:366–72.
27. Miura Y, Morita Y, Koizumi H, Shingai T. Effects of taste solutions, carbonation, and cold stimulus on the power frequency content of swallowing submental surface electromyography. Chem Senses. 2009;34(4):325–33.
28. Krival K, Pelletier C, Kelchner L. Effects of carbonated vs. thin and thickened liquids on swallowing in adults with stroke. Scientific paper presented at the Sixteenth Annual Dysphagia Research Society Meeting; 2008 Mar 5–8; Isle of Palms, SC.
29. Chi-Fishman G, Sonies BC. Kinematic strategies for hyoid movement in rapid sequential swallowing. J Speech Lang Hear Res. 2002;45(3):457–68.
30. Dantas RO, Kern MK, Massey BT, Dodds WJ, Kahrilas PJ, Brasseur JG, et al. Effect of swallowed bolus variables on oral and pharyngeal phases of swallowing. Am J Physiol. 1990;258(5 Pt.1):G675–6781.
31. Dantas RO, Dodds WJ, Massey BT, Kern MK. The effect of high- vs low-density barium preparations on the quantitive features of swallowing. AJR Am J Roentgenol. 1989;153(6):1191–5.
32. Lazarus C, Logemann JA, Rademaker AW, Kahrilas PJ, Pajak T, Lazar R, et al. Effects of bolus volume, viscosity, and repeated swallows in nonstroke subjects and stroke patients. Arch Phys Med Rehabil. 1993;74(10):1066–70.
33. Logemann JA, Gensler G, Robbins J, Lindbald A, Brandt D, Hind JA, et al. A randomized study of three interventions for aspiration of thin liquids in patients with dementia and Parkinson's disease. J Speech Lang Hear Res. 2008;51:173–83.
34. Miller JL, Watkin KL. The influence of bolus volume and viscosity on anterior lingual force during the oral stage of swallowing. Dsyphagia. 1996;11(2):117–24.
35. Nicosia MA, Hind JA, Roecker EB, Carnes M, Doyle J, Dengel GA, et al. Age effects on the temporal evolution of isometric and swallowing pressure. J Gerontol Biol Sci Med Sci. 2000;55(11):M634–40.
36. Reimers-Neils L, Logemann J, Larson C. Viscosity effects on EMG activity in normal swallow. Dysphagia. 1994;9(2):101–6.
37. Robbins J, Gensler G, Hind J, Logemann JA, Lindblad AS, Brand D, Baum H, Lilienfeld D, Kosek S, Lundy D, Dikeman K, Kazandjian M, Gramigna GD, McGarvey-Toler S, Miller Gardner PJ. Comparison of 2 interventions for liquid aspiration on pneumonia incidence a randomized trial. Ann Intern Med. 2008;148(1):509–18.

38. Shaker R, Cook IJ, Dodds WJ, Hogan WJ. Pressure-flow dynamics of the oral phase of swallowing. Dysphagia. 1988;3(2):79–84.
39. Steele CM, Van Lieshout PH. Influence of bolus consistency on lingual behaviours in sequential swallowing. Dysphagia. 2004;19(3):192–206.
40. Daniels SK, Huckabee M. Dysphagia following stroke. San Diego, CA: Plural Publishing, Inc.; 2008. 240–242.
41. Ekberg O. Posture of the head and pharyngeal swallowing. Acta Radiol Diagn. 1986;27(6):691–6.
42. Welch MV, Logemann JA, Rademaker AW, Kahrilas PJ. Changes in pharyngeal dimensions effected by chin tuck. Arch Phys Med Rehabil. 1993;74(2):178–81.
43. Shanahan TK, Logemann JA, Rademaker AW, Pauloski BR, Kahrilas PJ. Chin-down posture effect on aspiration in dysphagic patients. Arch Phys Med Rehabil. 1993;74:736–9.
44. Lewin JS, Hebert TM, Putnam JB, DuBrow RA. Experience with the chin tuck maneuver in postesophagectomy aspirators. Dysphagia. 2001;16:216–9.
45. Hori K, Tamine K, Barbezat C, Maeda Y, Yamori M, Muller F, Ono T. Influence of chin-down posture on tongue pressure during dry swallow and bolus swallows in healthy subjects. Dysphagia. 2011;26(3):238–45.
46. Bülow M, Olsson R, Ekberg O. Videomanometric analysis of supraglottic swallow, effortful swallow, and chin tuck in healthy volunteers. Dysphagia. 1999;14:67–72.
47. Nagaya M, Kachi T, Yamada T, Sumi Y. Videofluorographic observations on swallowing in patients with dysphagia due to neurodegenerative diseases. Nagoya J Med Sci. 2004;67:17–23.
48. Logemann JA, Kahrilas PJ, Kobara M, Vakil NB. The benefit of head rotation on pharyngoesophageal dysphagia. Arch Phys Med Rehabil. 1989;70(10):767–71.
49. Rasley A, Logemann JA, Kahrilas PJ, Rademaker AW, Pauloski BR, Dodds WJ. Prevention of barium aspiration during videofluoroscopic swallowing studies: value of change in posture. AJR Am J Roentgenol. 1993;160(5):1005–9.
50. Ohmae Y, Ogura M, Karaho T, Kitahara S, Inouye T. Effects of head rotation on pharyngeal function during normal swallow. Ann Otol Rhinol Laryngol. 1998;107:344–8.
51. Tsukamoto Y. CT study of closure of the hemipharynx with head rotation in a case of lateral medullary syndrome. Dysphagia. 2000;15:17–8.
52. Ertekin C, Keskin A, Kiylioglu N, Kirazli Y, Yagiz On A, Tarlaci S, Aydogdu I. The effect of head and neck positions on oropharyngeal swallowing: a clinical and electrophysiologic study. Arch Phys Med Rehabil. 2001;82:1255–60.
53. McCulloch TM, Hoffman MR, Ciucci MR. High-resolution manometry of pharyngeal swallow pressure events associated with head turn and chin tuck. Ann Otol Rhinol Laryngol. 2010;119(6):369–76.

Rehabilitative Treatment

Caryn Easterling

Abstract

Positive patient outcomes from rehabilitative treatment depend on keen differential diagnostic wisdom and ability. Choosing the appropriate rehabilitative treatment for a particular deglutitive disorder is based on a deglutologist's accuracy in evaluation and diagnosis of the deglutitive disorder. Appropriate choice of the best rehabilitative treatment comes from critical analysis and understanding of the available research evidence, clinical experience, and consideration of the patient objectives and goals. Rehabilitative treatment, in its adolescence, offers exciting approaches and regimens with positive scientific results and clinical success. The successes experienced thus far require careful and wise clinical application, definition, and, of course, further investigation and publication. Rehabilitative treatments for deglutitive disorders and the evidence supporting the use of each treatment are presented in this chapter.

Keywords

Deglutition disorders • Rehabilitative treatment • Evidence-based medicine • Deglutologist • Lingual strengthening • Expiratory muscle strength training

Prevalence of deglutitive disorders in adults over 50 years of age has been estimated to range from 7 % to 22 %, with a higher prevalence for adults who reside in long-term care facilities being 40–50 % [1–11]. Prevalence of swallowing disorders increases in older individuals as the incidence of head and neck cancer, frailty caused by a range of conditions such as polypharmacy and inadequate nutrition, and diseases of the central nervous system such as stroke and dementia increases compared to young adults [12–16]. Dysphagia in older adults cannot be attributed solely to disease and illness. Individuals over the age of 65 years experience normal age-related changes which, although not considered pathologic, may affect swallowing, including sensory, motor, and structural changes that affect swallowing. It is important to recognize the normal changes that occur to the swallow mechanism as

C. Easterling, PhD, CCC, BRS-S, ASHAF (✉)
Department of Communication Sciences and Disorders,
University of Wisconsin-Milwaukee, Milwaukee, WI, USA
e-mail: caryn@uwm.edu

R. Shaker et al. (eds.), *Principles of Deglutition: A Multidisciplinary Text for Swallowing and its Disorders*,
DOI 10.1007/978-1-4614-3794-9_55, © Springer Science+Business Media New York 2013

a consequence of healthy aging in order to accurately differentially diagnose and apply appropriate rehabilitation strategies to those changes that are pathologic. Sensory changes include a decrease in pharyngeal and supraglottic sensitivity, which may be a contributing factor in the development of swallowing problems and increased incidence of aspiration in healthy older adults [17]. Loss of dentition affects bolus manipulation and masticatory ability that contribute to altered oral perceptual and sensory awareness and may impact food selection patterns [18]. Decreased production of saliva and perception of oral dryness occurring with aging can be exaggerated by medication usage and disease and may affect food choices and oral bolus manipulation [19]. Other changes that interfere with oral bolus manipulation and movement include decreased tongue pressure during bolus transit, diminished tongue strength, and longer oral phase [20]. Healthy older adults experience slowed oral and pharyngeal bolus transit, delayed initiation of the pharyngeal swallow, diminished pharyngeal and laryngeal sensation, and reduced deglutitive anteroposterior upper esophageal sphincter (UES) opening [17, 20–22].

What Is Evidence-Based Practice?

Evidence-based practice (EBP) is defined as "the conscientious, explicit and judicious use of current best evidence in making decisions about the care of individual patients… [by] integrating individual clinical expertise with the best available external clinical evidence from systematic research" [23]. EBP "…allows clinicians to be accountable, ethical, and responsible, not only to their clients, but to their profession… [and] permits clinicians to account for their services when reporting to clients, their families, and third-party payers" [24]. EBP benefits both clinicians and clients.

When deciding on a rehabilitative treatment for a patient with dysphagia, deglutologists should choose treatment protocols for which efficacy or effectiveness has been established. Treatment efficacy yields "the probability of benefit to individuals in a defined population

from a medical technology applied for a given medical problem under ideal conditions of use" [25]. When reviewing a research article to determine efficacy of a treatment, one must determine if researchers controlled for variables so that only the effect of the independent variable that is the treatment protocol on the dependent variable or the clinical outcome reasonably accounts for the change in the outcome measure [26]. Treatment effectiveness is the likelihood that a given treatment will bring about change in a clinical setting [26]. Efficacy of treatment must be established before effectiveness of treatment can be assessed.

There are different levels of research evidence impacting the quality and value of published research [25] The highest levels of evidence, Level I and Level II, entail either meta-analysis of more than one randomized controlled trial (RCT) or a single well-designed RCT. Presently, there are few RCTs focused on dysphagia rehabilitative treatment techniques that have been conducted. RCTs usually take a long time to complete and are expensive to conduct.

Because of the limited number of RCTs for any particular rehabilitative dysphagia treatment, deglutologists need to use other levels of evidence. That is, Level III, well-designed controlled studies without randomization; Level IV, well-designed, non-experimental studies from more than one research group; and Level V, studies which are expert committee reports, consensus conference reports, and clinical experience from respected authorities.

For some rehabilitative treatment techniques, the only level of evidence may be Level V, an expert authority report. Clinicians then must employ logical reasoning based upon clinical experience, available outcomes, and patient goals. To rely solely on clinical experience or research evidence in clinical decision making is not sufficient [23]. EBP utilizes comparison of knowledge acquired from clinical experience and the best available evidence from published research. When published research confounds clinical experience, clinicians should re-evaluate therapy practices and make appropriate alterations. EBP provides a way to "…systematically improve …[their] efforts to be better clinicians, colleagues, advocates, and investigators-not by ignoring clinical experience and patient preferences but rather by considering these against a background of the highest quality scientific evidence that can be found" [27].

This chapter will review the evidence supporting the effectiveness of rehabilitative treatment for deglutitive disorders.

Rehabilitative Treatment

Rehabilitative treatment techniques alter the physiology of a specific aspect of the disordered deglutitive process [28]. Before applying specific rehabilitative treatment, one must accurately evaluate the deglutitive dysfunction using an instrumental technique such as endoscopy or fluoroscopy.

Rehabilitative treatment includes muscle strengthening, range of motion (ROM) exercise, and maneuvers. The change or outcome in the disordered deglutitive physiology is permanent because of the effect of the rehabilitative treatment. Rehabilitative treatment is indirect or direct. Indirect rehabilitative treatment employs specific exercise principles and techniques without food or liquid as part of the treatment. Direct rehabilitative treatment facilitates physiologic deglutitive change utilizing food and/or liquid as part of the treatment exercise regimen. Both types of rehabilitative treatment techniques require that the patient have adequate cognitive ability, that is, adequate attention, comprehension, and memory to appreciate the purpose of the treatment and to complete the regimen in order to derive benefit from the treatment [28].

Maneuvers

Swallow maneuvers included in rehabilitative treatment are the Mendelsohn Maneuver and the effortful swallow. These maneuvers demand increased muscular effort by the patient and have been shown to alter timing, bolus flow, and therefore the duration of physiologic swallow events. In order to perform maneuvers, one is required to expend increased muscular effort. Effectiveness of a maneuver on altering the deglutitive physiologic function or dysfunction varies and therefore should always be performed during the instrumental swallowing evaluation. Maneuvers are used temporarily with discontinuation of the maneuver as deglutitive function improves. Maneuvers require adequate cognitive abilities such as attention, comprehension, and memory. Patients with cognitive or linguistic disorders may not be able to comprehend or retain the sequential steps required to perform a maneuver. Because of the increased muscular effort required to perform maneuvers, patients who fatigue quickly during performance of the maneuver may not be appropriate candidates for the rehabilitative approach, or the approach may require a stepwise frequency and duration treatment design to overcome fatigue and be successful with the rehabilitative techniques.

The Mendelsohn Maneuver requires that the patient have the ability to identify the time during the swallow when there is maximal laryngeal elevation and be able to hold the larynx in that position for several seconds as the bolus is completely swallowed [28]. The effectiveness of this maneuver on normal swallow function has been studied [29, 30], as well as in patients with neurologic disease [31] and head and neck cancer [32]. When performed correctly, the Mendelsohn Maneuver increases the extent and duration of laryngeal excursion [30] and the extent and duration of deglutitive UES opening diameter [28, 30, 32]. The Mendelsohn Maneuver is applicable as a rehabilitative technique for patients with reduced deglutitive laryngeal elevation, and decreased deglutitive anteroposterior UES opening diameter. Prolonged duration of tongue base to posterior pharyngeal wall contact, improved bolus clearance, and elimination of aspiration have also been reported as beneficial outcomes of the Mendelsohn Maneuver [30, 32].

The effortful swallow also requires the patient to deliberately increase muscular effort to carry out the instruction to swallow hard. The effortful swallow has been shown to benefit patients with reduced tongue base retraction or decreased pharyngeal constriction during the swallow resulting in post-deglutitive residual in the pharynx.

The effectiveness of this maneuver has been studied in normal individuals [33–37] and in patients with neurologic dysfunction [38]. The effortful swallow results in greater exertion of oral and pharyngeal pressure for longer durations during the swallow [34–37, 39], reduced depth of laryngeal penetration, and increased base of tongue retraction during the pharyngeal swallow [37–39]. Also, it has been noted that the effortful swallow increases duration of maximum anterior hyoid excursion, laryngeal vestibule closure, and extent of superior hyoid excursion [38]. Contradictions in research findings underscore the necessity that the patient performs the specific maneuver during the instrumental evaluation to determine its effectiveness. (*Please refer to Chap. 54 by Maggie Lee Huckabee and Chap. 30 by Cathy Lazarus for more research and outcomes related to the efficiency and efficacy of the Effortful Swallow and Mendelsohn Maneuver for rehabilitation of deglutitive disorders*).

Exercise

Strength-training exercises for limb muscles alter the effects of muscle weakness that accompanies normal aging. Sarcopenia, the process accompanying aging that results in muscle weakness, is preventable and reversible. Muscle weakness is a result of decreased physical activity accelerated by disuse and acute or chronic illness [40–43]. Resistance training can increase muscle strength, coordination, and hypertrophy. Resistance training promotes an increase in the number of muscle fibers and muscle fiber area, resulting in increased neural activation of muscles. This body of research literature and our increased understanding and application of exercise principles have been inspirational in designing rehabilitative treatment regimens for deglutitive disorders.

Lingual Strengthening

Outcomes from lingual strengthening and ROM exercises have been studied in patients with head and neck cancer, stroke patients, and in healthy young and older adults. These studies have demonstrated that lingual resistance exercise results in increased tongue strength, resulting in decreased oral transit time, improved tongue pressure/strength during swallowing, and improved tongue base to posterior pharyngeal wall pressure [44–48]. Tongue strength is important for the efficient containment and movement of the bolus during deglutition. There is a correlation between tongue strength and oral transit time and efficient bolus clearance [49]. Isometric tongue exercises have been shown to improve the isometric pressure and lingual swallow pressure as well as tongue volume in healthy older adults who performed an 8-week tongue resistance exercise program [48]. In a study of ten stroke patients who were enrolled in an 8-week lingual isometric exercise regimen using a device that provided biofeedback as well as a pressure measurement for the exerciser, the stroke patients experienced significant increase in maximum isometric pressure generation and increased swallow pressures for tested bolus conditions after completion of the protocol [50]. Measureable changes noted in the videofluoroscopic evaluation after completion of the exercise program were decreased oral transit time and increased pharyngeal response duration. Although postdeglutitive pharyngeal residue was decreased for the bolus types tested, the changes noted after exercise did not reach significance [50] (*Please refer to Chapter 12 by JoAnne Robbins for more research and outcomes related to the efficiency and efficacy of the lingual exercise for rehabilitation of deglutitive disorders*).

Masako Maneuver

Tongue base to posterior pharyngeal wall contact during bolus transit through the pharynx creates pressure on the bolus as it moves through the pharynx. The pressure applied to the bolus from this structural contact results in a visual fluoroscopic image that resembles an inverted "v," previously described as the "tail" of the bolus moving from proximal to the distal hypopharynx. Tongue base to posterior pharyngeal wall contact is an important visual representation of the pressure exerted in the pharynx and measured using pharyngeal strain gauge manometry. If tongue base to posterior pharyngeal wall contact is not successful, the swallow would be inefficient, resulting in pharyngeal residuals.

The Masako Maneuver or "tongue hold" exercise is a resistance exercise that has been shown to improve tongue base to posterior pharyngeal wall contact in those who do not have ample contact during swallowing, resulting in bolus transit failure with post-deglutitive pharyngeal residue. The Masako Maneuver must be performed without food or drink as a safety precaution. If food or drink were used during the Maneuver, aspiration would likely occur because of the anterior tongue position during the resistance exercise. The Masako Maneuver is performed in the following manner: the patient secures the tongue between the teeth while performing a swallow. This maneuver or exercise is performed as many times as the patient can tolerate. There is no prescribed exercise regimen. This exercise has been shown to improve tongue base to posterior pharyngeal wall contact and pharyngeal pressure during swallowing [51, 52]. The exact protocol, that is, the number of times per session, duration of tongue hold, or number of swallows per exercise session has not been determined.

Shaker Exercise

The Shaker Exercise is an isometric and isokinetic exercise designed to strengthen suprahyoid muscles, thereby improving anterior laryngeal excursion and increasing deglutitive anteroposterior upper esophageal sphincter opening diameter. In the published research regarding the Shaker Exercise, it was performed three times per day for 6 weeks. The instructions for the two-part exercise are as follows: Part I: Lay flat on your back on the floor or bed. Hold your head off the floor or bed looking at your feet for 1 min (do not raise your shoulders), relax for 1 min, and repeat three times. Part II: Raise your head 30 times and look at your feet. Do not sustain these head lifts or raise your shoulders off the bed or floor.

Please remember to breathe while performing both steps of the Shaker Exercise [53, 54].

A randomized clinical trial was conducted in a heterogeneous group of tube-fed patients with dysphagia, including stroke patients and patients who had completed treatment for head and neck cancer [54]. All patients experienced post-deglutitive aspiration secondary to decreased A-P UES opening diameter and had pharyngeal residual in the pyriform sinuses. Results indicated improved physiologic and functional outcomes, including resumption of oral intake after completion of the exercise regime [53, 54]. The Shaker Exercise was found to significantly improve deglutitive biomechanical measures of anterior hyolaryngeal excursion related to deglutitive anteroposterior UES opening diameter, decreased post-deglutitive pyriform residuals, and elimination of post-deglutitive aspiration in all patients, regardless of etiology or duration of dysphagia. This research supported the appropriateness of the Shaker Exercise for patients who exhibit aspiration due to post-deglutitive residue and abnormal deglutitive UES opening. The Shaker Exercise is not appropriate for patients with dysphagia who experience aspiration pre- or intra-deglutitive aspiration. (*Please refer to Chapter 13 by Caryn Easterling for more specific research and outcomes related to the efficiency and efficacy of the Shaker Exercise for rehabilitation of deglutitive disorders*).

Electrical Stimulation

Promising rehabilitation treatments, such as neuromuscular or transcutaneous electrical stimulation, are being systematically studied. Before implementation of such techniques, one must carefully scrutinize the research related to the use of new technology, that is, devices and techniques. To date, published research employing different techniques and applications of electrical stimulation in rehabilitation of deglutitive disorders varies in quality and results. (*Please refer to Chapter 56 by Christy Ludlow for specific research and outcomes related to the efficiency and efficacy of Electrical Stimulation for rehabilitation of deglutitive disorders)*

Lee Silverman Voice Treatment

The Lee Silverman Voice Treatment program emphasizes training the patient to provide maximum respiratory drive during vocal use. This program requires the treating clinician to undergo a certification program in order to provide the protocol to patients. The effectiveness of this program has been studied in patients with Parkinson's disease only. Although the protocol was designed for treatment of voice disorders, it has been reported to have cross-system effects on temporal deglutitive measures. In a single subject study of a patient with mild idiopathic Parkinson's disease, use of the Lee Silverman Voice Treatment decreased oral residue and consequently the number of swallows required to clear residue from 3 to 5 mL liquid bolus as well as decreased pharyngeal transit time [55]. More research is needed to determine the efficacy of this technique in improving deglutitive disorders in patients with Parkinson's disease and the possible application to other diseases with co-occurring respiratory and swallowing disorders.

Expiratory Muscle Strength Training

Use of Expiratory Muscle Strength Training (EMST) was described in clinical respiratory science literature as a device-assisted protocol that could be used to improve expiratory pressure support in healthy young adults [56], patients with Parkinson's disease [57, 58], and patients with multiple sclerosis [49, 59]. Knowing the documented importance of the suprahyoid muscles in swallowing biomechanics, the use of EMST adjustable resistance device by patients as an activator of the suprahyoid muscle group has been studied [60]. The purpose of the study was to measure the maximum expiratory pressure (MEP) and the impact on deglutitive biomechanics by using sEMG to measure suprahyoid muscle

group activation pre- and post-EMST protocol in healthy young adults. The results of the study showed that EMST significantly improved MEP and significantly increased activation in the suprahyoid muscles when comparing pre- to post-sEMG data [60]. This emerging rehabilitative treatment is promising both for improved respiratory function and swallowing biomechanics in patients with Parkinson's disease. The application of this technique and its documented effect on voice and swallowing disorders in patients with other neurologic disease have not been studied.

Conclusions

The purpose of this chapter was to provide a review of research evidence for rehabilitative treatment for use by deglutologists. Table 55.1 provides an "At a Glance" summary reference for application of the rehabilitative treatments reviewed in this Chapter.

In order to best serve patients with dysphagia, we must utilize treatment techniques with sound theoretical, methodological, and analytical bases. A large body of research pertaining to treatment techniques for dysphagia currently exists, most studies have included relatively small numbers of subjects, and many have not controlled for effects of aging, disease, treatment dose effect on outcome, patient compliance issues, etc. These studies provide primarily evidence Levels III, IV, and V. Few published studies present Level II evidence, those reporting on the effectiveness of lingual strengthening and the Shaker Exercise rehabilitative treatments. Further research is needed to establish the efficacy of rehabilitative treatment for specific deglutitive disorders and to establish treatment dosage to ensure better cost effectiveness and positive patient deglutitive outcomes from rehabilitation programs.

As new treatment techniques are introduced, those treating deglutitive disorders should critically examine the rationale of the supportive research. Deglutologists should utilize rehabilitative treatment techniques only when there is reasonable knowledge, evidence, and expectation

Table 55.1 At a glance: application of rehabilitative treatment

Rehabilitative treatment	What symptom will the treatment rehabilitate?	What physiologic disorder was observed during instrumental evaluation?	Patient instruction
Mendelsohn Maneuver	Post-deglutitive pyriform sinus residue	Decreased deglutitive anterior hyolaryngeal excursion	As you swallow, feel your Adam's apple lift and hold that position at the highest point of your swallow for several seconds as you continue to swallow.
		Decreased duration and maximum deglutitive anteroposterior upper esophageal sphincter opening	(sEMG biofeedback can assist in learning this maneuver)
Supraglottic swallow	Aspiration during the swallow	Incomplete vocal fold closure	Inhale and hold your breath, swallow as you hold your breath. Cough before you take another breath and swallow again.
	Penetration or aspiration before the swallow	Delayed pharyngeal swallow	May require blood pressure and heart rate monitor during this maneuver
	Protects airway before and during swallow (may experience penetration because of insufficient laryngeal vestibule closure, see Super supraglottic swallow)		
Super supraglottic swallow	Aspiration during the swallow	Incomplete airway closure at laryngeal vestibule level	"Inhale and hold your breath tightly while bearing down. Swallow as you hold your breath and bear down. After you swallow and before you take another breath, cough and swallow again." Patient may require blood pressure and heart rate monitor during this maneuver.
	Penetration or aspiration before the swallow	Delayed pharyngeal swallow	*May require blood pressure and heart rate monitor during this maneuver
	Protects airway before and during swallow		
Oral motor exercise	Involuntary bolus loss—anterior oral cavity	Insufficient lingual control	Repetitive exercise performed over several week period includes: increasing tongue pressure against palate using pressure measurement device (e.g., Iowa oral pressure instrument, IOPI) or tongue depressor
	Insufficient bolus manipulation		
	Oral cavity residual post-swallow		
	Pre-deglutitive pharyngeal pooling		
Effortful swallow	Pharyngeal residual	Incomplete epiglottic inversion	Patient is instructed: swallow hard
		Incomplete tongue base to posterior pharyngeal wall contact	
		Decreased pharyngeal motility	

(continued)

Table 55.1 (continued)

Rehabilitative treatment	What symptom will the treatment rehabilitate?	What physiologic disorder was observed during instrumental evaluation?	Patient instruction
Masako Maneuver	Post deglutitive residue in the valleculae	Incomplete tongue base to posterior pharyngeal wall contact	Repetitive exercise performed without food or drink. Instruction: Hold tongue between your teeth and swallow while your tongue is securely held between your teeth
		Incomplete epiglottic inversion	
		Decreased pharyngeal motility	
Shaker Exercise	Post-deglutitive pyriform sinus residue	Decreased deglutitive anterior hyolaryngeal excursion	Part I: Lay flat on your back on the floor or bed. Hold your head off the floor or bed looking at your feet for 1 min (do not raise your shoulders), relax for 1 min, repeat three times
		Decreased deglutitive anteroposterior upper esophageal sphincter opening	Part II: Raise your head 30 times and look at your feet. Do not sustain these head lifts or raise your shoulders off the bed or floor. Remember to breathe while performing both steps of the Shaker Exercise. Exerciser works to target goals as tolerate
			Parts I and II of Shaker Exercise are performed three times daily for 6 weeks

that the patient will benefit from the treatment. Without research evidence coupled with clinical experience and patient's expectations, deglutologists have no assurance that their efforts will benefit the dysphagic patient.

References

1. Howden CW. Management of acid related disorders in patients with dysphagia. Am J Med. 2004;117:44S–8.
2. Sonies BC. Oropharyngeal dysphagia in the elderly. Clin Geriatr Med. 1992;8:569–77.
3. Feinberg MJ, Knebl J, Tully J. Prandial aspiration and pneumonia in an elderly population followed over 3 years. Dysphagia. 1996;11:104–9.
4. Lindgren S, Janzon L. Prevalence of swallowing complaints and clinical findings among 50–70 year old men and women in an urban population. Dysphagia. 1991;6:187–92.
5. Siebens H, Trupe E, Siebens A, Cook F, Anshen S, Hanauer R, et al. Correlates and consequences of eating dependency in institutionalized elderly. J Am Geriatr Soc. 1986;34:192–8.
6. Logemann JA. Effects of aging on the swallowing mechanism. Otolaryngol Clin North Am. 1990;23:1045–56.
7. Bloem BR, Lagaay AM, van Beek W, Haan J, Roos RA, Wintzen AR. Prevalence of subjective dysphagia in community residents aged over 87. Br Med J. 1990;300:721–2.
8. Locke GR, Talley NJ, Fett SL, Zinsmeister AR, Melton LJ. Prevalence and clinical spectrum of gastroesophageal reflux: a population-based study in Olmsted County, Minnesota. Gastroenterology. 1997;112:1448–55.
9. Horner J, Massey EW. Silent aspiration following stroke. Neurology. 1988;38:317–9.
10. Groher ME, Bukatman R. The prevalence of swallowing disorders in two teaching hospitals. Dysphagia. 1986;1:3–6.
11. Steele CM, Greenwood C, Ens I, Robertson C, Seldman-Carlson R. Mealtime difficulties in a home for the aged: not just dysphagia. Dysphagia. 1997;12:43–50.
12. Lieu PK, Chong MS, Seshadri R. The impact of swallowing disorders in the elderly. Ann Acad Med Singapore. 2001;30:148–54.
13. Nilsson H, Ekberg O, Olsson R, Hindfeldt B. Quantitative aspects of swallowing in an elderly nondysphagic population. Dysphagia. 1996;11:180–4.
14. Mann G, Hankey G, Cameron D. Swallowing disorders following acute stroke: prevalence and diagnostic accuracy. Cerebrovasc Dis. 2000;10:380–6.
15. Lovell SJ, Wong HB, Loh KS, et al. Impact of dysphagia on quality of life in nasopharyngeal carcinoma. Head Neck. 2005;27:864–72.
16. Kinney JM. Nutritional frailty, sarcopenia and falls in the elderly. Curr Opin Clin Nutr Metab Care. 2004;7:15.20.
17. Aviv JE, Martin JH, et al. Age related changes in pharyngeal and supraglottic sensation. Ann Otol Rhinol Laryngol. 1994;103:749–52.
18. Chauncey HH, Muench ME, Kapur KK, Wayler AH. The effect of the loss of teeth on diet and nutrition. Int Dent J. 1984;34:98–104.
19. Gilbert GH, Heft MW, Duncan RP. Mouth dryness as reported by older Floridians. Commun Dent Oral Epidemiol. 1993;21:390–7.
20. Nicosia MA, Hind JA, Roecker EB, et al. Age effects on the temporal evolution of isometric and swallowing pressure. J Gerontol A Biol Sci Med Sci. 2000;55: M634–40.
21. Shaker R, Lang IM. Effect of aging on the deglutitive oral, pharyngeal, and esophageal motor function. Dysphagia. 1994;9:221–8.
22. Shaker R, Ren J, Zamir Z, et al. Effect of aging, position, and temperature on the threshold volume triggering pharyngeal swallows. Gastroenterology. 1994;107:396–402.
23. Sackett DL, Rosenberg W, Muir Gray JA, Haynes R, Richardson W. Evidence-based medicine: what it is and what it isn't. Br Med J. 1996;312:71–2.
24. Apel K, Self T. Evidence-based practice: the marriage of research and clinical services. ASHA Leader. 2003;8(16):6–7.
25. Robey RR. A five-phase model for clinical-outcome research. J Commun Disord. 2004;37:401–11.
26. American Speech-Language-Hearing Association. Evidence-based practice in communication disorders [Position statement]. Rockville, MD: Author; 2005.
27. Belsey J, Snell T. What is evidence-based medicine? 2010. Available at: http://www.evidence-based-medicine.co.uk. Accessed 30 Nov 2010.
28. Logemann JA. Evaluation and treatment of swallowing disorders. 2nd ed. Austin, TX: Pro-Ed, Inc; 1998.
29. Ding R, Larson CR, Logemann JA, Rademaker AW. Surface electromyographic and electroglottographic studies in normal subjects under two swallow conditions: normal and during the Mendelsohn maneuver. Dysphagia. 2002;17:1–12.
30. Kahrilas PJ, Logemann JA, Krugler C, Flanagan E. Volitional augmentation of upper esophageal sphincter opening during swallowing. Am J Physiol. 1991;260: G450–6.
31. Logemann JA, Kahrilas PJ. Relearning to swallow after stroke—application of maneuvers and indirect biofeedback: a case study. Neurology. 1990;40: 1136–8.
32. Lazarus C, Logemann JA, Gibbons P. Effects of maneuvers on swallowing function in a dysphagic oral cancer patient. Head Neck. 1993;15:419–24.
33. Bulow M, Olsson R, Ekberg O. Videomanometric analysis of supraglottic swallow, effortful swallow, and chin tuck in healthy volunteers. Dysphagia. 1999;14:67–72.
34. Hind JA, Nicosia MA, Roecker EB, Carnes ML, Robbins J. Comparison of effortful and noneffortful swallows in healthy middle-aged and older adults. Arch Phys Med Rehabil. 2001;82:1661–5.

35. Hiss SG, Huckabee ML. Timing of pharyngeal and upper esophageal sphincter pressures as a function of normal and effortful swallowing in young healthy adults. Dysphagia. 2005;20:149–56.

36. Huckabee ML, Butler SG, Barclat M, Jit S. Submental surface electromyographic measurement and pharyngeal pressures during normal and effortful swallowing. Arch Phys Med Rehabil. 2005;86:2144–8.

37. Pouderoux P, Kahrilas PJ. Deglutitive tongue force modulation by volition, volume, and viscosity in humans. Gastroenterology. 1995;108:1418–26.

38. Bulow M, Olsson R, Ekberg O. Supraglottic swallow, effortful swallow, and chin tuck did not alter hypopharyngeal intrabolus pressure in patients with pharyngeal dysfunction. Dysphagia. 2002;17:197–201.

39. Huckabee ML, Steele CM. An analysis of lingual contribution to submental surface electromyographic measures and pharyngeal pressure during effortful swallow. Arch Phys Med Rehabil. 2006;87:1067–72.

40. Booth F, Weeden S, Tsong B. Effect of aging on human skeletal muscle and motor function. Med Sci Sports Exerc. 1994;26:556–60.

41. Harris T. Muscle mass and strength: relation to function in population studies. J Nutr. 1997;127:4S–6.

42. Lindle RS, Metter FJ, Linch NA, Fleg JL, Fozard JL, Tobin J. Age and gender comparisons of muscle strength in 654 women and men aged 20–93 years. J Appl Physiol. 1997;83:1581–7.

43. Porter MM, Vandervoort AA, Lexell J. Aging of human muscle: structure, function, and adaptability. Scand J Med Sci Sports. 1995;5:124–9.

44. Lazarus CI, Logemann JA, Huang CH, Rademaker AW. Effects of two types of tongue strengthening exercises in young normals. Folia Phoniatr Logop. 2003;55(4):199–205.

45. Veis S, Logemann JA, Colangelo L. Effects of three techniques on maximum posterior movement of the tongue base. Dysphagia. 2000;15:142–5.

46. Lazarus C, Logemann JA, Song CW, Rademaker AW, Kahrilas PJ. Effects of voluntary maneuvers on tongue base function for swallowing. Folia Phoniatr Logop. 2002;54:171–6.

47. Lazarus CL, Logemann JA, Pauloski BR, et al. Swallowing and tongue function following treatment for oral and oropharyngeal cancer. J Speech Lang Hear Res. 2000;43(4):1011–23.

48. Robbins J, Gangnon RE, Theis SM, Kays SA, Hewitt AL, Hind JA. The effects of lingual exercise on swallowing in older adults. J Am Geriatr Soc. 2005;53:1483–9.

49. Chiara T, Martin AD, Davenport PW, Bolser DC. Expiratory muscle strength training in persons with multiple sclerosis having mild to moderate disability: effect on maximal expiratory pressure, pulmonary function and maximal voluntary cough. Arch Phys Med Rehabil. 2006;87:468–73.

50. Robbins J, Kays SA, Gangnon RE, Hind JA, Hewitt AL, Gentry LR, et al. The effects of lingual exercise in stroke patients with dysphagia. Arch Phys Med Rehabil. 2007;88(2):150–8.

51. Fujiu M, Logemann JA, Pauloski BR. Increased postoperative posterior pharyngeal wall movement in patients with anterior oral cancer: preliminary findings and possible implications for treatment. Am J Speech Lang Pathol. 1995;4:24–30.

52. Fujiu M, Logemann JA. Effect of a tongue holding maneuver on posterior pharyngeal wall movement during deglutition. Am J Speech Lang Pathol. 1996;5:23–30.

53. Easterling C, Kern M, Nitschke T, et al. Effect of a novel exercise on swallow function and biomechanics in tube fed cervical dysphagia patients: a preliminary report. Dysphagia. 1999;14:119.

54. Shaker R, Easterling C, Kern M, et al. Rehabilitation of swallowing by exercise in tube-fed patients with pharyngeal dysphagia secondary to abnormal UES opening. Gastroenterology. 2002;122:1314–21.

55. Sharkawi AE, Ramig L, Logemann JA. Swallowing and voice effects of Lee Silverman voice treatment (LSVT): a pilot study. J Neurol Neurosurg Psychiatry. 2002;72(1):31–6.

56. Sapienza CM, Davenport PW, Martin AD. Expiratory muscle training increases pressure support in high school band students. J Voice. 2002;16:495–501.

57. Silverman EF, Cm S, Saleem A, Carmichael C, Davenport PW, Hoffman-Ruddy B, et al. Tutorial on maximum inspiratory and expiratory mouth pressures in individuals with idiopathic Parkinson disease (IPD) and the preliminary results of an expiratory muscle strength training program. NeuroRehabilitation. 2006;21:71–9.

58. Saleem AF, Sapienza CM, Okun MS. Respiratory muscle strength training: treatment and response duration in a patient with early idiopathic Parkinson's disease. NeuroRehabilitation. 2005;20:323–33.

59. Chiara T, Martin D, Sapienza C. Expiratory muscle strength training: speech production outcomes in patients with multiple sclerosis. Neurorehabil Neural Repair. 2007;21:239–49.

60. Wheeler KM, Chiara T, Sapienza CM. Surface electromyographic activity of the submental muscles during swallow and expiratory pressure threshold training tasks. Dysphagia. 2007;22:108–16.

Electrical Stimulation Treatment

56

Christy L. Ludlow

Abstract

This chapter reviews ongoing research using electrical stimulation in dysphagia. Neuromuscular stimulation on the skin overlying the throat area resists hyo-laryngeal elevation during swallowing and does not increase benefit over traditional dysphagia therapy. Sensory stimulation of the pharyngeal mucosa has benefits for early recovery of swallowing post stroke but requires catheter insertion into the pharynx. Functional electrical stimulation has been most useful for limb control rehabilitation and has not been applied in dysphagia but presents with several technical challenges before it can be implemented. The use of electrical stimulation for dysphagia is at an early stage in its development but has great potential for the future benefits in dysphagia rehabilitation.

Keywords

Dysphagia • Neuromuscular stimulation (NMES) • Electrical stimulation • Sensory stimulation • Functional electrical stimulation (FES)

Introduction: Applications of Electrical Stimulation for the Treatment of Motor Control Disorders

The use of electrical stimulation for assisting patients with motor control disorders has been explored for several decades, although its application to swallowing is relatively recent. When electrical stimulation is applied at rest to increase muscle power and prevent muscle atrophy [1], it is known as *neuromuscular stimulation*. Electrical stimulation to augment sensory input to the spinal, brain stem, or cortical control systems for the facilitation of patient movement [2] is known as *sensory facilitation*. Many applications use electrical stimulation of nerves and/or muscles applied at precise times to augment purposeful movement [3] known as *functional electrical stimulation*. These three types of electrical stimulation are summarized in Table 56.1.

C.L. Ludlow (✉)
Communication Sciences and Disorders Credentials,
James Madison University,
Harrisonburg, VA, USA
e-mail: ludlowcx@jmu.edu

R. Shaker et al. (eds.), *Principles of Deglutition: A Multidisciplinary Text for Swallowing and its Disorders*,
DOI 10.1007/978-1-4614-3794-9_56, © Springer Science+Business Media New York 2013

Table 56.1 Characteristics of different types of electrical stimulation

Type	Purpose	Frequency and duration of stimulation	Benefits
Neuromuscular stimulation (NMES)	Stimulate nerve or nerve endings innervating a muscle	30 Hz 3–5 s on, 10–15 s off	Prevents muscle atrophy or reduces atrophy in upper motor neuron disorders
Sensory stimulation	Increases sensory input to central nervous system	2 Hz Immediately prior to or during movement	Increases excitability in central nervous system and may increase neuroplasticity
Functional electrical stimulation	Augments a patient movement during behavior by stimulating a group of muscles during movement	Must be triggered to occur synchronous with the patient's target movement	Augments the patient's movement and has recently been shown to increase neuroplasticity

Neuromuscular Stimulation

Neuromuscular stimulation (NMES) uses a regular rate of stimulation of a nerve to maintain muscle activity. Stimulation is typically cycled "on" for short intervals with rest "off" intervals of no stimulation to prevent fatigue. A usual duty cycle is 5 s on and 10 s off to prevent muscle fatigue and injury. The rate of stimulation is usually similar to the rate of firing of motor neurons for that muscle, such as 30 Hz in most spinal muscles. There are a few exceptions; the eye muscles can fire more rapidly >100 Hz for short periods of 3–5 s without fatigue. Similarly some of the laryngeal muscles can fire more rapidly for short periods (>90 Hz). For most muscles, however, the usual rate is around 30 Hz for short periods of 3–5 s on interspersed with longer off periods of 10–15 s.

The type of electrical stimulation used is dependent upon the underlying mechanisms of a patient's motor control disorder. NMES is used to prevent disuse atrophy or reverse muscle atrophy. For NMES to be effective, the nerve innervating the muscle must be intact for the electrical stimulation to induce an action potential that will be transmitted along the nerve to the endplate and release acetylcholine at the neuromuscular junction to activate muscle fibers. Electrical stimulation does not activate muscle fibers directly; rather contractions occur as a result of action potentials induced in the nerve by changes in the electrical field that produce neurotransmission at the neuromuscular junction. For electrical stimulation to activate the muscle, the neural system controlling the muscle must be intact including the motor neuron, the axon, and the neuromuscular junction. Types of pathology that impact the neural system innervating a muscle include pathologies that affect lower motor neurons as occurs in some patients with amyotrophic lateral sclerosis, peripheral nerve injury that can result in distal nerve degeneration, loss of myelin sheath covering the axons affecting axonal conduction, or disruption of function at the neuromuscular junction. Neuromuscular abnormalities include a block in acetylcholine release into the neuromuscular junction after botulinum toxin poisoning or antibodies to acetylcholine as occurs in myasthenia gravis causing rapid depletion of acetylcholine at the neuromuscular junction resulting in fatigue.

Thus neuromuscular electrical stimulation is only useful when the peripheral nerve is intact. Patients with upper motor neuron injuries following stroke or traumatic brain injury where the peripheral nervous system is intact but communication from the central nervous system is impaired either at the cortex, involving the corticospinal tract, or above the level of the motor neurons in the brain stem or spinal cord are appropriate for NMES. NMES is most helpful when it is applied to peripheral nerves to activate a muscle when the patient can no longer activate the motor neurons due to a lesion above the level of the motor neurons in the spinal cord or when communication from the cortex to the motor neurons in the spinal cord or brain stem is lost. A typical use of NMES is when a person has a spinal cord injury and has lost the ability to use his or her legs but wants to maintain muscle bulk in their legs for appearance. Here surface stimulation over the thighs can be cycled to activate the muscle at regular intervals with intervening rest intervals.

Care must be taken not to stimulate at too fast a rate or for too long an interval to prevent muscle injury. Electrical stimulation that induces strong isometric contractions (that is, the length of the muscle is not reduced although the muscle is trying to shorten) at high rates such as 75 Hz has been shown to induce muscle damage [4]. Further, recent research compared maximum voluntary isometric contractions with electrical stimulation evoked isometric contractions when both were 4 s isometric contractions followed by 15 s rest and showed that damage was greater with electrical evoked isometric contractions [5].

Sensory Stimulation

When a low rate of electrical stimulation, usually between 2 and 5 Hz, sends nerve pulses in afferent nerve endings to the central nervous system, it can elicit increased excitability in corticobulbar and craniobulbar projections to the swallowing musculature [6] as well as in cortical regions involved in volitional movement control [7]. The sensory facilitation and inhibition of other systems in the body by electroacupuncture on different afferents are currently being elucidated [8]. The electrical stimulation of afferents has been examined to a lesser degree than vibrotactile and touch stimulation likely because electrical stimulation is more likely to become painful if the current is increased while pressure and vibrotactile stimulation rarely excite pain fibers and are confined to mechanoreceptors. Electrical stimulation of skin afferents on the limbs is relatively easy compared to the intra-oral, laryngeal, and

pharyngeal regions that contain both the glossopharyngeal and laryngeal afferents known to have excitatory input to the brainstem swallowing regions [6, 9, 10].

Electrical sensory stimulation is useful for increasing excitability of the central nervous system in regions that are normally involved in movement control. Many cutaneous afferents are rapidly adapting and will only respond to stimulation onset and offset [11]; therefore single short afferent stimuli can be effective. Sensory stimulation is most effective in aiding movement if it is provided immediately before the patient needs to move or during the movement to increase cortical activity in the relevant area [12]. As neural responses to sensory stimuli are fast, short-lived, and rapidly adapt, sensory stimuli should be short infrequent volleys (less than 3 Hz) and applied sparingly, that is, immediately before movement onset and during movement. Sensory stimuli are particularly beneficial when they are applied within 200 ms prior to movement [12].

Functional Electrical Stimulation

When the peripheral muscle contraction is induced by electrical stimulation coincident with the patients' motor behavior it can augment the patient's motor behavior and increase function. An example of this is the assistance of patients during walking by providing functional electrical stimulation to prevent foot drop during the lift and swing phase of walking. Here the patient is benefited by a system that corrects for a movement control deficit (foot drop) by electrically induced muscle stimulation that is activated during walking. Recent analysis has found that patients prefer such functional electrical stimulation (FES) systems to orthotic braces that prevent foot drop [13]. Recent evidence has also suggested that FES systems have a further rehabilitation benefit as they interact with the patients' central neural control by enhancing neuroplasticity. This was demonstrated by increased corticospinal conduction and muscle function in stroke patients [14]. A recent trial comparing cyclic NMES with a contralaterally controlled FES system found significantly greater benefits from the FES system in stroke patients [15]. The superiority of FES systems is exciting but challenging. These systems are much more complex than NMES which only requires placing a stimulator on a muscle and programming a duty cycle of a few seconds stimulation alternated with rest time. A FES system, on the other hand, needs to be triggered during the patient's movement, must be programmed to occur in synchrony with movement to augment it, and must target particular muscles to activate in order to augment a patient's movement.

To summarize, for rehabilitation purposes NMES is least beneficial as it only prevents muscle atrophy and maintains muscle bulk, while both sensory and FES can benefit the patient's ability to move and produce the target behavior thus altering cortical physiology with greater potential for neurorehabilitation.

Application of Electrical Stimulation Systems to Swallowing

Although electrical stimulation has received a great deal of attention in recent years in the swallowing literature, it is still in its infancy in contrast with limb control. Clinical applications currently in use are confined to neuromuscular stimulation.

Neuromuscular Stimulation for Deglutition

Vital Stim® is a commercially available transcutaneous neuromuscular stimulation system that is used today during swallowing therapy by allied health professionals (particularly speech pathologists). This is the only NMES system currently cleared for use on the human throat area by the Food and Drug Administration. This system uses surface electrical stimulation to produce muscle contraction in the neck. Two bipolar pairs of electrodes are placed in the submental region and over the laryngeal area on the neck. Each pair is placed on the patient and the current is increased until the patient feels a strong muscle tug indicating that muscles in the region are contracting. The muscles that are contracting are those that are in close proximity to the surface where nerve endings innervating the muscle are most likely to be in the electrical field. These are schematized in Fig. 56.1 and their actions are summarized in Table 56.2.

Several aspects of how this stimulation is applied are not congruent with usual methods of NMES. First the rate of stimulation is at 80 Hz which is fast for the neck muscles being stimulated which should normally be stimulated at 30 Hz. Second the duty cycle is likely to induce fatigue as the stimulator stays on for 59 s and cycles off for 1 s. Finally the training course instructs therapists to leave it turned on for 60 min during a therapeutic session.

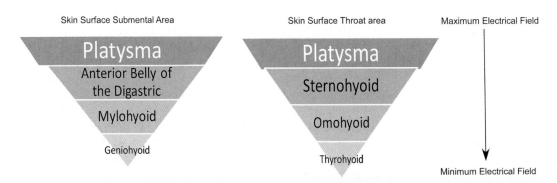

Fig. 56.1 A schematic illustration of the amplitude of the electrical field affecting muscles from the surface to layers beneath the skin in the submental and the throat areas

- Surface stimulation in the submental region does not raise the hyoid or larynx.
- Surface stimulation does not affect the intrinsic laryngeal muscles and does not change vocal fold opening or closing.
- Combined surface stimulation on the throat and submental regions resists hyo-laryngeal elevation during swallowing.

During electrical stimulation of the oral and pharyngeal mucosa:

- Stimulation should be at slow rates and at low current levels to avoid painful stimulation.
- Most appliances for providing intrinsic oral and pharyngeal electrical stimulation may interfere with swallowing behavior.
- For sensory stimulation to augment swallowing control it should be concurrent with volitional swallowing.

Functional electrical stimulation has not yet been applied to swallowing but may have greater potential for neurorehabilitation.

References

1. Morrissey MC, Brewster CE, Shields Jr CL, Brown M. The effects of electrical stimulation on the quadriceps during postoperative knee immobilization. Am J Sports Med. 1985;13(1):40–5.
2. Ng SS, Hui-Chan CW. Transcutaneous electrical nerve stimulation combined with task-related training improves lower limb functions in subjects with chronic stroke. Stroke. 2007;38(11):2953–9.
3. Mulcahey MJ, Betz RR, Smith BT, Weiss AA, Davis SE. Implanted functional electrical stimulation hand system in adolescents with spinal injuries: an evaluation. Arch Phys Med Rehabil. 1997;78(6):597–607.
4. Nosaka K, Aldayel A, Jubeau M, Chen TC. Muscle damage induced by electrical stimulation. Eur J Appl Physiol. 2011;111(10):2427–37.
5. Jubeau M, Muthalib M, Millet GY, Maffiuletti NA, Nosaka K. Comparison in muscle damage between maximal voluntary and electrically evoked isometric contractions of the elbow flexors. Eur J Appl Physiol. 2012;112(2):429–38.
6. Fraser C, Rothwell J, Power M, Hobson A, Thompson D, Hamdy S. Differential changes in human pharyngoesophageal motor excitability induced by swallowing, pharyngeal stimulation, and anesthesia. Am J Physiol Gastrointest Liver Physiol. 2003;285(1):G137–44.
7. Li G, Jack Jr CR, Yang ES. An fMRI study of somatosensory-implicated acupuncture points in stable somatosensory stroke patients. J Magn Reson Imaging. 2006;24(5):1018–24.
8. Kagitani F, Uchida S, Hotta H. Afferent nerve fibers and acupuncture. Auton Neurosci. 2010;157(1–2):2–8.
9. Jean A. Control of the central swallowing program by inputs from the peripheral receptors. A review. J Auton Nerv Syst. 1984;10:225–33.
10. Paterson WG. Alteration of swallowing and oesophageal peristalsis by different initiators of deglutition. Neurogastroenterol Motil. 1999;11(1):63–7.
11. Davis PJ, Nail BS. Quantitative analysis of laryngeal mechanosensitivity in the cat and rabbit. J Physiol. 1987;388:467–85.
12. Classen J, Steinfelder B, Liepert J, et al. Cutaneomotor integration in humans is somatotopically organized at various levels of the nervous system and is task dependent. Exp Brain Res. 2000;130(1):48–59.
13. Bulley C, Shiels J, Wilkie K, Salisbury L. User experiences, preferences and choices relating to functional electrical stimulation and ankle foot orthoses for foot-drop after stroke. Physiotherapy. 2011;97(3): 226–33.
14. Tarkka IM, Pitkanen K, Popovic DB, Vanninen R, Kononen M. Functional electrical therapy for hemiparesis alleviates disability and enhances neuroplasticity. Tohoku J Exp Med. 2011;225(1):71–6.
15. Knutson JS, Harley MY, Hisel TZ, Hogan SD, Maloney MM, Chae J. Contralaterally controlled functional electrical stimulation for upper extremity hemiplegia: an early-phase randomized clinical trial in subacute stroke patients. Neurorehabil Neural Repair. 2012;26(3):239–46.
16. Humbert IA, Poletto CJ, Saxon KG, et al. The effect of surface electrical stimulation on hyo-laryngeal movement in normal individuals at rest and during swallowing. J Appl Physiol. 2006;101:1657–63.
17. Ludlow CL, Humbert I, Saxon K, Poletto C, Sonies B, Crujido L. Effects of surface electrical stimulation both at rest and during swallowing in chronic pharyngeal dysphagia. Dysphagia. 2007;22:1–10.
18. Humbert IA, Poletto CJ, Saxon KG, Kearney PR, Ludlow CL. The effect of surface electrical stimulation on vocal fold position. Laryngoscope. 2008;118(1):14–9.
19. Park JW, Oh JC, Lee HJ, Park SJ, Yoon TS, Kwon BS. Effortful swallowing training coupled with electrical stimulation leads to an increase in hyoid elevation during swallowing. Dysphagia. 2009;24(3):296–301.
20. Logemann JA. Evaluation and treatment of swallowing disorders. 2nd ed. Austin, TX: Pro-Ed; 1998.
21. Logemann JA, Pauloski BR, Rademaker AW, Colangelo LA. Super-supraglottic swallow in irradiated head and neck cancer patients. Head Neck. 1997; 19:535–40.
22. Lim KB, Lee HJ, Lim SS, Choi YI. Neuromuscular electrical and thermal-tactile stimulation for dysphagia caused by stroke: a randomized controlled trial. J Rehabil Med. 2009;41(3):174–8.
23. Lin PH, Hsiao TY, Chang YC, et al. Effects of functional electrical stimulation on dysphagia caused by

radiation therapy in patients with nasopharyngeal carcinoma. Support Care Cancer. 2011;19(1):91–9.

24. Permsirivanich W, Tipchatyotin S, Wongchai M, et al. Comparing the effects of rehabilitation swallowing therapy vs. neuromuscular electrical stimulation therapy among stroke patients with persistent pharyngeal dysphagia: a randomized controlled study. J Med Assoc Thai. 2009;92(2):259–65.

25. Ryu JS, Kang JY, Park JY, et al. The effect of electrical stimulation therapy on dysphagia following treatment for head and neck cancer. Oral Oncol. 2009;45(8):665–8.

26. Bulow M, Speyer R, Baijens L, Woisard V, Ekberg O. Neuromuscular electrical stimulation (NMES) in stroke patients with oral and pharyngeal dysfunction. Dysphagia. 2008;23(3):302–9.

27. Dick TE, Oku Y, Romaniuk JR, Cherniack NS. Interaction between central pattern generators for breathing and swallowing in the cat. J Physiol. 1993; 465:715–30.

28. Gestreau C, Milano S, Bianchi AL, Grelot L. Activity of dorsal respiratory group inspiratory neurons during laryngeal-induced fictive coughing and swallowing in decerebrate cats. Exp Brain Res. 1996;108:247–56.

29. Chi-Fishman G, Capra NF, McCall GN. Thermomechanical facilitation of swallowing evoked by electrical nerve stimulation in cats. Dysphagia. 1994;9(3):149–55.

30. Yoshida Y, Tanaka Y, Hirano M, Nakashima T. Sensory innervation of the pharynx and larynx. Am J Med. 2000;108 Suppl 4a:51S–61.

31. Odom JL. Airway emergencies in the post anesthesia care unit. Nurse Clin N Am. 1993;28:483–91.

32. Power M, Fraser C, Hobson A, et al. Changes in pharyngeal corticobulbar excitability and swallowing behavior after oral stimulation. Am J Physiol Gastrointest Liver Physiol. 2004;286(1):G45–50.

33. Park CL, O'Neill PA, Martin DF. A pilot exploratory study of oral electrical stimulation on swallow function following stroke: an innovative technique. Dysphagia. 1997;12(3):161–6.

34. Fraser C, Power M, Hamdy S, et al. Driving plasticity in human adult motor cortex is associated with improved motor function after brain injury. Neuron. 2002;34(5):831–40.

35. Power ML, Fraser CH, Hobson A, et al. Evaluating oral stimulation as a treatment for dysphagia after stroke. Dysphagia. 2006;21(1):49–55.

36. Hamdy S, Aziz Q, Thompson DG, Rothwell JC. Physiology and pathophysiology of the swallowing area of human motor cortex. Neural Plast. 2001;8(1–2):91–7.

37. Jayasekeran V, Singh S, Tyrrell P, et al. Adjunctive functional pharyngeal electrical stimulation reverses swallowing disability after brain lesions. Gastroenterology. 2010;138(5):1737–46.

38. Leelamanit V, Limsakul C, Geater A. Synchronized electrical stimulation in treating pharyngeal dysphagia. Laryngoscope. 2002;112(12):2204–10.

39. Gay T, Rendell JK, Spiro J. Oral and laryngeal muscle coordination during swallowing. Laryngoscope. 1994;104:341–9.

40. Barkmeier JM, Bielamowicz S, Takeda N, Ludlow CL. Modulation of laryngeal responses to superior laryngeal nerve stimulation by volitional swallowing in awake humans. J Neurophysiol. 2000;83(3):1264–72.

41. Ludlow CL. Central nervous system control of interactions between vocalization and respiration in mammals. Head Neck. 2011;33 Suppl 1:S21–25

42. Burnett TA, Mann EA, Stoklosa JB, Ludlow CL. Self-triggered functional electrical stimulation during swallowing. J Neurophysiol. 2005;94(6):4011–8.

43. Burnett TA, Mann EA, Cornell SA, Ludlow CL. Laryngeal elevation achieved by neuromuscular stimulation at rest. J Appl Physiol. 2003;94(1):128–34.

Rationale for the Use of Botulinum Toxin in the UES for Dysphagia

The first use of Botox for cricopharyngeal dysfunction was reported by Schneider et al. [22]. They reported on seven cases with improvement in five using a variety of measures and no complications. The rationale for the intervention is supported by prior literature and experience with surgical myotomy treating similar clinical entities. The use of Botox is often times described as a chemical myotomy and is effective at producing weakness in the targeted muscle. It is dose dependent and will diffuse to surrounding tissues depending on the concentration and volume of fluid injected. The UES is a complex fibromuscular system which can develop increased muscle tone, resulting in dysphagia. When this is identified as the etiology, appropriately placed and dosed botulinum toxin will decrease the symptoms of and risks associated with dysphagia. Most cases of dysphagia, though, are multifactorial and the specific contribution of the UES is often questionable. As UES relaxation and opening rely on several factors, it is important to assess the function of all these potential problem areas before committing to treatment with Botox. Assessment should include an evaluation of hyolaryngeal excursion, oral and pharyngeal muscle strength, sensory function, and airway protection including laryngeal movement. It is also important to document the status of vocal fold motion and pharyngeal strength as diffusion of Botox can lead to laryngeal paralysis and pharyngeal weakness [24].

The importance and contributions of hyolaryngeal elevation and bolus volume to UES opening in normal subjects were well demonstrated by Cook et al. [19]; however, these relationships are lost or less obvious in patients with Zenker's diverticulum and in patients with failed UES relaxation [26]. The static UES would support an intervention directed at this level. The ideal patient for Botox injection is similar to that described by Kelly for cricopharyngeal myotomy [27]. The patient should have adequate hyolaryngeal elevation and tongue/pharyngeal propulsion. The patient should also be medically and neurologically stable. Additionally, the UES dysfunction should be myogenic at its root cause and not secondary to fibrosis or connective tissue changes such as fatty infiltration or inflammation.

Evidence Supporting the Use of Botulinum Toxin in the UES for Dysphagia

The use of botulinum toxin for treatment of dysphagia due to cricopharyngeal dysfunction has garnered regular interest since the initial description by Schneider et al. [22]. Most articles published since then are case reports or case series concluding that botulinum toxin injections are an effective treatment for cricopharyngeal hypertonicity. Moerman et al. [24] reviewed 16 articles published between 1994 and 2006 and found that 74 of 100 patients experienced improvement after injection. Of these 16 studies, seven reported an improvement rate of 100%, though this includes four case reports from the same authors presenting a total of eight patients with different disorders [28–31].

Alberty et al. [32] performed botulinum toxin injection in ten patients with mild to severe dysphagia caused by pure UES dysfunction. UES opening improved in all patients and hypopharyngeal retention and penetration was significantly reduced in four of seven patients. Clinical symptom scores improved in all subjects, but the degree of improvement varied. One patient experienced complete relief and was free of symptoms, while mild dysphagia persisted in six patients and moderate dysphagia persisted in three patients. This pattern of improvement is consistent with reports by Schneider et al. [22], Atkinson et al. [33], and Blitzer et al. [34], where most (if not all) patients experience a benefit from injection, but the degree of that benefit can vary considerably from restoration of normal function to only mild improvement.

Parameswaran and Soliman conducted a retrospective review of 12 patients receiving endoscopic botulinum toxin injections in the cricopharyngeus for dysphagia with cricopharyngeal spasm [35]. Eleven of the 12 patients experienced an improvement in their symptoms, with improvement lasting an average of approximately 4 months. Similar to the study by Alberty et al. [32], a range of improvement in swallowing function from 25 to 100% was observed. Patients reported less difficulty passing a bolus, decreased meal times, and less coughing and choking during meals.

In the largest published series on this topic, Zaninotto et al. [36] reported on 21 patients undergoing botulinum toxin injection to the cricopharyngeus for oropharyngeal dysphagia unresponsive to rehabilitation. Improvement after injection was reported in only 9 of the 21 patients (43%). Eight of 11 patients who did not improve with botulinum toxin improved after myotomy. Despite the relatively low success rate, the authors still advocate the use of botulinum toxin injection as a first-line option in the treatment of oropharyngeal dysphagia, as it is a safe and simple procedure. Multivariate analysis demonstrated that patients most likely to experience improvement have cricopharyngeal spasm on EMG and do not have severely impaired swallowing function on videofluoroscopy. Accordingly, the comparatively low success rate reported in this study may be due to differences in subject selection criteria, as most studies employ more strict criteria and include only subjects with isolated cricopharyngeal dysfunction.

Several themes are present in the majority of published case series on botulinum toxin injection for the management of UES dysfunction. First, relatively high success rates are reported consistently. While each report consists of a limited number of subjects, pooling the studies reveals fairly consistent improvement in symptoms for most patients. Second, the complication rate is low. In the review by Moerman et al. [37], nine complications were reported for 100 patients. This included one case of urinary retention caused by anesthesia, one case of neck cellulitis in a patient undergoing simultaneous excision of a thyroglossal duct cyst [35], and one patient dying from aspiration attributed to the underlying disease [36]. A low complication rate combined with the relative ease of performing the procedure compared to myotomy makes botulinum toxin injection an appealing therapeutic

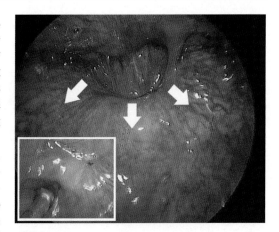

Fig. 57.5 Direct injection into UES at time of operative dilatation

option in appropriate patients. Third, there is a consistent call for studies evaluating treatment effects in a larger number of patients with longer duration of follow-up. While a meta-analysis could answer some questions regarding treatment efficacy, differences in outcome measures across studies preclude rigorous quantitative statistical analysis. Though larger studies evaluating duration of improvement and the benefit of repeat injections are warranted, the current literature provides support for the use of botulinum toxin injections in cases of cricopharyngeal spasm or hypertonicity.

Adding botulinum toxin injection to cricopharyngeal dilation can be strongly supported (Fig. 57.5). With direct access to the UES at the time of dilation, the agent can be guided precisely into the posterior two-thirds of the muscle in small volumes with high concentrations. Coupling chemical myotomy with physical dilation should increase the likelihood of long-term benefit by addressing both the muscular and connective tissue components of the UES.

Conclusion

Although there are no absolute criteria for the use of botulinum toxin in the management of dysphagia, most carefully selected patients will benefit from its addition to their treatment plan. When used correctly, the risk of harm is extremely low. Considering the pathophysiology of an individual patient's dysphagia is paramount when deciding whether to perform a botulinum toxin injection. As botulinum toxin is a paralytic agent, it is valuable for dysphagia caused by excessive muscle activity. The most favorable outcomes will be seen in patients with documented UES muscular hypertonicity identified by manometry and/or EMG; however, it is also likely to be beneficial to individuals with otherwise preserved pharyngeal function but evidence of persistent UES narrowing when swallowing a large bolus. There is no support for its use in patients with significant pharyngeal weakness, progressive neuromuscular disease, scar, or fibrosis. It should also not be used in the treatment of Zenker's diverticulum where complete surgical myotomy is known to be highly effective.

References

1. Erbguth FJ, Naumann M. Historical aspects of botulinum toxin: Justinus Kerner (1786–1862) and the "sausage poison". Neurology. 1999;53(8):1850–3.
2. Van Ermengem E. Ueber einen neuen anaeroben Bacillus und seine Beizehungen zum Botulismus. Zeitschrift Hygiene Infektionkrankheiten. 1897;26:1–56.
3. Burke GS. Notes of Bacillus botulinus. J Bacteriol. 1919;4:555–65.
4. Jankovic J, Hallett M. Therapy with botulinum toxin. New York, NY: Marcel Dekker; 1994.
5. Schantz EJ. Historical perspective. In: Jankovic J, Hallet M, editors. Therapy with botulinum toxin. New York: Marcel Dekker; 1994. p. xxii–vi.
6. Snipe PT, Sommer H. Studies on botulinus toxin. 3. Acid precipitation of botulinus toxin. J Infect Dis. 1928;43:152–60.
7. Schantz EJ, Johnson EA. Botulinum toxin: the story of its development for the treatment of human disease. Perspect Biol Med. 1997;40:317–27.
8. Scott AB, Rosenbaum A, Collins CC. Pharmacologic wakening of extraocular muscles. Invest Ophthalmol. 1973;12:924–7.
9. Scott AB. Botulinum toxin injection into extraocular muscles as an alternative to strabismus surgery. Ophthalmology. 1980;87:1044–9.
10. Terre R, et al. Long-lasting effect of a single botulinum toxin injection in the treatment of oropharyngeal dysphagia secondary to upper esophageal sphincter dysfunction: a pilot study. Scand J Gastroenterol. 2008;43:1296–303.
11. Montecucco C, Schiavo G. Mechanism of action of tetanus and botulinum neurotoxins. Mol Microbiol. 1994;13(1):1–8.
12. Montal M. Botulinum neurotoxin: a marvel of protein design. Annu Rev Biochem. 2010;79:591–617.
13. Borodic GE et al. In: Therapy with botulinum toxin. Jankovic J. and Hallett M (eds). New York: Marcel Dekker; 1994: 119–57.
14. Dressler D, Eleopra R. Clinical use of non-A botulinum toxins: botulinum toxin type B. Neurotox Res. 2006;9(2–3):121–5.
15. Brin MF, et al. Safety and efficacy of NeuroBloc (botulinum toxin type B) in type A-resistant cervical dystonia. Neurology. 1999;53(7):1431–8.
16. Pappert EJ, Germanson T. Botulinum toxin type B vs. type A in toxin-naïve patients with cervical dystonia: randomized, double-blind, noninferiority trial. Mov Disord. 2008;23(4):510–7.
17. Jackson CE, et al. Randomized double-blind study of botulinum toxin type B for sialorrhea in ALS patients. Muscle Nerve. 2009;39:137–43.
18. Shapiro J, Kelly J. Anatomy, histology, and clinical dysfunction of the cricopharyngeus muscle. Otolaryngol Head Neck Surg. 1994;2:52–4.
19. Cook IJ, et al. Opening mechanisms of the human upper esophageal sphincter. Am J Physiol. 1989;257:G748–59.
20. Lawson G, Remacle M. Endoscopic cricopharyngeal myotomy: indications and technique. Otolaryngol Head Neck Surg. 2006;14(6):437–41.
21. Brownlow H, Whitmore I, Willan PL. A quantitative study of the histochemical and morphometric characteristics of the human cricopharyngeus muscle. J Anat. 1989;166:67–75.
22. Schneider I, et al. Treatment of dysfunction of the cricopharyngeal muscle with botulinum A toxin: introduction of a new, noninvasive method. Ann Otol Rhinol Laryngol. 1994;103:31–5.
23. Dohlman G. Endoscopic operations for hypopharyngeal diverticula. Proceedings of the Fourth International Congress on Otolaryngology in London. 1949; 715–7.
24. Moerman MBJ. Cricopharyngeal Botox injection: indications and technique. Curr Opin Otolaryngol Head Neck Surg. 2006;14:431–6.
25. Murry T, et al. Injection of botulinum toxin A for the treatment of dysfunction of the upper esophageal sphincter. Am J Otolaryngol Head Neck Med Surg. 2006;26:157–62.
26. Williams RB, et al. Biomechanics of failed deglutitive upper esophageal sphincter (UES) relaxation in patients with neurogenic dysphagia. Am J Physiol. 2002;283:G16–26.
27. Kelly JH. Management of upper esophageal sphincter disorders: indications and complications of myotomy. Am J Med. 2000;108(Suppl 4a):43S–6.
28. Restivo D, et al. Successful botulinum toxin treatment of dysphagia in oculopharyngeal muscular dystrophy. Gastroenterology. 2000;119:1416.

29. Restivo D, et al. Successful botulinum toxin treatment of dysphagia in a young child with nemaline myopathy. Dysphagia. 2001;16:228–9.

30. Restivo D, Palmeri A, Marchese-Ragona R. Botulinum toxin for cricopharyngeal dysfunction in Parkinson's disease. N Engl J Med. 2002;346:1174–5.

31. Restivo D, Marchese-Ragona R. Botulinum toxin treatment for oropharyngeal dysphagia due to tetanus. J Neurol. 2006;253:388–9.

32. Alberty J, et al. Efficacy of botulinum toxin A for treatment of upper esophageal sphincter dysfunction. Laryngoscope. 2000;110:1151–6.

33. Atkinson SI, Rees J. Botulinum toxin for cricopharyngeal dysphagia: case reports of CT-guided injection. J Otolaryngol. 1997;26:273–6.

34. Blitzer A, Brin M. Use of botulinum toxin for diagnosis and management of cricopharyngeal achalasia. Otolaryngol Head Neck Surg. 1997;116:328–30.

35. Parameswaran M, Soliman A. Endoscopic botulinum toxin injection for cricopharyngeal dysphagia. Ann Otol Rhinol Laryngol. 2002;111:871–4.

36. Zaninotto G, et al. The role of botulinum toxin injection and upper esophageal sphincter myotomy in treating oropharyngeal dysphagia. J Gastrointest Surg. 2004;8:997–1006.

37. Haapaniemi J, et al. Botulinum toxin in the treatment of cricopharyngeal dysphagia. Dysphagia. 2001;16:171–5.

Open and Endoscopic Cricopharyngeal Myotomy

58

André Duranceau

Abstract

Cricopharyngeal myotomy is a recognized treatment for disorders of the pharyngoesophageal junction. The etiology of these disorders is either neurologic, muscular, idiopathic, iatrogenic or may result from distal esophageal dysfunction or obstruction. Independently of the cause for the abnormal function, the operation aims at improving bolus transport from pharynx to cervical esophagus. Indications investigation and the open approach technique are described with the rationale for the operation. The clinical and functional results are discussed for each category of dysfunction. The recent literature emphasizes the advent of minimally invasive surgery to remove the obstructive effects of the upper esophageal sphincter. The vast majority of these operations are now reported for the pharyngoesophageal diverticulum. However, endoscopic Cricopharyngeal myotomy has now been performed for Cricopharyngeal dysfunction. This chapter aims at reviewing the results of both the open or endoscopic Cricopharyngeal myotomy to treat oropharyngeal dysphagia.

Keywords

Endoscopic cricopharyngeal myotomy • Open cricopharyngeal myotomy • Postmyotomy care • Neurologic dysphagia • Myogenic dysphagia

Cricopharyngeal myotomy is a recognized treatment for disorders of the pharyngoesophageal junction [1–5]. The open cervical approach provides good exposure for this operation that aims at improving Bolus transport between pharynx and cervical esophagus [6]. Since the early 1990s, the advent of minimally invasive surgery has stimulated the development of less invasive techniques to remove the obstructive effects of the cricopharyngeus. This chapter aims to review the indications, the technique, and the documented results of cricopharyngeal myotomy when using the open or the endoscopic approaches to treat the dysfunction.

Independent of the approach, the indications to proceed with a surgical treatment are most

A. Duranceau, MD (✉)
Division of Thoracic Surgery, Department of Surgery,
Centre Hospitalier de l'Université de Montréal,
Université de Montréal, 1560, Sherbrooke Est,
Montréal, QC, Canada H2L 4M1
e-mail: andre.duranceau@umontreal.ca

important. The etiology of oropharyngeal symptoms related to disorders of the pharyngoesophageal junction can usually be categorized in five major sections [7].

Neurologic oropharyngeal dysphagia is seen in patients suffering neurological damage at any level of the afferent or efferent pathway or in the brainstem and the cerebral cortex, where integration of the information for swallowing takes place. Neurological disease, cerebrovascular lesions, tumors, or neurosurgical interventions may result in incapacitating oropharyngeal dysphagia [8].

Myogenic disorders occur at the motor endplate of the skeletal muscle or in the skeletal muscle itself. Myasthenia gravis is the characteristic disorder of the motor endplate but is rarely an indication for surgical treatment. Skeletal muscle diseases include muscular dystrophies, mostly its oculopharyngeal form, and inflammatory myositis. Metabolic myopathies as in hyperthyroidism are rare indications to treat the pharyngoesophageal dysphagia by cricopharyngeal myotomy [9].

Idiopathic cricopharyngeal muscle dysfunction is seen when abnormal function of the cricopharyngeus is documented without evident neurological or neuromuscular disease. The dysfunction resides in the sphincter itself which acts as an obstructive factor for the swallowing mechanism. The etiology of this idiopathic dysfunction remains unclear. Patients with a symptomatic cricopharyngeal bar, an upper esophageal sphincter that does not relax with or without pharyngoesophageal diverticulum are good examples of idiopathic cricopharyngeal muscle dysfunction. The management of pharyngoesophageal diverticulum is described in a separate chapter. It remains unclear if idiopathic dysfunction of the cricopharyngeus represents the same muscle pathology that might eventually evolve in the herniation of mucosa and submucosa through the muscular wall.

Iatrogenic causes may be responsible for oropharyngeal dysphagia. Transection or resection at the pharyngoesophageal level may result in dysfunction of the upper esophageal sphincter. The laryngectomized patient is a good example for such an etiology that is, any surgery affecting the elevation of the pharynx and or larynx may cause oropharyngeal dysphagia [10].

Distal causes. Distal obstruction, functional or mechanical, may cause oropharyngeal symptoms. Although reflux disease has been proposed by some as a cause for cricopharyngeal dysfunction, it is rarely an indication for cricopharyngeal myotomy.

The Indications

Independent of etiology, pharyngoesophageal dysfunction determined by objective instrumental diagnosis may require a cricopharyngeal myotomy. Patient symptoms must be quantified for their frequency duration and severity. Videofluoroscopy and pharyngoesophageal emptying scintigrams can be used to quantify the impact of the dysfunction. With new high resolution manometry, the concept of resistance can be added to these measurements. The correlation of symptoms with objectively measured functional abnormalities is important. These objective findings include lack of UES relaxation seen on videofluoroscopy and hypopharyngeal retention as recorded by a radionuclide scintigram. These objectively measured functional abnormalities constitute for us the best indication for offering a cricopharyngeous myotomy. These nuclear medicine recordings aim at quantifying with boluses of various viscosities, the abnormal retention or misdirection of swallowed boluses [11, 12].

Rationale for Open Cricopharyngeal Myotomy

The rationale for the 6-cm cricopharyngeal myotomy is explained by the illustration of the pressure profile reported by Sivarao et al. [2] (Fig. 58.1). The high pressure zone separating hypopharynx from cervical esophagus measures 2.5–4.5 cm in length. Within this zone is a shorter high pressure zone 1 cm long of maximally elevated pressure that corresponds to the location of the cricopharyngeus itself, identified by its attachment on the laminae of the cricoid cartilage. The cricopharyngeus, however, does not account totally for the 2–3 cm width of the high pressure

Fig. 58.1 Pressure profile
of the upper esophageal
sphincter [2]

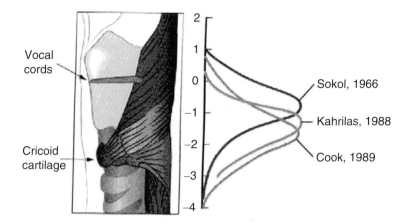

Fig. 58.2 Physiological effects of cricopharyngeal myotomy [13]

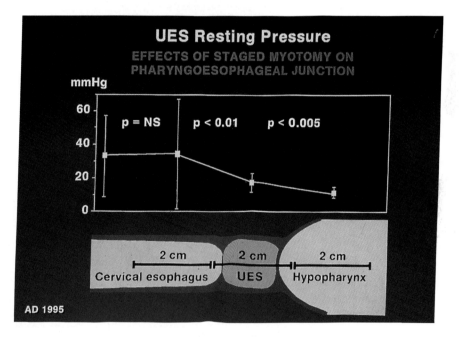

zone of the UES as reported in these three pressure profiles of the sphincter. A significant contribution to this pressure zone comes from the fibers of the inferior constrictor of the pharynx.

The physiological effects of open cricopharyngeal myotomy have been well documented. The UES pressure tone is reduced by approximately 50 % when dividing the cricopharyngeus, located during the operation by identifying the position of the cricoid cartilage. Pera [13] recorded the resting pressure of the pharyngoesophageal

junction during cricopharyngeal myotomy. They used a 6 cm manometric sleeve technique for pressure recording. Division of the muscle on the cervical esophagus does not change the resting pressures. When the muscularis is transected over the 2 cm in direct relation to its attachment to the cricoid cartilage a significant fall in resting pressures is recorded. Extension of the myotomy an additional 2 cm on the hypopharynx will result in a further significant decrease in the resting pressures (Fig. 58.2). As evidenced in Fig. 58.3, these

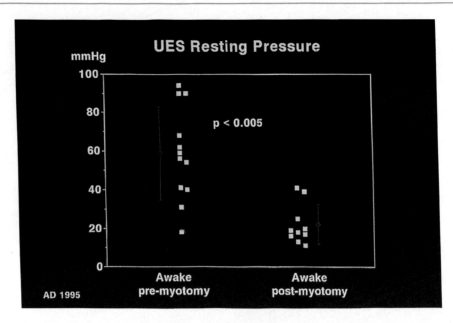

Fig. 58.3 Pressure recordings of the upper esophageal sphincter before and after cricopharyngeal myotomy [13]

effects of cricopharyngeal myotomy recorded under anesthesia remain significant when the patient is awake.

Open Cricopharyngeal Myotomy [13–15]

(a) Technique [6] (Figs. 58.4–58.10)

The muscle is transected transversely at the proximal and distal ends of the myotomized area. The muscle flap resulting is resected for histological analysis. After insuring meticulous hemostasis, the mucosal integrity is verified by passing a nasogastric tube to the level of the myotomy. Air is insufflated while the myectomized area is maintained under saline water.

(b) Postmyotomy care

The nasogastric tube is then descended toward the stomach to provide gastric decompression during the first 12–18 h.

– A modified liquid diet is started the next day and a pureed diet suggested for the first week.

– Patients are usually discharged after 48–72 h.

Outcomes of Open Cricopharyngeal Myotomy [13–15]

Cricopharyngeal myotomy is performed in order to reduce sphincteric tone and resistance to flow across the pharyngoesophageal junction. The abnormal opening of the upper esophageal sphincter must be classified relative to the etiology, as prognostic factors may vary with each category of dysfunction.

Neurologic Dysphagia

Neurologic dysphagia results from disruption of the swallowing mechanism in patients with central nervous system disease or with cranial nerve involvement. Cerebrovascular disease and stroke are most frequently responsible for the condition. The efficacy of myotomy in neurogenic dysphagia is extremely variable and influenced by the location and extent of damage. Intact voluntary swallow function, tongue movement, and protective airway closure should remain in order to achieve maximum improve-

Table 58.2 (continued)

References	Patient	Results	Morbidity	Mortality
Hurwitz and Duranceau	1	Poor		
Loizou et al. (1980)	20	15 Sustained improvement	(Limitation of coughing and breathing capacity)	
Gay et al. (1984)	8	5 Failures 2 Good 1 Temp. improvement		5 Deaths
Mitchell and Amanini (1975)	1	Improved		
Wilson (1990)	7	6/7 Improved (83 %)		

Table 58.3 Poliomyelitis, progressive bulbar palsy, and pseudobulbar palsy

References	Patient no.	Results
Lund (1968)	1	Improved
Mills (1964)	1	Improved
Bofenkamp (1958)	2	Improved
Schneider and Nagurney (1977)	1	Excellent
Van Overbeek and Betlem (1979)	1	–
Kaplan (1951)	1	Moderate
Loizou et al. (1980)	2	1 Improved 1 Unimproved
Bonavena et al. (1985)	1	–
Nanson (1974)	1	Failure
Millar (1973)	1	Improved
Calcaterra et al. (1975)	1	Improved

gies is needed to support surgical intervention. Positive clinical outcome postcricopharyngeal myotomy in this patient population is less than or equal to 60 % [8].

Myogenic Dysphagia

Primary and secondary muscular disorders may produce oropharyngeal dysphagia. Poor propulsive forces in the pharynx as well as poor relaxation of the upper esophageal sphincter result in misdirection of the swallowed bolus. Hypopharyngeal stasis with pharyngo-oral and nasal regurgitations and tracheobronchial aspirations are the most frequent symptoms. Aspiration pneumonia may result [9]. The extensive cricopharyngeal myotomy illustrated in this chapter has been described in the early 1970s by

Montgomery and Lynch. It remains in use to this day and has been most appropriate for patients with oculopharyngeal muscular dystrophy. The muscular strength of the pharyngeal contraction cannot be restored in muscle disease patients. The intact voluntary swallow coupled with a reduced resistance to pharyngoesophageal transit after removal of the posterior pharyngoesophageal junction is possibly responsible for the symptomatic improvement. Peterman (1974) initially described this improvement with its subsequent evolution. Our experience has documented significant improvement in esophageal and tracheobronchial symptoms but never to return to a normal function level. When patients are asked to quantify each of their symptoms on a numerical scale before and after surgery, the level of comfort obtained in swallowing rarely exceeds 65–75 % of the preoperative level.

Improvement in dysphagic symptoms has been most appreciated when patients attempt to swallow a solid bolus. Swallowing of liquids is frequently reported as more difficult after the myotomy. Tracheobronchial symptoms and nocturnal bronchorrhea seem to improve as well. The stage of the disease and the severity and extent of the muscular pathology influence the postsurgical outcomes. The presence of facial atony with dysphonia and the incapacity to generate a significant voice tone may have a prognostic influence with persistent aspiration. Hypothetically, the symptoms may result from advanced muscular disease from poor pronunciation and poor phonation from decreased control of facial muscles and vocal cord tensor muscles.

It is clear that in these patients cricopharyngeal myotomy provides palliation of the swallow

Table 58.4 Various neurological lesions

References	Patient no.	Results	Morbidity	Mortality
Parkinson's disease				
Gay et al. (1984)	3	Good		
West and Barker (1977)	1	Poor		
	1	Good		
Born (1996)		Improved	4/4 (2 with Zenkers)	0
Akl and Blackley (1974)	1	Improved		
Various central lesions				
Akl and Blakeley (1974)	1	Poor	Aspiration	1
Reichert et al. (1977)	2	Moderate		
Gay et al. (1984)	2	Good		
Loizou et al. (1980)	1	Improved		
Bonavena et al. (1985)	1	–		
Mitchell and Armanini (1977)	1	Improved		
Bergman and Lewicki (1977)	1	Failure		
Orringer (1980)	2	–		
Trauma				
Desaulty et al. (1975)	1	Improved		
Aubry et al. (1967)	1	Normal deglutition		
Van Overbeek and Betlem (1979)	4	–		
Gay et al. (1984)	1	Good		
Bonavena et al. (1985)	1	–		

Table 58.5 Peripheral nervous system lesions

References	Patient no.	Results
Mills (1973)	2	Excellent
Akl (1974)	3	Poor
Henderson et al. (1974)	3	Good
Bonavena et al. (1985)	6	–
Gagic (1983)	2	Improved

symptoms caused by muscle weakness. The reported results of cricopharyngeal myotomy for primary muscular disease are described in Table 58.6.

Following cricopharyngeal myotomy, pharyngeal emptying scintigrams have documented improvement in the clearing of a liquid bolus and hypopharyngeal stasis. Increased viscosity of the bolus used for radionuclide emptying studies seems to increase the validity of the observations of change postsurgically [11].

As for neurologic dysphagia most of the reported experiences at present are case series without randomized observations to other forms of treatment or medical management [5]. Despite the convincing clinical results suggesting improved swallowing, the scientific evidence suggests cricopharyngeal myotomy remains at the "C" level with all published reports being uncontrolled retrospective case series.

Idiopathic Dysfunction of the Upper Esophageal Sphincter

When no neurological or neuromuscular disease can be diagnosed, dysfunction of the cricopharyngeus is termed idiopathic. Mr. Belsey (1966) first described this condition describing the symptom "as recurrent attacks aggravated by generalized nervous tension." Although neurological disease or neuromuscular dysfunction has been never been thought to play an important role in the pathophysiology of the pharyngoesophageal diverticulum, psychological factors and high strung personalities associated with this condition have not been investigated. Idiopathic cricopharyngeal dysfunction without diverticulum formation may represent an earlier stage of the same condition but this has not been documented.

Table 58.6 Primary muscular disease

References	Patient no.	Results	Morbidity	Mortality
Melgar (1968)	1	Considerable improve		
Desaulty et al. (1975)	1	Spectacular improve		
Blakeley et al. (1968)	2	Excellent		
Akl and Blakeley (1974)	9	7 Marked relief		
		2 Satisfactory		
Mitchell and Armanini (1975)	1	Excellent		
Dayal and Freeman (1976)	1	Excellent		
Peterman et al. (1964)	1	Excellent for 1 year		
		Poor results		
		Following appearance of hoarseness		
Hurwitz et al. (1975)	2	–		
Montgomery and Lynch (1971)	8	7 Excellent		
		1 Partial failure (reported by Johnson (1974)		
Leonard and Smith (1970)	1	Complete relief		
Bender (1976)	1	Excellent		
Duranceau et al. (1978, 1980)	11	8 Excellent		
		3 Moderate		
Nanson (1974)	2	Marked improvement		
Weitzner (1969)	1	Poor	GI hemorrhage	Died
Taillefert				
Castell				

Cricopharyngeal myotomy for idiopathic upper esophageal sphincter dysfunction is frequently reported as surgery for cricopharyngeal bars. Table 58.7 summarizes some of these reports. Seventy of 80 patients showed excellent symptomatic improvement following their myotomy. As for other patients with oropharyngeal dysphagia, the difficulty in selecting those with significant clinical and radiological abnormalities and quantifiable malfunction of the cricopharyngeus that are sufficient to treat surgically require even more objectivity in the investigation. A strong psychological overlay to symptoms may make the decision more difficult.

Complication of Cricopharyngeal Myotomy

Cricopharyngeal myotomy for oropharyngeal dysphagia is performed to improve the patient's dysphagic symptoms and efficiency of swallowing. A strong exaggeration of symptoms from or by anxiety may make the decision more difficult.

The operation, however, can result in complications and even death.

In Brigand's reported series of 253 cricopharyngeal myotomies (2007), [16] 15 patients with neurologic dysphagia were included. One patient experienced complications related to the surgery that is, the surgical incision became infected requiring wide reopening and drainage of the cervical incision. Failure of aspiration control in this patient also required a permanent tracheostomy with laryngeal exclusion (Fig. 58.11).

The group of 139 patients undergoing cricopharyngeal myotomy for muscular dysphagia caused by oculopharyngeal muscular dystrophy (Table 58.8) also experienced complications. Those resulted in four hospital deaths after the operation, all from acute respiratory distress syndrome. Twelve mucosal tears occurred during the completion of the myotomy. They were all repaired primarily without infection or fistula formation. Failure to control postsurgical aspiration may require permanent tracheostomy and or laryngeal exclusion (Fig. 58.11).

Table 58.7 Idiopathic UOS dysfunction without PO diverticulum

Authors	Patients	Results	Morbidity
Hiebert (1976)	6	In 15 patients: 13 excellent 2 improved	
Calcaterra et al. (1975)	3	Excellent	
Leonard and Smith (1970)	1	Excellent	
Bingham (1963)	1	Excellent	
Parrish (1968)	1	Good	
Belsey (1966)	32	Excellent	
West and Baker (1977)	7	6 Excellent 1 Good	
Desaulty et al. (1975)	2	Poor	Fistula, stricture
Melgar (1968)	1	Improved	
Gagic (1983)	4	3 Excellent	
Chodosh (1975)	1	Excellent	
Mitchell and Armanini (1975)	1	Excellent	
Cruse et al. (1979)	6	–	
Ellis and Crozler (1981)	6	Excellent	
Sutherland (1962)	8	7 Excellent 1 Moderate	
Gay et al. (1984)	1	Poor	
Orringer (1980)	7	6 Excellent 1 Poor	

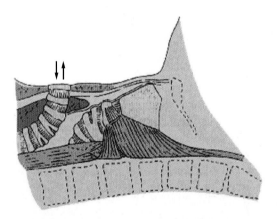

Fig. 58.11 Failure to control aspiration, following myotomy/myectomy, may require permanent tracheostomy with laryngeal exclusion

Endoscopic Cricopharyngeal Myotomy

Endoscopic treatment of oropharyngeal dysphagia was initially described by Dohlman and Mattson for patients with a pharyngoesophageal diverticulum. The introduction of the operating microscope, the refinement of the laryngoscope

Table 58.8 Complications of open cricopharyngeal myotomy

	n	Reoperation	Death
Pulmonary infection	8	0	4
Hematoma	2	1	0
Mucosal breaks	12	1	0
Wound infection	1	0	0
Fistula	1	1	0
Buccal floor infection	1	0	0
Pulmonary embolism	1	0	0
Hypertensive crisis	1	0	0
Stroke	1	0	0
Total no. with complications	16	2	4

into a diverticuloscope, and the availability of the CO_2 laser with surgical staplers have made these minimally invasive techniques available [17, 18]. Cricopharyngeal dysfunction without diverticulum formation can also be approached in the same way. In a number of case studies, patients with pharyngoesophageal dysfunction have been treated with the approach described and have reported clinical improvement without major complications [17, 19, 20].

Indications

The advantages of an intraoral approach seem to be the lack of morbidity reported with the procedure. Although rare with open surgery, use of intraoral approach decreases the occurrence of pharyngoesophageal fistula and recurrent laryngeal nerve injuries giving the intraoral approach an important hypothetical advantage. The intraoral approach also results in a reduction of patient complaints of pain and quicker return to oral eating. The adoption of laser-assisted cricopharyngeal myotomy has been tempered, however by the fear of mediastinitis that might result in mucosal disruption and penetration into the mediastinal space [18]. The rationale for endoscopic laser cricopharyngeal myotomy seems to be that it is "effective, safe, brief and prompt in restoring swallowing" [21].

The indications for this minimally invasive approach are the same as for the open approach, that is: neurologic dysphagia, the patient with a symptomatic cricopharyngeal bar and documented idiopathic dysfunction. Myogenic oropharyngeal dysfunction has also been approached with this technique. Transmucosal myotomy has even been proposed as a diagnostic tool by Halvorsen [22] in a selected group of patients without any definitive preoperative studies, based on "suspicion of the diagnosis." Most of the surgeons who have proposed endoscopic cricopharyngeal myotomy are ear, nose, and throat specialists using careful symptom evaluation. Functional outcome swallowing scale (FOSS) [23, 24] and the MDADI quality of life evaluation (Chen) [25] with the modified barium swallow and videofluoroscopy documentation of the cricopharyngeal dysfunction form the base of these evaluations.

Technique

The operation is completed under general anesthesia. A direct rigid esophagoscopy is completed initially. Exposure may be potentially difficult in patients with xyphosis or anterior cervical osteophytes. In addition, retrognathia, cervical spine fixation, or abnormal dentition may render the introduction of the endoscope difficult.

The Benjamen–Holinger or the Weerda distending diverticuloscopes can be introduced down to the upper edge of the cricopharyngeal muscle. At that point creation of an invagination or creation of a pseudodiverticulum posterior to the cricopharyngeus is realized (Fig. 58.12). If the endoscope is not placed deeply enough, the cricopharyngeus muscle may not be adequately exposed. It is then placed in suspension on a laryngeal holder to stretch the cricopharyngeal bar (Fig. 58.13). The endoscope is attached to an operating microscope with a 400 mm lens and CO^2 laser is used by most with a micromanipulator. The laser is set between 5 and 20 W with a focused or slightly defocused beam super pulsed at 0.5–0.8 mm spot size for a 0.2 s duration [21, 26].

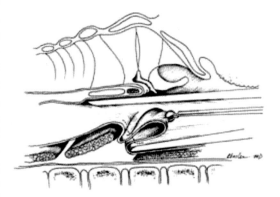

Fig. 58.12 The distending diverticuloscope, at the *upper edge* of the cricopharyngeus, creates a posterior pseudo diverticulum

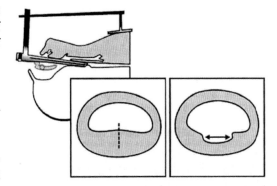

Fig. 58.13 When the cricopharyngeus is adequately exposed the diverticuloscope is placed in suspension on a laryngeal holder to stretch the cricopharyngeal bar

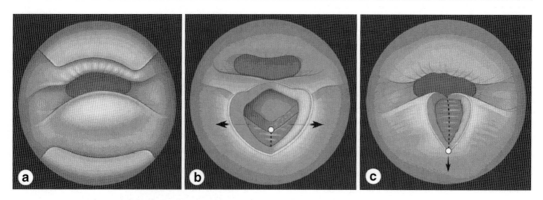

Fig. 58.14 (**a**) Stretched cricopharyngeus. (**b**) Mucosa and submucosa are incised vertically. (**c**) The cricopharyngeus is divided. Its fibers will retract laterally

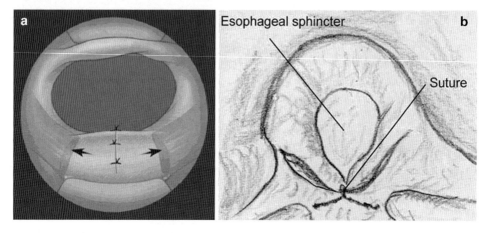

Fig. 58.15 (**a**) Vertical closure of the incised mucosa (Ho). (**b**) Horizontal closure of the vertical incision (Chitose)

The cricopharyngeal bar is incised vertically on the mid-line and the mucosal, submucosa, and the cricopharyngeus itself are divided. The divided fibers of the muscle retract laterally, resulting in a wedge-shaped incision (Fig. 58.14a–c). The cricopharyngeus is divided until the connective tissue of the buccopharyngeal fascia becomes apparent. A 0° and 70° rigid endoscope may be used to insure that all muscle fibers are cut and that the buccopharyngeal fascia is intact. Some suggest division of tissue down to the fat and areolar tissue overlying the prevertebral fascia (Brondbo [27], Takes [28]) while others prefer to leave a "last layer" of muscle fibers in place. Halvorson [22] also divides the inferior portion of the inferior constrictor by incising the posterior pharyngeal mucosa. Excisional biopsy specimen of muscle is taken by Ho [25]. Chitose [29] proceeds with a submucosal resection of the cricopharyngeus as widely as possible. The mucosa may be left open. Ho reapproximates the mucosa vertically with separate stitches (Fig. 58.15a) while Chitose closes the initial vertical incision horizontally, enlarging the esophageal introitus by doing so and avoiding dead space formation in the resected area (Fig. 58.15b).

Patients are usually observed for 48–72 h and given intravenous antibiotics for 24 h. A nasogastric tube is usually introduced after the myotomy and removed on the second or third day postoperatively. A clear liquid diet is started on the first day postoperatively if no free air is seen subcutaneously on the chest and lateral neck X-rays. A pureed diet is recommended for the first week. For some patients, the surgery can be performed as an outpatient. For the majority of patients, a 1–3 day hospital stay for observation is necessary.

Results

The clinical and functional results of endoscopic cricopharyngeal myotomy are summarized in Table 58.9. Most of the reported cases are small uncontrolled retrospective patient series with a short follow-up. The type of oropharyngeal dysphagia was heterogeneous and unclassified. A few patient series included Zenker's patients [26]. Pre- and postoperative assessment was by clinical examination and videoradiology.

Chang [30] demonstrated anatomically that the operation does divide the cricopharyngeus muscle while preserving the underlying buccopharyngeal fascia and leaving the retropharyngeal space intact. Most authors report significant improvement of the dysphagia. Lawson [21, 31], however, emphasizes that the benefits of the procedure may decrease over time, especially if the disease is progressive. Dauer [23] and Ozgursoy [24] both studied 14 patients before and after endoscopic cricopharyngeal myotomy. They assessed their patients with manofluorography and used the FOSS, an association of symptoms and functional findings. Five of the seven patients of Dauer were asymptomatic after division of their cricopharyngeal bar. In three patients where the results are less satisfactory, tongue base and hypopharyngeal weakness with decreased laryngeal elevation were observed, suggesting that the open approach might be more appropriate in patients with more complex swallowing problems. In another group, Ozgursoy also suggested the use of manofluorography to document strength abnormalities, outlet obstruction, and the effects of treatment on resistance across the pharyngoesophageal junction: Dauer [23] reported that when normal force was present in the pharynx cricopharyngeal myotomy results were satisfactory. Weak driving forces resulted in poorer results. In the subsequent report by Ozgursoy [24], cricopharyngeal myotomy provided a significant increase in the mean cross-sectional area of the upper esophageal sphincter. Intrabolus pressures across the pharyngoesophageal sphincter also decreased significantly from 25 to 13. Here again the weakest improvement was observed in neurologic patients with an abnormal function that remained decompensated.

Complications

As for any type of surgery, complications are reported after endoscopic cricopharyngeal myotomy. Bleeding, mediastinitis, supraglottic edema, esophageal perforations, and reclosure of the myotomy are mentioned in the available references. Subcutaneous emphysema and unexplained fever in the postoperative evaluation is always worrisome.

Summary and Conclusions

Cricopharyngeal myotomy offers excellent palliation to the patient with oropharyngeal dysphagia. When using the open approach or the endoscopic techniques current reports are based on clinical uncontrolled case series; most using poor investigation technology. Better planned clinical studies in well-identified and classified disease groups are essential as a first step. Objective quantification of the problems present, with their functional effects recorded by appropriate investigation methods, then becomes essential. Oropharyngeal dysphagia patients independently of their disease category can then be compared adequately for their treatment. The treatment can be surgical with open or endoscopic myotomy or nonsurgical with medication, dilatation or swallowing therapy techniques. Meaningful comparisons can then be made through adequately controlled trials and provide the basis for therapeutic recommendation for oropharyngeal dysphagia patients.

Table 58.9 Endoscopic cricopharyngeal myotomy

Authors	Patients	Pre-op	Post-op	Morbidity	Results	Follow-up
Herberhold [17]	32	History radiology	Clinical	1 Supraglottic edema 1 Mediastinitis 4 Repeat procedure	Improvement evident in all but 1	Up to 7 years
Lim [20]	44	History Endoscopy Videofluoroscopy	Clinical Videofluoroscopy	2 Esophageal perforations 4 Reclosed myotomy	100 % Improvement in stage I–III Stage IV: 0 % Stage V: 8/11 improved	2–22 months
Halvorsen [22]	18	History Videoradiology Modified BA swallow	Clinical	Nil	14/18 Complete response 4/18 Appreciable improvement	–
Brondbo [27]	17	Clinical Videoradiology	Clinical	Nil	13/17 Improved 3 Unrelated deaths 1 Not improved	–
Lawson [21]	29	Clinical Videoradiology	Clinical Videoradiology	Nil		21 months
Takes [28]	10	Clinical Videofluoroscopy	Clinical Videofluoroscopy	Hospit. 3–9 days Soft tissue air 4 pts Subout emphysema 1	Improved 9/10 Re-operation 1/10	3 months
Dauer [23]	14	Clinical Manofluorography	Clinical Manofluoroscopy	3 Complications 2 Fever unknown origin 1 Chest pain	7 Asymptomatic or minimally symptomatic with no functional impairment	–
Ozgursoy [24]	14	Clinical Manofluorography	Clinical Manofluorography	–		
Mortensen (2009)	8	–	–	1 Aborted operation (bleeding)	7/8 Improved dysphagia	–
Chitose et al. [29] 2011	1	Videoradiology	Same	–	Symptom free for 10 months	
Ho [25]	7	MDADI FOSS	Same	–	Improved	22 months

References

1. American Gastroenterological Association medical position statement on management of oropharyngeal dysphagia. Gastroenterology 1999;Feb;116(2):452–4.
2. Sivarao DV, Goyal RK. Functional anatomy and physiology of the upper esophgeal sphincter. Am J Med. 2000;108:275–375.
3. Asoh R, Goyal RK. Manometry and electomyography of the upper esophageal sphincter in the opposum. Gastroenterology. 1978;74:514.
4. Goyal RK, Martin SB, Shapiro J, Spechler SJ. The role of cricopharyngeus muscle in pharyngoesophageal disorders. Dysphagia. 1993;8:252–8.
5. Cook IJ, Kahrilas PJ. AGA technical review on management of oropharyngeal dysphagia. Gastroenterology. 1999;116:455–78.
6. Duranceau A. Treatment of Zenker's diverticulum. Tech Gen Surg. 1994;3(3):1–7.
7. Duranceau A. Oropharyngeal dysphagia. In: Jamieson GG, editor. Surgery of the esophagus. Edinburgh: Churchill Livingstone; 1988. p. 413–34. Chapter 45.
8. Poirier NC, Bonavina L, Taillefer R, Nosadini A, Peracchia A, Duranceau A. Cricopharyngeal myotomy for neurogenic oropharyngeal dysphagia. J Thorac Cardiovasc Surg. 1997;113:233–41.
9. Castell JA, Castell DO, Duranceau A, Topart P. Manometric characteristics of the pharynx, upper esophageal sphincter, esophagus and lower esophageal sphincter in patients with oculopharyngeal muscular dystrophy. Dysphagia. 1995;10:22–6.
10. Duranceau A, Jamieson GG, Hurwitz AL, Jones RS, Postlethwait RW. Alteration in esophageal motility after laryngectomy. Am J Surg. 1976;131:30.
11. Taillefer R, Duranceau A. Manometric and radionuclide assessment of pharyngeal emptying before and after cricopharyngeal myotomy in patients with oculopharyngeal muscular dystrophy. J Thorac Cardiovasc Surg. 1988;95:868–75.
12. Duranceau A (2002) Pharyngeal and cricopharyngeal disorders. In: Pearson's esophageal surgery. Churchill Livingstone, New York, NY, pp 477–506 (Chapter 30).
13. Pera M, Yamada A, Hiebert CA, Duranceau A. Sleeve recording of upper eso-phageal sphincter resting pressures during cricopharyngeal myotomy. Ann Surg. 1997;225:229–34.
14. Rocco G, Deschamps C, Martel E, Duranceau A, et al. Results of reoperation on the upper esophageal sphincter. J Thorac Cardiovasc Surg. 1999;117(1):28–30. discussion 30–31.
15. Orringer MB. Extended cervical esophagomyotomy for cricopharyngeal dysfunction. J Thorac Cardiovasc Surg. 1986;80:669.
16. Brigand C, Ferraro P, Martin J, Duranceau A. Risk factors in patients undergoing cricopharyngeal myotomy. Br J Surg. 2007;94:978–83.
17. Herberhold C, Walther EK. Endoscopic laser myotomy in cricopharyngeal achalasia. Adv Otorhinolaryngol. 1995;49:144–7.
18. Pitman M, Weissbrod P. Endoscopic CO^2 laser cricopharyngeal myotomy. Laryngoscope. 2009;119: 45–53.
19. Allen J, White CJ, Leonard R, Belafsky PC. Effect of cricopharyngeus muscle surgery on the pharynx. Laryngoscope. 2010;120:1498–503.
20. Lim RY. Endoscopic CO2 laser cricopharyngeal myotomy. J Clin Laser Med Surg. 1995;13:241–7.
21. Lawson G, Remacle M, Jamart J, Keghian J. Endoscopic CO^2 laser-assisted surgery for cricopharyngeal dysfunction. Eur Arch Otorhinolaryngol. 2003;260:475–80.
22. Halvorsen DJ. The treatment of cricopharyngeal dysmotility with a transmucosal myotomy using the potassium-titanyl-phosphate (KTP) Laser. Endoscopy. 1998;30:46–50.
23. Dauer E, Salassa J, Luga L, Kasper Bauer J. Endoscopic laser vs open approach for cricopharyngeal myotomy otolaryngology. Head Neck Surg. 2006;134:830–5.
24. Ozgursoy OB, Salassa JR. Manofluorographic and functional outcomes after endoscopic laser cricopharyngeal myotomy for cricopharyngeal bar. Otolaryngol Head Neck Surg. 2010;142:735–40.
25. Ho AS, Morzara S, Damrose EJ. CO^2-laser-assisted endoscopic cricopharyngeal myotomy with primary muscle closure. Ann Otol Rhinol Laryngol. 2011;120:33–9.
26. Mortensen M, Schaberg MR, Genden EM, Peak W. Trans-oral resection of short segment Zenker's diverticulum and cricopharyngeal myotomy: an alternative minimally invasive approach. Laryngoscope. 2010;120:17–22.
27. Brondbo K. Treatment of cricopharyngeal dysfunction by endoscopic laser myotomy. Acta Otolaryngol. 2000;543:222–4.
28. Takes RP, Van Den Hoogen FJA, Marres HAM. Endoscopic myotomy of the cricopharyngeal muscle with CO^2 laser surgery. Head Neck. 2005;27:703–9.
29. Chitose SI, Sato K, Hamakawa S, Umeno H, Nakashima T. A new paradigm of endoscopic cricopharyngeal myotomy with CO^2 laser. Laryngoscope. 2011;121:567–70.
30. Chang CWD, Liou SS, Netterville JL. Anatomic study of laser-assisted endoscopic cricopharyngeus myotomy. Ann Otol Rhinol Laryngol. 2005;114:897–901.
31. Lawson G, Remacle M. Endoscopic cricopharyngeal myotomy: indications and technique. Curr Opin Otolaryngol Head Neck Surg. 2006;14:437–41.

Surgical Treatment of Zenker's Diverticulum

59

Michele P. Morrison and Gregory N. Postma

Abstract

The purpose of this chapter is to review the most common surgical treatment options for Zenker's diverticulum (ZD).

Keywords

Zenker's diverticulum • Cricopharyngeus • Diverticulostomy • Cricopharyngeal myotomy • Dysphagia

Introduction

An esophageal diverticulum is a pouch created by herniation of the mucosa (false diverticulum) or all esophageal layers (true diverticulum) through the muscular esophageal wall. A diverticulum may be further classified based by its location (cervical, midesophageal, epiphrenic) or pathophysiology (pulsion vs. traction). A pulsion diverticulum is formed from increased intraluminal pressure, while traction diverticula are formed from external tethering. ZD is the most common type of pulsion diverticulum. Zenker and von Zeimsen in 1878 were the first to hypothesize that a cricopharyngeal diverticulum was due to increased hypopharyngeal pressure generated during deglutition [1].

Anatomy

Killian's dehiscence is a triangular weak spot located on the dorsal wall of the hypopharynx named after Gustav Killian who identified the area in 1908 [2, 3]. The area of weakness is formed between the inferior pharyngeal constrictor muscle and the cricopharyngeus muscle (Fig. 59.1). A recent study looking at morphometric and anthropometric measurements in cadavers demonstrated the incidence of Killian's dehiscence to be two times greater in men versus women; this is reflected in the greater incidence of ZD in men. An increased incidence of Killian's triangle was noted in people with taller body dimensions, and a longer larynx; more specifically, a greater distance between the thyroid and cricoid cartilages. This may explain the geographical differences in prevalence; ZD is more often seen in regions with taller people (i.e., Northern Europe,

M.P. Morrison, DO
Department of Otolaryngology, Naval Medical Center Portsmouth, Portsmouth, VA, USA

G.N. Postma, MD (✉)
Center for Voice, Airway and Swallowing Disorders
Department of Otolaryngology, Georgia Health Sciences University, 1120 15th St, Augusta, GA, USA
e-mail: gpostma@georgiahealth.edu

R. Shaker et al. (eds.), *Principles of Deglutition: A Multidisciplinary Text for Swallowing and its Disorders*, 847
DOI 10.1007/978-1-4614-3794-9_59, © Springer Science+Business Media New York 2013

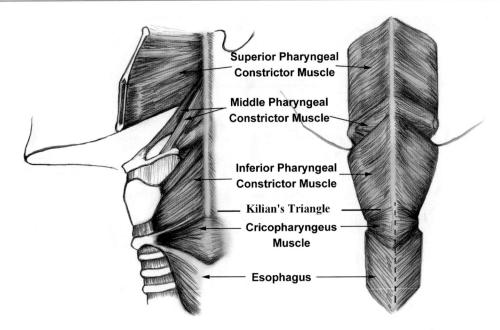

Fig. 59.1 Anatomical depiction of cricopharyngeus muscle and Killian's triangle

the United States, Canada, and Australia versus Japan and Indonesia) [2].

Pathophysiology

Patients with ZD have been found to have elevated intrabolus pressures due to restricted upper esophageal sphincter (UES) opening or compliance during bolus flow. This can occur from cricopharyngeal spasm, cricopharyngeal incoordination, fibrosis of muscle fibers, or a congenital weakness [4]. These patients show cricopharyngeus muscle fiber degeneration and fibroadipose tissue replacement. Studies suggest that the underlying etiology in Zenker's formation is poor cricopharyngeal muscle compliance; therefore, successful treatment *must* include a cricopharyngeal myotomy [5].

Clinical Features and Diagnosis

ZD is most prevalent between the seventh and eighth decades of life with an incidence between 0.01% and 0.11%, but can occur at nearly any age. Symptoms include dysphagia, regurgitation of undigested foods, halitosis, chronic cough, and hoarseness. With an increase in pouch size symptoms worsen to include weight loss, malnutrition, and aspiration pneumonia. A sudden worsening of symptoms (pain, hemoptysis) may indicate the presence of squamous cell carcinoma within the diverticulum (0.4–1.5% incidence) [4].

Findings on physical exam may include malnutrition, voice changes, neck mass, cervical borborygmi, or crepitus. Diagnosis is based mostly on history and confirmed by barium swallow (BaS) which will show a filling defect that does not move between films (Fig. 59.2). The diverticulum tends to be left sided due to the more lateral location of the left carotid artery and the curvature of the esophagus to the left. Barium swallow may miss a small diverticulum, although it is easier to discern on a lateral view, and a modified barium swallow (MBS) may be helpful. Flexible endoscopic evaluation of swallowing (FEES) may show pooling of secretions (more commonly unilateral) and regurgitation of food [4] (Fig. 59.3).

There are several classification schemes for ZD based on contrast radiographic findings (Table 59.1); however, clinical correlation is not strong and they are often not used.

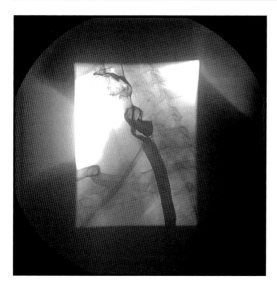

Fig. 59.2 Barium swallow demonstrating Zenker's diverticulum

Surgical Treatment of Zenker's Diverticulum

The current surgical options used to treat ZD include the use of an endoscopic stapler to perform a diverticulostomy (Endoscopic Staple-assisted Diverticulostomy, ESD), endoscopic diverticulostomy with laser, open diverticulopexy or diverticulectomy with cricopharyngeal myotomy, and finally the use of flexible esophagoscopy-assisted diverticulostomy.

Endoscopic Zenker's Diverticulostomy

The endoscopic approach for ZD involves division of the septum (containing the cricopharyngeus muscle) between the diverticulum and the

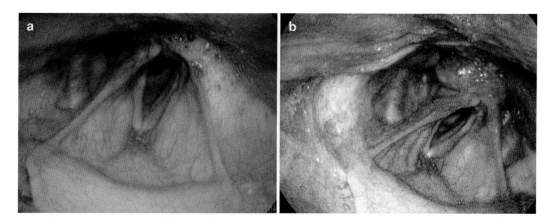

Fig. 59.3 (**a**) FEES showing frank pooling of secretions in patient with a Zenker's diverticulum. (**b**) FEES in same patient after swallowing applesauce with blue food coloring. Notice regurgitation

Table 59.1 Classification schemes for ZD

	Brombert classification	Morton and Bartley classification
Stage I	Longitudinal axis 2–3 mm, visible during UES contraction "Thorn-like diverticulum"	<2 cm
Stage II	Longitudinal axis 7–8 mm, visible during UES contraction "Club-like diverticulum"	2–4 cm
Stage III	Caudally oriented axis of >1 cm in length "Bag shaped diverticulum"	>4 cm
Stage IV	Compression of esophagus (displaced ventrally)	

UES upper esophageal sphincter [6]

cervical esophagus creating a common cavity between the diverticulum and esophagus; and obviously performing a cricopharyngeal myotomy [7]. The diverticular sac is not excised and is essentially marsupialized.

Endoscopic esophagodiverticulostomy to treat ZD was first attempted by Mosher using a knife to incise the common wall in 1917 [8, 9]. He subsequently stopped performing this procedure due to severe complications including bleeding and death from mediastinitis [8–11]. The procedure was reintroduced by Sieffert in 1937, but did not become well accepted until Dohlman and Mattson presented their case series of 100 patients undergoing endoscopic treatment of ZD using electrocautery without deaths or serious complications in 1960 [8, 12, 13]. The endoscopic procedure was modified by Collard in 1993 to include use of the endosurgical stapler to divide and seal the wall between the esophagus and the diverticulum, opening the pouch and dividing the cricopharyngeus muscle [14].

Benefits of the endoscopic approach include absence of skin incision, decreased complication rate, shorter operative time, minimal postoperative pain, quicker resumption of oral feeding, and shorter hospital stay resulting in a significant cost savings (Tables 59.2 and 59.3). This approach is particularly beneficial in patients who have undergone a previous open diverticulectomy, cricopharyngeal myotomy, or any previous neck surgery [7].

Contraindications to the endoscopic approach include severe medical comorbidities precluding general anesthesia or inability to endoscopically expose the diverticulum [15].

ESD is performed under general anesthesia with endotracheal intubation. A bivalved laryngoscope is placed with one valve in the diverticulum and one in the esophageal lumen. The septum between the diverticulum and esophagus is thus exposed and the diverticuloscope is secured using a suspension arm (Fig. 59.4). A 0° or 30° telescope is used for visualization. In patients with difficult exposure, an assistant may provide visualization with a small flexible endoscope. A stapler is placed with the anvil in the lumen of the diverticulum and the staple cartridge in the cervical esophageal lumen dividing the septum in the midline [7]. Repeat stapler applications may be needed depending on the size of the diverticulum. After completion the wound edges retract laterally [7] (Fig. 59.5). Scher et al. [8] describe a case series of 159 patients undergoing the endoscopic stapler technique on an outpatient basis and started on a clear liquid diet the day of treatment with a 98% successful relief of symptoms. The most common complication was chipped teeth (7.3%) followed by postoperative fever (4%); the overall complication rate was 12.7% with 2% considered major complications (perforation, aspiration pneumonia, and transient vocal fold paralysis). This approach reduces the risk of perforation because the mucosal edges are divided and closed with staples simultaneously; therefore, the mediastinum is not contaminated. If the surgeon is unable to expose the diverticular wall enough to insert the endo stapler, then a laser-assisted endoscopic diverticulostomy may be performed. The inability to endoscopically expose the pouch is approximately 3%.

Peracchia et al. [7] performed manometry before and after ESD as part of their study protocol finding a statistically significant decrease in mean hypopharyngeal intrabolus pressure after surgery, with normalization of UES compliance and decreased resistance to bolus flow. Manometry is not usually performed preoperatively in cases with a straightforward diagnosis of ZD based on symptoms and BaS [8].

Laser-assisted endoscopic diverticulostomy is performed with the patient under general anesthesia. The diverticulum is exposed endoscopically with a diverticuloscope and a myotomy is performed in the midline using a CO_2 laser. Of note, if exposure is difficult a thinner nonbivalved diverticuloscope can be used for exposure. The CO_2 laser has a higher complication rate compared to the endoscopic stapler technique; however, it allows for a good view of the diverticular wall throughout the procedure with similar success rate [8, 16, 17]. The most important technical consideration during performance of the laser-assisted diverticulostomy is that the entire cricopharyngeus muscle must be divided (Fig. 59.6).

Another endoscopic method involving transoral resection of diverticula has been described

Table 59.2 Comparison of endoscopic versus open approach for treatment of ZD

Method	Year	No.	Hospital stay in days: mean (range)	Days to oral diet: mean (range)	Complication rate: mean (range)[a]	Operative time (min): mean (range)	Mortality: mean (range)	Recurrence rate: mean (range)[b]
External	1990–2001	1,696	7.6 (2–10)	4.5 (0.8–8.1)	11.8% (0–38%)	83.2 (81–90)	1.6% (0–3.5%)	5.0% (0–19%)
Endoscopic[c]	1991–2002	1,678	2.7 (0.6–8.0)	1.3 (0.1–4.9)	5.5% (0–20%)	28.6 (14.3–60)	0.2% (0–1)[e]	6.6% (0–22%)
Cautery	1991–1999	160	4.3 (3.5–4.5)	2.6 (2–2.8)	8.1% (0–14.9%)	33.8 (20–60)	0%	3.4% (0–7.1%)
CO_2 laser	1993–2002	823	6.5 (5.2–8.0)	2.2 (1–4.9)	7.4% (1.4–20%)	NR	0.2% (0–1)[e]	11.5% (6.7–15.4%)
ESD[d]	1993–2002	695	1.8 (0.6–4.7)	1.0 (0.1–3)	2.6% (0–17%)	27.2 (14.3–34)	0.3% (0–1)[e]	6.0% (0–22%)

Reproduced with permission from John Wiley and Sons

Note: The total no. to calculate means used only those studies in which mean values were given

[a]Defined as mediastinitis, wound infection, fistula, significant bleeding requiring additional hospital stays, pneumomediastinum, vocal cord paralysis, perforation, aspiration pneumonia

[b]Caution on interpreting mean values is stressed as recurrence rates are useful only in the setting of follow-up time. Since follow-up times were not equal and inconsistently given, average numbers are particularly limited in value

[c]All endoscopic cases (cautery, CO_2 laser, and ESD) combined

[d]Includes all ESD reported in this table as well as the current study

[e]Range in absolute numbers

Table 59.3 Endoscopic approach for treatment of ZD from 1990 to 2002

Author	Year of publication	Method	Years of inclusion	No.	Unable to perform[a]	Symptom resolution[b]	Hospital stay in days (mean)	Days to oral diet (mean)	Significant complications[c]	Mean operative time (min)	Mortality[d]	Mean follow-up (mo)	Recurrence rate
Wayman	1991	Cautery	1978–1989	11	0	"all"[e]	3.5	2	0	60	0	24	NR
Ishioka	1995	Cautery[f]	1982–1992	42	0	92.9%/7.1%	NR	(3)[g]	4.8%	20	0	38.2	7.1%
Mulder	1995	Cautery[f]	1993–1995	20	0	"all"	NR	NR	0	NR	0	6.7	0
von Doersten	1997	Cautery	1985–1994	40	0	92.5%	4.5	2.8	10.0%	41	0	42	0
Hashiba	1999	Cautery[f]	"since 1978"	47	0	96%	NR	(1)	14.9%	NR	0	(Up to 12)	4%
Benjamin	1993	CO_2 laser	1987–1992	34	5.9%	97%	5.2	("within 1")	5.9%	(20–25)	0	NR	NR
van Overbeek	1994	CO_2/cautery	1964–1992	545	NR	90.6%/8.6%	NR	NR	6.7%	NR	1	(At least 10)	NR
Westrin	1996	CO_2 laser	"since 1987"	15	NR	"all"	(4-S)	(3)	NR	(40)	NR	NR	6.7%
Bradwell	1997	CO_2 laser	1985–1993	15	6.6%	73.3%	'less than 5'	("within 1")	20.0%	NR	0	(4–11)	13.3%
Lippert	1999	CO_2 laser	1984–1996	70	0	94.3%/4.3%	NR	1	1.4%	NR	0	(Minimum 12)	NR
Zbaren	1999	CO_2 laser	1987–1995	31	0	87%/9.7%	8.0	4.9	6.4%	NR	0	13	3.2%
Nyrop	2000	CO_2 laser	1989–1999	61	0	70%/22%	(Median 3)	(Median 2)	13.1%	NR	0	(Median 37)	13%
Mattinger	2002	CO_2/scissor	1974–1998	52	0	84.6%	NR	NR	13.5%	NR	1	NR	15.4%
Collard	1993	ESD	NR	6	0	83%/17%	NR	2	NR	NR	0	(Up to 16)	NR
Koay	1996	ESD	1994–1995	14	0	86%/14%	2.2	0.7	0	14.3	0	5.7	NR
Baldwin	1998	ESD	1993–1996	51	2.0%	NR	(2–4)	(1–7)	2.0%	NR	0	15.3	0
Burstin	1998	ESD	NR	3	0	100%	3	1	0	NR	0	(18)	0
Peracchia	1998	ESD	1992–1996	95	3.1%	92.2%/7.8%	(Median 3)	1	0	23	0	(Median 23)	5.4%
Name	1999	ESD	1992–1996	102	3.9%	"all"	(Median 4)	2	2.0%	(Median 20)	0	(Median 16)	0
Omote	1999	ESD	1996–1997	21	0	"all"	4.7	(1–2)	4.8%	22	1	12	0
van Eeden	1999	ESD	1990–1997	18	0	53%/35%	2.26	3	5.9%	NR	0	10.2	NR
Luscher	2000	ESD	1997–1998	23	0	87%/9%	(0)	(1)	4.3%	NR	0	12	4.3%
Philippsen	2000	ESD	1996–1999	14	14.3%	57%/21%	1.3	1	0	31	0	NR	NR
Sood	2000	ESD	"since 1992"	44	6.4%	94.6%	1.9	(0–7)	4.5%	NR	1	19	9%
Adams	2001	ESD	1997–1998	21	14.3%	NR	0.6	0.1	17.0%	NR	0	NR	NR

Jaramillo	2001	ESD	1996–1999	32	15.6%	80%	3.2	0.7	3.7%	20	0	(9–48)	7.4%
Stoeckli	2001	ESD	1997–2000	30	10.0%	96%	(2)	("after 24 h")	0	(5–15)	0	13.2	NR
Thaler	2001	ESD	1998–2001	23	30.0%	"all"	NR	(1)	0	NR	0	(1–24)	13%
Counter	2002	ESD	1993–1997	31	NR	84.2%/0%	4.1	1.9	9.7%	NR	0	61.2	22%
Smith	2002	ESD	NR	8	0	"all"	1.3	0.8	0	25.5	0	NR	NR
Current Study	2002	ESD	1995–2002	159	5.7%	73.6%/24.3%	0.76	0.25	2.0%	34.4	0	32.2	11.8%

Reproduced with permission from John Wiley and Sons

ZD Zenker's diverticulum, *No.* number of procedures, *NR* not reported, CO_2 carbon dioxide laser, *ESD* endoscopic staple diverticulostomy

aUnable to perform technique due to anatomical inaccessibility or difficulty in visualization of the common wall dividing the pouch from the esophagus

bIf one percentage is given, the paper gave only one percentage for symptom relief. If two percentages are given, the first percentage describes either "complete resolution" or "highly satisfied" outcome. The second percentage describes either "improved symptoms" or "satisfied" outcome

cSignificant complications include mediastinitis, wound infection, fistula, significant bleeding requiring additional hospital stays, pneumomediastinum, vocal cord paralysis, perforation, aspiration pneumonia, death

dDeaths is absolute numbers

eNo percentage nor distinction in patient outcome was given other than stating "all"

fNote: These studies were performed by gastroenterologists using a flexible endoscope

gValues within parentheses reflect information contained within the article, but not in averages. Either absolute, median, range, minimum, or maximum values were given instead. These values are not considered further in analyses

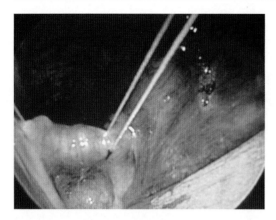

Fig. 59.4 Intraoperative endoscopic view of Zenker's diverticulum exposed using the Weerda bivalved rigid endoscope

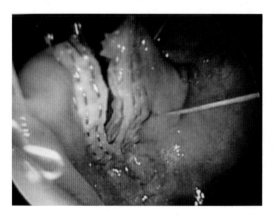

Fig. 59.5 Intraoperative view after endoscopic staple diverticulostomy of Zenker's diverticulum

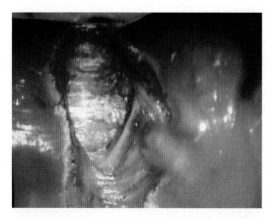

Fig. 59.6 Intraoperative view of CO_2 laser cricopharyngeal myotomy

by Woo et al. to address the small diverticulum. This procedure involves exposure of the diverticulum endoscopically as previously described; betadine is used to sterilize the area and the mucosa is injected under microscopic guidance with 1% lidocaine with 1:100,000 epinephrine. The pouch is everted with a cup forceps and the sack is removed with sharp endo-scissors. The cricopharyngeal muscle is exposed and divided with a laryngeal insulated cannula coagulation device. The mucosa is then sutured closed and covered with fibrin glue. The patient is kept NPO overnight and receives three doses of antibiotics. Patients may be started on a puree diet the next day and discharged if doing well. Of the six patients treated with this technique; all resumed an oral diet the morning after surgery with the average hospital stay of 1 day. Five of the six patients had resolution of their presurgical dysphagia [18].

Open Zenker's Diverticulectomy

Open diverticulectomy with cricopharyngeal myotomy is the classic operation performed for resection of a ZD and was first described by Wheeler [8]. Rigid esophagoscopy is traditionally performed at the start of the procedure allowing placement of a catheter into the esophagus or packing into the diverticulum. The esophagoscope is withdrawn and an endotracheal tube may be passed over the catheter to serve as a bougie [19]. A skin incision is made on the involved side at the level of the cricoid cartilage and subplatysmal flaps are raised. The sternocleidomastoid and carotid sheath are retracted laterally, while the larynx and thyroid gland are retracted medially exposing the pharynx and cervical esophagus. The omohyoid muscle, middle thyroid vein, and inferior thyroid artery are divided. The diverticulum is identified and retracted, dissecting off any loose connective tissue to identify its neck on the posterior pharyngeal wall. A cricopharyngeal myotomy is performed and the incision is extended through the inferior pharyngeal constrictor muscle. The diverticulum is transected using a knife and repaired with a multilayered closure or a surgical stapler may be employed depending on surgeon preference [20, 21].

An advantage of this procedure includes its use on all sizes of diverticula and eliminates any theoretical risk of carcinoma in the pouch. However, open diverticulectomy does have a higher complication rate including wound infection, hematoma, fistula formation, surgical emphysema, mediastinitis, and vocal fold paralysis [22] (Table 59.4). The complication rate is 11.8% for open diverticulectomy versus 5.5% for endoscopic surgery; the mortality rate is also higher at 1.6% versus 0.2%, respectively. Operating time is longer (83 vs. 30 min endoscopically), as well as an increased hospital stay. Resumption of oral diet is also delayed in the open versus endoscopic approach. However, the recurrence rate was slightly higher in the endoscopic group versus open (6.6% vs. 5.0%, respectively) [8] (Table 59.2).

A cost analysis was performed by Smith comparing open diverticulectomy versus endoscopic stapling technique. They found no statistical difference in actual procedure costs; although the endoscopic approach was shorter, the equipment is more expensive, thus balancing the expenses. The real cost differential came in postoperative hospital stay, which was reduced by a mean of 3.9 days in the endoscopic group saving a mean of $7,850 [23]. Of vital note, both the endoscopic and open procedures have similar success rates [8]. The National Institute for Clinical Excellence (NICE) from Great Britain issued procedure guidance in 2003 stating that ESD allows a more rapid recovery, requires a shorter hospital stay, and reduces operating time compared to open surgery. They also state that although ESD has a slightly higher recurrence rate compared to the open procedure it can be repeated, and they recommend that ESD should be performed by "super-specialists" in the procedure [24].

Open Zenker's Diverticulopexy

Diverticulopexy involves an open approach with a cricopharyngeal myotomy and instead of removing the diverticulum it is suspended superiorly to the prevertebral fascia. This eliminates the capability of saliva or food particles to accumulate in the sac and decreases the fistula rate. This is a good alternative if the sac is very large (>10 cm) or there are concerns for healing and fistula formation in a malnourished patient [21].

Flexible Esophagoscopy-Assisted Diverticulostomy

The most recent treatment method first published in 1995 by groups from the Netherlands and Brazil involves flexible endoscopy using a needle knife or argon plasma coagulator to divide the muscular septum [10, 25, 26]. This procedure may be beneficial to the elderly because it is performed under sedation versus general anesthesia, involves no neck extension, and can also be performed as an outpatient. It also has the possible added benefit of decreased cost [4].

The procedure involves performing a cricopharyngeal myotomy through the working channel of a gastroscope. Coagulation is the most commonly used method to divide the septum. An incision of 1.5–2.0 cm is adequate to treat a small diverticula (2 cm); however, for larger diverticula (>3 cm) a longer incision may be necessary and may require additional procedures. Manometric studies have shown a decrease in upper esophageal pressure after flexible endoscopic cricopharyngeal myotomy [4].

Complications of flexible endoscopic therapy include a 0–10% risk of bleeding, which can be controlled with electrocoagulation, injection of dilute epinephrine, or use of endoclips. Perforation is the dreaded complication which can lead to subcutaneous emphysema, mediastinal emphysema (uncomplicated in 0–23% with resolution of air in 2–5 days), cervical abscess, and mediastinitis. A post-procedure chest X-ray is routinely obtained to rule out mediastinal air [4].

Flexible endoscopic therapy for ZD results in symptomatic improvement and acceptable complication rates, but with significant recurrence rates (20%) leading to a high rate of repeated procedures [4, 10].

Table 59.4 Open approach for treatment of ZD since 1990

Author	Year of publication	Method	Years of inclusion	No.	Symptom resolution[a]	Hospital stay in days (mean)	Days to oral diet (mean)	Significant complications[b]	Mean operative time (min)	Mortality	Mean follow-up (mo)	Recurrence rate
Aggerholm	1990	D	1960–1984	115	91.3%/3.5%	NR	(about 7)[c]	21.0%	NR	0.9%	NR	16%
Barthlen	1990	DM, M	1982–1988	43	82%/18%	NR	NR	9.3%	NR	0	25	0
Lindgren	1990	M, DM, PM, VM	1976–1985	37	NR	NR	(1–7)	NR	NR	NR	NR	5.4%
Payne	1992	D, DM, M	1944–1978	888	93%	NR	NR	7.9%	NR	2%	NR	3.6%
Schmit	1992	M, EM	1977–1990	48	70%/17%	2.7	0.8	6.3%	NR	2.1%	64	19%
Louie	1993	DM+E	1987–1992	5	100%	10	NR	20%	NR	0	(6–48)	0
Morton	1993	DM, I	1982–1989	33	NR	(1–61)	NR	24.2%	(40–195)	3%	(40–60)	3.0%
Dorion	1994	DM	NR	11	NR	NR	(3)	0	("under 60")	0	NR	NR
Laccourreye	1994	DM, PM	1970–1991	43	100%	9.6	4.9	34.9%	81	2.3%	(6–24)	0
Laing	1995	DM	1979–1988	67	92.5%/7.5%	(Median 7)	(2–7)	16.4%	NR	NR	(24–144)	3.0%
Witterick	1995	DM	1987–1993	18	83%/17%	NR	(3–4)	5.6%	NR	0	30.3	0
Bonafede	1997	M, DM, PM	1976–1993	87	78%/13%	(1–76)	(1–47)	24%	NR	3.5%	(1–228)	NR
Nguyan	1997	D, DM, P, I, M	1975–1996	59	NR	7.4	4.1	15.3%	NR	0	2	6.8%
Cerdan	1998	M, DM, PM	1974–1995	32	100%	8.5	NR	6.3%	NR	0	(60)	0
Crescenzo	1998	DM, M, PM, D	1976–1996	75	88%/6%	(1–42)	NR	8.0%	NR	0	(Median 39.6)	6%
Walters	1998	DM	1989–1997	9	NR	NR	NR	"minimal"	NR	0	NR	NR
Feeley	1999	DM	1988–1998	24	NR	NR	NR	3.8%	NR	0	18	0
van Eeden	1999	D,DM,PM,VM,M	1990–1997	19	35%/35%	4	3.6	5.9%	NR	0	43	NR
Zbaren	1999	D,DM	1995–1997	66	77%/11%	11.4	8.1	15%	NR	1.5%	58.8	6.1%
Busaba	2001	DM	"past 2 years"	9	100%	2	1	0	90	0	5.6	0
Smith	2002	DM	NR	8	"all"	5.2	5.1	0	87.6	0	NR	NR

Reproduced with permission from John Wiley and Sons[7]

ZD Zenker's diverticulum, *No.* number of procedures, *D* diverticulectomy, *P* diverticulopexy, *I* imbrication, *M* cricopharyngeal myotomy, *V* diverticulum inversion, *E* cervical esophagostomy in a staged procedure, *NR* not reported

[a]If one percentage is given, the paper gave only one percentage for symptom relief. If two percentages are given, the first percentage describes either "complete resolution" or "highly satisfied" outcome. The second percentage describes either "improved symptoms" or "satisfied" outcome

[b]Significant complications include mediastinitis, wound infection, fistula, significant bleeding requiring additional hospital stays, pneumomediastinum, vocal cord paralysis, perforation, aspiration pneumonia

[c]Values within parentheses reflect information contained within the article, but not in averages. Either absolute numbers, median, range, minimum, or maximum values are given instead. These values are not considered further in analyses

Controversy

Controversy exists regarding treatment of small diverticular pouches with the endoscopic approach. There is a reported decrease in success rate with pouches less than 2 cm in size due to the common wall being too short to accommodate a full cartridge of staples; therefore, potentially leading to incomplete myotomy [20]. Of note, the smaller pouches are more likely to be asymptomatic. Kos and Miller note that diverticula less than 2 cm are difficult to expose and introduce the stapler [15, 27]. The use of the CO_2 laser in these individuals may be a better option. In our experience the use of stay sutures placed into the cricopharyngeus muscle has been very helpful in patients with small diverticular pouches. Using these traction sutures we have often been able to apply a full cartridge of staples into a small pouch, thereby performing a complete cricopharyngeal myotomy and opening the pouch without undue pressure placed at the base of the diverticulum. The assistant pulls the pouch and cricopharyngeus muscle up onto the stapler, thereby aiding the surgeon (Fig. 59.4). If this does not allow full placement of the staple cartridge, then the use of the CO_2 laser to divide the cricopharyngeus muscle in the midline would be performed. Richtsmeier discusses this issue as well as describing a modification of the staple device by shortening the anvil; however this creates a liability issue. He also describes cutting the left over ridge of tissue after using a securing suture at the apex of the pouch [28].

Conclusion

The current literature recommends ESD as the preferred approach to treat ZD over 2 cm in size. Reasons for this recommendation include decreased complication rate, shorter operative time, more rapid resumption of oral intake, excellent success rate, good long-term outcomes, and it can be performed on an outpatient basis leading to over $7,000 in cost savings [8, 23, 29–34].

References

1. Zenker FA, von Ziemmssen H. Dilatations of the esophagus. Cyclopaedia of the practice of medicine, vol. 3. London: Low, Marston, Searle and Rivington; 1878. p. 46–68.
2. Anagiotos A, Preuss SF, Koebke J. Morphometric and anthropometric analysis of Killian's triangle. Laryngoscope. 2010;120:1082–8.
3. Killian G. Ueber den mund der speiseroehre. Zeitschrift Fur Ohrenheilkunde Und Fur Die Krankheiten Der Luftwege. 1908;55:1–41.
4. Ferreira LEVVC, Simmons DT, Baron TH. Zenker's diverticula: pathophysiology, clinical presentation, and flexible endoscopic management. Dis Esopohagus. 2008;21:1–8.
5. Shaw DW, Cook IJ, Jamieson GG, Gabb M, Simula ME, Dent J. Influence of surgery on deglutitive upper oesophageal sphincter mechanics in Zenker's diverticulum. Gut. 1996;38:806–11.
6. Brombert M. Clinical radiology of the esophagus. Baltimore: Williams & Wilkins; 1961.
7. Peracchia A, Bonavina L, Narne S, Segalin A, Antoniazzi L, Marotta G. Minimally invasive surgery for Zenker diverticulum. Arch Surg. 1998;133:695–700.
8. Chang CY, Payyapilli RJ, Scher RL. Endoscopic staple diverticulostomy for Zenker's diverticulum: review of literature and experience in 159 consecutive cases. Laryngoscope. 2003;113:957–65.
9. Mosher HP. Webs and pouches of the esophagus: their diagnosis and treatment. Surg Gynecol Obstet. 1917;25:175–87.
10. Vogelsang A, Schumacher B, Neuhaus H. Therapy of Zenker's diverticulum. Dtsch Arztebl Int. 2008;105(7):120–6.
11. Hoffman M, Scheunemann D, Rudert HH, Maune S. Zenker's diverticulotomy with the carbon dioxide laser: perioperative management and long-term results. Ann Otol Rhinol Laryngol. 2003;112:202–5.
12. Sieffert A. Operation endoscopique d'un gros diverticule de pulsion. Bronchoscop Oesophageoscop Gastroscop. 1937;3:232–4.
13. Dohlman G, Mattson O. The endoscopic operation for hypopharyngeal diverticula. AMA Arch Otolaryngol. 1960;71:744–52.
14. Collard JM, Otte JB, Kestens PJ. Endoscopic stapling technique of esophagodiverticulostomy for Zenker's diverticulum. Ann Thorac Surg. 1993;56:573–6.
15. Peretti G, Piazza C, Del Bon F, Cocco D, De Benedetto L, Mangili S. Endoscopic treatment of Zenker's diverticulum by carbon dioxide laser. Acta Otorhinolaryngol Ital. 2010;30:1–4.
16. Kos MP, David EF, Mahieu HF. Endoscopic carbon dioxide laser Zenker's diverticulotomy revisited. Ann Otol Rhinol Laryngol. 2009;118(7):512–8.
17. Helmstaedter V, Engel A, Huttenbrink KB, Guntinas-Lichius O. Carbon dioxide laser endoscopic diverticulotomy for Zenker's diverticulum: results and

complications in a consecutive series of 40 patients. ORL J Otorhinolaryngol Relat Spec. 2009;71(1):40–4.
18. Mortensen M, Schaberg MR, Genden EM, Woo P. Transoral resection of short segment Zenker's diverticulum and cricopharyngeal myotomy: an alternative minimally invasive approach. Laryngoscope. 2009;120:17–22.
19. Jougon J, Dubois G, Delcambre F, Velly JF. Combination of surgical and endoscopic approach for Zenker's diverticulum. Interact Cardiovasc Thorac Surg. 2006;5:261–2.
20. Bonavina L, Bona D, Abraham M, Saino G, Abate E. Long-term results of endosurgical and open surgical approach for Zenker diverticulum. World J Gastroenterol. 2007;13(18):2586–9.
21. Feeley MA, Righi PD, Weisberger EC, et al. Zenker's diverticulum: analysis of surgical complications from diverticultomy and cricopharyngeal myotomy. Laryngoscope. 1999;109(6):858–61.
22. Siddiq MA, Sood S, Strachan D. Pharyngeal pouch (Zenker's diverticulum). Postgrad Med J. 2001;77: 506–11.
23. Smith SR, Genden EM, Urken ML. Endoscopic stapling technique for the treatment of Zenker diverticulum vs standard open-neck technique. Arch Otolaryngol Head Neck Surg. 2002;128:141–4.
24. National Institute for Clinical Excellence. ISBN: 1-84257-430-2. Nov 2003.
25. Mulder CJJ, den Hartog G, Robijn RJ, Thies JE. Flexible endoscopic treatment of Zenker's diverticulum: a new approach. Endoscopy. 1995;27:438–42.

26. Ishioka S, Sakai P, Maluf Filho F, Melo JM. Endoscopic incision of Zenker's diverticula. Endoscopy. 1995;27:433–7.
27. Miller FR, Bartley J, Otto RA. The endoscopic management of Zenker diverticulum: CO_2 laser versus endoscopic stapling. Laryngoscope. 2006;116: 1608–11.
28. Richtsmeier WJ. Myotomy length determinants in endoscopic staple-assisted esophagodiverticulostomy for small Zenker's diverticula. Ann Otol Rhinol Laryngol. 2005;114:341–6.
29. Aly A, Devitt PG, Jamieson GG. Evolution of surgical treatment for pharyngeal pouch. Br J Surg. 2004;91(6):657–64.
30. Brace M, Taylor SM, et al. Endoscopic stapling versus external transcervical approach for the treatment of Zenker diverticulum. J Otolaryngol Head Neck Surg. 2010;39(1):102–6.
31. Gross ND, Cohen JI, et al. Outpatient endoscopic Zenker diverticulotomy. Laryngoscope. 2004;114(2): 208–11.
32. Lang RA, Spelsberg FW, et al. Transoral diverticulostomy with a modified endo-Gia stapler: results after 4 years of experience. Surg Endosc. 2007;21(4):532–6.
33. Manni JJ, Kremer B, et al. The endoscopic stapler diverticulotomy for Zenker's diverticulum. Eur Arch Otorhinolaryngol. 2004;261(2):68–70.
34. Narne S, Cutrone C, et al. Endoscopic diverticulotomy for the treatment of Zenker's diverticulum: results in 102 patients with staple-assisted endoscopy. Ann Otol Rhinol Laryngol. 1999;108(8):810–5.

Dilation (UES, Esophagus, LES) Balloon Dilations, Bougies

60

Walter J. Hogan

Abstract

Benign esophageal strictures result from a variety of injuries causing local or diffuse narrowing of the lumen and compromising swallowing. Subsequently, nutritional health becomes impaired necessitating mechanical treatment (dilation) of the stricture.

Esophageal strictures are defined as simple or complex depending upon their structure and extent. The type and use of esophageal dilators often depends upon the nature of the stricture and the associated clinical situation. Some esophageal strictures respond predictably to dilations; others are more formidable or refractive to serial stretching.

This chapter details the appropriate use and technique of using the balloon or Bouginage dilating instruments. Stratification of the patient population ____clinical evaluation the risks and benefits of esophageal dilations and associated complications are detailed.

Potential new treatment with esophageal stenting is also discussed in light of recent early experience.

Appropriate endoscopic photographs are included to augment the teaching points.

Keywords

Dilation • Benign esophageal strictures • UES • Esophagus • LES • Balloon dilations • Bougie dilations

Introduction

A variety of injuries, acute or chronic, can cause irreversible damage to the wall of the esophagus, compromising normal elasticity and luminal diameter, resulting in the formation of a stricture. Depending upon the clinical situation, esophageal

W.J. Hogan, MD (✉)
Division of Gastroenterology and Hepatology,
Medical College of Wisconsin Froedtert Hospital,
9200 W. Wisconsin Ave, Milwaukee, WI 53226, USA
e-mail: whogan@mcw.edu

R. Shaker et al. (eds.), *Principles of Deglutition: A Multidisciplinary Text for Swallowing and its Disorders*, DOI 10.1007/978-1-4614-3794-9_60, © Springer Science+Business Media New York 2013

strictures may be localized, regional, or diffuse, impairing swallowing function. The purpose of primary treatment of these structural obstructions is to expand the esophageal diameter and improve or restore swallowing by esophageal dilation.

Esophageal dilation was first described in 1674 [1], although crude attempts may have occurred prior to this. The use of a whalebone with a sponge mounted on the tip was the dilator. The first bougienage dilator was described in the 1800s [2] and was the instrument used for esophageal dilation until the introduction of the balloon at the end of the twentieth century.

Pathogenesis of the Stricture/ Formation

The process of stricture formation in the gastrointestinal tract is a complex mechanism [3]. Injuries to tissue prompt activation of cell types to promote healing and repair damage so that tissue returns to full function. Improperly regulated healing causes fibrosis, whereby extracellular matrix and the fibroblasts replace parenchymal cells and impair organ function. Macrophages and fibroblasts are activated by CD_4 T cells which engage negative feedback loops that reduce fibrosis by restraining the immune process. Disruption of signals between macrophages and fibroblasts can promote or exacerbate the process of fibrosis.

Sources of Benign Esophageal Strictures

Acid reflux disease was the most common cause of benign esophageal strictures [4] prior to the introduction of proton pump inhibitor (PPI) therapy for this disorder [5, 6]. Subsequently, the frequency of peptic stricture formation has been markedly reduced. However, other sources of benign esophageal stricture formation arise from a variety of conditions which include Schatzki Ring formation, pill injury, surgical anastomosis, external beam radiation therapy, complications of photodynamic laser or radio-frequency ablation

treatments for Barrett's dysplasia, dermatology-associated diseases (e.g., pemphigoid and epidermal bullosum) (Fig. 60.1), nasogastric tube injury (Fig. 60.2), caustic ingestion (Fig. 60.3), and eosinophilic esophagitis (Fig. 60.4).

Stricture Classification

Esophageal strictures have been classified according to structure into two types: simple and complex [7]. Simple structures are symmetric or concentric in configuration, possess a luminal diameter ≥12 mm, and permit normal passage of the 9.5-mm adult endoscope. Complex strictures are often asymmetric, have a luminal caliber <12 mm, and restrict the passage of the adult endoscope.

The stricture may be compromised by other factors including distal esophageal tortuosity and angulation, concurrent active inflammation, or fragile mucosa (eosinophilic esophagus) which further influence safety and success of esophageal dilation.

Esophageal Dilators

Two basic types of instruments are currently available for dilation of the esophagus: the Bougie (or push type) and the balloon dilator.
1. Bougie (push type)
   - Maloney dilator (Medovations, Inc., Milwaukee, WI)
     This dilator is taper-tipped and has multiple progressive sizes to 60 Fr. This instrument is not passed over a guide wire and is used for simple strictures and self-dilation. A blunt-nosed form (Hurst) is seldom used today. The Maloney dilator was originally weighted with a mercury filling; it is now tungsten filled.
   - American dilator (C.R. Bard Interventional Products, Tewsbury, MA) and Savary–Gilliard dilator (Cook Medical, Bloomington, IL) (Fig. 60.5)
     This type of dilator is polyvinyl in construction with a hollowed center for passage over a guided wire. They are tapered

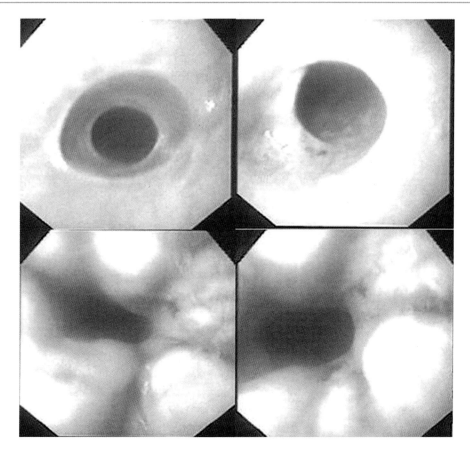

Fig. 60.1 Esophageal stricture associated with epidermolysis bullosa

at the end and have multiple progressive sizes to 60 Fr.

2. Hydrostatic balloon dilators (Fig. 60.6)
   - Through-the-scope (TTS) balloons (Boston Scientific, Natuck, MA; Cook Medical, Bloomington, IL)
     These balloons are passed directly through the endoscope and permit visualization during inflation. Each balloon expands to three progressive sizes, e.g., 10–12 mm and 16–20 mm.
   - Over-the-wire (OTW) balloon dilators (Boston Scientific, Natuck, MA)
     These dilators are passed over a wire and deliver three distinct pressure-controlled diameters (above) and are designed with rectilinear shoulders to enhance endoscopic visualization during inflation.

The Bougie dilators cause two mechanisms of force—radial and shearing effect. Balloon dilators provide only radial force. Bougie dilation is especially useful for dilating long or "refractive" strictures. They are the device of choice for dilating the small caliber esophagus encountered in patients with eosinophilic esophagitis. Balloon dilators are attached to the end of small diameter catheters and are deployed through the biopsy channel of the endoscope. These dilators are suitable for passage through "tight" localized strictures and permit visual placement of the balloon at the appropriate site (Fig. 60.7).

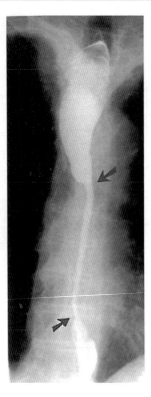

Fig. 60.2 Long esophageal stricture (demarcated by *arrows*), a complication of long-term nasogastric tube placement

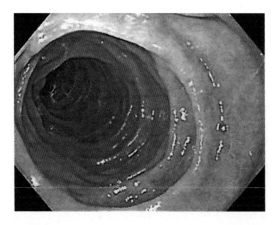

Fig. 60.3 Series of contiguous ring-like structures causing esophageal narrowing associated with lye ingestion

There is no scientific comparison study demonstrating consensus by experts on the clinical superiority of one type of dilator verses the other [9, 10]. The use of these devices depends upon the nature of the stricture, and the experience and personal preference of the physician.

Dilator Size: French Versus Millimeter

The nomenclature associated with the calibration (size) of the two types of dilators can often be confusing. Bougie dilators are numbered classically with the archaic "French gauge system" which measures the circumference of the dilator (π times diameter) [11]. Balloon dilators are measured by their diameters in millimeters. Conversion from one system to the other is often not stressed in our training programs. For example, three French (Fr) units equal 1 mm; a 20-mm dilator equals 60 French (Fr). On the other hand, a 15 Fr dilator is 5 mm in size.

Defining the Stricture

Esophageal dilation is the primary treatment for the patient with dysphagia caused by a stricture. Esophageal dilation in a patient with dysphagic complaints without evidence of a structural abnormality seldom solves the problem [12, 13]. However, a history of an impacted food bolus necessitating endoscopic removal in the emergency department is substantial evidence of a structural etiology. None the less, estimation of the type, location, and severity of the stricture requires objective definition. Several diagnostic studies are useful for this mission.

Barium Swallow (Esophagram)

A barium esophagram is the most accurate and safe diagnostic modality to assess the location, extent, and luminal diameter of the stricture. Furthermore, the esophagram defines the zone below the stricture, identifying malignancy or anatomic alterations which would preclude blind passage of a guidewire or balloon (Fig. 60.8).

The addition of a barium-soaked marshmallow swallow can provide clues to luminal narrowing and subtle ring formation. The barium esophagram has virtually no risks and is relatively inexpensive. Unfortunately, the contrast radiologic test is a "dying art" in many teaching and clinical institutions.

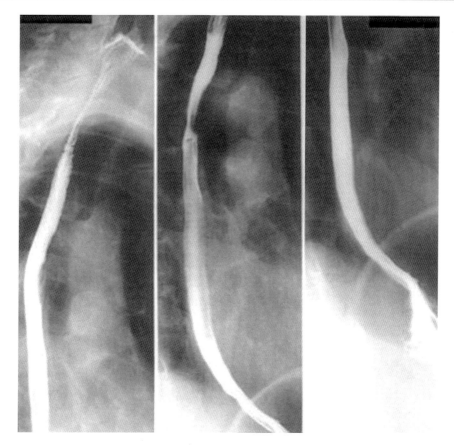

Fig. 60.4 "Small caliber" barium esophagram noting no change in basic configuration over a three photo sequence of 60 s. The lumen is small and "ring-like" forms are seen in the proximal esophagus on the *left*. These features are classic for eosinophilic esophagitis

Endoscopic Examination

Endoscopic inspection of the esophagus occurs prior to or at the time of dilation. The endoscopic view permits assessment of the diameter of the stricture opening, the presence of active inflammation, or Barrett's esophagus (Fig. 60.9). Inspection of the gastroesophageal junction from below (when a junctional stricture is present) aids in detecting a high fundic infiltrating malignancy (Fig. 60.10). Importantly, the endoscopic examination can provide tissue to help exclude a malignant stricture.

Inability to pass the standard 9.5-mm endoscope through the stricture helps define the simple versus complex stricture and provides

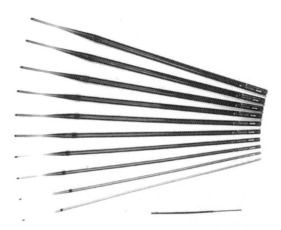

Fig. 60.5 A spread of American dilators ranging in size from 22 to 60 Fr. The wire guide (5 Fr) noted at the *bottom* of the picture for comparison

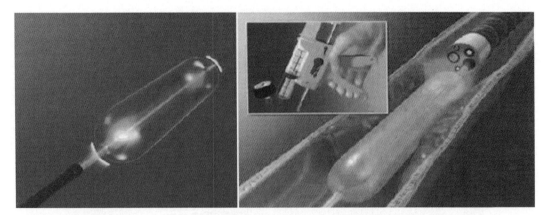

Fig. 60.6 A wire guided through the scope (TTS) balloon 18–20 mm diameter (*left*). Schema of endoscope and balloon in situ and pressure trigger (*right*) From http://www.bostonscientific.com/Device.bsci?page=HCP_Overview &navRelId=1000.1003&method=DevDetailHCP&id=10 004591&pageDisclaimer=Disclaimer.ProductPage &10602 with permission

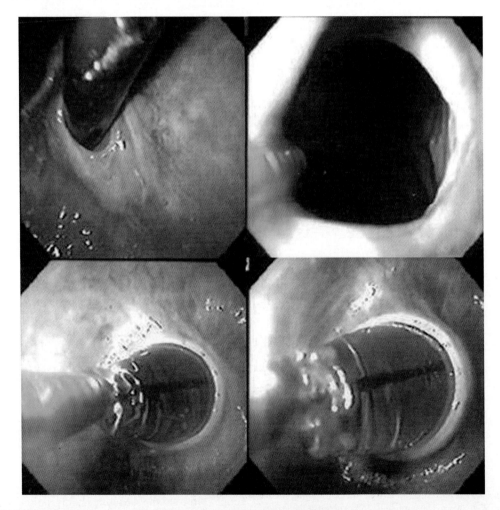

Fig. 60.7 A sequence of balloon dilation of a distal esophageal ring: (*top left*) retrograde endoscopic view of rings from within the stomach; (*top right*) catheter insertion through the ring zone; (*bottom* photos) adequate inflation of the balloon through the ring zone causing "ischemia" of the narrowed periphery

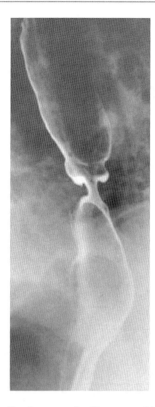

Fig. 60.8 Esophagram detailing a mid-esophageal Barrett's stricture. The stricture is immediately distal (beneath) to the pseudosacculations above

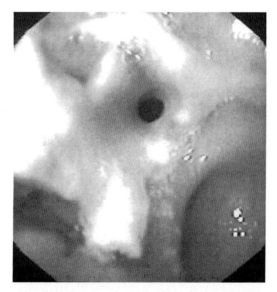

Fig. 60.9 Endoscopic appearance of distal esophageal stricture associated with active inflammation and ulceration

the clinician with a "starting point" in selecting the initial size and type of dilator. Additionally, the small diameter endoscope ≤5 mm is an excellent resource for passing the severe stricture and placing a guidewire or balloon.

Computerized Scan

The use of a chest computerized scan (CT scan) is not routinely used in evaluating esophageal strictures. CT scanning is useful in evaluating strictures that may have a possible malignant etiology, especially an infiltrating malignancy involving the cardioesophageal junction.

Contraindications to Esophageal Dilation

Esophageal dilation is contraindicated in the presence of significant esophagitis, impacted food bolus, or esophageal varices. Patients with pulmonary or cardiovascular conditions require appropriate pre-procedural evaluation and possible formal anesthesia administration. Patients with cervical deformities, postoperative pharyngeal malignancy surgery or external beam radiation treatment, Zenker's diverticulum, or chronic corticosteroid therapy require an extra-judicious approach to esophageal dilation.

Anticoagulants should be discontinued during the examination period and the patient may require heparin "bridging" over this time. Routine antibiotic prophylaxis coverage is not recommended for esophageal dilation [14].

Patient Preparation

Esophageal dilation is most frequently an outpatient procedure requiring an overnight fast. In situations where a significant narrowing has been identified, the patient should avoid solids for 1–2 days prior to the procedure. Anticoagulants should be suspended with heparin bridging if

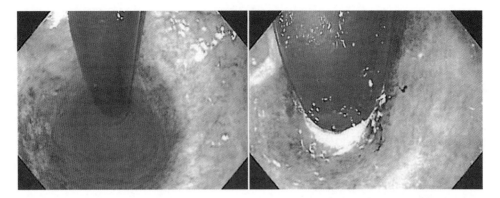

Fig. 60.10 Endoscopic retroflexed view of cardia (1) and gastroesophageal function (2) in a patient with distal esophageal stricture

needed. The patient should be well informed about the risks of complications, particularly perforation associated with esophageal dilations. Severe chest pain, hospitalization, and possible surgery are associated complications of esophageal perforation. The patient should be advised that a post-procedural esophagram may be necessary if a perforation is suspected. In addition, an appropriate communication channel should be in place as a contingency for delayed post-discharge complications or patient's concerns.

Progressive Dilation "Rules"

Esophageal Bouginage

There are traditional limits imposed on the number of tapered OTW dilators used at one time called the "rule of three" [15]. No more than three progressive sized dilators are passed based on "common sense" acquired decades ago. Despite newer dilator materials, guidewires, and fluoroscopic monitoring, this rule is accepted by the majority of physicians who use Bougies.

The dilator size for the initial dilator should be predicted on the assessment of the luminal diameter and structural characteristics of the stricture. Based on the resistance to passage of the first dilator, usually only two additional dilators are passed (Fig. 60.11). For example, if resistance occurs

with a 30-Fr dilator, using the rule of 3's, only two additional dilators (33 Fr and 36 Fr) are passed subsequently. Skipping to significantly higher dilator sizes and avoiding the traditional rule are considered by experts to increase the risk of perforation despite the lack of supportive evidence.

Esophageal Balloon Dilation

The introduction of the balloon dilator has altered the "rules" somewhat. Sets of individual balloons are constructed to expand in increments to a total of 3 mm diameters, e.g., 18–20 mm. There are no starting "guide lines" for using balloons for stricture dilations. However, balloon dilators are mounted on small-diameter catheters which readily pass through complex strictures, providing an approximation of the luminal diameter. For example, an estimated 6-mm stricture diameter suggests a 10–12-mm balloon as an initial size. Depending upon the size of the stricture and esophageal angulation and contraction activity, balloon expansion can be monitored visually through the endoscope. The ability to move the balloon through the stricture site during full inflation supplies evidence for higher diameter dilators. In addition, reexamination of the stricture site furnishes information about tissue trauma and the need to cease or continue with larger balloon diameters.

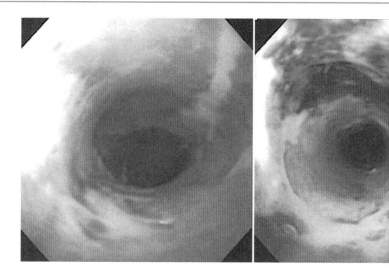

Fig. 60.11 Extensive, ulcerated peptic esophageal stricture with linear ulcerations (1); A portion of damage resulting from passage of a 21-Fr bougie associated with significant resistance. No further dilations were performed at initial procedure

Techniques of Dilation

Bougie Dilating

In preparation before Bouginage dilation, a guidewire is placed into the stomach through the endoscope. Care must be taken not to dislodge the wire during subsequent extraction of the endoscope and this is one advantage of radiologic monitoring of the procedure [8]. New guidewires have calibrations, but accuracy in securing appropriate gastric placement is difficult at times. Appropriate anatomic distances measured from the incisor teeth are helpful to remember (the antrum is 60 cm; the duodenum sweep is 90 cm).

The patient is customarily sedated following thorough anesthesia of the oral pharynx and is positioned in the regular left lateral position. A large mouth guard is used so that resistance to bougie passage is minimized. The operator should experience no appreciable sensation of resistance other than that caused by the stricture itself. For maximal ease in inserting the bougie through the oropharynx, the patient's head should be deflected to the thorax, chin down.

An experienced nurse or technician presents the first dilator after lubricating the inner core with water to ease wire insertion. As the bougie is inserted over the wire, the assistant holds the wire like a "clothesline" so there is no drag to the system. Lubrications should be confined to the proximal position of the dilator to avoid a slippery shaft which can compromise the operator's grip. Despite the wire track guidance, insertion through the oropharynx can be awkward and associated with resistance. One technique which may help is placement of the index finger into the mouth adjacent to the mouth guard to deflect the tip of the bougie down into the distal pharynx. The opposite hand of the operator holds the distal portion of the dilator assuming a "pool cue" grip. Grabbing the shaft with a "fist grip" prompts a more intense thrust rather than a graduated insertion of the dilator. Esophageal dilation with a bougie does not require one energetic ramming of the instrument down the esophagus. Gentle sustained insertion of the dilator into the esophagus affords the best tactile appreciation of resistance to passage and possible obstruction to that size of dilator.

A few caveats concerning wire-guided dilation of the esophagus are worthwhile. The sensation of "resistance" to bougie transit during insertion is considered a major factor in determining further progression to larger sized dilators. In the presence of active inflammation, the resistance factor is not present or appreciated by the operator. This should not be interpreted as a safety factor per se for passage of larger dilators. This feature is almost always a problem when dilating the eosinophilic esophagitis stricture.

The presence or absence of a coating of blood on the shaft of the extracted bougie following dilation is no specific indication for stopping or continuing with additional dilations. Endoscopic re-inspection of the esophagus provides more useful information in assessing tissue damage and providing clues concerning further dilations. This is especially helpful when dilating complex strictures, rings, and eosinophilic esophagitis.

Fluoroscopic Monitoring

The use of fluoroscopic monitoring during esophageal bouginage provides real-time information about bougie transit and wire guide position. Fluoroscopy is generally not necessary when dilating the simple stricture [16]. However, use of fluoroscopy may improve safety in situations involving a tortuous esophagus, a large hiatal hernia, or using a wireless bougie.

Maloney Dilators

Maloney (wireless) filiform dilators are useful in dilating certain simple strictures. Once the stricture has been characterized, "blind" passage can be successfully performed. One important caveat in using this dilator: avoid blind wireless insertion of the Maloney in the presence of a significant hiatal hernia. Impingement of the tip of the bougie into the wall of the hernia pouch can result in a gastric perforation.

Self-dilation after appropriate instruction has been performed at home using the Maloney dilator by a small subset of motivated patients [17].

Balloon Dilating

Current balloon dilators are designed to deliver three pressure-controlled diameters at one placement, e.g., 18–20 mm. The balloons are designed with rectilinear "rounded shoulders" which permit endoscopic observation during balloon expansion. This may not always be possible, however, when there is significant angulation of the distal esophagus or consistent esophageal motor activity. Balloon dilation is most frequently used for short, focal strictures. Stabilization of balloon during inflation can be a challenge because the esophagus shortens 1–1.5 cm during focal distention. Because of this feature, the (waist) of the balloon is positioned slightly above the stricture midpoint and the catheter is stabilized at the endoscope by the operator to prevent balloon migration. Successful balloon dilation to the desired diameter occurs when the balloon is "locked" against the wall of the stricture during the inflation process (Fig. 60.12). The ability of the operator to move the balloon through the stricture site at full volume suggests the site is

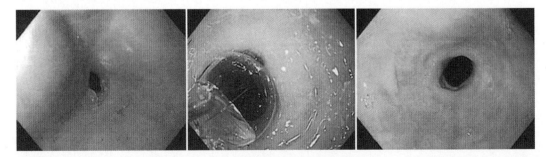

Fig. 60.12 Endoscopic view of a fully inflated (20 mm) balloon dilator securely "locked" into the stricture zone. The balloon could not be moved at this diameter indicating a successful "stretch" as noted on the *right* photo

not being effectively dilated; the lumen still exceeds the diameter of the balloon. The optimal duration of balloon inflation at any diameter is arbitrary, although 30–60 s is generally used by most physicians.

Therapeutic Goals of Esophageal Dilation

The goal of successful esophageal dilation (s) hinges upon two primary factors: (1) degree of luminal expansion and (2) need for subsequent dilations. It is generally accepted that dilation of the esophageal lumen to a diameter of 15 mm (45 Fr) allows the patient to tolerate a modified solid diet. Expanding the lumen to 18 mm (54 Fr) normalizes swallowing unless other factors exist [18].

However, there may be no predictable association between the magnitude of the luminal dilation and the patient's symptomatic improvement. For example, if the dysphagia for solids has been chronic, the patient has been conditioned to a modified diet despite the improvement in esophageal caliber. The patient is often reticent to challenge swallowing with larger solid foods. Additionally, it has been shown that the patient's symptomatic improvement may not correlate with objective swallowing tests (barium pill swallow) which indicated continuing obstruction of solid transit [19].

The interval between progressive dilations of the esophagus is not standardized. This cadence can range from several days to a few weeks. The presence of active inflammation and structural damage from the most recent series of dilations and the patient's rapid recurrence of symptoms will influence this interval time.

Some predictable features suggesting a poor response to esophageal dilation have been reported. Long stricture length and small luminal diameter are harbingers for ineffective balloon treatment [20]. A small diameter peptic stricture is often an indication that repetitive serial dilations will be necessary to accomplish adequate esophageal caliber. Radiation-induced strictures are typically difficult to dilate and may necessitate a repetitive series of dilations [21].

Refractive Strictures

Dilation of benign esophageal strictures has an immediate success ratio in relieving dysphagia of 80–90%. However, 30–40% of patients have symptomatic recurrence within the first year following initial dilations [18, 22]. The majority of these patients are treated with repeated dilations. When the sequence of dilations is necessarily repetitive or clinically ineffective, the stricture is considered "refractive" (Fig. 60.13).

In one series of 87 constrictive patients with benign esophageal strictures, significant predictors

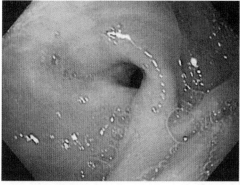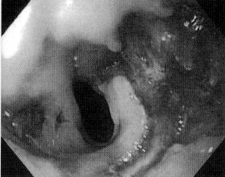

Fig. 60.13 Endoscopic appearance of a recurrent distal esophageal peptic stricture before (*left*) and after (*right*) dilation. The patient has required serial dilations (bougie) twice yearly

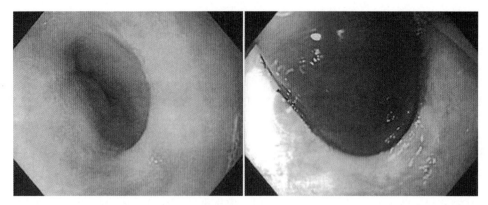

Fig. 60.14 The appearance of a "thickened, rubbery-like" nonpeptic stricture from within the esophagus (*left*) and from below (*right*) "hugging" the esophagus. The nature of this stricture is unknown but requires dilation (bougie) every 4 months with little evidence of mucosal trauma on endoscopic re-inspection

of early recurrence in peptic strictures included a hiatal hernia, persistence of heartburn, and the number of initial dilations to relieve dyspagias (>3 dilations). In the same study, multivariate modeling showed that a nonpeptic stricture was a significant predictor of earlier recurrence within 1 year of initial dilation [23].

Although each esophageal stricture poses its own challenge to dilation, certain categories of strictures present a more predictable recalcitrance. Esophageal strictures caused by radiation treatments of the neck and chest are notoriously difficult to maintain patency by dilations. Surgical anastomotic strictures encountered following subtotal esophagectomy are difficult to effectively expand. Strictures associated with certain skin disorders (pemphigoid and epidermolysis bullosa) respond poorly to dilation as do strictures resulting from caustic indigestion or prolonged nasogastric tube placement. The thickened, rubbery, doughnut-like stricture encountered at the gastroesophageal junction (nonpeptic?) offers particular resistance to repeated dilation (Fig. 60.14).

Several techniques/technology have been devised or are in clinical trials to more effectively treat refractive esophageal strictures. These include the use of intralesional corticosteroid infections, electrocautery incisions, and temporary placement of esophageal stents.

Coricosteroid Injection Treatment

Coricosteroid injection into esophageal stricture site(s) is based on the premise that there is subsequent disruption of collagen formation and disposition and reduction of the inflammatory response. A 5-year follow-up of a prospective randomized trial comparing the effects of savory dilation with or without intralesional steroid injections in a group of patients with peptic strictures demonstrated a prolonged benefit in improving dysphagia symptoms and decreasing the frequency of dilations among patients receiving steroid injections [24]. A more recent study involving 30 peptic stricture patients in a prospective, double-blind protocol compared steroid injection to sham injection [25]. In the patients who were followed for 1 year, two patients in the steroid group (13 %) and nine in the sham group (60%) required repeat dilation. PPIs were provided during this study to suppress potential acid injury.

Steriod Injection Technique

Endoscopic steroid injection is customarily performed using a standard 22-gauge sclerotherapy needle. Triamcinolone acetonide (Kenalog, 40 mg 50/mL) is administered in 1.0 mL aliquots (into four quadrants) at the narrowest region of the stricture.

We initially dilate the esophageal stricture prior to steroid injection. Subsequently repeat endoscopy examination discloses the site(s) of wall damage at the narrowest luminal points. Corticosteroid injections are directed into these trauma furrows to maximize spread into subcutaneous tissue.

Esophageal Stents

Conventional esophageal dilation per se occurs over a very short period of time. Theoretically, sustaining a dilator in the stricture zone for a prolonged time would enhance expansion and assure better fixation of the esophageal wall. To address this possibility, temporary placement of endoscopically delivered stents in the stricture zone has been used. There are now a variety of self-expanding plastic stents (SEPS) available for dilating refractive benign esophageal strictures. These stents are constructed to provide stronger radial forces to maintain patency, assure anchoring position, and have fluoroscopic visibility. These stents are safe, extractable, and can be cost effective. For example, a silicon-coated, expanding, plastic stent, Polyflex™ (Willy Rusch GIMH/Boston Scientific, Natuck, MA) has recently been approved by the US Food and Drug Administration (FDA) for use in patients with refractory benign esophageal strictures. The stent is covered with a polyester siliconized coat to avoid ingrowth of epithelial tissue, permit insertion, and, importantly, eventual removal from the stricture site. The stent is supplied in smaller diameter (18/23 mm) and larger diameter (21–25 mm).

Stricture Placement

The tight refractive stricture is dilated to capacity with Savary–Gilliard or American dilators prior to insertion of the plastic stent. After estimating the length of the stricture endoscopically, placement of radiopaque markers on the skin can mark the proximal and distal ends of the stricture to enhance the accuracy of stent placement under fluoroscopic observation.

The experience with the Polyflex™ stent for benign strictures has been varied and most often, unimpressive. A 4 weeks polyflex stent placement trial in 40 patients with a benign esophageal stricture demonstrated improvement (dysphagia free) in only 40% of patients [26]. Another study of 30 patients reported long-term improvement in just 6% of cases during long-term follow-up [27]. In a report of Polyflex™ stent placement in 13 patients with the majority demonstrating anastomotic strictures, 11 patients had satisfactory relief of dysphagia to solids while the SEPS was in place, but this persisted in only 3 patients after removal of the stents [28].

Biodegradable stents have recently been developed and used in a clinical trial in Europe. The device is an Ella BD stent (Ella-CS, Hradec Kralove, Czech Republic) made of polydioxanone. Polydioxanone is a semi-crystalline biodegradable polymer 25 mm in diameter. The BD stent degrades after 4–5 weeks by random hydrolysis. Stent material is partially absorbed and partially excreted through the GI tract. In a recent report, two groups of consecutive patients with benign strictures received temporary (6 weeks) placement of SEPS (20 patients) or biodegradable stents (18 patients) [29]. Placement of SEPS or biodegradable stents provided relief of dysphagia in 30% and 33%, respectively, in follow-up ranging from a mean of 6–12 months. Major complications occurred in four patients (22%).

Stent Complications

Although self-expandable fully covered plastic stents represent a potential future treatment for benign esophageal strictures, they are associated with significant complications and morbidity. Complications of insertion of the stent include aspiration and airway compromise and require removal of the device. The biggest problem is migration of the stent. Reports of stent migration range from 7 to 85% [30]. Other complications include bleeding, perforation, aorta-fistula formation, and new stricture development at the respective poles of the stent itself.

At the time of this writing, an effective durable stent therapy for refractive benign esophageal stricture remains elusive.

Alternative Therapies

Electroincision technique can be a therapeutic option in certain refractive strictures, particularly the post-op esphagogastric anastomosis which is short and shelf-like. Benign anastomotic strictures occur in 5–46% of patients after resection of the esophagus for cancer [31]. As many as 39% of patients with post-op esophagogastric anastomotic strictures require more than three dilations to achieve adequate results [32]. In a study of 62 patients with a post-op esophagogastric stricture randomized to electrocautery incision versus savary bouginage, there was no significant difference between the incision versus the dilation groups in mean number of dilations (2.9 versus 3.3) or the ultimate success rate (96.2 versus 80.8%), neither were there complications with either technique [33]. In this study, multiple longitudinal electroincisions were made around the circumference of the stenotic ring using an ERCP needle knife. The depth of the incision was estimated at approximately 4 mm—the end point was passage of the endoscope.

Self-Dilation

Esophageal self-dilation is a treatment option for patients with resistant benign esophageal strictures. The patient has to be motivated and the stricture has to be simple. Successful home dilation provided symptomatic improvement in 13 patients followed for a mean of 4.8 years [34]. A more recent report describes significant improvement in dysphagia in seven patients for a mean of 3 years [35].

The technique of self-dilation involves a detailed process of education, a minimum of three teaching sessions, and close supervision of passage of a Maloney dilator until all parties are satisfied [17].

Eosinophilic Esophageal Strictures

The incidence of eosinophilic esophageal (EoE) strictures has increased significantly over the last two decades. In one prospective report, the prevalence of EoE in adult population undergoing upper endoscopy was 6.5% [36]. The unique tissue remodeling associated with this disorder promotes subepithelial fibrosis which results in the formation of esophageal rings and strictures, causing solid food dysphagia. Many of these patients require esophageal dilation, but the mucosal fragility associated with this disorder predisposes to significant damage from standard dilation. Extensive mucosal sheering can be painful and perforation more problematic. However, in a review of 468 patients with EoE who underwent 671 dilations; the majority of cases had mucosal tears but only one perforation occurred [37].

Nonetheless, dilation of the EoE strictures requires additional caution by the physician. For example, on occasions, passage of the standard 9.7-mm endoscope may cause significant disruption of the esophageal lining. In addition, the esophageal wall involvement in EoE stricture patients causing dysphagia may be unevenly distributed. For that reason, bouginage may be the dilator of choice in these patients and the "rule of threes" is waived. Endoscopic reinspection after passage of the initial dilator is often rewarding in providing information about damage and need for further dilations. It should be pointed out that the dyspagia associated with mild to modest EoE strictures may respond to medical therapy negating the risk of esophageal dilation.

Proton Pump Acid Control

The introduction of PPI therapy to treat gastroesophageal reflux disease has made a dramatic impact in decreasing peptic strictures. This medication has been invaluable in preventing the recurrence of symptoms and reformation of strictures in patients with peptic disease. Prior to this potent antacid medication, repeated esophageal dilations were necessary in approximately 70% of patients with GERD strictures [38]. PPI use decreases stricture recurrence and the necessity for future dilations. In a prospective randomized study, long-term PPI therapy prevented the reformation of a Schatzke Ring after initial dilation [39]. Patients with strictures resulting from acid reflux may require prolonged proton pump therapy for an indefinite period in the future after appropriate response to dilation.

Upper Esophageal Strictures

Strictures encountered in the upper esophagus are most often the result of therapy (surgery, radiotherapy, or chemotherapy) for head and neck malignancy. The proximal esophagus is also the site for cervical webs (Plumer–Vinson syndrome); dermatology-associated lesions, e.g., epidermolysis bullosa and pemphigoid; tracheoesophageal repair site; and eosinophilic esophagitis strictures.

Barium contrast swallow is essential in defining the structural characteristics of a proximal stricture. The caliber of endoscopic passage further defines the severity, i.e., the need for a 5-mm diameter endoscope.

Strictures located beneath the upper esophageal sphincter preclude the use of balloon dilators because of placement issues. Fluoroscopy is important when dilating severe or angulated structures, and the "rule of three" depends on the clinical situation experienced with bougie passage. In one report on dilation upper esophageal strictures (UES), in situations when bougie dilation was impossible, the use of a "biliary" type guidewire and ERCP accessories eventually permitted progression to polyvinyl dilators [40].

In situations, especially following radiation therapy, when complete obstruction of the esophagus occurs, a combined antegrade/retrograde approach for dilation of the stricture has been used. The patients all have had a pre-existing gastrostomy tube. A neonate endoscope is inserted through the gastrostomy and maneuvered retrograde into the esophagus where the distal portion of the stricture can be examined. A spring-tipped guidewire introduced through a peroral endoscope and the proximal side of the stricture is gently probed while there is concurrent visualization from the distal side below. In one report using this method on 12 patients in conjunction with an otolaryngologist who employed a number of probing devices to open the upper portion of the stricture to allow guidewire passage, ten of the maneuvers were successful in opening the stricture for delivery of nutrition orally [41].

Complications of Dilation

Esophageal dilation can cause bleeding, chest pain, and the most concerning complication—perforation. The overall frequency of complications associated with dilations of the esophagus ranges from 0.1 to 0.4% [7]. However, the individual risk of esophageal perforation depends upon the complexity and location of the stricture and the nature of the disorder, e.g., eosinophilic esophagitis. Early recognition and management of an esophageal perforation is paramount for successful treatment.

Cervical and high esophageal perforations can often be treated conservatively with nasogastric suction to divert secretions and gram-positive antibiotic administration. In the past, surgical management of esophageal perforation has been the mode of treatment. Currently this is increasingly becoming a nonsurgical issue. When complications are immediately recognized, endoscopic placement of clips to close the perforation, or fully covered, removable, and expandable stents have been employed to cover larger perforations. If leakage from the perforation consists of air, not fluid, it will be absorbed as the stent closes. Both gastrograptric contrast swallow and computed tomography are important guidelines for directing conservative management of perforations caused by stricture dilation.

Conclusions

Esophageal stricture significantly impacts on the patient's ability to swallow, that is, impeding or prohibiting oral intake of food. Dysphagia resulting from an esophageal stricture can have a profound effect on nutrition and may be associated with pain, aspiration, impacted food bolus, life style disruption, and fear of eating.

Esophageal strictures are caused by a number of disorders ranging from primary physiologic disturbances like GERD to secondary causes from surgical procedures. This feature is the explanation for variation in stricture characteristics and response to therapy.

Because the esophageal food conduit possesses unique motor function which is irreplaceable, treatment is almost exclusively conservative (surgical treatment is the last resort), and efforts to mechanically re-open the lumen involve dilating the stricture with filiform or balloon dilators.

The equipment, technique, and appropriate use of dilating esophageal strictures have been reviewed in this chapter. The associated risks and goals related to esophageal dilation are outlined.

The success of esophageal dilation and maintenance of luminal potency is estimated to be over 80%. There are a significant minority of patients, however, with strictures that "defy" conventional dilation and subsequent improvement. These strictures are classified as "refractive" and require different techniques and instruments to expand the esophageal lumen. For example, a new cadre of plastic, covered, degradable, and expanding stents has been developed for prolonged placement within the zone of a refractive stricture.

Each esophageal stricture possesses basic structural characteristics, but other features including the severity, extent, on-going inflammation, and regional location compromise the lesion and treatment challenge. The approach to esophageal dilation requires a clinician who is careful, appropriately talented, and experienced.

Swallowing is an essential part of life. Restoring acceptable or normal esophageal food transit by esophageal dilation is a most worthy task.

References

1. Willis T. Pharmaceutice rationalis, sive, diatriba de medicamentorum operationibus in humano corpore. London: R Scott; 1675.
2. Hildreth CT. Stricture of the esophagus. N Engl J Med Surg. 1921;10:235–40.
3. Barron L, Wynn TA. Fibrosis is regulated by Th2 and Th17 responses and by dynamic interactions between fibroblasts and macrophages. Am J Physiol Gastrointest Liver Physiol. 2011;300(5):G723–8.
4. Richter JE. Peptic strictures of the esophagus. Gastroenterol Clin North Am. 1999;28(4):875–91. vi.
5. Barbezat GO, Schlup M, Lubcke R. Omeprazole therapy decreases the need for dilatation of peptic oesophageal strictures. Aliment Pharmacol Ther. 1999;13(8):1041–5.
6. Marks RD, et al. Omeprazole versus H2-receptor antagonists in treating patients with peptic stricture and esophagitis. Gastroenterology. 1994;106(4):907–15.
7. Hernandez LV, Jacobson JW, Harris MS. Comparison among the perforation rates of Maloney, balloon, and savary dilation of esophageal strictures. Gastrointest Endosc. 2000;51(4):460–2.
8. McClave SA, et al. Does fluoroscopic guidance for Maloney esophageal dilation impact on the clinical endpoint of therapy: relief of dysphagia and achievement of luminal patency. Gastrointest Endosc. 1996;43(2 Pt 1):93–7.
9. Saeed ZA, et al. Prospective randomized comparison of polyvinyl bougies and through-the-scope balloons for dilation of peptic strictures of the esophagus. Gastrointest Endosc. 1995;41(3):189–95.
10. Scolapio JS, et al. A randomized prospective study comparing rigid to balloon dilators for benign esophageal strictures and rings. Gastrointest Endosc. 1999;50(1):13–7.
11. Osborn NK, Baron TH. The history of the "French" gauge. Gastrointest Endosc. 2006;63(3):461–2.
12. Lavu K, Mathew TP, Minocha A. Effectiveness of esophageal dilation in relieving nonobstructive esophageal dysphagia and improving quality of life. South Med J. 2004;97(2):137–40.
13. Scolapio JS, et al. Dysphagia without endoscopically evident disease: to dilate or not? Am J Gastroenterol. 2001;96(2):327–30.
14. Banerjee S, et al. Antibiotic prophylaxis for GI endoscopy. Gastrointest Endosc. 2008;67(6):791–8.
15. Tulman AB, Boyce Jr HW. Complications of esophageal dilation and guidelines for their prevention. Gastrointest Endosc. 1981;27(4):229–34.
16. Wang YG, Tio TL, Soehendra N. Endoscopic dilation of esophageal stricture without fluoroscopy is safe and effective. World J Gastroenterol. 2002;8(4):766–8.
17. Dzeletovic I, Fleischer DE. Self-dilation for resistant, benign esophageal strictures. Am J Gastroenterol. 2010;105(10):2142–3.
18. Patterson DJ, et al. Natural history of benign esophageal stricture treated by dilatation. Gastroenterology. 1983;85(2):346–50.
19. Saeed ZA, et al. An objective end point for dilation improves outcome of peptic esophageal strictures: a prospective randomized trial. Gastrointest Endosc. 1997;45(5):354–9.

20. Chiu YC, et al. Factors influencing clinical applications of endoscopic balloon dilation for benign esophageal strictures. Endoscopy. 2004;36(7):595–600.

21. Spinelli P, et al. Endoscopic treatment of postradiation strictures. Tumori. 1993;79(1):34–6.

22. Smith PM, et al. A comparison of omeprazole and ranitidine in the prevention of recurrence of benign esophageal stricture. Restore Investigator Group. Gastroenterology. 1994;107(5):1312–8.

23. Said A, et al. Predictors of early recurrence of benign esophageal strictures. Am J Gastroenterol. 2003;98(6): 1252–6.

24. Dunne D. Five year followup of a prospective randsomized trial of Savary dilation with or without intralesional steriods for benign gastroesophageal reflux strictures. Gastroenterology. 1999;116:A152.

25. Ramage Jr JI, et al. A prospective, randomized, double-blind, placebo-controlled trial of endoscopic steroid injection therapy for recalcitrant esophageal peptic strictures. Am J Gastroenterol. 2005;100(11): 2419–25.

26. Dua KS, et al. Removable self-expanding plastic esophageal stent as a continuous, non-permanent dilator in treating refractory benign esophageal strictures: a prospective two-center study. Am J Gastroenterol. 2008;103(12):2988–94.

27. Holm AN, et al. Self-expanding plastic stents in treatment of benign esophageal conditions. Gastrointest Endosc. 2008;67(1):20–5.

28. Oh YS, et al. Clinical outcomes after self-expanding plastic stent placement for refractory benign esophageal strictures. Dig Dis Sci. 2010;55(5):1344–8.

29. van Boeckel PG, Vleggaar FP, Siersema PD. A comparison of temporary self-expanding plastic and biodegradable stents for refractory benign esophageal strictures. Clin Gastroenterol Hepatol. 2011;9(8): 653–9.

30. Barthel JS, Kelley ST, Klapman JB. Management of persistent gastroesophageal anastomotic strictures with removable self-expandable polyester siliconcovered (Polyflex) stents: an alternative to serial dilation. Gastrointest Endosc. 2008;67(3):546–52.

31. Pierie JP, et al. Incidence and management of benign anastomotic stricture after cervical oesophagogastrostomy. Br J Surg. 1993;80(4):471–4.

32. Honkoop P, et al. Benign anastomotic strictures after transhiatal esophagectomy and cervical esophagogastrostomy: risk factors and management. J Thorac Cardiovasc Surg. 1996;111(6):1141–6. discussion 1147–8.

33. Hordijk ML, et al. A randomized comparison of electrocautery incision with Savary bougienage for relief of anastomotic gastroesophageal strictures. Gastrointest Endosc. 2009;70(5):849–55.

34. Grobe JL, Kozarek RA, Sanowski RA. Self-bougienage in the treatment of benign esophageal stricture. J Clin Gastroenterol. 1984;6(2):109–12.

35. Kim CH, Groskreutz JL, Gehrking SJ. Recurrent benign esophageal strictures treated with self-bougienage: report of seven cases. Mayo Clin Proc. 1990;65(6):799–803.

36. Veerappan GR, et al. Prevalence of eosinophilic esophagitis in an adult population undergoing upper endoscopy: a prospective study. Clin Gastroenterol Hepatol. 2009;7(4):420–6.

37. Jacobs Jr JW, Spechler SJ. A systematic review of the risk of perforation during esophageal dilation for patients with eosinophilic esophagitis. Dig Dis Sci. 2010;55(6):1512–5.

38. Glick ME. Clinical course of esophageal stricture managed by bougienage. Dig Dis Sci. 1982;27(10):884–8.

39. Sgouros SN, et al. Long-term acid suppressive therapy may prevent the relapse of lower esophageal (Schatzki's) rings: a prospective, randomized, placebo-controlled study. Am J Gastroenterol. 2005;100(9):1929–34.

40. Ahlawat SK, Al-Kawas FH. Endoscopic management of upper esophageal strictures after treatment of head and neck malignancy. Gastrointest Endosc. 2008;68(1):19–24.

41. Dellon ES, et al. Outcomes of a combined antegrade and retrograde approach for dilatation of radiation-induced esophageal strictures. Gastrointest Endosc. 2010;71(7):1122–9.

Esophageal Stenting for Relief of Dysphagia

61

Kulwinder S. Dua

Abstract

The majority of the patients with esophageal cancer present with dysphagia and over 50% are unresectable at presentation. Some may also develop a trachea-esophageal fistula preventing them from oral intake. Self-expanding esophageal stents are now the most commonly used modality to palliate these patients since these stents are easy to place with minimally invasive techniques and the relief in symptoms is almost immediate. Plastic coating on the stents can also seal fistulae. Compared to chemoradiation, since the relief in symptoms with stents is immediate, these stents are also being considered for locally advanced esophageal cancer as a bridge to surgery for those requiring neoadjuvant therapy. This approach is not universally accepted since stents can be associated with serious complications that may delay therapy. With the availability of expandable stents that can be removed, there has been a great interest in using stents as long-term dilators for treating benign refractory esophageal strictures. Results have been mixed and several studies have reported significant complications. Hence stents for benign esophageal strictures should be used in carefully selected patients in centers with expertise to manage stent-related complications. Newer developments in design are needed. Biodegradable stents that get metabolized by the body and eventually absorbed are available in other countries and it will be interesting as to how they perform especially in those who need temporary esophageal stenting.

Keywords

Esophageal stenting • Dysphagia • Palliation • Malignant dysphagia • Refractory benign esophageal strictures

K.S. Dua (✉)
Division of Gastroenterology and Hepatology,
Medical College of Wisconsin,
Milwaukee, WI, USA
e-mail: kdua@mcw.edu

R. Shaker et al. (eds.), *Principles of Deglutition: A Multidisciplinary Text for Swallowing and its Disorders*,
DOI 10.1007/978-1-4614-3794-9_61, © Springer Science+Business Media New York 2013

Introduction

Dysphagia can result from either intrinsic lesions of the esophagus or from extrinsic compression. These lesions can either be benign or malignant in nature. Widely accepted grading for severity of dysphagia is Grade 0: no dysphagia; Grade 1: difficulty swallowing most solids; Grade 2: difficulty swallowing solids and semisolids; Grade 3: difficulty swallowing liquids also; and Grade 4: unable to swallow one's own saliva. Some consider patients with a trachea-esophageal fistula also as Grade 4. Due to the good compliance of the esophageal wall, patients generally do not complain of dysphagia until over 50% of the esophageal lumen is obstructed or in absolute terms, the luminal diameter has decreased to 12 mm or less in adults. Hence the majority of the patients with esophageal cancer presenting with dysphagia have advanced disease and carry a dismal 5-year survival rate of less than 20% with over 50% unresectable at presentation [1–3]. Despite this poor prognosis, palliating dysphagia is important for maintaining nutrition, preventing aspiration, and improving quality of life. Surgery for palliating malignant dysphagia can be associated with significant morbidity and mortality and similarly, palliative chemoradiation can be associated with significant side effects and do not relieve dysphagia immediately. In the recent past several endoscopic approaches have emerged and currently, self-expandable esophageal stents have become the most commonly used modality for immediate relief of dysphagia and for sealing trachea-esophageal fistula.

Dysphagia secondary to benign esophageal strictures, on the other hand is easy to manage with periodic endoscopic dilatations [4, 5]. However complex benign strictures can develop after corrosive injuries, radiation, surgery, and esophageal ablative treatments like photodynamic therapy and mucosal resections. These strictures are difficult to dilate, carry a high procedural complication rate, and tend to recur within weeks of the dilatation [6, 7]. Hence these strictures are considered as *Refractory Benign Esophageal Strictures (RBES)* defined as an anatomic fibrotic esophageal restriction, in the absence of inflammation or motility disorder, with the inability to achieve a diameter of ≥14 mm in five sessions of dilatations at 2-week intervals or the inability to maintain a diameter of ≥14 mm for 4 weeks once ≥14 mm diameter is achieved [8]. The role of using expandable esophageal stents in treating RBES is evolving.

Esophageal Stents

The concept of using hollow tubes for treating malignant dysphagia dates back to over 100 years ago. Charles J Symonds in 1885 for the first time introduced the concept of using stents to relieve dysphagia. These tubes were made of ivory or boxwood. Several decades later, semirigid plastic esophageal stents were introduced. These plastic stents were 16–18 mm in diameter, required preinsertion dilatation and were associated with high complication rates [9–12]. Hence besides stents, alternatives like laser, alcohol injection, and photodynamic therapy were also used for palliation of malignant dysphagia. With the introduction of self-expanding metal esophageal stents (SEMS) in the early 1990s, interest in using stents as a palliative option was revived and currently SEMS have virtually replaced the older plastic stents.

Although there are several types of FDA cleared SEMS available in the US (and many more varieties worldwide), the broad principle of design and placement remain the same (Fig. 61.1). The majority of the stents are made of a nickel titanium metal alloy (Nitinol) wire woven into a tubular structure that is constrained to a thin diameter (7–10 mm) on a delivery catheter. Once released, the stent expands to its preset diameter that can range from 16 to 25 mm. SEMS are available in various lengths. The upper and lower ends of the stent have flared flanges to prevent migration. Some of the advantages of SEMS over semirigid plastic stents are (1) thinner delivery system as the stent is constrained to a smaller diameter. Hence pre-insertion dilatation is not required in most patients. (2) Despite the thinner delivery system, the expanded stent can reach diameters larger than the plastic stent. (3) Expansion is gradual unlike the abrupt stretching from plastic stents. (4)

Botulinum Toxin for LES Spastic Disorders

62

Linda Nguyen and Pankaj J. Pasricha

Abstract

Botulinum toxin is one of the most potent neurotoxins available, blocking vesicular mediated neurotransmitter release from nerve endings and causing a paralysis or reduction in tone of the targeted muscle. Endoscopic injection of botulinum toxin has now been used for achalasia for nearly two decades, with grade I evidence for its efficacy. The experience with other spastic disorders of the esophagus is considerably more limited. Its main advantage is its simplicity and relative safety. On the other hand, its drawbacks include the limited duration of its effects and hence the requirement for repeat injections. Further, it is not very effective in younger patients. While not considered first-line therapy in most patients, it has nevertheless emerged as an alternative therapy for this condition in patients who are considered at high risk for more invasive methods of treatment such as pneumatic dilation or surgery. It is also of some value as a therapeutic trial in patients with equivocal clinical or manometric measures to assess the contribution of lower esophageal tone to symptoms.

Keywords

Botulinum toxin • LES spastic disorders • Neurotoxin • Muscle paralysis • Endoscopic injection

Introduction and Mechanism of Action

Botulinum toxin (BoNT) is a neurotoxin that causes muscle paralysis or relaxation. It is a protein produced by the bacterium Clostridium botulinum. There are seven different subtypes of BoNT (types A–G). All (except C2) block acetylcholine from nerve endings. This multifunctional protein has a complex yet extremely elegant mechanism of

L. Nguyen • P.J. Pasricha (✉)
Division of Gastroenterology and Hepatology,
Stanford University School of Medicine,
Stanford, CA, USA
e-mail: pasricha@stanford.edu

action, as recently reviewed [1]. The heavy chain binds to co-receptors specifically expressed by target cells: in the case of BoNT/A these are SV2 and a ganglioside (GD1b or GT1b); for BoNT/B the receptor is synaptotagmin, in addition to the ganglioside. Thereafter, the toxin becomes internalized by endocytosis into an endosome. The heavy chain then forms a channel across the endosomal membrane, through which the light chain is translocated to the cytoplasm. The light chain, which is a zinc-dependent endoprotease, then degrades critical proteins involved in neurotransmitter release. For BoNT/A, this protein is synaptosomal-associated protein 25 (SNAP-25), which is required to bind and fuse the synaptic vesicle (containing the neurotransmitter) to the presynaptic membrane; thereby, preventing acetylcholine release into the neuromuscular junction [2]. For the BoNT/B light chain, the target is synaptobrevin.

Commercial Preparations and Approved Uses

BoNT therapy is currently approved for many neurological diseases with several commercial preparations (BoNT/A: Botox®, Dysport®, and Xeomin®; BoNT/B: Myoblock®/Neuroblock®). There is little if any literature on the use of BoNT/B for spastic esophageal disorders and the rest of this discussion will be confined to BoNT/A. In 1993, Pasricha et al. [3] described the first therapeutic use of BoNT/A for a smooth muscle disorder as a treatment of achalasia and since then it has been used in hundreds of patients with "spastic" smooth muscle syndromes of the gut. However, it should be noted that although there are several gastrointestinal disorders for which BoNT is currently being used, none of these are approved indications by the FDA.

BoNT for Achalasia

The rationale for using BoNT/A in achalasia is based on our current understanding of the pathophysiology of achalasia, which is characterized by aperistalsis and impaired lower esophageal sphincter (LES) relaxation. The net LES tone/pressure results from a balance between excitatory cholinergic and inhibitory neurotransmitters for example VIP or nitric oxide. In achalasia, this balance is upset due to a selective loss of the inhibitory nerves. This results in an LES that may be hypertonic, but more importantly, also fails to relax [4]. Locally injected BoNT blocks the release of acetylcholine, thus lowering LES resting tone, as confirmed by initial animal and human studies [5, 6].

Method of Endoscopic Injection

The most commonly available commercial preparation of BoNT/A is supplied in vials containing 100 units of the lyophilized powder. For achalasia, this is diluted in 4 or 5 mL of normal saline to yield a solution containing 20–25 units/mL. Flexible upper endoscopy is performed using routine sedation or awake utilizing an ultrathin transnasal endoscope, and the LES is estimated endoscopically by identification of the sphincter rosette, typically seen right at the squamocolumnar junction (z-line). The solution containing the toxin is injected through a 5 mm sclerotherapy needle into the LES, approximately 1 cm above the z-line and slanting the needle approximately 45°. Aliquots of 1.0 mL (20–25 units BoNT/A/mL) are injected into each of four quadrants, for a total of 80–100 units. The procedure requires no fluoroscopy and typically takes no more than 15 min to complete (including the time for endoscopic examination) and patients are recovered and discharged as per any routine upper endoscopy or clinic procedure. Patients are allowed to eat as tolerated, later the same day with most responders noting improved swallowing by the next morning.

Other techniques have also been described including a "2×4" technique (the total dose is divided into eight injections: four quadrant injections are done at two different levels within the LES region) [7], injection from below the gastroesophageal junction using a retroflexed view [8], and endoscopic ultrasound (EUS) [9] or manometry [10] guided injection. However, there is no evidence that the actual technique determines efficacy and more sophisticated approaches may not be necessary as the toxin is capable of diffusion for a limited distance in tissue. In a small study, toxin location after injection was determined by EUS in five patients with Chagasic achalasia: approximately 85 % of the injections were found to be located inside the muscle layers and only about 15 % of injection points were found in the submucosa. However, even patients in the latter group reported improvement of their symptoms over a 6-month period [11].

Dose Considerations

The most common dose, as discussed earlier, is around 100 units. Smaller (50 IU) and larger (200 IU) generally show similar results, at least in the short term. However, one study showed that 100 IU given twice in a 30-day period produced the best long-term results with about 68 % patients remaining in remission for more than 24 months [7].

Efficacy and Duration of Response

Overall, 70–90 % of patients will show a clinically robust improvement after the first injection of BoNT/A [12–17]. However, by 6 months, only about two-thirds of patients remain in remission. The other one-third (nonresponders) appears to be resistant to further injections. Even in responders, the benefit will wane with time, but still lasts longer than it does in patients with skeletal muscle disorders. The median duration of remission after the first set of treatment varies greatly ranging from <1 to >15 months following a single injection [6, 7, 17, 18]. Annese et al. demonstrated that a second injection of BoNT/A 30 days later resulted in a lower relapse rate with 68 % of patients still in remission at 24 months [7]. We advise patients that if they do respond, they can usually expect to sustain this for about 6–9 months.

Clinical response is also accompanied by significant improvement in all objective tests of esophageal function, in a range that is similar to that reported for pneumatic dilation: LES pressure goes down by about 40 %, LES opening diameter increases by more than twofold, esophageal diameter decreases by 20 %, and 5-min retention on scintigraphy improving by 33 % [18].

Predictors of Response

A sustained response (beyond 3 months) was significantly more likely in patients older than age 50 (82 % vs. 43 %) and in patients with vigorous compared with classic achalasia (100 % vs. 52 %) [18]. Conversely, severe esophageal dilation is a negative predictor, with an odds ratio of 0.2 [19]. Other factors such as gender, duration of symptoms, symptom severity, and history of previous dilation do not predict response to BoNT therapy [10, 12, 18]. However, high-resolution esophageal manometry (HRM) appears to identify subtypes of achalasia that impact response to therapy. According to Pandolfino, HRM can be used to classify achalasia into three patterns: type I-classic achalasia without pressurization of the esophagus, type II-aperistalsis with esophageal compression and pressurization of the esophagus, type III-vigorous achalasia with spastic contractions of the distal esophagus [20]. Patients with type II achalasia are more likely to respond to any therapy with the response rate for BoNT being approximately 70 % (the comparable figures for pneumatic dilation and surgical myotomy being 91 % and 100 %) [19]. Patients with type III achalasia were the least likely to respond to any therapy (29 %); however, the greatest response was seen with the use of BoNT injection. These initial findings need to be validated by other centers but potentially represent an important advance.

Recurrent Therapy with BoNT

In our experience, the response to repeated BoNT injections may not be as robust as the initial one. Although, Annese et al. demonstrated in their series that 43 of 57 (75 %) of patients could be kept in remission for 4 years with repeat injections approximately every 10 months [21]. One concern is the formation of neutralizing antibodies. However, among a group of patients who were secondary treatment failures for various indications, neutralizing antibodies were found in less than 45 % [22].

Comparisons with Other Therapies

Although the initial clinical and manometric responses to BoNT/A injection are comparable to pneumatic dilation, the response rate 1 year after a single injection is markedly inferior for BoNT/A, which is to be expected given its pharmacological properties [16, 23–25]. A meta-analysis comparing various therapies for achalasia [26] revealed that intrasphincteric BoNT/A injection was inferior to pneumatic dilation and surgical myotomy in terms of initial response as well as duration of response. From a cost-effectiveness perspective, surgical myotomy has been estimated to be the most costly strategy (costing approximately $10,800 compared to $3,245 and $3,911 for pneumatic dilation and BoNT/A, respectively), despite higher short- and long-term efficacy [27]. Pneumatic dilation is less costly than BoNT/A so long as the rates of pneumatic dilation efficacy and perforation were >70 % and <10 %, respectively, and the cost of BoNT/A (including endoscopy) was >$450. A Canadian cost minimization analysis comparing BoNT/A to pneumatic dilation suggested that BoNT/A injections were less costly only if the life expectancy was less than 2 years [28].

Complications and Side Effects

An important advantage of BoNT therapy is its relative simplicity and safety. The risk of causing generalized neuromuscular blockade or paralysis at the dose used is negligible. The pooled complication rate of BoNT/A injection compared to pneumatic dilation is 4.5 % compared to 18.8 %. The most common side effects are chest pain and dysphagia [26]. The injection itself may cause transient and minor chest pain in up to 25 %;

heartburn, presumably due to reflux, may occur in up to 5 % patients [18, 26]. Chest pain appears related to the injection rather than to the toxin itself [12]. Paraesophageal tissue inflammation is rare [29]. There has been single case reports of a fatal heart block [30], nonfatal mediastinitis [31], esophageal mucosal ulceration and sinus tract formation [32, 33], and pneumothorax [33].

Impact of Endoscopic Treatment of Subsequent Myotomy

Inflammation and fibrosis of the muscle has been described in animals following both BoNT injection and pneumatic dilation [34]. This has raised the issue whether myotomy is more difficult and less likely to succeed following either of these endoscopic therapies [35–37]. However, this may have resulted from a selection bias where patients who failed prior endoscopic therapy were more likely to be refractory to any therapy. Other studies suggest that myotomy remains effective and safe after prior endoscopic therapy [38–40], although Horgan et al. did find that prior BoNT injection made surgery more technically difficult due to challenges in identifying the submucosal plane [38].

Summary and Recommendations for Current Use

There is level I evidence that a single injection of BoNT can result in short-term improvement of symptoms in patients with achalasia. There is also level I evidence that the duration of response is lower than pneumatic dilation. There is not enough evidence to draw conclusions about the efficacy or safety of repeated injections. Given this data, most experts do not recommend BoNT treatment as first-line therapy. BoNT should be reserved for the treatment of achalasia in patients who are not surgical candidates [41]. It can be used as an alternative in patients who fail to respond to medical therapy or first line in those who are intolerant of medical therapy. Intrasphincteric injection of BoNT into the LES can also be used as a diagnostic guide in patients with insufficient manometric criteria to make the diagnosis, or complicated cases such as those with significant anatomical distortion (i.e., large epiphrenic diverticula), in which it is unclear that more invasive procedures such as pneumatic dilation or surgical myotomy will be beneficial [42].

Other Spastic Conditions of the Esophagus

These include diffuse esophageal spasm, nutcracker esophagus, nonreflux related ineffective esophageal motility, Hypertensive LES, and isolated gastroesophageal junction dysfunction. The use of HRM has yielded a new diagnosis of spastic nutcracker which is defined as hypertensive (frequently repetitive) peristaltic contractions with a distal contractile integral (DCI) of >8,000 mmHg-cm-s [20]. This new classification of nutcracker esophagus may identify a subgroup of patients with nutcracker esophagus that may impact therapy. The pathogenesis of spastic esophageal motility disorders is not well understood. Diffuse esophageal spasm and nutcracker esophagus can be idiopathic (primary) or reflux associated (secondary). Herbella et al. found that 60 % of patients with DES and 69 % of patients with nutcracker esophagus had evidence of pathologic reflux on 24 h ambulatory pH monitoring [43]. Manometric patterns cannot help differentiate primary from secondary esophageal dysmotilities [44]. Patients with reflux-associated DES are more likely to have symptoms of heartburn than patients with idiopathic DES [45].

DES can overlap clinically with achalasia. In a group of patients with documented, symptomatic diffuse esophageal spasm, 65 % had evidence of LES dysfunction manifested by a bird's beak appearance on barium esophagram [46]. As is the case with achalasia, primary spastic disorders of the esophagus appear to be associated with a problem with the inhibitory regulation of esophageal motility, resulting in various forms of disordered contraction [47]. Furthermore, a subset (<5 %) of patients with diffuse esophageal spasm or nonspecific esophageal motor disorders have

been described to progress to achalasia [48–50]. A recent study utilizing simultaneous manometry and esophageal ultrasound found that patients with achalasia, diffuse esophageal spasm, or nutcracker esophagus had an increase in muscle thickness and cross sectional area [51]. It is unclear if this increased muscle thickness is idiopathic or secondary hypertrophy due to prolonged LES dysfunction and functional outlet obstruction. Little else is known about the pathophysiology, pathogenesis, or natural history of these disorders.

Clinically, there is poor correlation between manometric findings and patient symptoms [52–54]. Symptoms in these patients may result from an associated disorder of sensory perception [55], with the manometric abnormalities being markers for this syndrome rather than playing a central role in the pathogenesis. Symptoms of spastic esophageal motility disorders include heartburn, dysphagia, and/or chest pain.

Treatment of Spastic Esophageal Motility Disorders

A more detailed discussion of treatments for spastic esophageal motility disorders is described separately. In general, medical therapy includes diagnosing and treating reflux, calcium channel blockers [56], nitrates [57], and antidepressants (for their neuromodulatory effects). Studies evaluating the effects of medical therapy on symptoms and manometry are limited in number and high rates of side effects [56, 58, 59]. Antidepressants such as trazodone or imipramine improved symptoms of chest pain without impacting esophageal motility [60, 61].

The rationale for using BoNT/A in the treatment of other spastic esophageal disorders is similar to that for achalasia, with an added benefit of its possible effect on nociceptive signaling. BoNT/A injection presents an ideal therapeutic option due to the limited availability of medical therapy and safety profile of intrasphincteric BoNT injection as previously discussed. Similarly to achalasia, a subset of patients with diffuse esophageal spasm may require pneumatic dilation or surgical myotomy. Likewise, issues related to performing pneumatic dilation or myotomy following BoNT injection still apply.

Methods of Endoscopic Injection

Various methods have been described for injecting BoNT/A for the treatment of non-achalasia esophageal motility disorders. The most common is injection of 80–100 units of BoNT/A into the LES. The first report by Miller et al. [62] in 1996 used a method similar to that described initially for achalasia by Pasricha et al. [3]. The BoNT/A was injected in 1 mL aliquots (20 IU/mL) into four quadrants of the LES just above the z-line (total dose: 80 IU). Storr et al. [63] described a technique where patients with diffuse esophageal spasm were treated by injecting 100 IU of BoNT/A linearly along the posterior wall of the esophagus to mimic a surgical myotomy. One hundred units of BoNT/A were diluted in 10 mL of saline. The entire volume was injected endoscopically in 1 mL aliquots starting at the LES and moving proximally every 1–1.5 cm. Endoscopically visible contraction rings were also injected with 1 mL of BoNT/A.

Efficacy

Most of the reports in the literature deal predominantly with diffuse esophageal spasm. BoNT/A injection into the LES decreased symptom severity in patients in 55–100 % of patients with diffuse esophageal spasm [62, 64, 65]. In these studies, the duration of symptom response was at least 6 months with some patients having a response persisting up to 24 months [62]. The largest study of BoNT/A in the treatment of non-achalasia esophageal dysmotilities included 29 patients with noncardiac chest pain, diffuse esophageal spasm, nutcracker esophagus, non-specific esophageal motility disorder, hypertensive LES, and ineffective esophageal motility [64]. This study demonstrated a significant decrease in symptoms of dysphagia, regurgitation, and chest pain.

Summary and Recommendations for Current Use

The use of intrasphincteric BoNT/A injection for non-achalasia spastic esophageal dysmotilities has not been as well studied compared to achalasia. Three published uncontrolled studies involving 5–29 patients have demonstrated improvement in symptoms of chest pain and dysphagia [62–65]. These studies did not assess the effects of BoNT/A on esophageal function in these patients. In 2009, Vanuytsel et al. published a randomized sham-controlled study in abstract form. This was a double blind cross over study involving 22 patients with spastic non-achalasia esophageal disorders. Patients who received BoNT/A had a significant reduction in symptoms of dysphagia but not chest pain, regurgitation, or heartburn [66].

In the absence of a peer-reviewed randomized trial, there is only level III evidence for the efficacy of BoNT in non-achalasic spastic disorders. Our recommendation is that because most cases of idiopathic DES are associated with LES dysfunction and behave similarly, the approach to therapy including the use of BoNT should also be similar. For other spastic conditions, the link between symptoms and manometric abnormalities is more tenuous. Generally, in carefully considered cases, a therapeutic trial of local BoNT injection may help clarify the association between symptoms and the manometric findings, especially given the paucity of alternative treatments. Clearly, more studies need to be done in this group of conditions.

References

1. Montal M. Botulinum neurotoxin: a marvel of protein design. Annu Rev Biochem. 2010;79:591–617.
2. Montecucco C, Schiavo G. Mechanism of action of tetanus and botulinum neurotoxins. Mol Microbiol. 1994;13(1):1–8.
3. Pasricha PJ, Ravich WJ, Kalloo AN. Botulinum toxin for achalasia. Lancet. 1993;341(8839):244–5.
4. Mearin F, Mourelle M, Guarner F, et al. Patients with achalasia lack nitric oxide synthase in the gastro-oesophageal junction. Eur J Clin Invest. 1993;23(11):724–8.
5. Pasricha PJ, Ravich WJ, Kalloo AN. Effects of intrasphincteric botulinum toxin on the lower esophageal

sphincter in piglets. Gastroenterology. 1993;105(4):1045–9.

6. Pasricha PJ, Ravich WJ, Hendrix TR, Sostre S, Jones B, Kalloo AN. Treatment of achalasia with intrasphincteric injection of botulinum toxin. A pilot trial. Ann Intern Med. 1994;121(8):590–1.

7. Annese V, Bassotti G, Coccia G, et al. A multicentre randomised study of intrasphincteric botulinum toxin in patients with oesophageal achalasia. GISMAD achalasia study group. Gut. 2000;46(5):597–600.

8. Goldstein JA, Barkin JS. Botox injection for achalasia: a modified technique. Gastrointest Endosc. 1999; 49(2):272–3.

9. Hoffman BJ, Knapple WL, Bhutani MS, Verne GN, Hawes RH. Treatment of achalasia by injection of botulinum toxin under endoscopic ultrasound guidance. Gastrointest Endosc. 1997;45(1):77–9.

10. Wehrmann T, Schmitt T, Dietrich CF, Caspary WF, Seifert H. Manometrically-guided endoscopic injection of botulinum toxin for esophageal achalasia: a pilot trial. Z Gastroenterol. 2000;38(11):899–903.

11. Brant CQ, Nakao F, Ardengh JC, Nasi A, Ferrari Jr AP. Echoendoscopic evaluation of botulinum toxin intrasphincteric injections in Chagas' disease achalasia. Dis Esophagus. 1999;12(1):37–40.

12. Pasricha PJ, Ravich WJ, Hendrix TR, Sostre S, Jones B, Kalloo AN. Intrasphincteric botulinum toxin for the treatment of achalasia. N Engl J Med. 1995;332(12):774–8.

13. Cuilliere C, Ducrotte P, Zerbib F, et al. Achalasia: outcome of patients treated with intrasphincteric injection of botulinum toxin. Gut. 1997;41(1):87–92.

14. Rollan A, Gonzalez R, Carvajal S, Chianale J. Endoscopic intrasphincteric injection of botulinum toxin for the treatment of achalasia. J Clin Gastroenterol. 1995;20(3):189–91.

15. Fishman VM, Parkman HP, Schiano TD, et al. Symptomatic improvement in achalasia after botulinum toxin injection of the lower esophageal sphincter. Am J Gastroenterol. 1996;91(9):1724–30.

16. Muehldorfer SM, Schneider TH, Hochberger J, Martus P, Hahn EG, Ell C. Esophageal achalasia: intrasphincteric injection of botulinum toxin a versus balloon dilation. Endoscopy. 1999;31(7):517–21.

17. Kolbasnik J, Waterfall WE, Fachnie B, Chen Y, Tougas G. Long-term efficacy of botulinum toxin in classical achalasia: a prospective study. Am J Gastroenterol. 1999;94(12):3434–9.

18. Pasricha PJ, Rai R, Ravich WJ, Hendrix TR, Kalloo AN. Botulinum toxin for achalasia: long-term outcome and predictors of response. Gastroenterology. 1996;110(5):1410–5.

19. Pandolfino JE, Kwiatek MA, Nealis T, Bulsiewicz W, Post J, Kahrilas PJ. Achalasia: a new clinically relevant classification by high-resolution manometry. Gastroenterology. 2008;135(5):1526–33.

20. Pandolfino JE, Ghosh SK, Rice J, Clarke JO, Kwiatek MA, Kahrilas PJ. Classifying esophageal motility by pressure topography characteristics: a study of 400 patients and 75 controls. Am J Gastroenterol. 2008;103(1):27–37.

21. Annese V, Basciani M, Borrelli O, Leandro G, Simone P, Andriulli A. Intrasphincteric injection of botulinum toxin is effective in long-term treatment of esophageal achalasia. Muscle Nerve. 1998;21(11):1540–2.

22. Lange O, Bigalke H, Dengler R, Wegner F, deGroot M, Wohlfarth K. Neutralizing antibodies and secondary therapy failure after treatment with botulinum toxin type A: much ado about nothing? Clin Neuropharmacol. 2009;32(4):213–8.

23. Annese V, Basciani M, Perri F, et al. Controlled trial of botulinum toxin injection versus placebo and pneumatic dilation in achalasia. Gastroenterology. 1996;111(6):1418–24.

24. Vaezi MF, Richter JE, Wilcox CM, et al. Botulinum toxin versus pneumatic dilatation in the treatment of achalasia: a randomised trial. Gut. 1999;44(2):231–9.

25. Ghoshal UC, Chaudhuri S, Pal BB, Dhar K, Ray G, Banerjee PK. Randomized controlled trial of intrasphincteric botulinum toxin A injection versus balloon dilatation in treatment of achalasia cardia. Dis Esophagus. 2001;14(3–4):227–31.

26. Wang L, Li YM, Li L. Meta-analysis of randomized and controlled treatment trials for achalasia. Dig Dis Sci. 2009;54(11):2303–11.

27. Imperiale TF, O'Connor JB, Vaezi MF, Richter JE. A cost-minimization analysis of alternative treatment strategies for achalasia. Am J Gastroenterol. 2000;95(10):2737–45.

28. Panaccione R, Gregor JC, Reynolds RP, Preiksaitis HG. Intrasphincteric botulinum toxin versus pneumatic dilatation for achalasia: a cost minimization analysis. Gastrointest Endosc. 1999;50(4):492–8.

29. Eaker EY, Gordon JM, Vogel SB. Untoward effects of esophageal botulinum toxin injection in the treatment of achalasia. Dig Dis Sci. 1997;42(4):724–7.

30. Malnick SD, Metchnik L, Somin M, Bergman N, Attali M. Fatal heart block following treatment with botulinum toxin for achalasia. Am J Gastroenterol. 2000;95(11):3333–4.

31. Mac Iver R, Liptay M, Johnson Y. A case of mediastinitis following botulinum toxin type A treatment for achalasia. Nat Clin Pract Gastroenterol Hepatol. 2007;4(10):579–82.

32. Fitzgerald JF, Troncone R, Sukerek H, Tolia V. Clinical quiz. Sinus tract between esophagus and fundus. J Pediatr Gastroenterol Nutr. 2002;35(1):38–98.

33. Weusten BL, Samsom M, Smout AJ. Pneumothorax complicating botulinum toxin injection in the body of a dilated oesophagus in achalasia. Eur J Gastroenterol Hepatol. 2003;15(5):561–4.

34. Richardson WS, Willis GW, Smith JW. Evaluation of scar formation after botulinum toxin injection or forced balloon dilation to the lower esophageal sphincter. Surg Endosc. 2003;17(5):696–8.

35. Bonavina L, Incarbone R, Antoniazzi L, Reitano M, Peracchia A. Previous endoscopic treatment does not affect complication rate and outcome of laparoscopic Heller myotomy and anterior fundoplication for oesophageal achalasia. Ital J Gastroenterol Hepatol. 1999;31(9):827–30.

36. Smith CD, Stival A, Howell DL, Swafford V. Endoscopic therapy for achalasia before Heller myotomy results in worse outcomes than Heller myotomy alone. Ann Surg. 2006;243(5):579–84. discussion 84–6.

37. Finley CJ, Kondra J, Clifton J, Yee J, Finley R. Factors associated with postoperative symptoms after laparoscopic Heller myotomy. Ann Thorac Surg. 2010;89(2):392–6.

38. Horgan S, Hudda K, Eubanks T, McAllister J, Pellegrini CA. Does botulinum toxin injection make esophagomyotomy a more difficult operation? Surg Endosc. 1999;13(6):576–9.

39. Rakita S, Bloomston M, Villadolid D, Thometz D, Zervos E, Rosemurgy A. Esophagotomy during laparoscopic Heller myotomy cannot be predicted by preoperative therapies and does not influence long-term outcome. J Gastrointest Surg. 2005;9(2):159–64.

40. Deb S, Deschamps C, Allen MS, et al. Laparoscopic esophageal myotomy for achalasia: factors affecting functional results. Ann Thorac Surg. 2005;80(4): 1191–4. discussion 4-5.

41. Spechler SJ. American gastroenterological association medical position statement on treatment of patients with dysphagia caused by benign disorders of the distal esophagus. Gastroenterology. 1999;117(1):229–33.

42. Katzka DA, Castell DO. Use of botulinum toxin as a diagnostic/therapeutic trial to help clarify an indication for definitive therapy in patients with achalasia. Am J Gastroenterol. 1999;94(3):637–42.

43. Herbella FA, Raz DJ, Nipomnick I, Patti MG. Primary versus secondary esophageal motility disorders: diagnosis and implications for treatment. J Laparoendosc Adv Surg Tech A. 2009;19(2):195–8.

44. Campo S, Traube M. Manometric characteristics in idiopathic and reflux-associated esophageal spasm. Am J Gastroenterol. 1992;87(2):187–9.

45. Hayashi H, Mine K, Hosoi M, et al. Comparison of the esophageal manometric characteristics of idiopathic and reflux-associated esophageal spasm: evaluation by 24-hour ambulatory esophageal motility and pH monitoring. Dig Dis Sci. 2003;48(11):2124–31.

46. Prabhakar A, Levine MS, Rubesin S, Laufer I, Katzka D. Relationship between diffuse esophageal spasm and lower esophageal sphincter dysfunction on barium studies and manometry in 14 patients. AJR Am J Roentgenol. 2004;183(2):409–13.

47. Sifrim D, Janssens J, Vantrappen G. Failing deglutitive inhibition in primary esophageal motility disorders. Gastroenterology. 1994;106(4):875–82.

48. Robson K, Rosenberg S, Lembo T. GERD progressing to diffuse esophageal spasm and then to achalasia. Dig Dis Sci. 2000;45(1):110–3.

49. Paterson WG, Beck IT, Da Costa LR. Transition from nutcracker esophagus to achalasia. A case report. J Clin Gastroenterol. 1991;13(5):554–8.

50. Khatami SS, Khandwala F, Shay SS, Vaezi MF. Does diffuse esophageal spasm progress to achalasia? A prospective cohort study. Dig Dis Sci. 2005;50(9): 1605–10.

51. Dogan I, Puckett JL, Padda BS, Mittal RK. Prevalence of increased esophageal muscle thickness in patients with esophageal symptoms. Am J Gastroenterol. 2007;102(1):137–45.

52. Peters L, Maas L, Petty D, et al. Spontaneous noncardiac chest pain. Evaluation by 24-hour ambulatory esophageal motility and pH monitoring. Gastroenterology. 1988;94(4):878–86.

53. Breumelhof R, Nadorp JH, Akkermans LM, Smout AJ. Analysis of 24-hour esophageal pressure and pH data in unselected patients with noncardiac chest pain. Gastroenterology. 1990;99(5):1257–64.

54. Ghillebert G, Janssens J, Vantrappen G, Nevens F, Piessens J. Ambulatory 24 hour intraoesophageal pH and pressure recordings v provocation tests in the diagnosis of chest pain of oesophageal origin. Gut. 1990;31(7):738–44.

55. Richter JE, Barish CF, Castell DO. Abnormal sensory perception in patients with esophageal chest pain. Gastroenterology. 1986;91(4):845–52.

56. Thomas E, Witt P, Willis M, Morse J. Nifedipine therapy for diffuse esophageal spasm. South Med J. 1986;79(7):847–9.

57. Orlando RC, Bozymski EM. Clinical and manometric effects of nitroglycerin in diffuse esophageal spasm. N Engl J Med. 1973;289(1):23–5.

58. Blackwell JN, Holt S, Heading RC. Effect of nifedipine on oesophageal motility and gastric emptying. Digestion. 1981;21(1):50–6.

59. Nasrallah SM. Nifedipine in the treatment of diffuse oesophageal spasm. Lancet. 1982;2(8310):1285.

60. Clouse RE, Lustman PJ, Eckert TC, Ferney DM, Griffith LS. Low-dose trazodone for symptomatic patients with esophageal contraction abnormalities. A double-blind, placebo-controlled trial. Gastroenterology. 1987;92(4):1027–36.

61. Cannon 3rd RO, Quyyumi AA, Mincemoyer R, et al. Imipramine in patients with chest pain despite normal coronary angiograms. N Engl J Med. 1994;330(20): 1411–7.

62. Miller LS, Parkman HP, Schiano TD, et al. Treatment of symptomatic nonachalasia esophageal motor disorders with botulinum toxin injection at the lower esophageal sphincter. Dig Dis Sci. 1996;41(10): 2025–31.

63. Storr M, Allescher HD, Rosch T, Born P, Weigert N, Classen M. Treatment of symptomatic diffuse esophageal spasm by endoscopic injection of botulinum toxin: a prospective study with long term follow-up. Gastrointest Endosc. 2001;54(6):18A.

64. Miller LS, Pullela SV, Parkman HP, et al. Treatment of chest pain in patients with noncardiac, nonreflux, nonachalasia spastic esophageal motor disorders using botulinum toxin injection into the gastroesophageal junction. Am J Gastroenterol. 2002;97(7): 1640–6.

65. Bashashati M, Andrews C, Ghosh S, Storr M. Botulinum toxin in the treatment of diffuse esophageal spasm. Dis Esophagus. 2010;23(7):554–60.

66. Vanuytsel T, Bisschps R, Holvoet L, et al. A sham-controlled study of injection of botulinum toxin in non-achalasia esophageal motility disorder. Gastroenterology. 2009;136:P131.

Toshitaka Hoppo and Blair A. Jobe

Abstract

Achalasia is the most common primary esophageal motility disorder that is characterized by the inability of the LES to relax and by absence of esophageal body peristalsis due to the inflammatory loss of ganglion cells in the myenteric plexus of the esophageal body and LES, causing dysphagia for solids and liquids, regurgitation of retained food, and chest pain. Pharmacological treatments such as smooth muscle relaxants and botulinum toxin injection are mainly reserved for patients who cannot tolerate more invasive interventions due to severe comorbidities or as a bridge to a more definite treatment option. Pneumatic dilation and laparoscopic Heller myotomy with a partial fundoplication are the most commonly performed to treat achalasia. Recent randomized controlled study to compare these two treatment options demonstrated the similar efficacy in the therapeutic success during the short-term follow-up. However, further modifications of the treatment protocol have the potential for improvement in the outcomes of each option. Since the widespread acceptance of laparoscopic Heller myotomy, the efficacy of pneumatic dilation has been probably underestimated, and gastroenterologists should be trained to successfully perform pneumatic dilation. Note that all treatment options are palliative and none of the treatment options can restore the impaired muscle function of the esophageal body and LES, and it is more important to stratify patients to the optimal initial treatment to accomplish long-term symptom control rather than to simply achieve initial success. For this purpose, the predictors of treatment outcomes should be considered.

Other spastic esophageal motility disorders such as diffuse esophageal spasm (DES), nutcracker esophagus, and hypertensive LES are diagnosed based on well-defined manometric criteria. It is important to evaluate these

T. Hoppo, MD, PhD • B.A. Jobe, MD, FACS (*)
Department of Cardiothoracic Surgery, University of
Pittsburgh Medical Center,
Pittsburgh, PA, USA
e-mail: jobeba@upmc.edu

R. Shaker et al. (eds.), *Principles of Deglutition: A Multidisciplinary Text for Swallowing and its Disorders*,   897
DOI 10.1007/978-1-4614-3794-9_63, © Springer Science+Business Media New York 2013

patients for the presence of GERD as symptoms of spasticity may subside when reflux is properly treated. Myotomy should be considered when GERD has been adequately treated, and symptoms persist despite appropriate reassurance and medical therapy. The outcomes of surgical treatment in this setting are variable.

Keywords

Achalasia • High-resolution manometry • Laparoscopic Heller myotomy • Myenteric plexus • Pneumatic dilation • Pseudoachalasia • Spastic esophageal motility disorders

Introduction

Achalasia, DES, nutcracker esophagus (NE), and the hypertensive lower esophageal sphincter (HTN-LES) fall within the realm of primary esophageal motility disorders because they occur without an identifiable cause such as gastroesophageal reflux disease (GERD) [1]. Secondary esophageal motility disorders are associated with a wide range of disease processes such as GERD and connective tissue disease, and therapy is aimed at the underlying cause [2]. In this chapter, we focus on the diagnosis and surgical treatment of primary esophageal motility disorders including achalasia, DES, NE, and HTN-LES.

Achalasia

Diagnosis

Achalasia is the most common primary esophageal motility disorder and should be suspected for any patients with dysphagia for both solids and liquids, and regurgitation of undigested food and saliva. The differential diagnosis is listed in Table 63.1. It is crucial to exclude any anatomical lesions such as an esophageal malignancy, which can cause pseudoachalasia. The delay in the diagnosis of achalasia frequently occurs due to misinterpretation of typical findings by physicians rather than atypical clinical presentation of the disease [3].

Barium Esophagram

When achalasia is suspected, a barium esophagram with fluoroscopy is the best initial diagnostic test. A barium esophagram may show a symmetrical tapering at the gastroesophageal junction (GEJ) known as a "bird-beak" appearance, with a dilated, aperistaltic, sometimes tortuous esophageal body in the upright position (Fig. 63.1). An air-fluid level in the posterior mediastinum and absence of intragastric air bubble can sometimes be visualized. It should be noted that esophageal dilation may not be present and the "bird-beak" appearance can be misinterpreted as a peptic stricture in the early stage disease. Recently, the timed barium swallow has been introduced as a simple physiologic assessment of esophageal emptying for achalasia [4, 5]. Esophageal emptying is assessed in the upright position over 5 min. Most patients with achalasia have residual barium in the esophagus at the end of 5 min, whereas healthy subjects completely empty barium over 1–2 min. Furthermore, the height of the residual barium column correlates with the severity of regurgitation and the slope of esophageal emptying from 1 to 5 min with the degree of dysphagia. This test can be serially repeated following the treatments to objectively assess the efficacy of treatments performed [6].

Upper Endoscopy

Upper endoscopy may show a dilated esophagus with retained food and some increased resistance at the GEJ as a feeling of "pop," although the

Table 63.1 Differential diagnosis of achalasia

Malignancies (Pseudoachalasia)

Involving the gastroesophageal junction

  Adenocarcinoma (breast, gastric, prostate, and lung)

  Esophageal squamous cell carcinoma

  Lymphoma (gastric, esophageal)

  Esophageal lymphangioma

Remote from the gastroesophageal junction

  Brainstem metastasis

  Hodgkin's disease

  Hepatocellular carcinoma

  Gastric adenocarcinoma

  Poorly differentiated lung cancer

  Reticular cell sarcoma

  Peritoneal mesothelioma

Nonmalignant Esophageal Infiltrative Disorders

  Amyloidosis

  Leiomyomatosis

  Eosinophilic esophagitis

  Sarcoidosis

  Sphingolipidosis

Miscellaneous

  Chagas' disease

  Congenital lower esophageal diaphragmatic web

  Diabetes mellitus

  Familial adrenal insufficiency with alacrima

  Multiple endocrine neoplasia (type IIB)

  Pancreatic pseudocysts

  Postvagotomy

Reproduced from Birgisson et al.: Achalasia: What's new in diagnosis and treatment. Dig Dis 1997;15(Suppl):1–27. Copyright: S. Karger AG, Basel

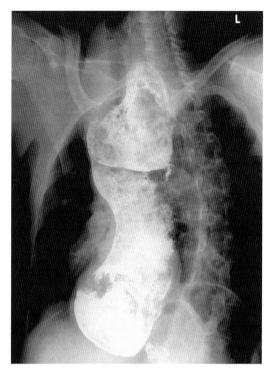

Fig. 63.1 Barium esophagram in the patient with end-stage achalasia. Barium esophagram showed a massive dilated, tortuous esophagus with a sharp narrowing at the gastroesophageal junction

endoscopy usually can be passed through the GEJ. The main role of upper endoscopy is to exclude any anatomical lesions in the upper gastrointestinal tract, which can cause pseudoachalasia. Pseudoachalasia is a clinical syndrome similar to achalasia, being observed in approximately 2–4 % of patients with a suspicious diagnosis of achalasia [7]. In general, patients with pseudoachalasia are older and have a shorter history of dysphagia and remarkable weight loss, although these characteristics are associated with poor specificity [8]. The most common cause of pseudoachalasia is a malignancy infiltrating the GEJ. If pseudoachalasia is still suspicious after the meticulous endoscopic examination, endoscopic ultrasound and/or CT scan should be con-

sidered. Pseudoachalasia can occur as a part of paraneoplastic syndromes, and the treatment of the primary tumor leads to improvement in symptom of achalasia [9, 10].

High-Resolution Manometry

Esophageal manometry has been the gold standard for the diagnosis of achalasia, and it is essential to establish the diagnosis of achalasia by performing manometry prior to the initiation of any treatments. Upper endoscopy is diagnostic in about 1/3 and a barium esophagram in about 2/3 of patients, whereas manometry can establish the accurate diagnosis in over 90 % of patients [11]. Manometric characteristics of achalasia include incomplete relaxation of the LES at deglutition and an aperistaltic esophageal body, sometimes with elevated intraesophageal pressure due to retained food and saliva. Absent or incomplete LES relaxation with wet swallows

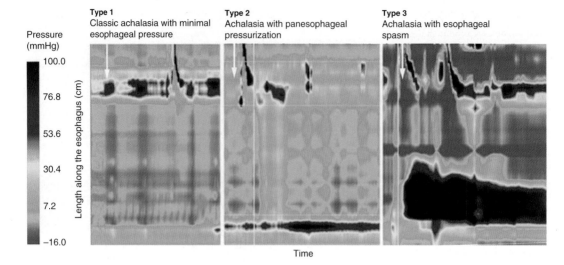

Fig. 63.2 Subclassification of achalasia using high-resolution manometry. High-resolusion manometry showed three types of achalasia: classic achalasia with minimal esophageal pressure (type I), achalasia with panesopha-geal pressurization (type II), and achalasia with esophageal spasm (type III). From V.F. Eckardt et al. Nat Rev Gastroenterol Hepatol 2011;8:311–19 with permission

can be observed in approximately 80 % of patients, whereas the remaining patients may have complete but shortened LES relaxation (<6 s). The resting LES pressure may be elevated in approximately 50 % of patients with achalasia. The aperistalsis is characterized by low amplitude (usually <30 mmHg), simultaneous mirror image (isobaric) waves due to a common cavity phenomenon. The low amplitude wave pattern represents simultaneous fluid movement in a fluid-filled esophagus. "Vigorous" achalasia has been recognized as an achalasia variant when the pressure waves have a higher amplitude and different morphology, indicating simultaneous contractile activity in the esophageal body [12].

Recently, Pandolfino et al. categorized patients with achalasia into three groups based on the new subclassification using high-resolution manometry: achalasia with minimal esophageal pressurization (type I, classic), achalasia with esophageal compression or compartmentalization in the distal esophagus >30 mmHg (type II), and achalasia with spastic contractions (type III) (Fig. 63.2) [13]. In addition, logistic regression analysis demonstrated that type II is a predictor of positive treatment response, whereas type III is associated with negative treatment response, suggesting this subclassification may be useful to predict the outcomes and tailor the treatment options.

Treatment

None of treatments can restore the impaired muscle activity of esophageal body and LES, and all therapeutic approaches are palliative to improve esophageal outlet obstruction. The ultimate goal of treatment is to eliminate dysphagia by opening the LES while preventing gastroesophageal reflux and to achieve long-term symptom control. Since the first report of achalasia which was treated with dilation using a whalebone by Willis in 1674 [14], several treatment options have been introduced. The most commonly performed treatment options are endoscopic pneumatic dilation (see Chap. 39) and surgical myotomy. Pharmacological treatments (see Chaps. 39 and 62) are mainly reserved for patients who cannot tolerate more invasive interventions or as a bridge to a more definite treatment option.

Pneumatic Dilation

The purpose of pneumatic dilation is to widen the LES by forceful stretching using balloons.

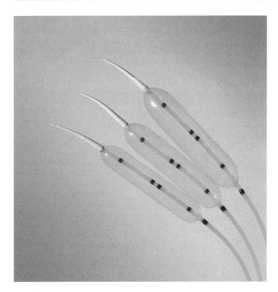

Fig. 63.3 Rigiflex balloon dilation system

Pneumatic dilation is routinely performed in an outpatient setting using the Microinvasive Rigiflex balloon system (Boston Scientific Corp, Natik, MA) (Fig. 63.3). This system includes three different sizes of flexible, polyethylene balloons (3.0, 3.5, and 4.0 cm). The balloon is placed across the GEJ over a guide wire, and the proper position of balloon is confirmed by fluoroscopy or endoscopy. The balloon is gradually inflated following the distension protocol, which varies among centers. To minimize dilation-related complications such as perforation, a graded dilation protocol starting with 3.0 cm, followed by 3.5 cm, and then 4.0 cm balloon in subsequent sessions has been commonly used [15]. A recent review including 24 studies published up to 2009 has demonstrated that the short- or intermediate-term success rates (mean follow-up, 37 months) of 74 %, 86 %, and 90 % were achieved when balloon sizes of 3.0 cm, 3.5 cm, and 4.0 cm were used, respectively [16]. On the other hand, a recent meta-analysis has demonstrated that success rates of pneumatic dilation steadily decline with longitudinal follow-up: 84.8 % at 1 month, 73.8 % at 6 months, 68.2 % at 12 months, and 58.4 % at ≥36 months [17]. Therefore, some have proposed repeated on-demand pneumatic dilations, which can achieve the long-term maintenance of

symptomatic relief in ≥90 % of patients. For the proper patient selection, some risk factors for relapse after pneumatic dilation have been defined as follows: young age (<40 years), male gender, single dilation with a 3.0 cm balloon, postdilation LES pressure > 10–15 mmHg, and poor esophageal emptying on a timed barium swallow [18, 19]. Similar to Botox injection, pneumatic dilation causes submucosal microhemorrhage, leading to submucosal fibrosis and thereby increase the risk of mucosal perforation during a subsequent myotomy.

Surgical Treatment

The first successful surgical treatment of achalasia was described by the German surgeon Ernest Heller in 1913 [20]. With the advances in minimally invasive surgical techniques, Pellegrini et al. introduced a minimally invasive Heller myotomy in 1992 [21]. Currently, laparoscopic Heller myotomy combined with a partial antireflux procedure (Dor or Toupet fundoplication) has been most commonly performed since the randomized controlled study conducted by Richards et al. [22] demonstrated that an additional partial fundoplication significantly reduced postoperative gastroesophageal reflux from 47.6 % to 9.1 % (p=0.005). Surgical myotomy involves a longitudinal incision of the circular and longitudinal muscular layers of the esophagus and extension of this incision onto the stomach across the GEJ. A previous comparison study demonstrated less postoperative dysphagia when the myotomy was extended to 3 cm on to the stomach compared to a group with a 1–2 cm proximal gastric myotomy [23]. Based on this, it has been emphasized that the myotomy must be extended 5–7 cm proximal to the GEJ and at least 2–3 cm distally onto the stomach to adequately divide the gastric sling fibers, thus further decreasing LES pressure and improving dysphagia (Fig. 63.4). Partial fundoplication is preferred to 360° Nissen fundoplication because it results in significantly lower postoperative dysphagia rates (2.8 % vs. 15 %, p=0.001) [24]. Recently, a multicenter, prospective, randomized-controlled trail to compare Dor (Fig. 63.5) vs. Toupet fundoplication (Fig. 63.6) following Heller myotomy for

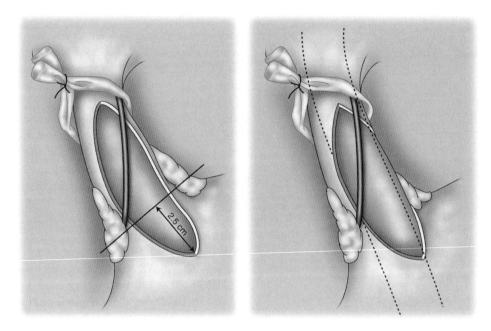

Fig. 63.4 The scheme of Heller myotomy. The complete myotomy should be performed, extending 5–7 cm proximal to the gastroesophageal junction and 2–3 cm onto the gastric cardia

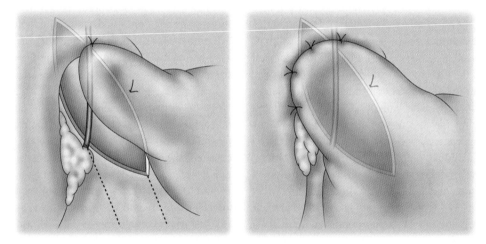

Fig. 63.5 Dor fundoplication (anterior partial fundoplication)

achalasia demonstrated that Heller myotomy provides significant improvement in dysphagia and regurgitation in patients with achalasia regardless of the type of partial fundoplication, and there was a trend towards higher percentage of abnormal postoperative pH testing in patients with Dor compared to those with Toupet, although there was no significant difference [25]. It is extremely important to apply cricoid pressure (Sellick's maneuver) during the induction of general anesthesia in order to prevent aspiration of gastric and intraesophageal contents as patients with achalasia may have retained food or fluid in the esophagus even after a 3-days liquid diet for the attempt to reduce the amount of intraesophageal contents prior to surgery.

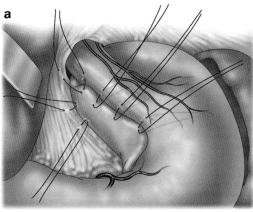

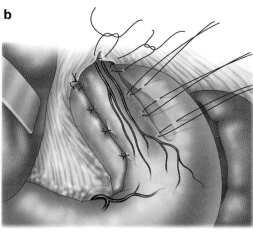

Fig. 63.6 AB Toupet fundoplication (posterior partial fundoplication). From N. Katkhouda et al. Ann Surg 2002;235(4):591–9 modified with permission

In a recent meta-analysis of 39 studies involving nearly 3,100 patients, the good-to-excellent symptom relief with laparoscopic Heller myotomy was achieved in 89.3 % of patients during a mean follow-up of 35 months [17]. Surgical myotomy can be successfully performed after failed pneumatic dilation or botulinum toxin injection; however, this may be associated with lower success rate probably due to submucosal fibrosis [26, 27]. Younger male patients and patients with higher LES pressure more likely have an excellent response to surgical myotomy [28]. In contrast, patients with severe preoperative dysphagia, progressive esophageal enlargement, and low preoperative LES pressures (<30–35 mmHg) are associated with poor outcomes of surgical myotomy [1, 2, 26]. Recent studies to evaluate the long-term outcomes have demonstrated the

consistent efficacy of laparoscopic Heller myotomy even after 10 years [28–30].

Complications of laparoscopic Heller myotomy include death (0.1 %), esophageal perforation (7–15 %), and chronic gastroesophageal reflux (5–55 %) [16]. Esophageal perforation usually can be identified and repaired during the procedure. Reflux symptoms can be controlled by antisecretory medications such as proton pump inhibitors and H2 blockade. The main cause of postoperative dysphagia is an incomplete myotomy, especially on the gastric side. Other etiology of postoperative dysphagia includes submucosal fibrosis, esophageal outlet obstruction due to tight fundoplication, megaesophagus, or gastroesophageal reflux-related complications such as esophagitis and peptic stricture. Redo-myotomy can be considered if the initial myotomy fails to achieve sufficient symptomatic improvement, and a repeat myotomy can be successfully performed on the opposite location to the initial myotomy [31]. Also, pneumatic dilation could be an alternative to redo-myotomy especially for patients who have severe comorbidities or are reluctant to undergo further surgical interventions [32]. Esophagectomy is the last resort for patients who do not respond to any treatment options [33]. In addition, the surgical outcomes of patients who have a sigmoid-shaped megaesophagus have been conflicting [27, 34, 35], and this population may eventually require esophagectomy.

Pneumatic Dilation vs. Surgical Myotomy

With the widespread acceptance of laparoscopic Heller myotomy, surgical myotomy has been most commonly performed and is considered by many to be superior to pneumatic dilation, being supported by recent three meta-analyses which favored surgery as the best treatment to achieve long-term success [17, 36, 37]. However, publication bias and heterogeneity in study designs and technique coupled with the relative rarity of achalasia have caused inadequately powered studies and have not allowed us to make a final conclusion. Recently, Boeckxstaens et al. performed a multicenter, randomized controlled trial involving 14 hospitals in five European countries to compare pneumatic dilation with laparoscopic Heller myotomy with Dor fundoplication [38]. In this study, a total of 201 patients with a new diagnosis of achalasia and an Eckardt symptom score greater than three were randomly assigned to pneumatic dilation ($n = 95$) or laparoscopic Heller myotomy group ($n = 106$). Patients with recurrent symptoms in the dilation group were allowed to undergo repeat on-demand dilation up to a maximum of three series of dilations. There was no significant difference in therapeutic success as defined by the Eckardt score ≤3 at both 1 and 2 years follow-up between pneumatic dilation and myotomy groups (90 vs. 93 % at 1 year and 86 vs. 90 % at 2 years, respectively). Furthermore, there was no significant difference in quality of life or esophageal function as measured by validated questionnaires such as SF-36 and QLQ-OES24 between the two groups. On the other hand, preexisting daily chest pain was identified as a predictor of treatment failure requiring reintervention in both groups, and younger patients (<40 years) in the dilation group required more dilations for recurrent symptoms. In the dilation group, 4 % did not respond to the initial dilations, and 24 % required an additional dilation for the recurrent symptoms. In contrast, 14 % of patients in the myotomy group required dilation due to treatment failure. Esophageal perforation occurred in 4 % in the dilation group and 12 % in the myotomy group. This study concluded that laparoscopic Heller myotomy was not associated with superior rates of therapeutic success compared to pneumatic dilation at least during the short-term period.

There are still several limitations. Therapeutic success rate would vary depending on the criteria used. In this study, the need for subsequent intervention or number of reinterventions was not taken into consideration. In addition, the myotomy was extended from 1 to 1.5 cm on to the stomach, which may have been inadequate to divide the entire bundle of sling fibers, potentially affecting the therapeutic success of myotomy group. It has been reported that the efficacy of pneumatic dilation declines over time, and the long-term follow-up (>5 years) is therefore required. It should be noted that none of treatments can restore the impaired muscle activity of esophageal body and LES, and the ultimate goal of treatment is to accomplish long-term symptom control rather than simply initial success. Therefore, it is important to stratify patients to the optimal initial treatment, which will likely achieve long-term excellent outcome.

Posttreatment Assessment and Management

Currently, there is no consensus on optimal protocols for follow-up and surveillance after the treatment of achalasia. It is important to objectively assess the efficacy of treatment not only for the therapeutic success but also for the early detection of clinical remission and/or complications by using the scoring system, postprocedure manometry, and timed barium swallow, although the efficacy of treatment can be assessed symptomatically. Eckardt et al. have introduced a simple scoring system (Eckardt score), which is the sum of the symptom scores for weight loss [0 (no loss) to 3 (>10 kg loss)], dysphagia, retrosternal pain, and regurgitation [0 (absence of symptoms) to 3 (severe symptoms)] (Tables 63.2 and 63.3) [39]. A postdilation LES pressure less than 10–15 mmHg is generally considered to be a predictor of a good long-term response [18, 19], and a >50 % improvement over baseline in the height of the barium column 1 min after timed barium swallow in conjunction with symptomatic improvement is also a predictor of treatment success [4, 40]. On the other hand, posttreatment surveillance can contribute to detect or prevent long-term complications such as megaesophagus, cancer development, and GERD. A sigmoid-shaped esophagus or megaesophagus occurs in approximately 10 % of patients with a long-standing achalasia (>10 years after the initial diagnosis), especially in patients who have been inadequately treated for years [41]. Furthermore, it is well known that a long-standing achalasia is associated with

Table 63.2 Clinical scoring system for achalasia (Eckardt score)

Score	Symptom			
	Weight loss (kg)	Dysphagia	Retrosternal pain	Regurgitation
0	None	None	None	None
1	<5	Occasional	Occasional	Occasional
2	5–10	Daily	Daily	Daily
3	>10	Each meal	Each meal	Each meal

Reproduced from Eckardt et al. Treatment and surveillance strategies in achalasia: an update. Nat Rev Gastroenterol Hepatol 2011;8:311–19

Table 63.3 Clinical staging of achalasia based on Eckardt score

Stage	Eckardt score[a]	Clinical implication
0	0–1	Remission
I	2–3	Remission
II	4–6	Treatment failure
III	>6	Treatment failure

Reproduced from Eckardt et al. Gastroenterology 1992;103:1732–38

[a]See Table 63.2 for details regarding the Eckardt score

the development of squamous cell carcinoma [42, 43]. A recent prospective study with long-term follow-up of patients who had undergone regular surveillance at 3-years intervals demonstrated a hazard ratio of 28 for developing esophageal squamous cell carcinoma, and cancers occurred at a mean age of 71 years (24 years after the onset of symptoms and 11 years after the diagnosis of achalasia), although a survival benefit from surveillance was observed in only 13 % of patients who developed cancer [44]. The most common long-term complication is GERD, which occurs in up to 25 % of patients who are followed up for more than 30 years [45]. The guideline proposed by the American Society of Gastrointestinal Endoscopy states that there are still insufficient data to support routine endoscopic (cancer) surveillance for patients with achalasia [46]; however, the long-term impact of esophageal mucosal injury, such as esophagitis and Barrett's esophagus, due to GERD on quality of life should not be underestimated, and it should be noted that Barrett's esophagus may progress to adenocarcinoma. Further studies are required to determine the optimal surveillance protocol.

Future Therapy: Peroral Endoscopic Myotomy

With the advances in endoscopic technique and devices, more aggressive endoscopic procedures such as endoscopic submucosal dissection have been invented and performed. Recently, Inoue et al. introduced a new endoscopic approach to treat achalasia, peroral endoscopic myotomy (POEM) [47]. The POEM procedure uses endoscopic submucosal dissection technique to create a submucosal tunnel with CO_2 insufflation. After the injection of saline mixed with indigo carmine into the submucosal space approximately 13 cm proximal to the GEJ, a 2-cm longitudinal small mucosal incision is made to create the entry to the submucosal space (Fig. 63.7a). Then, cap-attached endoscope is inserted into the submucosal space, and submucosal dissection is performed using a specialized endoscopic needle knife distally 2–3 cm on to the gastric cardia across the GEJ (Fig. 63.7b). At the completion of submucosal tunnel creation, only the circular muscular layer is then divided on the entire length of submucosal tunnel (Fig. 63.7c, d). Following the myotomy, adequate opening of the LES is confirmed by passing the endoscope, and the mucosal entry is closed by deploying EndClips (Fig. 63.7e). In the initial report ($n=17$), the dysphagia score and the resting LES pressure were significantly reduced from 10 to 1.3 ($p<0.001$) and from 52.4 to 19.9 mmHg ($p<0.001$), respectively. No complications occurred. During a mean follow-up of 5 months, only one patient developed LA grade B esophagitis requiring PPI. In the follow-up to this study ($n=43$), all patients had an excellent symptomatic relief postoperatively, and the resting LES pressure was reduced from 52.1 to

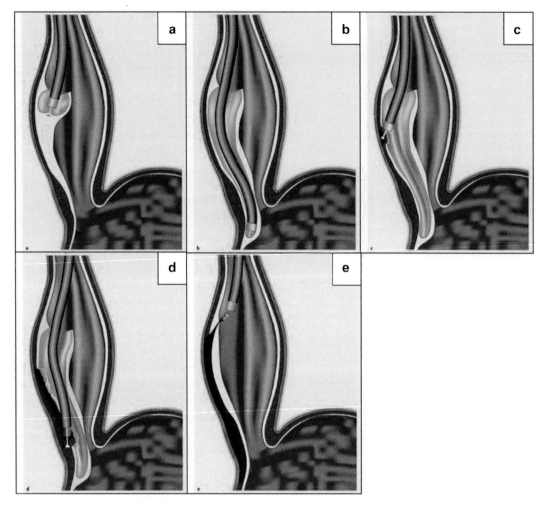

Fig. 63.7 The scheme of peroral endoscopic myotomy (POEM). (**a**) Creation of the entry to submucosal space, (**b**) creation of submucosal tunnel all way down to the gastric cardia, (**c**) beginning of myotomy, (**d**) myotomy is extended onto the gastric cardia, (**e**) the entry is closed by endoclips. From H. Inoue et al. Endoscopy 2010;42(4): 265–71 with permission

18.8 mmHg. No specific complications occurred [48]. Although the initial results of POEM procedure is encouraging, the long-term outcome will be required to meet the widespread acceptance.

Spastic Esophageal Motility Disorders: DES, NE, and HTN-LES

Diagnosis

Most patients with DES and HTN-LES present primarily with dysphagia whereas chest pain is the most common primary symptom in patients with NE [49]. It is important to exclude the presence of coronary artery disease as an integral component of the initial evaluation. As for achalasia, these spastic esophageal motility disorders are diagnosed based on the specific manometric criteria, which are summarized in Table 63.4 [1]. DES is present when more than 20 % of esophageal contractions are simultaneous rather than peristaltic. However, if 100 % of the contractions are simultaneous, the diagnosis is achalasia. Unlike achalasia, the LES profile is typically normal in patients with DES. NE is characterized by high-pressure esophageal contractions, usually in excess of 180 mmHg, and prolonged duration (>6 s) with normal

Table 63.4 Manometric findings of spastic esophageal motility disorders

	Manometric findings
Diffuse esophageal spasm	Simultaneous contractions ≥20 % of wet swallows Intermittent peristalsis Contraction amplitude >3 mmHg but usually not high amplitude Can have repetitive or multipeak contractions (≥three peaks) Can have spontaneous contractions not associated with swallows
Nutcracker esophagus	Increased mean distal amplitude >180 mmHg Normal peristalsis Can be of increased distal duration >6 s
Hypertensive lower esophageal sphincter (HTN-LES)	Resting lower esophageal sphincter pressure >45 mmHg May be incomplete lower esophageal sphincter relaxation

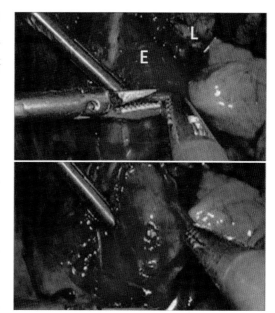

Fig. 63.8 Extended myotomy through a right thoracoscopic approach. (*Upper*): Myotomy is started by cutting the muscle layer of esophagus. *L* lung, *E* esophagus. (*Lower*): Completed myotomy

peristalsis. HTN-LES is defined as a hypertensive LES resting pressure of greater than 45 mmHg; which, LES relaxation may be incomplete in patients with HTN-LES, however they exhibit normal esophageal body peristalsis.

Radiographic findings in patients with DES can be highly variable. Many of these patients have a normal appearing esophagram whereas some show disruption of peristalsis with tertiary activity producing a "corkscrew" or "rosary bead" esophagus [50]. Radiographic findings can be normal in patients with NE and similar to achalasia in patients with HTN-LES. In patients with spastic disorder of the esophagus, ambulatory pH testing is particularly important to perform in order to evaluate for a diagnosis of GERD, which is associated with many of these conditions [2].

Treatment

It is noted that many patients with spastic esophageal motility disorders respond well to confident reassurance that their chest pain is not cardiac in origin or life threatening [51]. If GERD is present, the medical and/or surgical treatment of GERD should be implemented; many of these patients will have resolution of spastic symptoms when the GERD has been appropriately treated. Patients who have not responded to reassurance and medical

therapy should be considered candidates for the surgical treatment, which is myotomy and partial fundoplication. The myotomy is usually extended more proximally than in patients with achalasia and can be tailored to cover the region of spastic smooth muscle as defined by preoperative manometry. When the access to the intrathoracic esophagus is needed, we prefer a right thoracoscopic approach, in which extended myotomy on the entire length of thoracic esophagus from the thoracic inlet to diaphragm can be performed (Fig. 63.8). Several studies have demonstrated excellent results of myotomy in patients with DES [49, 52, 53]. Patti and colleagues reported that dysphagia was relieved in 80 % of patients after thoracoscopic myotomy and in 86 % after laparoscopic myotomy while chest pain was relieved in 75 % and 80 % of patients, respectively. The symptom of regurgitation is also significantly improved in patients with DES [49]. Patients with DES and a primary symptom of chest pain should be counseled that long myotomy may be less likely to relieve this symptom and that the results of surgery are difficult to predict [54]. The outcomes of surgical treatment in patients with NE and chest pain are unpredictable. Patti and colleagues reported that chest pain was relieved only in 50 % of patients with NE whereas dysphagia was improved in 80 % of patients. These authors proposed a myotomy for patients with NE only when the primary symptom is dysphagia [49]. The surgical treatment of HTN-LES is similar to that of achalasia and should be employed when patients present with dysphagia.

Conclusion

Achalasia is the most common primary esophageal motility disorder that is characterized by the inability of the LES to relax and by absence of esophageal body peristalsis due to the inflammatory loss of ganglion cells in the myenteric plexus of the esophageal body and LES, causing dysphagia, regurgitation of retained food, and chest pain. Pneumatic dilation and laparoscopic Heller

myotomy with a partial fundoplication are most commonly performed to treat achalasia. Recent randomized controlled study to compare these two treatment options demonstrated the similar therapeutic efficacy during the short-term follow-up. However, further modifications of the treatment protocol have the potential for improvement in the outcomes of each treatment option. Since the widespread acceptance of laparoscopic Heller myotomy, the efficacy of pneumatic dilation has been probably underestimated, and gastroenterologists should be trained to successfully perform pneumatic dilation. Note that none of the treatment options can restore the impaired muscle function of the esophageal body and LES, and it is more important to stratify patients to the optimal initial treatment to accomplish long-term symptom control rather than to simply achieve initial success by considering the predictors of treatment outcome (Table 63.5) [55].

Table 63.5 Predictors of treatment outcomes in patients with achalasia

Treatment option	Positive predictors	Negative predictors
Botulinum toxin injection	Vigorous achalasia	High initial LES pressure
	Advanced age	Lack of response to first treatment
Pneumatic dilation	Age >40 years	Male gender
	Type II pattern of achalasia on HRM	Incomplete obliteration of the balloon waist or small balloon size (<30 mm)
	Early disease	High postdilation LES pressure
	Postinterventional LES pressure <10 mmHg	Type I or type III patterns of achalasia on HRM
	>50 % improvement over baseline in barium column height 1 min after initiation of a timed barium swallow	Features of advanced disease (e.g., an enlarged esophagus)[a]
		Postinterventional LES pressure >10–15 mmHg
		<50 % improvement over baseline in barium column height 1 min after initiation of a timed barium swallow
Surgical myotomy	Age <40 years	Severe preoperative dysphagia
	Type II pattern of achalasia on HRM	Low initial LES pressure
	Postinterventional LES pressure <10 mmHg	Prior endoscopic treatment (primarily Botox injection)
	>50 % improvement over baseline in barium column height 1 min after initiation of a timed barium swallow	Type I or type III patterns of achalasia on HRM
		Features of advanced disease (e.g., an enlarged esophagus)[a]
		Postinterventional LES pressure >10–15 mmHg
		<50 % improvement over baseline in barium column height 1 min after initiation of a timed barium swallow

Reproduced from Eckardt et al. Treatment and surveillance strategies in achalasia: an update. Nat Rev Gastroenterol Hepatol 2011;8:311–19
[a]A negative predictor in most studies. *HRM* high-resolution manometry, *LES* lower esophageal sphincter

Other spastic esophageal motility disorders such as DES, NE, and HTN-LES are diagnosed based on specific manometric criteria. It is important to evaluate for GERD as an underlying cause as symptoms may subside when GERD is properly treated. The surgical treatment, myotomy and partial fundoplication, should be considered when a diagnosis of GERD has been excluded, and reassurance and medical therapy fail. However, the outcomes of surgical treatment in this setting are variable.

References

1. Richter JE. Oesophageal motility disorders. Lancet. 2001;358(9284):823–8.
2. Herbella FA, Raz DJ, Nipomnick I, Patti MG. Primary versus secondary esophageal motility disorders: diagnosis and implications for treatment. J Laparoendosc Adv Surg Tech A. 2009;19(2):195–8.
3. Eckardt VF, Kohne U, Junginger T, Westermeier T. Risk factors for diagnostic delay in achalasia. Dig Dis Sci. 1997;42(3):580–5.
4. Vaezi MF, Baker ME, Achkar E, Richter JE. Timed barium oesophagram: better predictor of long term success after pneumatic dilation in achalasia than symptom assessment. Gut. 2002;50(6):765–70.
5. de Oliveira JM, Birgisson S, Doinoff C, et al. Timed barium swallow: a simple technique for evaluating esophageal emptying in patients with achalasia. AJR Am J Roentgenol. 1997;169(2):473–9.
6. Andersson M, Lundell L, Kostic S, et al. Evaluation of the response to treatment in patients with idiopathic achalasia by the timed barium esophagogram: results from a randomized clinical trial. Dis Esophagus. 2009;22(3):264–73.
7. Gockel I, Eckardt VF, Schmitt T, Junginger T. Pseudoachalasia: a case series and analysis of the literature. Scand J Gastroenterol. 2005;40(4):378–85.
8. Sandler RS, Bozymski EM, Orlando RC. Failure of clinical criteria to distinguish between primary achalasia and achalasia secondary to tumor. Dig Dis Sci. 1982;27(3):209–13.
9. Hejazi RA, Zhang D, McCallum RW. Gastroparesis, pseudoachalasia and impaired intestinal motility as paraneoplastic manifestations of small cell lung cancer. Am J Med Sci. 2009;338(1):69–71.
10. Liu W, Fackler W, Rice TW, Richter JE, Achkar E, Goldblum JR. The pathogenesis of pseudoachalasia: a clinicopathologic study of 13 cases of a rare entity. Am J Surg Pathol. 2002;26(6):784–8.
11. Howard PJ, Maher L, Pryde A, Cameron EW, Heading RC. Five year prospective study of the incidence, clinical features, and diagnosis of achalasia in Edinburgh. Gut. 1992;33(8):1011–5.
12. Richter JE. Achalasia: an update. J Neurogastroenterol Motil. 2010;16(3):232–42.
13. Pandolfino JE, Kwiatek MA, Nealis T, Bulsiewicz W, Post J, Kahrilas PJ. Achalasia: a new clinically relevant classification by high-resolution manometry. Gastroenterology. 2008;135(5):1526–33.
14. Cohen S, Parkman HP. Treatment of achalasia—whalebone to botulinum toxin. N Engl J Med. 1995;332(12):815–6.
15. Kadakia SC, Wong RK. Graded pneumatic dilation using Rigiflex achalasia dilators in patients with primary esophageal achalasia. Am J Gastroenterol. 1993;88(1):34–8.
16. Richter JE. Update on the management of achalasia: balloons, surgery and drugs. Expert Rev Gastroenterol Hepatol. 2008;2(3):435–45.
17. Campos GM, Vittinghoff E, Rabl C, et al. Endoscopic and surgical treatments for achalasia: a systematic review and meta-analysis. Ann Surg. 2009;249(1):45–57.
18. Eckardt VF, Aignherr C, Bernhard G. Predictors of outcome in patients with achalasia treated by pneumatic dilation. Gastroenterology. 1992;103(6):1732–8.
19. Hulselmans M, Vanuytsel T, Degreef T, et al. Long-term outcome of pneumatic dilation in the treatment of achalasia. Clin Gastroenterol Hepatol. 2010;8(1):30–5.
20. Heller S. Prophylactic measures for people growing blind. Cal State J Med. 1913;11(2):63–4.
21. Pellegrini C, Wetter LA, Patti M, et al. Thoracoscopic esophagomyotomy. Initial experience with a new approach for the treatment of achalasia. Ann Surg. 1992;216(3):291–6. discussion 296–299.
22. Richards WO, Torquati A, Holzman MD, et al. Heller myotomy versus Heller myotomy with Dor fundoplication for achalasia: a prospective randomized double-blind clinical trial. Ann Surg. 2004;240(3):405–12.
23. Wright AS, Williams CW, Pellegrini CA, Oelschlager BK. Long-term outcomes confirm the superior efficacy of extended Heller myotomy with Toupet fundoplication for achalasia. Surg Endosc. 2007;21(5):713–8.
24. Rebecchi F, Giaccone C, Farinella E, Campaci R, Morino M. Randomized controlled trial of laparoscopic Heller myotomy plus Dor fundoplication versus Nissen fundoplication for achalasia: long-term results. Ann Surg. 2008;248(6):1023–30.
25. Rawlings A, Soper NJ, Oelschlager B, et al. Laparoscopic Dor versus Toupet fundoplication following Heller myotomy for achalasia: results of a multicenter, prospective, randomized-controlled trial. Surg Endosc. 2012;26(1):18–26.
26. Schuchert MJ, Luketich JD, Landreneau RJ, et al. Minimally-invasive esophagomyotomy in 200 consecutive patients: factors influencing postoperative outcomes. Ann Thorac Surg. 2008;85(5):1729–34.
27. Snyder CW, Burton RC, Brown LE, Kakade MS, Finan KR, Hawn MT. Multiple preoperative endoscopic interventions are associated with worse outcomes after laparoscopic Heller myotomy for achalasia. J Gastrointest Surg. 2009;13(12):2095–103.
28. Costantini M, Zaninotto G, Guirroli E, et al. The laparoscopic Heller-Dor operation remains an effective treatment for esophageal achalasia at a minimum 6-year follow-up. Surg Endosc. 2005;19(3):345–51.

29. Bonatti H, Hinder RA, Klocker J, et al. Long-term results of laparoscopic Heller myotomy with partial fundoplication for the treatment of achalasia. Am J Surg. 2005;190(6):874–8.

30. Gockel I, Junginger T, Eckardt VF. Long-term results of conventional myotomy in patients with achalasia: a prospective 20-year analysis. J Gastrointest Surg. 2006;10(10):1400–8.

31. Gockel I, Junginger T, Eckardt VF. Persistent and recurrent achalasia after Heller myotomy: analysis of different patterns and long-term results of reoperation. Arch Surg. 2007;142(11):1093–7.

32. Guardino JM, Vela MF, Connor JT, Richter JE. Pneumatic dilation for the treatment of achalasia in untreated patients and patients with failed Heller myotomy. J Clin Gastroenterol. 2004;38(10):855–60.

33. Duranceau A, Liberman M, Martin J, Ferraro P (2010). End-stage achalasia. Dis Esophagus. doi: 10.1111/j.1442-2050.2010.01157.x.

34. Mineo TC, Ambrogi V. Long-term results and quality of life after surgery for oesophageal achalasia: one surgeon's experience. Eur J Cardiothorac Surg. 2004;25(6):1089–96.

35. Patti MG, Feo CV, Diener U, et al. Laparoscopic Heller myotomy relieves dysphagia in achalasia when the esophagus is dilated. Surg Endosc. 1999;13(9):843–7.

36. Wang L, Li YM, Li L. Meta-analysis of randomized and controlled treatment trials for achalasia. Dig Dis Sci. 2009;54(11):2303–11.

37. Wang L, Li YM, Li L, Yu CH. A systematic review and meta-analysis of the Chinese literature for the treatment of achalasia. World J Gastroenterol. 2008;14(38):5900–6.

38. Boeckxstaens GE, Annese V, des Varannes SB, et al. Pneumatic dilation versus laparoscopic Heller's myotomy for idiopathic achalasia. N Engl J Med. 2011;364(19):1807–16.

39. Eckardt VF. Clinical presentations and complications of achalasia. Gastrointest Endosc Clin North Am. 2001;11(2):281–92. vi.

40. Oezcelik A, Hagen JA, Halls JM, et al. An improved method of assessing esophageal emptying using the timed barium study following surgical myotomy for achalasia. J Gastrointest Surg. 2009;13(1):14–8.

41. Mattioli S, Di Simone MP, Bassi F, et al. Surgery for esophageal achalasia. Long-term results with three different techniques. Hepatogastroenterology. 1996;43(9):492–500.

42. Chuong JJ, DuBovik S, McCallum RW. Achalasia as a risk factor for esophageal carcinoma. A reappraisal. Dig Dis Sci. 1984;29(12):1105–8.

43. Sandler RS, Nyren O, Ekbom A, Eisen GM, Yuen J, Josefsson S. The risk of esophageal cancer in patients with achalasia. A population-based study. J Am Med Assoc. 1995;274(17):1359–62.

44. Leeuwenburgh I, Scholten P, Alderliesten J, et al. Long-term esophageal cancer risk in patients with primary achalasia: a prospective study. Am J Gastroenterol. 2010;105(10):2144–9.

45. Csendes A, Braghetto I, Burdiles P, Korn O, Csendes P, Henriquez A. Very late results of esophagomyotomy for patients with achalasia: clinical, endoscopic, histologic, manometric, and acid reflux studies in 67 patients for a mean follow-up of 190 months. Ann Surg. 2006;243(2):196–203.

46. Hirota WK, Zuckerman MJ, Adler DG, et al. ASGE guideline: the role of endoscopy in the surveillance of premalignant conditions of the upper GI tract. Gastrointest Endosc. 2006;63(4):570–80.

47. Inoue H, Minami H, Kobayashi Y, et al. Peroral endoscopic myotomy (POEM) for esophageal achalasia. Endoscopy. 2010;42(4):265–71.

48. Inoue H, Kudo SE. Per-oral endoscopic myotomy (POEM) for 43 consecutive cases of esophageal achalasia. Nihon Rinsho. 2010;68(9):1749–52.

49. Patti MG, Gorodner MV, Galvani C, et al. Spectrum of esophageal motility disorders: implications for diagnosis and treatment. Arch Surg. 2005;140(5):442–8. discussion 448–449.

50. Hewson EG, Ott DJ, Dalton CB, Chen YM, Wu WC, Richter JE. Manometry and radiology. Complementary studies in the assessment of esophageal motility disorders. Gastroenterology. 1990;98(3):626–32.

51. Ward BW, Wu WC, Richter JE, Hackshaw BT, Castell DO. Long-term follow-up of symptomatic status of patients with noncardiac chest pain: is diagnosis of esophageal etiology helpful? Am J Gastroenterol. 1987;82(3):215–8.

52. Almansa C, Hinder RA, Smith CD, Achem SR. A comprehensive appraisal of the surgical treatment of diffuse esophageal spasm. J Gastrointest Surg. 2008;12(6):1133–45.

53. Leconte M, Douard R, Gaudric M, Dumontier I, Chaussade S, Dousset B. Functional results after extended myotomy for diffuse oesophageal spasm. Br J Surg. 2007;94(9):1113–8.

54. Henderson RD, Ryder D, Marryatt G. Extended esophageal myotomy and short total fundoplication hernia repair in diffuse esophageal spasm: five-year review in 34 patients. Ann Thorac Surg. 1987;43(1):25–31.

55. Eckardt AJ, Eckardt VF. Treatment and surveillance strategies in achalasia: an update. Nat Rev Gastroenterol Hepatol. 2011;8(6):311–9.

56. Katkhouda N, Khalil MR, Manhas S, et al. Andre Toupet: surgeon technician par excellence. Ann Surg. 2002;235(4):591–9.

Vocal Fold Medialization, Arytenoid Adduction, and Partial Pharyngectomy

64

C. Blake Simpson

Abstract

Multiple operative techniques have been designed to address dysphonia and dysphagia that results from unilateral vocal fold paralysis (VFP). This chapter addresses three main procedures: silastic medialization laryngoplasty, arytenoid adduction, and hypopharyngeal pharyngoplasty. Silastic medialization laryngoplasty (ML) is an excellent long-term solution for repositioning a paralyzed vocal fold near the middle to correct glottic insufficiency and minimize aspiration. In patients with unilateral VFP who have a lack of vocal process contact during phonation (large posterior gap), shortened immobile vocal fold, and those with vocal folds at different levels, Arytenoid Adduction (AA) should be considered in addition to ML. The improved posterior glottic closure afforded by an AA can result in better voice and less aspiration in select cases. For "high vagal palsy", Hypopharyngeal Pharyngoplasty (HPPP) is a surgical procedure that can be used in conjunction with ML and AA. It tightens the paralyzed inferior constrictor and reduces the size of the pyriform sinus to limit the buildup of secretions. In addition, a cricopharyngeal (CP) myotomy in often performed in conjunction with the HPPP to facilitate opening of the CP, which often fails to relax as a result of CN X injuries.

Keywords

Arytenoid adduction • Aspiration • Dysphonia • Partial pharyngectomy • Symptomatic glottic insufficiency • Vocal fold medialization

Introduction

Multiple operative techniques have been designed to address dysphonia and dysphagia that result from unilateral vocal fold paralysis. This chapter addresses three main procedures [1]: silastic medialization laryngoplasty, arytenoid adduction, and hypopharyngeal pharyngoplasty.

C.B. Simpson, MD (✉)
Department of Otorhinolaryngology—Head and Neck
Surgery, Medical Arts and Research Center,
San Antonio, TX, USA
e-mail: simpsonc@uthscsa.edu

R. Shaker et al. (eds.), *Principles of Deglutition: A Multidisciplinary Text for Swallowing and its Disorders*, DOI 10.1007/978-1-4614-3794-9_64, © Springer Science+Business Media New York 2013

911

Silastic Medialization Laryngoplasty

It is important to note that silastic medialization laryngoplasty (ML) is designed to be a long-term treatment for symptomatic UVFP. Experimental and clinical evidence supports the efficacy of silastic ML over a prolonged period of time. However, it should be noted that silastic ML is fully reversible, that is, the implant can be removed if return of vocal fold mobility occurs, or if a revision surgery needs to be performed at a later date. There is minimal tissue reactivity to silastic over time; generally a thin fibrous capsule surrounding the implant is all that is seen months to years following ML.

Indications

- Symptomatic Glottic Insufficiency (Dysphonia, Aspiration), especially if there is little to no chance of return of vocal fold motion

Contraindications

- Previous history of radiation therapy to the larynx (relative)
- Malignant disease overlying the laryngotracheal complex
- Poor abduction of the contralateral vocal fold (due to airway concerns)
- Presence of lesion on the vocal folds

No single implant material is superior to the others for performing ML. It is really a matter of surgeon preference and experience. The author advocates hand carving of a medium-grade Silastic block (available from Medtronic ENT) using the surgical technique described by Netterville [2]. This leads to precise medialization, superior voice results, and a better understanding of the dynamics of vocal fold medialization. However, other systems (such as the preformed implants in the Montgomery Thyroplasty Implant System [Boston Medical Products, Inc, Westborough, Massachusetts]) or strip Gore-Tex (William L. Gore, Flagstaff, Arizona) and VoCoM Hydroxyapatite (Smith and Nephew, Bartlett, Tennessee) can be employed successfully as well.

Surgical Procedure [1–3]

The surgical region is liberally infiltrated with 1 % lidocaine with 1:100,000 epinephrine, from the hyoid down to the cricoid cartilage, on the side of the intended surgery. Typically 15 ccs are used. Preoperative IV Decadron (10 mg) is administered. Four percent lidocaine and oxymetazoline nasal spray is applied to the most patent nasal cavity. Placement of an indwelling nasolaryngeal fiberptic scope with videomonitoring of the larynx is employed during the entire surgical case. The visual feedback of the larynx is invaluable when performing this surgery. One inch tape is used to secure the fiberoptic scope to a modified IV pole hanging above the patient's head. The neck is then prepped and drapped, including a clear overdrape to allow manipulation of the scope during the case (Fig. 64.1). A horizontal incision is placed in a skin crease at the level of the mid-thyroid cartilage, typically 5–6 cm in length. Subplatysmal flaps are raised to the hyoid superiorly and the upper portion of the cricoid below; retention hooks are used to secure the flaps out of the way. The midline raphae are divided between the strap muscles with cautery, exposing the laryngeal cartilage. A single prong hook is placed under the thyroid notch, and the larynx is retracted to the side opposite the paralysis, bringing the entire hemilaryngeal cartilage into view (Fig. 64.2). The outer perichondrium of the thyroid cartilage is then

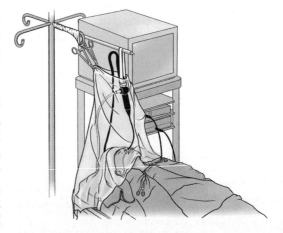

Fig. 64.1 Diagram of typical prep/drape for medialization laryngoplasty

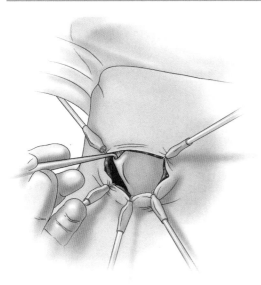

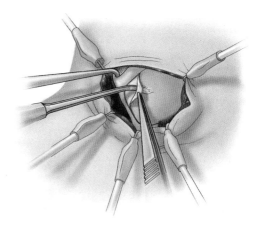

Fig. 64.3 Posteriorly based outer perichondrial flap elevation

Fig. 64.2 Single prong hook under the thyroid notch to gain exposure to thyroid ala

incised with a 15-blade, and a posteriorly based flap is raised with a cottle or freer elevator. This requires serial release of the perichondrium superiorly and inferiorly (Fig. 64.3). The inferior border of the thyroid ala has muscle fibers from the cricothyroid muscle inserting onto it, so these must be divided (typically with bipolar cautery followed by 15-blade division). This exposes the inferior border, so that the correct orientation of the window can be properly determined (Fig. 64.4).

The exposure of the inferior thyroid cartilage border must extend posterior to the muscular tubercle (an inferior-projecting extension of the thyroid ala), as the angulation of this process can cause mistaken orientation of the medialization window. The downward projection of the muscular tubercle must be ignored when determining the horizontal plane of the inferior border of the thyroid cartilage (Fig. 64.5).

A window is outlined in the thyroid cartilage, measuring 6×13 mm using the window size gauge instrument. The window is placed 3 mm above the inferior border of the thyroid cartilage. Placement of the window any higher (superior) may result in medialization of the false vocal fold or ventricular mucosa, with poor voice results. The window is "set back" from the midline of the thyroid cartilage by a distance of 5 mm in women and 7 mm in men. This set back helps avoid medialization of the anterior

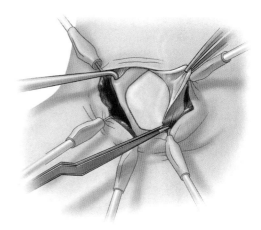

Fig. 64.4 Bipolar cautery and sharp dissection are used to expose the inferior border of the thyroid ala

vocal fold, which may result in "pressed" voice (Fig. 64.6). The window of cartilage is then removed (with a 15-blade, Kerrison rongeur, or drill, depending on laryngeal calcification). In younger patients, the cartilage is soft, and can be removed with a 15-blade, being cautious to avoid penetration of the cartilage with resultant paraglottic bleeding. Often, a triangle of cartilage can be incised and then removed from the posterior superior aspect of the window using a Woodson elevator. Once an entry point through the thyroid cartilage is established, a Kerrison rongeur can be used to complete the window (Fig. 64.7). When drilling the window, a 2–3 mm cutting burr is used. The inner perichondrium that lies deep to the window is removed,

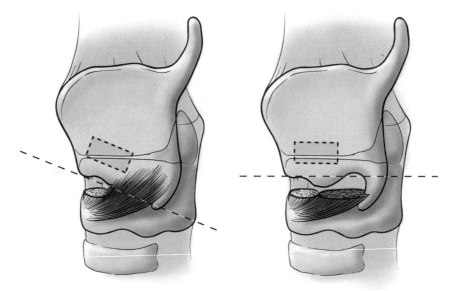

Fig. 64.5 Diagram showing the incorrect (*left*) and correct (*right*) method of exposing the inferior thyroid ala.
On the *left*, the cricothyroid fibers have not been divided
from the inferior border, and an incorrect, downwardly
sloping line is used to trace the proposed horizontal plane

of the vocal fold. On the *right*, a thorough dissection of the
inferior thyroid ala allows the true horizontal plane of
the vocal fold to be outlined, insuring correct window
placement. In this case, the inferior muscular tubercle is
ignored when determining the plane

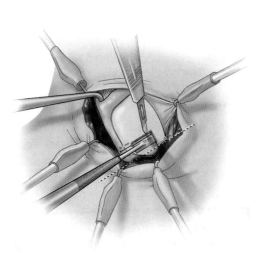

Fig. 64.6 Correct placement of the medialization window, 5–7 mm from the midline of the thyroid ala (5 mm—
females, 7 mm—males) and 3 mm above the inferior
border. The window size gauge instrument is 6 × 13 mm in
dimension

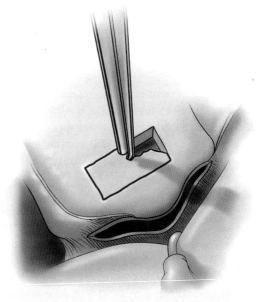

Fig. 64.7 A Kerrison rongeur is then used to remove the
remainder of the cartilage, after gaining entry with a
15-blade or drill

exposing the thyroarytenoid muscle fascia. Often this inner perichondrium is removed piecemeal with the Kerrison rongeur during primary cartilage removal of the window. However if it is intact, it may be incised superiorly, posteriorly, and inferiorly (Fig. 64.8). A surgical plane is then developed with the right angle elevator within the paraglottic space (just superficial to the TA fascia) in all directions around the window except anterior (Fig. 64.9). Dissection anterior to the window may result in perforation into the airway through the very thin (and closely adherent) ventricular mucosa and should be avoided. Incising the inner perichondrium and establishing a surgical plane in the paraglottic space is important to successful medialization. An intact perichondrium remains tightly bound to the thyroid cartilage (even with undermining) and often provides great resistance to medialization; it is analogous to trying to displace a trampoline. In contrast, the paraglottic space allows for unencumbered medialization, once the inner perichondrium is incised. The inferior paraglottic surgical plane should extend developed below the inferior strut of the thyroid ala. This can be achieved by undermining from below the strut, using the long elevator. The TA fascia in the window should be displaced medially to avoid perforation/penetration of the TA muscle fibers. The TA muscle is then displaced within the window while visualizing the effects on vocal fold displacement on the videomonitor. This helps establish the correct plane of medialization. Within the window, the inferior aspect generally is the most desirable for medialization and corresponds to the free edge of the vocal fold. Displacement within the superior aspect

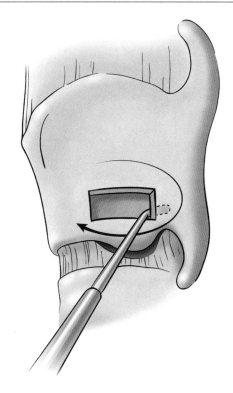

Fig. 64.9 Undermining within the paraglottic space (deep to the inner perichondrium) superiorly, posteriorly, and inferiorly

of the window usually medializes the false vocal fold or ventricular mucosa, and results in suboptimal results in most cases. A depth gauge is used to displace the paralyzed TA muscle medially, while the patient counts to 10 (Fig. 64.10). A combination of visual feedback from the videolaryngoscopy monitor and the patient's vocal quality is used to judge the correct amount of medialization needed. Ideally, the paralytic vocal fold will assume a straight contour in the midline, allowing for complete glottic closure and significant voice improvement. Two principal measurements are obtained: the distance from the anterior window to the point of maximal displacement (i.e. the tip of the depth gauge), which is referred to as the "A" measurement in the corresponding illustration. This is often 10–13 mm in length, as posterior medialization most often is used (in women this measurement is typically at the mid aspect of the window, 6–8 mm. However, it is not uncommon for the point of maximal displacement to be at the anterior portion of the window in females) (Fig. 64.11). The other measurement is the depth of

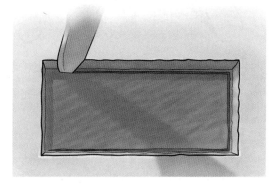

Fig. 64.8 Release of the inner perichondrium, with a 15-blade superiorly, posteriorly, and inferiorly

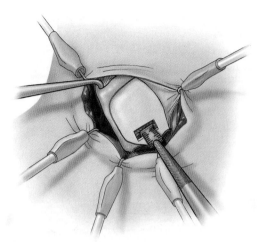

Fig. 64.10 Displacement of TA muscle with the depth gauge. Note the displacement is generally at the posterior, inferior border of the window

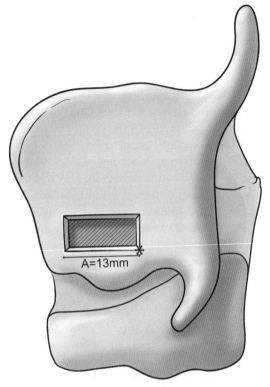

medialization and is read off of the depth gauge instrument. The measurement is taken off the inner table of the cartilage, not the outer table (Fig. 64.12). Typically, 5–7 mm of medialization are needed at the posterior aspect of the window. It is rare that any medialization is needed at the anterior aspect of the window. Once the appropriate measurements are made, $3 \times 1/2$ cottonoids soaked in 1:10,000 epinephrine are placed inside the window to aid in hemostasis while the implant is carved. An implant is then carved out of medium-grade Silastic wedge on the back table to meet the specifications provided by the depth gauge measurements. A preformed 20-mm wedge block ("silicone strip" by Medtronic ENT, Jacksonville, FL) simplifies this task and shortens surgical time. This section describes its proper preparation for implantation.

The distance from the anterior edge of the window to the point of maximal medialization (typically 11–13 mm in males and 6–10 mm in females) is measured along the block (measurement "A" on the diagram), and a dot is placed with a marking pen (Fig. 64.13). From the dot, a line is extended into the substance of the block (measurement "B" in the diagram) which corresponds to the depth of medialization (Fig. 64.14). This measurement was obtained using the depth gauge and is typically 5–7 mm in most patients. Lines are then drawn connecting the tip of line B with both the anterior and posterior portions of the block (measurement "C" and "D," respectively) (Fig. 64.15). This creates a character-

Fig. 64.11 Distance from the anterior window to the point of maximal displacement of the depth gauge. This is generally 10–13 mm in males and 6–8 in females. This is referred to as the "A" length during implant carving

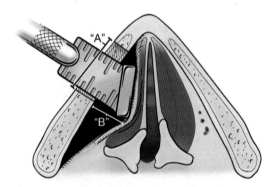

Fig. 64.12 Measuring the depth of medialization using the depth gauge. This is typically 5–7 mm. The measurement should be taken of the inner (deep) aspect of the cartilage. This is referred to as the "B" measurement during implant carving

istic triangular shape of the implant, with the edge "C" corresponding to the portion of the implant which displaces the vocalis muscle medially, and segment "D" corresponding to the posterior extension of the implant which helps to hold it in place.

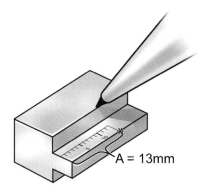

Fig. 64.13 Carving a left-sided implant. A mark is made on the implant corresponding to the point of maximal medialization ("A" length from Fig. 64.11)

A 10-blade is used to cut along lines C and D, removing the excess portion of the block (Fig. 64.16). One must be careful to make these cuts at 90° angles to maintain the integrity of the depth of the implant. The implant is placed in a customized implant holder for further shaping. The plane of medialization (lower, middle, or upper portion of the window) which corresponds to the plane of the true vocal fold is marked with a line along the implant border (Fig. 64.17). In general, this is the inferior or lower

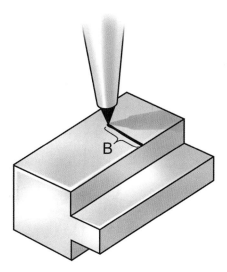

Fig. 64.14 A line is drawn perpendicular, beginning from the "A" mark, extending the distance determined by the depth of medialization ("B" length from Fig. 64.12)

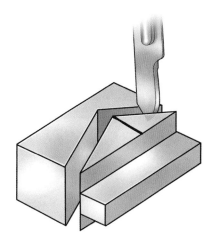

Fig. 64.16 Trimming excess silastic using a 10-blade

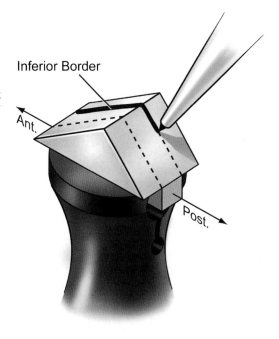

Fig. 64.17 Marking the plane of medialization (corresponding to the inferior border in most implants)

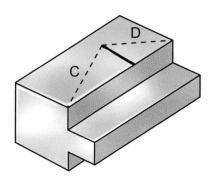

Fig. 64.15 A triangular implant is then created

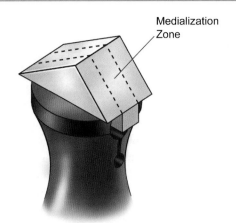

Fig. 64.18 Medialization should only occur within the "medialization zone" indicated. The implant material above and below this zone is strictly used as flanges to hold the implant in place

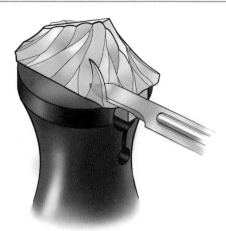

Fig. 64.20 Sculpting the final implant contour. Note the line of medialization is at the inferior aspect of the medialization zone

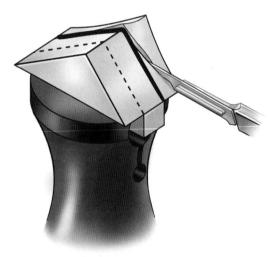

Fig. 64.19 Removal of silastic using a 15-blade

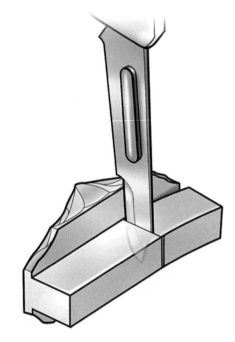

Fig. 64.21 Posterior 7-mm slot is removed from the implant to allow placement

border of the window space. The line must be drawn along the medialization "zone" in the middle of the implant, not on the upper or lower "flange" portions of the implant (Fig. 64.18). Using a 15-blade, the excess silastic is removed superior and inferior to the plane of medialization, preserving an approximately 3 mm strip of material along the indicated line (Figs. 64.19 and 64.20). The extreme upper and lower edges of the implant must be thinned considerably to make the flanges flexible. This will facilitate easier placement of a large implant through the window. The A and B measurements are rechecked for accuracy.

Finally, the implant is removed from the holder, and the posterior 7 mm of the "slot" is removed from the implant (Fig. 64.21). The implant is now ready for placement.

The implant is placed through the window using two addson forceps with teeth. The posterior inferior part of the implant should be advanced into the paraglottic space first.

Once the implant is in place, the patient's voice should be rechecked, and the laryngoscopic image should be observed to insure that the medialization recreates what was achieved with the depth gauge. If the voice sounds "pressed" or "strained," the anterior portion of the implant should be grasped and pulled out of the window slightly. If this improves the voice, then there is too much medialization anteriorly, and the implant should be removed, and reduced an appropriate amount. On the other hand, if the voice sounds breathy, the implant can be displaced at the posterior aspect of the window. If the voice improves, an implant with a greater depth of medialization may be necessary. The excess implant lateral to the thyroid ala is then trimmed to make it flush with the cartilage (Fig. 64.22). The implant is then secured to the thyroid cartilage with permanent sutures (4.0 prolene) around the inferior "strut" of cartilage (Fig. 64.23). Hemostasis is obtained and all layers are closed including outer perichondrium, strap muscles, platysmal, and skin. In general, a drain is not necessary, but may be placed depending on the surgeon's preference.

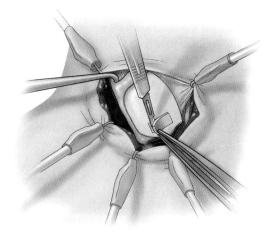

Fig. 64.22 Trimming of excess implant

Postoperative care after medialization is as follows:

- Overnight 23 h observation
- Pain management
- IV steroids at q8 h intervals (Decadron 8 mg, then 4 mg)
- Elevation of the head of bed
- A return to clinic is scheduled 2–4 weeks after surgery
- In general, the patient's voice is poor within 6–8 h after surgery due to edema

Complications/Common Surgical Errors can occur. A common mistake includes medialization too far superiorly within the window. In this instance, the indwelling laryngoscopic image will show a medialized false vocal fold or bulging of the ventricular mucosa—sometimes a subtle finding. Another common mistake is excess medialization of the anterior commissure. In this case the voice has a distinctive "pressed" or "strained" quality. Implant extrusion or exposure is another potential complication. Implant extrusion probably arises due to unrecognized tear in the ventricular mucosa and soiling of the wound with respiratory secretions. The implant may extrude

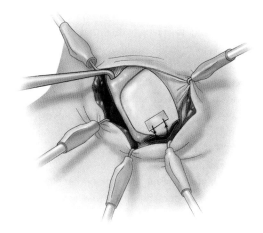

Fig. 64.23 Securing the implant to the lower strut with two 4–0 prolene sutures

through the skin incision or into the airway, possibly precipitating an airway foreign body emergency. Securing the implant with sutures significantly reduces the risk of this complication.

Yet another complication is undermedialization. This probably occurs when excessive edema of the vocal fold occurs prior to placement of the implant. The patient is noted to have an excellent voice interoperatively when the implant is placed, but the voice begins to fade 1–2 weeks postoperatively, as the edema resolves. In cases where a prolonged period of time elapses between the opening of the window, and final placement of the implant, one must anticipate the vocal fold will be slightly overmedialized, and the voice slightly strained to account for this edema.

Most outcomes studies for ML have focused on improvement in the voice, but a study by Flint et al. showed that approximately 70 % of patients with vocal fold paralysis and PEG tube dependency were able to be advanced to oral alimentation after ML [4]. More study in this area is needed.

Arytenoid Adduction

Fundamentals of Arytenoid Adduction

Arytenoid adduction (AA) is used in the treatment of glottal insufficiency [5]. Unlike medialization larygnoplasty, AA, acts through direct traction on the arytenoid cartilage at the muscular process, mimicking the action of the lateral cricoarytenoid muscle. Arytenoid adduction is an important adjunct in selected cases of vocal fold paralysis. The physiologic effects of AA include the following [6, 7]:

- Lowers the position of the vocal process
- Medializes and stabilizes the vocal process
- Rotates the arytenoid cartilage

In patients with VFP who have a lack of vocal process contact during phonation (large posterior gap), shortened immobile vocal fold, and those with vocal folds at different levels, AA should be considered in addition to ML. Videostroboscopy often provides valuable information about vocal process contact, vocal fold height and length, and therefore is useful preoperatively in assessing whether a patient may need an AA. A maximal phonation time (MPT) of less than 5 s has also been identified as a predictor of the need for AA in cases of VFP [8].

Indications

Unilateral vocal fold paralysis, especially in the following cases:
1. Posterior glottic gap/lateralized vocal fold during phonation
2. Vertical height differences (generally the paralyzed vocal fold is superiorly located)
3. Inability to achieve good voice or swallowing results with ML alone

Contraindications

1. Intact vocal fold mobility
2. VFP with the chance of recovery of motion ("early" paralysis)
3. Limited abduction of contralateral vocal fold

Surgical Procedure [1, 9]

Arytenoid adduction (AA) is almost always performed in conjunction with the ML procedures. In general, if the surgeon is unable to achieve good voice/proper correction of glottic insufficiency, an AA is performed. At this point, certain additional steps are needed to help achieve adequate exposure of the posterior laryngeal framework and arytenoid complex. A right-sided AA is illustrated as follows:

After the midline raphae are divided between the strap muscles, approximately 1 cm of the medial aspect of the sternohyoid muscle is sectioned below its insertion onto the hyoid. The step is necessary to improve posterior exposure of the laryngeal framework for AA (Fig. 64.24). Unlike in the ML procedure, the outer periochondrial flap is extended all the

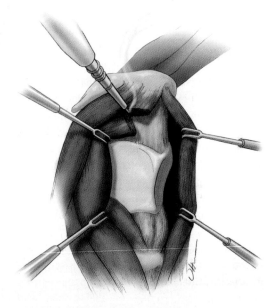

Fig. 64.24 Partial division of sternohyoid muscle 1 cm below its insertion

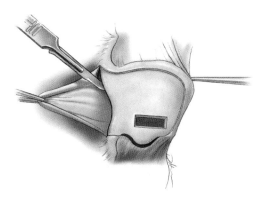

Fig. 64.25 A posteriorly based flap is separated away from the posterior cartilaginous border

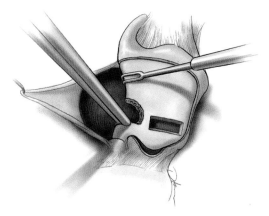

Fig. 64.27 Posterior "cookie-bite" window is created with a Kerrison ronguers

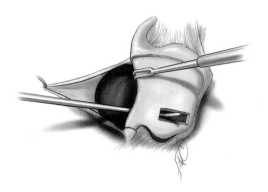

Fig. 64.26 The paraglottic space is connected between the posterior cartilage border and the ML window

way to the posterior border of the thyroid ala. The outer perichondrium is incised with a 15-blade along the posterior border of the cartilage to prevent elevation of the inner perichondrium on the medial side of the thyroid ala. The incision is continued to the level of the superior cornu above and the inferior cornu below (Fig. 64.25). The surgical plane of the medialization window (paraglottic space) is then connected to the posterior laryngeal dissection, so that there is one continuous surgical plane. A cottle or freer elevator is used to achieve this (Fig. 64.26). A skin hook is placed on the posterior border of the cartilage to aid in posterior retraction. Access to the arytenoid can then be achieved with one of two methods.

Creation of a Window in the Posterior Thyroid Ala

A window of cartilage is removed from the posterior border of the thyroid cartilage using a 2-mm Kerrison rongeur. The cartilage is removed until

the muscular process of the arytenoid is palpable and the anterior extension of the pyriform sinus can be visualized (Fig. 64.27). The size of the window ranges from 10 to15 mm in height and extends approximately 10 mm anteriorly, although the dimensions vary. The posterior aspect of this window should be located on the same level of the anterior window. It is important not to allow the anterior and posterior windows to "connect," as this will likely lead to framework instability.

Separation of the Cricothyroid Joint

Another way to gain exposure is by separation of the cricothyroid joint along with lateral thyroid ala retraction. A small dissection scissor (tenotomy) is used to separate the cricothryoid joint. Skin hook retractors are placed, and the thyroid ala is gently retracted laterally. Often, additional muscular or perichondrial attachments along the inferior and superior cornu must be divided to facilitate lateral alar retraction (Fig. 64.28). The pyriform sinus mucosa must be identified and retracted posteriorly before the muscular process of the arytenoid is identified. Great care must be taken with this step to avoid perforation of this delicate mucosa. The pyriform mucosa can be seen extending anteriorly onto the posterior cricoarytenoid (PCA) muscle. To aid in its identification, the patient is asked to blow against pursed lips (blow out the birthday candles), which results in distension and easy identification of the pyriform mucosa.

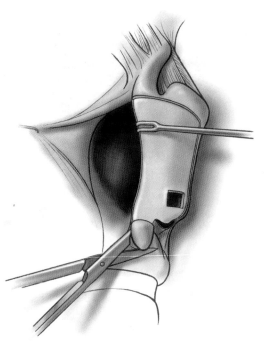

Fig. 64.28 Alternately, the CT joint can be divided for posterior exposure

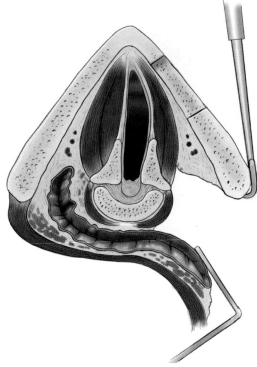

Fig. 64.30 Axial representation of larynx after posterior pyriform mucosa dissection/protection with Sewell retractor

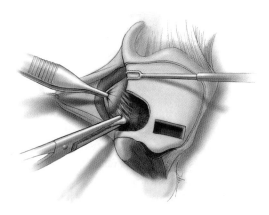

Fig. 64.29 The pyriform mucosa is dissected posteriorly using a Kitner

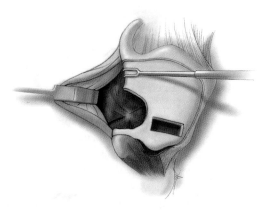

Fig. 64.31 Muscular process of the arytenoid is identified

The mucosa is grasped and dissected posteriorly, using blunt dissection with a Kitner dissection instrument (Fig. 64.29). The pyriform can then be shielded under a Sewell retractor (Fig. 64.30). The muscular process must then be identified using a number of landmarks.

The muscular process is usually at the same vertical height of the vocal fold and found by tracing the fibers of the PCA muscle anterior/superiorly to its tendinous insertion (Fig. 64.31). The muscular process is small (about the size of a grain of rice), but can be palpated. In addition, if the CT joint is separated as in step 5B, this can be used as a nearby landmark, as the muscular

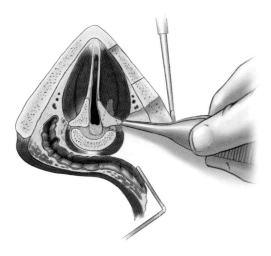

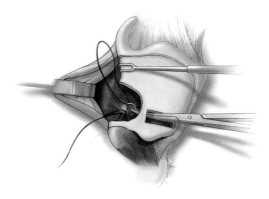

Fig. 64.34 Passage of the suture through the ML window

Fig. 64.32 Axial representation of manual traction on the muscular process to demonstrate adduction of the vocal fold

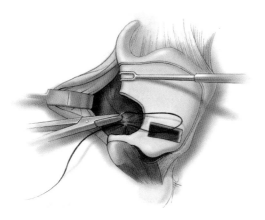

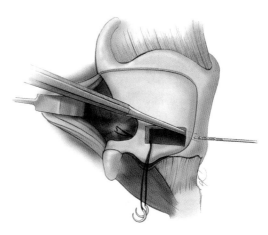

Fig. 64.35 A 1-mm wire-passing drill bit is used to create an anterior passage for one arm of the AA suture near the midline

Fig. 64.33 A 4–0 double armed prolene suture is passed through the muscular process in a figure of 8 fashion

process can be reliably found within 1 cm above this point. By grasping the muscular process with a toothed forceps, and rotating the arytenoid (anteriorly), one should be able to easily rotate the arytenoid into a medial position while confirming this with the endolaryngeal image on the monitor (Fig. 64.32). In order to obtain a secure purchase on the muscular process, a 4–0 monofilament suture (double armed) is passed through the lateral edge of the muscular process in a figure of 8 fashion (Fig. 64.33).

Both needles are brought through the dissected paraglottic space into the medialization window,

taking great care not to inadvertently catch any tissue with the needle tips, which could adversely affect the vector of pull for the AA stitch. Generally, the needles are passed with the dull end as the leading edge (Fig. 64.34). One of the needles is passed through the cartilage anterior to the medialization window, using a 1-mm wire-passing drill bit if the cartilage is calcified (Fig. 64.35). The other needle is passed underneath the inferior strut and is secured anteriorly through the anterior cricothyroid membrane (Fig. 64.36). The two ends of the suture are then marked with hemostats. The sutures are gently pulled anteriorly to adduct the arytenoid and the effect on the voice is tested by having the patient

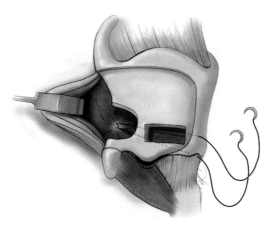

Fig. 64.36 After successful passage of both arms of the AA suture through the midline

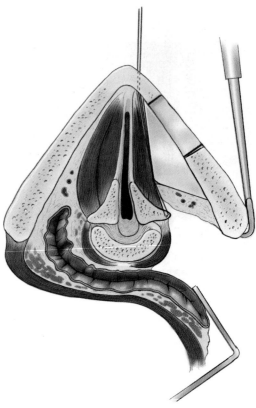

Fig. 64.37 Axial representation of AA sutures deep to ML implant

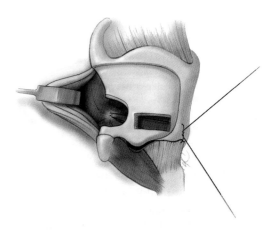

Fig. 64.38 Final tying of a surgeon's knot over the midline thyroid ala

count from 1 to 10. In addition, at this time the effects of medialization, using the previously mentioned depth gauge instrument are tested both in isolation, and with the addition of tension of the AA suture. Once the implant is created, it is placed through the window, taking care to keep the AA suture lines deep to the implant (Fig. 64.37).

Finally, the AA suture tension is adjusted and the knot is secured over the anterior thyroid cartilage, again assessing the voice. In general, only a small amount of tension is required for this (Fig. 64.38).

Complications/Common Surgical Errors

Airway problems are more common with framework surgery that involves AA. The additional retraction and dissection necessary for exposure and manipulation of the arytenoid complex results in increased paraglottic and arytenoid edema postoperatively. Additional corticosteroids may be warranted in patients undergoing ML+AA.

Pharyngocutaenous fistula is a possible complication with AA, although it is quite uncommon. Careful handling of the pyriform mucosa and protection of the mucosa with a retractor should prevent this complication. If an injury to the mucosa is suspected, the field can be irrigated and the patient instructed to valsalva. If air bubbles occur during this maneuver, the pyriform muscosa should be repaired with absorbable

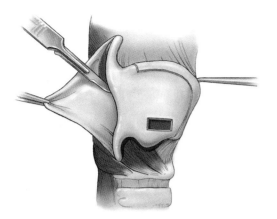

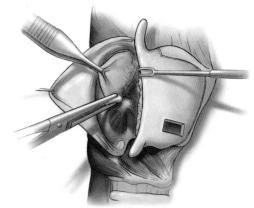

Fig. 64.39 A posteriorly based musculoperichondrial flap is raised, which includes the inferior constrictor muscle

Fig. 64.40 The cricothyroid joint is disarticulated and the pyriform mucosa is bluntly dissected posteriorly and superiorly, exposing the muscular process

suture, and the patient should be retested for air leakage. One should consider whether to proceed with the ML and/or AA at this point [9].

Excessive tension on the AA suture can create over-rotation of the arytenoid and worsening of the voice. The tension needed on this suture is actually minimal in most cases; therefore the surgeon should err on the side of light tension on the AA suture.

Hypopharyngeal Pharyngoplasty

In addition to ML and AA, there is a third procedure that may be added to enhance deglutition.

Indications and Contraindications

This procedure, designed by Peak Woo, is referred to as a "hypopharyngeal pharyngoplasty" (HPPP) and is best suited as an adjuvant procedure in cases of high vagal nerve paralysis [10]. Dysphagia experienced after a high vagal nerve injury is complicated by not only glottic incompetence, but also pharyngeal phase dysfunction including paralysis of the ipsilateral pharyngeal constrictors and poor relaxation of the cricopharyngeus. This results in a patulous hypopharynx that creates a reservoir for phyarngeal sections in the pyriform sinus and an increased risk of aspi-

ration. The HPPP was designed to address these issues.

The ML and AA are performed in conjunction with a HPPP. The HPPP has two main goals: (1) address the paralyzed inferior constrictor muscles by an advancement and plication of the muscle anteriorly and (2) reduction of the size of the pyriform sinus mucosa with the goal of eliminating a potential reservoir for secretions. In addition, a cricopharyngeal (CP) myotomy in often performed in conjunction with the HPPP to facilitate opening of the CP, which often fails to relax as a result of CN X injuries.

The steps of the procedure are as follows:
1. A posteriorly based musculoperichondrial flap is raised, which includes the inferior constrictor muscle (Fig. 64.39). Note that the medialization window has already been created.
2. The cricothyroid joint is disarticulated and the thyroid ala is retracted to gain access for an arytenoid adduction. The pyriform mucosa is bluntly dissected posteriorly and superiorly, exposing the muscular process (Fig. 64.40).
3. A 1 × 2-cm section of pyriform mucosa is then resected after stapling it with an autosuture-stapling device (Fig. 64.41).
4. Roughly one-third of the posterior thyroid ala is resected (1.5 cm) (Fig. 64.42). This will allow additional tightening of the pharyngeal wall after plication of the musculoperichondrial flap.

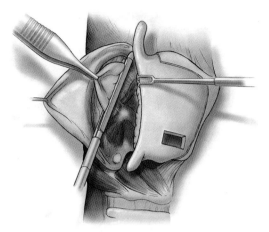

Fig. 64.41 1 × 2-cm section of pyriform mucosa is then resected with an autosuture-stapling device

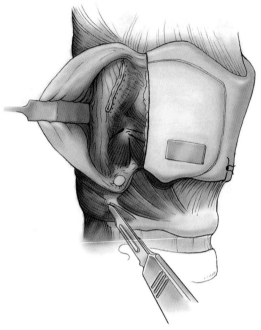

Fig. 64.43 CP myotomy is carried out. Note that ML and AA have already been completed

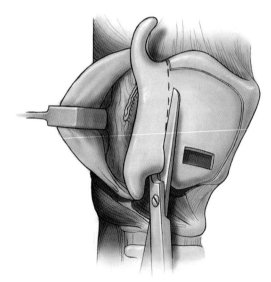

Fig. 64.42 A portion of the posterior thyroid ala is resected

5. A standard ML and AA are then performed, as well as a CP myotomy (Fig. 64.43).
6. The musculoperichondrial flap is then advanced anteriorly and secured to the thyroid ala with permanent sutures (Fig. 64.44).

The purpose of the HPPP is to increase the intra-bolus pressure, reduce pooling in the pyriform sinus, and increase the rate of hypopharyngeal transit, particularly in patients with high vagal injuries. According to Mok et al. [10] in a retro-spective review, the HPPP in conjunction with

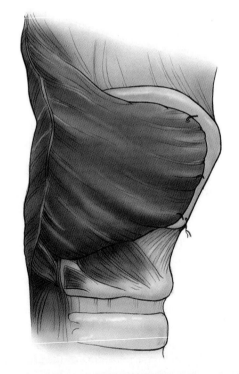

Fig. 64.44 The musculoperichondrial flap is then advanced anteriorly and secured to the thyroid ala with permanent sutures

ML and AA resulted in subjective and objective improvement in swallowing in 7 out of 8 subjects, five of which progressed to unrestricted diets. All of the patients had high vagal injuries and 3/8 had multiple cranial nerve involvement.

Although it adds potential additional morbidity, the HPPP is a useful surgical adjunct in carefully selected patients with high vagal injuries and severe dysphagia.

References

1. Rosen CA, Simpson CB. Operative techniques in laryngology. 1st ed. Heidelberg: Springer; 2008. p. 241–62.
2. Netterville JL, Stone RE, Luken ES, Civantos FJ, Ossoff RH. Silastic medialization and arytenoid adduction: the Vanderbilt experience. A review of 116 phonosurgical procedures. Ann Otol Rhinol Laryngol. 1993;102(6):413–24.
3. Wanamaker JR, Netterville JL, Ossoff RH. Phonosurgery: silastic medialization for unilateral vocal fold paralysis. Oper Techn Otolaryngol Head Neck Surg. 1993;4:207–17.
4. Flint PW, Purcell LL, Cummings CW. Pathophysiology and indications for medialization thyroplasty in patients with dysphagia and aspiration. Otolaryngol Head Neck Surg. 1997;116(3):349–54.
5. Isshiki G. Arytenoid adduction for unilateral vocal cord paralysis. Arch Otolaryngol. 1978;104: 555–8.
6. Noordzij JP, Perrault DF, Woo P. Biomechanics of combined arytenoids adduction and medialization laryngoplasty in an ex vivo canine model. Otolaryngol Head Neck Surg. 1998;119:634–42.
7. Woodson GE, Picerno R, Yeung D, et al. Arytenoid adduction: controlling vertical position. Ann Otol Rhinol Laryngol. 2000;109:360–4.
8. Woo P. Arytenoid adduction and medialization laryngoplasty. Otolaryngol Clinic North Am. 2000;33(4):817–39.
9. Miller FR, Bryant GL, Netterville JL. Arytenoid adduction in vocal fold paralysis. Oper Techn Otolaryngol Head Neck Surg. 1999;10:36–41.
10. Mok P, Woo P, Schaefer-Mojica J. Hypopharyngeal pharyngoplasty in the management of pharyngeal paralysis: a new procedure. Ann Otol Rhinol Laryngol. 2003;112:844–52.

Laryngohyoid Suspension

65

Hans F. Mahieu, Martijn P. Kos, and Ingo F. Herrmann

Abstract

In patients with chronic severe aspiration and recurrent pneumonia often a strict percutaneous endoscopic gastrostomy (PEG) feeding policy, a total laryngectomy, or any other type of permanent anatomical or functional separation of airway and digestive tract, is performed. However in selected cases it is possible to preserve or restore oral intake with a functional larynx by a laryngohyoid suspension procedure in combination with a UES myotomy. This procedure should be considered if aspiration is caused by a combination of deficient deglutitive laryngeal elevation and anterior movement, lack of pharyngeal constrictor activity, and insufficient opening of the esophageal inlet.

By suspending the laryngohyoid complex antero-cranially to the mandible the airway is pulled away from the bolus and is partially covered by the epiglottis diverting the bolus around it. The repositioning of the laryngohyoid complex also pulls the esophageal inlet open providing better drainage in the esophagus and less chance of aspiration from stasis.

Keywords

Laryngohyoid suspension • Life-threatening aspiration • Preservation laryngeal function • Surgical treatment • Restoration oral intake

H.F. Mahieu, MD, PhD (✉)
Department of Otorhinolaryngology, Meander Medical Center, Amersfoort, The Netherlands
e-mail: hans.mahieu@planet.nl

M.P. Kos, MD, PhD
Department of Otorhinolaryngology, Waterland Hospital, Purmerend, The Netherlands

I.F. Herrmann, MD, PhD
ENT Department, Reflux Center Düsseldorf, Düsseldorf, Germany

R. Shaker et al. (eds.), *Principles of Deglutition: A Multidisciplinary Text for Swallowing and its Disorders*,
DOI 10.1007/978-1-4614-3794-9_65, © Springer Science+Business Media New York 2013

Introduction

Once dysphagia has lead to chronic aspiration and/or recurrent pneumonia, this condition can no longer be qualified as "merely" a troublesome, socially debilitating and quality of life diminishing nutritional problem, but in addition to all this the patient is now also facing a potentially life-threatening condition. Often in such circumstances one of the first measures taken will include a strict tube feeding nutritional regimen, either by means of a nasogastric tube or a percutaneous gastrostomy (PEG) tube. This will however not always result in complete abolishment of the chronic aspiration, because the production of saliva and the need to swallow this saliva will still continue. Life time tube feeding is often considered unacceptable by many patients; therefore other means to prevent chronic aspiration and restore the ability for oral intake have been sought over the years. Such other means will entail surgical intervention; of course, the procedure will depend on the patient's disease or disorder underlying their dysphagia.

In cases of dysphagia with mild aspiration as a result of diminished pharyngeal constrictor activity, upper esophageal sphincter (UES) dysfunction, or laryngeal (and/or pharyngeal) hemiparesis, procedures that include UES myotomy, laryngeal framework surgery, and partial pharyngectomy can have a very successful outcome for the patient.

If, however, the aspiration is more severe, the laryngeal elevation and anterior movement during the pharyngeal phase is deficient, laryngeal sensation is diminished, or the coordination of deglutition is inadequate, more drastic procedures will usually be required to enable a safe oral intake without aspiration. The most drastic procedures involve total laryngectomy, or some other type of intervention resulting in a permanent anatomic separation of airway and digestive tract, with the invariable loss of normal voice and respiration.

In between the above-mentioned surgical interventions for mild aspiration and the latter procedures described with more drastic consequences there is a need for a surgical procedure which, despite more severe aspiration and

oropharyngeal dysphagia, the aim is for preservation of voice, respiration, and restoration of oral intake or at least the prevention of aspiration of saliva. Such a procedure is the laryngohyoid suspension, which is invariably combined with an open UES myotomy. This procedure should especially be considered if aspiration is caused by a combination of deficient deglutitive laryngeal elevation and anterior movement, lack of pharyngeal constrictor activity, and insufficient opening of the esophageal inlet.

The reason why UES myotomy alone is often insufficient to prevent aspiration is easy to understand given the fact [1] that the most important factor responsible for opening of the esophageal inlet in normal deglutition is not relaxation of the UES, nor passive opening as a consequence of the propulsion of the bolus being pushed downward by the peristaltic contraction of the pharyngeal constrictor muscles, but deglutitive laryngeal elevation and anterior movement (Fig. 65.1). Because the UES is attached to the larynx, anterior and cranial displacement of the larynx during the pharyngeal phase of the swallowing act results in opening of the esophageal inlet. Simultaneous relaxation of the UES facilitates the opening of the esophageal inlet, and propulsive activity of the tongue base and of the pharyngeal musculature improves the passage of the food bolus.

In addition to being the most important factor in opening of the esophageal inlet and thus facilitating rapid and complete passage of the food bolus, the anterior and cranial displacement of the larynx also results in other mechanisms that help to protect the airway from aspiration:

1. The larynx is pulled out of the way of the food bolus' path
2. The epiglottis is lowered over the laryngeal entrance protecting the airway
3. The larynx is pulled under the base of the tongue, thus providing a partial cover of the laryngeal inlet

Such a situation can be obtained surgically by means of a laryngohyoid suspension, in which the larynx is permanently fixed in the position that would normally be obtained during the pharyngeal phase of swallowing. True and false vocal fold closure is not necessary for the success of

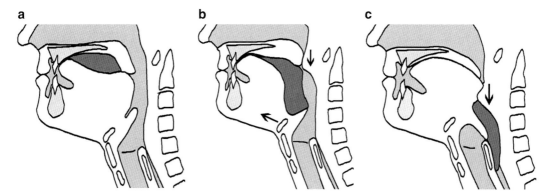

Fig. 65.1 Schematic presentation of normal deglutition. (**a**) Oral phase of deglutition. Note low position of larynx. (**b**) Early pharyngeal phase of deglutition. Masticated solid food is collected in the valleculae during respiration without risk of aspiration. When the bolus touches the Pharyngo-epiglottic folds, the swallowing act is triggered. Only hasty eaters will jump over this phase of bolus collection. When drinking this phase of collection in the vallecula is also skipped. That's why simultaneous respiration while drinking is not possible. Note anterior and superior displacement of hyoid and descending propulsive activity of constrictor pharyngeal muscles during deglutition. (**c**) Late pharyngeal phase of deglutition. Note anterior and superior displacement of larynx, in protected position under base of tongue; epiglottis tilted over laryngeal entrance; opened esophageal inlet; and pharyngeal constrictor muscle + tongue base propelling bolus in esophagus

this surgical procedure but would provide a better outcome.

Laryngohyoid suspension or laryngeal suspension has been described several times in the past [2–7] as an integral part of major ablative surgery with loss of the mandibular-hyoid integrity or extended partial laryngectomy to restore the continuity between the laryngeal-hyoid complex and the mandible and/or floor of the mouth musculature.

Employing this procedure as one of the surgical options for severe aspiration is less well known [8–11].

Procedure Laryngohyoid Suspension

Aim of Procedure

The primary aim of the laryngohyoid suspension in combination with the UES myotomy is prevention or reduction of aspiration of saliva as well as food or drink, while maintaining normal laryngeal function. Secondarily, dysphagia may be positively influenced by the permanent open esophageal inlet, but since the mechanism for bolus propulsion is not improved, complete normalization of deglutition is not feasible.

Indication

Patients are considered eligible for laryngeal suspension and a UES myotomy procedure on the basis of all of the following three factors:
1. Long-standing history of severe aspiration or recurrent aspiration pneumonia
2. Failed extensive nonsurgical swallowing rehabilitation
3. Videofluoroscopic examination or endoscopic examination of the function—swallowing drinks or food—demonstrating severe aspiration as a result of severely impaired pharyngeal constrictor muscle or tongue base activity, incomplete UES opening, and impaired laryngeal elevation/anterior movement during the pharyngeal phase of swallowing (Fig. 65.1b)

Contraindication

Patients are considered ineligible for laryngeal suspension and a UES myotomy procedure on the basis of all of the following five factors:
1. Poor general condition with high anesthesiological risk
2. Airway compromise

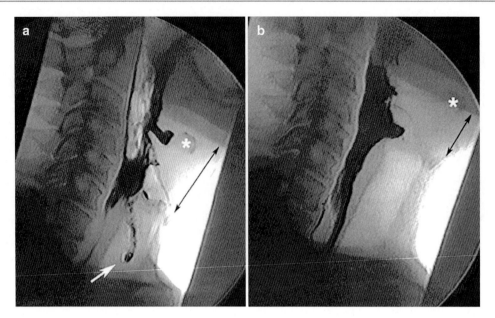

Fig. 65.2 Preoperative and postoperative videofluoros- copy. *Asterisks*—body of hyoid bone. (**a**) Videofluoroscopic frame shows aspiration (*white arrow*) in mid-pharyngeal phase in the situation before laryngeal suspension and UES myotomy. Note absent pharyngeal constrictor activity and absent laryngeal elevation. Distance between anterior commissure of vocal folds and mandible depicted by *black arrow*. (**b**) Videofluoroscopic frame in late pharyngeal phase after laryngeal suspension and UES myotomy shows no aspiration. Note position of suspended larynx and epi- glottis. Distance between anterior commissure of vocal folds and mandible (*black arrow*) much shorter than in A

3. Severe gastroesophageal reflux or lower esophageal sphincter (LES) insufficiency
4. Rapid progressive neuromuscular disease
5. History of radiochemotherapy involving lar- ynx and mandible with severe fibrosis

Preoperative Workup

To determine the eligibility for laryngohyoid sus- pension the following workup is required:
– Laryngeal function: to determine by means of videolaryngostroboscopic examines the motil- ity during phonation and respiration
– Regarding deglutition:
– Videofluoroscopy (Fig. 65.2) to determine the closure of the rhinopharynx, the laryngohyoid movement, the movement of the tongue base, the pharyngeal contraction wave, the UES opening, and the aspiration.
– Functional fiberoptic evaluation of swallow- ing. The aim is to determine the function of the pharynx, the larynx, and the UES; the upper digestive tract; and the bolus-transport without radiological overlapping of different structures (pooling in the hypopharynx and aspiration).
– Esophageal and pharyngeal manometry: to measure the tonicity, to determine contraction and relaxation of UES and LES, as well as the propulsion of the esophagus.
– On indication, e.g., positive history of GER or insufficiency of LES on manometry, 24-hour double-probe esophageal pH-metry (if neces- sary with impedance registration) to exclude preexisting reflux.
– Esophagoscopy to exclude strictures or other pathology in UES or LES.
– In case of history of airway compromise: assessment of the airway and pulmonary function.

Patient Counseling

Often patient expectations can be unrealistic. It is therefore essential that the patient is aware that the laryngohyoid suspension does not result in normal deglutition. Therefore the following issues are discussed during patient counseling:

- Emphasize that the goal of the procedure is not to normalize the swallowing act, but to prevent life-threatening aspiration with preservation of a functional larynx.
- The reported long-term success rate (in limited patient series) is between 50% and 60%. (Success meaning oral intake without the need for tube feeding, but with possible adjustments in food consistency).
- Should the outcome of the procedure be unsuccessful, in the sense that aspiration is inadequately addressed, other solutions such as tube feeding or surgical procedures involving anatomical separation of the aerodigestive tract remain possible options.
- Minor aspiration may still occur.
- Temporary tracheotomy is required to secure the airway during the first postoperative days.
- Influx of air in the esophagus during inspiration is possible because the UES is in a permanent open position and may result in belching.
- The UES as barrier against reflux and regurgitation is no longer functional; therefore it is advisable not to lie down within 2 h following meals.
- The anterior laryngeal position following laryngohyoid suspension may make it difficult for an anesthesiologist to visualize the larynx for intubation.
- Swelling of the submental area is an esthetic consequence of the high position of the larynx.
- Usual head and neck surgical risks including hemorrhage and infection.

Surgical Procedure

The surgical procedure includes orotracheal intubation as a means of administering general anesthesia. The patient's head is initially in retroflexion, at the moment the laryngohyoid complex is suspended from the mandible the head is put in anteflexion.

Skin Incisions and Exposure of UES and Larynx

A U-shaped incision is made along the anterior border of the sternocleidomastoid muscle bilaterally and the horizontal part of the incision approximately 2–3 cm above the sternum. The upper part of the incision is taken up to the level of the hyoid. A skin-platysma flap is developed in cranial direction all the way up to the submental area. The strap muscles of the larynx and hyoid are exposed and transected just below the larynx, including the omohyoid muscle and if necessary also the superior thyroid artery, in order to achieve a good exposure and freedom to elevate the laryngohyoid complex later on.

A horizontal submental skin incision is made through which the mandible can be approached, thus avoiding the need for a more extensive visor flap or degloving approach (Fig. 65.3).

Open UES Myotomy

The technique for open UES myotomy has been described in one of the previous chapters and will not be repeated here. The sole remark to be made here is that we generally prefer the use of an inflatable balloon within the UES lumen and a "leak test" at the end of the procedure [12].

Approximation of Thyroid Cartilage and Hyoid Bone

The crucial point is to make sure that all strap muscles have been severed (including the omohyoid muscles) below the level of the thyroid cartilage to prevent muscular down-pull later on.

The thyroid cartilage and hyoid bone are approximated by two mattress sutures on each side, one of strong but resorbable material Vicryl size 0 (Ethicon, Somerville, New Jersey, USA) to withstand the initially strong traction forces and the second of permanent polytetrafluoroethylene (Gore-Tex; Gore Medical, Newark, Delaware, USA) sutures size CV-2. All stitches on the thyroid cartilage are made in the supraglottic part of the

H.F. Mahieu et al.

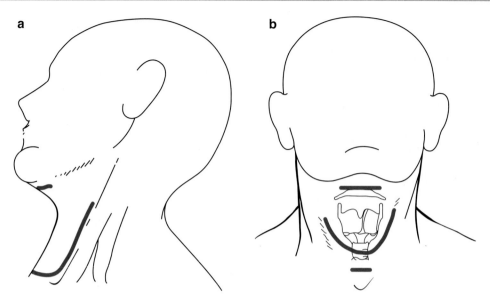

Fig. 65.3 Skin incisions (**a**) lateral view (**b**) frontal view

thyroid cartilage, staying well above the vocal fold line, yet taking a sufficient large bite of cartilage to decrease the risk or the suture tearing through the cartilage. In strongly calcified larynges it may be necessary to use a drill to perforate the thyroid.

The first stitch on the thyroid cartilage (either Vicryl or Gore-Tex) is made inside-out several millimeters in front of the oblique line on the thyroid. The stitch is then passed (inside out–outside in) through a 2 mm thick sheet of polytetrafluoroethylene (Gore-Tex; Gore Medical, Newark, Delaware, USA) to prevent rupturing of the thyroid cartilage. A few millimeters from the anterior border of the thyroid the stitch is then passed outside in through the thyroid ala. The stitch is then passed around the body of the hyoid bone, passing from the front to the back. All four sutures 2 Vicryl and 2 Gore-Tex are performed in this way. Before tying the sutures over the hyoid bone and thus approximating the thyroid and the hyoid, 2 Ethibond size 1 sutures (Ethicon, Somerville, New Jersey, USA) are passed behind the body of the hyoid, to later suspend the thyro-hyoid complex from the mandible. The four thyro-hyoid sutures can now be tied creating a firmly interconnected thyro-hyoid complex. Do not cut the sutures at this moment but leave them long for

the time being. Further anterior displacement and cranial displacement will follow the suspension of the thyro-hyoid complex from the mandible.

Suspension of Thyro-Hyoid Complex from Mandible

In order to be able to suspend the thyro-hyoid complex from the chin, two holes are drilled in the mandible just posterior to the angle of the chin and anterior to the foramen of the mental nerve. These holes should be sufficiently large to enable the passage of both ends of the ethibond sutures as well as the Gore-Tex sutures which are attached to the thyro-hyoid complex. The Vicryl sutures will only be used in case one of the other sutures breaks. Drilling of the holes should be done slightly oblique downwards and in the anterior direction from the lateral surface of the mandible, in order to facilitate the passage of the sutures. Sometimes a hollow needle is required to pass both ends of the sutures through the drill holes, one from inside out and the other from outside in. The head should now be put in anteflexion and an assistant should manually support the suspension of the laryngohyoid complex (Figs. 65.4–65.6).

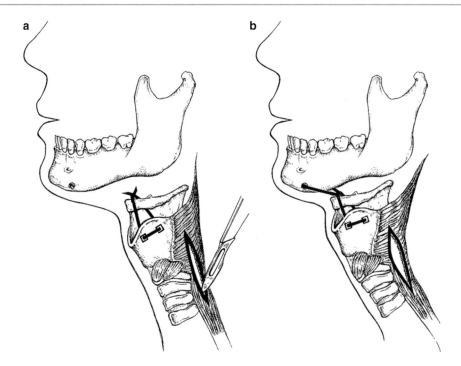

Fig. 65.4 Schematic presentation of UES myotomy and laryngeal suspension procedure. (**a**) UES myotomy performed; thyrohyoid approximation by 0-Vicryl and Gore-tex sutures tied as mattress sutures over Gore-tex bolsters on thyroid cartilage and around body of hyoid bone. (**b**) Thyrohyoid complex suspended to mandible by 0-Ethibond and Gore-tex sutures, which have been passed around body of hyoid bone and through holes drilled in mandible

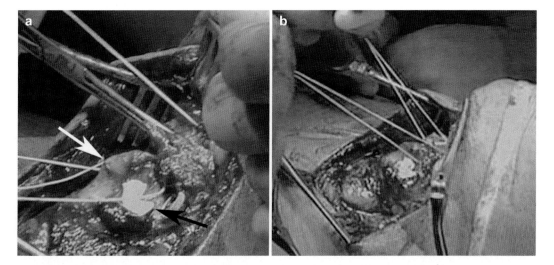

Fig. 65.5 Approximation of thyroid cartilage and hyoid bone. Before (**a**) and after (**b**) approximating the thyroid and hyoid with the sutures. The *white arrow* indicates the thyroid notch and the *black arrow* the sheet of polytetrafluoroethylene (Gore-Tex; Gore Medical, Newark, Delaware, USA)

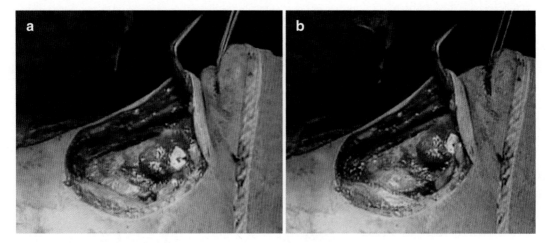

Fig. 65.6 Suspension of the larynx. (**a**) The thyroid cartilage has already been approximated towards the hyoid and therefore already higher located in the neck. (**b**) Pulling at the suspension sutures towards the mandible results in further displacement of the larynx anterocrani-ally. Note that the head is still in retroflexion. Changing the head position to anteflexion will further reduce the distance between chin and laryngohyoid complex. The larynx will then disappear under the skin flap

Tracheotomy

The tracheotomy should be performed, through a separate skin incision, with the larynx held in the high position. The tracheotomy will support the high positioned larynx during the first days. The oro-tracheal tube can then be replaced by a tracheal cannula.

Endoscopy

Before making the suspension permanent it is advisable to perform an endoscopy either with a flexible scope or with a 70° angled scope to evaluate the situation in the larynx. If the arytenoids are firmly pulled into the base of tongue, the suspension is probably too tight. The epiglottis will close the laryngeal entrance during inspiration. In this case the sutures to the mandible have to be slightly released. Fine-tuning of the larynx position under endoscopic view is necessary. Before the local edema starts, a test with spontaneous respiration passing a deflated cuff might be helpful. The aim is to decannulate after several days. Be aware that the patient is under muscle relax-ation and that the base of tongue will passively drop down and backward, so do not misinterpret a consequently blocked laryngeal entrance as a too tightly suspended larynx. The difference between both conditions is that in the latter situation you can lift the base of tongue slightly and pass into the larynx with a scope or probe. Within the first days, the sutures will become slightly slacker anyway because of slight tearing into the cartilage and remaining musculature around the hyoid and this will create a larger laryngeal entrance. The suspending sutures on the mandible can be tied permanently at this point in the procedure.

Feeding Tube Placement

If the patient does not have a PEG it is wise to insert a nasogastric feeding tube before closure of the neck. The feeding tube can be carefully guided through the pharynx and UES by external palpation and gentle pressure of the surgeon's finger in the opened neck. At this point, the neck can be closed and a vacuum drain left in place.

Postoperative Protocol

The protocol followed postsurgically includes a strict nonoral intake policy for the first four postoperative days. Swallowing rehabilitation under guidance of specialized Speech Language Pathologist starts on the fifth postoperative day if no signs of perforation or local infection have occurred. In the first days of the rehabilitation process, edema can interfere with swallowing but prolonged delay of swallow training is not considered favorable because of the possible development of local fibrosis and consequently stenosis of the UES. Patients are discharged from the hospital after a safe and adequate oral intake had been achieved. If they failed to accomplish safe oral intake despite extensive postoperative swallowing rehabilitation, PEG feeding or adequate dietary adjustments may be necessary to ensure safety at home.

The cuffed tracheacannula is usually replaced after 2 days for a cannula without cuff. If the cannula can be occluded for 48 h consecutively without dyspnea, the cannula is removed and the tracheotomy opening is closed. As long as a nasogastric feeding tube is in place, proton-pump inhibitors are prescribed.

Postoperative Evaluation

The recovery period and the required period of intensive swallowing rehabilitation is dependent upon the progress made and the nature of the underlying disease. Before discharge, a videofluoroscopy and usually a functional fiberoptic evaluation of swallowing is performed to evaluate possible aspiration. To assess the patient's laryngeal function a videolaryngostroboscopy is performed.

Description of Patient Outcomes from Personal Series of First Author (HM)

In the period 1996 to 2007, 19 patients who were evaluated in for dysphagia were eligible for laryngeal suspension in combination with an open UES myotomy procedure. The patient group included 13 men and 6 women, with a mean age of 55.8 years (range, 21–78 years). Fifteen patients were unable to manage any oral intake and were completely feeding tube dependent (PEG or nasogastric). The other four had chosen to remain on oral nutrition despite several episodes of aspiration pneumonia.

Preoperative manometry was performed in 15 patients; two patient refused manometry, and the manometric examination failed in two others because the catheter could not be tolerated. Absence of pharyngeal contraction was noted in the manometric registrations of all patients but one. The only patient who had weak but manometrically definable pharyngeal contractions first underwent UES myotomy, which failed to prevent the aspiration. Two of the 15 patients showed manometric signs suggestive of LES insufficiency. Three patients had severe nocturnal episodes of dyspnea because of aspiration of saliva. Neither had any oral intake and spent the whole day spitting out their saliva. Four patients had a tracheotomy in the past combined with extensive head and neck cancer surgery. One patient presented with a persistent tracheotomy. His swallowing problems due to muscular dystrophy became apparent after general anesthesia for an elective mandibular surgery. This procedure was performed in combination with a tracheotomy.

The cause of the dysphagia was muscular dystrophy or myositis in four patients; muscular atrophy as a late sequelae of radiotherapy in four patients; intracranial, central nervous system, and/or skull base surgery in six patients; and extensive head and neck cancer surgery in combination with radiotherapy in five patients (see Table 65.1).

Outcome Measure

The outcome was considered a complete success, a partial success, or a failure. A complete success meant that a patient was able to totally fulfill his or her nutritional needs by oral intake without clinically significant aspiration. A partial success meant that oral intake without clinically significant aspiration was possible but not sufficient for nutritional needs and that PEG

Table 65.1 Patient characteristics

Patient	Cause of aspiration	Preoperative intake	Postoperative intake	Postoperative fluoroscopy	Preoperative state of LES	Postoperative reflux	Outcome at 6 months	Outcome at >1 jr
1	OPMD	Oral	Oral, normal consistency	No aspiration	Normal	No	Complete success	Complete success
2	OPMD	Oral	Oral, modified consistency	No aspiration[a]	Normal	Yes	Failure	Failure, TLE
3	Myotonic dystrophy	Nasogastric TF	Oral, normal consistency	Minor aspiration	Unknown	No	Complete success	Complete success
4	Myositis	Oral	Oral, normal consistency	No aspiration	Normal	No	Complete success	Complete success
5	RTx nasopharyngeal cancer (>10 year)	PEG	PEG	No aspiration	Insufficient	Yes	Failure	Failure (aspiration of refluxate), TLE
6	RTx nasopharyngeal cancer (>10 year)	Oral	Oral, modified consistency, later PEG	Minor aspiration	Normal	Yes	Complete success	Partial success
7	RTx nasopharyngeal cancer (>10 year)	Nasogastric TF	PEG	Minor aspiration[a]	Insufficient	Yes	Failure	Failure, TLE
8	RTx nasopharyngeal cancer (>10 year)	PEG	Oral, modified consistency	Minor aspiration	Normal	Yes	Complete success	Complete success
9	CNS and/or Skullbase surgery + RTx	PEG	Oral, normal consistency	No aspiration	Normal	No	Complete success	Complete success
10	CNS and/or Skullbase surgery	Nasogastric TF	PEG, later oral, modified consistency	Moderate aspiration	Normal (on esophagoscopy no reflux)	No	Failure	Partial success
11	CNS and/or Skullbase surgery	PEG	PEG	Significant aspiration	Normal	Yes	Failure	Failure
12	CNS and/or Skullbase surgery	PEG	Oral, normal consistency	Minor aspiration	Normal	No	Partial success	Complete success
13	CNS and/or Skullbase surgery	Nasogastric TF	Oral, normal consistency	Minor aspiration	Normal	No	Complete success	Complete success
14	CNS and/or Skullbase surgery	Nasogastric TF	Oral, modified consistency	No aspiration	Normal	No	Complete success	Complete success
15	Posterior pharynx resection + RTx	PEG	Oral, normal consistency	No aspiration	Unknown	No	Complete success	Complete success

16	Commando + 2 x flap reconstruction + RTx	PEG	Oral, modified consistency	Minor aspiration	Unknown	No	Partial success	Complete success
17	Supraglottic laryngectomy + partial resection base of tongue + RTx	PEG	PEG	Significant aspiration	Normal	No	Failure	Failure
18	Commando resection + flap reconstruction + RTx	PEG	Oral, modified consistency, later PEG	Minor aspiration	Normal	No	Partial success	Partial success
19	Commando resection + flap reconstruction + RTx	PEG	Oral, modified consistency	Minor aspiration	Unknown	No	Partial success	Lost to follow-up

LES lower esophageal sphincter, *OPMD* oculopharyngeal muscular dystrophy, *TLE* total laryngeal excision, *TF* tube feeding, *RTx* radiotherapy, *PEG* percutaneous endoscopic gastrostomy, *CNS* central nervous system

[a]Eventually significant aspiration because of progressive muscular dysfunction

feeding was still required for adequate nutrition. A failure meant that there was very restricted or no oral intake possible without aspiration.

Results

The mean follow-up for all patients was 4.4 years (range, 1.2–8.0 years). The initial results after 6 months showed complete success in nine patients, partial success in four patients, and failure in six patients. The long-term outcome, after a follow-up period of more than 1 year, was considered a complete success in ten patients (56%). Seven of these patients were able to have a diet with a normal consistency, and three were only able to have a diet with a modified consistency. A long-term partial success was seen in three patients (17%). These three were only able to have an oral diet with a modified consistency. One patient who was considered a short-term partial success after 6 months died of a third primary tumor slightly over a year after her laryngohyoid suspension. Although she allegedly was able to get along without any nutritional support through her (dormant) PEG tube during her last months she refused further evaluation and treatment following the diagnosis of her third primary tumor. Five patients had a very restricted or no oral intake at all, and their cases were considered failures in long-term follow-up.

The need to constantly spit out saliva improved for all patients (10) who experienced this problem preoperatively.

During the follow-up of patients with partial or complete success, two patients again developed one single episode of pneumonia without obvious aspiration, which was adequately treated with antibiotics. The other 11 patients have remained completely free of any sign of pulmonary sequelae of aspiration.

Three of the five patients in whom the procedure failed eventually underwent total laryngectomy. Two of these were initially able to rely on oral intake for their nutritional needs without significant aspiration, but after approximately half a year they had recurrent episodes of aspiration and septicemia. Repeated videofluoroscopy

was suggestive of progressive muscular dysfunction in both. The larynx was still in the elevated position, ruling out the possibility of slipping of the sutures. One patient showed progressive insufficiency of the velum, and the other developed problems with opening of the esophageal inlet without evidence of mechanical obstruction on pharyngoesophagoscopy.

Of six patients who had postoperative signs of reflux, only two had shown preoperative manometric signs suggestive of LES insufficiency. These two cases are both considered failures, and the patients eventually underwent total laryngectomy. In one of them laryngectomy had to be performed, despite a markedly improved pharyngeal phase of swallowing after laryngeal suspension and UES myotomy, because the patient repeatedly had aspiration pneumonias from secondary aspiration following gastroesophageal reflux. Postoperative videofluoroscopy excluded primary aspiration. Furthermore, the aspiration pneumonias recurred despite prolonged periods of strict PEG feeding, suggesting secondary aspiration from gastroesophageal reflux. In this particular case, the preoperative history had been negative for gastroesophageal reflux, but preoperative manometry of the LES had shown abnormally low LES pressure over a short segment. One of the two other patients who eventually underwent total laryngectomy also showed preoperative manometric signs suggestive of LES insufficiency.

Two of the five patients in whom the procedures failed over the long term did not undergo total laryngectomy. Although they tolerated no more than a very restricted oral intake, they found the laryngeal suspension and UES myotomy to be an improvement in the sense that they no longer aspirated saliva and no longer needed to go around with a container to spit their saliva in. Both had PEG feeding. One of these patients had previously undergone extended horizontal laryngectomy with partial base-of-tongue resection and postoperative radiotherapy. Although the esophageal inlet was widely opened in this patient, aspiration persisted because of the lack of tissue bulk in the base of the tongue. Augmentation of the base of the tongue was performed, but unfortunately, this did not improve the swallowing act.

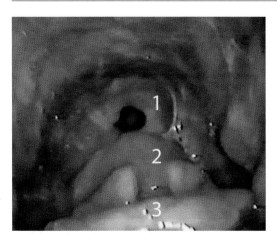

Fig. 65.7 View of larynx and esophageal inlet following laryngeal suspension, obtained with 90° telescope during spontaneous respiration. (1) Wide-open esophageal inlet; (2) posterior surface of cricoid plate; (3) epiglottis

In 12 patients, preoperative and postoperative voice range profiles were determined and showed no significant difference in dynamic or melodic range.

In three patients a second myotomy had to be performed to further improve deglutition, in two of them after 1 month and in the other after 3.5 years.

All temporary tracheotomies were closed within 5 weeks, with the exception of two patients who underwent decannulation, respectively, 1 and 4 years later, after correction for their preexistent impaired laryngeal mobility. Both had neurosurgical causes of aspiration.

In one patient, the laryngeal suspension was overcorrected initially. At the laryngoscopic examination during the procedure, it was estimated that sufficient space would still be available between the base of tongue and the arytenoids, but during the postoperative examination, the laryngeal inlet was seen to be completely obstructed. Initially, this obstruction was considered to be a consequence of postoperative swelling, but when after 2 weeks the patient was still unable to speak or block her cannula, revision surgery was performed by slightly loosening the sutures between the thyroid and hyoid cartilages. After this revision, she underwent successful decannulation and regained normal phonation (Fig. 65.7).

Discussion

Various surgical procedures have been described to deal with life-threatening aspiration. None of these studies have included large numbers of patients. Most procedures entail a permanent separation of airway and food passage, resulting in functional deficits, e.g., permanent tracheostomy and/or loss of normal voice.

Laryngohyoid suspension can fill the void between on the one hand procedures such as UES myotomy preserving as much function as possible and on the other disruptive procedures such as total laryngectomy or other means of permanent separation of food path and airway which inevitably interfere with normal breathing and normal voice.

A flow chart for treatment of aspiration without apparent anatomical cause or obstruction is presented in Fig. 65.8. Essentially the first treatment strategy should be extensive rehabilitation by an experienced SLP trained in swallowing rehabilitation. If this fails, the aspiration is no more than mild, and there are signs of UES dysfunction or constrictor pharyngeal weakness, a UES myotomy can be considered. In case of failure a larngo-hyoid suspension can then be considered. If the aspiration is more severe and a serious lack of laryngeal elevation and anterior movement exists, it is best to immediately take laryngohyoid suspension into consideration if conservative treatment measures fail.

In case of severe fibrosis in the neck following radiotherapy or radiochemotherapy and fixation of the larynx in the neck by this fibrosis, there is a risk that a laryngohyoid suspension procedure will lead to chondronecrosis. Therefore it is probably better in such circumstances to consider total laryngectomy or another method of permanent separation of food path and airway if conservative measures fail. Also in case of overt gastroesophageal reflux pathology laryngohyoid suspension is not the treatment of choice because the expected increase of reflux and consequently possible aspiration of the refluxate following this procedure.

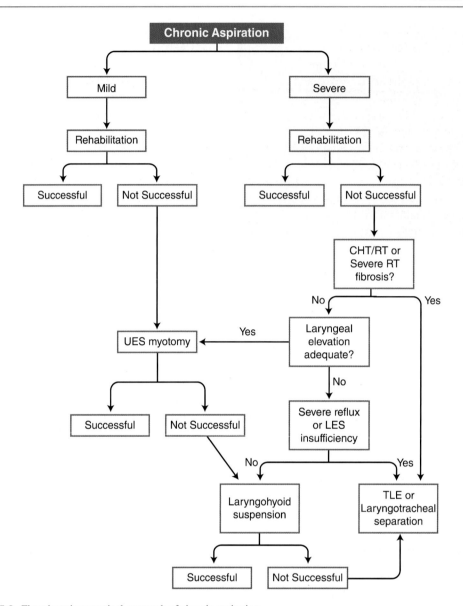

Fig. 65.8 Flowchart therapeutical approach of chronic aspiration

Laryngeal suspension is a procedure that can only partly compensate for the functional deglutitive deficiency and thus hopefully prevent aspiration. Patients who are unable or unwilling to accept these uncertainties in the outcome are not good candidates for the procedure. To avoid unrealistic expectations, patients have to be made aware that the goal of the surgical procedure is primarily to prevent aspiration, and not to normalize the swallowing act. Normal deglutition will never be obtained. Especially in patients who, because of loss of sensation, did not notice their aspiration (silent aspiration) before the operation, the postoperative situation can be disappointing, because the propulsion of the food bolus is still not normalized. These patients fail to notice the improvement with respect to the aspiration.

Efficacy of Intervention

Improvement of the conditions that contribute to life-threatening aspiration is obtained in almost three-fourths of the cases following laryngohyoid suspension. Complete fulfillment of nutritional needs through oral intake alone is realized in slightly more than one half of the cases. Although laryngohyoid suspension can by no means be considered minor surgery, all other surgical alternatives have major impact on the patient's quality of life as respiratory and phonatory functions are sacrificed. These functions are preserved in a laryngohyoid suspension procedure.

Strength of Evidence

We have to realize that the strength of the evidence for efficacy of laryngohyoid suspension as a treatment to prevent aspiration is weak. This is a consequence of the fact that the life-threatening condition of severe aspiration ethically precludes formation of an untreated control group. Furthermore the relatively small number of treated patients and the diversity of underlying conditions causing the dysphagia and aspiration are incompatible with providing strong statistical evidence.

Summary

Laryngeal suspension combined with UES myotomy can be considered a reasonable alternative to total laryngectomy or laryngeal diversion procedures in a selected group of patients with severe aspiration problems. Just more than half of the patients treated were able to restore oral intake with a normal or near normal diet without clinically significant aspiration, but some needed a diet with a modified consistency and/or additional PEG feeding to fulfill their nutritional needs. The need to spit out saliva improved on all of those patients who experience this problem preoperatively

Overt gastroesophageal reflux disease (GERD), hiatal hernia, and other signs of LES insufficiency should be considered absolute contraindications to laryngeal suspension and UES myotomy. This type of surgery will result in a permanently opened esophageal inlet, which will facilitate the aspiration of gastric contents.

For some of patients with severe aspiration, surgical laryngohyoid suspension in combination with open UES myotomy provides a less mutilating alternative than most other procedures which interfere with normal phonation and respiration.

References

1. Kahrilas PJ, Dodds WJ, Dent J, et al. Upper esophageal sphincter function during deglutition. Gastroenterology. 1988;95:52–62.
2. Edgerton MT, Duncan MM. Reconstruction with loss of the hyomandibular complex in excision of large cancers. Arch Surg. 1959;78:425–36.
3. Desprez JD, Kiehn CL. Method of reconstruction following resection of the anterior oral cavity and mandible for malignancy. Plast Reconstr Surg. 1959;24:238–49.
4. Calcatarra T. Laryngeal suspension after supraglottic laryngectomy. Arch Otol. 1971;94:306–9.
5. Goode RL. Laryngeal suspension in head and neck surgery. Laryngoscope. 1976;86:349–55.
6. Tiwari R, Karim ABM, Greven AJ, et al. Total glossectomy with laryngeal preservation. Arch Otolaryngol Head Neck Surg. 1993;119:945–9.
7. Fujimoto Y, Hasegawa Y, Yamada H, et al. Swallowing function following extensive resection of oral or oropharyngeal cancer with laryngeal suspension and cricopharyngeal myotomy. Laryngoscope. 2007;117:1343–8.
8. Herrmann IF. Surgical solutions for aspiration problems. J JPN Bronchoesophageal Soc. 1992;43:72–9.
9. Herrmann IF, Arce Recio S. Special techniques for resolving aspiration problems. Op Tech Otolaryngol Head Neck Surg. 1998;9:180–92.
10. Mahieu HF, de Bree R, Westerveld GJ, et al. Laryngeal suspension and upper esophageal sphincter myotomy as a surgical option for treatment of severe aspiration. Op Tech Otolaryngol Head Neck Surg. 1999;10: 305–10.
11. Kos MP, David EF, Aalders IJ, et al. Long-term results of laryngeal suspension and upper esophageal sphincter myotomy as treatment for life-threatening aspiration. Ann Otol Rhinol Laryngol. 2008;117:574–80.
12. Kos MP, David EF, Klinkenberg-Knol EC, et al. Long-term results of external upper esophageal sphincter myotomy for oropharyngeal dysphagia. Dysphagia. 2010;25:169–76.

Surgical Management of Life-Threatening Aspiration

66

Kaicheng Lawrence Yen and D. Gregory Farwell

Abstract

Intractable aspiration as a result of glottal insufficiency is a life-threatening medical condition. The choice of therapy is dictated by the level and severity of pathology resulting in aspiration and the likelihood of patient recovery. However, many dysphagia-associated disease conditions are not amenable to conservative treatment, and will lead to intractable aspiration and life-threatening pneumonia. Total laryngectomy and laryngotracheal separation are the two surgical options with optimal results, and decisions should be carefully weighed for each individual patient in making the appropriate selection.

Keywords

Dysphagia • Cricopharyngeal dysfunction • Aspiration pneumonia • Medialization thyroplasty • Narrow-field laryngectomy • Laryngotracheal separation

Introduction

Intractable aspiration as a result of glottal insufficiency is a life-threatening medical condition. This can be seen in patients with progressive neurological disease, stroke, and head and neck cancer, with stroke as the leading cause in the United States. The clinical scenario of a neurologically debilitated patient admitted to the

K.L. Yen, MD, PhD • D.G. Farwell, MD, FACS (✉)
Department of Otolaryngology Head and Neck Surgery,
University of California, Davis, 2521 Stockton Blvd.,
Suite 7200, Sacramento, CA 95817, USA
e-mail: dgfarwell@ucdavis.edu

medical intensive care unit with aspiration pneumonia is a common occurrence in modern day hospitals. In the United States, about 500,000 patients suffer from cerebrovascular accident (CVA) every year, and among them, around 50 % present with some degree of aspiration on swallow evaluation [1]. The odds ratio of pneumonia after stroke is 6.5 times higher if aspiration is demonstrated on video swallow study. The mortality rates from aspiration in the acute stages of CVA have been reported to be as high as 25 %, with 6 % of CVA patients dying from aspiration pneumonia in the first year. Patients who suffer from multiple strokes, brainstem strokes, and subcortical strokes suffered the highest incidence of aspiration pneumonia.

R. Shaker et al. (eds.), *Principles of Deglutition: A Multidisciplinary Text for Swallowing and its Disorders*, 945
DOI 10.1007/978-1-4614-3794-9_66, © Springer Science+Business Media New York 2013

The clinical characteristics of severe dysphagia are different between adults and children. Adults develop and acquire medical problems throughout their life, and after an acute event such as trauma or a CVA, they may develop de novo swallowing difficulties that lead to various morbidities. Whereas in the pediatric population, patients may sustain a single insult either in utero or perinatally that results in numerous medical problems leading to dysphagia. As in the adult, impairment of swallow function leads to repeated pulmonary insults such as aspiration pneumonia or to micro-aspiration and chronic lung damage. Aspiration of organic material into the tracheobronchial tree leads to several adverse effects described by Bartlett as the "triple threat," that is, chemical pneumonitis, bacterial pneumonia, and mechanical obstruction of the airways [2].

Airway Patency and Nutrition: Tracheostomy Tubes and Feeding Tubes

Patients with signs of aspiration should be evaluated by a medical professional trained and specializing in the evaluation and treatment of swallowing disorders. In the severe patient with suspected life-threatening aspiration, the first step is to perform a tracheotomy and a percutaneous endoscopic gastrostomy (PEG) to protect the airway from further aspiration and establish nutritional support. The placement of a cuffed tracheotomy tube will help protect the airway from further aspiration by preventing passage of the secretions to the lower airways and assisting with pulmonary hygiene [3]. Detailed assessment of respiratory and swallow function is made as the patient's condition allows.

For the selected patients, compensatory swallow therapy, selective use of drying agents (scopolamine/glycopyrrolate/botulinum toxin) [4], diet modifications [5], fundoplication [6], and proton pump inhibitors (PPI) [7] may be of benefit in lessening and/or alleviating the aspiration risks. The choice of therapy depends on a multitude of factors, including the likelihood of spontaneous recovery, the anticipated time of recovery, the

degree of the swallowing impairment, the patient's pulmonary reserve, cognitive status, cooperation, medical conditions, and overall prognosis. However, while pharmacologic treatment and placement of a tracheotomy may lessen the morbidity from chronic aspiration, it does not eliminate it [8]. Nasogastric and PEG tubes are commonly used to deliver nutrition directly into the stomach and small intestines and to avoid contact with the common upper aerodigestive tract, averting further possible aspiration. However, studies have shown that aspiration is not totally preventable. Refluxate from the stomach may still be aspirated through the hypopharynx [9, 10].

Controversy continues around the impact of a tracheotomy on dysphagia and aspiration. Some argue that tracheotomies increase the risks of aspiration by altering the laryngeal elevation and swallow reflex by anchoring the larynx [11–13]. Other studies of trauma patients and of patients with head and neck cancer in the early postsurgical period show that a tracheotomy neither increases nor decreases incidence of aspiration [14, 15].

The use of tracheal occlusion in reducing aspiration has also been controversial. Clinical studies have not shown that occlusion of the tracheotomy tube decreases aspiration in the early postsurgical periods in patients with head and neck cancer [16]. A physiologic study has shown that an occluded tracheotomy promotes an increase in subglottic pressure during swallow as opposed to the unoccluded tracheotomy tubes [17, 18].

Coffman and colleagues have shown that the use of either continuous or intermittent subglottic suction in specially designed proximal suction tracheotomy tubes significantly decreased aspiration of saliva distal to the cuff when compared to conventional tracheotomy tubes without the suction capability [19]. For ventilator-dependent patients, it has been shown that the risk of ventilator-associated pneumonia (VAP) may be significantly reduced with the use of intermittent subglottic suction drainage, from as much as 4 to 16 % [20]. Studies of the late postsurgical period have actually demonstrated an increase in aspiration in patients with the unoccluded tracheotomy tubes [21]. Numerous theories have been postulated to explain the discrepancy in early and late postsurgical periods, including differences in dysphagia over time and the progressive decline of the adductor laryngeal reflexes in patients with prolonged tracheal intubation [22, 23]. Clearly, well-designed studies are needed to clarify this phenomenon. For practical purposes, tracheotomy should be considered a respiratory treatment and not as a tool for the management of dysphagia. The insertion of a cuffed tracheotomy tube may be considered as the first-line care of aspiration, but is inappropriate for long-term control, as prolonged use may cause tracheomalacia, resulting in bolus and secretion leakage into the bronchi.

Surgical Options for the Treatment of Vocal Cord Paralysis with Chronic Aspiration

The airway is guarded by three levels of protection: the epiglottis, the false vocal folds, and the true vocal folds. The latter two are controlled by the recurrent laryngeal nerve on the corresponding side and close the airway upon swallow.

Several surgical options are available for the management of chronic aspiration from vocal paralysis. The choice of surgical therapy is dictated by the level and severity of pathology resulting in aspiration, the severity of dysphagia, the effect on quality of life, the likelihood of patient recovery, and the patient's preference.

For patients with glottic insufficiency from unilateral recurrent laryngeal nerve or vagal nerve injury and poor compensation from the normally functioning vocal cord, a vocal fold medialization procedure may provide enough glottic competence to improve the quality of voice and closure to prevent aspiration.

Popularized by Isshiki, medialization thyroplasty has become the standard technique for managing patients with a paretic vocal cord [24]. Several authors have demonstrated significant improvement in dysphagia after the definitive intervention with medialization thyroplasty. This relatively straightforward laryngeal framework surgical procedure may provide a lasting remedy for dysphagia and aspiration in patients with permanently paralyzed vocal folds and glottal incompetence [25, 26], as well as for patients who fail to achieve satisfactory relief from the less invasive medialization injections [27].

Medialization injection or injection thyroplasty may be performed under local anesthesia, and as an office-based procedure. It is an alternative to the more invasive open technique laryngeal framework surgery and more suited to the debilitated patient. In this technique, a percutaneous or endoscopic injection of a filler material is made into the true vocal fold to medialize the cord to a more midline position on the paralyzed side, thus allowing adequate glottal closure on phonation and swallow [28]. Gelfoam, hyaluronic acid, collagen, and methylcellulose are some of the materials available commercially for injection thyroplasty and may provide short-term relief [29, 30]. They are often utilized for conditions where the recurrent laryngeal nerve is still intact and there is the possibility of recovery of function over time. Fat, fascia, and calcium hydroxyapatite (CaHA) are more permanent substances used and offer a longer lasting effect [31].

In a report of a series of gastrostomy-dependent patients with glottal incompetence, 55 % were able to discontinue their gastrostomy tube use after medialization laryngoplasty, with another 25 % who discontinued g-tube use with additional swallowing therapy [32]. For those patients with severe chronic aspiration and unwilling to lose their voice use, a bilateral medialization thyroplasty has been attempted and successful in three patients. Some patients regained the ability to tolerate some oral diet consistency, while all of the patients required a permanent tracheostomy [33].

Bhattacharyya et al. [25] has demonstrated that approximately one-third of the patients with unilateral vocal fold paralysis had significant aspiration or penetration on videofluroscopic swallowing studies. Their prospective study of 27 patients showed improved glottal competence with intervention, but demonstrates no significant advantage when comparing medialization thyroplasty and injection procedures.

Medialization may also be considered in children with aspiration and phonatory disturbance. In a series of 15 patients, injection laryngoplasty, thyroplasty, or nerve reinnervation was performed with good subjective outcome [34]. It is recommended that framework thyroplasty be attempted in those with greater aspiration concerns and older adolescents able to tolerate a procedure performed under local anesthesia. Injection medialization is appropriate for younger patients and those who have a greater chance for spontaneous recovery. The nerve reinnervation procedure is performed when there is known permanent nerve injury and no chance of spontaneous recovery of recurrent laryngeal nerve function.

Surgical Options for the Treatment of Chronic Aspiration

Many disease conditions associated incidence of dysphagia are not amenable to these procedures and adjuvant treatments. Inadequate treatment may lead to repeated and intractable aspiration, and the added risks of malnutrition and life-threatening pneumonia. Such clinical entities often are progressive neuromuscular disorders or neurological diseases, such as amyotrophic lateral sclerosis, stroke, and severe cerebral palsy [23].

A second group of patients are those recovering from treatment for head and neck malignancies. Head and neck cancer patients who have undergone extensive surgery such as tongue resection, partial laryngectomy, or high-dose radiation therapy, especially in the era of organ-preservation concurrent chemoradiation therapy (CCRT), are especially prone to developing severe long-term toxicities. In a recent report of a series of patients with advanced laryngeal and hypopharyngeal cancers, 23 % experienced significant long-term toxicity, and 8.5 % required permanent tracheostomy [35]. The previously treated upper aerodigestive tract may have resulted in an immobile tongue, an insensate and immobile larynx and pharynx, or patients may have had already lost the anatomical structures necessary for speech and swallowing function. Unfortunately, a significant percentage of these patients are totally reliant on the gastrostomy tube for nutrition and recovery is not anticipated or delayed. These patients often have very complex medical and social issues that also must be considered in the treatment recommendations.

Attempts at managing glottal insufficiency with laryngeal framework preservation have been described. Montgomory [36] described in 1975 a glottic closure technique via an anterior thyrotomy approach. In this technique, the mucosa is stripped off the true and false cords, and the opposing cords are approximated using permanent sutures. Others have attempted closure of the supraglottic larynx via an infrahyoid approach. In this method, the edges of the epiglottis, the aryepiglottic folds, and arytenoids mucosa are denuded and the epiglottis is then sutured back to the arytenoids and the aryepiglottic folds [37]. However, such procedures were troubled by dehiscence and recurring aspiration. While some patients may be neurologically impaired, the laryngeal muscles still retain some function and pull apart the mucosal suture lines. In an attempt to overcome this muscular pull and allow healing, preoperative botulinum toxin injections to paralyze the larynx and cricopharyngeus muscle were introduced to achieve complete laryngeal paralysis. The effects of neuromuscular blockade persist for months and allow healing of the sutured mucosa. In a small series of six patients, only one developed a small fistula at the posterior commissure [38]. This however adds to the treatment complexity and time by the need of an additional procedure.

If the prevention of aspiration and its complications is the main therapeutic goal, the two operative options with optimal results are laryngectomy and laryngotracheal separation (LTS). Total laryngectomy involves the removal of the larynx, thereby completely separating the upper digestive tract from the respiratory system, and is definitive in eliminating aspiration. This is the treatment of choice for nonverbal patients with life-threatening aspiration and irreversible recovery of laryngeal function [39]. Additionally, it is an appropriate option for patients where multiple interventions to control aspiration have been unsuccessful and the patient's condition is deteriorating [40]. The main reason for consideration of diversion procedure such as an LTS is essentially to allow for potential reversal surgery [41]. This would only be appropriate in patients with the potential for recovery through elimination of their aspiration risk, and return of swallowing function.

Narrow-Field Laryngectomy

Cannon and McLean [42] advocated narrow-field laryngectomy for intractable aspiration. This procedure involves removal of the laryngeal skeleton, but spares the hyoid bone, strap muscles, and hypopharyngeal mucosa. This technique allows a tension-free closure, thereby minimizing fistula formation (Fig. 66.1).

Because most patients have a preexisting tracheotomy, a vertical incision may be made from the upper end of the tracheostoma to the hyoid bone, and the strap muscles elevated off the laryngeal framework at the midline to expose the thyroid and cricoid cartilages. The trachea may be transected at the first or second ring, and the cricoid is lifted upward and separated from the post-cricoid mucosa. The pharynx is entered at the level of the arytenoids cartilages, and a limited infrahyoid pharyngotomy is performed, preserving as much mucosa as possible. After the larynx is removed, the pharynx is then approximated together and supported with the strap muscles as a second layer. A permanent tracheostoma is formed in the usual manner. For some patients, an apron neck incision may be the incision of choice, to allow for a wider field of resection and primary reconstruction with a more acceptable scar. The horizontal incision also allows broader access for pedicled or free flaps to reconstruct the alimentary tract as necessary. However, such invasive procedures are not without risks, such as increased rate of fistulas and infection.

In their series of patients undergoing narrow-field laryngectomy, Krespi and Blitzer [44] reported that the majority were performed under local anesthesia and intravenous sedation. No fistula developed in these patients, and oral feeding began 5–11 days after the laryngectomy. For selected patients, tracheoesophageal puncture and placement of voice prosthesis devices may further allow speech rehabilitation.

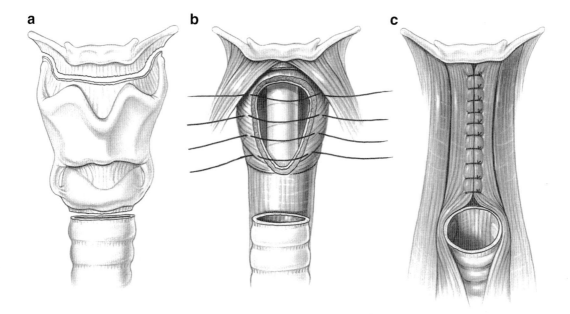

Fig. 66.1 (**a**) Narrow-field laryngectomy outlined (**b**) Pharyngeal mucosa spared (**c**) Strap muscles used as second layer closure [25]. From G. Wisdom et al. Oper Tech Otolaryngol Head Neck Surg 1997;8:200 with permission from Elsevier

This procedure may have specific utility in head and neck cancer survivors who have perichondritis and chondronecrosis of the laryngeal framework [45] resulting from previous radiation [35] or laser [46] treatment. By removing the affected soft tissue and cartilage, the patients' symptoms may improve significantly. However, cancer persistence or recurrence should always be considered a possibility, and extensive preoperative workup and operative pathology control utilized.

Laryngotracheal Separation

LTS involves the complete separation of the airway from the upper digestive tract. It is a more challenging technique than narrow-field laryngectomy, and is associated with more complications but has the advantage of being reversible.

As such, it may be a more acceptable choice for patients or families that are unwilling to consider a laryngectomy for definitive treatment. In 1975, Lindeman [47] described a procedure in which the trachea is separated at the third or fourth tracheal ring, and the distal end brought out to the skin as a tracheotomy (Fig. 66.2). The proximal tracheal stump is then anastomosed end-to-side to the anterior esophagus. However, as many patients had already undergone a higher placed tracheotomy, Lindeman et al. [48] later proposed a modified procedure where the proximal stump is merely sewn together in layers and the closure reinforced with rotated sternohyoid muscle flaps (Fig. 66.3). Some surgeons have found the concept of maintaining a proximal blind pouch that is chronically filled with saliva and food debris conceptually imprudent. Tucker [49] later introduced a procedure where both the proximal and distal tracheal stumps are sutured to the skin.

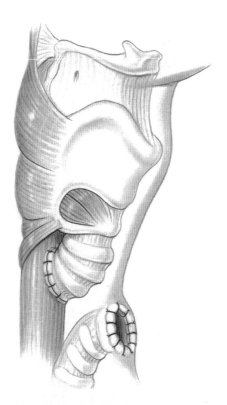

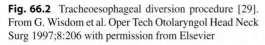

Fig. 66.2 Tracheoesophageal diversion procedure [29]. From G. Wisdom et al. Oper Tech Otolaryngol Head Neck Surg 1997;8:206 with permission from Elsevier

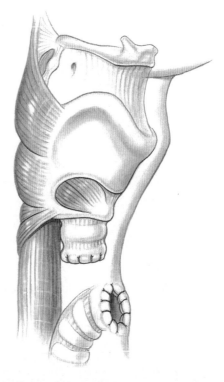

Fig. 66.3 Laryngotracheal separation procedure [30]. From G. Wisdom et al. Oper Tech Otolaryngol Head Neck Surg 1997;8:206 with permission from Elsevier

The proximal stump was passed through a split in the sternocleidomastoid muscle, and onto the neck skin. This results in a stoma that requires frequent hygiene for the chronic secretions. This can be somewhat controlled by a small stoma bag in some patients.

Krespi et al. [50] described a technique of carefully removing the anterior tracheal cartilages from the short proximal stump, as well as the inferior half of the cricoid cartilage. The more pliable tracheal mucosal stump is then sewn to the anterior esophagotomy in the end-to-side fashion to allow for the diversion of secretions back to the alimentary tract (Fig. 66.4). He reported relief of aspiration of all five patients, and four of these patients were able to resume oral feeding.

From a series of 34 patients over a 9-year period, Eibling noted that with LTS, aspiration was effectively controlled in every patient [51]. Thirteen patients developed postoperative fistula, and of these, 11 resolved with conservative management. Prior tracheotomy was associated with

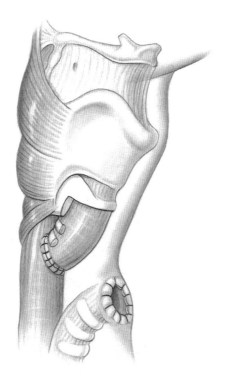

Fig. 66.4 Modified tracheoesophageal diversion procedure [32]. From G. Wisdom et al. Oper Tech Otolaryngol Head Neck Surg 1997;8:207 with permission from Elsevier

fistula formation, and the authors recommend that whenever possible, LTS be considered before a tracheotomy procedure to reduce the risk of a wound healing complication. The postoperative nursing care was decreased and most patients were discharged or transferred to a chronic care facility within 2–3 weeks following the LTS procedure. In the end, 43 % of patients were able to tolerate regular or liquid diet, while the rest required feeding with nasogastric or gastrostomy tube due to their underlying neurological disease. In a review of a series of 21 pediatric patients, 88 % had fewer hospitalizations or were discharged for the first time after their LTS [8]. The number of pneumonias decreased, and care requirements decreased in all but one patient. More importantly, the parents reported satisfaction and improved quality of life. A subsequent report of 56 consecutive LTS patients over an 18-year period showed a reduced average number of diagnosis related groups (DRGs) per months ($p < 0.001$) as well as work relative value units (wRVUs), translating to reduced healthcare costs and social burden for these patients [52]. Transient fistula formation (11 %) was the most common complication, followed by wound infection (9 %). While most reports of complications were minor, a patient died from a lethal tracheo-innominate artery fistula (TIAF) some months after the operation [53]. Juxtaposition of the innominate artery against the trachea is often seen in patients with chest deformity in the setting of severe scoliosis, and an alternative procedure should be attempted for these patients [54].

In a series of seven patients, of which six received laryngectomy and one with LTS, all were able to resume oral feeding after surgery in an average of 18 days. Not only was the control of pneumonia and albumin levels improved significantly, the grade of depression and mood of patients and their families also improved significantly [39]. It is important to understand that separation of the airway and the digestive tract does not necessarily mean patients will be able to eat orally. There is an obvious decrease in the proportion of patients resuming oral feeding with LTS than those with laryngectomy. Studies have demonstrated that the risk of laryngeal penetration and aspiration in these patients may be due to absent laryngeal adductor reflex (LAR) and impaired pharyngeal contraction [55, 56]. The separation of the trachea from the larynx does not address this underlying problem. For these patients, the opening at the pharyngoesophageal segment may be further augmented by cricopharyngeal myotomy, dilation, or injection of botulinum toxin [57, 58]. Cricopharyngeal myotomy has been shown to normalize the upper esophageal sphincter relaxation pattern, thus allowing a more normal swallow [59]. This has been shown to be the more effective treatment modality [57] and may be performed at the time of LTS surgery.

LTS has been proven to be a reliable solution to treat chronic aspiration. During the procedure, if the recurrent laryngeal nerves were carefully preserved, successful reversal of separation procedure with return in swallow and phonation has been reported in selected patients [41]. This reversal procedure is performed under general anesthesia. The original apron flap is raised and both the tracheostoma and mucous fistula/stump are incised circumferentially. The ends of the tracheal openings are freshened and mobilized. Anastomosis is performed by suturing the circumferential mucosa, and the closure reinforced with non-absorbable stay sutures between adjacent tracheal rings to relieve tension on the mucosal anastomosis. In a series of eight adult patients who underwent reversal of their LTS, the operation was successful in six [60]. Four patients had postoperative complications, ranging from mild to moderate transient aspiration in two, tracheal stenosis in one, and severe aspiration with tracheal stenosis in one. Surgical reversal was not successful in the last two patients. Patients whose surgery was successful were able to maintain oral feeding and comprehensible speech. However, the high incidence of complication and failure rates should be weighed carefully before committing to surgical reversal. In the pediatric population, severe neurological deficit and developmental delay are some of the major factors that preclude reversal attempts. Pediatric reversal procedures have only recently been reported in the literature. In four patients,

only two proved to be successful. Both of these children can now tolerate an oral diet and their speech and language development is in congruence with their developmental level [61].

Summary

Detailed evaluation of dysphagia will elucidate conditions that may benefit from surgery for protection of the airway. It will also help identify patients who will potentially have significant improvement in their quality of life. Surgical separation of the airway and digestive tracts, such as narrow-field laryngectomy and LTS, is appropriate for some patients but may be controversial in others. Decisions should be tailored on an individual basis, taking into account the underlying disease, the neurological and medical comorbidities, the prognosis for recovery, and patient and family expectations. These surgical procedures, when indicated, have been shown to be safe and effective in the management of life-threatening aspiration, with a much improved quality of life in exchange of loss of verbal communication. Family benefits with reduced medical complications, and less intense care requirements are significant and should be considered in the ultimate treatment decision. For patients whose underlying causes for aspiration are reversible, the LTS procedure allows the opportunity for reversal to regain laryngeal function.

References

1. Ding R, Logemann JA. Pneumonia in stroke patients: a retrospective study. Dysphagia. 2000;15:51–7.
2. Bartlett LG. Treatment of postoperative pulmonary infections. Surg Clin North Am. 1975;55:1355–60.
3. Boyd SW, Benzel EC. The role of early tracheotomy in the management of the neurosurgical patient. Laryngoscope. 1992;102:559–62.
4. Fry EN. Postoperative gastric aspirations reduced by glycopyrrolate during upper abdominal surgery. J R Soc Med. 1986;79:334–5.
5. Garcia JM, Chambers 4th E. Managing dysphagia through diet modifications. Am J Nurs. 2010;110: 26–33.
6. Oelschlager BK, Chan MM, Eubanks TR, Pope 2nd CE, Pellegini CA. Effective treatment of rumination

with Nissen fundoplication. J Gastrointest Surg. 2002;6:638–44.

7. Rantanen TK, Sihro EI, Rasanen JV, Salo JA. Gastroesophageal reflux disease as a cause of death is increasing: analysis of fatal cases after medical and surgical treatment. Am J Gastroenterol. 2007;102: 246–53.

8. Lawless ST, Cook S, Luft J, et al. The use of a laryngotracheal separation procedure in pediatric patients. Laryngoscope. 1995;105:198–202.

9. Metheny NA, Schallom L, Oliver DA, Clouse RE. Gastric residual volume and aspiration in critically ill patients receiving gastric feeding. Am J Crit Care. 2008;17:512–9.

10. Manning BJ, Winter PC, McGreal G, Kirwan WA, Redmond HP. Nasogastric intubation causes gastroesophageal reflux in patients undergoing elective laparotomy. Surgery. 2001;130:788–91.

11. Sharma OP, Oswanski MF, Singer D, Buckley B, Courtright B, Raj SS, Waite PJ, Tatchell T, Gandaio A. Swallowing disorders in trauma patients: impact of tracheostomy. Am Surg. 2007;73:1117–21.

12. Smith Hammond CA, Goldstein LB. Cough and aspiration of food and liquids due to oral-pharyngeal dysphagia: ACCP evidence-based clinical practice guidelines. Chest. 2006;129:154S–68.

13. Nash M. Swallowing problems in the tracheotomized patient. Otolaryngol Clin North Am. 1988;21:701–9.

14. Leder SB, Joe JK, Ross DA, Coelho DH, Mendes J. Presence of a tracheotomy tube and aspiration status in early, postsurgical head and neck cancer patients. Head Neck. 2005;27:757–61.

15. Leder SB, Ross DA. Investigation of the causal relationship between tracheotomy and aspiration in the acute care setting. Laryngoscope. 2000;110:641–4.

16. Leder SB, Ross DA, Burrell MI, Sasaki CT. Tracheotomy tube occlusion status and aspiration in early postsurgical head and neck cancer patients. Dysphagia. 1998;13:167–71.

17. Gross RD, Mahlmann J, Grayhack JP. Physiologic effects of open and closed tracheostomy tubes on the pharyngeal swallow. Ann Otol Rhinol Laryngol. 2003;112:143–52.

18. Young PJ, Burchett K, Harvey I, Blunt MC. The prevention of pulmonary aspiration with control of tracheal wall pressure using a silicon cuff. Anaesth Intensive Care. 2000;28:660–5.

19. Coffman HM, Rees CJ, Sievers AE, Belafsky PC. Proximal suction tracheotomy tube reduces aspiration volume. Otolaryngol Head Neck Surg. 2008;138: 441–5.

20. Smulders K, van der Hoeven H, Weers-Pothoff I, Vandenbroucke-Grauls C. A randomized clinical trial of intermittent subglottic secretion drainage in patients receiving mechanical ventilation. Chest. 2002;121: 858–62.

21. Muz J, Hamlet S, Mathog R, Ferris R. Scintigraphic assessment of aspiration in head and neck cancer patients with tracheostomy. Head Neck. 1994;16:17–20.

22. Sasaki CT, Suzuki M, Horiuchi M, Kirchner JA. The effect of tracheostomy on the laryngeal closure reflex. Laryngoscope. 1977;87:1428–33.

23. Shama L, Connor NP, Ciucci MR, McCulloch TM. Surgical treatment of dysphagia. Phys Med Rehabil Clin North Am. 2008;19:817–35.

24. Isshiki N, Okamura H, Ishikawa T. Thyroplasty type I (lateral compression) for dysphonia due to vocal cord paralysis or atrophy. Acta Otolaryngol. 1975;80: 465–73.

25. Bhattacharyya N, Kotz T, Shapiro J. Dysphagia and aspiration with unilateral vocal cord immobility: incidence, characterization, and response to surgical treatment. Ann Otol Rhinol Laryngol. 2002;111(8): 672–9.

26. Carrau RL, Pou A, Eibling DE, Murry T, Farguson BJ. Laryngeal framework surgery for the management of aspiration. Head Neck. 1999;21:139–45.

27. Yung KC, Likhterov I, Courey MS. Effect of temporary vocal fold injection medialization on the rate of permanent medialization laryngoplasty in unilateral vocal fold paralysis patients. Laryngoscope. 2011;121: 2191–4.

28. Arviso LC, Johns 3rd MM, Mathison CC, Klein AM. Long-term outcomes of injection laryngoplasty in patients with potentially recoverable vocal fold paralysis. Laryngoscope. 2010;120:2237–40.

29. Song PC, Sung CK, Franco Jr RA. Voice outcomes after endoscopic injection laryngoplasty with hyaluronic acid stabilizing gel. Laryngoscope. 2010;120 Suppl 4:S199.

30. Tan M, Woo P. Injection laryngoplasty with micronized dermis: a 10-year experience with 381 injections in 344 patients. Laryngoscope. 2010;120:2460–6.

31. Rees CJ, Mouadeb DA, Belafsky PC. Thyrohyoid vocal fold augmentation with calcium hydroxyapatite. Otolaryngol Head Neck Surg. 2008;138:743–6.

32. Hendricker RM, de Silva BW, Forrest LA. Gore-Tex medialization laryngoplasty for treatment of dysphagia. Otolaryngol Head Neck Surg. 2010;142: 536–9.

33. Thevasagayam MS, Willson K, Jennings C, Pracy P. Bilateral medialization thyroplasty: an effective approach to severe, chronic aspiration. J Laryngol Otol. 2006;120:698–701.

34. Sipp JA, Kerschner JE, Braune N, Hartnick CJ. Vocal fold medialization in children: injection laryngoplasty, thyroplasty, or nerve reinnervation? Arch Otolaryngol Head Neck Surg. 2007;133:767–71.

35. Lambert L, Fortin B, Soulieres D, et al. Organ preservation with concurrent chemoradiation for advanced laryngeal cancer: are we succeeding? Int J Radiat Oncol Biol Phys. 2010;76:398–402.

36. Montgomery WW. Surgery to prevent aspiration. Arch Otolaryngol Head Neck Surg. 1975;101: 679–82.

37. Habal MB, Murray JE. Surgical treatment of life-endangering aspiration. Arch Otolaryngol Head Neck Surg. 1983;109:809–11.

38. Thumfart WF, Pototschnig CA, Schneider I, et al. Repeated by successful closure of the larynx for the treatment of chronic aspiration with the use of botulinum toxin A. Ann Otol Rhinol Laryngol. 1996;105: 521–4.

39. Takano Y, Suga M, Sakamoto O, Sato K, Samejima Y, Ando M. Satisfaction of patients treated surgically for intractable aspiration. Chest. 1999;116:1251–6.

40. Eisele DW. Surgical approaches to aspiration. Dysphagia. 1991;6:71–9.

41. Synderman CH, Johnson JT. Laryngotracheal separation for intractable aspiration. Ann Otol Rhinol Laryngol. 1988;97:466–70.

42. Cannon CR, McLean WC. Laryngectomy for chronic aspiration. Am J Otolaryngol. 1982;3:145–9.

43. Wisdom G, Krespi YP, Blitzer A. Surgical therapy for chronic aspiration. Oper Tech Otolaryngol Head Neck Surg. 1997;8:199–208.

44. Krespi YP, Blitzer A. Laryngectomy for aspiration: narrow field technique. Oper Tech Otolaryngol Head Neck Surg. 1997;8:227–30.

45. Hunter SE, Scher RL. Clinical implications of radionecrosis to the head and neck surgeon. Curr Opin Otolaryngol Head Neck Surg. 2003;11:103–6.

46. Steiner W, Vogt P, Ambrosch P, Kron M. Transoral carbon dioxide laser microsurgery for recurrent glottic carcinoma after radiotherapy. Head Neck. 2004;26: 477–84.

47. Lindeman RC. Diverting the paralyzed larynx: a reversible procedure for intractable aspiration. Laryngoscope. 1975;85:157–80.

48. Lindeman RC, Yarington CT, Sutter D. Clinical experience with the tracheoesophageal anastomosis for intractable aspiration. Ann Otol Rhinol Laryngol. 1976;85:609–13.

49. Tucker HM. Management of the patient with an incompetent larynx. Am J Otolaryngol. 1979;1: 47–56.

50. Krespi YP, Quatela VC, Sisson GA, et al. Modified tracheoesophageal diversion for chronic aspiration. Laryngoscope. 1984;94:1298–301.

51. Eibling DE, Snyderman CH, Eibling C. Laryngotracheal separation for intractable aspiration: a retrospective review of 34 patients. Laryngoscope. 1995;105:83–5.

52. Cook SP. Candidate's thesis: laryngotracheal separation in neurologically impaired children: long-term results. Laryngoscope. 2009;119:390–5.

53. Shima H, Kitagawa H, Wakisaka M, et al. The usefulness of laryngotracheal separation in the treatment of severe motor and intellectual disabilities. Pediatr Surg Int. 2010;26:1041–4.

54. Tatekawa Y, Hosino N, Hori T, Kaneko M. Closure of the larynx for intractable aspiration in neurologically impaired patients. Pediatr Surg Int. 2010;26:553–6.

55. Aviv JE, Spitzer J, Cohen M, Ma G, Belafsky P, Close LG. Laryngeal adductor reflex and pharyngeal squeeze as predictors of laryngeal penetration and aspiration. Laryngoscope. 2002;112:338–41.

56. Setzen M, Cohen MA, Perlman PW, Belafsky PC, Guss J, Mattucci KF, Ditkoff M. The association between laryngopharyngeal sensory deficits, pharyngeal motor function, and the prevalence of aspiration with thin liquids. Otolaryngol Head Neck Surg. 2003;128:99–102.

57. Allen J, White CJ, Leonard R, Belafsky PC. Effect of cricopharyngeus muscle surgery on the pharynx. Laryngoscope. 2010;120:1498–503.

58. Belafsky PC, Rees CJ, Allen J, Leonard RJ. Pharyngeal dilation in cricopharyngeus muscle dysfunction and Zenker diverticulum. Laryngoscope. 2010;120: 889–94.

59. Yip HT, Leonard R, Kendall KA. Cricopharyngeal myotomy normalizes the opening size of the upper esophageal sphincter in cricopharyngeal dysfunction. Laryngoscope. 2006;116:93–6.

60. Zocratto OB, Savassi-Rocha PR, Paixao RM. Long-term outcome of reversal of laryngotracheal separation. Dysphagia. 2011;26(2):144–9.

61. Young O, Cunningham C, Russell JD. Reversal of laryngotracheal separation in paediatric patients. Int J Pediatr Otorhinolaryngol. 2010;74:1251–3.

Anti-Reflux Surgery

67

Candice L. Wilshire and Jeffrey H. Peters

Abstract

New onset post fundoplication dysphagia is among the most significant potential adverse events following antireflux surgery. Although this occurs in a small number of patients, its prevention is important and largely possible. Importantly, the majority of patients with preoperative dysphagia, report an improvement in swallowing postoperatively. Early postoperative dysphagia is common and well tolerated; however, persistent or new onset dysphagia occurs in approximately 5–10% of patients. Patient selection, preoperative abnormalities and accurate construction of a short, loose fundoplication will help minimize the incidence of persistent postoperative dysphagia. Although adequate esophageal body contractility has received the vast majority of attention, careful study suggests that hiatal outflow resistance is among the most common reasons for new onset dysphagia. When persistent dysphagia causing severe dietary limitations or significant weight loss prompts treatment bougie dilation may be attempted, although its benefit remains untested in controlled studies. Most patients will improve with time. Remedial surgical correction including takedown of hiatal closure, reclosure and conversion to partial fundoplication may be occasionally necessary.

Keywords

Gastroesophageal reflux disease • Postoperative dysphagia • Anti-reflux surgery • Fundoplication • Dilation • Reoperative antireflux surgery

C.L. Wilshire, MD (✉)
Division of Thoracic and Foregut Surgery,
University of Rochester School of Medicine
and Dentistry, Rochester, NY, USA
e-mail: candice.wilshire@gmail.com

J.H. Peters, MD
Division of Thoracic and Foregut Surgery,
University of Rochester School of Medicine
and Dentistry, Rochester, NY, USA

R. Shaker et al. (eds.), *Principles of Deglutition: A Multidisciplinary Text for Swallowing and its Disorders*, 955
DOI 10.1007/978-1-4614-3794-9_67, © Springer Science+Business Media New York 2013

Prevalence of Dysphagia in Patients with Gastroesophageal Reflux Disease

Dysphagia is uncommon as the primary or most severe symptom in patients with gastroesophageal reflux disease (GERD). When it is the primary symptom, alternate diagnoses such as achalasia or eosinophilic esophagitis should be entertained, as well as a mechanical obstruction including stricture, neoplasm, or paraesophageal hernia. On the other hand, dysphagia as a component of the symptom complex is more common than often recognized, occurring in up to 40–50% of patients. Most studies report the prevalence of dysphagia proportional to disease severity, ranging from 3% in uncomplicated GERD to 47% in patients with a reflux-induced esophageal stricture or ulcerative esophagitis [3–7].

The presence of dysphagia is also related to the degree of esophageal body dysmotility associated with GERD. Previous reports have identified peristaltic dysfunction with decreased wave amplitudes in up to 50% of patients with moderate to severe reflux-induced esophagitis. Díaz de Liaño and colleagues manometrically demonstrated the presence of peristaltic dysfunction in 71% of patients with GERD and concomitant symptoms of dysphagia [8]. Similarly, Fumagalli et al. [6] found dysphagia to be significantly more common among patients with altered esophageal motility (27%) than among patients with normal esophageal motility (7%) preoperatively.

Dysphagia and Antireflux Surgery

A large cohort of outcome studies, including several prospective randomized trials, confirm relief of typical reflux symptoms post-fundoplication in 80–95% of patients at follow-up intervals of 5–10 years [4, 9–12]. Dysphagia occurs postoperatively in a small proportion of patients and can either be persistent or new onset. The risk factors and causes of each of these circumstances may be quite different and as such, we consider them separately.

Persistent Dysphagia Post-antireflux Surgery

Despite the fact that antireflux surgery may induce dysphagia, in the vast majority of patients in whom dysphagia was present before surgery, it resolves following fundoplication. Reports have shown that up to 68% of patients with preoperative dysphagia experience an improvement in swallowing following laparoscopic fundoplication [5, 12]. Tsuboi et al. [5] recently demonstrated that relief of dysphagia may be as high as 87%.

Persistent dysphagia post-antireflux surgery is likely related to factors present prior to fundoplication. Thus, the decision to proceed with surgical intervention should be based upon both subjective (a careful symptom assessment) and objective (specific diagnostic) findings. Although adequacy of esophageal motility prior to antireflux surgery has been among the most widely of studied risk factors, there is not one but three key components that should be considered:

1. The presence of dysphagia as a preoperative symptom.
2. Esophageal motility, including both percent peristalsis and contractile wave amplitudes.
3. The adequacy of esophageal bolus transport.

The presence of dysphagia as the primary or a prominent symptom in a patient being considered for antireflux surgery not only deserves careful contemplation but should trigger the vigilant clinician to think twice prior to proceeding with surgical correction of reflux. When prominent, dysphagia should prompt either consideration of a nonoperative approach or an alternative operative approach, such as a partial fundoplication.

The presence of dysphagia prior to surgery is among the most significant risk factors for its presence after surgery. Tsuboi et al. [5] recently reported a multivariate logistic regression analysis of 219 patients post-primary antireflux surgery identifying risk factors predisposing to dysphagia post-fundoplication. The presence of preoperative dysphagia was found to be a significant risk factor for dysphagia 1 year postoperatively. Similar results have been reported by other groups, including Montenovo and colleagues who reported that patients with postoperative dysphagia were much more likely to have had dysphagia prior to surgery (77%) than those who had no preoperative dysphagia (23%; $p<0.01$) [7].

Further, although abnormal esophageal motility in and of itself correlates poorly with the risk of postoperative dysphagia, the presence of abnormal esophageal body contractility in concert with dysphagia preoperatively may indeed affect the risk of postoperative dysphagia. Díaz de Liaño and colleagues reported that patients in whom preoperative dysphagia persisted after surgery had significantly less improvement in esophageal body motor function as reflected in percent primary peristalsis and mean distal esophageal contraction amplitudes following fundoplication, when compared to patients in whom preoperative dysphagia resolved (30% versus 82%, $p<0.01$) [8]. Thus, persistent esophageal dysmotility may account for a component of the etiology for persistent dysphagia postoperatively.

Other potential risk factors including the grade of esophagitis and inadequate LES relaxation preoperatively have been studied, with little evidence supporting any correlation to the incidence of postoperative dysphagia [3, 5, 13, 14]. While manometric evidence of peristaltic dysfunction was traditionally considered a contraindication to total fundoplication, numerous studies have failed to demonstrate that preoperative manometric and/or impedance findings taken in isolation are reliable predictors of postoperative dysphagia. In fact, disordered peristalsis often improves following fundoplication [5, 7]. As such, in contrast to common misunderstandings, the primary utility of manometry prior to antireflux surgery is to evaluate characteristics of the LES and to identify patients with complete aperistalsis or those with achalasia for whom other treatment options are preferable.

The third component likely predisposing to dysphagia post-antireflux surgery is the adequacy of preoperative bolus transport. The assessment of esophageal function for either solid or liquid bolus material is often ignored and can be difficult to quantify. Historically it has relied on subjective assessment of barium transport when viewing a video esophagram or, less commonly, nuclear medicine esophageal emptying studies. The recent introduction of impedance assessment of bolus transport to esophageal motility studies has provided a more reproducible and quantifiable method of assessing transport function, although few studies to date have related it to the risk of dysphagia after antireflux surgery. Using nuclear studies, Montenovo's group reported that patients with worsened dysphagia postoperatively had lower liquid bolus clearance rates and longer liquid bolus transit times than patients whose postoperative dysphagia was the same or improved from what it was preoperatively [7]. Tsuboi et al. [5] identified in a multivariate analysis as a risk factor for persistent postoperative dysphagia, delayed esophageal emptying on preoperative video barium esophagram.

New Onset Dysphagia Post-fundoplication

Up to 70% of patients experience some degree of early postoperative dysphagia following fundoplication [13]. Persistence greater than 6–12 months affects between 3 and 30% of patients, with the incidence being highly dependent on measurement parameters such as dysphagia scoring systems, surgical techniques, and length of follow-up [3–5, 7, 13, 15]. Clinically relevant rates, however, have been reported in the range of 2–6% [4, 6].

Since the introduction of fundoplication into surgical practice by Rudolph Nissen in 1956, several important modifications of Nissen's original technique, focusing on minimizing postoperative dysphagia, have been described. Among the most important was the introduction of the concept of a short, loose fundoplication (as compared to the original snug 4–6 cm wrap) by both DeMeester and Donahue in the 1980s [3]. Furthermore, the introduction of the laparoscopic approach in 1991 revolutionized the surgical treatment of GERD, minimizing the pain and complications associated with open laparotomy and the disability of a major surgical procedure. Laparoscopic fundoplication is now recognized as the preferable surgical approach.

Mechanisms responsible for early postoperative dysphagia are not well understood and the majority has no identifiable cause. Hypotheses include esophageal inflammation and edema with spasm of the esophageal wall, temporary hypomotility, reduced axial motion, decreased transit time at the LES, and impaired deglutitive relaxation [3, 7, 9]. The majority of these patients will improve with dietary advice and reassurance alone, usually by 2–3 months following surgery.

For symptoms persisting beyond 2–3 months, the precise etiology may be difficult to elicit. Reports have shown that several detail nuances may be related to the incidence of new onset postoperative dysphagia. Whether the geometry or location of the fundic wrap versus persistent mechanical obstruction at the hiatus is responsible for postoperative dysphagia remains a topic of debate. Granderath and colleagues attempted to make this distinction by radiographically identifying the morphologic cause of dysphagia in 50 patients following laparoscopic fundoplication. The authors demonstrated that subtleties in hiatal closure causing either hiatal stenosis (excessively tight) or intrathoracic migration of the wrap (excessively loose) were more problematic than a tight, twisted, or slipped fundoplication (90% versus 10%, respectively), although wrap migration was more frequently seen [15]. Poor esophageal body function may compound circumstances further, ultimately leading to surgical revision.

Open Versus Laparoscopic Surgical Approach

Although studies have shown that relief of GERD symptoms following laparoscopic versus an open antireflux procedure is comparable, some reports suggest that the prevalence of postoperative dysphagia is higher following laparoscopic when compared to open surgery [10]. Technical factors thought to be responsible include a reduced posterior window, fibrosis of the esophageal hiatus as a result of liberal diathermy use, adhesions, and faulty geometry of the wrap.

Limitations in the study design of the trials included in these series may be the fact that most reported early dysphagia. Rantanen et al. [3] reported a 3-year follow-up study of 57 patients with erosive esophagitis treated with fundoplication. They found a significant difference in early dysphagia (open 41% versus laparoscopic 67%; $p = 0.05$) but not long-term dysphagia (open 18% versus laparoscopic 20%). Further, there have been many trials reporting no difference or a nonsignificant difference between the two approaches [3, 4, 10, 16].

Adequate Fundic Mobilization

Many surgeons advocate division of the short gastric vessels to obtain greater mobility of the gastric fundus allowing careful construction of the fundoplication. Conflicting results have been reported, with good outcomes reported after both laparoscopic and open procedures, with and without division of the short gastric vessels [12]. Dalenbaack and colleagues demonstrated a significant reduction in dysphagia following fundic mobilization, and similar conclusions have been drawn by DeMeester et al. in their experience with fundic mobilization in 100 consecutive fundoplications [3, 16]. However, many report the construction of tension free wraps without the division of the short gastric vessels. The consensus is that the geometry of the fundoplication is important, which may be improved by division of the short gastric vessels. Table 67.1 indicates the range of outcomes following fundoplication as reported by various authors, with and without division of the short gastric vessels.

Hiatal Closure

Herbella et al., among others, noted accentuation of the esophageal anteroposterior angle following antireflux surgery and hiatal repair in some patients. This led them to hypothesize that a long posterior repair may predispose to esophageal angulation and increase in the incidence of

Table 67.1 Outcomes following fundoplication, with and without division of short gastric vessels.

Author	Morbidity		Length (min)		Dysphagia		Recurrence	
	DSGV	ND	DSGV	ND	DSGV	ND	DSGV	ND
Luostarine et al.	NR	NR	NR	NR	5/26	8/23	1/26	1/23
Watson et al.	7/52	6/50	95	71	15/52	17/50	3/52	5/50
Bloomqvist et al.	15/52	5/47	120	104	11/39	15/41	1/52	1/47
Chrysos et al.	2/24	3/32	100	60	4/24	5/32	1/24	0/32
Total	24/128	14/122	105	78	35/141	45/146	6/154	7/152
	18.7%	11.5%			24.5%	30.8%	3.9%	4.6%

DSGV Division of short gastric vessels, *ND* Nondivision. Modified from Wills et al. [3]

postoperative dysphagia [3, 13, 15]. Although plausible, most data suggest that this is an unlikely cause of dysphagia. The evaluation of 32 patients post-laparoscopic fundoplication and hiatoplasty in Herbella's study revealed no significant change in the esophageal anteroposterior angle pre- and postoperatively, as well as no correlation with dysphagia [13]. This was subsequently confirmed by prospective randomized trials concluding that hiatal repair may be performed anteriorly, posteriorly, or a combination of both with no significant effect on postoperative dysphagia.

The Need for Bougie Placement

Most experts believe that postoperative dysphagia is reduced by calibrating the fundoplication around a large-caliber bougie (56–60 French), thus ensuring a floppy Nissen. In a classic report of 100 consecutive patients, DeMeester et al. [3] showed that the prevalence of postoperative dysphagia was reduced when the size of the bougie used during fundoplication was increased from 36 to 60 French. A significant reduction in persistent dysphagia, both severity and frequency, was also observed by Swanström et al. [4] when the use of an intraoperative 56 French bougie (17%) versus no bougie (31%) was compared in 171 patients, $p = 0.047$. The potential benefit should still be weighed against the risk of bougie-related esophageal perforations, which have been reported in approximately 1% of laparoscopic fundoplications [4].

Partial Versus Complete Fundoplication

Partial fundoplication has been used as an alternative to a 360° Nissen fundoplication with the intent to minimize the prevalence of postoperative dysphagia, particularly in patients with esophageal peristaltic dysfunction. Examples of partial fundoplication include the posterior Toupet, Lind, or Guarner fundoplications; the transthoracic Belsey Mark IV procedure; anterior Dor, Watson, or Thal fundoplication; and the Hill repair. The rationale for this approach is the reduction in the resistance to bolus passage afforded by partial fundoplication, with a consequent decrease in the risk of dysphagia. The use of partial fundoplication is supported by many studies which suggest long-term symptomatic improvement comparable to those following total fundoplication, but fewer side effects [15, 17]. In fact, a recent meta-analysis of 11 trials comparing partial versus total fundoplication in 991 patients identified a significantly higher incidence of postoperative dysphagia following total fundoplication [17]. However, poor methodological quality and validity of this meta-analysis limit its usefulness [15].

Fundoplication Length and Extent

The only technical modification conclusively and repetitively shown to reduce postoperative dysphagia is the construction of a loose, short (1–2 cm) fundoplication [3, 10]. Figure 67.1 shows an intra-

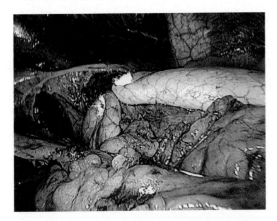

Fig. 67.1 Intraoperative laparoscopic photograph of a loose, short Nissen fundoplication constructed over a 60 French bougie

operative laparoscopic view of a short fundoplication, constructed over a 60 French bougie.

Prosthetic Crural Repair

The use of a prosthetic mesh in hiatal hernia repair is widely debated, particularly with type III hiatal hernias. Granderath et al. demonstrated a significantly higher rate of dysphagia within the first 3 months following surgery in 170 patients with a prosthetic crural repair than in 361 patients without mesh placement (35.3% versus 19.8%, p <0.05). This difference was no longer evident at 1 year after fundoplication (4.9% versus 4.4%) [16]. Thus, the use of prosthetic hiatal repair may increase the risk of postoperative dysphagia, although its long-term effects are not clear. Few authors advocate the routine use of mesh when treating GERD.

Physiology of Fundoplication

The goal of fundoplication is to restore an anatomic and functionally competent antireflux barrier. This occurs with correction of the axial and radial crural defects of the associated hiatal hernia, re-approximation of the diaphragmatic crura to allow contact with the lower abdominal esophagus, and enhancement in the pressure and length of

the neo high pressure zone at the esophagogastric junction (EGJ) via the extrinsic effect of the fundic wrap. These combined effects restore compliance and limit the opening dimensions at the EGJ ideally toward normal, and not supra-normal, values [9, 18, 19].

Pandolfino and colleagues compared the manometric characteristics and distensibility of the EGJ between three groups: eight normal subjects, nine GERD patients, and eight postfundoplication patients. A custom-made manometry catheter was utilized, combined with a distally placed overlying barostat bag designed to determine EGJ compliance. Once the EGJ opening pressure was established and noted fluoroscopically, swallows were recorded at 5 mmHg barostat distension pressure increments up to a pressure of 30 mmHg. EGJ diameter and intraluminal distensive pressures regulated by the barostat were plotted and their relationship determined. The mean basal LES and opening pressures during the interswallow period of patients following fundoplication were comparable with those of normal subjects, and both groups had significantly higher pressures than those recorded in patients with GERD ($p < 0.05$). In addition, they showed that following fundoplication the EGJ opening diameter approximated normal values, along with a greater overall length [18].

This decreased compliance and reduction in opening diameter at any given distention force following fundoplication has also been reported by Scheffer et al. This study included 12 patients pre- and postoperatively evaluated with concurrent high-resolution manometry (HRM) and fluoroscopy during swallows of both liquid and solid boluses. The authors reported an increase in resistance to flow as a consequence of the altered EGJ dimensions post-fundoplication, along with reduced axial bolus length, an elevated intrabolus pressure, and a prolonged EGJ transit time for both liquids and solids ($p < 0.05$). This prolonged transit time was found to have a proportional relationship to higher dysphagia symptom scores [9].

Historically it has been suggested that the vagally mediated reflex, transient lower esophageal sphincter relaxation (TLESR), is associated with gastroesophageal reflux, and that distension and stimulation of stretch receptors, particularly in the gastric cardia, trigger these TLESRs. Scheffer and colleagues sought to evaluate the effect of fundoplication on the TLESR reflex. Twenty GERD patients were studied before and after fundoplication. Twenty normal subjects served as controls. HRM and pH monitoring were performed 1 h before and 2 h following ingestion of a liquid meal, while three-dimensional ultrasonographic images of the stomach were constructed prior to and every 15 min postprandially for up to 2 h. The study confirmed that patients with GERD prior to surgical correction have significantly larger proximal gastric volumes when compared to control subjects ($p < 0.001$). This may promote meal-induced altered fundic relaxation and an increased rate of TLESRs. Proximal gastric distention was significantly reduced post-fundoplication ($p < 0.001$), although no relationship to the rate of TLESRs was found. Further, neither reflux frequency nor duration was found to correlate with gastric volumes in any patient group, suggesting a mechanism other than proximal gastric distension may be responsible for transient sphincter loss following fundoplication [19]. As previously discussed, this study provided further confirmation

that fundoplication alters transsphincteric pressure profiles, leading to an overall decrease in EGJ compliance preventing reflux during periods of gastric distention [19].

Treatment of Dysphagia Following Antireflux Surgery

Dysphagia post-fundoplication is common and perhaps even desirable in the early postoperative period (1–2 weeks up to 2–3 months). Patients are generally sent home with a soft solid diet minimizing bulky foods such as bread and meat, while maximizing softer foods such as soups, fish, eggs, and anything with a pudding consistency. With such instructions, generally lasting 2–4 weeks, dysphagia is minimal in most patients. If dysphagia emerges or persists following this early postoperative time, generally accepted as more than 3 months after surgery, and particularly if it is severe enough to require significantly limited solid food intake or results in a >10–15 lb weight loss, it is considered a complication of the fundoplication.

Most patients will improve with time (Fig. 67.2) and do not require specific treatment. When severe dietary limitations or

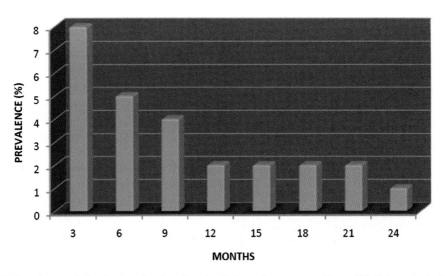

Fig. 67.2 Prevalence of dysphagia related to length of time after surgery. From J.H. Peters et al. Ann Surg 1998;228(1):40–50 with permission

Table 67.2 Incidence of pre- and persistent postoperative dysphagia, with subsequent intervention

Reference	Year	# Patients	Incidence of dysphagia (%)		Intervention for dysphagia (%)	
			Pre-op	Persistent post-op (>3 months)	Dilatation[a]	Reoperation
Patterson et al.	2000	171	33	10	9[b]	0
Blom et al.	2002	163	37	8	NR	NR
Sato et al.	2002	139	33	6	6	4
Fumagalli et al.	2008	276	9	9	1	5
Montenovo et al.	2009	74	43	17	NR	NR
Tsuboi et al.	2010	208	26	9	NR	NR

Modified from Wills et al. [3]
[a]Dilatation for persistent dysphagia >3 months
[b]>10 weeks postoperatively

significant weight loss prompts treatment (usually well less than 1–2% of patients) options include bougie or pneumatic dilation, and occasionally reoperation (Table 67.2). The choice of intervening at all, as well as what specific treatment to pursue, will depend upon a review of the operative technique used, both pre- and postoperative esophageal motility findings, evidence of outflow resistance on motility and video barium upper gastrointestinal study, the severity of symptoms, alimentary ability, weight loss, and treatment risk.

Most patients are able to maintain their weight with modest dietary changes and continue to improve with time over the course of 12–24 months postoperatively. Dilation utilizing 50–60 French Savary guide wire bougienage is often carried out and improvement may follow. No controlled studies have shown its efficacy although uncontrolled case series have suggested there may be some benefit. A literature review by Wills et al. evaluating dysphagia, post-fundoplication over a 15-year period reported that approximately 50% of patients responded to initial attempts at dilation [3]. A similar proportion of dilation success was found in the group of patients that Granderath et al. [15] identified as having postoperative hiatal stenosis possibly benefiting from pneumatic dilation. On the other hand, 45% of these patients did not respond to the first attempt at dilation and 17% required redo surgery following multiple attempts.

Dysphagia and Reoperative Antireflux Surgery

Approximately 5–17% of patients will undergo reoperation following the primary antireflux procedure [15, 21]. Although recurrent heartburn/reflux is the most common reason for repair, a substantial minority undergo reoperation for persistent, new, or recurrent dysphagia, most of whom will have concomitant anatomic abnormalities such as recurrent hiatal hernia, slipped or spiral fundoplication. First time reoperation is generally more technically demanding than primary fundoplication, requires longer operating time, and is associated with greater morbidity. Successful outcomes occur in 80–90% of patients with recurrent heartburn and 70–80% of patients operated upon for dysphagia. A systematic review of 17 series representing 1,167 re-operative fundoplications identified dysphagia as the second leading indication for reoperation (30%), while recurrent heartburn/reflux was the most prevalent (59%). The authors identified similar complication rates and outcome scores to initial fundoplication, with a weighted average success rate of 81% (range, 65–100%) [21].

Summary and Conclusions

The majority of GERD patients with dysphagia improve following antireflux surgery. Early postoperative dysphagia is common and generally well tolerated. Persistent or new onset dysphagia occurs in 5–10% of patients. Patient selection, preoperative abnormalities, and accurate construction of a short, loose fundoplication can lead to a decrease in the incidence of persistent postoperative dysphagia.

References

1. Sato K, Awad ZT, Filipi CJ, et al. Causes of long-term dysphagia after laparoscopic Nissen fundoplication. JSLS. 2002;6(1):35–40.
2. Grudell AB, Alexander JA, Enders FB, et al. Validation of the mayo dysphagia questionnaire. Dis Esophagus. 2007;20(3):202–5.
3. Wills VL, Hunt DR. Dysphagia after antireflux surgery. Br J Surg. 2001;88(4):486–99.
4. Patterson EJ, Herron DM, Hansen PD, Ramzi N, Standage BA, Swanstrom LL. Effect of an esophageal bougie on the incidence of dysphagia following nissen fundoplication: a prospective, blinded, randomized clinical trial. Arch Surg. 2000;135(9):1055–61.
5. Tsuboi K, Lee TH, Legner A, Yano F, Dworak T, Mittal SK. Identification of risk factors for postoperative dysphagia after primary anti-reflux surgery. Surg Endosc. 2011;25(3):923–9.
6. Fumagalli U, Bona S, Battafarano F, Zago M, Barbera R, Rosati R. Persistent dysphagia after laparoscopic fundoplication for gastro-esophageal reflux disease. Dis Esophagus. 2008;21(3):257–61.
7. Montenovo M, Tatum RP, Figueredo E, et al. Does combined multichannel intraluminal esophageal impedance and manometry predict postoperative dysphagia after laparoscopic Nissen fundoplication? Dis Esophagus. 2009;22(8):656–63.
8. Diaz de Liano A, Oteiza F, Ciga MA, Aizcorbe M, Trujillo R, Cobo F. Nonobstructive dysphagia and recovery of motor disorder after antireflux surgery. Am J Surg. 2003;185(2):103–7.
9. Scheffer RC, Samsom M, Haverkamp A, Oors J, Hebbard GS, Gooszen HG. Impaired bolus transit across the esophagogastric junction in postfundoplication dysphagia. Am J Gastroenterol. 2005;100(8):1677–84.
10. Le Blanc-Louvry I, Koning E, Zalar A, et al. Severe dysphagia after laparoscopic fundoplication: useful-ness of barium meal examination to identify causes other than tight fundoplication—a prospective study. Surgery. 2000;128(3):392–8.
11. Granderath FA, Kamolz T, Schweiger UM, Pointner R. Long-term follow-up after laparoscopic refundoplication for failed antireflux surgery: quality of life, symptomatic outcome, and patient satisfaction. J Gastrointest Surg. 2002;6(6):812–8.
12. Catarci M, Gentileschi P, Papi C, et al. Evidence-based appraisal of antireflux fundoplication. Ann Surg. 2004;239(3):325–37.
13. Herbella FA, Nipomnick I, Patti MG. Esophageal angulation after hiatoplasty and fundoplication: a cause of dysphagia? Dis Esophagus. 2009;22(1):95–8.
14. Tatum RP, Shi G, Manka MA, Brasseur JG, Joehl RJ, Kahrilas PJ. Bolus transit assessed by an esophageal stress test in postfundoplication dysphagia. J Surg Res. 2000;91(1):56–60.
15. Granderath FA, Schweiger UM, Kamolz T, Pointner R. Dysphagia after laparoscopic antireflux surgery: a problem of hiatal closure more than a problem of the wrap. Surg Endosc. 2005;19(11):1439–46.
16. Granderath FA, Schweiger UM, Kamolz T, Pasiut M, Haas CF, Pointner R. Laparoscopic antireflux surgery with routine mesh-hiatoplasty in the treatment of gastroesophageal reflux disease. J Gastrointest Surg. 2002;6(3):347–53.
17. Varin O, Velstra B, De Sutter S, Ceelen W. Total vs partial fundoplication in the treatment of gastroesophageal reflux disease: a meta-analysis. Arch Surg. 2009;144(3):273–8.
18. Pandolfino JE, Curry J, Shi G, Joehl RJ, Brasseur JG, Kahrilas PJ. Restoration of normal distensive characteristics of the esophagogastric junction after fundoplication. Ann Surg. 2005;242(1):43–8.
19. Scheffer RC, Gooszen HG, Hebbard GS, Samsom M. The role of transsphincteric pressure and proximal gastric volume in acid reflux before and after fundoplication. Gastroenterology. 2005;129(6):1900–9.
20. Peters JH, DeMeester TR, Crookes P, et al. The treatment of gastroesophageal reflux disease with laparoscopic Nissen fundoplication: prospective evaluation of 100 patients with "typical" symptoms. Ann Surg. 1998;228(1):40–50.
21. van Beek DB, Auyang ED, Soper NJ. A comprehensive review of laparoscopic redo fundoplication. Surg Endosc. 2011;25(3):706–12.

Tube Feeding: Indications, Considerations, and Technique

68

William L. Berger

Abstract

Tube feeding, as an alternative to eating, conveys nutrition, fluid, and medications safely and reliably to the intestinal tract. This chapter reviews the many ways of establishing and maintaining tube feeding. For a satisfactory outcome, the requesting provider, patient, family, and consultant must understand the indication, purpose, and expectations of this approach. Because tube position determines function, proper selection and placement are discussed in detail. Special attention is given to surgical and percutaneous endoscopic and radiological approaches. Long-term complications are reviewed in detail and a comprehensive approach to management is outlined, with emphasis on the role of a multidisciplinary enteral nutrition team. Position papers and core references are provided.

Keywords

G–J Tube • Nasoenteric • Open G-tube • PEG • Tube feeding

When the patient becomes a deglutitive failure, our focus shifts from the cause to the consequences of dysphagia. Unlike therapies in prior chapters, tube feeding does not correct deglutition, it bypasses swallowing altogether. Tube feeding, as an alternative to eating, conveys nutrition, fluid, and medications safely and reliably to the intestinal tract. This chapter reviews the many ways of establishing and maintaining tube feeding.

Indications

The indication is the problem for which artificial feeding is a solution. Although dysphagia is the topic of this book, it is not the only indication for artificial feeing. The consultant is responsible for confirming that tube feeding is an appropriate solution and that alternatives have been considered. In practice, a consultant is more

W.L. Berger, MD (⊠)
Division of Gastroenterology and Hepatology,
Medical College of Wisconsin, Clement J. Zablocki
VA Medical Center, Milwaukee, WI, USA
e-mail: wberger@mcw.edu

R. Shaker et al. (eds.), *Principles of Deglutition: A Multidisciplinary Text for Swallowing and its Disorders*,
DOI 10.1007/978-1-4614-3794-9_68, © Springer Science+Business Media New York 2013

comfortable answering a request to evaluate a "feeding disorder"[1] than for "PEG tube placement," a request with a predetermined solution. It is best if the requesting provider and consultant collaborate on a solution, possibly including a PEG tube but open to reevaluation of the problem and creative alternative solutions. Blindly following a procedural request is to blindly accept the judgment of the requesting provider and to close the door to other options.

In considering the appropriate type of tube feeding, start with physiology. Feeding disorder can be the result of many different processes (including, but not limited to dysphagia) just as dysphagia can result from many different diseases. These underlying diseases may have collateral effects influencing prognosis and approaches to treatment. Similarly, other medical and psychosocial issues may uniquely permit or limit therapeutic options. The provider and patient are well served by considering these potential implications, possible obstacles to placement and maintenance, and likely complications before starting artificial nutrition. What are the nature of the feeding disorder and its range of appropriate solutions? Is permanently bypassing oral nutrition the only or best solution? Consider cause and nature of the feeding disorder, other comorbidities, and psychosocial context.

The nature of the feeding disorder depends on more than its proximate cause. To say that a patient is dysphagic after a cerebral hemorrhage is only partially helpful. This does not tell us what the exact deficit is or what the prognosis for recovery might be. To define the best approach, we need to delineate as precisely as possible the type of impairment, its severity, and whether it is expected to progress or recover. The expected duration of artificial feeding is also important. Do not allow a patient to suffer inadequate nutrition for more than a week in the hopes of avoiding

artificial feedings. Rarely is one criticized for initiating nutritional support too early. Everyone needs nutrition, and this is especially true of sick patients. If the underlying condition cannot be corrected or will take >30 days to resolve, a more permanent, stable, percutaneous tube should be considered. Sometimes only enteral supplementation of oral feeding is necessary, if the feeding disorder is incomplete or if metabolic requirements simply outstrip the patient's ability to eat. Some special diets or medications may simply be too unpalatable to take orally, especially for children.

As a general rule, when the gut works, but cannot be accessed by eating, get a tube. This is typically the case with deglutitive failure, but not for all causes of feeding disorder. If the underlying disease includes a bowel obstruction, for instance, parenteral nutrition might be more appropriate. The underlying disease and other comorbidities (e.g., cancer, CVA, or a variety of neurodegenerative diseases) can define the prognosis as well as the type of nutrition required. If the prognosis is severely limited, a temporary solution (even just IV hydration) may be most appropriate. An albumin <3.0 g/dl, advanced age, urinary tract infection, a documented history of aspiration, COPD, and incurable cancer all predict early mortality after feeding tube insertion. In fact, half of patients with more than three of these risk factors are dead at 3 weeks. Additional risk factors include BMI <18.5 and CRP >10. One recent study showed that 89 % of those who die within the 30 days after PEG are from a cohort with both low albumin and high CRP. Acute and chronic diseases with special metabolic requirements include brittle diabetes, acute postoperative recovery, acute infection, preexisting malnutrition, and obesity. Such circumstances may influence not only what nutrition is given, but how it is supplied. Pay special attention to any intrinsic gastrointestinal disease that interferes with digestion, absorption, transport, or excretion. Mechanical obstruction is the only absolute contraindication to enteral nutrition, but there are many conditions that would affect *how* tube feeding is best administered.

[1] "Feeding Disorder" ICD-9 code 783.3 is universally accepted as an indication for tube feeding and encompasses any problem preventing adequate oral nutrition, including severe anorexia, deglutitive failure, or even coma. It does not specify the source of the problem, just its existence. "Feeding disorder" is not "Eating disorder."

The psychosocial context needs to be carefully considered in defining feeding goals. Select those options that best align with the goals of the patient and—as applicable—their family.[2] Is the disposition after hospitalization expected to be self-care, home care with family, institutional care, or palliative? Unfortunately, such questions may never have been explicitly considered before. The frequent clash between expectations, desires, and reality can be hard for everyone. It is important here to define both what the patient and family wish for and expect as well as to clearly determine what physiology, logistics, family involvement, insurance, and reality will support. Dignity, autonomy, and body image issues are different for every individual and can all be affected by different feeding solutions. The option to do nothing and to "let nature take its course" is always on the table. Although this was the only choice from the dawn of humanity until 1849,[3] today many patients and their families need permission to consider this option.

Nutrition is a basic physiological and human function. Loss of oral feeding and the insertion of an artificial tube can carry with them not only the loss of taste and food enjoyment, but changes in lifestyle, altered body image, and even the specter of impending mortality. Not surprisingly, rationalization and denial can often complicate such cases. Few other clinical circumstances in gastroenterology come burdened with as many ethical and political issues. Occasionally, religious and even legal forces may enter the arena. Ethically unambiguous solutions agreeable to all parties cannot always be found. Advanced directives, living wills, and durable powers of attorney do not always provide direction and clear answers [1]. Although ethics consultation can bring a certain level of clarity and objectivity, abstract concepts such as medical futility are often unhelpful in resolving the often conflicting medical goals of prolonging life and reducing suffering. A feeding tube trial with withdrawal at a specified future date has often been advocated, but we have rarely seen this attempted. Even less often does it end as anticipated. Unfortunately, lacking a satisfactory consensus, the best outcome usually involves graceful acceptance of the informed decisions of the individual with legal authority. This being said, navigating such anxiety to bring peace to a patient and their family can be one measure of success. Patience, flexibility, experience, and clear communication are keys. Through a process of education and defining values, truly informed consent (or informed refusal) can take place.

Tube feeding is life support. Normally, our body autoregulates by stimulating us to eat when we are hungry and drink when we are thirsty. Shifting control of intake to an external caregiver carries a certain amount of risk. The consequences of not being able to deliver nutrition to the gut include not only starvation, but dehydration and lack of medications. These functions could be given over to central venous access, but the risk and cost of parenteral nutrition are much higher and the implications are the same. In addition, enteral feeding serves to maintain gut epithelial integrity and health. In general, if the gut works use it.

Do not start down a road you cannot support. Deciding that tube feeding is appropriate and technically possible is only the beginning. Placing a tube in a patient is a commitment. Think several steps ahead. Not only is someone—possibly you—responsible for acute postinsertion complications and planning, but someone must also manage the tube and the patient long term. The patient or a caregiver will be using this device daily for the rest of this patient's life and needs to know basic care of the tube. But a medical professional has long-term responsibility including, but not limited to, optimizing nutritional effectiveness, arranging logistics, and managing complications of tube feeding. As with any form of life support, the goal is not to drop the ball. If you and the patient are lucky, all this effort will improve quality of life, modify disease outcome,

---

[2] A dependent person is rarely isolated; illness brings family; family brings issues. This may be an asset (or not) but it is not going away. The consultant is well advised to address any issues early and openly.

[3] Charles Se'dillot, a French surgeon, is the first to report a surgical gastrostomy in a human. Unfortunately, the first long-term survivor of this procedure was not reported until 1870 by LL Staton, a surgeon in North Carolina.

and potentially prolong survival. Since one caregiver cannot be reliably there 24/7, alternative caregivers must be available and trained. Eventually, the tube will malfunction, and urgent or emergent attention may be required. Incompetence needs to be anticipated, and education only reduces this potential. Some patients, caregivers, and even medical professionals will always seem "unclear on the concept." The purpose of this chapter is to help the reader not be that person.

Tube Selection

Tube materials and design are myriad and changing. There are many different materials (polyvinyl chloride, polyurethane, and silicone rubber), diameters (8–28 Fr; 2.7–9 mm), lengths (1.8–119 cm), and options (multilumen, thin walled, weighted, side holes, etc.). To avoid "dislodgement"—the term for when a tube is partially or completely pulled out—there are many different mechanisms for fixing the device in position ("Mushroom Tip," balloon, suture, and nasal "bridle"). Skin-level devices ("Buttons") are useful in reducing the risk of dislodgement or in patients with concerns about body image. We cannot exhaust all conceivable combinations, but would note some features that are to be avoided in a feeding tube. Multiple side holes near the tip, for example, are useful for preventing obstruction during suction but are unnecessary for feedings. Moreover, they functionally shorten the tube and—counterintuitively—increase the risk for clogging and kinking. Tube weights are another useless feature. [4] There is no reason to use these holdovers from the era of the mercury-filled balloon on the Miller–Abbott tube, since they do not help move the tube forward or increase the

probability of small bowel intubation after gastric placement.

Feeding methods include push bolus, slow bolus, continuous, and nocturnal infusions. Each has their specific indications. It may be helpful to think of tube feeding as a liquid, "predigested" diet. Commercial feedings are designed to flow through a narrow tube and to forego mastication and gastric digestion. In fact, one method of supplemental tube feeding is to puree food left on the patient's plate after a meal with a blender and infuse it into the gastric tube. There are also specially formulated feedings, designed for patients with a wide variety of specific metabolic needs.

Tube position determines function. A feeding tube generally has two ends. Nutrition goes into the *external end* of the tube and out the *internal tip*. The tube enters at the *intubation point* on the outside of the body and ends inside the body at the *infusion point*, where delivery from the tube tip into the gastrointestinal tract is intended. In carrying fluids from one end of the tube to another, these fluids bypass dysfunctional anatomy. There are several possible placement combinations and these delimit the tube type and feeding method required (Fig. 68.1).

The intubation point will be either at a "natural orifice" or an "artificial access point," typically a stoma. Nasal or oral access to the GI system can be considered "natural orifice" sites for intubation. These are "natural" not because it is normal to eat through one's nose. Rather, we use the term to differentiate such access points from "artificial" access points, specifically, ostomies or stomas.[5] The GI tract can be accessed through a stoma either to the esophagus as it passes

---

[4] Because weighted tubes are still sold one might assume that the weight is effective in moving these tubes forward. The weighting of tubes was an unproven but common feature of tubes made before 1976, the date the FDA began regulating such medical devices. Such "grandfathered" or "preamendment devices" do not require proof of safety or efficacy.

[5] An "-ostomy" [*Greek, stoma*: mouth] is *a procedure* (surgical, endoscopic, or radiological) to create an opening (e.g., "a colostomy was performed for diverticular disease"). A "-stoma" (pl. stomata) is *the opening* from the skin into an interior hollow organ, but one rarely hears the terms "gastrostoma" or "colostoma." These openings are typically referred to simply as "a gastrostomy" or "a colostomy." Though not strictly correct, this has become the common usage and will be employed here. Similarly, we anglicize the plural to "stomas" or "-ostomies" instead of *stomae* or *–ostomae*.

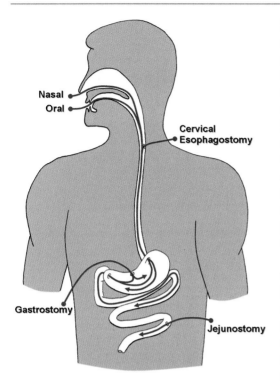

Fig. 68.1 Tube schema. Infusion points (*arrow heads*) are gastric or jejunal

through the neck (cervical esophagostomy) or to the stomach (gastrostomy) or to the proximal small intestine (jejunostomy) via the anterior abdominal wall. The major determinant in the choice between *natural orifice* and *stoma* is that the length of time tube feeding will be required. In general, if artificial nutrition will be required for more than 30 days, a stoma should be considered. One guideline is that if a tracheostomy is being considered, so should a gastrostomy. Stoma formation is an investment. It costs time and money; it involves discomfort and risk; and it carries the stigma of permanence. It also offers several advantages. A stoma is short, stable, and big; inevitable tube replacement is generally much simpler; and it avoids the problems inherent in long-term use of nasal tubes.

Nasal tubes—nasogastric or nasoenteric—are safe, effective, and useful. For some conditions, especially those with a reasonable possibility of rapid improvement, early nutritional treatment, beginning with nasal access, is encouraged.

Potentially reversible causes for dysphagia include almost all metabolic diseases and some neurologic conditions. Norton, however, showed that early Percutaneous Endoscopic Gastrostomy (PEG) was superior to nasogastric tube feedings in the setting of acute dysphagic stroke [2]. Improvement in nutrition and reduction in aspiration apparently accounted for the marked difference in mortality, which brought the study to an early conclusion. Although the risk of creating a stoma outweighs the risk of NG tube placement, the risk of having a stoma is much less. When it becomes clear that percutaneous access is unavoidable, it should be undertaken expeditiously.

Using suction tubes for feeding should be discouraged. It is disconcerting how often a Salem sump (large, multilumen, hard plastic tube designed not to collapse during nasogastric suction) is used for feeding. Presumably, these are used because they are readily available and easy to place. Their use is sometimes rationalized as a way to check for gastric residuals. Unfortunately, in addition to patient complaints of throat discomfort, these tubes can be dangerous. Nasal, sinus, cricopharyngeal, and esophageal complications are common. Pressure ulcers can occur throughout the course of a tube, but most concerning is posterior cricoid. This unique injury may not be apparent until days after the tube is removed and is particularly likely to occur in patients with diabetes, laying supine in the ICU, with the tube in the midline. Sofferman's triad of NG tube, pain, and impaired phonation are predictive, but because this is a spectrum of injury and the area involved is not readily visualized, exact incidence is unknown [3]. The most severe sequelae of the tissue necrosis are a posterior abscess and damage to local structures with permanent impairment of voice. Side effects increase with increasing length of use, tube size, and tube hardness (Fig. 68.2).

The ideal nasal tube should be as soft and small as possible, an 10–12 Fr tube of polyurethane works well. Soft feeding tubes collapse under suction, so these cannot be used for decompression or to reliably check residuals. Additional considerations for any natural orifice intubation include body image, dignity, social interaction,

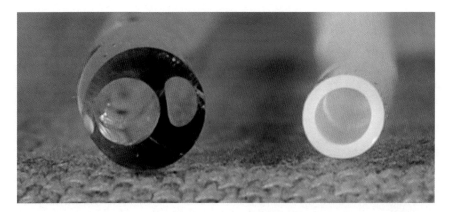

Fig. 68.2 Salem sump and polyurethane nasojejunal tube. Note that the polyurethane tube is much softer and more pliable than the thick-walled polyvinyl Salem sump

and inconvenience. This is particularly true of oral tubes, which cause more gagging and impair speech. An oral tube is probably only justified when an endotracheal tube is already in place or when very temporary, intermittent intubation is used for supplemental feedings or medications.

The infusion point at the internal tube tip may be placed in either the stomach or small bowel. Feeding the stomach should be the same as feeding the small bowel, but this is not always the case. The stomach is generally preferred and has many advantages. It is designed to sterilize, store, and digest ingested food, subsequently emptying nutrients in a controlled, autoregulated fashion into the small bowel for optimal absorption.

Sterility of tube feedings on a shelf does not prevent inoculation of the digestive tract. The tube itself is a foreign body from which microorganisms are poorly cleared. Thus it can act as a nidus for inoculation of the gut, particularly with jejunal tubes. Microbial activity is encouraged by the coincidence of a foreign body, a warm, moist environment, and ample nutrients. Surprisingly, this rarely causes overt bacterial overgrowth, but recurrent bouts of *Clostridium difficile* and other organisms have been reported [4], and failure of silicon tubes is often precipitated by actual infiltration and growth of *Candida* into the material of the tube.

A gastric infusion point has several advantages: gastric storage and emptying make intermittent, gastric bolus feeding possible. The stomach is designed to hold food and mete it out to the small bowel at a controlled and manageable rate. Failure to properly empty may be reflected in high gastric residuals (>200 ml). Too rapid emptying or bolus feeding directly into the small bowel can cause "dumping" syndrome. In this scenario, feedings overload the bowel causing fluid shifts, hyperglycemia followed by hypoglycemia, malabsorption, and voluminous diarrhea. An infusion pump can mimic this gastric function by delivering feedings to the small bowel at a controlled rate (150 ml/h or less), but this approach is high maintenance. The acid milieu in the stomach aids in chemical digestion, acts as a barrier to microbial contamination, and chemically reduces elemental metals in preparation for absorption. In addition, gastric intrinsic factor enables B_{12} absorption. Easier tube placement is another advantage. The stomach is a larger, more proximal, and less mobile target, more easily accessed either per stoma or transluminally for primary or replacement tubes. Finally, feeding the stomach means fullness and satiety can be appreciated. Feeding to the stomach can give the sensation of being fed. Gastric feeding, however, may also enable nausea and emesis.

Jejunal access is indicated if the stomach does not empty well for mechanical or motility reasons or cannot function. Since the purpose of tube feeding is to bypass nonfunctional anatomy, placing the tube tip into the jejunum can address gastric dysfunction. Jejunal feedings can be more reliable in critically ill patients and will reduce

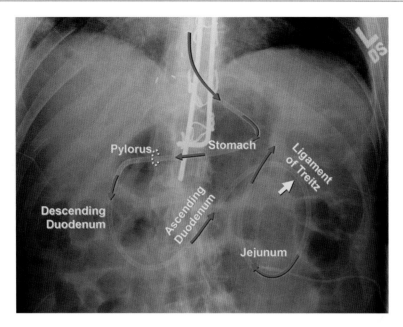

Fig. 68.3 Finding the ligament of Treitz. Note that the infusion point in the bowel cannot be confirmed by the radiological position of the tube tip in the abdomen, but only by tracing the path of the tube. From the stomach the tube proceeds to the patient's right, crossing the midline as it enters the duodenum through the pylorus.
Then the tube turns caudally, as the duodenum descends along the right side of the spine before returning back across the midline and ascending to the ligament of Treitz (LoT), where the tube turns into the jejunum. A tube must navigate the entire duodenum and pass the LoT for its tip to be in the jejunum

gastroesophageal reflux. Intuitively, this should reduce aspiration, although the literature has not shown a direct correlation. Since we have all seen an individual in whom jejunal feeding clearly reduced aspiration, and almost identical patients who were not helped, trial of a jejunal tube seems prudent if even the potential for benefit exists.

Duodenal placement is *not* jejunal placement. Intuitively, simply getting the tube tip out of the stomach solves the problems associated with gastric feedings. In fact, the terms "postpyloric," "small bowel" (or sometimes even "jejunal placement") imply duodenal placement. Physiologically, there is a huge difference. The duodenal–jejunal junction is at the Ligament of Treitz (LoT). This landmark is radiologically distinct [5] (Fig. 68.3) and physiologically important [6]. Infusion beyond this point leads to significantly less reflux to the stomach and (especially >20 cm beyond the LoT) less stimulation of upper gastrointestinal (gastric, duodenal, pancreatic, and—possibly—salivary) secretion. Additional benefits may include reduction in pulmonary aspiration and

tube back-migration. In short, if there is good reason to bypass gastric infusion, then the infusion point should be distal to the LoT. There is simply no reason to feed into the duodenum.

Techniques of Tube Placement

Intubating a body orifice is easy, but getting the internal tip to the appropriate infusion point may be quite difficult. Some tubes we place blindly, some we must guide into position, and for some we even create a new body orifice. Each approach brings unique indications, techniques, and risks. Below, we review what is unique about each approach.

Blind Tube Placement: Natural Orifice or Preexisting Stoma

There are two potential challenges to blind introduction of a feeding tube. The first is the frequent need to place the infusion point quite distally to the intubation point. This is the case for all natural orifice introductions as well as for esophagostomy and transgastrostomic jejunal (PEG-J) tube placement. The second challenge involves introduction immediately through an artificial stoma. The risk here is an unstable stoma. This is particularly true of a fresh stoma (<14 days), where dehiscence or separation of the gut and abdominal wall can occur. NGT placement is a basic clinical skill taught to physicians and nurses. Misplacement is rare, but serious. Radiographs showing NG tubes coiled in the mouth, lung, or even brain are dramatic reminders of how easily one can go through the larynx or cribiform plate especially with a Salem Sump. In addition, dislodgement is common, but can be minimized with use of a nasal bridle.[6]

Creating a New Stoma: PEG as a Prototype

1. *Percutaneous endoscopic gastrostomy* (PEG) was first described in 1980 by Gauderer and Ponsky [7]. Prior to this new technique for percutaneously creating a tube gastrostomy with endoscopic assistance, only surgical placement had been possible. There were several revolutionary aspects of this procedure. Instead of cutting individual holes in the abdominal wall and stomach and then manually aligning and fixing them together, as is done surgically, the percutaneous endoscopic tract is defined by a needle stick from the skin into an air-distended stomach. This single motion creates a hole through the abdominal and gastric walls simultaneously. This new tract is then developed by wire-guided dilation from 2 mm to 6–9 mm by passing a conical dilator, which separates muscle fibers and tears mucosa and serosa rather than cutting them. Only the skin is cut, because only it will not easily stretch or tear. The dilator trails a tube as it passes through the tract, simultaneously

dilating the tract and placing the tube gastrostomy. Later, this same percutaneous approach was applied to jejunostomy and esophagostomy (Fig. 68.4).

Eventually, three methods of percutaneous gastrostomy evolved. The "Pull" (original Gauderer–Ponsky method) technique uses a string or wire to pull the dilator and tube through the abdominal wall from the inside of the stomach. The "Push" (Sacks-Vine or overwire) technique positions a guidewire in position through the abdominal wall into the stomach and then up the esophagus and out the mouth. A dilator and tube are then slid over this wire like a clothesline. The "Introducer" (Russell) method can be employed endoscopically, but will be discussed in detail as a technique for radiological placement.

Almost immediately after publication, the technique came under criticism, particularly by surgeons sincerely convinced that this could lead only to disaster. PEG seemingly violated every surgical principle by blindly crossing facial planes, randomly poking holes in hollow viscera, and relying on a "sutureless approximation." On top of that, a foreign body is then coated it in saliva and implanted into a fresh wound across a previously sterile peritoneal cavity. This seemed frankly insane. In spite of these initial concerns PEG proved itself, safely creating reliable, stable access possible without an operating room, general anesthesia, or open abdominal surgery. Acceptance eventually followed the data, but also shifted gastrostomy placement to a new set of providers, the gastroenterologists. Costs and other barriers plummeted, and utilization and optimism skyrocketed (Fig. 68.5).

2. *Alternative uses for percutaneous stomas* are worth noting here. PEG can be used for:
   (a) Infusion of feedings, hydration, medications, etc., is the most common
   (b) Decompression or drainage for bowel obstruction or severe motility disorder
   (c) Fixation of a mobile intraabdominal organ, typically to prevent volvulus
   (d) Access for instrumentation, especially with new ultrathin scopes.

[6] http://www.amtinnovation.com/bridle.html cashed by http://www.google.com at Nov 18, 2011 12:31:03 GMT

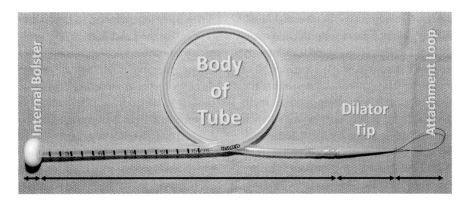

Fig. 68.4 PEG tube assembly. The Ponsky-type tube shown consists of four parts. The attachment loop by which the dilator and tube are pulled into position through the tract; the dilator; the tube body; and the internal bolster, which keeps the tube from pulling all the way through and falling out

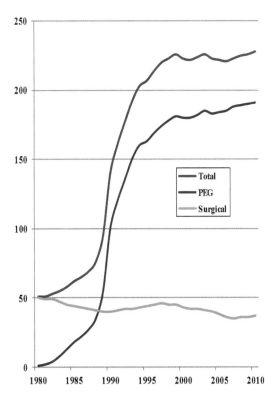

Fig. 68.5 U.S. Gastrostomy Utilization (in thousands)

A combination of uses (e.g., drainage of refluxed bile from the stomach above an obstructed GI tract combined with subsequent reinfusion of the bile beyond the obstruction) can also be employed. Different uses may mandate different technical needs. Access and drainage

usually need a larger bore tube. Fixation may require two points to prevent revolvulation

3. *Acute complications* became apparent as experience with the new technique grew and reality expressed herself. While in theory, there is no difference between theory and practice, it seems that in practice, there is.[7] Subsequently, procedural modifications arose to control these new risks. Although complications are usually discussed *after* discussing the procedure, we bring them up before presenting a detailed protocol, because many important specifics of the technique are rooted in complication avoidance. The end result of this evolution of method and device is reflected in many critical differences from how PEG was initially described.

(a) *Infection* is, not surprisingly, the most significant acute risk, presenting 1–3 days after placement in ~5 % of patients. This occurs in the tissue surrounding the tract and appears as redness, induration, and tenderness. Occasionally, purulent drainage will develop around the tube. Often, this will respond to hot packs and lengthening the skin incision to allow better drainage. If the infection is severe, unresponsive, or rapidly developing, IV antibiotics should

---

[7]These words have been variously attributed to Jan LA van de Snepschuet, Chuck Reid, and even Yogi Berra.

(c) *Call a "Time Out"* immediately before the procedure so that everyone involved in the procedure is "on the same page." With the entire team assembled, we verbally confirm the following: [abbreviated *"PPAACE"*]
   – *Patient*—there is no excuse for doing a procedure on the wrong patient, yet it happens.
   – *Procedure*—performing the wrong procedure is just as bad and happens just as often.
   – *Allergies*—no excuse for missing this, especially regarding anesthetics and antibiotics.
   – *Antibiotics*—confirm administration of this powerful tool for reducing post-PEG infection.
   – *Consent*—should have been completed before arrival and documented on the chart.
   – *Equipment*—everything you might possibly need is immediately available.

(d) *Position, prep, and sedate* the patient. An IV should already be running for antibiotics. Some endoscopists would swab the mouth with antiseptics at this point in an effort to reduce bacterial load, but there is no good evidence that this is of more than a theoretical benefit. We use wrist restraints even in patients who are fully oriented to prevent them from moving their hands into the prepped area when under sedation. It often works best for the two proceduralists to have access to opposite sides of the cart. With the patient in supine position, obstructive sleep apnea is more likely to occur with sedation. We often remove the pillow for this reason. Airway issues during sedation often benefits from a temporary nasopharyngeal airway without interfering with endoscopy.

(e) *Evaluate the oropharynx* carefully during endoscopic introduction. These patients are well known for having the most cluttered airways imaginable. We have seen foreign bodies, pills, 3-day-old scrambled eggs, heavy, inspisated mucous, and even partial laryngeal obstruction. Such material can fall into the airway during the procedure. It should be deliberately and completely removed before esophageal intubation. It is not uncommon to see impaired baseline oxygenation improve dramatically after clearance. The endoscope and Yankauer suction can be good tools for this, but occasionally, McGill forceps are needed. Once the airway is fully cleared, examine the upper GI tract to the duodenum. Any unexpected pathology (e.g., gastric ulcer or pyloric stenosis) may put the entire procedure in a new light. Be open to acute modification of your treatment plan.

(f) *Confirm and localize the site endoscopically* by (1) transilluminating the abdominal wall from inside the stomach using the light from the endoscope (this will give a red glow to the skin, confirming that no optically dense organ (i.e., liver) is between the stomach and skin) and (2) making "finger circles" on the abdominal wall at the intended point of gastrostomy (this will precisely define where the endoscopist should look for the needle to come in. Simply "poking" does not always clearly define a spot). Make sure the stomach is fully insufflated to bring it into apposition with the anterior abdominal wall. The ideal location is ~2 cm left of the midline (avoid the linea alba, if possible) and ~2 cm below the costal margin (the tube may cause periosteal pain if too close to the rib margin) if this falls within the transilluminated region (Fig. 68.6).

(g) *Prep and drape* the site identified on the abdominal wall. Shaving the site is no longer felt to be helpful in decreasing infection, but in some individuals may be necessary for practical reasons. Since PEG actually involves taking a foreign body, coating it in saliva, and dragging it into an open wound, this is not actually a sterile procedure (in fact, it would technically be considered "clean-contaminated").

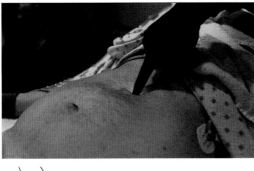

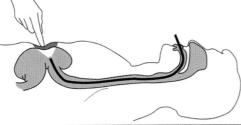

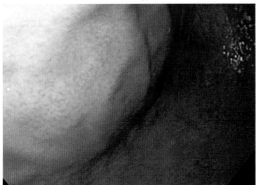

Fig. 68.6 Localization of the PEG site depends on (**a**) good transillumination, confirming that the optically dense liver is avoided; (**b**) good finger indentation, indicating that the gastric and abdominal walls are closely approximated; and (**c**) "Safe Tract" (see below)

As such, sterile gloves may not actually be better than clean, disposable gloves from a box. Their use must also be weighed against the latex restrictions often in place in GI labs.

(h) *"Safe-Tract" technique* [8] makes use of the small gauge needle supplied for local skin anesthesia to "sound out" the intended tract of the percutaneous tube. After re-targeting with finger circles, the needle is slowly advanced under continuous aspiration until bubbles suddenly appear in the syringe. This instant should coincide exactly with the needle tip penetrating the gastric mucosa as seen by the endoscope. If gas, stool, or blood appear before this point, the needle tip can be assumed to have encountered an intervening organ, and the tract is not safe (Fig. 68.7).

(i) *Incise the skin* horizontally (in line of skin tension) and large (at least 1.0 cm for a 20 Fr tube). An incision that is too small or is not all the way through the skin and into the subcutaneous fat will cause pressure necrosis of the skin. Not only is this necrotic tissue directly adjacent to an inoculated foreign body (i.e., PEG tube), but some feel the tight approximation may serve to retain a hematoma or an abscess and thereby increase the risk of infection (Fig. 68.8).

(j) *Position the snare* under endoscopic guidance. The anticipated site of puncture

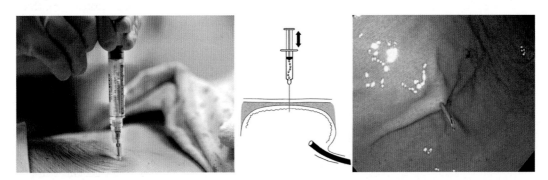

Fig. 68.7 Safe tract technique

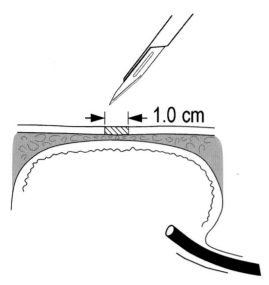

Fig. 68.8 Skin incision

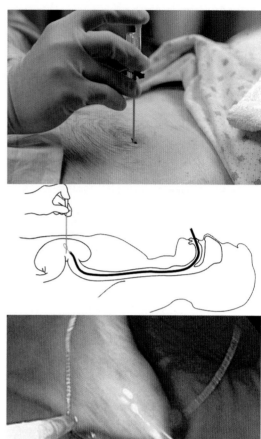

Fig. 68.9 Inserting the trochar

may already be evident if the Safe Track finder needle left a gastric mucosal mark. In any event, it is always good to re-target with finger circles. Open the snare completely to incorporate this area. The trochar should enter the snare directly in most circumstanced.

(k) *Stab the trochar[8] through the incision* and into the gastric lumen under direct endoscopic visualization. If the stomach is not fully insufflated, the trochar may only tent but not pierce the gastric mucosa. Nevertheless, care should be taken not to be too aggressive in this maneuver, since it is possible to actually pierce through the back wall of the stomach and into the pancreas or aorta. Once the cannula is well into the stomach, pull the trochar tip back into the cannula to prevent laceration of the mucosal or scope (Fig. 68.9).

(l) *Close the snare on the cannula.* This may require repositioning the snare or even tipping the cannula to facilitate encirclement. The endoscopist should remember that the snare closes to the tip of the snare sheath, not to the middle of the loop. If improperly placed, the snare will pull off of the cannula as it closes. Once the trochar–cannula assembly is snared, the trochar is removed from the cannula and a wire is passed through the cannula and into the stomach. Opening the snare slightly releases the cannula so

---

[8] Classically, the *trochar* is a metal rod sharply pointed at one end by three cut angles (from Fr. *trois+carre*). Once placed inside a sheath or *cannula* the *trochar–cannula* assembly can push through tissue into a body cavity. When the trochar is removed, the hollow cannula provides an opening into the cavity for access or drainage. The trochar–cannula assembly is typically referred to simply as a trochar.

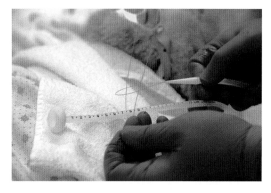

Fig. 68.10 Capturing the cannula and wire

the snare can be repositioned onto the wire alone. Close the snare on the wire firmly and pull the snare sheath to the tip of the scope—but NOT into the biopsy channel (Fig. 68.10).

(m) *Slowly withdraw the endoscope* and wire through the esophagus and out the mouth. Make sure the wire feeds smoothly without tension from below to avoid "cheese-wiring."

(n) *Attach the PEG tube to the wire.* The wire in most Ponsky "Pull" kits is typically blue in color and doubled over into a long loop which attaches to the loop on the dilator end of the PEG tube. To connect these loops, run the wires "blue through, then through blue" (Fig. 68.11) or as directed by the individual kit. The Saks-Vine "Push" technique uses a standard angiography guidewire, and the tip of the dilator has a hole for the wire to go through. It will exit through the internal bolster on the other end of the tube.

(o) *To facilitate reintroduction* of the scope into the upper esophagus, 30 cm of snare sheath may be pulled out the tip of the scope and inserted fully into the free end of the PEG tube. The internal bolster of the PEG tube then encompasses the scope tip. At this point, the snare should be opened inside the tube to avoid trauma from the blunt snare sheath on esophageal mucosa. As the tube is pulled through the upper esophageal sphincter, so is the snare. The sheath then guides the scope

Fig. 68.11 Attaching the tube to the wire

easily through the sphincter into the upper esophagus. Once the scope is past the upper esophageal sphincter, the snare is withdrawn. If an easy reintroduction is anticipated, this step can be eliminated.

(p) *Pull the wire out through the abdominal wall* until the cannula spontaneously pulls out, indicating the knot has encountered the incision. At this point, firmly pull with a circular motion to facilitate dilation of the tract until the tube body is delivered into the new tract. Look for the depth marks on the tube and continue to withdraw the tube until ~5–10 cm of depth remains (Fig. 68.12).

(q) *Endoscopically reevaluate the stomach* to confirm appropriate placement of the internal bolster against the gastric wall. Under direct visualization, pull the tube through the tract until the internal bolster is brought into gentle contact with the gastric mucosa. Check and record skin

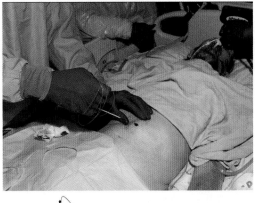

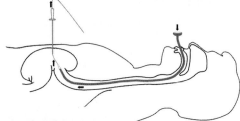

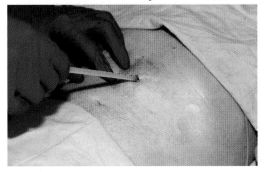

Fig. 68.12 Pulling the PEG tube into position

position by the depth marks on the tube at the abdominal wall. Avoid excessive traction (Fig. 68.13).

(r) *Attach the external bolster* fixing this at 0.5 cm above the skin position. There are often two options for external bolsters. The disk is most stable for bedridden patients, but the bar is more comfortable for ambulatory, active patients. Cut the tube leaving all markings possible. Attach the feeding connector, and drain the open tube to a small, but appropriate, decompression bag (e.g., a clear vinyl glove or small biohazard bag). A single layer of small, thin dressing can be applied under the bolster until this is checked the next morning. After that, no dressing should normally be used. If the patient is disoriented and tends to pull out tubes (NGT, IVs, etc.), using an abdominal binder to cover the tube for the first 2 weeks might be wise. If this continues to be a problem, change to a button after tract maturation.

(s) *Postcare* begins at discharge from the endoscopy unit. Orders are written to resume prior oral or NGT medications with a small flush of water. There are studies suggesting that feedings can also be safely initiated within hours of a PEG, but unless nutrition has deteriorated to an urgent degree, we wait 1 day. In the

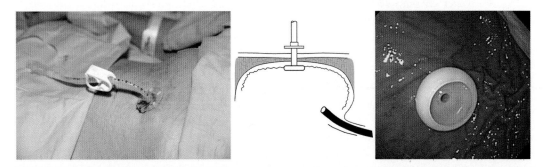

Fig. 68.13 Final check

unlikely event of gastric stasis or other cause for emesis, a sedated, supine patient is at increased risk for aspiration. Also, infection, hematoma, or visceral perforation might be more apparent the next day. Careful clinical assessment the following day is mandatory. Although the site may be slightly tender to tube manipulation, it should not be frankly painful or display erythema, induration, or discharge. There should be no new fever or leukocytosis. Ideally, the patient will be hungry. A water test flush can be given. Only begin feedings if there are no concerns at this point.

Percutaneous Radiological Gastrostomy

The "Introducer" (Russell) method places a 14 Fr balloon tube through a peel-away sheath introduced into the stomach from the skin using the Seldinger technique. This technique does not actually require an endoscope since an NGT can be used to inflate the stomach for fluoroscopically guided placement. The radiological approach, however, requires T-fasteners and foregoes endoscopic examination of the upper gastrointestinal tract, endoscopic assistance in site selection, and direct observation of a safe placement. T-fasteners are additional fixation devices used to help minimize separation or the abdominal wall and gastric wall during placement. The inward, distracting force of serial dilation might otherwise simply push the stomach away from the abdominal wall resulting in peritoneal placement. T-fasteners also help prevent later separation in the event the balloon tube is dislodged before tract maturation. Although a small pneumoperitoneum is not uncommon after any percutaneous gastrostomy, it is virtually assured after the "Introducer" technique. This method is used endoscopically in cases where an internal bolster should not be dragged through the mouth and esophagus during placement. One such case is cancer of the oropharynx or esophagus that may "seed" the tube resulting in tumor implantation at the gastrostomy site. In addition, some esophageal strictures are too tight to allow reliable passage of the tube. So, if

the procedure takes the new tube directly past malignant tissue, if the esophagus requires dilation, or if a pediatric endoscope is required to do the procedure, consider the introducer technique.

Surgical Stoma

The four most common ways to surgically access the gut for feedings are the Stamm gastrostomy, Janeway gastrostomy, Witzel gastrostomy, or the needle catheter jejunostomy. Generally, one of these would be placed in conjunction with a procedure that had already necessitated opening the abdomen. The Stamm is the most simple and straightforward of these: (1) the surgeon makes a stab wound in the abdominal wall and another in the anterior gastric wall. (2) through these, a feeding tube is placed and held in position by a purse-string suture of the gastric wall, and (3) then the gastric wall is attached to the anterior abdominal wall, aligning theses holes. The Janeway and Witzel gastrostomies are more complicated, but also more stable and less leak prone. In needle-catheter jejunostomy an IV catheter through the abdominal wall is then inserted into the small bowel lumen for immediate, but temporary postoperative feeding.

Is Surgical, Endoscopic, or Radiological Gastrostomy superior? The literature is replete with studies by endoscopists "showing" PEG is superior to radiologically or surgically placed tubes and studies by radiologists "showing" PRG is better than PEG or surgical tubes. There are essentially no studies showing that surgical tubes are better, because they have been repeatedly shown to have a higher complication rate, a longer length of stay, and higher cost. As gastroenterologists, we have an obvious preference, but frankly, if your institution has particularly capable endoscopic or radiologic expertise, this probably outweighs the technical advantages of one approach over the other. All things being equal, specific anatomical considerations (e.g., tight stricture, which might interfere with the passage of PEG bolster, an ENT cancer that might seed the tube to implant in the new stoma, or prior upper

Printed in the United States of America